BIOMEDICAL ENGINEERING AND DESIGN HANDBOOK

ABOUT THE EDITOR

Myer Kutz, founder and president of Myer Kutz Associates, Inc., is the author and editor of many books, handbooks, and encyclopedias.

BIOMEDICAL ENGINEERING AND DESIGN HANDBOOK

Volume 2: Applications

Myer Kutz Editor

Second Edition

McGraw Hill

New York Chicago San Francisco Lisbon London Madrid
Mexico City Milan New Delhi San Juan Seoul
Singapore Sydney Toronto

The McGraw-Hill Companies

Cataloging-in-Publication Data is on file with the Library of Congress

1 2 3 4 5 6 7 8 9 0 DOC/DOC 0 1 5 4 3 2 1 0 9

ISBN: P/N 978-0-07-149839-5 of set 978-0-07-149840-1
MHID: P/N 0-07-149839-7 of set 0-07-149840-0

Sponsoring Editor
Stephen S. Chapman

Editing Supervisor
Stephen M. Smith

Production Supervisor
Pamela A. Pelton

Project Manager
Vastavikta Sharma, International Typesetting and Composition

Copy Editor
Megha RC, International Typesetting and Composition

Proofreader
Priyanka Sinha, International Typesetting and Composition

Indexer
WordCo Indexing Services, Inc.

Art Director, Cover
Jeff Weeks

Composition
International Typesetting and Composition

Printed and bound by RR Donnelley.

This book is printed on acid-free paper.

For Arlene, forever

CONTENTS

CONTRIBUTORS

Ronald S. Adrezin *United States Coast Guard Academy, New London, Connecticut* (Chap. 16)

Jorge F. Arinez *General Motors, Research and Development Center, Warren, Michigan* (Chap. 22)

Shilditya Bhattacharya *Thomas J. Long School of Pharmacy and Health Science, University of the Pacific, Stockton, California* (Chap. 6)

Barrett S. Caldwell *Purdue University, West Lafayette, Indiana* (Chap. 27)

M. Cenk Cavusoglu *Case Western Reserve University, Cleveland, Ohio* (Chap. 13)

Breet Clippingdale *University of Michigan, Ann Arbor, Michigan* (Chap. 18)

Albert M. Cook *University of Alberta Edmonton, Alberta, Canada* (Chap. 15)

Daniela Crivianu-Gaita *The Hospital for Sick Children, Toronto, Canada* (Chap. 25)

John Michael Currie *EwingCole, Washington, DC* (Chap. 26)

Alfred Dolan *University of Toronto, Toronto, Canada* (Chaps. 23, 24)

Laurie L. Fajardo *University of Iowa, Iowa City, Iowa* (Chap. 12)

Tom Filburn *University of Hartford, West Hartford, Connecticut* (Chap. 28)

Kenneth L. Gage *University of Pittsburgh, Pittsburgh, Pennsylvania* (Chap. 3)

Sandra K. Garrett *Clemson University, Clemson, South Carolina* (Chap. 27)

Joe Genovese *Hamilton Sundstrand (retired), Windsor Locks, Connecticut* (Chap. 28)

John Graf *NASA Johnson Space Center, Houston, Texas* (Chap. 28)

Mark Hodges *University of Michigan, Ann Arbor, Michigan* (Chap. 18)

Bhaskara R. Jasti *Thomas J. Long School of Pharmacy and Health Science, University of the Pacific, Stockton, California* (Chap. 6)

Arthur T. Johnson *University of Maryland, College Park, Maryland* (Chap. 4)

Leo Joskowicz *School of Computer Science and Engineering Computer-Aided Surgery and Medical Image Processing Laboratory, The Hebrew University of Jerusalem, Israel* (Chap. 14)

Robert Klepinski *Fredrikson & Byron, PA, Minneapolis, Minnesota* (Chap. 2)

Xiaoling Li *Thomas J. Long School of Pharmacy and Health Science, University of the Pacific, Stockton, California* (Chap. 6)

Mark Madsen *University of Iowa, Iowa City, Iowa* (Chap. 11)

Stan Mastrangelo *Center for Applied Health Science, Virginia Tech, Blacksburg, Virginia* (Chap. 24)

Mohsen Mosleh *Howard University, Bethesda, Maryland* (Chap. 22)

Patrick J. Nolan *DDL, Inc., Eden Prairie, Minnesota* (Chap. 7)

James P. O'Leary *Tufts University, Medford, Massachusetts* (Chap. 1)

Martha Pollack *University of Michigan, Ann Arbor, Michigan* (Chap. 18)

Narender P. Reddy *University of Akron, Akron, Ohio* (Chap. 5)

David J. Reinkensmeyer *University of California, Irvine, California* (Chap. 19)

Peter Rockett *Oxford University, Oxfordshire, England* (Chap. 10)

Blair A. Rowley *Wright State University, Dayton, Ohio* (Chap. 17)

Daniel J. Schaefer *MR Systems Engineering, Milwaukee, Wisconsin* (Chap. 8)

Jonathon W. Sensinger *Mahidol University, Nakhon Pathom, Thailand* (Chap. 20)

David M. Shade *Johns Hopkins Hospital, Baltimore, Maryland* (Chap. 4)

Steve I. Shen *Thomas J. Long School of Pharmacy and Health Science, University of the Pacific, Stockton, California* (Chap. 6)

M. Barbara Silver-Thorn *Marquette University, Milwaukee, Wisconsin* (Chap. 21)

John M. Smith *Consultant, Gormley, Canada* (Chap. 25)

Russell Taylor *Department of Computer Science Center for Computer-Integrated Surgical Systems and Technology, The Johns Hopkins University, Baltimore, Maryland* (Chap. 14)

Kai E. Thomenius *GE Corporate Research and Development, Schenectady, New York* (Chap. 9)

William R. Wagner *University of Pittsburgh, Pittsburgh, Pennsylvania* (Chap. 3)

Ge Wang *University of Iowa, Iowa City, Iowa* (Chap. 10)

Julie S. Weber *University of Michigan, Ann Arbor, Michigan* (Chap. 18)

Richard F. Weir *Rehabilitation Institute of Chicago, Chicago, Illinois* (Chap. 20)

Mark B. Williams *University of Virginia, Charlottesville, Virginia* (Chap. 12)

VISION STATEMENT

The First Edition of this handbook, which was called the *Standard Handbook of Biomedical Engineering and Design*, was published in the fall of 2002. It was a substantial reference work, with 39 chapters spread over the major areas of interest that constitute the discipline of biomedical engineering—areas in which biomedical engineering can exert its greatest impact on health care. These areas included biomedical systems, biomechanics of the human body, biomaterials, bioelectronics, medical device design, diagnostic equipment design, surgery, rehabilitation engineering, prosthetics design, and clinical engineering. Coverage within each of the areas was not as broad as I would have liked, mainly because not all of the assigned chapters could be delivered in time to meet the publication schedule, as is often the case with large contributed works (unless the editor keeps waiting for remaining chapters to stagger in while chapters already received threaten to become out-of-date). So, even as the First Edition was being published, I looked forward to a Second Edition when I could secure more chapters to fill in any gaps in the coverage and allow contributors to add greater depth to chapters that had already been published.

The overall plan for the Second Edition of what is now called the *Biomedical Engineering and Design Handbook* was to update 38 chapters that were in the First Edition (one chapter of a personal nature was dropped) and add 14 new chapters, including chapters with topics that were assigned for the First Edition but were not delivered, plus chapters with entirely new topics. Because of the size of the Second Edition, I recommended splitting it into two volumes, with 24 chapters in Volume 1 and 28 chapters in Volume 2. The split is natural: the first volume covers fundamentals, and the second volume covers applications.

The two volumes have been arranged as follows:

Volume 1: Fundamentals

- Part 1: Biomedical Systems Analysis
- Part 2: Biomechanics of the Human Body
- Part 3: Biomaterials
- Part 4: Bioelectronics

Volume 2: Applications

- Part 1: Medical Device Design
- Part 2: Diagnostic Equipment Design
- Part 3: Surgery
- Part 4: Rehabilitation Engineering and Prosthetics Design
- Part 5: Clinical Engineering

Overall, more than three-quarters of the chapters in the Second Edition are new or updated—a quarter cover topics not included in the First Edition and are entirely new, and over half have been updated. The Preface to each volume provides detail about the parts of the handbook and individual chapters.

The intended audience for the handbook is practicing engineers, physicians, and medical researchers in academia, hospitals, government agencies, and commercial, legal, and regulatory organizations, as well as upper-level students. Many potential readers work in the field of biomedical engineering, but they may also work in a number of other disciplines—mechanical, electrical, or materials engineering, to name just three—that impinge on, for example, the design and development of medical devices implanted in the human body, diagnostic imaging machines, or prosthetics. Depending on the topic being addressed, the audience affiliation can be closely aligned with the discipline of biomedical engineering, while at other times the affiliation can be broader than biomedical engineering and can be, to a substantial degree, multidisciplinary.

To meet the needs of this sometimes narrow, sometimes broad, audience, I have designed a practical reference for anyone working directly with, in close proximity to, or tangentially to the discipline of biomedical engineering and who is seeking to answer a question, solve a problem, reduce a cost, or improve the operation of a system or facility. The two volumes of this handbook are not research monographs. My purpose is much more practice-oriented: it is to show readers which options may be available in particular situations and which options they might choose to solve problems at hand. I want this handbook to serve as a source of practical advice to readers. I would like the handbook to be the first information resource a practitioner or researcher reaches for when faced with a new problem or opportunity—a place to turn to before consulting other print sources, or even, as so many professionals and students do reflexively these days, going online to Google or Wikipedia. So the handbook volumes have to be more than references or collections of background readings. In each chapter, readers should feel that they are in the hands of an experienced and knowledgeable teacher or consultant who is providing sensible advice that can lead to beneficial action and results.

Myer Kutz

PREFACE

Volume 2 of the Second Edition of the *Biomedical Engineering and Design Handbook* focuses on applications. It is divided into five parts:

Part 1: Medical Device Design, which consists of seven chapters and covers general design principles, FDA requirements for devices sold and used in the United States, devices used in major organs and systems in the human body, and design and development of systems for precisely delivering drugs, as well as packages for storing and shipping medical devices

Part 2: Diagnostic Equipment Design, which consists of five chapters and presents detailed information on machines and systems used for imaging diagnosis, including MRI, ultrasound, and x-ray tomography, as well as on applications involving nuclear medicine and the special problem of breast imaging

Part 3: Surgery, which consists of two chapters and covers both surgical simulations and computer-integrated and robotic surgery

Part 4: Rehabilitation Engineering and Prosthetics Design, which consists of eight chapters and treats a variety of topics, including technology that assists people with disabilities, design and development of artificial arms and legs, and wear of artificial knees and hips

Part 5: Clinical Engineering, which consists of six chapters and covers topics involving technology development and application in healthcare facilities, organizations, and systems, as well as space travel life-support systems

In all, Volume 2 contains 28 chapters. Eight chapters are entirely new to the handbook, 15 have been updated from the First Edition, and five are unchanged from the First Edition. The purpose of these additions and updates is to expand the scope of the parts of the volume and provide greater depth in the individual chapters.

The eight new chapters in Volume 2 are

Two chapters in Medical Device Design—FDA Medical Device Requirements and Design of Artificial Kidneys

One chapter in Surgery—Surgical Simulation Technologies

Two chapters in Rehabilitation Engineering and Prosthetics Design—Intelligent Assistive Technology and Wear of Total Hip and Knee Joint Replacements

Three chapters in Clinical Engineering—Risk Management in Clinical Engineering, Healthcare Systems Engineering, and Enclosed Habitat Life Support

The 15 chapters that contributors have updated are

Four chapters in Medical Device Design—Overview of Cardiovascular Devices, Design of Respiratory Devices, Design of Controlled-Release Drug Delivery Systems, and Sterile Medical Device Package Development

Four of the five chapters in Diagnostic Equipment Design—Design of Magnetic Resonance Systems, Instrumentation Design for Ultrasonic Imaging, Nuclear Medicine Imaging Instrumentation, and Breast Imaging Systems: Design Challenges for Engineers

One chapter in Surgery—Computer-Integrated Surgery and Medical Robotics

Three chapters in Rehabilitation Engineering and Prosthetics Design—Technology and Disabilities, Applied Universal Design, and The Design of Artificial Arms and Hands for Prosthetic Applications

Three chapters in Clinical Engineering—Clinical Engineering Overview, Technology Planning for Health Care Institutions, and An Overview of Health Care Facilities Planning

Three-quarters of the chapters in Volume 2 were written by academics, and a quarter by contributors working in hospitals or industry. All contributors work in North America, except for one, who works in Israel. I would like to express my heartfelt thanks to all of them for working on this book. Their lives are terribly busy, and it is wonderful that they found the time to write thoughtful and complex chapters. I developed the handbook because I believed it could have a meaningful impact on the way many engineers, physicians, and medical researchers approach their daily work, and I am gratified that the contributors thought enough of the idea that they were willing to participate in the project. I should add that a majority of contributors to the First Edition were willing to update their chapters, and it's interesting that even though I've not met most of them face to face, we have a warm relationship and are on a first-name basis. They responded quickly to queries during copy editing and proofreading. It was a pleasure to work with them—we've worked together on and off for nearly a decade. The quality of their work is apparent. Thanks also go to my editors at McGraw-Hill for their faith in the project from the outset. And a special note of thanks is for my wife Arlene, whose constant support keeps me going.

Myer Kutz
Delmar, New York

PREFACE TO THE FIRST EDITION

How do important medical advances that change the quality of life come about? Sometimes, to be sure, they can result from the inspiration and effort of physicians or biologists working in remote, exotic locations or organic chemists working in the well-appointed laboratories of pharmaceutical companies with enormous research budgets. Occasionally, however, a medical breakthrough happens when someone with an engineering background gets a brilliant idea in less glamorous circumstances. One afternoon in the late 1950s, the story goes, when an electrical engineer named Wilson Greatbatch was building a small oscillator to record heart sounds, he accidentally installed the wrong resistor, and the device began to give off a steady electrical pulse. Greatbatch realized that a small device could regulate the human heart, and in two years he had developed the first implantable cardiac pacemaker, followed later by a corrosion-free lithium battery to power it. In the mid-1980s, Dominick M. Wiktor, a Cranford, New Jersey, engineer, invented the coronary stent after undergoing open heart surgery.

You often find that it is someone with an engineer's sensibility—someone who may or may not have engineering training, but does have an engineer's way of looking at, thinking about, and doing things—who not only facilitates medical breakthroughs, but also improves existing healthcare practice. This sensibility, which, I dare say, is associated in people's consciousness more with industrial machines than with the human body, manifests itself in a number of ways. It has a descriptive component, which comes into play, for example, when someone uses the language of mechanical engineering to describe blood flow, how the lungs function, or how the musculoskeletal system moves or reacts to shocks, or when someone uses the language of other traditional engineering disciplines to describe bioelectric phenomena or how an imaging machine works.

Medically directed engineer's sensibility also has a design component, which can come into play in a wide variety of medical situations, indeed whenever an individual, or a team, designs a new healthcare application, such as a new cardiovascular or respiratory device, a new imaging machine, a new artificial arm or lower limb, or a new environment for someone with a disability. The engineer's sensibility also comes into play when an individual or team makes an application that already exists work better—when, for example, the unit determines which materials would improve the performance of a prosthetic device, improves a diagnostic or therapeutic technique, reduces the cost of manufacturing a medical device or machine, improves methods for packaging and shipping medical supplies, guides tiny surgical tools into the body, improves the plans for a medical facility, or increases the effectiveness of an organization installing, calibrating, and maintaining equipment in a hospital. Even the improved design of time-released drug capsules can involve an engineer's sensibility.

The field that encompasses medically directed engineer's sensibility is, of course, called biomedical engineering. Compared to the traditional engineering disciplines, whose fundamentals and language it employs, this field is new and rather small, Although there are now over 80 academic programs in biomedical engineering in the United States, only 6500 undergraduates were enrolled in the year 2000. Graduate enrollment was just 2500. The U.S. Bureau of Labor Statistics reports total biomedical engineering employment in all industries in the year 2000 at 7221. The bureau estimates this number to rise by 31 percent to 9478 in 2010.

The effect this relatively young and small field has on the health and well being of people everywhere, but especially in the industrialized parts of the world that have the wherewithal to fund the field's development and take advantage of its advances, is, in my view, out of proportion to its age and size. Moreover, as the examples provided earlier indicate, the concerns of biomedical engineers are very wide-ranging. In one way or another, they deal with virtually every system and part in the human body. They are involved in all phases of healthcare—measurement and diagnosis, therapy and repair, and patient management and rehabilitation. While the work that biomedical engineers do involves the human body, their work is engineering work. Biomedical engineers, like other engineers in the more traditional disciplines, design, develop, make, and manage. Some work in traditional engineering settings—in laboratories, design departments, on the floors of manufacturing plants—while others deal directly with healthcare clients or are responsible for facilities in hospitals or clinics.

Of course, the field of biomedical engineering is not the sole province of practitioners and educators who call themselves biomedical engineers. The field includes people who call themselves mechanical engineers, materials engineers, electrical engineers, optical engineers, or medical physicists, among other names. The entire range of subjects that can be included in biomedical engineering is very broad. Some curricula offer two main tracks: biomechanics and bioinstrumentation. To some degree, then, there is always a need in any publication dealing with the full scope of biomedical engineering to bridge gaps, whether actually existing or merely perceived, such as the gap between the application of mechanical engineering knowledge, skills, and principles from conception to the design, development, analysis, and operation of biomechanical systems and the application of electrical engineering knowledge, skills, and principles to biosensors and bioinstrumentation.

The focus in the *Standard Handbook of Biomedical Engineering and Design* is on engineering design informed by description in engineering language and methodology. For example, the Handbook not only provides engineers with a detailed understanding of how physiological systems function and how body parts—muscle, tissue, bone—are constituted, it also discusses how engineering methodology can be used to deal with systems and parts that need to be assisted, repaired, or replaced.

I have sought to produce a practical manual for the biomedical engineer who is seeking to solve a problem, improve a technique, reduce cost, or increase the effectiveness of an organization. The Handbook is not a research monograph, although contributors have properly included lists of applicable references at the ends of their chapters. I want this Handbook to serve as a source of practical advice to the reader, whether he or she is an experienced professional, a newly minted graduate, or even a student at an advanced level. I intend the Handbook to be the first information resource a practicing engineer reaches for when faced with a new problem or opportunity—a place to turn to even before turning to other print sources or to sites on the Internet. (The Handbook is planned to be the core of an Internet-based update or current-awareness service, in which the Handbook chapters would be linked to news items, a bibliographic index of articles in the biomedical engineering research literature, professional societies, academic departments, hospital departments, commercial and government organizations, and a database of technical information useful to biomedical engineers.) So the Handbook is more than a voluminous reference or collection of background readings. In each chapter, the reader should feel that he or she is in the hands of an experienced consultant who is providing sensible advice that can lead to beneficial action and results.

I have divided the Handbook into eight parts. Part 1, which contains only a single chapter, is an introductory chapter on applying analytical techniques to biomedical systems. Part 2, which contains nine chapters, is a mechanical engineering domain. It begins with a chapter on the body's thermal behavior, then moves on to two chapters that discuss the mechanical functioning of the cardiovascular and respiratory systems. Six chapters of this part of the Handbook are devoted to analysis of bone and the musculoskeletal system, an area that I have been associated with from a publishing standpoint for a quarter-century, ever since I published David Winter's book on human movement.

Part 3 of the Handbook, the domain of materials engineering, contains six chapters. Three deal with classes of biomaterials—biopolymers, composite biomaterials, and bioceramics—and three deal with using biomaterials, in cardiovascular and orthopedic applications, and to promote tissue regeneration.

The two chapters in Part 4 of the Handbook are in the electrical engineering domain. They deal with measuring bioelectricity and analyzing biomedical signals, and they serve, in part, as an introduction to Part 5, which contains ten chapters that treat the design of therapeutic devices and diagnostic imaging instrumentation, as well as the design of drug delivery systems and the development of sterile packaging for medical devices, a deceptively robust and complex subject that can fill entire books on its own. Imaging also plays a role in the single-chapter Part 6 of the Handbook, which covers computer-integrated surgery.

The last two parts of the Handbook deal with interactions between biomedical engineering practitioners and both patients and medical institutions. Part 7, which covers rehabilitation engineering, includes chapters that treat not only the design and implementation of artificial limbs, but also ways in which engineers provide environments and assistive devices that improve a person's quality of life. Part 8, the last part of the Handbook, deals with clinical engineering, which can be considered the facilities-planning and management component of biomedical engineering.

Acknowledgments

The contributors to this Handbook work mainly in academia and hospitals. Several work in commercial organizations. Most work in the United States and Canada; a few work in Israel. What they all have in common is that what they do is useful and important: they make our lives better. That these busy people were able to find the time to write chapters for this Handbook is nothing short of miraculous. I am indebted to all of them. I am additionally indebted to multiple-chapter contributors Ron Adrezin of the University of Hartford and Don Peterson of the University of Connecticut School of Medicine for helping me organize the biomechanics chapters in the handbook, and for recruiting other contributors, Mike Nowak, a colleague at the University of Hartford and Anthony Brammer, now a colleague at the University of Connecticut Health Center. Also, contributor Alf Dolan of the University of Toronto was especially helpful in recommending contributors for the clinical engineering chapters.

Thanks to both of my editors at McGraw-Hill—Linda Ludwig, who signed the Handbook, and Ken McCombs, who saw the project to its completion. Thanks also to Dave Fogarty, who managed McGraw-Hill's editing process smoothly and expeditiously.

I want to give the final word to my wife Arlene, the family medical researcher and expert, in recognition of her patience and support throughout the life of this project, from development of the idea, to selection and recruiting of contributors, to receipt and editing of manuscripts: "It is our hope that this Handbook will not only inform and enlighten biomedical engineering students and practitioners in their present pursuits, but also provide a broad and sturdy staircase to facilitate their ascent to heights not yet scaled."

Myer Kutz
Albany, New York

P · A · R · T · 1

MEDICAL DEVICE DESIGN

CHAPTER 1
MEDICAL PRODUCT DESIGN

James P. O'Leary
Tufts University, Medford, Massachusetts

1.1 INTRODUCTION/OVERVIEW

The design of a medical product is a complex task. All design activities involve the resolution of conflicts and compromise among the desired features, but in medical products the conflicts tend to be more intense, the stakes are often higher, and the background information is often more uncertain. This section describes a process that has been found to be useful in bringing successful products to market. It is based on an approach to design that has recently been described as *concurrent engineering*.

This section opens with some groundwork on getting a program started, follows that with a somewhat specific set of steps to be carried out as the design is developed (Fig. 1.1), and then examines some issues that pervade the entire process, reviewing how these concerns might affect a design and in particular the design of a medical device. Figure 1.1 shows the steps in the process to be described.

In order to be more specific about some of the details, an example is sometimes necessary. In this section that product is an improved system of exterior fixation of long bone fractures. In exterior fixation, pins of some type are attached through the skin to the bones above and below the fracture and these pins are in turn attached to an external structure that maintains the position of the bone segments during healing. This is a problem that is easy to picture and understand, which makes it a good example for this document. It is a difficult area in which to make progress, however, and none will be made here. It will only serve as an illustration.

Everything has to start somewhere, and a medical product may emanate from a variety of originating events, but at some point a decision is made to pursue a certain need, question, request, or

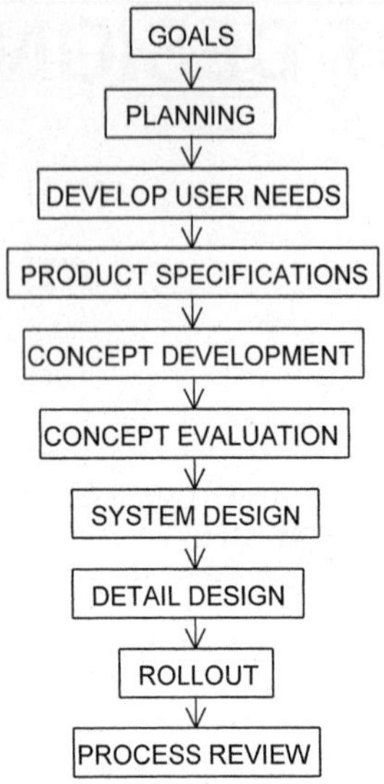

FIGURE 1.1 Elements of the medical device design process.

idea, and to devote some resources toward that effort. At that point there is an embryonic project, and the device development effort has begun. A preliminary examination is made, a goal is defined, perhaps a report is prepared, some estimates are made of the market, the cost of development, the time to market, the fit with the existing organization plans, and the competition. If the aggregate of these estimates is attractive, a decision is made to develop a new product, and a planning stage is funded. The process here will start with that planning activity.

Sometime before, after, or during the planning process, the development team is assembled. Even though it may not follow in that sequence, the process of building the team will be discussed even before the planning phase. The steps in building the team are probably as important as any in a serious development task. Even if it is to occur later, it must be considered carefully in laying out the plan.

With a plan and a team in place, the next step is to carefully define the characteristics that the product is to have. A medical product fulfills a set of needs, which are referred to here as the user needs. It is most important that the product does indeed fill a legitimate and clearly defined need. A process is described here for arriving at and documenting the need, through contact with potential users, medical professionals, patients, and others who will be affected by the device.

With a clear vision of the desired outcome, the team can then proceed to converting the desires of the various parties into a set of specifications for the design. These requirements are to be stated in measurable terms, allowing for careful evaluation of ideas in the early stages and progress as the design is solidified.

The next step in the process is to generate concepts. Although it is frequently the case that a program starts with a solution, all too often the starting idea is not the best one. A concerted effort must be made to seek the best possible idea or concept to exploit. The approach taken is to generate as long and broad a set of alternatives as possible. The logic and some processes for doing this will be discussed.

With a large set of alternatives in hand, the list must be winnowed down to a number that can be pursued. This may be a single idea, but it is preferred that several are taken through the next few steps. There are selection tools or methodologies that can help in this process. A great deal of judgment is required, and great care is advised here.

With the concept selection completed, a design must be executed. This is accomplished in the system and detail design phases. Elements here are highly dependent on the nature of the product, so that the process here is less explicitly described than the previous steps. This activity is greatly influenced by several of the issues mentioned previously, so a framework will be laid here and then these ancillary issues will be discussed along with ways they might interact with the design itself.

With a medical product designed, it must be tested thoroughly, not just to verify its efficacy and safety, but to assure that it has those characteristics that embody a successful product. There are strategies for managing the prototyping and testing process in ways that enhance the product's likelihood of success.

The last activity in the process is the start-up of manufacturing and the product rollout. This event is the result of careful planning done though the duration of the project, often starting on the very first day! Some of the special considerations discussed here cannot be allowed to wait, but are integrated into all the activities. Nonetheless, it will be discussed as a phase near the end of the section.

The last part of this discussion will be devoted to some overarching issues: documentation, the roll of design tools and other resources, and regulatory issues and their impact on the design activity.

1.2 SCOPE

The term *medical product* can describe things that vary in size, scope, complexity, importance, and cost by several orders of magnitude. All of the material covered here is applicable over virtually all of that range, but the relative importance of and effort spent in various elements will vary in the same way. A stage that requires a year in the development of one product may be completed as part of a single meeting on another. The reader is cautioned to exercise judgment in this regard. Judgment will be found to play a major role throughout any product development effort.

1.3 QUALITIES OF SUCCESSFUL PRODUCT DESIGN

Before proceeding it may be useful to define the objectives of this section more specifically. Eppinger and Ulrich[1] suggest that there are five aspects to the quality of a product design effort:

- Product quality
- Product cost
- Development cost
- Development time
- Enhanced development capability

Product quality in this context is the overall accumulation of desired characteristics—ease of use, precision, attractiveness, and all of the other things that one finds attractive in artifacts. Cost is, of course, the cost to manufacture. In general, the market determines a product's selling price, while the cost is determined by the design. There are differing opinions about where in the design process cost becomes locked in—in the conception, the details, or the manufacturing start-up—and it no doubt differs for various products, but it is always within the scope of the material discussed here. The profitability of the project depends on the difference between the two, the gross margin. That difference must cover the other expenses of the enterprise with something left over. In the medical device business, those other expenses are much higher than in most sectors. Costs of selling, tracking, providing customer service, etc., are higher for medical devices than for other products of equivalent function. The development cost of the product is another of those expenses that must be covered by the margin. (It is also one that is higher in the medical device sector.) It represents an investment and is apportioned over the life of the product. Development time is often tightly related to development cost, as projects tend to have a spending rate. In addition, the investment in development cost must be recovered in a timely way, which only begins when the product begins to sell. Furthermore, it is generally accepted that the product will eventually be replaced by another in the market, and that the "window" of opportunity opens when the product is introduced and begins to close when its successor appears. The design team can widen the window by an earlier introduction.

The last of these qualities needs some explanation. The process used here results in good documentation of the design activities. This results in an opportunity for those engaged to re-evaluate the work done and to learn from that effort. Coming out of a design effort with an organization better equipped to undertake the next task is an important benefit of doing it well. Design of medical products is always done in a rapidly changing milieu where the rate of learning is very important.

1.4 CONCURRENT ENGINEERING

Although a recently coined term, concurrent engineering embodies an approach that has been around for a very long time. Simply stated, it asks that a design be developed from the outset by a team that is capable of respecting all aspects of the problems faced. This has been contrasted with the style of design organization sometimes described as the waterfall scheme, where a group does part of the design task and then passes their results on to another group, which makes its contribution and in turn passes the result on again. The most popular image of this is someone throwing a document package "over a wall" to the next phase. Concurrent engineering is based on assembling a complete design team at the time the project is begun, and having it work as a unit throughout the design cycle. A great deal of the success of this technique depends on the composition of the team.

1.5 GOALS

The preliminary efforts should have defined a goal. In the corporate world, this must usually be well defined in order to be approved, but it's a good idea to step back at the beginning and be sure that the goal is clearly defined and agreed on by all parties. There are times when the goal of the project starts out as an assignment or charge from a higher point in the organization or it might originate within the group. Regardless of origin, it's a good idea to critique it, edit it, and turn it into a single sentence, often with a few important adjectives. When sufficiently polished, it should be displayed in some way that assists the team in remaining focused.

In the case of the external fixation system, the goal might be: *Develop an external fixation system, that can be quickly installed at all of the common long bone fracture sites, using as few as possible distinct elements.*

1.6 TEAM/TALENT

There are two important aspects to building or recruiting a product design team: covering all of the specialties required to accomplish the task, and assembling a group of individuals who can work together effectively and efficiently. It is much easier to discuss the first of these. Although every function within a corporation will have some impact on how successful the effort is, the product design team is usually built around a core of people representing marketing, engineering, and production. In the case of a medical device, an additional specialty in regulatory affairs is important. The size of this group, the core team, will depend on the nature of the project and could be from four people, each at one-quarter time, to several dozen full-time key people.

The team will have a working relationship with one or more clinicians who are expected to be heavy users of the product. Very often this will be an individual who suggested the product opportunity. This person can be categorized as an expert user, but plays a different role than the users that the team will deal with later. In almost every case, this is a small part of this person's professional activity. He or she has an active practice and is involved here for reasons of intellectual pride or curiosity. The help of these individuals is vital in formulating the problem and sometimes in maintaining a correct focus. Finding high-caliber practitioners who are effective in this role can be very difficult. Many find the give and take of the product design and evolution process frustrating, or do not find the design team environment very comfortable. Recruiting a knowledgeable clinician who is helpful in this regard should be an early priority.

The team leader, who might carry the title product manager or some variation of that, may come from any of the four specialties mentioned earlier, but must be capable of providing insight in each of them and leadership to the entire team. If possible, the leader should have some control over the membership of the core team. The effectiveness of communication among the core team will have much to do with the success of the program, so the leader must feel that the team will be candid, both with the leader and with each other as problems and challenges arise.

Another position often mentioned in the product design literature is the "champion." This is an individual who is high enough in the organization to influence the spending of resources at the level required and who is personally committed to the project. In some cases the champion may be the team leader, but more often is the person the leader reports to. Regardless of the titles and terminology, the champion is a vital part of the team. If this person doesn't exist, the project will not weather the first storm.

The team leader will carry the primary project management responsibilities. This includes drafting the original plan, defining schedule and resource requirements, assessing the various risks that things will not proceed as planned, and watching the progress of the plan in all of its details. Much has been written about the role of the leader, and most professionals with some experience recognize the importance of the leadership, management, and technical skills required for a successful program.

If there are team members new to the medical device field, they should bear in mind that many of the rules of thumb that are useful in managing a product design effort need to be recalibrated in this sector. Things take longer, cost more, and are more difficult to pin down. The same items are important but the parameters are often different.

1.7 PLANNING/RESOURCES

Before the project gets underway, a fairly detailed plan must be put into place. A good plan is the best possible start for the project. The team leader along with the core team should compile a document that spells out the schedule, the people and other assets required to accomplish the various tasks.

The plan should identify gating events. These are the points in the project where an evaluation of progress and potential outcomes is made. The plan is held to, changed, or abandoned on the basis of the gating events. These points should be well defined at the planning stage. The level of formality at the gate points depends on the nature of the product and the corporate culture. The need for meeting regulatory requirements will guide the choice of some of these gates, but other issues will also play a role. The points where the rate of spending increases or when other commitments must be made are good choices.

The planning process also involves the setting of targets. If the five measures of success mentioned earlier are considered, there is at least one target imbedded in each of them. First there is a product of high quality, with quality measured in market acceptance, performance, and perhaps other attributes. Target values should be spelled out and serve as a focus throughout the project. Likewise there are manufacturing cost, development cost, and development time targets that should be delineated. These should be aggressive without being absurd. In the current business environment, there is little room for any but the best of products. To be successful, the product must have a strong advantage over its competition. It will have to offer something unattainable elsewhere. A strong focus on the advantage to be attained is very important. If the thing is worth doing, it is worth doing well.

It is difficult to set measures for the enhancement of capabilities that is the final measure of success. One set of objectives could be the establishment and documentation of procedures if the group is doing things in a really new way. A second approach is to challenge the time and cost schedules. In a larger, more mature organization, a formal benchmarking process can be used to measure the strength and effectiveness of the development team. See Ref. 2 for an overview of this approach.

1.8 DEVELOPING USER NEEDS

Before proceeding to design a product, it is extremely important to establish clearly what it is that the product will do. It is important that this sequence be understood and respected. First the function required of the device will be defined, and only then are the means to accomplish the function sought. Many design efforts have resulted in failure because the object was defined first and the major effort was aimed at proving the device was needed, trying to make the market fit the design.

It doesn't work that way unless a team is extremely lucky. The place to start is to define what is referred to here as the need, with no regard to the means of meeting the need.

Before digging into the need definition process, the term *stakeholder* must be introduced. In this context, the stakeholders are all of the individuals who are going to be affected by the introduction of this product. There are often a large number of individuals represented here. They range from the those who work in the manufacturing facility where the device is produced, to the patient who benefits most directly, to the organization responsible for disposing of it when it is no longer functional, with many people in between. All of these people have some interaction with the product, will influence its effectiveness, and will in some way contribute to the success or failure of the venture. The definition of need begins with the identification of the stakeholders and an evaluation of the contribution each can make to the process.

The actual user of the device obviously heads the list of those who must be consulted, and this discussion will focus on this individual first. This might be a surgeon, a therapist, a nurse, an operating room technician, or some other member of the health-care delivery system. Regardless of the role, the purpose of the device under development is to in some way assist that individual, to do something that could not be done before, to make something easier to do, to make it safer, less invasive, less traumatic, or in some other form more desirable. A chronic problem with designers is that they try to make things better from their own point of view, rather than that of the user.

The knowledge that is sought from these stakeholders concerns the desired characteristics of the product. What would make it a good or attractive device from their point of view? It is important to maintain a separation here from any particular design or solution, and not to ask the individual to "design" the device. (Although often they will wish to do just that.) As an example, a useful piece of knowledge is that "the device should weigh as little as possible." Some stakeholders will want to suggest making the product out of aluminum or foamed plastic, in essence jumping over the issue, toward a design solution. We know that choosing a low-density material is not always the best way to attain a lighter weight in the finished product. By exploring the rationale for the suggestion, the developer can get a clearer understanding of the user's desires. Try to understand the attitude and try and get it into functional requirements in the user's own words.

In medical products the stakeholder group also includes the patient, and sometimes the patient's family. If we consider the external fixation device, the person most interested in keeping the weight down is the patient who may be encumbered by it for a period of months. That is probably not the only problem, however. In this instance, an effort should be made to locate a number of patients who have had external fixations and gather the available information.

The patients never see many medical devices, so that the potential contribution from this source must be evaluated for each product. Examine the circumstances carefully. The error that is often made is to rely on the clinician to present the patient's point of view. If the patient is conscious of interacting with the device, he or she should be spoken to directly.

There are a variety of techniques for soliciting the opinion of the stakeholder in this context; questionnaires, interviews, focus groups, and direct observations have all been used effectively. The best choice in a particular situation will depend on many circumstances. It is important that the choice not be based on convenience, cost, or time constraints, but on the nature of the product, the state of development of products of this type, the user group itself, and a myriad of other issues.

There are some concerns in selecting the individual users for this process. Von Hipple[3] has identified a group of individuals he calls "lead users." These are the pacesetters in the area in which they work. They are always looking for new ideas and new ways to do things. Lead users should be part of the user group studied for two reasons. They are often critical of ideas and are very helpful in identifying new directions. In addition, these individuals are often the first to be willing to try out new products and their peers will look to them for guidance in this regard. It is also important that those queried include representatives of average users of a product. It is possible to design a product that can only be used by or is only useful to the a few practitioners at the very top of their field. Producing a product of this kind can be prestigious, but it is seldom a good business decision. (There are many examples of prototype and custom-built devices, particularly surgical instruments, made for these individuals, that were successful in the hands of the target user but were not commercialized because there was no expectation of a sizable market.)

An additional concern that should be recognized here is that many aspects of medical practice vary, often geographically and sometimes in more complex patterns. A procedure may be done frequently in one facility and rarely in another, which would seem to have a similar patient base. At the international scale, the variations can be striking. Rutter and Donaldson[4] provide an interesting examination of some of these issues. In assessing the needs for a device, patterns of treatment that are relative to the problem should be examined carefully.

The material collected from this exercise should be sorted, characterized, and summarized into a document that is the first real step toward the design. Individual statements from stakeholders should be preserved verbatim. Condensation should only remove redundancy. If we have seven people telling us that the design must be such that it can be operated with one hand, at least one of them should be quoted in the needs document. At a later point in the process, it will be important to examine whether the request was met, and it should be tested against the user's words, not the developer's interpretation of the user's need.

When a list of the needs has been established, the team should assign weights to each item. This can be done on a scale of 1 to 5 or 1 to 10, or even a three-level scale of "highly," "moderately," and "minimally" important.

This is the first time that the team doing numerical evaluations has been mentioned, and it brings up several potential problems. In this instance, there may be some tendency to bias the scores according to what is perceived to be obtainable. If we know that keeping the weight of the product down is going to be difficult, we know that we will feel better if somehow it is not so important. Unfortunately, how we feel has little to do with how important it might be, so the team must gather itself up and evaluate things from the point of view of the user, regardless of the difficult position into which it may put itself.

The second risk in team scoring is team members who strategize. Typically, this takes the form of stating a position that is different and more extreme than that which is held, in order to offset the position of another team member. If I think the item is a 6, and I think you want to score it an 8, I would give it a 4 to offset your opinion. Some individuals have difficulty resisting the desire to do this, and some may even do it unconsciously. It is one of the responsibilities of the team leader to recognize that this is happening and to deal with it. One measure of an effective team is the absence of this effect. If it were to happen frequently, the team could be considered dysfunctional.

The most highly developed and detailed processes for obtaining user input have been described under the title *quality function deployment* (QFD). For a more detailed description of this process, see Hauser and Clausing.[5]

1.9 PRODUCT SPECIFICATIONS

The document that clarifies the needs is expressed in the language of the user. The next step in our process is to transform these needs into specifications that can be used to guide the design decisions. These product specifications become the targets for the product development and as such they need to be measurable. In general there should be a specification for each identified need, but there are exceptions to this that run in both directions.

The important characteristic of specifications is that they must be expressed in measurable terms, for example, "The device must weigh less than 2.3 lb," or "The power consumption must be less than 350 W." While the user needs were often qualitative, the purpose now is to write requirements that can be used to evaluate the ideas and designs produced. Before proceeding to define the specifications, the metric or unit of measure for each of the needs must be identified. These are often obvious, but sometimes require some thought. Most requirements will state maximum or minimum values, like weight and power consumption. Sometimes there are actual target values that are desired, such as "Must fit in size B front end."

The metrics selected for each requirement should be considered carefully. They should be the common measures for simple characteristics. The difficulty of making the measurements must be considered. These specifications could easily turn into quality assurance requirements in the product, necessitating numerous repetitions of the measurement. It will be much more convenient to have easily determined objectives. It is almost always possible to reduce the issue to easily examined variables. One exception would be a reliability specification where many units would have to be tested to arrive at an acceptable failure rate.

Once the list of metrics has been set, the values to be required must be determined. Here we have several leads to go on. We have the results of our user studies, which might have set some specific guidelines. We have the existing products that our competitors or we market and products that will be perceived to fall into the same category. These must be examined for similar user characteristics, sizes, operating forces, etc. What are the current accepted values? What are the values we hope to achieve? It is a good idea to obtain samples of all these products if it has not yet been done, even those that are in no way competitive, if they are going to be thought of by the user as in the same class. If there is a range of quality here, the level that is being aimed for must be determined and the values set accordingly. Having reviewed all the pertinent information available, specification values should be set. (See Table 1.1.)

TABLE 1.1 Idealized Example of Some User Needs Translated to Specifications for the External Fixation System

User comment	Specification	Units	Value
Make it from aluminum or carbon fiber	The system mass will be no more than X	Kilograms	0.75
It must be easy to install	Installation time will be less than X	Minutes	20
It must not weaken the bone too much	Holes in bones must have diameters no more than X	Millimeters	4.0

The documentation of this process is important because in most cases the target specifications arrived at here will be unobtainable. (You find that you cannot make the laproscopic tool strong enough and still fit it through a 7-mm port!) Later in the project there will be an effort to reach some compromises and having at hand the details of how the existing values were chosen will save more than half of the discussion time and, more often, allow the discussion to proceed in a more civilized manner, preserving the team morale.

1.10 CONCEPT DEVELOPMENT

With the specifications in place, it is now time to seriously look for solutions. The concept development phase is the time to search out ideas that will meet the need. Much has been written about ways to generate new ideas, and some of them will be touched on here, but more important than method is motivation. The objective is to generate an absolutely superb product, one that meets all the requirements in a cost-effective, safe, elegant way, and to do it quickly and efficiently. Unfortunately, at this stage of the process, quickly and efficiently often dominate the first part of that sentence in a manner that is very shortsighted. There is a tendency to proceed with the first idea that appears to have merit. In the general scheme of things, a little extra time at this stage might very well produce a much better idea, or perhaps even a scheme that is only slightly better. Consider the trade-off.

Time spent on concept generation is relatively inexpensive. Prototypes are not being built, clinical trials aren't being conducted. A great deal of paper may get expended and even some computer time, but if one looks at the rate at which resources are consumed, the concept phase of a development project is on the lower end of the scale. If one thinks of the concept phase as a search for the best idea, it's not like searching for a needle in a haystack, but perhaps something slightly larger than a needle. If we search for a while, we may find an attractive idea. If we search further, we may find a better idea. If we walk away from the haystack, someone else may come along and find a better idea than the best one that we found and bring it to market shortly after we bring ours—and our product will be obsolete.

The primary argument for shortening the development time, or the "time to market" as it is thought of, is that eventually another product will displace ours. If we think of that product's introduction as an event over which we have no control, we lengthen our market window by an early introduction. If, however, we pass up the best product to get to market a short time earlier, we are inviting the early arrival of product termination.

Generating a long list of alternative design ideas is a very difficult task, requiring creativity, resourcefulness, energy and, most importantly, stamina. It is for this reason that so much emphasis has been placed on the quantity of concepts. After a short time and a few seemingly credible ideas, it is hard to continue to dig for alternatives. Different teams and leaders advocate different modes of idea generation, each having worked well for them. A starting point is to ask each team member to spend some time alone making a concept list. A comfortable place to work undisturbed, a pad of paper, and a few hours should produce many more ideas than each had at the outset. These lists can be brought together in a team meeting or brainstorming session. (Brainstorming has two working definitions. One is a formal process developed to produce ideas from a group. It has a clear procedure and set of rules.[6] The word is also used to describe any group working together to find a problem solution. Either definition could be applied here.)

At this point in our project we do not want to discard ideas. It is widely believed that some of the really good ideas are stimulated by some less sane proposals, so the objective is to lengthen the list, and hold off on criticism or selectivity.

There are some techniques that can assist when things begin to slow down here. One is to break out some characteristic of the device and make a list of all of the ways one could supply that function. For example, an active device requires energy. Ways to supply energy would include electric power from the utility, batteries, springs, pneumatics, hydraulics, hand power, and foot power. Trying to think up design ideas that use each of these functions will often lead to some different kinds of solutions. Other types of characteristics are specific material classes, cross-section shapes, etc.

It is also fruitful to look at the ways that analogous medical devices function. Is there an equivalent functionality that has been used in a different medical problem? One example of this is access ports that might function for feeding in one instance, as a drug-delivery mode in another, and as a monitoring channel in a third. All have similar problems to overcome. Surgical instruments can provide many examples of devices that are variations of previous designs.

Another means of expanding the list is to combine ideas with features from other ideas. Look especially at the ideas that seem novel and find as many permutations on them as possible.

Some means of compiling the concept list is necessary. Index cards, spreadsheets, or even Post-it Notes® may be used. It helps if the scheme allows the ideas to be sorted and rearranged, but the importance of this will vary a great deal with the situation. Ultimately, you should emerge from this phase with a list of ideas to be considered. The list should be long, have many ideas that are of little value, and hopefully have several that have the potential to turn into world class products.

1.11 CONCEPT EVALUATION

Having spent a great deal of time and effort developing an extended set of concepts, the team must now select those that will be developed further. There are several important points to keep in mind as this process begins. The first is to have an even-handed approach. It is unwise to compare an idea that has been sketched out in 30 s to one that has had many hours of development, and discard the first because it isn't understood. As much as is reasonably possible, concepts should be compared at an equal state of development. That having been said, there will be ideas brought up that can be recognized immediately as inappropriate. (This is particularly true if the team is diligent about seeking ideas.) The notably bad ideas should be quickly but carefully (and sometimes even gently) culled out and discarded.

The second issue revolves around selection criteria. The process will (or should) pick the idea that provides to the team and the organization the best opportunity to develop a successful product. In making that selection, the capabilities of the organization come into consideration. What kind of products is the group experienced with? What kind of manufacturing facilities does it have at hand? What are the core competencies of the corporation? The concern here is the good idea that doesn't fit. As a simplistic example, if the organization builds mechanical things, and the best concept for the product under discussion is an electronic solution, there is an impasse. The kind of design available is second rate, and will fail in the marketplace. (Someone will market the electronic version!) The options are (1) abandon the product plan, (2) acquire the needed skills and competency, or (3) partner with one or more organizations that can provide the talent. Contracting with a design firm for development and an outside manufacturing organization might accomplish the latter. This decision will probably be made at a higher level in the organization, on the basis of the evaluation of concept potential done within the team.

Having reduced the list to ideas that have real possibilities, a selection process should be used that rates the concepts on all-important criteria. The specification document will provide not only the list of criteria but also some guidance as to the importance of each item. This list should be used in a two-step process; the first step will screen the concepts, and the second will select those to be developed further.

For the screening we will use a method called Pugh concept selection.[7] Place a list of the criteria to be used in the first column of a matrix, use the list of the remaining concepts as the headings for the adjacent columns. A spreadsheet program will be very useful for this purpose. Choose one of the concepts as a reference. This should be a well-understood idea, perhaps embodied in a current product, yours or a competitor's. Now compare each concept against the reference concept for each criterion and score it with a plus sign if it does better and a minus sign if it is inferior. Use a zero if there is no clear choice. When all the cells are full, add the number of pluses and subtract the number of minuses to get the score for each idea. Many of the scores will be close to zero, and of course the reference idea will get exactly zero. (See Table 1.2.)

TABLE 1.2 Partial Scoring of Concepts for External Fixation

Criteria	Concept A	Concept B	Concept C	Baseline concept
Weight	+	–	+	0
Installation time	–	+	+	0
Weakening	+	0	–	0
Totals	+#	–#	+#	0

At this point the number of concepts under consideration should be cut back to about 10 or 15. The first criterion for the reduction is the score on the requirements sheet. Before discarding any of the ideas, however, examine each one to determine why it has done so poorly. See if the idea may be modified to increase its potential. If so, retain it for the next cycle.

With the field narrowed to a reasonable number of candidates, it is now possible to devote a little effort to refining each of them, get to understand them better, and then construct a new matrix. This time a weighting factor should be agreed to for each of the criteria. A range of 5 for very important and 1 for minimally important will suffice. Now score each of the concepts on a basis of 1 to 10 on each criterion and compute the sums of the weighted scores. This will allow the ideas to be ranked and a selection made of the ideas to be seriously developed.

The major decision remaining here is how many concepts should be pursued in depth. This is another judgment decision, to be guided by a number of factors: How much confidence is there in the first two or three ideas? How long will it take to prove out the uncertainties? What resources are available? It is highly probable that the idea that emerges from the selection process with the highest score will have some yet-to-be-discovered flaw. This stage is much too early to commit all of the resources to a single concept. It is a time when options should be kept open.

Conclude this process by documenting the selection. Include all of the scoring sheets, concept descriptions, and related data. This will become part of the medical device master file, and perhaps play a role in getting product approval and it will be useful when concepts need to be reconsidered later in order to make final decisions.

1.12 ARCHITECTURE/SYSTEM DESIGN

It was mentioned early that the term *medical device* describes a wide variety of products. The process of proceeding from concept through system design and detail design will vary greatly thoughout the spectrum of products. Design development should in general follow a path similar to that of physically similar nonmedical items. The major accommodation is in documentation. It is important to maintain a detailed record of the decisions made and their basis. This will be important through the product's manufacturing start-up and afterward, when alterations are proposed for manufacturing reasons, to accommodate later product upgrades, etc. The ability to return to well-kept documentation and follow the original logic will provide guidance, sometimes supporting the change, often indicating its inappropriateness. There is a tendency in these situations to repeat the same mistakes. A change in a medical device is a much more expensive undertaking than it would be in other objects of equivalent complexity because of the qualification, verification, and testing that is so often required. Good documentation can often prevent the initiation of some misguided efforts.

The objective in the system-level design is to deconstruct the product into separate elements that can be considered independently. Once this has been done, the various team members can proceed to define the elements of the product. The system design must define the interfaces where the separate elements meet. This includes shapes, dimensions, and connection characteristics, such as currents, digital signals, fluid pressures, and forces. Decisions made at this stage have a profound effect on the complete design. The team and the leader must exercise judgment here. In a sense these decisions are allocating a budget. In certain examples this is obvious, as in space allocated or power consumption limits. Sometimes it may be subtler than this, but much of the budgetary sense will remain.

The actual relationships defined in the system design are called the architecture. There are two extremes that are considered in system architecture, integrated and modular. Modular systems are made up of components or modules that have clear interfaces with each other, and are easily visualized as systems. Integrated products, on the other hand, appear to be a single element, with what interfaces exist being so soft and blurred as to be hard to identify. Each of these styles has its advantages. Integration allows the device to be technically more efficient. With the overall device optimized, there is no loss due to inefficiencies of connections, etc.

Modularity provides flexibility at several levels, which is often extremely desirable. As mentioned earlier, it can make the design effort simpler. It also allows for modifications and upgrades. If a system component is changed, one can test the new component for performance more efficiently than testing the entire system. All of the engineering issues tend to be less challenging in this modular environment. In addition, a modular design enables element replacement. This is important in several ways. An element of the system can be designed with the expectation that its life will be shorter than that of the system, and it will be replaced when needed. The clearest case of this in medical devices is a single-use or disposable element such as a blade. An appropriate architecture allows a very efficient design, replacing the elements that cannot be reused without wasting those that can.

Modularity also enables variety in design by permitting variation in one or more components. This is a way to provide devices in various sizes, or sometimes at various levels of performance. In some cases, this is accomplished by selling the components of the system separately, in others the unit can be thought of as a platform product with several different products, all based on the same system and sharing a large number of elements.[8]

In addition to the economic and technical reasons that support modularity, it can assist in a medical product gaining acceptance. If the product can be viewed by the clinician as having a number of modules that are familiar, along with some new functionality, it may be easier to introduce than a system that is viewed as an entirely new approach. Most medical professionals are somewhat conservative and like to be on ground that is at least somewhat familiar. This could be a consideration in choice of architecture and even in the details of the deconstruction process.

In many designs, the layout of the system is obvious. Similar products have been broken out the same way to everyone's satisfaction, and no other arrangement seems possible. On the other hand, it is good practice to ask if this is indeed the optimum architecture for the given product, and explore the advantages and disadvantages of altering the architecture.

1.13 DETAIL DESIGN

The detail design phase is where the individual components of the system are fully defined. Again, the issues here vary greatly across the product spectrum, but primarily the issue is function against the various penalties of weight, space, cost, etc. None of these are unique to the medical device area, but the costs tend to be higher, the penalty for error much higher, and therefore the need for care very intense.

It is good practice to use commercially available components as much as possible as long as they do not compromise the design functionality in any way. Each and every part that is unique to the product will require careful specification, manufacturing study, shape, and manufacturing documentation, manufacturing qualification, etc. It is difficult to estimate the cost of adding a part to a medical product production system, but Galsworthy[9] quotes a source from 1994 stating that the average in the commercial world is no less than $4000. The medical product equivalent must be an order of magnitude larger.

As the parts are designed, consideration must be given to not only the manufacturing process to be used, but also the method of testing and verifying functionality. Some foresight at the detail level can provide "hooks" that enable the initial testing of the part, the system, and even the ongoing quality assurance testing that good manufacturing practice mandates. Providing an electrical contact point or flat on which to locate a displacement probe can make what would otherwise be a project into a routine measurement.

1.14 DESIGN FOR MANUFACTURE

The need for design for manufacture goes without saying, since one of the primary measures of success in product development is cost to manufacture. There is a strong belief among developers that the cost to manufacture a product is largely determined at the concept-selection stage, but there is a great deal of evidence that indicates details of design based on selection of manufacturing methods are the real determining factors. The major stumbling block here is that so many manufacturing processes are volume sensitive. The design of parts for the same physical function and annual volumes of 1000, 100,000, and 10 million would call for three totally different manufacturing processes. In detailing the part, it is important to know the production targets. Things can be designed to transition from low volume to high volume as the product gains market, but it needs careful planning and good information. This is one of the places that the team's skills in marketing, design, and manufacture can pay large dividends.

1.15 ROLLOUT

Bringing the product out of the trial phase and into manufacturing and the marketplace is the last responsibility of the team. The initial product planning should have defined target sales volumes, and the marketing function of the team should have been updating these estimates throughout the development and trials. Products are often introduced at shows, resulting in a national or even international introduction. This means that there should be sufficient quantities of product "on the shelf" to meet the initial round of orders. It is difficult to recover from a product scarcity that develops in the initial launch. All of the stakeholders become disenchanted.

The arrangements for product sales and distribution are not within the scope of this book, but the plan for this should be understood by the development team well in advance of the introduction. Issues like training the sales staff, providing printed materials, and samples should have been worked out well in advance.

1.16 PROCESS REVIEW

This is also the time for the team to evaluate the job it has done, the lessons it has learned, and specifically how it performed against the five objectives set forth at the start of this section. Quality, cost to manufacture, time to market, and cost to develop will be well recognized. The fifth objective of improving the capability of the organization will require some thought. An effort should be made to determine what aspects of the process did not work as well as they should have. A team meeting may be the best way to do this, or the team leader may choose to meet members individually.

The basis for assessment should be the plan and the process. Were the plan and the process followed closely? If not why? Should the plan have been different on the basis of the knowledge at the time it was drawn? Is the process, as laid out, the best approach for this group? How should it be altered? Were the resources and external support adequate? If not, in what way?

The answers to these and related questions should be compiled into a report and that document circulated in a way that maximizes the learning function of the project. It is important to review this document again as the next product development project is being proposed.

1.17 PROTOTYPING

Making prototypes is so much a part of device development that it is often taken for granted. Prototyping plays a very important part in the process but it must be thought out and planned, if the maximum benefit is to be derived. Clearly the size and scope of the product and the effort will control to some extent this activity. In some cases, many prototypes will be built before the design is frozen while in other projects one or two may be an efficient plan. Of course, a clinical trial will require many copies of the prototype design in most cases.

In planning the project, the goals of each prototyping effort should be defined. They are often associated with milestones in the plan. A prototype having particular working characteristics is to be functional by a particular date. In setting that goal, the purpose of that prototype should be understood and stated. We generally think of the prototype as proving the feasibility of the design, but close examination often shows that not to be the case. Clausing[10] describes situations where the effort that should be focused on the design is going into debugging prototypes that have already become obsolete. We need to have focus.

In many situations a partial prototype, one that might be more properly termed a test bed, is in order. This is a device that mimics some part of the proposed design, and allows critical characteristics of the design to be altered and tested. This system may bear little resemblance to the final product; it really only needs to have the significant physical characteristics of the segment under study. This might be the working parts of a transducer or the linkage of some actuator. It may be constructed to evaluate accuracy, repeatability, durability, or some other critical feature. It should be thought of as an instrument. If it is worth the trouble, time, and effort to build it, then an experiment should be designed to garner as much information as it has to offer.

With partial medical device experiments, usually called bench testing, an often-encountered problem is the replication of the biological materials that the device interacts with. If we return momentarily to the external fixation device, it requires that the pins be affixed to the fractured bone. In considering the need, it is recognized that the fracture might represent an athletic injury to a young healthy person with very strong bones, or it may have resulted from a mild impact to an individual with relatively weak bones. We would like our device to function over this range, and must choose test media accordingly. We would start with commercial bone emulation material (e.g., Sawbones®), but then probably move to some animal models. Careful analysis of this situation is important. Why is the test carried out? Are we interested in failure mode to better understand the device or are we proving that this design is superior? Caution is called for.

1.18 TESTING

The testing and evaluation of the final device is a most important activity. This is dealt with here separately from the prototyping activity because it reaches beyond the design team in many respects and because the process and attitude required are more distinct from nonmedical products here than in the prototyping activities that are really internal to the design process.

Once the design is finalized, all of the evaluation and test data become important in the regulatory approval process, so each step should be carefully planned, executed, and documented. Each test should be done with the clear objective of validating some aspect of the design. The level of performance required should be established in advance. The test conditions should be carefully spelled out.

Bench or laboratory testing should measure the integrity, precision, and other "engineering" aspects of the device. They can also verify the production techniques, as at this stage the units being tested should come from the manufacturing processes that will be used in full production. Besides testing for normal performance, it is wise to test devices to failure at this stage, to ascertain that there are no unforeseen failure modes or collateral effects.

Many products move next to cadaver testing, where the biologically driven uncertainties cause complications. Sometimes it is possible to use animal models first in this phase, which allows for much more consistent conditions. Human cadaver tests require careful notation of the history and condition of the cadavaric materials. Results may be correlated with this data if there are anomalies that require explanation.

Clinical trials with human subjects require extensive documentation. They are most often done in institutions that have in place extensive procedures to ensure the subjects are informed about any experimental activities that they participate in. A committee reviews the forms and procedures for doing this along with the details of the study before institutional approval is granted. These things require long lead times in many cases, so the planning of the experiments ought to be done well in advance.

It is common practice to run clinical trials in several settings, often distant from each other. The point was made earlier that the device should be usable by an average practitioner, not just the ultra-highly skilled. The trials should include the opportunity to evaluate this aspect, as well as to evaluate training materials and other ancillary items that contribute to product function. Care and forethought continue to be the watchwords.

1.19 DOCUMENTATION

Documentation of a medical device design is critical. This applies not only to the usual drawings and manufacturing documents that accompany commercial products, but also to the needs and requirements documents that have been discussed earlier, as well as test data, evaluation reports, results of clinical trials, and any other pertinent information about the device, its history, or experience.

The U.S. Food and Drug Administration requires that for each device there be a device master file. The length and breadth of that rule becomes clearer when it is explained that the "file" need not be in one place! It is the collection of all the material just mentioned and it could be in several states, or even on several continents. The need to provide all of this documentation and to have it accessible requires that the project have someone in the role of librarian. If the project gets too far along and too much material is generated before a document control system is in place, it may be a situation from which there is no recovery. Document control should be part of the initial project planning. If the organization has experience in device development, it probably has already established formats and templates to handle the materials and data, and a new master file can probably be built around existing standards. If the current project is a first, an experienced person will be needed to take charge of these matters and will need to have the power to demand that procedures are followed.

1.20 TOOLS

There are a number of software products and related items that can be very useful in various aspects of product development. These include computer-aided design (CAD), computer-assisted manufacturing (CAM), various engineering analysis tools for things like finite-element stress analysis or circuit analysis, planning tools, scheduling products, systems that generate rapid prototypes, and a vast number of other things that have the potential to save effort, and more important, time. Most if not all of these tools have associated with them a learning process that requires time and effort. It is wise to develop at the outset of the project a clear picture of what tools of this kind will be needed and to be sure that the team includes members who have experience in their use.

As alluded to above, the choice to make use of a particular tool is an investment decision, and should be dealt with in that way. Software and hardware will have to be acquired, and individuals may require training in their use. The selection of these tools from the outset allows training to be done early when it will have the longest-term benefit. (It also requires the expenditure of the corresponding funds at a time that the project may appear to be overspending!) In most categories, there are competing products from which to choose. Once the requirements are met, the most desirable characteristic is familiarity. If the people on the team have used it (that might include venders and others you need to exchange information with), you are well ahead selecting that product. The purchase price can't be disregarded, but the cost in time spent learning to use a computer tool is usually higher than its price.

With most tools and particularly with CAD and similar products, there is a more or less continuous version upgrade problem. If at all possible, this is to be avoided. If you select a product that fills your needs at the outset, you should be able to get along without the three new "hotkeys" and the six new plotter interfaces that have been added to version 37.3. Installing a new release will cost time that you do not have, increase the likelihood of losing data, and will not pay off in a productivity increase that is noticeable.

The previous paragraphs presume an intense design effort on a single product. If a group is spread out continuously over a large number of projects, upgrades are a fact of life. One can, and many do, skip some of them. With some products, installing every third or fourth version will keep the group's tools sufficiently up-to-date.

1.21 REGULATORY ISSUES

Manufacturing and marketing a medical product in the United States must be done under the regulations of the Food and Drug Administration (FDA). Medical devices are handled by the agency's Center for Devices and Radiological Health (CDRH). Complying with these requirements constitutes one of the major resource requirements in the development process. As with so many other topics in this section, the extent of effort will vary greatly, depending on the nature of the product, the potential of it causing harm, and the history of similar products and devices in similar areas. Having available a person knowledgeable about the agency's dealings with similar products is a must.

Under the law granting the FDA jurisdiction over devices, products already on the market were permitted to continue. Products "equivalent to" products on the market require only a formal notification of the intent to market, but the agency is the arbiter of what is "equivalent." (Note also that the required notification documents can constitute a large package!) Devices without a predicate product are held to much more stringent controls, usually requiring a series of clinical trials, showing statistically that the device is safe and effective.

The agency has a responsibility to monitor organizations producing and distributing devices, to see that they do business in ways that do not endanger the public. This includes assuring that quality is adequately monitored, that complaints about device performance are promptly investigated, that steps are taken to correct any potential problems, etc.

The FDA has a very large and difficult responsibility and, given the resources it has to work with, carries it very well. Those who carefully design products so that they are safe and effective tend to resent having to explain the way they have gone about it, as they view the effort as unproductive. Nonetheless, this will continue to be a problem and the team must prepare for it and accept the burden.

In keeping with its responsibility, the FDA publishes documents that can be very helpful to those developing products. Most of the useful documents are in the category of "guidance." Available on many topics, including specific categories of products, these publications aim to assist people to understand what the agency expects. It is important to understand that these documents do not carry the force of law as do the regulations, but they are much more readable and can be very helpful. A suggested example is the Design Control Guidance for Medical Device Manufacturers.[11] These documents are indexed on the Web site www.accessdata.fda.gov/scripts/cdrh/cfdocs/cfTopic/topicindex/topindx.cfm.

1.22 CLOSURE

This is clearly a very short introduction to the topic of medical device design. It has been only recently that design process activities have been written on extensively, and with a few exceptions where the process is easily codified, most of what has been written is very general. All of the books in the references address the broader questions, but they provide strategy and advice that is useful to the medical product designer. All can be read with great benefit. In addition to those cited previously, attention can be paid to Cooper[12] on planning, to Leonard and Swap[13] for concept generation and teamwork. The remaining three: Otto and Wood,[14] Patterson,[15] and Wheelwright and Clark[16]; all provide deep insight into the product design world.

REFERENCES

1. Ulrich, Karl T., and Eppinger, Steven D., *Product Design and Development*, 2d ed., Irwin/McGraw-Hill, 2000.
2. Tucker, Frances G., Zivan, Seymour M., and Camp, Robert C., "How to Measure Yourself Against the Best," *Harvard Business Review*, January–February 1987, p. 8.
3. Von Hipple, Eric, *The Sources of Innovation*, Oxford University Press, 1988.
4. Rutter, Bryce G., and Donelson, Tammy H., "Measuring the Impact of Cultural Variances on Product Design," *Medical Device and Diagnostic Industry*, October 2000.
5. Hauser, John, and Clausing, Don, "The House of Quality," *Harvard Business Review*, vol. 66, no. 3, May–June 1988, pp. 63–73.
6. Osborn, Alex F., *Applied Imagination*, 3d ed., Scribners, 1963.
7. Pugh, Stuart, *Total Design*, Addison Wesley, 1991.
8. Meyer, Mark H., and Lehnerd, Alvin P., *The Power of Product Platforms*, The Free Press, 1997.

9. Galsworthy, G. D., *Smart Simple Design*, Oliver Wight Publications, Wiley, 1994.
10. Clausing, Don, *Total Quality Development*, ASME Press, 1994.
11. "Design Control Guidance for Medical Device Manufacturers," FDA Center for Devices and Radiological Health.
12. Cooper, Robert G., *Product Leadership*, Perseus Books, 2000.
13. Leonard, Dorothy, and Swap, Walter, *When Sparks Fly*, Harvard Business School Press, 1999.
14. Otto, Kevin, and Wood, Kristin, *Product Design*, Prentice Hall, 2001.
15. Patterson, Marvin L., with Lightman, Sam, *Accelerating Innovation*, Van Nostrand Reinhold.
16. Wheelwright, Steven C., and Clark, Kim B., "*Revolutionizing Product Development*," Free Press, 1992.

CHAPTER 2
FDA MEDICAL DEVICE REQUIREMENTS

Robert Klepinski
Fredrikson & Byron, PA, Minneapolis, Minnesota

2.1 INTRODUCTION

Engineers will find that working with medical devices is a different experience from dealing with other projects. While many areas of engineering involve extensive regulation, such as in nuclear products, it is difficult to imagine an area with more pervasive government control than the design, production, and sale of medical products. Regulation is simply inherent in the medical area, and it is a necessary part of engineering practice to be aware of the complexities and nuances of working in this environment.

While the primary focus of this chapter is on medical devices, engineers may now be exposed to many other types of regulation. The current trends toward combining technologies will bring engineers into contact with products that include combinations of drugs, biologics, and medical devices.

This chapter discusses the cradle-to-grave nature of U.S. medical device regulations, as well as a look at the comparable European Union (EU) regulatory scheme.

2.2 WHAT IS A MEDICAL DEVICE?

The term *medical device* covers an extremely broad range of products. Medical devices range from the simplest over-the-counter health aids to complex implantable life-supporting devices.

Any device that diagnoses, cures, mitigates, treats, or prevents disease in a human or animal is included.

> (h) The term "device" (except when used in paragraph (n) of this section and in sections 331 (i), 343 (f), 352 (c), and 362 (c) of this title) means an instrument, apparatus, implement, machine, contrivance, implant, in vitro reagent, or other similar or related article, including any component, part, or accessory, which is—
>
> (1) recognized in the official National Formulary, or the United States Pharmacopeia, or any supplement to them,
> (2) intended for use in the diagnosis of disease or other conditions, or in the cure, mitigation, treatment, or prevention of disease, in man or other animals, or
> (3) intended to affect the structure or any function of the body of man or other animals, and
>
> which does not achieve its primary intended purposes through chemical action within or on the body of man or other animals and which is not dependent upon being metabolized for the achievement of its primary intended purposes.
>
> 21 U.S.C. § 321(h)

In contrast, drugs are defined in wording almost identical to devices, except that drugs achieve their effectiveness by chemical interaction with the body or by being metabolized. Usually devices act by mechanical, electrical, magnetic, or some other physical interaction with the body. Sometimes this boundary between drugs and devices is not clear.

It is further complicated by the boundary between drugs and cosmetics. *Cosmetics* are articles intended to be rubbed, poured, sprinkled, or sprayed on, introduced into, or otherwise applied to the human body for cleansing, beautifying, promoting attractiveness, or altering the appearance.*

How does this affect your morning toothbrushing? When you brush your teeth you are using a medical device—the brush. The brush works in a mechanical manner on your teeth to remove unwanted material. The toothpaste you use could be a cosmetic in that it is applied to the teeth to cleanse. However, if you choose a fluoride toothpaste you are using a drug, since the fluoride is metabolized by the body in order to prevent tooth decay. If you choose to use an oral rinse to reduce adhesion of plaque to your teeth before you brush, you are using a medical device. The oral rinse loosens plaque that is then removed by your brushing.

Do not assume that the form of the product, liquid versus mechanical, determines whether it is a device. You must look through the sometimes arcane rules and consider its interaction with other products to determine the nature of any object designed to affect the human body.

The single most important determinant of the legal status of any item is what it is intended to be. As is discussed below, "claims" as to what a product is or does determine its legal category. A device can be a nonmedical consumer product or a medical device, depending on how you label it.

2.3 WHAT IS FDA?

While medical devices and other medical products are regulated by many government agencies, the U.S. Food and Drug Administration (FDA) is the primary regulator.

*21 U.S.C. § 321(i).

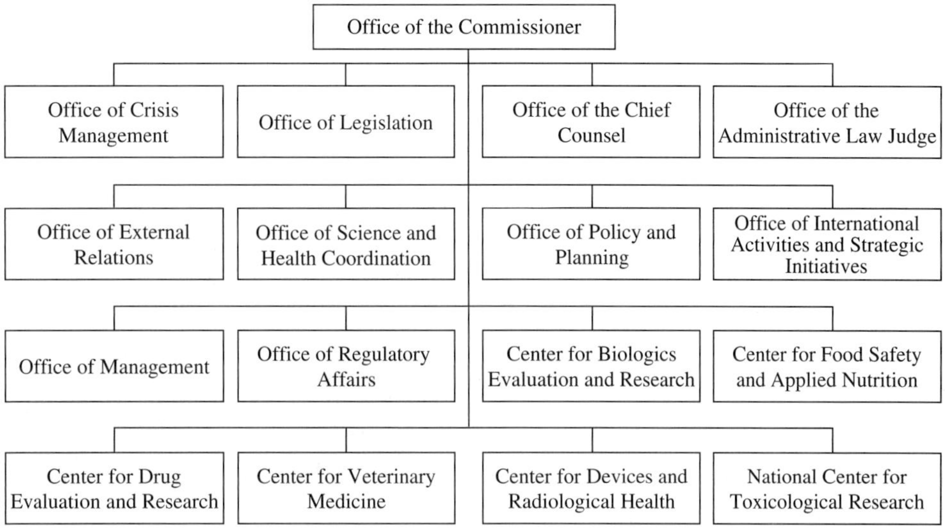

FIGURE 2.1 FDA commissioner's office.

FDA is a consumer protection organization that is part of the U.S. Department of Health and Human Services (HHS), the entity that includes many other health organizations, such as Medicare and the National Institutes of Health (NIH).

FDA is not a monolithic agency with only one face to the public. As a device engineer, you may have to interact with very disparate parts of the agency. The two major functional parts of FDA you will encounter are the headquarters organization in the suburbs of Washington, D.C., and the field organization spread throughout the country.

FDA is led by a commissioner, which is a position appointed by the President of the United States. The commissioner's office is shown in Fig. 2.1.

The rest of FDA headquarters is divided into centers, most of which have subject-matter jurisdiction (see Fig. 2.1 for centers).

The Office of Regulatory Affairs (ORA) runs the field organization. ORA divides the United States into five regions, which are further divided into district offices (refer to Fig. 2.2). These district offices are the main point of interaction between companies and FDA. District offices perform the field investigations that gather the information for almost all FDA compliance activity.

2.4 STATUTE AND REGULATIONS

While engineers generally resist the intrusion of the law into the practice of engineering, it is important to have at least rudimentary knowledge of the legal scheme that controls medical devices. The hierarchy of FDA law is

U.S. Constitution
Federal statutes (United States Code or U.S.C.)
Federal regulation (Code of Federal Regulation or C.F.R.)
Laws regulating a state or political subdivision of a state if—

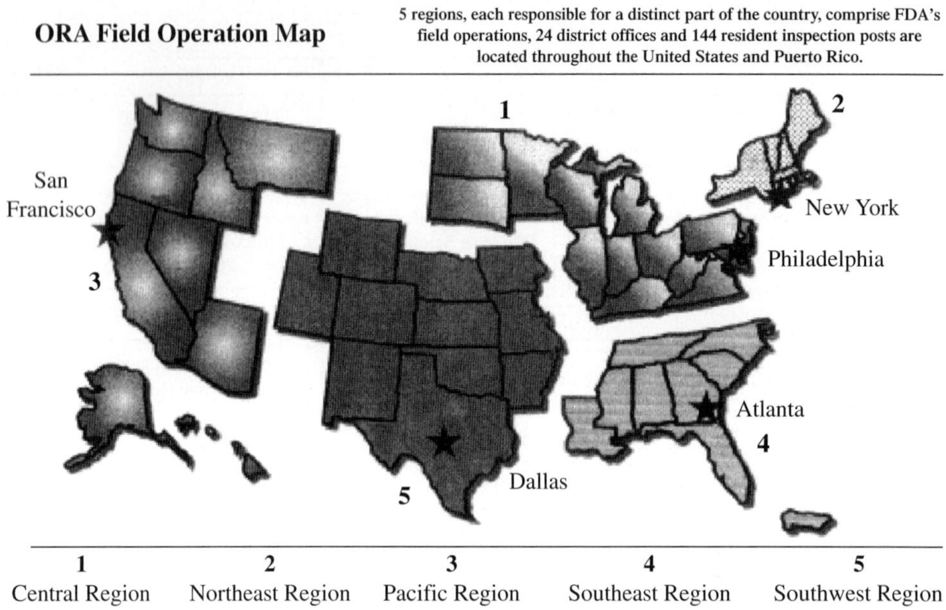

> (1) the requirement is more stringent than a requirement under this chapter which would be applicable to the device if an exemption were not in effect under this subsection; or
> (2) the requirement—
>   (A) is required by compelling local conditions, and
>   (B) compliance with the requirement would not cause the device to be in violation of any applicable requirement under this chapter.
>
> *Id.* § 360k.

FIGURE 2.2 ORA field operations.

This hierarchy is important in that one working with medical devices may be consulting any of these sources of law. The Constitution is the highest law of our land. You may think that constitutional law is too arcane for the engineer to comprehend. However, recent Supreme Court cases have rejected federal laws on constitutional grounds, limiting action by the FDA. For example, FDA's control of commercial speech has been limited by constitutional interpretation, as discussed below. This can have a direct impact on device companies.

The more usual level of attention is at the level of statute or regulation. Federal statutes are enacted by Congress. The prevalent one for the medical device industry is the Federal Food, Drug, and Cosmetic Act (FDCA). The FDCA was first enacted in 1938 in reaction to public demand for federal action to control the food supply.

After a crisis in which a poisonous substance was used as the delivery liquid for a drug, Congress changed the FDCA to require prior approval of drugs before they could be sold. However, the modern era of control of medical devices did not arrive until 1976, when the FDCA was amended to include the basic structure of how medical devices arrive in the marketplace. Before that, FDA had the authority to remove unsafe devices from the market, but no clearance authority. The Medical Device Amendments in 1976 enacted a comprehensive scheme of control of devices.

As a federal agency, FDA has the authority to enact regulations to flesh out the mandates of the FDCA through regulation. Occasionally, Congress will require that regulations be drafted. More normally, it is a permissive authority, with no direct obligation for FDA to act. Therefore, there are still areas where it is necessary to consult the FDCA directly. When FDA does promulgate regulations, they must follow the procedure mandated in federal law. Once regulations have been promulgated following this procedure, they have the force and effect of law. Violation of an FDA regulation is the same as violation of the FDCA.

It should be noted that the FDCA is a criminal enforcement act. Violation of the FDCA is a misdemeanor punishable by up to a year in jail and fines. Repeated violation may be a felony.

2.5 WORKING WITH FDA

It should be noted that working with FDA on medical devices can be an extremely interactive personal experience. It is not like the anonymous interaction with the Internal Revenue Service or other U.S. agencies. In work relating to medical devices, you may continually run into the same FDA personnel. This builds a continuing relationship unlike the normal conduits into government.

For example, your company may have its product clearance applications reviewed by the same group for a decade. You will learn their likes and dislikes in style. You will learn their particular view of what the regulations mean. You may grow to personally like or dislike them as individuals. In most cases, however, you must learn to manage this long-term, long-range relationship in a professional manner that advances the cause of your company.

FDA personnel are dedicated to the mission of consumer protection. This devotion may occasionally lead individuals to leap to conclusions about you or your company. You must be prepared for zealous advocacy by FDA personnel in accomplishment of their mission. At times it will seem unfair and arbitrary. You must learn how to work within this system and keep up the working relationship.

2.6 SCOPE OF REGULATION

FDA regulates the entire life cycle of a medical device, from cradle-to-grave. The examples below demonstrates the major regulations affecting a device through its life:

• Design stage (post research)	• Quality System Regulation (QSR) Design Control
• Bench testing	• QSR Design Control
• Animal testing	• Good Laboratory Practices (GLP)/Design Control
• Human testing	• Investigational Device Exemption (IDE)/Design Control
• Market clearance	• 510(k)/PMA
• Manufacturing	• QSR Process Control, etc.
• Distribution	• QSR Traceability
• Postmarket	• Complaint handling/QSR/Corrective and Preventive Action (CAPA)/Medical Device Reports (MDR)

2.7 MARKETING CLEARANCE OF MEDICAL DEVICES

There are basically two paths through the FDA system to arrive at marketing of a product: Premarket Approval and 510(k) (sometimes called Premarket Notification). In order to understand these paths, it is best to learn the history behind them, starting from the Medical Device Amendments of 1976.

Congress was faced with creating a comprehensive plan for the wide range of medical devices. It had to establish a system that could regulate both dental floss and implantable heart valves. It was faced with public pressure to address problems perceived with some devices, such as intrauterine devices (IUDs) for birth control, while not disturbing the great mass of low-risk products that appeared to be successful and safe.

Class I	Class II	Class III
Low risk	Moderate risk	High risk
General controls	General controls/special controls	General controls
Exempt	510(k)	PMA

FIGURE 2.3 Medical device class hierarchy.

Congress decided to control this wide range of medical devices by a classification system. A hierarchy of three classes was established (Fig. 2.3).

Note that the classes are always referenced by their Roman numerals, for example, Class III medical devices.

The classes are risk based, with Class I being the lowest risk and Class III the highest. The statutory definitions are as follows:

Class III

(C) Class III, Premarket Approval.—A device which because—

- **(i)** it
  - **(I)** cannot be classified as a Class I device because insufficient information exists to determine that the application of general controls are sufficient to provide reasonable assurance of the safety and effectiveness of the device, and
  - **(II)** cannot be classified as a Class II device because insufficient information exists to determine that the special controls described in subparagraph (B) would provide reasonable assurance of its safety and effectiveness, and
- **(ii)**
  - **(I)** is purported or represented to be for a use in supporting or sustaining human life or for a use which is of substantial importance in preventing impairment of human health, or
  - **(II)** presents a potential unreasonable risk of illness or injury,

is to be subject, in accordance with section 360e of this title, to Premarket Approval to provide reasonable assurance of its safety and effectiveness.

If there is not sufficient information to establish a performance standard for a device to provide reasonable assurance of its safety and effectiveness, the Secretary may conduct such activities as may be necessary to develop or obtain such information.

(2) For purposes of this section and sections 360d and 360e of this title, the safety and effectiveness of a device are to be determined—
- **(A)** with respect to the persons for whose use the device is represented or intended,
- **(B)** with respect to the conditions of use prescribed, recommended, or suggested in the labeling of the device, and
- **(C)** weighing any probable benefit to health from the use of the device against any probable risk of injury or illness from such use.

(3)
- **(A)** Except as authorized by subparagraph (B), the effectiveness of a device is, for purposes of this section and sections 360d and 360e of this title, to be determined, in accordance with regulations promulgated by the Secretary, on the basis of well-controlled investigations, including 1 or more clinical investigations where appropriate, by experts qualified by training and experience to evaluate the effectiveness of the device, from which investigations it can fairly and responsibly be concluded by qualified experts that the device will have the effect it purports or is represented to have under the conditions of use prescribed, recommended, or suggested in the labeling of the device.
- **(B)** If the Secretary determines that there exists valid scientific evidence (other than evidence derived from investigations described in subparagraph (A))—
  - **(i)** which is sufficient to determine the effectiveness of a device, and
  - **(ii)** from which it can fairly and responsibly be concluded by qualified experts that the device will have the effect it purports or is represented to have under the conditions of use prescribed, recommended, or suggested in the labeling of the device,

then, for purposes of this section and sections 360d and 360e of this title, the Secretary may authorize the effectiveness of the device to be determined on the basis of such evidence.

(C) In making a determination of a reasonable assurance of the effectiveness of a device for which an application under section 360e of this title has been submitted, the Secretary shall consider whether the extent of data that otherwise would be required for approval of the application with respect to effectiveness can be reduced through reliance on postmarket controls.

(D)

(i) The Secretary, upon the written request of any person intending to submit an application under section 360e of this title, shall meet with such person to determine the type of valid scientific evidence (within the meaning of subparagraphs (A) and (B)) that will be necessary to demonstrate for purposes of approval of an application the effectiveness of a device for the conditions of use proposed by such person. The written request shall include a detailed description of the device, a detailed description of the proposed conditions of use of the device, a proposed plan for determining whether there is a reasonable assurance of effectiveness, and, if available, information regarding the expected performance from the device. Within 30 days after such meeting, the Secretary shall specify in writing the type of valid scientific evidence that will provide a reasonable assurance that a device is effective under the conditions of use proposed by such person.

(ii) Any clinical data, including one or more well-controlled investigations, specified in writing by the Secretary for demonstrating a reasonable assurance of device effectiveness shall be specified as result of a determination by the Secretary that such data are necessary to establish device effectiveness. The Secretary shall consider, in consultation with the applicant, the least burdensome appropriate means of evaluating device effectiveness that would have a reasonable likelihood of resulting in approval.

(iii) The determination of the Secretary with respect to the specification of valid scientific evidence under clauses (i) and (ii) shall be binding upon the Secretary, unless such determination by the Secretary could be contrary to the public health.

Id. § 360c.

Class III includes active implantables such as pacemakers, implantable cardioverter/defibrillators, neurological spine brain stimulators, and implantable brain stimulators. It also includes passive implantables, such as heart valves.

Class II

(B) Class II, Special Controls.—A device which cannot be classified as a Class I device because the general controls by themselves are insufficient to provide reasonable assurance of the safety and effectiveness of the device, and for which there is sufficient information to establish special controls to provide such assurance, including the promulgation of performance standards, postmarket surveillance, patient registries, development and dissemination of guidelines (including guidelines for the submission of clinical data in Premarket Notification submissions in accordance with section 360 (k) of this title), recommendations, and other appropriate actions as the Secretary deems necessary to provide such assurance. For a device that is purported or represented to be for a use in supporting or sustaining human life, the Secretary shall examine and identify the special controls, if any, that are necessary to provide adequate assurance of safety and effectiveness and describe how such controls provide such assurance.

Id.

Class II includes the vast bulk of diagnostic and external therapeutic devices. The wide array of monitors, IV pumps, etc., seen walking down a hospital corridor are mostly Class II devices.

Class I

(A) Class I, General Controls.—

(i) A device for which the controls authorized by or under section 351, 352, 360, 360f, 360h, 360i, or 360j of this title or any combination of such sections are sufficient to provide reasonable assurance of the safety and effectiveness of the device.

> **(ii)** A device for which insufficient information exists to determine that the controls referred to in clause (i) are sufficient to provide reasonable assurance of the safety and effectiveness of the device or to establish special controls to provide such assurance, but because it—
> **(I)** is not purported or represented to be for a use in supporting or sustaining human life or for a use which is of substantial importance in preventing impairment of human health, and
> **(II)** does not present a potential unreasonable risk of illness or injury, is to be regulated by the controls referred to in clause (i).
>
> *Id.*

Class I includes a myriad of medical supplies and low-risk devices. This is where FDA has classified the toothbrushes discussed above. Everything from bedpans to Q-tip swabs is found in this class.

As Fig. 2.3 shows, Congress chose a level of marketing clearance requirements and control based upon the perceived risk.

At the high end of risk, Congress created the Premarket Approval (PMA) process. This was to be the route to market for devices in Class III. FDA was instructed to call for PMAs on all devices in Class III or downclass them to Class II. The downclass procedure was so complex that FDA did not want to use up vast resources on downclassing. They immediately called for PMAs on what they viewed as the most serious Class III devices but left some devices in Class III without PMAs. To this day, there are lingering devices in Class III that do not require a PMA.

At the opposite end of the risk spectrum is Class I. Congress believed this class needed minimal control. The big question was what to do with the vast middle area. Congress believed that current devices were performing adequately, and that there was no need to rashly require a marketing clearance for everything on the market, so Congress grandfathered in devices that were already on sale at the time of the Medical Device Amendments in 1976. There are still devices on sale today that were grandfathered in.

The next question was what to do if another company wanted to produce a product like the ones grandfathered in. It would not be fair to allow the first company to sell the product, but not allow follow-ons. Therefore, Congress created the 510(k) process, which got its name from its section of FDCA. Section 510(k) said that if you wanted to sell a device substantially equivalent to one on the market before 1976, you just had to notify FDA. If FDA did not tell you within 90 days that you could not sell your device on the market, you could proceed and market. New products were to go automatically into Class III, until FDA acted to downclass them.

It did not take FDA long to realize that this was an impractical scheme. If Section 510(k) were read too narrowly, any improvements in medical devices would end up in Class III. It would take enormous resources to process PMAs on new products and it would be too expensive to downclass them. The FDCA required that FDA write a performance standard before moving a device out of Class III and into Class II. FDA never did this.

Instead FDA rethought the 510(k) process. FDA turned the 510(k) process into a de facto approval process, while still calling it notification. If FDA determined that a device belonged in class II, even if it was a technological advancement, it worked to find a predicate device to find the device equivalent to. It never required the performance standards mentioned in the statute. The process generally worked. Finally, in 1990, Congress modified the FDCA to remove the need for performance standards and to adopt FDA's definition of substantial equivalence.

2.8 PREMARKET APPROVAL (PMA)

A PMA is a detailed scientific review of a product. As discussed above, this is required for all new Class III products. The FDA is required by statute to find, based upon valid scientific evidence, that the device is safe and effective for the use for which it is labeled.

Remember that the labeling is of paramount importance. For example, take a device that is already on the market as a Class II device under general use labeling, such as an ablation device; if you label it for a specific use in treating a disease state, you can move it into a different range of risk. This may make it a Class III device, requiring a PMA. This is true even if the identical hardware is on sale under different labeling in Class II.

A PMA submission is a complex procedure, both for FDA and the industry. The regulatory requirements include

(1) The name and address of the applicant.
(2) A table of contents that specifies the volume and page number for each item referred to in the table. A PMA shall include separate sections on nonclinical laboratory studies and on clinical investigations involving human subjects. A PMA shall be submitted in six copies each bound in one or more numbered volumes of reasonable size. The applicant shall include information that it believes to be trade secret or confidential commercial or financial information in all copies of the PMA and identify in at least one copy the information that it believes to be trade secret or confidential commercial or financial information.
(3) A summary in sufficient detail that the reader may gain a general understanding of the data and information in the application. The summary shall contain the following information:
  (i) Indications for use. A general description of the disease or condition the device will diagnose, treat, prevent, cure, or mitigate, including a description of the patient population for which the device is intended.
  (ii) Device description. An explanation of how the device functions, the basic scientific concepts that form the basis for the device, and the significant physical and performance characteristics of the device. A brief description of the manufacturing process should be included if it will significantly enhance the reader's understanding of the device. The generic name of the device as well as any proprietary name or trade name should be included.
  (iii) Alternative practices and procedures. A description of existing alternative practices or procedures for diagnosing, treating, preventing, curing, or mitigating the disease or condition for which the device is intended.
  (iv) Marketing history. A brief description of the foreign and U.S. marketing history, if any, of the device, including a list of all countries in which the device has been marketed and a list of all countries in which the device has been withdrawn from marketing for any reason related to the safety or effectiveness of the device. The description shall include the history of the marketing of the device by the applicant and, if known, the history of the marketing of the device by any other person.
  (v) Summary of studies. An abstract of any information or report described in the PMA under paragraph (b)(8)(ii) of this section and a summary of the results of technical data submitted under paragraph (b)(6) of this section. Such summary shall include a description of the objective of the study, a description of the experimental design of the study, a brief description of how the data were collected and analyzed, and a brief description of the results, whether positive, negative, or inconclusive. This section shall include the following:
    (A) A summary of the nonclinical laboratory studies submitted in the application;
    (B) A summary of the clinical investigations involving human subjects submitted in the application including a discussion of subject selection and exclusion criteria, study population, study period, safety and effectiveness data, adverse reactions and complications, patient discontinuation, patient complaints, device failures and replacements, results of statistical analyses of the clinical investigations, contraindications and precautions for use of the device, and other information from the clinical investigations as appropriate (any investigation conducted under an IDE shall be identified as such).
  (vi) Conclusions drawn from the studies. A discussion demonstrating that the data and information in the application constitute valid scientific evidence within the meaning of Sec. 860.7 and provide reasonable assurance that the device is safe and effective for its intended use. A concluding discussion shall present benefit and risk considerations related to the device including a discussion of any adverse effects of the device on health and any proposed additional studies or surveillance the applicant intends to conduct following approval of the PMA.
(4) A complete description of:
  (i) The device, including pictorial representations;
  (ii) Each of the functional components or ingredients of the device if the device consists of more than one physical component or ingredient;
  (iii) The properties of the device relevant to the diagnosis, treatment, prevention, cure, or mitigation of a disease or condition;
  (iv) The principles of operation of the device; and

(v) The methods used in, and the facilities and controls used for, the manufacture, processing, packing, storage, and, where appropriate, installation of the device, in sufficient detail so that a person generally familiar with current good manufacturing practice can make a knowledgeable judgment about the quality control used in the manufacture of the device.

(5) Reference to any performance standard under section 514 of the act or the Radiation Control for Health and Safety Act of 1968 (42 U.S.C. 263b et seq.) in effect or proposed at the time of the submission and to any voluntary standard that is relevant to any aspect of the safety or effectiveness of the device and that is known to or that should reasonably be known to the applicant. The applicant shall—
   (i) Provide adequate information to demonstrate how the device meets, or justify any deviation from, any performance standard established under section 514 of the act or under the Radiation Control for Health and Safety Act, and
   (ii) Explain any deviation from a voluntary standard.

(6) The following technical sections which shall contain data and information in sufficient detail to permit FDA to determine whether to approve or deny approval of the application:
   (i) A section containing results of the nonclinical laboratory studies with the device including microbiological, toxicological, immunological, biocompatibility, stress, wear, shelf life, and other laboratory or animal tests as appropriate. Information on nonclinical laboratory studies shall include a statement that each such study was conducted in compliance with part 58, or, if the study was not conducted in compliance with such regulations, a brief statement of the reason for the noncompliance.
   (ii) A section containing results of the clinical investigations involving human subjects with the device including clinical protocols, number of investigators and subjects per investigator, subject selection and exclusion criteria, study population, study period, safety and effectiveness data, adverse reactions and complications, patient discontinuation, patient complaints, device failures and replacements, tabulations of data from all individual subject report forms and copies of such forms for each subject who died during a clinical investigation or who did not complete the investigation, results of statistical analyses of the clinical investigations, device failures and replacements, contraindications and precautions for use of the device, and any other appropriate information from the clinical investigations. Any investigation conducted under an IDE shall be identified as such. Information on clinical investigations involving human subjects shall include the following:
      (A) A statement with respect to each study that it either was conducted in compliance with the institutional review board regulations in part 56, or was not subject to the regulations under Sec. 56.104 or Sec. 56.105, and that it was conducted in compliance with the informed consent regulations in part 50; or if the study was not conducted in compliance with those regulations, a brief statement of the reason for the noncompliance.
      (B) A statement that each study was conducted in compliance with part 812 or part 813 concerning sponsors of clinical investigations and clinical investigators, or if the study was not conducted in compliance with those regulations, a brief statement of the reason for the noncompliance.

(7) For a PMA supported solely by data from one investigation, a justification showing that data and other information from a single investigator are sufficient to demonstrate the safety and effectiveness of the device and to ensure reproducibility of test results.

(8)
   (i) A bibliography of all published reports not submitted under paragraph (b)(6) of this section, whether adverse or supportive, known to or that should reasonably be known to the applicant and that concern the safety or effectiveness of the device.
   (ii) An identification, discussion, and analysis of any other data, information, or report relevant to an evaluation of the safety and effectiveness of the device known to or that should reasonably be known to the applicant from any source, foreign or domestic, including information derived from investigations other than those proposed in the application and from commercial marketing experience.
   (iii) Copies of such published reports or unpublished information in the possession of or reasonably obtainable by the applicant if an FDA advisory committee or FDA requests.

(9) One or more samples of the device and its components, if requested by FDA. If it is impractical to submit a requested sample of the device, the applicant shall name the location at which FDA may examine and test one or more devices.

(10) Copies of all proposed labeling for the device. Such labeling may include, e.g., instructions for installation and any information, literature, or advertising that constitutes labeling under section 201(m) of the act.

(11) An environmental assessment under Sec. 25.20(n) prepared in the applicable format in Sec. 25.40, unless the action qualifies for exclusion under Sec. 25.30 or Sec. 25.34. If the applicant believes that the action qualifies for exclusion, the PMA shall under Sec. 25.15(a) and (d) provide information that establishes to FDA's satisfaction that the action requested is included within the excluded category and meets the criteria for the applicable exclusion.
(12) A financial certification or disclosure statement or both as required by part 54 of this chapter.
(13) Such other information as FDA may request. If necessary, FDA will obtain the concurrence of the appropriate FDA advisory committee before requesting additional information.

21 C.F.R. § 814.20, as amended, 71 Fed. Reg. 42,048 (July 25, 2006).

This can result in a submission, including the six copies, as large as a refrigerator.

2.9 PREMARKET NOTIFICATION [PMN OR 510(k)]

Unlike a PMA, where there is a requirement of begin safe and effective, there is no statutory standard of review for Class II and I devices. Rather, one uses the 510(k) process to show substantial equivalence to a product legally marketed in the past.

This previously marketed product is known as a *predicate.* A predicate can be either a device legally marketed before 1976 or a product brought onto the market thereafter through the 510(k) process. The predicate cannot be an illegal or banned device. A PMA product cannot be used for a 510(k) predicate.

So, the first step in clearing a product through a 510(k) is to locate the proper predicate. This may involve more than one device. Each of the elements of the algorithm for substantial equivalence must be found in the devices used as the predicate. Therefore, a predicate is needed for the intended use and for safety evidence. For example, it is common to create a new device to accomplish an old use, using new technology. In this case, a predicate for the intended use is necessary. Next, a search for predicates will have to be made that use some form of your technology if there are safety issues to be satisfied.

A 510(k) is submitted to FDA containing the following information:

(a) Form FDA-2891 and Form FDA-2891(a) are the approved forms for initially providing the information required by the act and for providing annual registration, respectively. The required information includes the name and street address of the device establishment, including post office code, all trade names used by the establishment, and the business trading name of the owner or operator of such establishment.
(b) The owner or operator shall identify the device activities of the establishment such as manufacturing, repackaging, or distributing devices.
(c) Each owner or operator is required to maintain a listing of all officers, directors, and partners for each establishment he registers and to furnish this information to the Food and Drug Administration upon request.
(d) Each owner or operator shall provide the name of an official correspondent who will serve as a point of contact between the Food and Drug Administration and the establishment for matters relating to the registration of device establishments and the listing of device products. All future correspondence relating to registration, including requests for the names of partners, officers, and directors, will be directed to this official correspondent. In the event no person is designated by the owner or operator, the owner or operator of the establishment will be the official correspondent.
(e) The designation of an official correspondent does not in any manner affect the liability of the owner or operator of the establishment or any other individual under section 301(p) or any other provision of the act.
(f) Form FD-2892 is the approved form for providing the device listing information required by the act. This required information includes the following:
    (1) The identification by classification name and number, proprietary name, and common or usual name of each device being manufactured, prepared, propagated, compounded, or processed for commercial distribution that has not been included in any list of devices previously submitted on form FDA-2892.

> (2) The Code of Federal Regulations citation for any applicable standard for the device under section 514 of the act or section 358 of the Public Health Service Act.
> (3) The assigned Food and Drug Administration number of the approved application for each device listed that is subject to section 505 or 515 of the act.
> (4) The name, registration number, and establishment type of every domestic or foreign device establishment under joint ownership and control of the owner or operator at which the device is manufactured, repackaged, or relabeled.
> (5) Whether the device, as labeled, is intended for distribution to and use by the general public.
> (6) Other general information requested on form FDA-2892, i.e.,
> (i) If the submission refers to a previously listed device, as in the case of an update, the document number from the initial listing document for the device,
> (ii) The reason for submission,
> (iii) The date on which the reason for submission occurred,
> (iv) The date that the form FDA-2892 was completed,
> (v) The owner's or operator's name and identification number
> (7) Labeling or other descriptive information (e.g., specification sheets or catalogs) adequate to describe the intended use of a device when the owner or operator is unable to find an appropriate FDA classification name for the device.
>
> *Id.* § 807.25, as amended, 69 Fed. Reg. 11,312 (Mar. 10, 2004).

Note that there is no FDA form or required format for this filing. Over time, tools have been developed, both by FDA and by regulatory personnel, so that 510(k)s look similar. However, it is not an FDA-regulated format. FDA has published a checklist that many filers actually include in the submission.

The heart of the 510(k) process is to show substantial equivalence. After you submit your 510(k), FDA reviews it. The statute requires that it be finished in 90 days. FDA has rarely had the resources to meet this statutory agenda, but had recently come close to 90-day review periods. FDA may send a letter finding your submission substantially equivalent (SE) or not substantially equivalent (NSE). An SE letter will contain a 510(k) number for your product which is the letter K followed by two digits indicating the year and four digits indicating the numerical place in which your 510(k) was issued in that year.

Note that this is not a legal order, like a PMA letter. FDA has far less authority to place any conditions on a 510(k). It is basically a form letter finding your submission SE.

The heart of this process is substantial equivalence. The statutory algorithm for showing substantial equivalence to a predicate is

> (i) Substantial Equivalence
> (1) (A) For purposes of determinations of substantial equivalence under subsection (f) and section 520(l), the term "substantially equivalent" or "substantial equivalence" means, with respect to a device being compared to a predicate device, that the device has the same intended use as the predicate device and that the Secretary by order has found that the device—
> (i) has the same technological characteristics as the predicate device, or
> (ii) (I) has different technological characteristics and the information submitted that the device is substantially equivalent to the predicate device contains information, including appropriate clinical or scientific data if deemed necessary by the Secretary or a person accredited under section 523, that demonstrates that the device is as safe and effective as a legally marketed device, and (II) does not raise different questions of safety and effectiveness than the predicate device. (B) For purposes of subparagraph (A), the term "different technological characteristics" means, with respect to a device being compared to a predicate device, that there is a significant change in the materials, design, energy source, or other features of the device from those of the predicate device.
>
> 21 U.S.C. 360c.

This algorithm has allowed science to march on, producing improved technologies for medical devices without resorting to the PMA process unnecessarily. When one works through the Boolean algebra, you can see that it results in a standard with remarkable flexibility.

There are two basic steps connected by an AND. First, you need a predicate with the same intended use. Second, you need to deal with the possibility of technology.

For intended use, the easiest way is to show that the intended use on the 510(k) for the predicate is the same. You can also use labeling or advertisements from the predicate to show it had the intended use.

The second step has two paths connected by an OR. If your device uses the same technology as the predicate, showing equivalence is easier, of course. The more interesting path, and the one most often used as technology improves, is the second. Here there is a two-part requirement: you must show that your device is as safe and effective as the predicate and that there are no new questions of safety.

Note that FDA has no statutory authority to ask for proof of safety and effectiveness, but it has backed requiring such proof to show that new technologies are equivalent. This is the step in the process where FDA sometimes calls for clinical data as part of the evidence. As Class II devices become more complex and embody new technologies, the requirements for human clinical data increases.

A common engineering example of the foregoing is an EKG machine. Take as an example, a vacuum-tube powered machine of the era before 1976. At some point a 510(k) was filed for a new EKG machine with transistors. There was no change in the intended use. However, new technology was used. The applicant had to show that the transistor version was as safe and effective. Then, a succeeding applicant wanted to use solid-state electronics. This applicant probably picked the transistor unit as a predicate and then showed the new one was as safe and effective. Then a software-driven EKG machine arrived. It might pick any of the previous as a predicate, but probably picked the more recent. It then had to show that the software method was as safe and effective as the chosen predicate.

In this manner, technology can be used to solve medical problems and improve performance, while using the magic of the 510(k) substantial equivalence algorithm.

2.10 COMPARISON TO EU REGULATION

Medical device regulation in the EU has taken a path dramatically different from the U.S. model. The European system is a standards-driven model which heavily depends upon nongovernmental organizations (NGOs) for operation of the system.

A summary knowledge of the structure of the EU is needed in order to understand the medical device scheme. The EU does not have a central federal government enacting statutes, as we do in the United States. Rather the EU enacts Directives. These Directives do not act as law in themselves. Rather, the member states of the EU are required to harmonize their country laws so they conform to the Directives. Therefore, medical device laws that are used to prosecute violations exist in each country; however, they must be consistent with the Directives.

A loose analogy can be found in the 55-mph speed limit enacted during the 1970s in the United States. Speed limits were a state law issue, and the federal government did not really have authority to establish a national speed limit. Instead, Congress tied highway appropriations to a 55-mph limit. If a state wished to benefit from federal highway money, it had to enact a 55-mph limit. Similarly, if a country wishes to be in the EU, it has to harmonize its laws to the Directives.

Two different types of entities must be understood. Before the EU established its medical device scheme through Directives, each country had a governmental unit that approved medical devices and controlled their manufacture. These were usually called something like the Ministry of Health. Once the Directive scheme was established, these governmental units were called *Competent Authorities.* They still had jurisdiction for protecting the health of their citizens. They still enforced the law and took regulatory action such as recalls of devices. However, the Competent Authorities gave up two of their roles: (1) inspecting and certifying manufacturers and (2) approving devices.

A new set of NGOs took over these two important roles. These were called *Notified Bodies.* Most of these NGOs were former standards organizations. For example, one of them had begun as a steam boiler inspection authority in the nineteenth century. Under the new scheme, such an NGO could apply to the competent authority in its country to become a certifying organization. If approved, it was notified that it could now grant the CE mark. It became know as a Notified Body. Entities from outside the EU, such as from the United States, have since become notified.

The Directive system employs the CE (Conformite Europeene) mark as the indication that a product may be freely sold throughout the EU, without being subject to laws differing from the Directive. In effect, it is an indication of free movement within the EU. You may have seen the CE mark on children's toys, which were the subject of an early Directive.

Notified Bodies have the key role in the application of the CE mark in the area of medical Devices. A company intending to market a medical device within the EU hires one of these entities to act as its Notified Body. So there is a vendor/customer relationship between the Notified Body and the Device company, as well as the regulator/regulated relationship. At the same time, the Notified Body has a responsibility to the EU and to its competent authority to properly enforce the Directives. It is a tension that promotes both dedication to the Directive and understanding of the needs of the regulated.

The Notified Body then inspects the Device company, auditing against the standards that have been adopted by the EU (called EN for European Norms). The Notified Body then provides a certificate of compliance to the company. The audits are designed to test the entire quality system of the company. First the broadest parts of the system, such as the quality manual, are inspected. As part of its work with the company, the Notified Body regularly conducts audits. Each of these usually digs deeper into the details of the quality system. The Notified Body is the implementer of the EU philosophy—a well-controlled quality system will produce compliant products.

Once certified, the company may begin to use the CE mark on products. For lower-risk products, the company just keeps records, which are then inspected by the Notified Body. For high-risk products, such as active implantables, the company must apply to the Notified Body for permission to apply the CE mark, much in the same manner as a company would apply to FDA for a PMA.

The use of standards in the EU are very different from the United States. One need not follow the ENs. However, if choosing that path, the company would have to convince the EU that the product satisfied everything required by the Directives. The more normal route is to comply with the ENs. Then the route to the CE mark is assured.

One way to casually characterize this system is that it is more engineering-oriented than in the United States. Notified Bodies examine devices primarily to see if they act as they are claimed to act: if they meet specification. In comparison, the FDA system is more therapy-oriented. The main FDA question is not: does it work as it says. Rather, the FDA asks if the device provides a medical benefit.

2.11 MARKETING CLEARANCE OF COMBINATION PRODUCTS

The path toward marketing for devices is no longer sufficient for engineers. Technology has resulted in an increased mix of drugs and biologics with devices. These are known as *combination products* (or combos in our shorthand). This is not a statutory term, but one established by FDA in order to deal with how to regulate them.

Combos are not new. Drugs were combined with devices before the term combination products existed. For example, steroids were applied to the tips of cardiac pacing lead electrodes to reduce inflammation in difficult cases so the tip would achieve good electrical contact. Asthma drugs were dispensed by metered dose inhalers, spray cans that became a part of kids' school life. Implantable drug dispensers were approved for specific drug delivery rather than as general tools. Biologics were used early on devices. Some catheters had heparin coatings.

In the early days, there was uncertainty as to how to regulate combos. As discussed earlier, FDA was divided into centers. Which center regulated a product was important, since the regulations varied widely. Calling a product a drug, rather than a device, could result in a drastically different path to market.

FDA established an Office of Combination Products (OCP) under the Office of the Commissioner, so that it was not in any center. This office was to provide guidance on how to regulate combos. The guidance employs the concept of primary mode of action. If the primary mode of action is physical, like a device, then the combo is a device. If the primary mode of action is chemical, metabolized by the body, then the combo is a drug. This is easy in some cases. Take a stent, designed to keep an artery open, which is also coated with a drug to help prevent restentosis within the artery. This has a strong device orientation due to its physical effects. These have been regulated as devices. The metered dose inhaler acts primarily through drug action on the lungs. The device is more of a delivery method. So this was, and will continue to be, regulated as a drug. Some cases are less clear. The implantable drug pump was regulated as a device, since all the new technology was electromechanical. If such a new device came along today, would it be a device? The primary mode of action on the patient seems to be the drug that is delivered. Would this shift such delivery devices to the Center for Drug Evaluation and Research (CDER)? We will see as technology advances.

Regulatory professionals work to have a combination product reviewed by the center with which they are most comfortable and which has the most favorable procedures. No matter what center controls, they will commonly ask for consultative review by the other centers that have skills and experience related to the product. For example, in review of a drug-coated device by the Center for Devices and Radiological Health (CDRH), it is common to have a review of the drug component by CDER. However, all CDRH procedures apply as opposed to those of CDER. One can ask OCP for a determination of which center will control. The more normal path is to discuss it in advance with the center you prefer and submit it to them.

2.12 TESTING MEDICAL DEVICES ON NONHUMAN ANIMALS AND LIFE FORMS

It is usual for FDA to require testing of devices on animal models before introduction into human testing. This is generally referred to as preclinical or nonclinical testing. It should be noted that political and ethical concerns continually press for reduction in testing on animals. However, it remains a standard step in medical device development.

Preclinical testing is regulated by FDA under the regulations know as Good Laboratory Practices (GLP).* GLP applies to any nonclinical testing studies that support or are intended to support a research or marketing application to FDA. This is not just for human devices or drugs. GLP applies to applications for food or color additives, animal food additives, animal drugs, biologics, and electronic products. Any nonclinical study used to support a PMA, 510(k), or Investigational Device Exemption (IDE) is to be done under GLP.

Note that GLP does not apply to any testing, such as bench testing, that does not involve a live organism. Any test that uses a test system involving an animal, plant, microorganism, or subparts thereof is covered by GLP.

Research studies not intended to be submitted to FDA fall outside GLP. This raises a practical problem. Often research studies are done without GLP controls, only to find later that the data are needed in an FDA submission. Then it must be argued and explained that the original purpose was for research but that it is acceptable to use the data for a submission. It is often a financial trade-off to decide whether to conduct early studies under GLP in order to have the data more easily available later for submission.

There are two general classes of controls in GLP: animal care and data integrity. FDA has joint jurisdiction with the U.S. Department of Agriculture (USDA) over the care of the animals. Both inspect, but USDA is usually viewed as the prime regulator of animal treatment. FDA has, of course, a keen interest in the accuracy, completeness, and truthfulness of the data resulting from a GLP study. This part of GLP has a three-part basis. First, GLP requires a protocol that lays out the purpose of the testing, the end points to be tested, the data forms for collection, and the description of the data to be collected. Second, there must be a quality assurance unit that oversees and audits the study to make sure that the protocol and regulations are followed. Third, there must be a final report presenting the data found, the study results, and any conclusions.

GLP studies are audited and investigated by FDA, just as human clinical trials are. Precision and care must be exercised so that a GLP study produces data acceptable to FDA.

---

*21 C.F.R. pt. 58.

2.13 TESTING MEDICAL DEVICES ON HUMAN SUBJECTS

The key issues in regulation of research involving human subjects are parallel to those in preclinical studies: protecting the rights of subjects and assuring the integrity of the study data.

The current body of ethical standards for medical research on humans grew out of abuses ranging from fiendishly evil to benevolent condescension. In all cases, however, the abuses resulted in an international consensus that human subjects be given the free choice whether or not to participate in a study and be fully aware of the risks and benefits of the research.

The most striking examples of neglect of these principles were experiments on prisoners during World War II. For example, prisoners were submerged in icy water to determine how long they could survive. This had a supposedly sound scientific purpose in that it determined how long downed German pilots could survive in the North Sea. However, the cruelty to the prisoner/subjects so outraged humanity that a body of ethical thought and purpose developed from it. The Institute of Medicine organized an international meeting on the topic, which resulted in the Declaration of Helsinki, the touchstone of medical research ethics. The Declaration of Helsinki has been amended over the years, but survives as a base level ethical guide for the treatment of human research subjects.

The United States does not have a unified regulatory scheme to cover all human research; rather the control is segmented by functional purpose. For example, HHS has promulgated regulations governing human research conducted under government sponsorship, such as through NIH. This is sometimes known as the Common Rule. Some academic research is not regulated at all on the federal level. The research of concern in this chapter is that which is directed to testing products for submission to FDA. This research is heavily regulated by FDA.

There are three sets of regulations encompassing the FDA control of clinical studies:

(1) The informed consent process*

(2) Institutional review boards (IRBs)†

(3) The conduct of clinical studies‡

As discussed above, the process that distinguishes modern clinical research from its checkered past is called *informed consent.* It is important to understand this as a process. Although we are tempted to use the common shorthand and use the term informed consent to refer to a piece of paper signed by a subject, this paper is not the essence of informed consent. The signed document is but a record in which the subject recognizes that the process has occurred. FDA views the entire process of screening and informing the subject to be informed consent.

The elements of informed consent, which are all normally included in a written document, are

> (a) Basic elements of informed consent. In seeking informed consent, the following information shall be provided to each subject:
> (1) A statement that the study involves research, an explanation of the purposes of the research and the expected duration of the subject's participation, a description of the procedures to be followed, and identification of any procedures which are experimental.
> (2) A description of any reasonably foreseeable risks or discomforts to the subject.
> (3) A description of any benefits to the subject or to others which may reasonably be expected from the research.
> (4) A disclosure of appropriate alternative procedures or courses of treatment, if any, that might be advantageous to the subject.
> (5) A statement describing the extent, if any, to which confidentiality of records identifying the subject will be maintained and that notes the possibility that the Food and Drug Administration may inspect the records.
> (6) For research involving more than minimal risk, an explanation as to whether any compensation and an explanation as to whether any medical treatments are available if injury occurs and, if so, what they consist of, or where further information may be obtained.

**Id.* § 50.

†Id. pt. 56.

‡Id. pt. 812.

   (7) An explanation of whom to contact for answers to pertinent questions about the research and research subjects' rights, and whom to contact in the event of a research-related injury to the subject.
   (8) A statement that participation is voluntary, that refusal to participate will involve no penalty or loss of benefits to which the subject is otherwise entitled, and that the subject may discontinue participation at any time without penalty or loss of benefits to which the subject is otherwise entitled.

(b) Additional elements of informed consent. When appropriate, one or more of the following elements of information shall also be provided to each subject:
   (1) A statement that the particular treatment or procedure may involve risks to the subject (or to the embryo or fetus, if the subject is or may become pregnant) which are currently unforeseeable.
   (2) Anticipated circumstances under which the subject's participation may be terminated by the investigator without regard to the subject's consent.
   (3) Any additional costs to the subject that may result from participation in the research.
   (4) The consequences of a subject's decision to withdraw from the research and procedures for orderly termination of participation by the subject.
   (5) A statement that significant new findings developed during the course of the research which may relate to the subject's willingness to continue participation will be provided to the subject.
   (6) The approximate number of subjects involved in the study.

(c) The informed consent requirements in these regulations are not intended to preempt any applicable Federal, State, or local laws which require additional information to be disclosed for informed consent to be legally effective.

(d) Nothing in these regulations is intended to limit the authority of a physician to provide emergency medical care to the extent the physician is permitted to do so under applicable Federal, State, or local law.

Id. § 50.25.

These elements are orally presented to the subject. This is commonly done by the investigator. The subject then signs the document to verify that the information transmittal has occurred and that the subject is enrolling of his/her own free will. Some sites even videotape the informed consent session as a record showing that the process was followed.

The guardian of this informed consent process is the IRB. In countries other than the United States, this entity is commonly known as an *ethics committee*. The IRB is a committee charged with protecting study subject rights. The IRB is constituted under federal regulations, both FDA regulations (21 C.F.R. pt. 56) for FDA studies and HHS rules for government studies.

FDA rules specify the membership, the purpose, the processes, and the record-keeping of the IRB. The IRB's overall charge is to approve human research. Usually an IRB is associated with a hospital or medical practice. There are also independent IRBs that review and approve research for hospitals without IRBs or for multiple-site studies.

The FDA requirements for IRB approval of a study are

(a) In order to approve research covered by these regulations the IRB shall determine that all of the following requirements are satisfied:
   (1) Risks to subjects are minimized: (i) By using procedures which are consistent with sound research design and which do not unnecessarily expose subjects to risk, and (ii) whenever appropriate, by using procedures already being performed on the subjects for diagnostic or treatment purposes.
   (2) Risks to subjects are reasonable in relation to anticipated benefits, if any, to subjects, and the importance of the knowledge that may be expected to result. In evaluating risks and benefits, the IRB should consider only those risks and benefits that may result from the research (as distinguished from risks and benefits of therapies that subjects would receive even if not participating in the research). The IRB should not consider possible long-range effects of applying knowledge gained in the research (for example, the possible effects of the research on public policy) as among those research risks that fall within the purview of its responsibility.
   (3) Selection of subjects is equitable. In making this assessment the IRB should take into account the purposes of the research and the setting in which the research will be conducted and should be particularly cognizant of the special problems of research involving vulnerable populations, such as children, prisoners, pregnant women, handicapped, or mentally disabled persons, or economically or educationally disadvantaged persons.

(4) Informed consent will be sought from each prospective subject or the subject's legally authorized representative, in accordance with and to the extent required by part 50.
(5) Informed consent will be appropriately documented, in accordance with and to the extent required by Sec. 50.27.
(6) Where appropriate, the research plan makes adequate provision for monitoring the data collected to ensure the safety of subjects.
(7) Where appropriate, there are adequate provisions to protect the privacy of subjects and to maintain the confidentiality of data.

(b) When some or all of the subjects, such as children, prisoners, pregnant women, handicapped, or mentally disabled persons, or economically or educationally disadvantaged persons, are likely to be vulnerable to coercion or undue influence additional safeguards have been included in the study to protect the rights and welfare of these subjects.
(c) In order to approve research in which some or all of the subjects are children, an IRB must determine that all research is in compliance with part 50, subpart D of this chapter.

Id. § 56.111.

The IRB review of research involves

(a) An IRB shall review and have authority to approve, require modifications in (to secure approval), or disapprove all research activities covered by these regulations.
(b) An IRB shall require that information given to subjects as part of informed consent is in accordance with Sec. 50.25. The IRB may require that information, in addition to that specifically mentioned in Sec. 50.25, be given to the subjects when in the IRB's judgment the information would meaningfully add to the protection of the rights and welfare of subjects.
(c) An IRB shall require documentation of informed consent in accordance with Sec. 50.27 of this chapter, except as follows:
  (1) The IRB may, for some or all subjects, waive the requirement that the subject, or the subject's legally authorized representative, sign a written consent form if it finds that the research presents no more than minimal risk of harm to subjects and involves no procedures for which written consent is normally required outside the research context; or
  (2) The IRB may, for some or all subjects, find that the requirements in Sec. 50.24 of this chapter for an exception from informed consent for emergency research are met.
(d) In cases where the documentation requirement is waived under paragraph (c)(1) of this section, the IRB may require the investigator to provide subjects with a written statement regarding the research.
(e) An IRB shall notify investigators and the institution in writing of its decision to approve or disapprove the proposed research activity, or of modifications required to secure IRB approval of the research activity. If the IRB decides to disapprove a research activity, it shall include in its written notification a statement of the reasons for its decision and give the investigator an opportunity to respond in person or in writing. For investigations involving an exception to informed consent under Sec. 50.24 of this chapter, an IRB shall promptly notify in writing the investigator and the sponsor of the research when an IRB determines that it cannot approve the research because it does not meet the criteria in the exception provided under Sec. 50.24(a) of this chapter or because of other relevant ethical concerns. The written notification shall include a statement of the reasons for the IRB's determination.
(f) An IRB shall conduct continuing review of research covered by these regulations at intervals appropriate to the degree of risk, but not less than once per year, and shall have authority to observe or have a third party observe the consent process and the research.
(g) An IRB shall provide in writing to the sponsor of research involving an exception to informed consent under Sec. 50.24 of this chapter a copy of information that has been publicly disclosed under Sec. 50.24(a)(7)(ii) and (a)(7)(iii) of this chapter. The IRB shall provide this information to the sponsor promptly so that the sponsor is aware that such disclosure has occurred. Upon receipt, the sponsor shall provide copies of the information disclosed to FDA.
(h) When some or all of the subjects in a study are children, an IRB must determine that the research study is in compliance with part 50, subpart D of this chapter, at the time of its initial review of the research. When some or all of the subjects in a study that is ongoing on April 30, 2001 are children, an IRB must conduct a review of the research to determine compliance with part 50, subpart D of this chapter, either at the time of continuing review or, at the discretion of the IRB, at an earlier date.

Id. § 56.109.

The other major parties to a clinical study are the sponsor and the investigator. The sponsor is the party responsible for the study, which usually involves funding the study. In normal commercial studies designed to get products approved by FDA, a commercial entity, the medical device manufacturer, is the sponsor. The investigators are experienced medical practitioners with whom the sponsor contracts to do the study. However, any combination is possible. For example, it is common to have a medical researcher be both a sponsor and investigator of an academic research study. The key issue is that the sponsor and the investigator must be identified and it must be made clear who is satisfying the requirements of the various regulations.

Federal regulations control the sponsor and investigator in their conduct of the study. For medical devices the main rule is in 21 C.F.R. 812. There is no name for this regulation, as we saw for GLP. Some use the term Good Clinical Practices (GCP) but it is an informal term, covering the mélange of regulations we have discussed.

Part 812 lays out the duties of the sponsor:

> Sec. 812.40 General responsibilities of sponsors.
>
> Sponsors are responsible for selecting qualified investigators and providing them with the information they need to conduct the investigation properly, ensuring proper monitoring of the investigation, ensuring that IRB review and approval are obtained, submitting an IDE application to FDA, and ensuring that any reviewing IRB and FDA are promptly informed of significant new information about an investigation. Additional responsibilities of sponsors are described in subparts B and G.
>
> Sec. 812.42 FDA and IRB approval.
>
> A sponsor shall not begin an investigation or part of an investigation until an IRB and FDA have both approved the application or supplemental application relating to the investigation or part of an investigation.
>
> Sec. 812.43 Selecting investigators and monitors.
>
> (a) Selecting investigators. A sponsor shall select investigators qualified by training and experience to investigate the device.
> (b) Control of device. A sponsor shall ship investigational devices only to qualified investigators participating in the investigation.
> (c) Obtaining agreements. A sponsor shall obtain from each participating investigator a signed agreement that includes:
>   (1) The investigator's curriculum vitae.
>   (2) Where applicable, a statement of the investigator's relevant experience, including the dates, location, extent, and type of experience.
>   (3) If the investigator was involved in an investigation or other research that was terminated, an explanation of the circumstances that led to termination.
>   (4) A statement of the investigator's commitment to:
>   (i) Conduct the investigation in accordance with the agreement, the investigational plan, this part and other applicable FDA regulations, and conditions of approval imposed by the reviewing IRB or FDA;
>   (ii) Supervise all testing of the device involving human subjects; and
>   (iii) Ensure that the requirements for obtaining informed consent are met.
>   (5) Sufficient accurate financial disclosure information to allow the sponsor to submit a complete and accurate certification or disclosure statement as required under part 54 of this chapter. The sponsor shall obtain a commitment from the clinical investigator to promptly update this information if any relevant changes occur during the course of the investigation and for 1 year following completion of the study. This information shall not be submitted in an Investigational Device Exemption application, but shall be submitted in any marketing application involving the device.
> (d) Selecting monitors. A sponsor shall select monitors qualified by training and experience to monitor the investigational study in accordance with this part and other applicable FDA regulations.
>
> Sec. 812.45 Informing investigators.
>
> A sponsor shall supply all investigators participating in the investigation with copies of the investigational plan and the report of prior investigations of the device.

Sec. 812.46 Monitoring investigations.

(a) Securing compliance. A sponsor who discovers that an investigator is not complying with the signed agreement, the investigational plan, the requirements of this part or other applicable FDA regulations, or any conditions of approval imposed by the reviewing IRB or FDA shall promptly either secure compliance, or discontinue shipments of the device to the investigator and terminate the investigator's participation in the investigation. A sponsor shall also require such an investigator to dispose of or return the device, unless this action would jeopardize the rights, safety, or welfare of a subject.
(b) Unanticipated adverse device effects. (1) A sponsor shall immediately conduct an evaluation of any unanticipated adverse device effect.
    (2) A sponsor who determines that an unanticipated adverse device effect presents an unreasonable risk to subjects shall terminate all investigations or parts of investigations presenting that risk as soon as possible. Termination shall occur not later than 5 working days after the sponsor makes this determination and not later than 15 working days after the sponsor first received notice of the effect.
(c) Resumption of terminated studies. If the device is a significant risk device, a sponsor may not resume a terminated investigation without IRB and FDA approval. If the device is not a significant risk device, a sponsor may not resume a terminated investigation without IRB approval and, if the investigation was terminated under paragraph (b)(2) of this section, FDA approval.

Id. §§ 812.40-46.

Part 812 also delineates the duties of the investigator:

Sec. 812.100 General responsibilities of investigators.

An investigator is responsible for ensuring that an investigation is conducted according to the signed agreement, the investigational plan and applicable FDA regulations, for protecting the rights, safety, and welfare of subjects under the investigator's care, and for the control of devices under investigation. An investigator also is responsible for ensuring that informed consent is obtained in accordance with part 50 of this chapter. Additional responsibilities of investigators are described in subpart G.

Sec. 812.100 Specific responsibilities of investigators.

(a) Awaiting approval. An investigator may determine whether potential subjects would be interested in participating in an investigation, but shall not request the written informed consent of any subject to participate, and shall not allow any subject to participate before obtaining IRB and FDA approval.
(b) Compliance. An investigator shall conduct an investigation in accordance with the signed agreement with the sponsor, the investigational plan, this part and other applicable FDA regulations, and any conditions of approval imposed by an IRB or FDA.
(c) Supervising device use. An investigator shall permit an investigational device to be used only with subjects under the investigator's supervision. An investigator shall not supply an investigational device to any person not authorized under this part to receive it.
(d) Financial disclosure. A clinical investigator shall disclose to the sponsor sufficient accurate financial information to allow the applicant to submit complete and accurate certification or disclosure statements required under part 54 of this chapter. The investigator shall promptly update this information if any relevant changes occur during the course of the investigation and for 1 year following completion of the study.
(e) Disposing of device. Upon completion or termination of a clinical investigation or the investigator's part of an investigation, or at the sponsor's request, an investigator shall return to the sponsor any remaining supply of the device or otherwise dispose of the device as the sponsor directs.

Id. §§ 812.100 and 812.110.

The process under which research is conducted on humans under Part 812 is called an *Investigational Device Exemption* (IDE). It is called an exemption because it allows a device to be transported in commerce for testing without being approved. Without this exemption, the device would be adulterated (a violation of the FDCA). The exemption is granted on a limited basis to allow testing of the device to gather evidence for FDA submissions.

There are three paths through Part 812 for conducting research: (1) exempt studies; (2) abbreviated IDE (nonsignificant risk) studies; and (3) IDE studies.

(1) Exempt studies

There are various types of studies that are exempt from Part 812 and need no FDA interaction:

(a) Preamendment devices which were on sale before 1976 and are used under their original indications.

(b) 510(k) devices, used under their cleared indications for use. Using a device in its normal commercially labeled manner is not a clinical test.

(c) Diagnostic devices, if the testing is noninvasive: does not require an invasive sampling procedure; does not, by design or intention, introduce energy into a subject; and is not used as a diagnostic without confirmation of the diagnosis by another medically established diagnostic product or procedure.

(d) Devices undergoing consumer preference testing if they are not for purposes of determining safety or effectiveness and does not put subjects at risk. This sounds at first to be a broad category, but actually most tests are, in some way, designed to determine safety or effectiveness.

(e) Devices for veterinary use.

(f) Devices for animal testing.

(g) Custom devices.

(2) IDE studies

These are for the highest risk devices. This requires a full submission to FDA.

(3) Abbreviated IDE studies or nonsignificant risk (NSR) studies

These are studies of devices that do not present significant risk, that is, the device is not an implant, does not present a serious risk to health, and is not for curing or preventing a disease or impairment to human health. You must have a determination from the relevant IRB that the device is not a significant risk.

You still have to follow some basic requirements of Part 812, such as monitoring, but you do not have to apply to FDA for an IDE.

The IDE process involves a sponsor submitting an application to FDA including

(1) The name and address of the sponsor.
(2) A complete report of prior investigations of the device and an accurate summary of those sections of the investigational plan described in 812.25(a) through (e) or, in lieu of the summary, the complete plan. The sponsor shall submit to FDA a complete investigational plan and a complete report of prior investigations of the device if no IRB has reviewed them, if FDA has found an IRB's review inadequate, or if FDA requests them.
(3) A description of the methods, facilities, and controls used for the manufacture, processing, packing, storage, and, where appropriate, installation of the device, in sufficient detail so that a person generally familiar with good manufacturing practices can make a knowledgeable judgment about the quality control used in the manufacture of the device.
(4) An example of the agreements to be entered into by all investigators to comply with investigator obligations under this part, and a list of the names and addresses of all investigators who have signed the agreement.
(5) A certification that all investigators who will participate in the investigation have signed the agreement, that the list of investigators includes all the investigators participating in the investigation, and that no investigators will be added to the investigation until they have signed the agreement.
(6) A list of the name, address, and chairperson of each IRB that has been or will be asked to review the investigation and a certification of the action concerning the investigation taken by each such IRB.
(7) The name and address of any institution at which a part of the investigation may be conducted that has not been identified in accordance with paragraph (b)(6) of this section.
(8) If the device is to be sold, the amount to be charged and an explanation of why the sale does not constitute commercialization of the device.
(9) A claim for categorical exclusion or an environmental assessment.
(10) Copies of all labeling for the device.
(11) Copies of all forms and informational materials to be provided to subjects to obtain informed consent.
(12) Any other relevant information FDA requests for review of the application.

Id. § 812.20.

FDA is required to respond within 30 days, if not, the sponsor may proceed. FDA may approve, disapprove, or approve with conditions and modifications. This means that FDA may conditionally approve the IDE so that the sponsor may proceed, although requiring that certain conditions be met.

Once IDE approval is received for a study, a sponsor may begin the difficult process. The sponsor must establish a protocol for the study. This is a daunting document which may run to over a hundred pages. The protocol describes the methodology for the study and includes a detailed analysis of why the study is scientifically sound. This is a pivotal document in the study. It must be followed by the sponsor and all investigators.

The sponsor must enroll sites at which investigators will conduct the study under the protocol. An IRB must approve the study for the site, including approving the wording of the informed consent document. The sponsor must enter into contracts with the site and the investigator. The investigator and study coordinator must be trained. A process must be put in place for recording all needed data on forms provided by the sponsor.

During the study, the sponsor must monitor the investigation to ensure that it is compliant with the regulations and the protocol. This usually involves periodic visits to the site. This is not to be confused with auditing. Auditing a study is a retroactive activity which looks at data to determine if the study was run properly. Monitoring is a continuing function during the study to ensure compliance.

Once a study is complete, the data are assembled and may be used for whatever the purpose of the study was (FDA submission, reimbursement submission, publication, etc.).

2.14 QUALITY SYSTEM REGULATION

The Quality System Regulation (QSR) is a comprehensive control for the entire life cycle of a medical device. The statutory basis is in what is known in the FDCA as good manufacturing practices (GMP). The FDCA gives authority to FDA to regulate many products by prescribing GMP for their manufacture. Different centers have implemented differing types of GMP, sometimes with differing names. For example, GMP for pharmaceuticals are called cGMP, the small "c" meaning "current." This was to indicate that cGMPs are not a static standard. What is expected of a manufacturer changes over the years as quality assurance practices improve and more is known about what to consider "best practices."

When CDRH entirely revised GMPs for medical devices in 1997, it chose to use a new name indicative of the new theory. The new language for device GMP was harmonized, to large extent, with the then-current international standard for quality for devices: ISO 9001. Even though FDA regulations were still based upon criminal law, unlike the EU standards-based theory, FDA chose to harmonize the language of the regulation to achieve international consistency. The ISO standard was based upon a pyramid of quality principles and controls known as a quality system. If one followed the quality system, then quality product would logically flow. To indicate this harmonization, FDA named the new system the QSR. Some within FDA tried to discourage the use of the acronym QSR, since it already stood for a particular record within the system. However, these attempts have not quelled the instant and complete adoption of the acronym QSR for the regulation.

The QSR had a scope much broader than the manufacturing controls of the old GMP. To harmonize with ISO standards, FDA encompassed the entire design process into the QSR, so that it now covers a product from cradle-to-grave.

(1) Who is covered?

Anyone who performs a manufacturing step, as defined by the QSR is covered. A manufacturer is defined as

> any person who designs, manufactures, fabricates, assembles, or processes a finished device. Manufacturer includes but is not limited to those who perform the functions of contract sterilization, installation, relabeling, remanufacturing, repacking, or specification development, and initial distributors of foreign entities performing these functions.

Id. § 820.3(o).

Note that this covers foreign entities who perform these functions. The significant exception is that manufacturers of components or parts are not covered. The easy case is when a company manufactures its own product and puts its name on it. In this way, the manufacturer is clearly identified. Outsourcing has changed this picture. Now there may be many different manufacturers involved in one product.

A company who designs or partially designs a product and then has it built by another company is known as a *specification manufacturer.* It is primarily responsible for quality and for conformance with QSR. Whatever company actually assembles the finished product is also a manufacturer. The companies that provide components are not manufacturers. However, a contractor who packs or sterilizes the product would be a manufacturer. Each of these "manufacturers" is responsible for the performance of the portions of the QSR that relate to their task. At the top of the pyramid, the specification manufacturer remains responsible for everything.

(2) What does the QSR require?
The QSR covers all phases of a product from design to traceability to customers. The significant areas of coverage are

- Design
- Manufacturing
- Packaging
- Storage
- Installation
- Servicing

In order to comply with the QSR you must have a system. Most sections of the QSR require that you "establish" systems. This means that there must be written procedures, along with documentary evidence that you are working under the procedures. The old FDA canard is: "If it's not written down, it didn't happen."

The sections of the QSR are as follows:

Subpart A: General Provisions. This introductory subpart contains some important provisions. The scope of the QSR is defined here. This is where component manufacturers are exempted from QSR compliance.*

This subpart explains the flexible nature of QSR in that it only requires compliance for those activities you actually perform. For example, if you do not distribute, you do not have to show compliance to that part of the QSR. It also explains the term where appropriate. This means that you can excuse yourself from an irrelevant portion of the QSR if you properly document it.

Subpart A also include the definitions for the QSR.† This is a pivotal set of information. The real context of the regulation often lies in the definition. For example, the definition of manufacturer really determines who is covered by QSR. Most of the important design control records are defined here. The important definition of validation is found here. When interpreting a section of the QSR, remember to look back into these definitions to see if relevant meaning is found here.

Subpart A also includes the important overall requirement to establish and maintain a quality system.‡

Subpart B: Quality System Requirements. Management responsibility§ is a key concept in the QSR. FDA views this as the heart of the system, upon which all other modules depend. The main obligations of management are

**Id.* § 820.1(a).
†*Id.* § 820.3.
‡*Id.* § 820.5(c).
§*Id.* § 820.20.

(1) Establish a quality policy and ensure it is understood.

(2) Establish an organizational structure to assure compliance.

(3) Provide adequate resources.

(4) Appoint a management representative with executive responsibility to ensure that the quality system is established and to report on its performance.

(5) Conduct management reviews, including review of the suitability and effectiveness of the quality system.

Subpart B also defines the concept of quality audits* which are an ongoing part of an operating quality system. FDA wished to encourage self-correction through the audit system, so it decided not to inspect the records of such audits. This allows a company to aggressively search into its systems without fear that an investigator will use the findings against them. Investigators will look for records proving that the audit system is in place and is working.

This subpart also defines the need for sufficient personnel with the background and training to operate under the quality system.†

Subpart C: Design Controls. The inclusion of design controls, a major concept harmonized from ISO standards, into device GMPs was one of the most important steps in creating the QSR. This was a major departure from the previous concept of device GMPs, which focused on manufacturing. This extended the control of QSR over virtually the entire device life cycle.

Design controls cover all Class III and Class II devices.‡ Class I devices are generally exempt from design controls, except for a handful of specifically listed devices.

Design controls require that manufacturers have a documented design control system:

> Each manufacturer shall establish and maintain plans that describe or reference the design and development activities and define responsibility for implementation. The plans shall identify and describe the interfaces with different groups or activities that provide, or result in, input to the design and development process.
>
> *Id.* § 820.30(b).

Many manufacturers are adopting software control systems to ensure that all steps in the process are completed and documented. This overall planning and control is an essential part of an ISO-style, top-down quality system.

This system must include design review procedures. The QSR states

> Each manufacturer shall establish and maintain procedures to ensure that formal documented reviews of the design results are planned and conducted at appropriate stages of the device's design development. The procedures shall ensure that participants at each design review include representatives of all functions concerned with the design stage being reviewed and an individual(s) who does not have direct responsibility for the design stage being reviewed, as well as any specialists needed.
>
> *Id.* § 820.30(e).

These reviews must be documented in a Design History File (DHF).

The major steps in the design control process are

(1) Design input

(2) Design output

(3) Design verification

**Id.* § 820.22.
†*Id.* § 820.25.
‡*Id.* § 820.30(a).

(4) Design validation

(5) Design transfer

A major difference in philosophy from previous GMP systems is that these five stages are not one-time events. Each time a change in design occurs, it must be analyzed to determine whether certain of these steps must be repeated. Different types of changes may require different loops through the system. It must be determined, for example, if verification or validation must be repeated on the parts of testing that are affected by a change. This makes the design control process a living system that is always being probed, rather than a single historical process.

(1) Design input
This phase covers the gathering and specifying of all the requirements for the product:

> Each manufacturer shall establish and maintain procedures to ensure that the design requirements relating to a device are appropriate and address the intended use of the device, including the needs of the user and patient. The procedures shall include a mechanism for addressing incomplete, ambiguous, or conflicting requirements.
>
> *Id.* § 820.30(c).

Note that the needs of the user and patient are to be considered. This does not make a customer-focused system a matter of law, but it does create a requirement to do analysis of the needs of all the audiences. Device companies use various procedures to amass and document the inputs. Some companies start with a general functional list of features, which is sometimes called marketing requirements. This may be followed by a more detailed list of the engineering requirements needed to implement them. Some companies merge these two into one process. In any case, the needs of all users must be considered and the functional and engineering requirements must be documented, reviewed, and approved.

FDA guidance says to include

Functional requirements—what the device does
Performance requirements—how well the device performs
Interface requirements—compatibility with external systems

One way to look at design inputs is that this is the first manifestation of what the company's marketing claims will look like years later when the product is approved and commercially released. The user needs and benefits built into the design inputs are the very things the company will want to tout in the commercial environment.

(2) Design output
This section of the design controls regulation essentially includes the specifications that define the medical device. The output is the package of documentation that is used to clear the product with FDA and to manufacture it.

The manufacturer must establish and maintain procedures for defining and documenting the output. The QSR states:

> Design output procedures shall contain or make reference to acceptance criteria and shall ensure that those design outputs that are essential for the proper functioning of the device are identified.
>
> *Id.* § 820.20(d).

The output contains things such as

- Design specification
- Testing against standards, such as biocompatibility, toxicity, and electrical

- Detailed assembly drawings
- Manufacturing flowcharts
- Software code
- Packaging specifications
- Labeling specifications

The many interactions of a design project, including prototyping and testing, all go into a design package that is the basis for the device master record.*

(3) Design verification

Design verification is the testing of the design output to ensure that it meets all the requirements in the design input.† Of course, this has to be done in using written procedures established and maintained by the manufacturer.

It is important to differentiate this use of the term verification from the use of the term in manufacturing. Here, it is the design output that is being verified. This is commonly done by all the bench testing that goes into proving the concept of the design. Each requirement must be tested to show conformance, for example, pull testing to show tensile strength. Later in the manufacturing process, verification and validation are alternate paths to qualifying a manufacturing process. Here in the design arena, both verification and validation of a design are required.

(4) Design validation

Once all requirements in the design output are verified, the device goes on to the validation phase. *Validation* is the process of ensuring that the device works for the purpose for which it was designed, in the environment for which it was intended. This must be distinguished from the term *process validation,* which is used in the manufacturing area as an optional way of qualifying a process. Design validation must be done on every design. The QSR states:

> Design validation shall be performed under defined operating conditions on initial production units, lots, or batches, or their equivalents. Design validation shall ensure that devices conform to defined user needs and intended uses and shall include testing of production units under actual or simulated use conditions. Design validation shall include software validation and risk analysis, where appropriate.
>
> *Id.* § 820.30(g).

As usual, this must be done under a written set of procedures. The results become part of the DHF.

Methods of validation differ with the type of device. Most lower-risk Class II devices may be validated in simulated environments on the bench. Some of these Class II devices are validated in relatively simple user tests in a hospital or doctor's office. In the type of higher-risk devices for which FDA expects human clinical data for clearance/approval, the validation is done as part of the clinical testing. The successful use in a clinical trial validates that the design meets the defined user needs.

Software validation, a term built into the FDA design validation definition cited above, is yet a third use of the term validation. This involves establishing a test plan and thoroughly testing the software. This testing involves a combination of tools which resemble both what are call verification and validation in the manufacturing regulation. FDA has issued guidance on software validation which has established some fairly common techniques and procedures used by the industry.

Once again, the results documenting the successful completion of design validation become part of the DHF.

**Id.* § 820.181.
†*Id.* § 820.30(f).

(5) Design transfer
Design transfer is the process of translating the device design into production specifications. This must be done under controlled written procedures. This step in the design control process is meant to avoid what engineer's jokingly call "throwing the design over the wall" to manufacturing compatriots. In the regulated FDA environment, this step is critical in ensuring that no requirements are lost in the transfer. It is critical that the manufacturing procedures and the attendant tests, actually confirm the elements of the design output.

Subpart D: Document Controls. The many references above to written procedures and records show the importance of controlling documents within a quality system. An essential element of your quality system is a procedure to control your procedures. Such a system includes a numbering method for documents, a revision control method for tracking changes and identifying the current version, and an approval method for review and approval of the original document and changes.

First, you need personnel and a system:

> Each manufacturer shall designate an individual(s) to review for adequacy and approve prior to issuance all documents established to meet the requirements of this part. The approval, including the date and signature of the individual(s) approving the document, shall be documented.
>
> *Id.* § 820.40(a).

Then you need a process for making the documents available where needed, and to update as needed:

> Documents established to meet the requirements of this part shall be available at all locations for which they are designated, used, or otherwise necessary, and all obsolete documents shall be promptly removed from all points of use or otherwise prevented from unintended use.
>
> *Id.*

Traditionally, procedures were made available in paper copy. This required vigilance in replacing manuals as they were updated. Many companies have moved to electronic systems that automatically update controlled documents so that users can only access the current version preventing mishaps.

Updating the documents can be a time-consuming, and perhaps thankless task, but is required:

> Changes to documents shall be reviewed and approved by an individual(s) in the same function or organization that performed the original review and approval, unless specifically designated otherwise. Approved changes shall be communicated to the appropriate personnel in a timely manner.
>
> *Id.* § 820.40(b).

The critical part of system design is to create a change-control system wherein the entire history of changes to a document can be recorded for later reconstruction:

> Each manufacturer shall maintain records of changes to documents. Change records shall include a description of the change, identification of the affected documents, the signature of the approving individual(s), the approval date, and when the change becomes effective.
>
> *Id.*

Subpart E: Purchasing Controls. Purchasing controls are growing more important since companies are outsourcing more activities. The modern virtual company is still responsible for its quality system and the quality of its products. The actual work involved in creating those products may be outside the corporate structure. Purchasing controls are what tie together the responsibilities for QSR compliance.

A purchasing system must have procedures to

(1) Evaluate and select potential suppliers, contractors, and consultants on the basis of their ability to meet specified requirements, including quality requirements. The evaluation shall be documented.
(2) Define the type and extent of control to be exercised over the product, services, suppliers, contractors, and consultants, based on the evaluation results.
(3) Establish and maintain records of acceptable suppliers, contractors, and consultants.

Id. § 820.50(a).

You must establish contracts controlling the suppliers that include your quality requirements. These contracts must specify that the supplier will notify you of any changes that might affect quality. These supplier contracts are a major link between your quality system and the place of actual production. It is critical that they correctly lay out responsibilities.

Subpart F: Identification and Traceability. You must have a way to follow your product during all stages of receipt, production, distribution, and installation to prevent mix-ups. Usually this is done by either lot control or by individual serial numbers on product. While higher-risk PMA products usually carry serial numbers, the vast majority of medical devices are traced by lot.

The importance of lot control becomes apparent the first time you have an issue in manufacturing. If you later discover, for example, that you have received a shipment of raw material or components that does not meet specifications, it is necessary to trace back and find every product in which it was used. Without identification procedures this could be impossible. If a recall is needed due to a bad lot of raw material, you would have to recall all of your product unless you could narrow it down through your lot-control process.

While the regulation only requires such control for "a device that is intended for surgical implant into the body or to support or sustain life and whose failure to perform when properly used in accordance with instructions for use provided in the labeling can be reasonably expected to result in a significant injury to the user,"* it is recommended for all products so that you can trace any problems back to a limited lot of goods.

Subpart G: Production and Process Controls. This is the part of the QSR with which most lay people are aware. It is the heart of the old GMP. This subpart controls the actual manufacturing of devices.

The underlying principle of subpart G is that a manufacturer has to establish and maintain production processes that produce devices that meet specification. This control is built into the system to prevent deviations from specification. Process controls include

(1) Documented instructions, standard operating procedures (SOPs), and methods that define and control the manner of production;
(2) Monitoring and control of process parameters and component and device characteristics during production;
(3) Compliance with specified reference standards or codes;
(4) The approval of processes and process equipment; and
(5) Criteria for workmanship which shall be expressed in documented standards or by means of identified and approved representative samples.

Id. § 820.70(a).

This system of procedures must include a controlled method for making changes, including doing all the testing needed to verify or validate a change before it is implemented.

Id. § 820.65.

Subpart G includes a list of requirements that look very broad and general. These are interpreted by FDA to require a company to use what is viewed as the current standard of care in the industry. That is, the requirements grow and change as technology advances. Among the requirements are

- Environmental control—The manufacturer must control environmental conditions that could affect product quality. This includes inspecting and verifying that the equipment is adequate and functioning properly.
- Personnel—You need requirements for the health, cleanliness, personal practices, and clothing of personnel if they can affect product quality.
- Contamination—You need to prevent contamination of equipment or product.
- Buildings—Buildings must be suitable for manufacturing your product and must contain sufficient space to manufacture without mix-ups.
- Equipment—Your equipment must meet process specifications and must be designed, constructed, placed, and installed to facilitate maintenance, adjustment, cleaning, and use.
- Maintenance schedule—You need documented schedules for adjustment, cleaning, and other maintenance of equipment.
- Inspection—There must be scheduled periodic inspections to ensure that maintenance has been done according to procedure.
- Adjustment—Limitations or allowable tolerances must be posted on equipment that requires periodic adjustment.
- Manufacturing material—Any manufacturing material that could negatively affect product quality must be removed from the manufacturing area.
- Automated processes—Any software used in computers or automated processing must be validated. Any changes must be validated before implementation.

While these requirements may look general, there is a whole history of industry meaning built into every one. Most of these requirements vary with the complexity of the device being manufactured and the risk to the end user. Great flexibility is built into the QSR so that manufacturers may develop processes appropriate to the product. The QSR is a little more precise and prescriptive when it comes to calibration:

> Each manufacturer shall ensure that all inspection, measuring, and test equipment, including mechanical, automated, or electronic inspection and test equipment, is suitable for its intended purposes and is capable of producing valid results. Each manufacturer shall establish and maintain procedures to ensure that equipment is routinely calibrated, inspected, checked, and maintained. The procedures shall include provisions for handling, preservation, and storage of equipment, so that its accuracy and fitness for use are maintained.
>
> *Id.* § 820.72(a).

There must be

- Calibration procedures that set limits for accuracy and precision, along with remedial action to be taken if the equipment is out of calibration.
- Calibration standards must be derived from accepted national or international standards.
- Calibration records must be near the equipment so that the current state of calibration is readily available.

Finally, this subpart requires either verification or validation of processes.* As discussed above, the terms verification and validation can have different meanings in different contexts. The definitions show the way in which the two terms are used in the different contexts. Verification is defined as

**Id.* § 820.75

> *Verification* means confirmation by examination and provision of objective evidence that specified requirements have been fulfilled.
>
> *Id.* § 820.3(aa).

While validation is defined as

> *Validation* means confirmation by examination and provision of objective evidence that the particular requirements for a specific intended use can be consistently fulfilled.
>
> (1) *Process validation* means establishing by objective evidence that a process consistently produces a result or product meeting its predetermined specifications.
> (2) *Design validation* means establishing by objective evidence that device specifications conform with user needs and intended use(s).
>
> *Id.* § 820.3(z).

This shows that verification is based upon testing of results, while validation is based upon statistical prediction of future performance. While design controls require that design output be both verified and validated, process controls follow a different algorithm. A process may be either verified or validated. The regulation states that if a process cannot be verified, it must be validated.

A process can be verified if the results of that process can be consistently tested to show conformance with specification. For example, if a process step is to paint a part blue, it can be verified on the line for every part. An inspector can hold the part up to a paint chip sample, and then look for chips or missed spots. Total verification can be accomplished by inspection.

Many processes are more complex and defy verification. For example, a weld cannot be visually inspected. It is possible that all specifications for a weld cannot be satisfied without destructive testing. Since you would have no product if you destructively tested each one, you need a predictive method of producing quality product. These processes must be validated.

You validate by determining what statistical sample size is needed to predict that quality results will occur within the percentage level of success you specify. For example, how many parts do I need to test to predict meeting specification at the 99 percent confidence level? The FDA default for sampling for validation is to do three runs of 30 products each. Of course, there is flexibility based upon the type of product and how you validate each process. For example, if your process is the final step in producing a $10,000 medical device, you do not want to do destructive testing on 90 (3 runs of 30) products. That would cost near a million dollars. You would then validate previous processes and argue for a smaller sample on the final test. In any case, you need to develop a statistical rationale for the sampling size that can provide a "high degree of assurance" for each process to be validated. Then you need to put the designated runs of product through the process and test them for meeting specification. Upon this, you can project the successful future results of the process. As in all QSR activities, this validation must be conducted under a controlled written procedure.

Of course, this predictive validation is only valid if the process runs according to specification. You must establish and maintain control of your processes to make sure that they continue to meet specification. Tools such as statistical process control are usually employed to assure continuing compliance.

As with other things established under the QSR, a change to any process must be evaluated as to its effect on the specification. Revalidation my be required. Your procedure must have a robust method of evaluating changes.

Subpart H: Acceptance Activities. The acceptance activities required in subpart H suffuse the entire manufacturing process, from raw material to finished product. This is not just a section for accepting product from outside the company. Rather it controls acceptance of product or work at every step. Subpart H has taken on new significance in the era of the virtual manufacturer. If significant subassemblies or whole finished product is being outsourced, it is critical that these acceptance activities either be performed on receipt or delegated to the supplier under the purchasing controls discussed in subpart E.

Acceptance activities, including "inspections, test, or other verification activities"* must be performed, under established procedures, throughout the manufacturing cycle. First, of course, is incoming product:

> Incoming product shall be inspected, tested, or otherwise verified as conforming to specified requirements. Acceptance or rejection shall be documented.
>
> *Id.* § 820.80(b).

Note that this covers all incoming product: raw material, components, subassemblies, finished product, packaging, etc. This activity may be delegated to a supplier under contract if you have established quality standards, through vendor qualification, contract, and audit.

Work in progress must also be accepted under this subpart. Your procedures must

> ensure that in-process product is controlled until the required inspection and tests or other verification activities have been completed, or necessary approvals are received, and are documented.
>
> *Id.* § 820.29(c).

Whatever control system you employ on the manufacturing line, whether paper travelers or an integrated software system, you need to have processes for acceptance at process steps.

This control continues through the final steps to complete a finished device. You need final acceptance criteria to ensure that each run, lot, or batch meets specification. Finished devices must be controlled, sometimes called *quarantine,* until the final acceptance occurs. The finished product may not be released into distribution until

> (1) The activities required in the DMR are completed;
> (2) the associated data and documentation is reviewed;
> (3) the release is authorized by the signature of a designated individual(s); and
> (4) the authorization is dated.
>
> *Id.* § 820.80(d).

For each of these types of acceptance you need records showing

> (1) The acceptance activities performed;
> (2) the dates acceptance activities are performed;
> (3) the results;
> (4) the signature of the individual(s) conducting the acceptance activities; and
> (5) where appropriate the equipment used. These records shall be part of the DHR.
>
> *Id.* § 820.80(e).

The term "signature" is a holdover from the days of paper travelers. On paper records, a signature can be initials or some other designator. On electronic systems, the signature must comply with the electronic records rules in 21 C.F.R. Part 11.

All material passing through the process must be marked to show its status:

> Each manufacturer shall identify by suitable means the acceptance status of product, to indicate the conformance or nonconformance of product with acceptance criteria. The identification of acceptance status shall be maintained throughout manufacturing, packaging, labeling, installation, and servicing of the product to ensure that only product which has passed the required acceptance activities is distributed, used, or installed.
>
> *Id.* § 820.86.

**Id.* § 820.80(a).

Subpart I: Nonconforming Product. Procedures must be established for dealing with any product found not to meet specification under acceptance procedures. Once again, as in subpart H, this covers the entire manufacturing process from raw material through finished goods. These procedures must "address the identification, documentation, evaluation, segregation, and disposition of nonconforming product."* The procedure must provide for determining whether an investigation is needed and whether to notify the persons responsible for the nonconformity.

Your procedure must identify the person or group that reviews the nonconforming product and determines its disposition, for example, destruction, rework, salvage of parts, etc. The disposition must be documented.

You must have a procedure controlling rework. It is important to distinguish rework from a multiple-try process. Some processes call for multiple tries, "polish and inspect up to three times until product meets specification." On the other hand, when a product finishes the manufacturing process and fails, then sending it back is called *rework.* The specification should state if there is a limit on the number of times a product can be reworked. Reworked product must meet all tests and acceptance criteria.

Subpart J: Corrective and Preventive Action (CAPA). This subpart is critical because it is one of the most heavily inspected activities by FDA. It is considered a major module in an inspection of a quality system because these procedures are where nonconformities are corrected and, perhaps more importantly, examined to see if preventive action can be taken to preclude other future nonconformities.

The difference between Corrective and Preventive Action is sometimes not clear. In general it might be said that corrective action is that which prevents the same nonconformity from recurring. For example, if the pull test of a gluing step was missing nonconforming the product, corrective action might be changing the test to one that can find all errors, such as by increasing the pull weight or duration. Preventive action could be to look around your manufacturing process for other steps where similar tests are done to see if any similar processes should be upgraded. Corrective action looks back at an error to prevent recurrence; preventive action tries to use what was learned to prevent other types of errors.

CAPA procedures covers a wide range of nonconformities. CAPA procedures analyze input from "processes, work operations, concessions, quality audit reports, quality records, service records, complaints, returned product, and other sources of quality data to identify existing and potential causes of nonconforming product, or other quality problems."† This is a wide area of data input. This has led some FDA inspectors to incorrectly treat CAPA as a "system" that must receive input from all sources. Actually the CAPA procedures need not be one enterprise-wide system, but there must be a way to determine if data concerning nonconformities found in different areas are related. Statistical methods may be required to analyze the multiple data inputs to detect recurring problems. Some inspectors have misread this section to mean that corrective action related to audit reports must be in your one, unified CAPA system. This is incorrect. Internal audit results may be handled in a separate audit CAPA process. Nevertheless, the scope of CAPA is immense. Modern quality theory is expanding CAPA procedures beyond manufacturing to areas such as clinical trial compliance.

Once you have events in the CAPA procedure, subpart J requires

(2) Investigating the cause of nonconformities relating to product, processes, and the quality system;

(3) Identifying the action(s) needed to correct and prevent recurrence of nonconforming product and other quality problems;

(4) Verifying or validating the Corrective and Preventive Action to ensure that such action is effective and does not adversely affect the finished device;

(5) Implementing and recording changes in methods and procedures needed to correct and prevent identified quality problems;

**Id.* § 820.90(a)

†*Id.* § 820.100(a)(1).

(6) Ensuring that information related to quality problems or nonconforming product is disseminated to those directly responsible for assuring the quality of such product or the prevention of such problems; and
(7) Submitting relevant information on identified quality problems, as well as Corrective and Preventive Actions, for management review.

Id. § 820.100(a).

FDA file personnel look to CAPA first to see the state of your business. CAPA tells what your problems are, how you fixed them, and the quality of your processes for finding future issues.

Subpart K: Labeling and Packaging Control. The labeling of a medical device is as important a component as any piece of hardware. The labeling defines what the product is. Remember there is a distinction between the label and labeling. A *label* is what is affixed to the product or its container. What you stick on the box is a label. That label plus whatever instructions go to the customer, constitute *labeling*. All labeling is controlled. The QSR is concerned with two major aspects of labeling: (1) is the content correct and (2) is the correct labeling applied to the product? Labeling requirements state

(a) *Label integrity.* Labels shall be printed and applied so as to remain legible and affixed during the customary conditions of processing, storage, handling, distribution, and where appropriate use.
(b) *Labeling inspection.* Labeling shall not be released for storage or use until a designated individual(s) has examined the labeling for accuracy including, where applicable, the correct expiration date, control number, storage instructions, handling instructions, and any additional processing instructions. The release, including the date and signature of the individual(s) performing the examination, shall be documented in the DHR.
(c) *Labeling storage.* Each manufacturer shall store labeling in a manner that provides proper identification and is designed to prevent mixups.
(d) *Labeling operations.* Each manufacturer shall control labeling and packaging operations to prevent labeling mixups. The label and labeling used for each production unit, lot, or batch shall be documented in the DHR.
(e) *Control number.* Where a control number is required by 820.65, that control number shall be on or shall accompany the device through distribution.

Id. § 820.120.

Labeling errors result in many recalls of product. Putting the wrong label on a box or inserting the wrong instructions-for-use in a box is a simple human error. It can, however, result in risk to patients and interference with the provision of medical care. FDA investigators look to see if your labeling and labels are carefully sorted and marked to prevent incorrect application. They also commonly look for crowded or poorly laid out labeling stations that confuse the personnel and increase the risk of error.

Subpart L: Handling, Storage, Distribution, and Installation. While the handling and storage provisions of this subpart apply to all processes, the most significant thing in the subpart is the extension of the QSR all the way through manufacturing to distribution.

Handling procedures must be in place throughout your system for preventing "mixups, damage, deterioration, contamination or other adverse effects."* You must also have adequate storage at all steps along the manufacturing process to prevent these errors.†

Your distribution must be under a controlled procedure that ensures that goods which have deteriorated or are beyond their shelf-life are not distributed.‡ You must also keep records of

(1) The name and address of the initial consignee;
(2) The identification and quantity of devices shipped;

**Id.* § 820.140.
†*Id.* § 820.150
‡*Id.* § 820.160(a).

(3) The date shipped; and
(4) Any control number(s) used.

Id. § 820.160(b).

If you perform installation of your product, you must establish procedures for installation.* This continues the QSR right into your customer location.

Subpart M: Records. Since records are the lifeblood of a quality system, this subpart contains some important issues. It defines that records must be legible and accessible, including for FDA inspectors. This can be an issue if you are using paper records. If your manufacturing is not done at the same location as design, you may have difficulty having all applicable records available for inspection. The modern era of electronic systems prevents this by having one record, accessible by all.

This subpart also contains the statement that you can mark these records as confidential, limiting FDA's release of them to the public. Virtually all QSR records should be marked as confidential.

Records under the QSR must be kept for the expected life of the device, but in no case less than 2 years after commercial release.

Important exceptions to FDA's access to QSR records are "reports required by 820.20(c) Management review, 820.22 Quality audits, and supplier audit reports used to meet the requirements of 820.50(a) Evaluation of suppliers, contractors, and consultants."† FDA wants to encourage robust internal questioning of your quality system. FDA's inspection of these records could cause hesitancy to be forthright. Therefore they are placed off-limits for FDA investigators. Once a legal proceeding begins, however, this limitation is no longer in effect.

This subpart defines a few of the most important QSR records, such as the device master record, the device history record, and the quality system record. The most important definition is the section on complaint files. A complaint is

> any written, electronic, or oral communication that alleges deficiencies related to the identity, quality, durability, reliability, safety, effectiveness, or performance of a device after it is released for distribution.

Id.§ 820.3(b).

A manufacturer must maintain complaint files, along with a procedure that ensures they are processed in a timely manner, documented even if oral, and evaluated to see if they must be reported as Medical Device Reports (see the following paragraph). Then each complaint must be evaluated to determine whether an investigation is necessary. Such an investigation must be done if there is a possible failure of the device, labeling or packaging to meet specification.‡

Complaints usually are put into the CAPA system when investigation is needed. A record of the investigation must include

(1) The name of the device;
(2) The date the complaint was received;
(3) Any device identification(s) and control number(s) used;
(4) The name, address, and phone number of the complainant;
(5) The nature and details of the complaint;
(6) The dates and results of the investigation;
(7) Any corrective action taken; and
(8) Any reply to the complainant.

Id. § 820.198(e).

**Id.* § 820.170.
†*Id.* § 820.180(c).
‡*Id.* § 820.198.

Complaint records must be available at the manufacturing site. If your complaint analysis is done at a different location, the records must be made available. In paper records this often meant duplicating the paper records at the manufacturing site. With electronic systems, it is easier to provide access to complaint records at all site.

Subpart N: Servicing. If servicing is part of your device requirements, you must establish servicing procedures.* Servicing interacts with other areas of the QSR. For example, service reports must be analyzed to see if they must be analyzed under a CAPA procedure, including statistical analysis for frequency, etc. Some service reports may be reportable as MDRs. These automatically are classified as complaints under subpart L.

Records must be kept of each service including

(1) The name of the device serviced;
(2) Any device identification(s) and control number(s) used;
(3) The date of service;
(4) The individual(s) servicing the device;
(5) The service performed; and
(6) The test and inspection data.

Id. § 820.200(d).

Subpart O: Statistical Techniques. Manufactures must establish procedures for "identifying valid statistical techniques required for establishing, controlling, and verifying the acceptability of process capability and product characteristics."† Sampling plans must be based upon a valid statistical rationale and must be adequate for the intended use.

2.15 MEDICAL DEVICE REPORTING

Medical Device Reporting (MDR)‡ is a reporting system for collecting serious adverse events related to commercially used devices. This regulation does not cover clinical devices. Adverse events for clinical trials are reported as part of the IDE system.

Congress established MDR reporting so that FDA would be aware of serious events in the field. The MDR system requires reporting from user facilities, importers, and manufacturers. These reports are done on an FDA form called MedWatch.

The events that must be reported are

- Deaths.
- Serious injury, meaning one that is life-threatening, results in permanent impairment of a body function, or permanent damage to a body structure.
- Malfunctions of a device that, if it were to recur, would be likely to cause or contribute to a death or serious injury.

FDA has taken a fairly expansive view of these definitions in an attempt to get broad reporting. For example, the practical usage of the term "would be likely" is "might."

The definitions of who must report are also wide:

**Id.* § 820.200.
†*Id.* § 820.250.
‡*Id.* pt. 803.

- A *user facility* means a hospital, ambulatory surgical facility, nursing home, outpatient diagnostic facility, or outpatient treatment facility, which is not a physician's office. School nurse offices and employee health units are not device user facilities.
- An *importer* means any person who imports a device into the United States and who furthers the marketing of a device from the original place of manufacture to the person who makes final delivery or sale to the ultimate user, but who does not repackage or otherwise change the container, wrapper, or labeling of the device or device package. If you repackage or otherwise change the container, wrapper, or labeling, you are considered a manufacturer as defined in this section.
- A *manufacturer* means any person who manufactures, prepares, propagates, compounds, assembles, or processes a device by chemical, physical, biological, or other procedure.

  The term includes any person who

  (a) Repackages or otherwise changes the container, wrapper, or labeling of a device in furtherance of the distribution of the device from the original place of manufacture.

  (b) Initiates specifications for devices that are manufactured by a second party for subsequent distribution by the person initiating the specifications.

  (c) Manufactures components or accessories that are devices that are ready to be used and are intended to be commercially distributed and intended to be used as is, or are processed by a licensed practitioner or any other qualified person to meet the needs of a particular patient.

  (d) Is U.S. agent of a foreign manufacturer.

These entities must report when they "become aware" of one of the reportable events. To become aware means that an employee of the entity required to report has acquired information that reasonably suggests a reportable adverse event has occurred:

- If you are a device user facility, you are considered to have become aware when medical personnel who are employed by or otherwise formally affiliated with your facility, obtain information about a reportable event.
- If you are a manufacturer, you are considered to have become aware of an event when any of your employees becomes aware of a reportable event that is required to be reported within 30 calendar days or that is required to be reported within 5 work days because reports had been requested in accordance with 803.53(b). You are also considered to have become aware of an event when any of your employees with management or supervisory responsibilities over persons with regulatory, scientific, or technical responsibilities, or whose duties relate to the collection and reporting of adverse events, becomes aware, from any information, including any trend analysis, that a reportable MDR event or events necessitates remedial action to prevent an unreasonable risk of substantial harm to the public health.
- If you are an importer, you are considered to have become aware of an event when any of your employees becomes aware of a reportable event that is required to be reported by you within 30 days.

  This casts a very wide net. Awareness by any employee may trigger a statutory obligation. Who must report to whom may be summarized by

  (a) If you are a device user facility, you must submit reports as follows:
    (1) Submit reports of individual adverse events no later than 10 work days after the day that you become aware of a reportable event:
      (i) Submit reports of device-related deaths to FDA and to the manufacturer, if known; or
      (ii) Submit reports of device-related serious injuries to the manufacturers or, if the manufacturer is unknown, submit reports to FDA.
    (2) Submit annual reports to FDA.

(b) If you are an importer, you must submit reports as follows:
   (1) Submit reports of individual adverse events no later than 30 calendar days after the day that you become aware of a reportable event:
      (i) Submit reports of device-related deaths or serious injuries to FDA and to the manufacturer; or
      (ii) Submit reports of device-related malfunctions to the manufacturer.

(c) If you are a manufacturer, you must submit reports (described in subpart E of this part) to FDA, as follows:
   (1) Submit reports of individual adverse events no later than 30 calendar days after the day that you become aware of a reportable death, serious injury, or malfunction.
   (2) Submit reports of individual adverse events no later than 5 work days after the day that you become aware of:
      (i) A reportable event that requires remedial action to prevent an unreasonable risk of substantial harm to the public health, or
      (ii) A reportable event for which we made a written request.
   (3) Submit annual baseline reports.
   (4) Submit supplemental reports if you obtain information that you did not submit in an initial report.

Id. § 803.10.

This massive data collection exercise has resulted in a huge database of events. Because it is so immense and the data so varied, it has not been as useful as Congress hoped. Attempts have been made by FDA to get better reports, but the mass of data continues to grow. It is difficult for FDA to craft an enforcement program that catches every required report, without inducing companies to over-report just to avoid FDA confrontation.

CHAPTER 3
OVERVIEW OF CARDIOVASCULAR DEVICES

Kenneth L. Gage and William R. Wagner
University of Pittsburgh, Pittsburgh, Pennsylvania

3.1 INTRODUCTION

Despite almost a 25 percent reduction in the mortality rate between 1994 and 2004, cardiovascular disease (CVD) remains the leading cause of death in the United States, with one in three adults living with some form of CVD (Rosamond et al., 2008). The economic impact of CVD is equally staggering. It is estimated that the total cost (direct and indirect) for CVD in the United States was almost 450 billion USD in 2008 (Rosamond et al., 2008). The burden of CVD is not limited to developed nations; with almost 17 million fatalities in 2002 (Mackay and Mensah, 2004), CVD is also the leading cause of death worldwide and is projected to remain so for decades (Mathers and Loncar, 2006). Clearly, technological advancements in cardiovascular devices have an impact that cannot be understated.

Many biomedical engineers have focused their careers on the study of cardiovascular disease and the development of devices to augment or replace function lost to the disease process. The application of engineering principles to device design has improved device function while minimizing the detrimental side effects, allowing complex, challenging cardiovascular surgical procedures (e.g., open-heart surgery) and medical therapies (e.g., dialysis) to become routine. In this chapter, eight major categories of cardiovascular devices are addressed, including cardiac valves and related technologies, stents and stent grafts, pacemakers and implantable defibrillators, vascular grafts, hemodialyzers, indwelling catheters, circulatory support devices, and blood oxygenators. Taken together, these categories span from the most basic equipment used in healthcare to cutting-edge devices still undergoing rapid change in both development and application.

For each topic the market size, indications for device use, device design, complications and patient management, and future trends are covered. The intent is to provide a brief introduction to the current status of cardiovascular device development and application and to identify challenges that remain in the field.

3.2 ARTIFICIAL HEART VALVES AND RELATED TECHNOLOGIES

3.2.1 Market Size

The number of valve replacement operations performed in the United States rose from an estimated 60,000 during 1996 (Vongpatanasin et al., 1996) to more than 78,000 in 2005 (DeFrances et al., 2007). Worldwide, over 350,000 valves are implanted each year, with over 50 percent being mechanical, or purely artificial, in design (Butany and Collins, 2005). As access to cardiac surgery becomes more widespread in developing nations, it is expected that the need for durable, safe, low-cost valves will grow considerably (Zilla et al., 2008).

3.2.2 Indications

The medical indications for valve replacement are thoroughly described in a report from the American College of Cardiology/American Heart Association Task Force on Practice Guidelines that addresses the management of patients with valve disease (Bonow et al., 2006). The etiology of valve disease differs, depending on the patient group and the valve location, as does the preferred corrective treatment. In developed nations, the young suffer from congenital valve defects, while older adults exhibit acquired valve disease. Valve replacement can be performed upon all valves of the heart but most cases involve the aortic or mitral valves. Common reasons for native valve replacement are severe stenosis and regurgitation with or without symptoms, which may include chest pain, shortness of breath, and loss of consciousness. The reduction in effective orifice size associated with a stenotic lesion results in a large transvalvular pressure gradient that may exceed 50 mmHg in the aortic position for severe cases (Bonow et al., 1998). In regurgitation, the blood pumped forward into the recipient vessel or ventricle spills back into the adjacent pumping chamber through an incompetent valve, minimizing forward movement. The end effects of chronic stenosis or regurgitation are compensatory anatomic changes that accommodate, for a limited time, the reduced pumping efficiency due to restricted blood movement. In general, heart valve replacement is performed when repair is not possible, as the implantation of an artificial heart valve brings with it another set of problems. Total replacement and removal of native valve components in the mitral position is particularly limited, as the mitral valve is anatomically and functionally integral to the left ventricle (David et al., 1983; Yun et al., 1999). Concomitant illnesses such as congestive heart failure, atrial fibrillation, and coronary artery disease can alter the indication for valve replacement, as can the surgical need to correct other cardiac disease.

3.2.3 Current and Historical Device Design

Artificial heart valve design has a long and colorful history, with more than 80 different versions of valve being introduced since the 1950s (Vongpatanasin et al., 1996). The two general types of replacement valves, mechanical and biologic, each have their own set of indications, complications, and performance factors. The mechanical valve can be further categorized into three major design lines: caged-ball, single-tilting-disc, and bileaflet (Vongpatanasin et al., 1996). Caged-ball valves have been largely supplanted by the more modern single-tilting-disc and bileaflet valves. Biologic valves are divided based on the source of the tissue material, with the term bioprosthetic reserved for valves constructed from nonliving, animal-source tissue. Homograft biologic valves are preserved human aortic valves, and autografts are pulmonary valves surgically moved to the aortic location within the same patient (Bonow et al., 2006). Heterograft bioprosthetic valves consist of porcine heart valves or bovine pericardial tissue formed into a valve over a support structure (Vongpatanasin et al., 1996). Because mechanical and bioprosthetic valves have different design considerations, the categories are discussed separately.

Mechanical Valves. The assorted mechanical valve designs use different approaches to achieve the same functional goal. Caged-ball valves use a free-floating polymeric sphere constrained by a metal

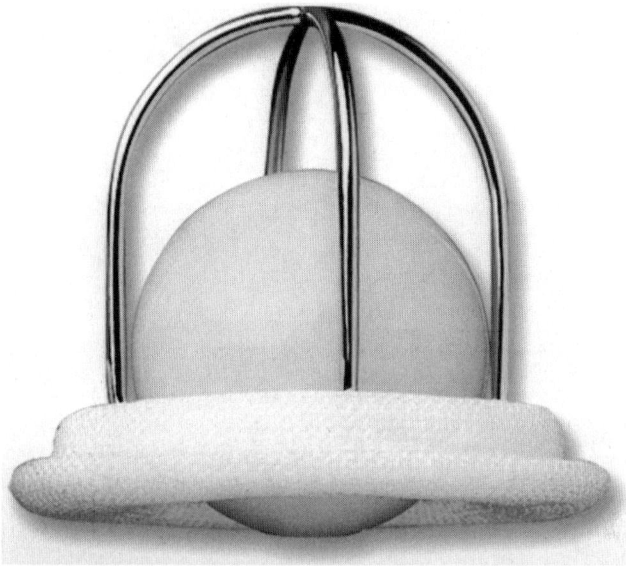

FIGURE 3.1 A caged-ball prosthetic heart valve is shown (Starr-Edwards Model 61.20). The simple and durable design is still in use for new implantations. (*Butany and Collins, 2005.) (Image courtesy of Edwards Lifesciences, Irvine, CA*).

cage to periodically occlude the valve orifice. Single-disc valves possess a central disc occluder that is held in place by struts projecting from the housing ring. The disc opens through a combination of tilting and sliding over the struts to reveal a primary and secondary orifice. Bileaflet valves feature leaflets that are hinged into the housing ring. The opened valve presents three orifices; two along the housing ring edge and one central orifice between the leaflet mount points. A caged-ball valve is shown in Fig. 3.1, while Fig. 3.2 demonstrates orifice and profile views of representative tilting disc and bileaflet mechanical valves.

Mechanical valves are expected to perform flawlessly for decades with minimal patient burden. Criteria used to evaluate designs during development and clinical use can be divided into *structural* and *hemodynamic* groups, although there is considerable overlap. *Structural* considerations involve fatigue and device integrity, valve profile, rotatability, and occluder interference (Akins, 1995). To accommodate the wear associated with operating hundreds of millions of times, current mechanical valves are manufactured with durable metal and carbon alloys (Helmus and Hubbell, 1993; Vongpatanasin et al., 1996), and include a polymer fabric sewing ring for surgical placement. Rotatability of the valve is desirable as evidence suggests that optimum orientations minimizing turbulence and microembolic signals exist for mechanical heart valves in vivo (Laas et al., 1999; Kleine et al., 2000). Concerns regarding valve profile and occluder interference focus on possible negative interactions between the valve, adjacent ventricular structures, native valve remnants, or surgical suture material. The impingement of these structures into the valve could prevent complete closure or cause binding of the occluder. It is believed that overgrowth of adjacent tissue in particular is an underappreciated cause of valve failure (Zilla et al., 2008). Although not a structural requirement, devices tend to be radiopaque to aid in visualization during radiographic procedures.

Hemodynamic performance factors that should be considered during functional evaluation of a valve design are the transvalvular pressure gradient, rate and duration of valve opening, dynamic regurgitant fraction, and static leak rate (Akins, 1995). The transvalvular pressure gradient is a function of the effective orifice area of the valve and the flow regime (turbulent or laminar) encountered.

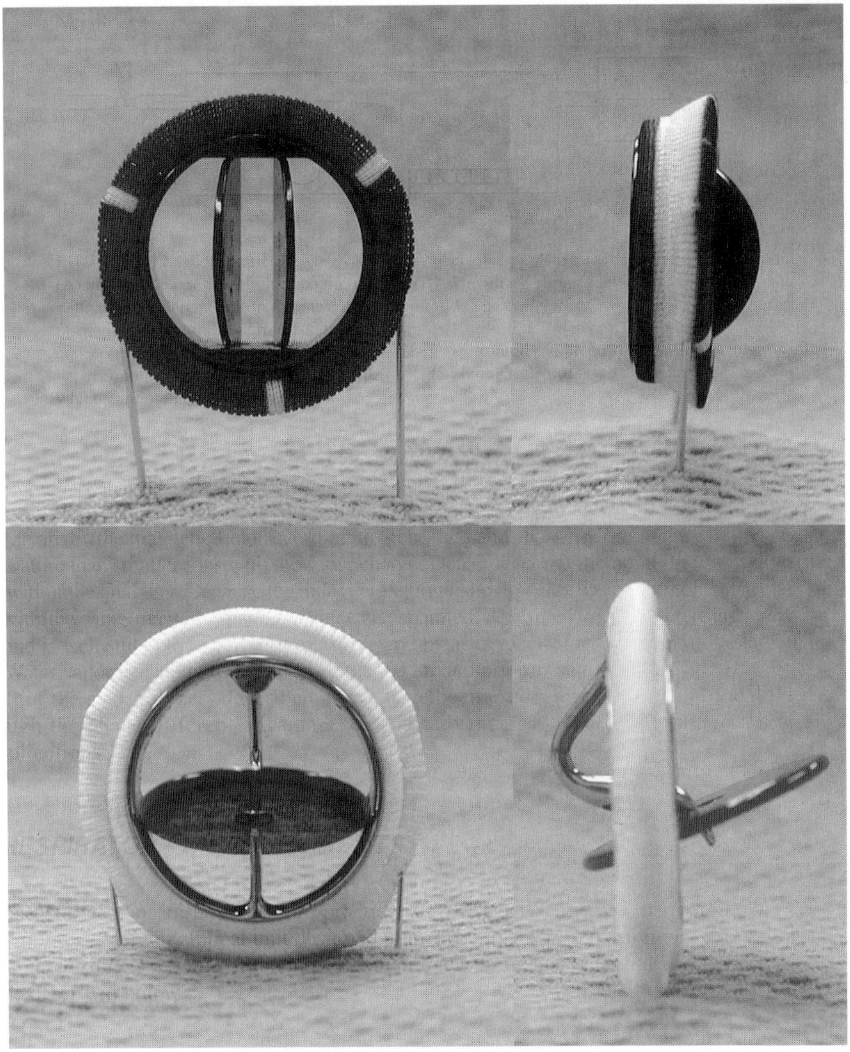

FIGURE 3.2 Orifice and profile views of representative bileaflet and tilting-disc valves are provided in the upper and lower halves of the figure. Note the larger percentage of open orifice area present in the bileaflet valve. The tilting disc projects farther into the downstream ejection zone than the leaflets on the bileaflet valve.

The mass of the occluder and mechanism of action play a significant role in the rate and duration of valve actuation, and similarly in the dynamic regurgitant fraction, which represents the percentage of blood that flows back into the originating chamber prior to valve closure. Finally, some leak is expected in the closed valve position. Consistent convective flow over these surfaces is believed to aid in the minimization of thrombotic deposition.

Bioprosthetic Valves. Engineering design concerns have little influence on homograft valves due to their anatomic origin, thereby limiting the focus to heterograft bioprostheses. The bioprosthetic tissue found in heterografts is treated with glutaraldehyde to cross-link the proteins that make up the tissue structure. The treatment is cytotoxic, disrupts the antigenic proteins that can cause an immune

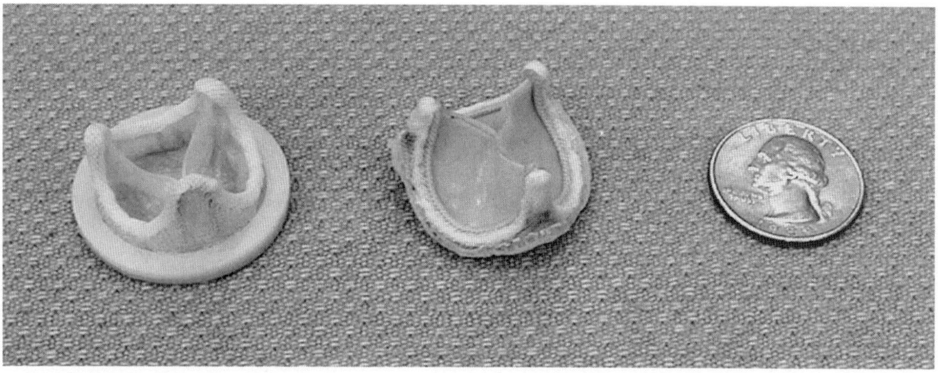

FIGURE 3.3 Two tissue-based artificial heart valves are shown above with a U.S. quarter dollar for size comparison. The valve on the far left is a porcine heart valve, while the other valve is constructed of bovine pericardium. Both valves are intended for aortic placement.

response, and improves the toughness of the tissue by cross-linking the structural collagen (Bonow et al., 1998). Some bioprosthetic valves are further treated with surfactants, diphosphonates, ethanol, or trivalent metal cations to limit the rate of calcification and associated structural deterioration (Schoen and Levy, 1999).

Porcine heterograft valves can be mounted on a support scaffold with sewing ring, although unmounted designs have been introduced to improve flow characteristics and structural endurance. Heterograft valves constructed of bovine pericardium are formed over a scaffold with sewing ring to mimic an anatomic valve shape. Because the pericardial valves are constructed to design criteria rather than harvested, the orifice size can be made larger to improve flow characteristics, while the higher collagen content may allow improved graft resilience when cross-linked (Bonow et al., 1998). Figure 3.3 shows representative porcine and bovine pericardial heterograft valves.

Design Performance Evaluation. The design of artificial heart valves has benefited from the advent of computational fluid dynamics and other computationally intensive modeling techniques. Simulations have been used to predict the performance of both bioprosthetic (Makhijani et al., 1997) and mechanical (Krafczyk et al., 1998) valve designs. Results from computer modeling can be compared with findings from experimental studies using such methods as particle image velocimetry (PIV) (Lim et al., 1998) and high-speed photography of valve structure motion (De Hart et al., 1998). Such comparisons provide necessary model validation, revealing inadequacies in the numerical model and capturing phenomena not predicted using existing model assumptions.

3.2.4 Complications and Patient Management

Mechanical and bioprosthetic valves suffer from complications that dictate follow-up care and preventive measures. Possible complications facing heart valve recipients include thromboembolism, hemolysis, paravalvular regurgitation, endocarditis, and structural failure of the valve (Vongpatanasin et al., 1996). Some preventive measures are indicated for both mechanical and biologic valve recipients, such as the use of antibiotics during dental surgery and invasive procedures to avoid infective endocarditis (Wilson et al., 2007). Other preventive treatments, such as long-term anticoagulation, are administered differently, depending on the type of valve implanted.

Because of the high incidence of thromboembolic complications associated with mechanical artificial heart valves, chronic anticoagulation is required. Anticoagulation with warfarin and an antiplatelet agent, such as aspirin, is indicated for both mechanical and heterograft bioprosthetic valves for the first 3 months after implantation (Bonow et al., 2006), with the level of anticoagulation depending on the valve type and anatomic location. After that time warfarin is discontinued for heterograft bioprosthetic valves, unless the patient possesses a risk factor that increases their susceptibility to thromboembolic complications (Bonow et al., 2006). Despite the use of chronic anticoagulant therapy, between 0.4 and 6.5 percent of mechanical heart valve recipients will experience a thromboembolic event per year, a range that is dependent upon valve type, number, placement, and other risk factors (Salem et al., 2004). The long-term risk of thromboembolism in bioprosthetic heart valve recipients is comparatively low, ranging from 0.2 to 5.5 percent per year (Salem et al., 2004).

In contrast to the anticoagulation requirement associated with mechanical valves, the largest problem facing patients with bioprosthetic valves is progressive structural deterioration due to calcification, which can eventually require valve replacement and the risks of a reoperation (Schoen and Levy, 1999; Hammermeister et al., 2000). Heterograft bioprosthetic valves and homograft (allograft) valves exhibit accelerated deterioration in younger patients, which promotes the use of mechanical valves in this age group (Bonow et al., 2006).

Although the literature is rife with comparisons between valve designs in regard to their complication rates, the general lack of large randomized trials using standardized methods makes valid comparisons problematic (Horstkotte, 1996). To reduce some of the confusion surrounding outcomes reporting in heart valve studies, the Society of Thoracic Surgeons and the American Association of Thoracic Surgery developed guidelines for reporting common surgical and nonsurgical artificial valve complications (Edmunds et al., 1996). The guidelines distinguish between structural and nonstructural valve deterioration, thrombosis, embolism, bleeding events, and infection. In addition, various types of neurologic events are graded, and methods of statistical data analysis are suggested based on the type of data being collected and analyzed. Adherence to such guidelines should allow valid comparisons to be made between manuscripts reporting on outcomes with different valve types and clinical approaches (Edmunds et al., 1996).

3.2.5 Future Trends

There are two major areas of development in artificial heart valves that are poised to change the field in the near term: percutaneous or minimally invasive valve implantation and valvular tissue engineering. Recent developments in both areas will be reviewed below.

Percutaneous valve implantation represents a natural progression toward minimal invasive therapies wherever lesion characteristics permit such an approach or the patient's clinical condition demands it. Percutaneous valvular prostheses have been implanted in the aortic (Cribier et a1., 2002; Grube et al., 2005) position within the native valve and in the analogous pulmonic position (Bonhoeffer et al., 2000) in right ventricular outflow tracts (RVOT) used in congenital heart repair. These devices and other novel designs are undergoing extensive trials at the time of writing and continue to advance at a rapid rate (Babaliaros and Block, 2007). An example of a percutaneous valvular prosthesis is shown in Fig. 3.4.

Tissue engineering holds great promise for the development of replacement valves with improved long-term function and viability. As reviewed in a recent article, approaches under investigation involve the use of synthetic scaffolds or decellurized tissue with cell seeding (Mendelson and Schoen, 2006). Efforts to produce artificial valves de novo using harvested endothelial cells and fibroblasts grown on a biodegradable scaffold have resulted in functional pulmonary valve leaflets in a lamb model (Shinoka et al., 1996). A biohybrid trileaflet pulmonary valve has also been successfully tested in lambs for a limited period (Sodian et al., 2000). More recently, decellurized valves seeded with autologous cells and matured in a bioreactor have been used as a pulmonic valve replacement in humans with good midterm results (Dohmen et al., 2007). These efforts show much promise, although challenges in creating valves with ideal performance characteristics remain. Successful development of a viable autologous biologic valve capable of long-term stability and growth would likely revolutionize the management of heart valve disease through a reduction of implant-related morbidity and mortality, with particular applicability to pediatric patients.

In addition to efforts to grow artificial valves, researchers have attempted to stimulate the growth of endothelial cells on existing bioprosthetic valves to limit valve degradation and thromboembolic

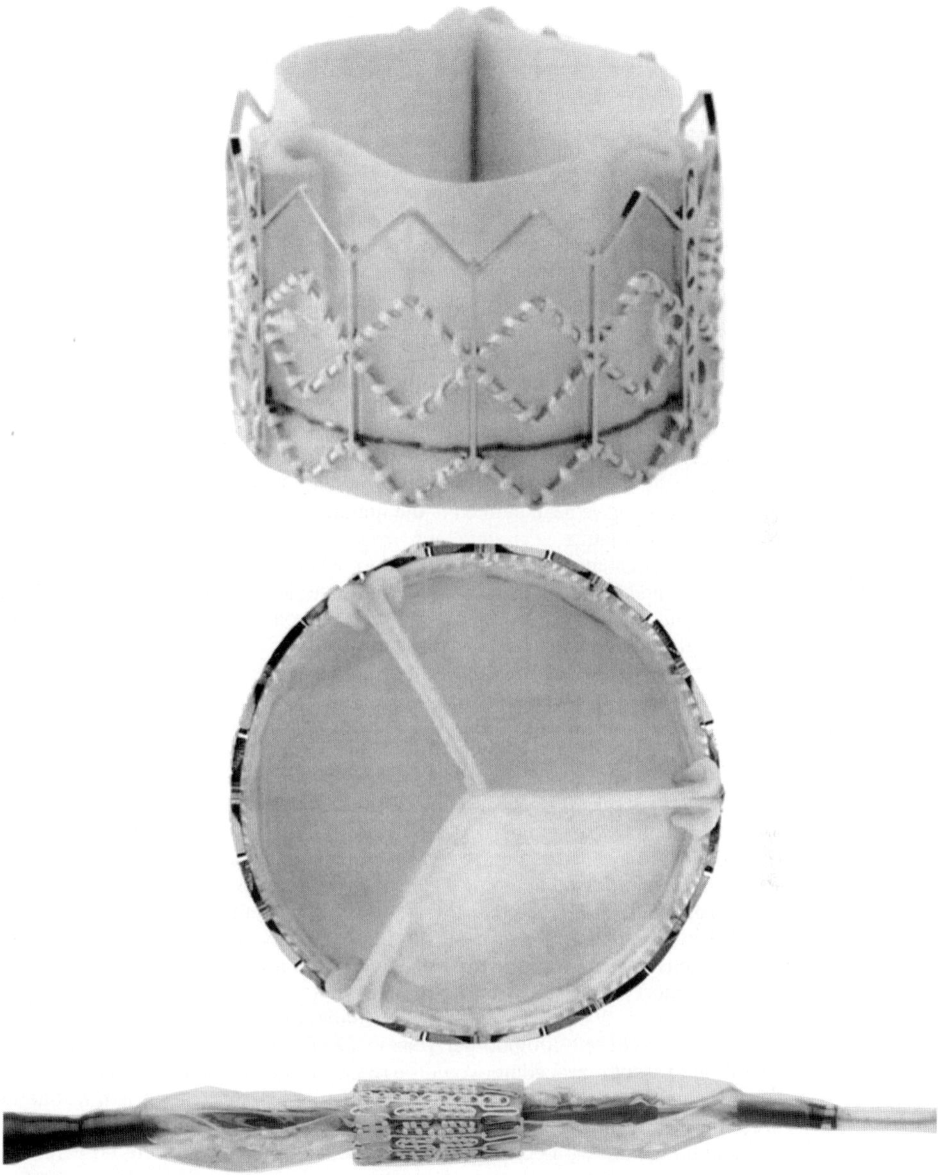

FIGURE 3.4 An example of a bioprosthetic valve designed for percutaneous implantation is shown (Edwards SAPIEN). (*a*) Side view (*b*) Top view. The valve is expanded via an inflatable balloon in a manner analogous to stenting. (*c*) The crimped valve is shown in place on the inflation balloon, (*images courtesy of Edwards Lifesciences, Irvine, CA*).

complications. Endothelialization of commercial bioprosthetic valve tissue is hampered by the cytotoxic aftereffects of glutaraldehyde fixation (Eybl et al., 1992), directing efforts toward alternate fixation techniques and coatings to improve cell adhesion and growth. Although results for endothelialized bioprosthetic valves have been mixed in some in vivo experiments (Lehner et al., 1997), development continues with promising results in animal models (Gulbins et al., 2006).

3.3 STENTS AND STENT-GRAFTS: PERCUTANEOUS VASCULAR THERAPIES

3.3.1 Market Size

According to Taber's Cyclopedic Medical Dictionary, the term *stent* refers to "any material used to hold tissue in place or provide a support for a graft or anastomosis while healing is taking place" (Thomas, 1989). As this broad definition would suggest, stents are indicated for a wide range of disease states in the genitourinary, hepatobiliary, gastrointestinal, reconstructive, and vascular fields. The focus of the current section is limited to those devices used in the vasculature, primarily the peripheral and coronary arteries.

Many patients suffering from atherosclerotic vascular disease possess focal narrowings inside their blood vessels. These narrowed regions, termed *stenoses*, are made up of fatty, and sometimes calcified, plaques (atheromas) that can restrict the movement of blood to downstream tissue, resulting in sequelae ranging from pain upon physical exertion to tissue breakdown. One dangerous scenario is thrombus formation at the lesion site with the potential for distal embolization. Thrombosis and thromboembolization can directly lead to tissue ischemia (oxygen starvation) and possible tissue death. Two categories of interventions to treat coronary stenoses and obstructions (e.g., thrombus) have been defined in the literature, with similar definitions for interventions in the peripheral vasculature. *Percutaneous transluminal coronary angioplasty* (PTCA), otherwise known as balloon angioplasty, is a procedure wherein a catheter-mounted balloon is moved to the lesion site and inflated, displacing the tissue and creating a wider lumen in the vessel. Percutaneous coronary intervention (PCI) is a broad definition that encompasses PTCA and a wide-ranging group of procedures, including atherectomy, thrombolysis, intravascular radiation, and the placement of stents. Stents are designed to keep the PTCA-treated lesion open through forceful opposition with the vessel wail; in essence, the stent braces the disrupted lesion in an expanded position. Stent-grafts consist of a polymer fabric or sheet coating mounted on a stenting device that excludes the vessel wall from the flowing blood, thus reducing its exposure to the pulse pressure wave and minimizing blood contact with the damaged endothelium. At present, stent-grafts have widespread application in the aorta and its major tributaries, with stents being applicable in almost all areas of the vasculature. Given the immense burden of CVD, stents and stent-grafts are widely used to treat vascular lesions and are being employed in a growing number of cases, expanding into anatomic areas once considered off-limits. In 2005, it was estimated that more than 2 million PCIs were performed worldwide (Smith et al., 2006), with more than 1.2 million in the United States (DeFrances et al., 2007). Stents are placed during most of these coronary interventions either as a primary or adjunct therapy (Al Suwaidi et al., 2000), and registry datasets report that less than 30 percent of interventions are now comprised of PTCA alone (Anderson et al., 2002). Estimates for the number of interventional procedures in the peripheral vasculature exceeded 200,000 per year in 1997, with the expectation that up to 50 percent of traditional vascular procedure would be replaced with an endovascular analog in the near future (Krajcer and Howell, 2000). One such endovascular intervention is the abdominal aortic stent-graft and its use in abdominal aortic aneurysm (AAA) repair, which is traditionally a high-risk surgical procedure with perioperative mortalities ranging from 5 to 60 percent, depending upon patient characteristics (Krajcer and Howell, 2000). In 2000, it was estimated that 4000 abdominal aortic stent-grafts had been placed since their introduction (Krajcer and Howell, 2000). However, recent data indicate that 21,000 stent-grafts were used in 2005 *alone* (DeFrances et al., 2007), suggesting a dramatic rise in the use of these devices. Simple stenting is also a major modality in the peripheral and central circulation. In 2005, it was estimated that almost 60,000 nondrug-eluting stents were placed in the peripheral vasculature, with an additional 10,000 carotid stent placements (DeFrances et a1., 2007). The clear shift toward endovascular repairs is significant enough to have led to changes in the training of vascular surgeons as their traditional caseload of open procedures diminishes (Sullivan et al., 2002; Diethrich, 2003).

3.3.2 Indications

Consensus documents developed through the collaboration of cardiovascular societies (American College of Cardiology, American Heart Association, and the Society for Cardiovascular Angiography and Interventions) detail coronary stenting indications currently supported by literature findings (Smith et al., 2006). Data suggest that most stents (at least 95 percent) are placed with a clear indication that follows the clinical standard of care (Anderson et al., 2002). Stents are most often placed in nonemergent (or elective) settings to optimize outcome and improve patency of vessels that have undergone balloon angioplasty (Al Suwaidi et al., 2000). An ideal PCI outcome has various classifications, but a residual vessel diameter stenosis of less than 20 percent along with TIMI 3 flow [defined as no visible reduction in the speed of contrast transit with good perfusion bed runoff (TMI Study Group, 1985)] has broad acceptance as defining an ideal outcome in the poststent era (Smith et al., 2006). Stents are also placed emergently in patients undergoing a myocardial infarction due to coronary obstruction, a procedure termed primary PCI (Smith et al., 2006). Other less well-established indications include stent placement for the treatment of chronic total vessel occlusion, saphenous vein bypass graft lesions, gradual tissue overgrowth in an existing stent, and lesions with difficult morphology, such as long, diffuse stenoses, stenoses in small vessels, and lesions at a bifurcation or vessel opening (Holmes et al., 1998). Ongoing randomized trials continue to delineate the optimal treatment of various coronary pathologies.

There has been considerable advancement in recognizing which patients and pathologies are amenable to either traditional open revascularization or endovascular treatment (Hirsch et al., 2006; Norgren et al., 2007). Reported indications for peripheral, noncoronary vascular stent placement include immediate treatment of balloon angioplasty complications such as intimal dissection and flap formation; the correction of unsatisfactory angioplasty outcomes such as residual stenosis, spasm, recoil or occlusion; treatment of complicated, chronic lesions or occlusions; and as a routine, combination treatment with angioplasty (Mattos et al., 1999). The most common reason for placement of a stent in the peripheral vasculature is an unsatisfactory result from angioplasty (Mattos et al., 1999).

3.3.3 Vascular Stent Design

The ideal stent would possess a number of characteristics designed to ease handling and permit stable, long-term function. Desired handling characteristics include a simple, effective deployment method, high radiopacity for visualization under fluoroscopy, flexibility to ease passage through tortuous vessels, limited shortening during expansion so placement is optimal, high expansion ratio to allow smaller profiles, and ease of retrievability or removal, if misplaced (Mattos et al., 1999; Henry et al., 2000). Preferred functional characteristics include a high hoop strength to counteract arterial spasm, biocompatibility that minimizes short-term and long-term complications, and durability in the stressful, corrosive environment of the human body (Mattos et al., 1999; Henry et al., 2000). Despite the large number of stent designs, with additional models under development, no one stent possesses all these particular characteristics (Henry et al., 2000).

Stents can be divided into two main groups based on the method of expansion. *Balloon-expandable* stents either arrive premounted on a balloon angioplasty catheter or are mounted by the doctor prior to the procedure. A balloon catheter with inflation apparatus is shown in Fig. 3.5. While mounted, the stent is moved into place and the balloon inflated to expand the stent to the desired diameter. Figure 3.6 illustrates the placement and inflation procedure for balloon-expandable stents. In contrast, *self-expanding* stents come premounted or sheathed. Once deployed to the treatment area, the sheath is pulled back, allowing the stent to expand to its predetermined diameter. Balloon-expandable stents can be further subdivided into slotted-tube and coil-based designs (Oesterle et al., 1998).

Each stent type possesses particular advantages and disadvantages. Self-expanding stents can experience shortening during deployment which may complicate placement, although more recent stent designs are able to mitigate this effect to a significant degree (Oesterle et al., 1998). Balloon-expandable stents exhibit a greater stiffness than the self-expanding models, which can cause difficulty navigating long or tortuous lesions and anatomy (Mattos et a1., 1999). In general, coil design

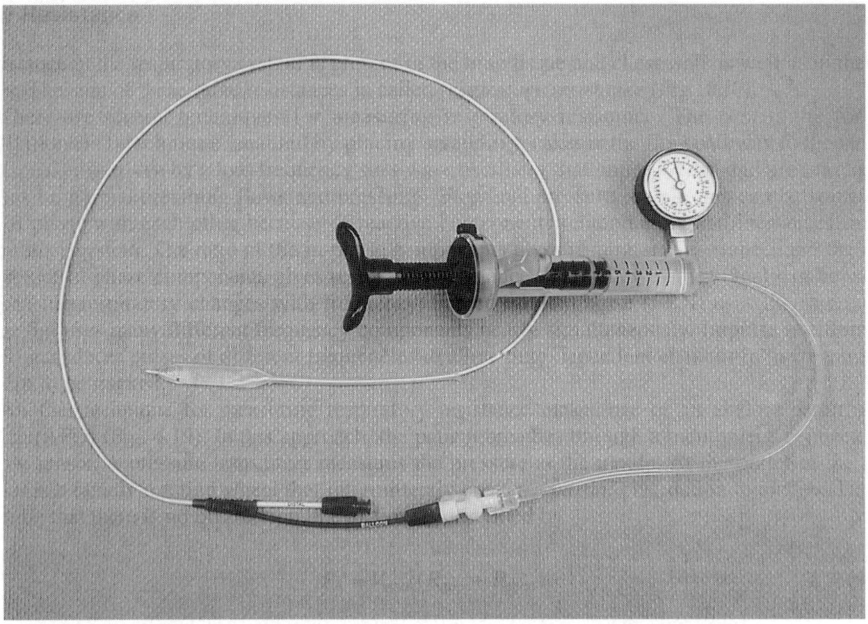

FIGURE 3.5 A balloon catheter and inflation pump are shown. Balloon catheters are used to widen stenosed or narrowed vessels and to expand stents. The balloon is often inflated with a mixture of saline and contrast agent to aid radiographic visualization.

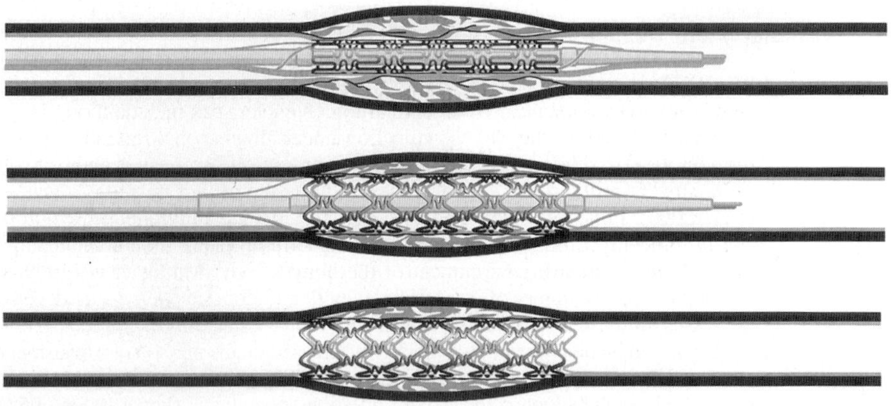

FIGURE 3.6 The stent implantation procedure for a balloon-expandable stent is demonstrated in the figure. The balloon-mounted stent is first guided into place inside a damaged vessel under fluoroscopy. The balloon is then inflated, expanding the stent to lie in opposition to the vessel wall. The balloon is then deflated and withdrawn, leaving the stent in place to prevent constriction of the vessel. (*Compliments of Cordis Corporation, Miami Lakes, FL*).

stents have greater flexibility than the slotted tube models, making them attractive for more complex and difficult to reach lesions such as those found at bifurcations and inside branches (Oesterle et al., 1998). Some more recent stent designs combine features of slotted tube and coil models. Both stent types usually undergo further balloon expansion to optimize the resulting placement (Oesterle et al., 1998). Figure 3.7 illustrates the flexibility that can be achieved by a modern stent.

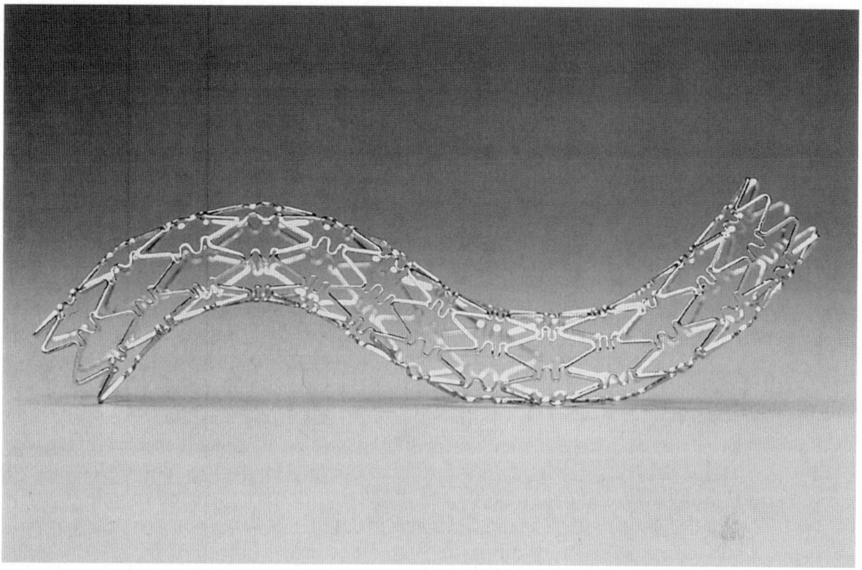

FIGURE 3.7 The flexibility of a modern stent design (Cordis Corporation 7-cell BX Velocity) is demonstrated in the figure. (*Compliments of Cordis Corporation, Miami Lakes, FL*).

Most stent designs use metal as a construction material. Traditional alloys include tantalum and certain stainless steels (304 and 316L) (Mattos et al., 1999). Nitinol, a nickel-titanium alloy, has been used in self-expanding stent designs due to its shape memory properties (Mattos et al., 1999). Both biodegradable and nondegradable polymeric stents have been developed, but the positive results of metallic stents over the long term, coupled with the technical challenges of producing a mechanically viable polymeric stent, have limited efforts in this area (Bertrand et al., 1998).

To accommodate the variety of arterial pathologies encountered, stents come in an ever-increasing array of sizes. Coronary stent diameters span from 2.5 to 4 mm, with lengths ranging from 8 to 38 mm (Al Suwaidi et al., 2000). Stents for the peripheral vasculature are of a considerably greater size due to the much larger vessels in the thorax, abdomen, and proximal extremities. The various stent designs appear to differ in their ability to maintain postexpansion lumen size (Okabe et al., 1999), which could affect clinical outcomes such as long-term patency (Fischman et al., 1994).

3.3.4 Management and Complications

As of 1997, incidence rates for complications following coronary stenting were under 1 percent for thrombosis when treated with antiplatelet agents, less than 25 percent for repeated arterial narrowing, and fewer than 15 percent of patients required an additional procedure on the stented lesion during the follow-up period (Oesterle et al., 1998). *Restenosis* is a term referring to the repeated narrowing or closure experienced in stented lesions typically due to an overgrowth of smooth muscle cells. Affecting up to a full quarter of patients, restenosis is a common complication following coronary stent placement and remains the major stumbling block in the long-term success of stenting (Virmani and Farb, 1999). Evidence from animal studies suggests that the amount of restenosis is related to the amount of damage incurred at stent implantation (Schwartz et al., 1992), while other evidence implicates the stent design as affecting the rate of restenosis and thrombosis (Rogers and Edelman, 1995). Additional causes implicated in restenosis include excessive thrombosis, inflammation, poor stent apposition, and the presence of large amounts of necrotic tissue or ruptured plaque

(Oesterle et al., 1998). Restenosis is not limited to stented lesions, but actually occurs at a higher rate in lesions receiving PTCA only (Serruys et al., 1994) and is a significant contributor to stent placement in previously treated lesions.

A large assortment of potential stent coatings and materials has been evaluated in an effort to reduce the number of complications associated with stent implantation. Approaches have included both degradable and nondegradable polymeric coatings for surface passivation and drug elution, coating with the anticoagulant heparin to limit platelet activation, endothelial cell seeding to create a "natural" surface, and using radioactive sources to inhibit cellular proliferation (Bertrand et al., 1998). Of these various approaches, two deserve further mention: drug-eluting stents (DES) and vascular brachytherapy (VBT).

Drug-eluting stents (DES) developed as an approach to combat in-stent restenosis (Serruys et al., 2006), a common problem plaguing traditional bare-metal stents (BMS). Potent antiproliferative agents are incorporated into a substrate (often a polymer) and coated onto the stent to guarantee local delivery of the drug (Serruys et al., 2006). Numerous clinical trials demonstrated the superior performance of drug-eluting stents over bare-metal designs for limited follow-up periods (Morice et al., 2002; Moses et al., 2003; Stone et al., 2004), and these devices gained widespread acceptance. However, it was later determined that DES have a higher rate of very late stent thrombosis (defined as occurring >1 year after the procedure) when compared to bare-metal designs (Windecker and Meier, 2007). A recent review article evaluating the various potential causes of very late stage stent thrombosis highlighted the fact that delayed development of an endothelial surface (which would reduce procoagulant tendencies) and inflammatory reactions to the bare polymer could both contribute to the risk of thrombosis (Van Belle et al., 2007). Although research into the root cause of very late stent thrombosis continues, these findings bring home the message that one must consider all ramifications of a particular treatment or modification; inhibiting cellular-proliferation limited restenosis but may have set the stage for later thrombosis with an unhealed, inflammatory surface.

Radiation treatment of the vessel area receiving PTCA has been attempted with both gamma- and beta-type radiation sources being delivered via catheter or radioactive stent to reduce cell proliferation (Waksman, 1999). Beta irradiation of lesions treated with PTCA without concomitant stent placement has been shown to reduce restenosis in a dose-dependent manner (Verin et al., 2001). The use of a gamma radiation source has shown improved rates of clinical and angiographic restenosis in patients treated for in-stent restenosis; unfortunately, the treatment was associated with a higher rate of late thrombosis and subsequent heart attack (Leon et al., 2001). Although the late incidence of thrombosis is likely due to the same prolonged denudation that affects DES, the widespread acceptance of DES by the interventional community, combined with a lack of access to vascular brachytherapy, has led to an almost complete cessation of radiation treatment (Thomas, 2005).

3.3.5 Future Developments

Progress in stent technology will undoubtedly focus on reducing the incidence of restenosis and on the improvement of stent outcomes in challenging vascular lesions. Treatment of restenosis in saphenous vein grafts (SVGs) is a particular challenge as these conduits often exhibit diffuse atherosclerotic disease and high complication rates when stented (Oesterle et al., 1998). Although initial enthusiasm for the use of PTFE-coated stents (Baldus et al., 2000) for SVG lesions has waned in light of recent data (Schachinger et al., 2003; Stankovic et al., 2003; Turco et al., 2006), both coated and drug-eluting stents continue to be evaluated. Drug-eluting stents show promise for mitigating neointimal formation and late-phase restenosis as high local concentrations of therapeutic and preventative agents may be achieved. It is not difficult to envision a stent capable of minimizing vessel injury during deployment, sealing the injured site when expanded, and releasing radiation, drugs, or other factors in a manner responsive to the particular characteristics of the lesion involved. Wound-responsive "smart" stents could result in improved patency rates even in difficult lesions where enhanced thrombotic deposition or neointimal proliferation is likely to occur. Improved knowledge regarding the pathobiologic causes of stent complications is required, as is additional insight into technical details such as elution rates, radiation dosing, and other responsive features.

3.4 PACEMAKERS AND IMPLANTABLE DEFIBRILLATORS

3.4.1 Market Size

The market for pacemakers and other cardiac electrophysiologic (EP) devices has grown over the past five decades due to improved device function, advances in technology and implantation techniques, and a rapidly expanding set of clinical indications. Approximately 1 million patients in the United States had permanent pacemakers in 1996 (Kusumoto and Goldschlager, 1996), many of whom will need either a lead or generator replacement sometime in the future. Recent incidence data from the CDC suggest that at least 167,000 permanent cardiac pacemakers were implanted in United States in 2005, with a minimal estimate of 79,000 automatic implanted cardioverter-defibrillator (AICD) units being placed during the same year (DeFrances et al., 2007). An additional 39,000 combination devices intended for coordinated contraction of the ventricles, termed *cardiac resynchronization*, were also implanted in 2005 (DeFrances et al., 2007). This last group in particular is expected to have significant future growth.

3.4.2 Indications

The American College of Cardiology/American Heart Association/Heart Rhythm Society consensus practice guideline lists current indications for artificial pacemaker and implanted cardioverter-defibrillator use (Epstein et al., 2008). In general, the purpose of a pacemaker is to deliver an electrical impulse of sufficient magnitude to depolarize the heart chamber in a spreading, coordinated fashion as occurs in a normal heartbeat. In contrast, defibrillators are used to depolarize the entire heart at once in an effort to terminate uncoordinated contractions. The natural refractory period of the myocardial tissue usually prevents erratic residual electrical activity from propagating for a short period of time, restoring coordinated muscular contraction.

In general, a pacemaker is warranted in certain cases where electric impulse conduction or initiation in the heart is blocked, slowed, or triggered in an irregular, variable fashion. Specific diseases for which pacemaker therapy is employed include certain forms of atrioventricular and fascicular conduction block, sinus node dysfunction, and some forms of neurocardiogenic syncope (Gregoratos et al., 1998). The most popular indications for first time implantation of cardiac pacemakers have changed over time. In 1997, almost 50 percent of new pacemakers were placed to treat sinus node dysfunction, the most common indication for pacemaker implantation in the United States (Bernstein and Parsonnet, 2001). Congenital or acquired atrioventricular (AV) conduction block was second, accounting for approximately 30 percent of primary implantations, followed by AV block secondary to radiofrequency ablation, drug-induced bradycardia, neurocardiogenic causes, and tachyarrhythmia (Bernstein and Parsonnet, 2001). Emerging indications, particularly pacemaker treatment of congestive heart failure, could significantly alter the percentages indicated above (Cazeau et al., 2001; Gerber et al., 2001). Worldwide results indicate fewer implantations for sinus node dysfunction when compared to U.S. data, with a significant percentage implanted for atrial fibrillation (Mond et al., 2004).

The indications for implantation of a cardioverter-defibrillator are based primarily on the past presence of a potentially fatal ventricular arrhythmia due to nontransient causes, regardless of the specific illness (Gregoratos et al., 1998). Three indications, spontaneous ventricular tachycardia (VT) or fibrillation (VF), aborted sudden death, and syncope with inducible VT or VF accounted for around 95 percent of the devices implanted in the United States for which an indication was reported (Bernstein and Parsonnet, 2001).

3.4.3 Device Design

The wide range of electrophysiologic disorders treated with pacemakers and defibrillators require devices with various capabilities and settings. Generic classification codes have been developed to ease the identification of the different pacemakers, defibrillators, and associated leads presented both in the literature and medical practice. One such code is the North American Society for Pacing and Electrophysiology/British Pacing and Electrophysiology Group Generic Pacemaker Code, which contains five positions and defines the chambers that are paced and sensed, the potential electrical

TABLE 3.1 The Five-Position NASPE/BPEG Generic Pacemaker Code

Positions and description	I. Chamber(s) paced	II. Chamber(s) sensed	III. Pacemaker response	IV. Rate modulation	V. Multisite pacing
	Atrium	Atrium	Triggered	Rate Modulation	Atrium
	Ventricle	Ventricle	Inhibited	NOne	Ventricle
	Dual	Dual	Dual		Dual
	NOne	NOne	NOne		NOne

The purpose of the code is to allow medical practitioners to recognize the basic features and capabilities of a given pacemaker. The code alone does not provide a complete description of device features, but is clear and simple to use.
Source: Adapted from Bernstein et al. (2002).

response to sensed rhythms, rate modulation functions, and whether multisite pacing is present (Bernstein et al., 2002). Table 3.1 summarizes the possible features for each location. The code represents a simplification of previous generic classification schemes (Bernstein et al., 1987) with antitachyarrythmia functions being represented with the analogous defibrillator classification code (Bernstein et al., 1993). A similar classification code exists for pacing leads (Bernstein and Parsonnet, 1996a). More than 60 percent of pacemakers implanted in 1997 were of the DDDR type, possessing dual chamber sensing and pacing with both excitatory and inhibitory functions, with additional rate adaptive features (Bernstein and Parsonnet, 2001). A similar trend toward dual chamber units was seen worldwide (Mond et al., 2004).

Pacemaker and defibrillator systems consist of two implanted and one external component: the generator, cardiac leads, and programmer, respectively (Morley-Davies and Cobbe, 1997). Although the clinical function of pacemakers and defibrillators differ, the desired component characteristics are similar and include low complication rates coupled with small size, durability, and longevity.

Generators. Despite enhanced functional performance and an ever-increasing array of features, current ICD generators displace less than half the volume of those devices implanted a short time ago due to improved circuit, packaging, and power storage technology (Morris et al., 1999). Similarly, modern pacemaker generators are small, thin, and weigh only 20 to 30 g (Kusumoto and Goldschlager, 1996). Generator and battery technology allows pacemakers to last approximately 5 to 9 years in the body (Morley-Davies and Cobbe, 1997), with the more complex dual chamber designs having shorter lifespans than the simpler, single chamber units (Kusumoto and Goldschlager, 1996). An example of a pacemaker and implantable defibrillator generator are shown in Fig. 3.8.

Power technology has steadily improved since the first mercury acid batteries of the 1960s, with modifications in other generator components and usage algorithms further increasing battery endurance (Jeffrey and Parsonnet, 1998). Novel power supplies have included the nuclear slug and biokinetic sources, but the advent of the lithiurn-based power source allowed for increased generator longevity over mercury acid types and was amenable to being hermetically sealed (Jeffrey and Parsonnet, 1998). The current batteries used in pacemakers and defibrillators differ in formulation. Pacemakers utilize lithium-iodine batteries (Kusumoto and Goldschlager, 1996) while ICDs utilize lithium-silver-vanadium batteries and a capacitor network for discharges (Morris et al., 1999).

Electrical Leads. The pacing lead consists of five components: the connector, conductor, insulating material, electrode(s), and fixation mechanism. Electrical leads have to fulfill a number of conflicting requirements, although reliable performance remains the dominant criteria (de Voogt, 1999). Leads should possess a small diameter, be flexible enough to place but durable enough to resist wear, possess favorable power consumption characteristics, anchor in place to prevent migration, and enjoy good biocompatibility.

Pacing leads can be subdivided into a number of groups based on the area of placement and method of stimulation. Leads can be placed either on the epicardium (external surface) of the heart or, by a transvenous route, onto the endocardium (internal surface) of the right heart atrium or ventricle. Epicardial leads are used for permanent pacing in pediatric cases, where size considerations or congenital defects prevent transvenous placement, and in patients who have undergone tricuspid valve replacement (Mitrani et al., 1999). Percutaneous transvenous placement of the lead is the preferred route in most patients.

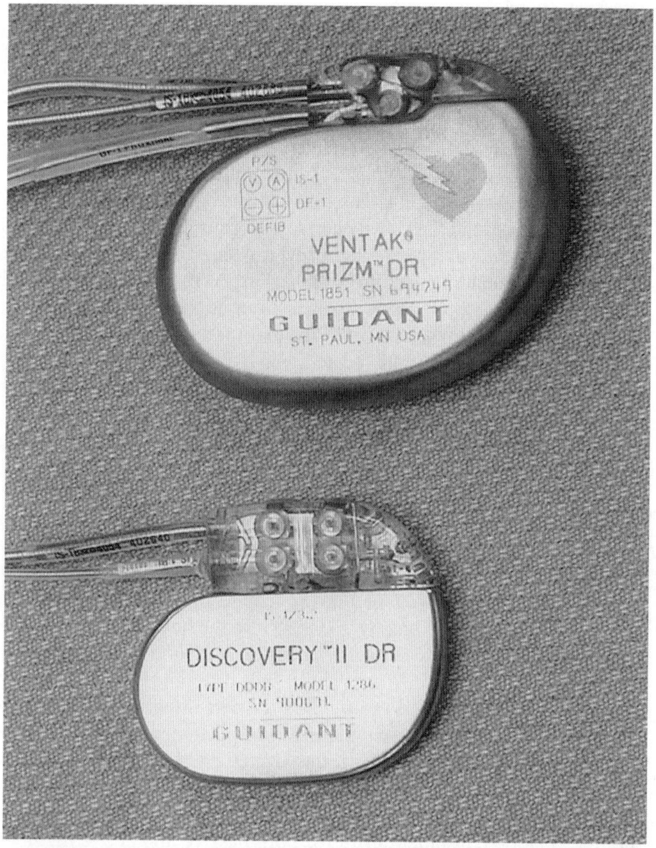

FIGURE 3.8 The generators of a modern cardioverter-defibrillator (Ventak Prizm DR, Guidant Corporation, Minneapolis, MN) and pacemaker (Discovery II DR, Guidant Corporation, Minneapolis, MN) are shown in the figure. Both are dual chamber devices, with the cardioverter-defibrillator possessing pacing features in addition to the core cardioversion hardware. The added hardware and power requirements demand a larger housing for this device in comparison to the pacemaker.

The depolarization shock can be delivered either through a *unipolar* or *bipolar* lead. Most older leads utilize the unipolar design (Morley-Davies and Cobbe, 1997) in which a single insulated electrode is placed near the myocardium of the heart and acts as a cathode (Morley-Davies and Cobbe, 1997; Tyers et al., 1997). The generator shell acts as the anode of the resulting circuit. Modern leads use a bipolar design where the cathode and anode are both in the lead and spaced a short distance apart (Morley-Davies and Cobbe, 1997). Three general approaches have been developed for placing two insulated conducting wires within the lead body for the bipolar design. The original bipolar leads were fabricated with two conducting wires alongside one another, enclosed in a large silicone rubber sheath (Tyers et al., 1997). These designs gave way to coaxial systems where a layered approach was used. Here, a conducting wire at the center is sheathed in an insulator, surrounded by another conducting layer and a final layer of insulation. Coaxial pacing leads tend to be smaller than the side-by-side models (Tyers et al., 1997). The most recent approach to bipolar lead design is described as a coradial pacing lead. The two conducting wires are coated with a thin layer of insulation and wound in a helical manner along the length of the pacing lead (Schmidt and Stotts, 1998). The wound helix is also sheathed in another layer of insulation to improve handling characteristics and provide some insulation redundancy. The compact nature of the coradial inner structure results in a very small lead.

To avoid the incompatibilities in mating technologies that arise from having a large number of electrophysiology (EP) device manufacturers, internationally accepted standards have been developed to define the mating connection between pacemakers and leads, thus allowing leads from one manufacturer to be mated to the generator of another. Originally developed by the British Standards Institution as the IS-1 specification for low-profile connectors for implantable pacemakers, the standard has been revised and re-released in 2000 as the ISO 5841-3 standard from the International Standards Organization as part of their publications governing the design of cardiac pacemakers. A similar standard (DF-1) exists for ICD shock leads (Morris et al., 1999).

A number of materials have been used for insulation in cardiac pacing leads, including polyethylene, polysiloxanes, polyurethanes, and poly(ethylene-co-tetrafluoroethylene) (ETFE). Polyethylene was the original lead insulation material but poor long-term performance has eliminated its use in the pacing lead market (Crossley, 2000). Polysiloxanes are used in modern electrophysiology leads but have undergone an evolution in performance and formulation over the years. A limited resistance to tearing required a relatively thick layer until newer, high-performance polysiloxanes were released (Crossley, 2000). Polyurethanes possess a high tear strength and, in contrast to early polysiloxane formulas, a low coefficient of friction, both of which served to popularize polyurethane use; leads could be made smaller and possessed improved placement characteristics, especially in multiple-lead applications (Schmidt and Stotts, 1998; Crossley, 2000). The newest coradial bipolar leads utilize a thin layer of ethylene tetrafluoroethylene (ETFE) as an insulation coating for the interior, helically wound leads, with a redundant layer of exterior polyurethane insulation (Schmidt and Stotts, 1998; Crossley, 2000). The coradial leads are small and appear to have a reduced complication rate compared to coaxial designs (Tyers et al., 1997).

To prevent migration, lead tips are fitted with either passive or active fixation mechanisms. Passive devices use hooks or tines to secure the line into place, while active fixation methods rely upon a screw like tip to burrow the lead into the heart tissue. Although active fixation leads have been considered less likely to dislodge or suffer from complications than passive leads, few major studies have been performed and some doubt that differences in performance exist in the hands of an experiened implanter (Mitrani et al., 1999). Some situations do warrant active fixation leads, however. Congenital heart disease may require lead placement in an odd area, which can make active fixation useful (Mitrani et al., 1999). In the United States, active fixation leads appear to be preferred for atrial placement, while passive fixation leads are the overwhelming choice when leads are placed in the ventricle (Mond et al., 2004). Figure 3.9 provides a close-up view of a variety of lead tips, revealing the fixation equipment used for both passive and active methods.

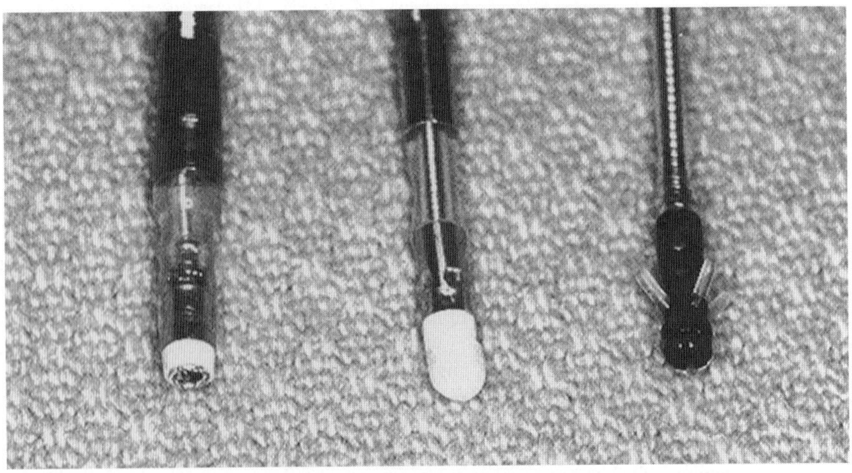

FIGURE 3.9 Close-up views of three pacemaker and/or cardioverter-defibrillator leads. The lead on the far left is an active fixation lead with a retractable screw embedded in the lead tip. It can be extended after implantation to attach the lead to the heart wall. The middle lead possesses a soluble cap that dissolves within a few minutes inside the body to reveal a hook or screw for tip fixation. A tined passive fixation lead is shown on the right. The soft tines become lodged in the irregular inside surface of the heart, preventing lead migration.

Rate-adaptive pacing requires some method of rate modulation, preferably without patient intervention, that mimics as closely as possible the normal behavior of the intact sinus node during exertion (Leung and Lau, 2000). A very large number of sensors, control techniques, and algorithms have been proposed in an effort to provide optimal rate responses to exercise and activity in those patients unable to generate an adequate heart rate increase (Leung and Lau, 2000). Because no single sensor and associated circuitry can perfectly replace the sinus node, dual sensor systems have been introduced to accommodate for particular deficiencies in either sensor (Mitrani et al., 1999). The most popular sensors are mechanical devices that measure vibration, which roughly indicates that body movement is taking place (Morley-Davies and Cobbe, 1997; Leung and Lau, 2000). These units have the benefit of being compatible with existing lead technology (Leung and Lau, 2000).

The current standard pacemaker lead utilizes many of the innovations described above and possesses a low coil resistance coupled with a high electrode impedence and is encased in a steriod-eluting covering (de Voogt, 1999). The steroid reduces the inflammatory reaction to the implanted lead that can increase the stimulation threshold over time (Mitrani et al., 1999; Crossley, 2000).

Programmer. The programmer allows the physician to adjust pacemaker and defibrillator settings to meet the particular needs of the patient. Modern microcomputer-based systems use radiofrequency waves or magnetic fields to communicate with the EP device noninvasively (Kusumoto and Goldschlager, 1996; Morley-Davies and Cobbe, 1997). The programmer can retrieve device settings and performance data, including failure episodes, electrocardiograms, and battery function, allowing the physician to optimize device performance or analyze an existing problem (Kusumoto and Goldschlager, 1996). A recent review divided the most common programmable features into six categories, including pacing mode selection, energy output and characteristics, electrical sensitivity, rate limits, refractory periods and their duration, and the various rate-adaptive features and functions (Kusumoto and Goldschlager, 1996). The ever-growing range of features and functions on the modern EP device complicates patient management but does allow tailored therapy.

3.4.4 Complications

Complications associated with electrophysiology devices can be divided into those that are a consequence of device failure or malfunction and complications secondary to device implantation, extraction, or patient care. In general, complications are reported to occur at a greater rate with those physicians who implant pacemakers less frequently (Bernstein and Parsonnet, 1996b; Bernstein and Parsonnet, 2001). Clinically significant perioperative complications such as hemothorax (blood in the chest cavity), pneumothorax (air in the chesty cavity), infection, and hematoma (blood collection around insertion site) are relatively rare at l to 2 percent (Morley-Davies and Cobbe, 1997; Bernstein and Parsonnet, 2001).

Generators. Approximately 20 percent of generator sales are for replacement of an existing device (Bernstein and Parsonnet, 2001). Although there are a number of problems that could necessitate generator replacement, the most common reason is a depleted battery at the end of its service life, which indicates that proper generator function and longevity is the norm rather than the exception. According to recent surveys, electrical component failure continues to decline as an indication for generator replacement (Bernstein and Parsonnet, 2001).

Electrical Leads. Pacing (de Voogt, 1999) and defibrillator electrical leads are the most problematic components in their respective electrophysiology systems. As a common site of malfunction and a significant factor in device power consumption, the electrical pacemaker lead has been subject to a variety of design and usage improvements (de Voogt, 1999). A recent survey of cardiac pacing revealed that the most common reason for lead replacement was insulation failure, followed by a high stimulation threshold for cardiac depolarization and displacement of the lead electrode itself (Bernstein and Parsonnet, 2001). Bipolar leads suffered from a higher complication rate in both the atrial and ventricular positions, and ventricular leads secured with passive fixation devices also experienced a higher reported complication rate (Bernstein and Parsonnet, 2001). Results from the Danish Pacemaker Register (Moller and Arnsbo, 1996) revealed significantly lower reliability in bipolar leads versus unipolar leads, but unipolar leads do have shortcomings. Unipolar sensing units suffer from electrical interference due to extracardiac muscle activity or electromagnetic interference (EMI), which can cause pacemaker malfunction (Morley-Davies and Cobbe, 1997; Mitrani et al., 1999). Because of this shortcoming, unipolar pacemaker leads are incompatible with implantable defibrillator devices (Mitrani et al., 1999).

Among common lead-insulation materials, polyurethane 80A, a polyetherurethane (PEU), is known to suffer from higher rates of degradation and failure and is responsible for a large proportion of lead malfunctions (Tyers et al., 1997; Crossley, 2000). The PEU 80A degrades via three mechanisms: environmental stress cracking, metal-ion–catalyzed oxidation, and calcification (Schmidt and Stotts, 1998; Crossley, 2000). The use of alternate polymers such as ETFE, polycarbonateurethanes, and more durable formulations of PEU are being used to overcome the limitations of PEU 80A (Schmidt and Stotts, 1998). These materials do not suffer from the same mechanisms of failure, or at least exhibit increased resilience to degradation via those pathways (Schmidt and Stotts, 1998).

3.4.5 Future Developments

Up to a fifth of all patients with implanted cardioverter-defibrillators have also demonstrated a pacemaker requirement (Pinski and Trohman, 2000). The dual requirement for pacemakers and ICDs has led to the development of units combining the two technologies on an advanced level, complete with dual chamber activity (Morris et al., 1999; Pinski and Trohman, 2000). The benefits of a combined EP device is the elimination of separate costs for each system and potential harmful interactions between pacemakers and ICDs, including a reduction in the number of leads (Morris et al., 1999; Pinski and Trohman, 2000).

Steady improvements in microelectronics and software will further expand the capabilities of EP devices toward the analysis and treatment of other pathologic heart conditions currently on the fringe of electrophysiology, such as atrial arrhythmias (Morris et al., 1999; Boriani et al., 2007). These enhanced units will monitor a wide variety of patient and system data to optimize performance to a greater extent than current systems. There is room for improvement in power technology and lead design, as well as improved algorithms able to perform advanced rhythm discrimination (Morris et al., 1999). As suggested in the literature, the development of a universal programmer capable of interfacing with any EP device would be a significant advance both in cost and ease of use for providers now faced with a multitude of different programming units (Kusumoto and Goldschlager, 1996). Improved and simplified programmer interfaces would also benefit the implanting physicians, who are now overwhelmed with feature-heavy and highly adjustable systems (Morris et al., 1999).

3.5 ARTIFICIAL VASCULAR GRAFTS

3.5.1 Market Size

The market for artificial vascular grafts is in a state of transition due to technological and clinical advancements. The advent of successful endovascular therapies (angioplasty, stenting, stent-grafting, etc.) has led to a shift toward less-invasive interventions for vascular repair and reconstruction, with a concomitant reduction in traditional open excision and replacement. Although changes in procedure classification limit direct comparison, data from nonfederal acute-care hospitals estimate that the total number of blood vessel resections with graft placement declined from at least 66,000 in 1997 (Owings and Lawrence, 1999) to 35,000 in 2005 (DeFrances et al., 2007), with an even greater shift toward endovascular repair of the abdominal aorta, once the dominant area for artificial graft usage. When less invasive approaches are unsuccessful or impractical, the limited availability of biologic tissues with the proper size and length for the replacement of large vessels often necessitates the use of an artificial vascular prostheses (Brewster, 2000).

In contrast to the technological changes identified above, prioritization of arteriovenous fistula (AVF) creation through various clinical initiatives is reducing the need for vascular access grafts in hemodialysis (HD) treatment, a major area for the use of artificial vascular prosthesis. Since 1991, the percentage of prevalent (existing) HD patients receiving treatment through an artificial graft has fallen more than half to around 35 percent in 2004 (US Renal Data System, 2007). Through the

"Fistula First" initiative, the Centers for Medicaid and Medicare (CMS) has a near-term goal to raise AVF use from around 40 percent at the end of 2005 to 66 percent of prevalent HD patients, and ultimately to between 70 and 80 percent (Centers for Medicare and Medicaid Services, 2005). Although treatment guidelines from the National Kidney Foundation still advocate the use and placement of an artificial graft for permanent vascular access when a native fistula cannot be created (Besarab et al., 2006), it is clear that this access mode is in decline.

3.5.2 Indications

A number of situations can necessitate the placement of an artificial vascular graft. Vascular grafts can be placed for primary diseases of the vasculature, such as aneurysms or severe atherosclerotic narrowing; for secondary causes, such as trauma; or for chronic vascular access issues, such as hemodialysis. In the case of primary disease or injury, the indications for placement are dependent upon the level of the vascular tree in which the lesion or damage is located, as well as the etiology of the illness. The choice of interventional therapy also varies, depending on whether the target vascular lesion is cardiac, thoracic, carotid, or peripheral. Replacement or bypass of a native vascular conduit is a procedure that lies on one end of the interventional spectrum for treatment of vascular insufficiency. The initial approach to addressing a case of vascular insufficiency (stenosis, occlusion, etc.) is usually a percutaneous intervention, such as balloon angioplasty and stenting, followed by surgical repair or replacement of the native vessel, if necessary. Practice guidelines have been developed that outline the preferred approach to repair (excisional vs. endovascular) in view of current medical outcomes and lesion characteristics (Norgren et al., 2007). Even when an excisional approach is indicated, some vascular patients with severe coexisting conditions are unable to tolerate the profound sedation required to directly excise and replace a damaged blood vessel. For these patients, long tunneled extra-anatomic grafts placed outside the path of the existing diseased vessel are the preferred therapy, despite poorer long-term outcomes and patency rates compared to traditional excisional grafting (Connolly et al., 1984; Foster et al., 1986; Biancari and Lapantalo, 1998).

3.5.3 Current Graft Designs

Vascular grafts or prostheses can be classified as originating primarily from biologic or synthetic sources. Biologic grafts can be harvested from other species (xenograft), from other humans (allograft), or the vasculature of the patient (autograft). As the focus of the present section is on the engineering aspects of vascular grafts, the following discussion will be limited to conduits of synthetic origin. Tissue-engineered biologic grafts will be discussed in the section covering future trends.

The ideal synthetic vascular graft would possess a number of characteristics designed to mimic native conduits, ease surgical placement, and limit manufacturing complexity and cost (Brewster, 2000). A number of features supporting these design goals are listed in Table 3.2. Initially, vascular graft research focused upon the development of completely passive conduits that would not elicit a biological response when exposed to blood. More recent research has focused on the development of grafts that generate a favorable biological response from the body as it has been recognized that a perfectly inert surface may be an unattainable goal (Greisler, 1991), and that a complex set of interactions between graft and host exists, along with a limited window for healing (Zilla et al., 2007).

TABLE 3.2 Desirable Characteristics of Prosthetic Vascular Grafts

Biologic features	Handling and implant features
Biocompatible	Range of sizes
Infection-resistant	Ease of sterilization
Antithrombotic	Flexible without kinking
Compliant	No blood leakage
Durable	Good suturability

Source: Adapted from Brewster (2000).

Current commercial polymeric graft designs can be divided into both *textile* and *nontextile* forms (Brewster, 2000). Textile-based grafts are generally composed of woven or knitted polyethylene terephthalate (Dacron), while the nontextile grafts are usually fashioned from expanded polytetrafluoroethylene (ePTFE). Other polymeric materials investigated or used in the manufacture of vascular grafts include polyamides or nylons, nonexpanded PTFE, polyvinyl alcohol (Ivalon), vinyl chloride-vinyl acetate copolymers (Vinyon-N), polyacrylonitrile (Orlon), and polyurethanes (Greisler, 1991; Eberhart et al., 1999; Brewster, 2000). Although the majority of these materials have been abandoned, polyurethanes have enjoyed continued interest as a source material, especially for small diameter vascular grafts, despite concerns over their long-term degradation performance (Eberhart et al., 1999). The polyurethaneurea Vectra graft (Thoratec Corp, Pleasanton, CA) is in clinical use in the United States for vascular access, and there are a number of improved polyurethane formulations on the horizon that should address the limitations of early generation polyurethane polymers (Kannan et al., 2005; Kapadia et al., 2008).

The preferred graft material differs for both implantation site and use, and selection is based upon patency rates, absence of complications, convenience or handling characteristics, and cost (Brewster, 2000). Large-diameter grafts for use in the aorta and major arteries have generally been made of Dacron, while medium-size grafts are primarily constructed of ePTFE. Smaller vessels located in the infrainguinal region (below the area where the legs connect with the torso) represent a significant challenge due to the traditionally poor patency rates with artificial grafts in these vessels (Veith et at., 1986; 1988; Londrey et al., 1991). Current evidence suggests that replacement of the damaged vessel with an autogenous vein or artery graft is the procedure of choice rather than implantation of an artificial graft (Faries et al., 2000). Unfortunately, preexisting disease, anatomic or size limitations, and other factors may rule out an autogenic source for vessel replacement, thereby forcing the use of an artificial (usually ePTFE) vascular graft or allograft, such as a human umbilical vein (HUV) graft (Harris, 2005). It is in these smaller vessels that the promise of tissue-engineered prosthesis are expected to have the greatest impact.

The different construction techniques used to manufacture textile grafts have an effect on the final device properties. Graft porosity is considered to be a prime factor determining a number of handling, performance, and outcome (Wesolowski et al., 1961) characteristics for textile implants. Knitted textile grafts possess a high porosity and generally require a special yet simple procedure called *preclotting* prior to implantation to prevent excessive leakage of blood through the graft wall. Traditionally, preclotting is performed with a sample of the patient's blood; coagulation is initiated to fill the open pores and interstices with fibrin. As of 1997, most (>80 percent) implanted grafts came presealed with collagen, gelatin, or other biological compounds (e.g., albumin) directly from the manufacturer in an effort to reduce time spent on graft preparation (Brewster, 2000) and limit surface thrombogenicity (Greisler, 1991). In contrast, woven textile grafts do not generally require preclotting but possess less desirable handling properties, such as increased stiffness (Brewster, 2000) and a tendency to fray when cut (Greisler, 1991). Examples of woven and knitted polyester aortic grafts are shown in Fig. 3.10. Nontextile PTFE grafts can possess differing levels of porosity, depending on the processing technique employed. This feature may influence the extent of the healing process (Golden et al., 1990; Kohler et al., 1992; Contreras et al., 2000).

3.5.4 Complications and Management

Graft "healing" or incorporation into the vasculature is a complex process that is the subject of numerous studies and reviews (Greisler, 1991; Davids et al., 1999; Zilla et al., 2007). Graft healing is affected by the graft material, the graft microstructure and surface characteristics, hemodynamic and biomechanical factors, and eventually the interplay between these characteristics and the cellular and humoral components involved in the ongoing incorporation of the graft (Greisler, 1991). Incorporation of the graft into the vasculature can occur through ingrowth of tissue from the anastomotic ends, from tissue growth through the graft wall, and from deposition of circulating cells onto the vessel surface (Zilla et al., 2007). Humans, in contrast to many animal models, usually fail to fully endothelialize the inner surface of a vascular graft, possessing instead some near-anastomic endothelialization and scattered islands of endothelial cells on a surface rich in fibrin and extracellular matrix (Berger et al., 1972; Sauvage et al., 1974; Sauvage et al., 1975; Pasquinelli et al., 1990). The lack of full healing has prompted extensive research into the mechanism of endothelialization and methods to improve it in the clinical setting.

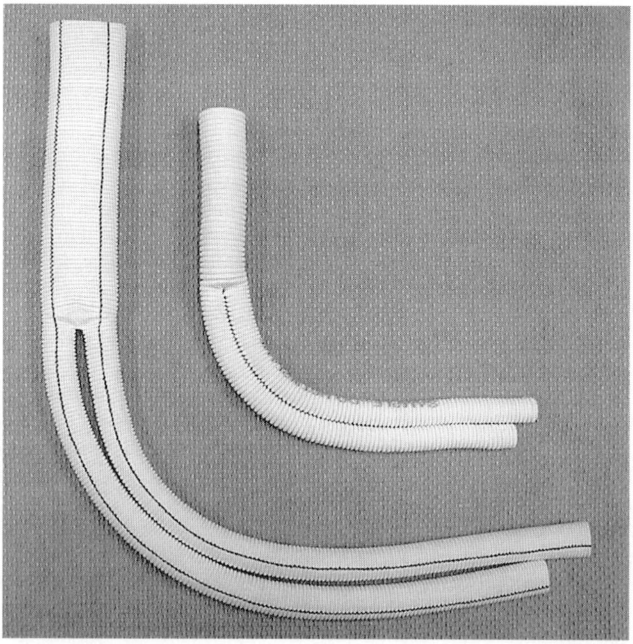

FIGURE 3.10 Two polyester aortobifemoral grafts (Meadox Division, Boston Scientific Corporation, Natick, MA) are shown. These large grafts are used to repair abdominal aortic aneurysms and other lesions affecting the distal aortic segment. The larger graft on the left is made of woven polyester, while the smaller graft is of knit construction. The knitted graft is significantly more elastic and can be stretched to a greater extent than the corresponding woven graft.

Graft complications can be split into those that occur with high or low frequency. High-frequency complications include graft thrombosis and anastomotic pseudointimal hyperplasia, a condition of cellular overgrowth that occurs at the site where the artificial graft meets the remaining native vessel.

Less-frequent complications include prosthesis infection and structural changes such as graft dilatation, a problem more prevalent in knitted Dacron prostheses than other graft types (Robinson et al., 1999).

Because of their grave consequences, graft thrombosis and infection are of particular concern to the implanting surgeon. Thrombosis in vascular grafts is a function of surface characteristics, hemodynamic properties, and the patient's hemostatic system, and represents a common cause of early graft failure. In hemodialysis patients, for whom vascular access is critical, the thrombosis rate of ePTFE access grafts averages 45 percent per year (Kaufman, 2000) and is often secondary to venous stenosis (Palder et al., 1985). Although treatment differs by graft location, results from a randomized clinical trial involving thrombosed lower extremity grafts revealed that catheter-based thrombolytic therapy with urokinase or tPA (tissue plasminogen activator) restores patency in most patients for whom catheter access is successful. This treatment can also reduce the extent of surgical revision if such revision is subsequently required (Comerota et al., 1996).

Graft infection occurs in less than 1 percent of cases as an early (<30 days) complication, but may afflict as many as 5 percent of graft recipients over the longer term (Bandyk and Esses, 1994). The usual culprit is a staphylococcal species, but many other species have been known to infect vascular grafts (Bunt, 1983), with different complications and rates of progression (Bandyk and Esses, 1994). Although there is some leeway in regards to the level of therapy, infections can often be fatal unless aggressive surgical means are coupled with antibiotic treatment. Because residual infection is a common cause of therapeutic failure, extensive debridement and graft excision with in situ or extra-anatomic prosthetic replacement is warranted in most cases (Calligaro and Veith, 1991; Seeger, 2000). Even with aggressive therapy and placement of an extra-anatomic bypass, graft infections result in amputation rates up to 30 percent and a mortality rate approaching 40 percent (Bandyk and Esses, 1994).

3.5.5 Future Trends

Much current research is focused on improving the performance of existing vascular graft designs (Kapadia et al., 2008). Novel coatings have been developed to steer the biological response to an implanted vascular graft toward endothelialization and improved biocompatibility, while moving away from the proliferation of cellular components linked to vessel narrowing and failure (Greisler, 1996). Various approaches to improve graft performance, healing, and long-term patency include endothelial cell seeding (Park et al., 1990; Williams et al., 1992) and the use of antithrombotic and antibiotic coatings (Devine et al., 2001). Clinical experiences with some of these approaches (endothelialization) have shown promising results (Deutsch et al., 1999) compared to traditional grafts, while others, such as antibiotic coatings, lack definitive outcomes (Earnshaw, 2000).

One area of vascular graft research with significant future promise is the development of tissue-engineered blood vessels (TEBV). Early efforts to create TEBV (L'Heureux et al., 1998; Niklason et al., 1999) have matured and begun to bear fruit, with tissue-engineered vascular conduits currently undergoing clinical trials in patients with congenital heart defects (Shin'oka et al., 2005), and for high-pressure applications such as arteriovenous bypass for hemodialysis and arterial revascularization (L'Heureux et al., 2007a; L'Heureux et al., 2007b). Initial results indicate that complex host-graft interactions such as size changes with flow volume (Shin'oka et al., 2005) and improved compliance (L'Heureux et al., 2007b) are present in these constructs. Although long-term results are needed, the potential applications for TEBV are broad and could result in solutions for problems that have plaqued cardiovascular surgeons since the field's beginning.

3.6 ARTIFICIAL KIDNEY

3.6.1 Market Size

According to the U.S. Renal Data System, the number of Americans in end-stage renal disease (ESRD) is expected to rise from around 485,000 current patients in 2005 to almost 800,000 by 2020 (US Renal Data System, 2007). The aggregate cost for treating ESRD is staggering, with approximately 32 billion USD expended in 2005, of which more than 21 billion USD came from Medicare (US Renal Data System, 2007). Treatment modalities used to replace the failing kidney are few, including hemodialysis with an artificial kidney or hemodialyzer, peritoneal dialysis, or kidney transplantation. With about 341,000 ESRD patients supported in 2005, hemodialysis remains the dominant therapy for ESRD in the United States and is predicted to expand to over half a million patients by 2020 (US Renal Data System, 2007). Hemodialysis is also the dominant therapy worldwide, with only a few countries showing high rates of peritoneal dialysis use (US Renal Data System, 2007). In the United States, kidney transplantation follows hemodialysis in number of patients treated, but a limited donor pool prevents dramatic expansion of this option. The percentage of U.S. ESRD patients receiving peritoneal dialysis continues to decline, falling from 13.5 percent in 1998 (US Renal Data System, 2000) to less than 6 percent in 2005 (US Renal Data System, 2007). The present section focuses on the use of hemodialyzers as a cardiovascular device addressing kidney failure.

3.6.2 Indications

Two physical processes, diffusion and convection, are in widespread use as methods to mimic the excretion functions of the native kidney. Therapies utilizing predominantly convective transport are accurately termed *hemofiltration*, while diffusion-dependent methods are grouped under *hemodialysis*. Both hemodialysis and hemofiltration are used in the inpatient and outpatient setting to treat renal and nonrenal diseases. In general, the purpose of these therapies is to either remove toxins circulating in the blood or reduce the blood volume by removal of water.

The indications to initiate hemodialysis for ESRD are variable but involve clinical and symptomatic manifestations related to uremia, a buildup of metabolic toxins in the blood. Indications requiring immediate initiation of therapy include encephalopathy or a change in mental status, disturbances in either the sensory or motor pathways, effusions in the pericardial space or pleura due to uremic irritation, uncontrollable metabolic derangements such as high serum potassium and low pH, and excessive water retention (Denker et al,, 2000). Because of evidence suggesting improved outcomes in patients receiving early dialysis intervention, patient symptoms resulting in a reduced quality of life (fatigue, cognitive changes, itching, and malnutrition) can be considered as indications for the initiation of dialysis (Hakim and Lazarus, 1995).

Indications for renal-replacement therapy in the acute setting and for other disease processes are different from those for ESRD. A common mode of ESRD therapy in the outpatient setting is intermittent hemodialysis (IHD) where a patient receives intense treatment over the course of a few hours several times a week. Acute renal failure in the inpatient setting is often treated with continuous renal-replacement therapy (CRRT), which is applied for the entire duration of the patient's clinical need and relies upon hemofiltration to a higher degree than IHD (Meyer, 2000). Other nonrenal indications for CRRT are based on the theoretical removal of inflammatory mediators or toxins and elimination of excess fluid (Schetz, 1999). These illnesses include sepsis and systemic inflammatory response syndrome, acute respiratory distress syndrome, congestive heart failure with volume overload, tumor lysis syndrome, crush injury, and genetic metabolic disturbances (Schetz, 1999).

3.6.3 Device Design

Three physical processes determine the removal rate for uremic toxins through membrane-based devices. *Convection* results in toxin removal through a semipermeable membrane that separates blood from dialysate and can be used to remove excess fluid. A pressure gradient across the membrane is responsible for the solvent flow, and toxins are removed as a function of their concentration in solution, the ultrafiltration rate or rate of fluid removal, and the seiving coefficient of the particular toxin across the membrane barrier. Membranes for convection-based therapies exclude molecules larger than their pore size but permit improved removal of the middle molecules (500 to 5000 Daltons) implicated in uremia (Meyer, 2000). Depending on the amount of fluid removed, replacement electrolyte solution may be required to maintain adequate hemodynamic volume. *Diffusion*-based solute removal primarily affects smaller molecules with high diffusion coefficients and possessing a favorable concentration gradient from the blood to the dialysate. *Adsorption* is the third and least characterized method of solute removal in renal-replacement therapies (Klinkmann and Vienken, 1995). Controlled by electrostatic and van der Waals forces between solute and membrane, adsorption-based removal can be beneficial or harmful, depending on the compound involved, such as removal of proinflammatory cytokines versus a needed anticoagulant (Klinkmann and Vienken, 1995). Convection and diffusion remain the dominant physical processes by which membranes and devices are designed.

Although hemodialysis and hemofiltration are often considered separate therapies, some clinical treatments rely on a combination of the two and therefore can be classified as hemodiafiltration procedures. Treatment techniques can be further stratified as to whether they are intermittent or continuous in nature, and whether the vessels accessed are both venous, or arterial and venous. Due to a lack of definitive prospective randomized trials (Bagshaw et al., 2008), the relative advantage of continuous versus intermittent treatment is unknown, although continuous administration is felt to be more "gentle" in some circles, allowing greater time for toxin equilibration and removal (Meyer, 2000) with a possible reduction in blood pressure fluctuation (Bagshaw et al., 2008).

Unit and Membrane Design. Hemodialysis units have undergone a variety of changes since the first practical design, a rotating drum dialyzer, was introduced in the 1940s (Kolff et al., 1944). As reviewed by Clark, subsequent unit designs have progressed through coil and parallel flow dialyzers to the current dominant design of the hollow fiber dialyzer, which was introduced to address performance and use limitations inherent in the earlier devices (Clark, 2000). Subsequent to the introduction of the hollow fiber dialyzer, much of the improvement and development in artificial kidney

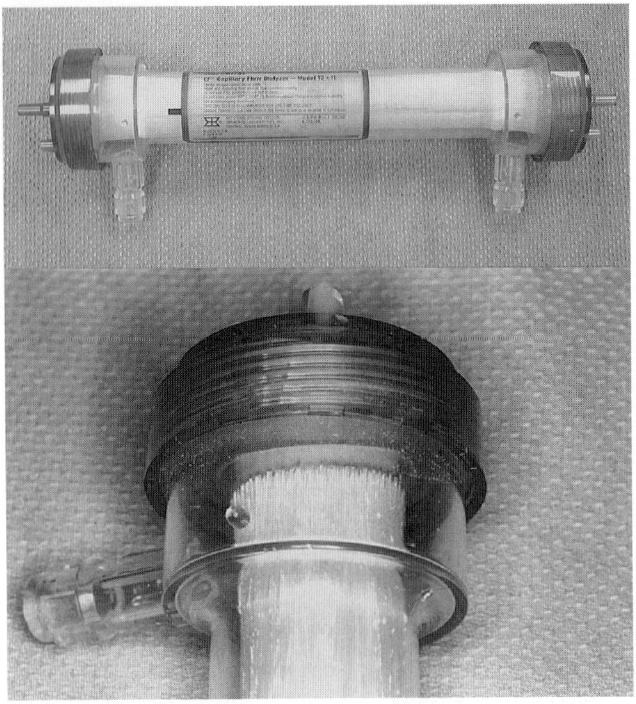

FIGURE 3.11 Hemodialysis exchangers are disposable units similar to membrane oxygenators in construction, (*a*) Note the simple design of the device as shown in the upper portion of the figure (Artificial Organs Division, Travenol Laboratories, Inc., Deerfield, IL). (*b*) Close-up view of hollow fibers used to separate the patient's blood from the dialysate fluid. Toxins in the blood diffuse through the fiber walls to the dialysate fluid.

devices has focused on the membrane barrier materials and device operating conditions. An example of a standard hollow fiber dialyzer is shown in Fig. 3.11, and there have been few major changes in the design since its introduction decades ago (Ronco et al., 2000).

As of 1995, more than 30 different polymer blends were being used in the manufacture of membranes for hemodialysis and hemofiltration (Klinkmann and Vienken, 1995). The various membrane types used for renal replacement therapy can be divided into membranes derived from cellulose (32 percent of 2004 worldwide total) and from synthetic materials (the remaining 68 percent) (Grassmann et al., 2005). The use of cellulose and its derivatives continues to shrink worldwide (Grassmann et al., 2005). Synthetic membranes have been constructed from such materials as polyacrylonitrile (PAN), polysulfone, polyamide, polymethylmethacrylate, polycarbonate, and ethylvinylalchohol copolymer (Klinkmann and Vienken, 1995). In the United States, use of synthetic materials for membrane construction predominates at around 88 percent of the total number of membranes used (Grassmann et al., 2005).

Membrane material selection is dependent upon the mode of therapy employed. Convective therapies such as hemofiltration require a high hydraulic permeability and a large pore size, which might permit large molecules such as cytokines to pass through the fiber wall. Synthetic membranes are well suited for this role and are desired for most continuous, convective techniques (Jones, 1998).

Design Performance Evaluation. Removal of uremic toxins and excess fluid is the central purpose of an artificial kidney. A proposed artificial kidney design should undergo transport testing that encompasses the spectrum of molecules encountered in an uremic state at the appropriate flow conditions. Mock circulatory circuits can approximate hemofiltration and hemodialysis flow environments, generating ultrafiltration rates, sieving coefficients (larger molecules), and clearances (smaller molecules) for sample fluids as simple as salt solutions up to uremic human blood (Leypoldt and Cheung, 1996). Many of the toxins responsible for uremia are unknown and are approximated with marker molecules spanning a large-size spectrum, including small solutes, middle molecules, and albumin (Leypoldt and Cheung, 1996). Small solutes used for in vitro studies include the clinically relevant compounds urea and creatinine, while middle molecules such as 2 microglobulin can be approximated with inulin and dextrans (Leypoldt and Cheung, 1996). Albumin is used to approximate high-molecular-weight oncotic substances in the blood, and its clearance is believed to be negligible (Leypoldt and Cheung, 1996). The transport properties derived using mock circulatory loops may not reflect clinical performance due to complex solute—carrier protein interactions and membrane surface fouling by plasma proteins (Leypoldt and Cheung, 1996).

Computational and *in silico* experiments have also been used for the design and analysis of both artificial kidneys (Eloot et al., 2004) and their associated access devices (De Wachter and Verdonck, 2002; Mareels et al., 2004). Researchers continue to develop computational models of various devices, complete with experimental validation (Mareels et al., 2007). Although validation of computational findings remains important, progress in the area of artificial organ simulation could reduce the need for exhaustive experimental testing.

3.6.4 Complications and Patient Management

Complications that occur during hemodialysis and hemofiltration can be divided into problems related to vascular access and those due to exposure of the blood to the exchange circuit. Depending upon the method used, most vascular access problems associated with renal replacement therapy are similar to those experienced in patients with vascular grafts or catheters and are covered in those respective sections. However, patients with progressive renal disease require particular consideration as a lack of vascular access leads to rapid patient demise.

The complications associated with blood exposure to the dialysis or filtration membrane are related to the activation and upregulation of various homeostatic systems. Inflammatory and hemostatic cascades can become activated by protein adsorption onto the significant surface area that these devices necessarily present to the blood. As part of the inflammatory response to dialyzer perfusion, activation of the complement system results in the generation of anaphylatoxins C3a and C5a and can potentiate activation of polymorphonuclear leukocytes and monocytes (Johnson, 1994; Grooteman and Nube, 1998). These activated leukocytes release cytotoxic compounds and inflammatory mediators that normally would be reserved for the killing of bacteria and infectious agents. The release of these inflammatory mediators is implicated in sequelae such as fever, cardiovascular instability, and increased catabolism of muscle protein (Pertosa et al., 2000). Since the nature and extent of protein adsorption impacts the inflammatory response, the surface properties of dialyzer membranes are of interest as a means to limit this response. In studying surface properties and complement activation, the presence of surface hydroxl groups has been implicated as a potential trigger for pathway activation (Chenoweth, 1984).

Activation of the coagulation cascade and platelet deposition in the artificial kidney circuit are obviously undesirable, leading to reduced device performance or failure. To minimize this phenomena, patients on hemodialysis are usually anticoagulated with heparin during the dialysis session on either a systemic or regional (extracorporeal circuit only) level (Denker et al., 2000). Patients with a sensitivity or contraindication to heparin therapy can be anticoagulated regionally with citrate as well (Denker et al., 2000). Minimizing the potential of membrane surfaces to activate both the hemostatic and inflammatory pathways is of interest to device manufacturers as they seek to reduce complications associated with artificial kidney use.

3.6.5 Future Trends

Artificial kidney designs will likely continue to experience incremental improvements in the materials and hemodynamic areas. New developments in biocompatible materials, superior transport methods for toxin removal, and improved patient management techniques will allow further maturation of hemodialysis and hemofiltration therapy. For example, considerable benefits could be realized from selective toxin removal without concomitant elimination of beneficial proteins. It has been suggested that future devices might utilize the absorption removal pathway with affinity methods as a primary technique to eliminate specific uremic toxins (Klinkmann and Vienken, 1995).

The promise of a true revolution in artificial kidney design comes from the area of tissue engineering. The living kidney performs a number of important metabolic, endocrine, and active transport functions that are not replaced with current hemofiltration and hemodialysis therapy. An artificial kidney that successfully replaces these functions could be a significant improvement when used in conjuction with existing therapies. Researchers have developed a bioartificial renal tubule assist device that successfully reproduces many of the homeostatic functions of the native kidney during in vitro studies, and that responds in the proper manner to known physiologic regulators of the various homeostatic functions (Humes et al., 1999). Efforts have progressed through animal studies (Humes et al., 2002a; Humes et al., 2002b) to a recently completed phase II clinical trial with promising results (Tumlin et al., 2008). Although a larger phase III clinical trial is needed, tissue-engineered artificial kidneys offer the hope of an eventual end to traditional dialysis methods.

3.7 INDWELLING VASCULAR CATHETERS AND PORTS

3.7.1 Market Size

Catheters, in their simplest form, are merely tubes inserted into a body cavity for the purpose of fluid removal, injection, or both (Thomas, 1989), The term *catheter* has been expanded to include a number of tubing-based percutaneous interventional devices used for tasks such as stent delivery and deployment, clot-removal, atherectomy, radiofrequency ablation, and intra-aortic balloon cardiac support. Because of their prevalence and representative uses, the present section will be limited to vascular infusion catheters and access ports. Stenting and cardiac support applications utilizing catheter-based techniques are discussed elsewhere in this chapter.

In 1991 it was estimated that more than 150 million intravascular catheters were being procured in the United States each year (Maki and Mermel, 1998). Of this number, more than 5 million were central venous catheters (Maki and Mermel, 1998). Catheters have a critical role in modern health care and are used in increasing numbers for central access of the major arteries and veins, as well as for an ever-expanding array of invasive procedures (Crump and Collignon, 2000). Given the ubiquitous nature of catheters, even minor design improvements can have a broad clinical and market impact.

3.7.2 Indications

Catheters are placed when there is a clinical need for repeated sampling, injection, or vascular access, usually on a temporary basis. In kidney failure, catheters allow emergent blood access for hemodialysis and hemofiltration (Canaud et al., 2000), and provide temporary access as more permanent sites such as arteriovenous fistulas or grafts mature (Trerotola, 2000). Placement of a catheter or access port is routine for the administration of chemotherapeutic agents and intravenous nutritional supplements. Catheters are often placed when frequent, repeated doses of medication are to be injected, blood samples are to be taken, and for monitoring of hemodynamic performance in critically ill patients (Pearson, 1996).

The anatomic location for temporary central venous catheter (CVC) insertion and placement can be dictated by certain patient or disease restrictions, but the most common sites are the internal jugular vein (neck), the femoral vein (groin), and the subclavian position (upper chest). The internal jugular approach is the first choice for placement of a hemodialysis CVC, while femoral placement is favored when rapid insertion is essential (Canaud et al., 2000). Subclavian vein access has fallen from favor due to a higher incidence of thrombosis and stenosis associated with this site, which can ultimately prevent use of the veins in the downstream vascular tree for high-flow applications such as dialysis (Cimochowski et al., 1990; Schillinger et al., 1991). Some experts suggest the use of the external jugular vein prior to the use of the subclavian, particularly when chronic use is anticipated (Weeks, 2002; Hoggard et al., 2008).

3.7.3 Device Design

Design considerations for vascular access devices include ease of handling, insertion and use, minimal thrombotic and other biocompatibility-related complications, structural and operational reliability over time, and optimization for application-specific performance issues (Canaud et al., 2000). Three different catheter tips are shown in Fig. 3.12 to illustrate these variations in design and structure. Due to the distinct characteristics of the different treatments and agents deployed through catheters, it is not practical to provide specific values for flow rates, pressure drops, viscosities, and other important transport properties.

Catheter device selection is based on a number of factors, including the planned application and placement site, duration of implantation, composition of fluids infused, and frequency of access (Namyslowski and Patel, 1999). Vascular catheters can be divided into two general groups: short-term, temporary catheters that are placed percutaneously; and long-term, indwelling vascular catheters that usually require a surgical insertion. Temporary catheters include short peripheral venous and arterial catheters, nontunneled central venous and arterial catheters, and peripherally inserted central catheters (Pearson, 1996). Tunneled central venous catheters and totally implantable intravascular devices (i.e., ports) are used for therapies requiring long-term vascular access (Pearson, 1996). The term *tunneled* refers to the placement of the catheter exit site at a location away from the area where the vasculature is penetrated, with the portion of the catheter between these two locations lying in a subcutaneous position. Peripheral venous catheters are the most common devices used for intravascular access, while the nontunneled central venous catheter is the most common central catheter (Pearson, 1996). Subcutaneous ported catheters are the

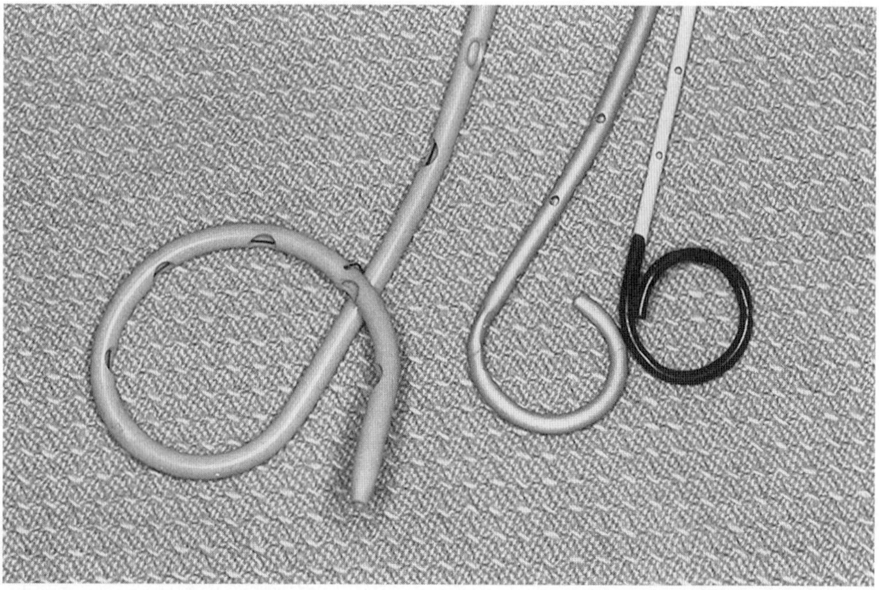

FIGURE 3.12 A selection of catheter tips is shown. The large number of applications for catheters requires differences in hole size, number and placement, along with changes in materials, coatings, and number of lumens.

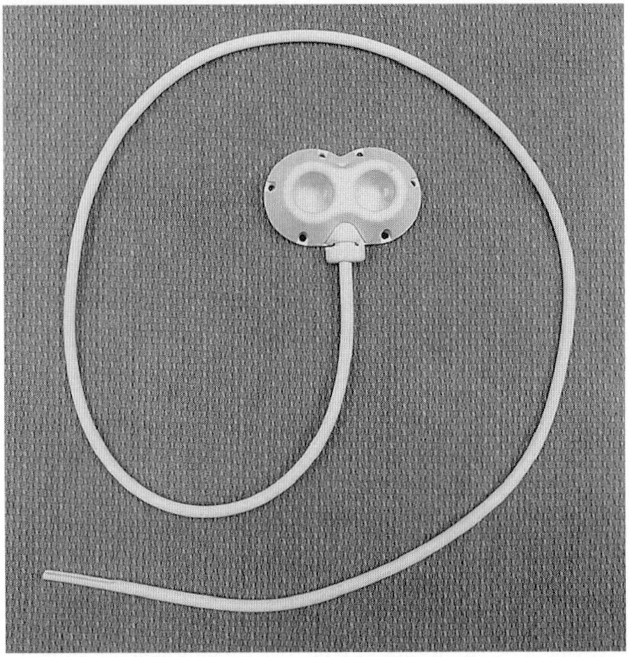

FIGURE 3.13 An implantable vascular access port is shown. The port is accessed through the skin via needle and is resilient enough to allow hundreds of punctures and infusions before needing to be replaced.

preferred long-term route, given an infrequent need for vascular access (Namyslowski and Patel, 1999). Figure 3.13 contains an example of a double-ported, fully implantable catheter used for longer-term access.

As mentioned previously, access for hemodialysis and related therapies is a common indication for catheter placement. Polysiloxane-tunneled central venous catheters and, more recently, totally implantable intravascular port devices have been utilized in hemodialysis for long-term vascular access (Schwab and Beathard, 1999). Temporary central venous catheters for hemodialysis access are further subdivided into different groups based on catheter flexibility and the length of time the device will be in use (Canaud et al., 2000). The longer the catheter will be in place, the more supple the material used for construction. Short-term use catheters possess a high stiffness and are fabricated from polytetrafluoroethylene, polyethylene, polyvinyl chloride, and polyurethane (Schwab and Beathard, 1999; Canaud et al., 2000), although the use of polyethylene and polyvinyl chloride is dropping due to concerns over bacterial adherence in vitro (O'Grady et al., 2002). Medium-term (8 to 30 days) catheters are primarily contructed of polyurethane, while catheters implanted for longer periods of time are usually based on polysiloxane, although polyurethane can be used (Canaud et al., 2000).

Catheters have been permeated, coated, or surface-modified with a variety of compounds in an effort to minimize thrombosis, infection, and friction (Triolo and Andrade, 1983b; Marin et al., 2000). The ultimate goal is an improvement in catheter-handling characteristics and long-term performance. Some of the more common strategies for imparting microbial resistance include saturating the catheter material with silver sulfadiazine and chlorhexidine (Maki et al., 1997), coating the surface with antibiotics (Raad et al., 1997), or bonding heparin to the exterior of the catheter (Appelgren et al., 1996). Results with antibacterial and antiseptic coatings have been mixed, but a recent meta-analysis involving several randomized controlled trials has shown a significant reduction in hospital-acquired infections when catheters modified for bacterial resistance are used

(Marin et al., 2000). The meta-analysis revealed a significant decrease in the number of catheter-related infections for all experimental catheters versus standard devices, plus a significant reduction in infections for catheters employing antimicrobial systems *other* than silver sulfadiazine and chlorhexadine when compared to those systems (Marin et al., 2000). A randomized trial comparing bacterial colonization and catheter-related bloodstream infection rates associated with two antimicrobial catheters came to a similar conclusion, with minocycline- and rifampin-coated catheters being linked with significantly fewer events than chlorhexidine- and silver-sulfadiazine–coated catheters (Darouiche et al., 1999). In an effort to improve handling characteristics, radiofrequency glow discharge has been used to alter the surface properties of common catheter materials to increase hydrophilicity (Triolo and Andrade, 1983a) and reduce friction. This latter property is important in the double catheter systems used for some interventional procedures (Triolo and Andrade, 1983a).

3.7.4 Management and Complications

Infection and thrombosis are common across a variety of catheter designs and applications, while other complications arise due to the particular nature of the therapy being administered, such as recirculation in hemodialysis. Catheter malfunction and related morbidity and mortality represent an area where significant strides are currently being made.

Infection is a common complication associated with intravenous catheters and represents the primary cause of hospital-acquired bloodsteam infection (Valles et al., 1997), resulting in significant morbidity, mortality, and consequent increase in healthcare expenditures. It has been estimated that 250,000 CVC-related blood stream infections occur each year in the United States (O'Grady et al., 2002). The preventable nature of most catheter-related blood stream infections (CRBSI) has led to the Centers for Medicare and Medicaid Services (CMS) to limit reimbursement when such infections occur during a hospitalization (Rosenthal, 2007). This approach should increase the demand for engineered solutions to common problems plaguing health care. Proper care and maintenance is essential for the continued functioning of a catheter, and a number of strategies have been implemented in an effort to minimize infection risk. The use of special coatings and antimicrobial saturated devices was discussed above in the area on device design. Careful exit site management with a dedicated catheter-care team, antibiotic flushes, and possibly catheter tunneling can lower the risk of infection (Raad, 1998), as can the use of a totally implantable intravascular device, which has the lowest infection rate among standard vascular access devices (Maki et al., 2006). Tunneled catheters are fitted with a Dacron cuff that stimulates accelerated healing and ingrowth of tissue distal to the insertion site, thereby providing a host barrier to pathogen migration. In addition, antiseptic cuffs have been placed on catheters to inhibit bacterial migration (Maki et al., 1988; Hasaniya et al., 1996) but overall results are mixed, suggesting that infecting organisms often migrate through the luminal route or that the cuff loses its antibiotic function over time (Sitges-Serra, 1999). In a recent meta-analysis, tunneled and cuffed CVCs had significantly fewer CRBSIs when compared to nontunneled and noncuffed devices (Maki et al., 2006). Once a catheter-related infection is detected, the approach to care is dependent upon the patient condition, the number of remaining access sites, and other factors such as the suspect organism, but the catheter is usually removed and antibiotic therapy initiated (Mermel et al., 2001).

Thrombotic complications are common with catheter use. The development of a fibrin sheath is a near universal occurrence on intravascular devices such as central venous (Hoshal et al., 1971) and hemodialysis catheters, and can have a profound effect upon blood flow in the device (Trerotola, 2000). This sheath can be removed either by stripping (Crain et al., 1996; Rockall et al., 1997) or fibrinolytic medical therapy (Twardowski, 1998), or the catheter can be replaced to restore adequate flow performance. Recent randomized controlled clinical trials have revealed improved long-term outcomes with catheter exchange versus fibrin sheath stripping (Merport et al., 2000), while no outcome differences were realized in patients randomized to either fibrin sheath stripping or thrombolytic therapy (Gray et al., 2000).

3.7.5 Future Trends

Improvements in catheter design are likely to be evolutionary, representing progress in materials, surface treatments, and functional monitoring as catheters are expected to perform for increasingly extended periods. Surfaces with active antithrombotic and antimicrobial activity will continue to be developed and evaluated as will surfaces designed to minimize protein and cellular adhesion. The risk of reduced reimbursement in light of the Center for Medicare and Medicaid's new policies regarding hospital-acquired infections will spur and accelerate development of low-cost, low-risk catheter designs.

3.8 CIRCULATORY SUPPORT DEVICES

3.8.1 Market Size

Heart disease remains the leading cause of death in the United States (Rosamond et al., 2008) and worldwide (Mathers and Loncar, 2006). The devices discussed in the current section provide cardiac support for a spectrum of indications and durations, spanning damage due to an acute myocardial infarction to the long-term decline that accompanies chronic congestive heart failure. The section excludes therapies such as extracorporeal membrane oxygenation and the use of cardiopulmonary bypass pumps as a support method since these are described in the following section on artificial lungs.

The most commonly used means of mechanical circulatory support is the intra-aortic balloon pump (IABP). In 1990, it was estimated that IABP therapy was provided to 70,000 patients annually (Kantrowitz, 1990); recent CDC data indicate at least 40,000 patients were supported via IABP in the United States in 2005 (DeFrances et al., 2007). As described below, the IABP can provide only limited cardiovascular support as its effects are limited to pressure unloading of the ventricle, in contrast to artificial hearts and ventricular assist devices, which provide volume unloading (Mehlhorn et al., 1999). To be effective, the IABP requires that the patient maintains some native pumping capacity as the movement of blood due to the balloon is minimal.

Unlike the IABP, ventricular assist devices (VADs) and total artificial hearts (TAHs) aid or replace the function of the native organ for an extended period of time. A cardiac transplant is the last resort for many patients who fail other medical and surgical therapy. Unfortunately, donor organs remain limited, creating the market for both temporary and extended cardiac support. It has been estimated that up to 100,000 patients in the United States alone would benefit from the implantation of a long-term cardiac support device, with between 5000 and 10,000 requiring biventricular support (Willman et al., 1999). However, existing designs are imperfect due to mechanical and biocompatibility limitations, falling far short of meeting the clinical need for mechanical support. These inherent limitations continue to spur development of novel approaches to chronic cardiac support.

3.8.2 Indications

The indications for IABP placement have changed over the years, as has the insertion method (Torchiana et al., 1997; Mehlhorn et al., 1999). Current indications can be divided into *hemodynamic indications,* due to cardiogenic shock, congestive heart failure, and hypotension, which are characterized by low cardiac output and systemic perfusion, or *ischemic indications* such as those caused by coronary artery disease, which result in poor cardiac perfusion and dysfunction (Torchiana et al., 1997). Current trends indicate an increased use of IABP support for ischemia in patients undergoing percutaneous cardiac therapies such as balloon angioplasty, with a dramatic shift from almost 100 percent surgical implantation to percutaneous implantation in 95 percent of cases (Torchiana et al., 1997; Ferguson et al., 2001). The number of IABPs placed for ischemic indications now exceeds those placed for hemodynamic concerns, with the trend for hemodynamic causes staying relatively flat (Torchiana et al., 1997).

The indications for implantation of TAHs and VADs remain similar to those for the IABP, but are usually reserved for patients who have failed balloon pump support and/or maximal medical therapy. Since the last edition of this chapter (Gage and Wagner, 2002), some VADs have been approved as an alternative to transplantation in specific patient populations, a practice otherwise known as "destination therapy" (Rose et al., 2001). VADs approved for destination therapy include the Heartmate XVE in the United States and the Novacor LVAS within Europe. Current FDA-approved VADs are placed for postcardiotomy support or as a bridge to either transplantation or recovery (Willman et al., 1999).

3.8.3 Current Device Design

Intra-Aortic Balloon Pump. The first clinical use of the intra-aortic balloon pump (IABP) was reported in 1968 (Kantrowitz et al., 1968). Although updated with electronics and computer control, the basic equipment of the modern IABP system remains similar to units introduced decades ago. An IABP system consists of an external pump control console which monitors physiologic patient variables (electrocardiogram and blood pressure) and delivers a bolus of gas to a catheter-mounted balloon located within the patient's aorta (Bolooki, 1998a). Figure 3.14 demonstrates the approximate location of the balloon inside the patient along with the exit site in the femoral artery. Gas delivery is controlled via a solenoid valve and is timed to correspond with the onset of diastole, during which the left ventricle is filling with blood and the aortic valve is closed (Bolooki, 1998a). Inflation of the balloon at this time, as demonstrated in Fig. 3.15*a*, results in blood being pushed back toward the heart and forward to the systemic vasculature, allowing improved perfusion of the target tissues. Figure 3.15*b* demonstrates active collapse (via vacuum) of the balloon during systole or ventricular contraction, which results in a reduction of the pressure the ventricle must work against and eases blood ejection. The reduced workload lowers myocardial oxygen consumption, reducing angina and other more serious consequences of a heart oxygen deficit (Bolooki, 1998c).

The intra-aortic balloon consists of a single, long (approximately 20 cm) inflatable polyurethane sac mounted circumferentially upon a polyurethane catheter (Bolooki, 1998b). Multichambered balloons have been investigated (Bai et al., 1994) but failed to enter clinical use despite potential theoretical advantages. Because of its lower viscosity and better transport speeds, helium is used as the shuttle gas to inflate modern balloons, although carbon dioxide and even air were used in older models (Bolooki, 1998a).

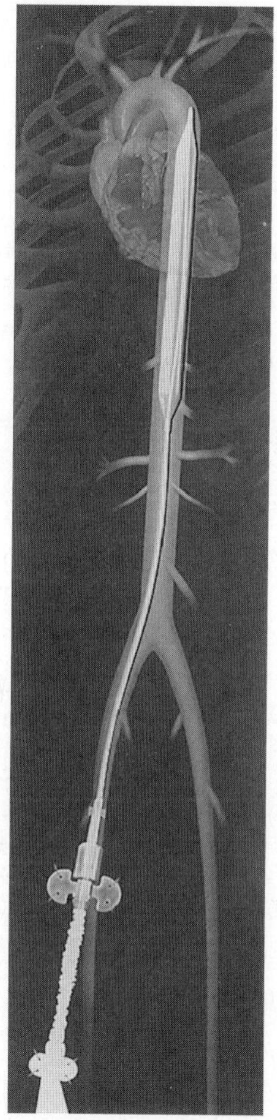

FIGURE 3.14 The anatomical placement of an intra-aortic balloon is shown. The balloon portion of the catheter is located in the aorta distal to the main vessels supplying the head and upper extremities. The catheter providing gas to the balloon is threaded through the iliac artery and aorta, emerging from a puncture site in the femoral artery in the groin. (*Compliments of Datascope Corporation, Cardiac Assist Division, Fairfield, NJ*).

Ventricular Assist Device and Total Artificial Heart. Ventricular assist devices (VADs) can be classified based on whether the device is placed internally (*intracorporeal*) or externally(*extracorporeal*), generates *pulsatile* or *nonpulsatile* flow, and whether it is intended for *bridge-to-recovery, bridge-to-transplant,* or *destination therapy.* Intracorporeal pulsatile LVADs available for commercial use in the United States

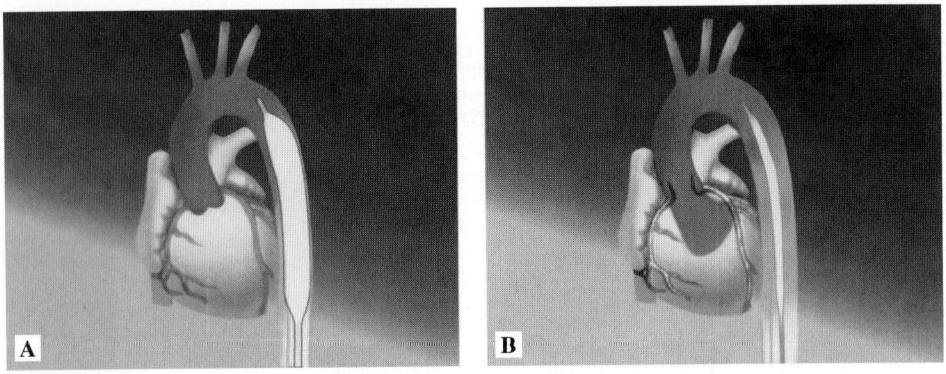

FIGURE 3.15 The balloon inflation-deflation cycle is demonstrated. (*a*) Balloon inflation occurs during diastole, or filling of the ventricle. At this point in the cardiac cycle, the aortic valve is closed. Inflation of the balloon forces blood back toward the heart and into the systemic circulation. The increased pressure developed by the balloon allows better perfusion of the heart muscle during the filling phase. (*b*) Balloon deflation coincides with systole, or ejection of blood from the heart. Deflating the balloon at this time decreases the pressure in the aorta, reducing the effort required by the heart to eject blood. (*Compliments of Datascope Corporation, Cardiac Assist Division, Fairfield, NJ*).

include the following: the Novacor electric pump (World Heart Corp., Ottawa, ON), the pneumatic and vented electric Heartmate pumps (Thoratec Corp., Pleasanton, CA) (McCarthy and Hoercher, 2000), and the Thoratec IVAD (Thoratec Corp., Pleasanton CA), which has the additional benefit of providing biventricular support, if required (Slaughter et al., 2007b). The Heartmate and Novacor devices utilize pusher-plate technology, with the Novacor using opposing, electrically activated plates to compress a smooth polyurethane sac, and the Heartmate using one moving plate to compress a polyurethane sheet into a housing coated with sintered titanium. The force comes from compressed air in the case of the pneumatic Heartmate device, and from an electrically driven cam mechanism in the vented-electric model. Each device requires a percutaneous lead for power and device monitoring (McCarthy and Hoercher, 2000). Figure 3.16 demonstrates the anatomic placement of the Heartmate VE and other current intracorporeal pulsatile VAD designs. All four devices are approved for bridge-to-recovery and bridge-to-transplant, with the Heartmate and Novacor devices approved for destination therapy in some countries.

Available extracorporeal pulsatile VAD designs include the ABIOMED BVS-5000 and AB5000 (ABIOMED, Inc., Danvers, MA) and Thoratec (Thoratec Corp., Pleasonton, CA) VADs (Dowling and Etoch, 2000). The potential advantages of extracorporeal systems include the ability to be implanted in smaller patients (<1.5 m^2 body surface area), multiple sites for cannulation of the heart, and reduced surgical time (Dowling and Etoch, 2000). Drawbacks include large percutaneous cannulation sites with a potential for infection, plus limited patient mobility due to the larger console size that is required for the pneumatic drivers of both devices (Dowling and Etoch, 2000). Figure 3.17 presents a sampling of current FDA-approved intra- and extracorporeal VAD designs and demonstrates the relative size differences between the intracorporeal (Heartmate VE and Novacor) and extracorporeal (Thoratec) designs. Both the Thoratec and Abiomed devices consist of polyurethane blood sacs housed in rigid plastic shells that are compressed with air provided by a driver console. For all practical purposes, the BVS-5000 does not allow patient mobility because of the large driver console and the need for gravity filling for the artificial ventricles. The Thoratec dual driver console is a wheeled, dishwasher-sized unit that is not intended for extensive mobile use; however, the Thoratec II portable pneumatic driver console allows much more patient freedom and is being used for patients discharged to home (Sobieski et al., 2004; Slaughter et al., 2007a).

A number of continuous flow devices have entered clinical use in recent years, with more to reach maturity in the near future. Of the nonpulsatile or continuous flow designs, there are two general categories: axial flow pumps and centrifugal pumps. Implantable axial flow devices in investigational device trials for bridge-to-transplant in the United States include the Jarvik 2000 (Jarvik Heart Inc.,

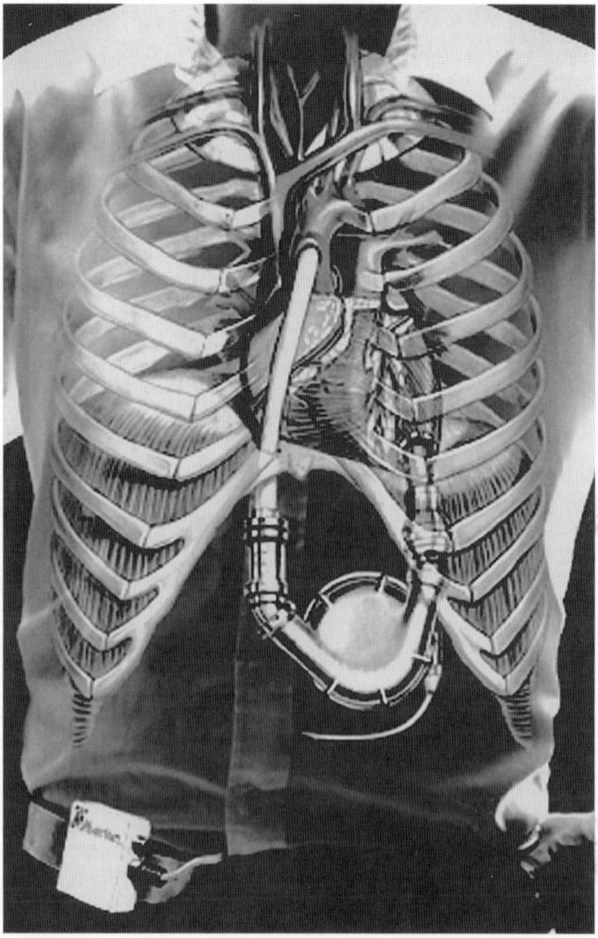

FIGURE 3.16 The anatomic placement of a Heartmate VE (Thoratec Corporation, Pleasanton, CA) left ventricular assist device (LVAD) is shown. The left ventricular apex is cannulated to allow the blood to drain from the ventricular chamber into the assist device during filling. The outflow graft is connected to the aorta, where the pump contents are discharged during the pump ejection phase. The pump itself lies in an abdominal pocket, with the inflow and outflow grafts penetrating into the thoracic cavity. A number of implantable LVADs use the anatomic placement and cannulation sites described here. (*Compliments of Thoratec Corporation, Pleasanton, CA*).

New York, NY) and the MicroMed DeBakey (MicroMed Technology Inc., Houston, TX) VADs. The Heartmate II axial flow VAD (Thoratec Corp., Pleasanton, CA) recently obtained FDA approval for bridge-to-transplant use; an early example of the latter device is displayed Fig. 3.18. Centrifugal pumps in various stages of clinical evaluation throughout the world include the VentrAssist (Ventracor, Sydney, Australia); CorAide (Arrow Intl, Redding, PA); DuraHeart (Terumo Heart, Ann Arbor, MI); and EvaHeart (EvaHeart Medical USA, Pittsburgh, PA) VADs (Kirklin and Holman, 2006). Two novel percutaneous assist devices deserve further mention. The centrifugal flow TandemHeart

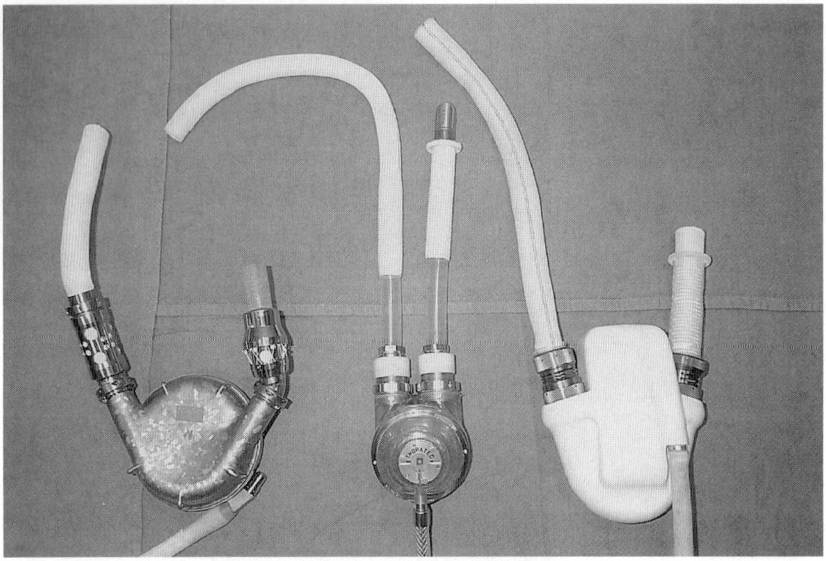

FIGURE 3.17 Some of the FDA-approved ventricular assist devices are displayed. On the left is the implantable Heartmate vented electric VAD (Thoratec Corporation, Pleasanton, CA). It uses a single moving plate to push a polyurethane disk into the rigid titanium pumping chamber. The middle device is the paracorporeal Thoratec VAD (Thoratec Corporation, Pleasanton, CA), which is capable of providing left or right heart support. The rigid pumping chamber contains a polyurethane sac that is compressed pneumatically. The final VAD on the right is the Novacor left ventricular assist system (Baxter Healthcare Corporation, Berkeley, CA). The Novacor device uses opposing plates actuated with a solenoid to compress a polyurethane blood sac.

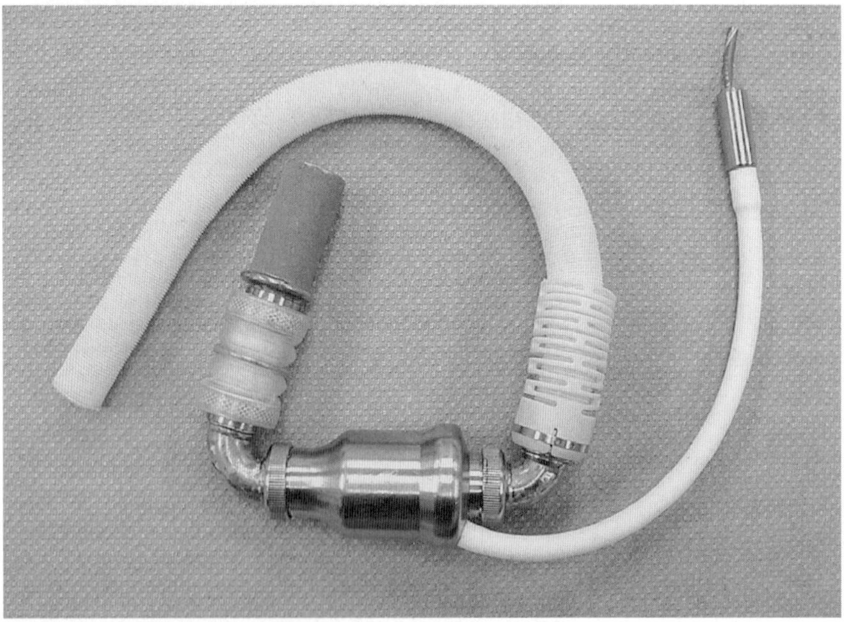

FIGURE 3.18 The Heartmate II (Thoratec Corporation, Pleasanton, CA) is an axial flow ventricular assist device. Unlike the pusher plate and pneumatic sac designs shown in Fig. 3.15, the Heartmate II provides continuous flow support without pulsatile pressure changes. The Heartmate II is much smaller than the Novacor, Thoratec, and Heartmate VE VADs.

percutaneous VAD (CardiacAssist, Inc., Pittsburgh, PA) shown in Fig. 3.19 and the axial flow Impella percutaneous cardiac assist system (Abiomed, Danvers, MA) are both suitable for rapid insertion within a catheterization lab, obviating the need for a thoracotomy in patients with short-term support needs (Windecker, 2007). The potential advantages of the nonpulsatile VADs include smaller size (with correspondingly smaller patient size requirements, fewer moving parts (increased reliability and lifespan), and reduced power requirements. The lack of valves could reduce the likelihood of thrombotic complications involving these sites, which have been shown to be problem areas in previous studies (Wagner et al., 1993). However, the bearings used to support the rotors in most continuous flow devices could act as a nidus for thrombus formation (Stevenson et al., 2001). Hemolysis due to the high shearing forces is of some concern, and the effect of chronic nonpulsatile flow in vivo is not completely understood.

Like VADs, total artificial hearts (TAHs) have been in development for decades. The presence of biventricular support devices has likely limited the progress of TAHs as the two technologies largely compete for the same patient group. Two major TAH designs in the U.S. include the CardioWest system (Syncardia, Tucson, AZ) and the AbioCor TAH (Abiomed, Danvers, MA). The CardioWest device was approved for bridge-to-transplant therapy in 2004 (Kirklin and Holman, 2006) after demonstrating an impressive clinical record (Copeland et al. 2004) in this patient population. The Abiocor TAH was designed for destination therapy as a completely implantable device and received FDA approval under a humanitarian device exemption in 2006 (Abiomed Inc., 2007). Development of a next-generation device is currently ongoing (Abiomed Inc., 2007).

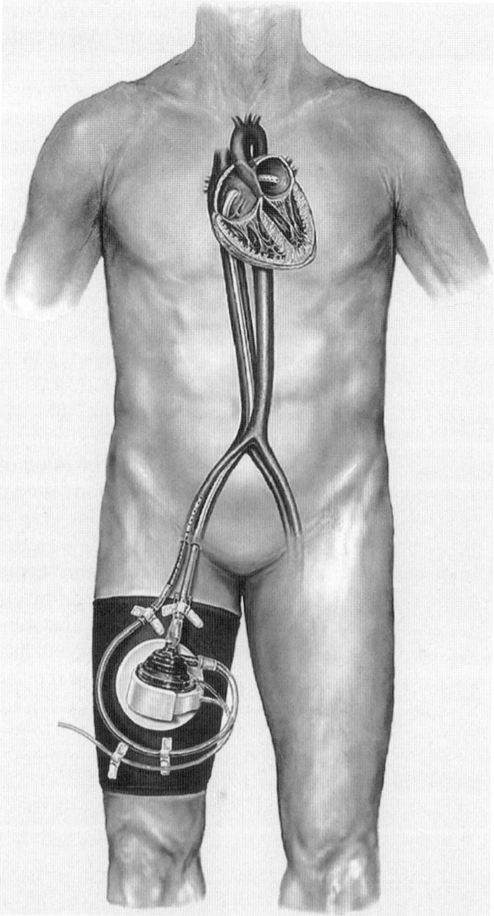

FIGURE 3.19 The TandemHeart percutaneous VAD (Cardiac Assist, Inc., Pittsburgh, PA) is shown. Intended as a short-term support device, the TandemHeart has the advantage of not requiring a major surgical procedure for implantation, and can be placed by interventional cardiologists in a catheterization laboratory. It is a centrifugal pump with novel integrated anticoagulation system that discharges into the pump chamber. (*Compliments of CardiacAssist, Inc., Pittsburgh, PA*).

3.8.4 Management and Complications

IABP support remains an invasive procedure not without risks and complications. However, recent data from a large international registry on IABP use suggest that overall complication rates have dropped from the 12 percent to 30 percent cited in most reports (Cohen et al., 2000) to 7 percent, with the incidence of major complications falling to around 3 percent (Ferguson et al., 2001). The most common complications seen during balloon pump support are vascular in nature, with limb ischemia remaining the dominant problem (Busch et al., 1997). Other vascular complications include bleeding and hematoma formation (Busch et al., 1997), aortic dissection (Busch et al., 1997), embolism (Kumbasar et al., 1999), and rare events such as paraplegia due to spinal infarction (Hurle et al., 1997). Nonvascular complications include infection and mechanical or device-related failures such as balloon rupture (Stavarski, 1996; Scholz et a1., 1998). Factors increasing the risk of complications vary among different studies, but generally include peripheral vascular disease, diabetes, female sex (Busch et al., 1997; Arafa et al., 1999; Cohen et al., 2000), small patient size (BSA <l.65 m^2) and advanced age (≥75 years) (Ferguson et al., 2001). Results have been mixed as to whether smaller catheter sizes and shorter periods of support can limit complication rates (Scholz et al., 1998; Arafa et al., 1999; Cohen et al., 2000) but a recent comparison of 8 Fr to 9.5 Fr IAB catheters revealed a lower rate of limb ischemia with smaller catheters (Cohen et al., 2002).

Complications associated with TAH and VAD use can be divided into those experienced shortly after implantation and events occurring later in the implant period. Postoperatively, the major concerns include hemorrhage, and in the case of isolated left ventricular VAD support, right heart failure or dysfunction, resulting in low pump outputs (Heath and Dickstein, 2000). Bleeding management can include infusion of blood products, but in some cases surgical intervention may be required. Right heart performance can often be improved through reduction of the pulmonary vascular resistance with various drug infusions and inhalants (Heath and Dickstein, 2000). Long-term VAD complications include infection, thromboembolism, and device failure (Kasirajan et al., 2000); the latter was found to be the second most common cause of death during the REMATCH trial and led to design changes and improvements (Rose et al., 2001). Infection can involve the percutaneous connections of the pump, the pump interior or exterior surfaces, or can be systemic in nature (Holman et al.,1999). Management includes antibiotics, debridement, and in severe cases involving the pump pocket, removal or replacement of the pump (Holman et a1., 1999; Kasirajan et al., 2000). Thromboembolism is limited through the use of anticoagulant medications such as heparin perioperatively and warfarin in the long term, although not all pumps require such therapy (Kasirajan et al., 2000). Antiplatelet regimens, such as aspirin, are also used to prevent emboli (Kasirajan et al., 2000).

3.8.5 Future Trends

Improvements in electronics and software development will undoubtedly be incorporated into future IABP designs. Closed loop designs requiring minimal operator intervention have been investigated (Kantrowitz et al., 1992) and results suggest that independent device control could be achieved. Catheters coated with antithrombotic agents have been shown to reduce thrombosis and thrombotic deposition even in immobile (noninflating) balloons when compared to similar uncoated designs (Lazar et al., 1999; Mueller et al., 1999). Hydrophilic coatings have also been placed on balloon catheters, providing a 72 percent reduction in ischemic vascular complications when modified devices are used (Winters et al., 1999). Antibiotic coatings for indwelling catheters could be used to coat intra-aortic balloons if such treatment is proven to be efficacious.

Recent animal data suggest a combination of percutaneous cardiac therapies (VAD and IABP) could produce better outcomes (Sauren et al., 2007) and eliminate the need for a surgical implantation in critical patients. As cardiac support becomes more mainstream, combination products such as the iPulse console (Abiomed Inc., Danvers, MA) are being developed, which can provide cardiac support through either an IAB or artificial external ventricles.

In contrast to the evolution of the IABP, VADs are undergoing a revolution in design and indications for use. The current rush of devices entering clinical trials show improvements in a variety of areas, including power transmission (transcutaneous vs. percutaneous), method of propulsion (electric centrifugal and axial flow vs. pneumatic pulsatile), and size reduction. The largest obstacle to the widespread use of these devices on a scale commensurate with heart disease are the complications that face these patients over the long term. The most critical future developments will focus on patient management issues with a significant impact on morbidity and mortality, such as infection control and thromboembolism, as well as device issues affecting quality of life and durability.

3.9 ARTIFICIAL LUNG

3.9.1 Market Size

According to the National Hospital Discharge Survey, approximately 220,000 membrane oxygenators were used in the United States in 2005 (DeFrances et al., 2007) for acute surgical cardiopulmonary bypass, representing over a 25 percent drop from the 300,000 used in 1997 (Owings and Lawrence, 1999). The number of oxygenators required for acute cardiopulmonary bypass use still dwarfs the number used for extended support of the failing lung, a modality termed *extracorporeal membrane oxygenation (ECMO)*. Changing ECMO demographics suggest new developments in alternative medical therapies might be causing a reduction in the number of neonatal patients supported via ECMO therapy, a standard of care for respiratory support for decades (Roy et al., 2000).

3.9.2 Indications

The indications for cardiopulmonary bypass are surgical in nature, and are based on whether the procedure requires the heart to be stopped. Currently, most cardiac surgical procedures fall into this category (McGiffin and Kirklin, 1995). Cardiopulmonary bypass provides the surgeon with a stable, blood-free field to perform intracardiac repairs and procedures such as coronary artery bypass grafting. Recent trends in minimally invasive surgery have led to surgical systems that allow some procedures such as coronary artery bypass grafting to be performed in the absence of oxygenator support (Svennevig, 2000).

In contrast to cardiopulmonary bypass, medical criteria are the primary indicators for ECMO support. Conventional treatment of acute respiratory failure calls for high-pressure mechanical ventilation with an elevated percentage of oxygen in the ventilation gas. Unfortunately, the high oxygen concentration can result in oxidative damage to lung tissue (oxygen toxicity) and, in the case of the newborn, proliferation of blood vessels in the retina leading to visual damage (retinoproliferative disorder) (Anderson and Bartlett, 2000). The high pressures used to achieve maximum ventilation area also cause lung damage through a process known as *barotrauma*. In essence, the lungs are being subjected to further damage by the therapy employed, preventing the healing necessary to restore proper lung function. The purpose of ECMO is to take over the burden of gas exchange and allow the native lung tissue time to heal.

ECMO is considered a standard therapy for the treatment of respiratory failure in neonatal patients (Anderson and Bartlett, 2000). In adult and pediatric patients, it is a treatment of last resort for individuals who would otherwise die despite maximal therapy (Anderson and Bartlett, 2000; Bartlett et al, 2000). Even in neonatal cases, ECMO is a therapy reserved for those patients with severe respiratory compromise and a high risk of death who are failing traditional ventilator-based interventions. Common causes of respiratory failure in the neonatal population that are treatable with ECMO support include pneumonia or sepsis, meconium aspiration syndrome, respiratory distress syndrome, persistent fetal circulation, and congenital diaphragmatic hernia (Anderson and Bartlett, 2000). Contraindications to ECMO support include root causes that are unresolvable, such as a major birth defect or genetic abnormality, and comorbid conditions such as intracranial hemorrhage or fetal underdevelopment that suggest a poor outcome (Anderson and Bartlett, 2000). Indications for ECMO use in the pediatric and adult populations are not dissimilar from those of the neonate, but the causes for respiratory or cardiopulmonary failure are different, and many individuals suffer from comorbid conditions. Indications include pneumonia, aspiration pneumonitis, acute respiratory distress syndrome, and recoverable heart failure as caused by infection or postsurgical complications (Anderson and Bartlett, 2000). Despite the current limited application of ECMO in adults, a randomized controlled trial (RCT) is recruiting in the United Kingdom to evaluate the cost-effectiveness and clinical benefit of modern ECMO technique in this population (Peek et al., 2006). The RCT will be one of the first RCTs performed in adults (Peek et al., 2006) since the benchmark NIH trial during the 1970s (Zapol et al., 1979) and could reveal if technical and clinical advancements improve outcomes.

3.9.3 Device Design

Although the first oxygenators were described in the late 1800s, it would not be until 1951 that total cardiopulmonary bypass would be performed on a human patient (Stammers, 1997). Oxygenators, or artificial lungs, have undergone a dramatic evolution in the five decades since the first total CPB operation. The initial clinical units are described as *film oxygenators* because a rotating cylinder was used to generate a large, thin film of blood on the cylinder surface where it contacted the exchange gas (Wegner, 1997). Although effective, these early film oxygenators suffered from a number of failings that eventually led to their replacement. The direct gas-blood interface allowed for adequate gas exchange but extensive cellular damage and protein denaturation resulted from the blood-gas interface (Wegner, 1997). The large blood-priming volume and time-consuming, complicated maintenance and use procedures characteristic of film oxygenators were addressed through the advent of *bubble oxygenators* (Stammers, 1997). Direct gas-blood contact remained in bubble oxygenators, but the large surface area of the dispersed oxygen bubbles resulted in greater mass transfer and a reduction in priming volume (Wegner, 1997). In addition, these devices were simple and disposable, consisting of a bubbling chamber, defoaming unit, and a return arterial reservoir (Stammers, 1997; Wegner, 1997). However, the blood damage seen with film oxygenators was not corrected with the new bubbling technology, and concerns regarding blood trauma during longer perfusions contributed to the movement toward *membrane oxygenators* (Stammers, 1997; Wegner, 1997). The use of a semipermeable membrane to separate the blood and gas phases characterizes all membrane oxygenator designs. Membrane oxygenators can be further divided into flat sheet/spiral wound and hollow fiber models. The flat sheet designs restrict blood flow to a conduit formed between two membranes with gas flowing on the membrane exterior; these systems were the first membrane oxygenators to enter use (Wegner, 1997). Spiral wound oxygenators use membrane sheets as well but are arranged in a roll rather than the sandwich formation of the original flat sheet assemblies. Polymers such as polyethylene, cellulose (Clowes et al., 1956), and polytetrafluoroethylene (Clowes and Neville, 1957) were used for membranes in these early designs as investigators searched for a material with high permeability to oxygen and carbon dioxide but that elicited mild responses when in contact with blood. The introduction of polysiloxane as an artificial lung membrane material in the 1960s provided a significant leap in gas transfer efficiency, particularly for carbon dioxide (Galletti and Mora, 1995). These membranes remain in use today for long-term neonatal ECMO support.

Development of the microporous hollow fiber led to the next evolution in lung design, the hollow fiber membrane oxygenator (Stammers, 1997). Increased carbon dioxide permeability compared to solid membranes, coupled with improved structural stability, has secured the standing of these devices as the market leader (Stammers, 1997; Wegner, 1997). The current, standard artificial lung is constructed of hollow microporous polypropylene fibers housed in a plastic shell. An extraluminal crossflow design is used for most models and is characterized by blood flow on the exterior of the fibers with gas constrained to the the fiber interior. Intraluminal flow designs utilize the reverse blood-gas arrangement, with blood constrained to the fiber interior. The laminar conditions experienced by blood flowing inside the fibers result in the development of a relatively thick boundary layer that limits gas transfer. Extraluminal flow devices are less susceptible to this phenomena, and investigators have used barriers and geometric arrangements to passively disrupt the boundary layer, resulting in large gains in mass transfer efficiency (Drinker and Lehr, 1978; Galletti, 1993). Extraluminal flow hollow fiber membrane oxygenators have come to dominate the market because of their improved mass transfer rates and decreased flow resistance, the latter of which minimizes blood damage (Wegner, 1997). Figure 3.20 presents a collection of commercial extraluminal flow membrane oxygenators demonstrating a diversity of design arrangements.

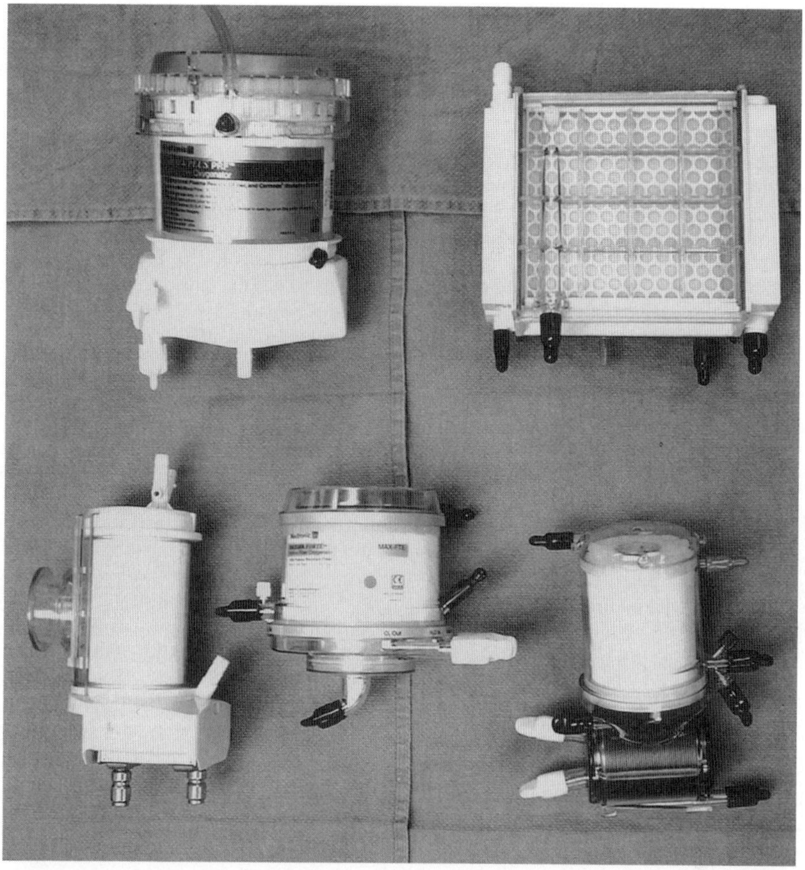

FIGURE 3.20 An assortment of commercial membrane oxygenators are shown to provide an indication of the possible arrangements and designs that can be used. Beginning with the upper left, the Maxima Plus (Medtronic, Inc., Minneapolis, MN) membrane oxygenator is shown. The bottom portion of the device is a heat exchanger for regulating blood temperature, while the upper portion contains a helically wound gas exchange fiber bundle. On the upper right is the rectangular William Harvey HF-5000 (C.R. Bard, Haverhill, MA) oxygenator. The bottom row displays the Cobe Optima (Cobe Cardiovascular, Arvada, CO) oxygenator on the left, with the Maxima Forte and Affinity oxygenators (Medtronic, Inc., Minneapolis, MN) following on the right. Note the smaller size of these designs compared to the oxygenators at the top.

3.9.4 Management and Complications

Despite the major advances in surgical and supportive therapy engendered by the introduction of the artificial lung, substantial limitations remain. The complications faced by patients on oxygenator support are not infrequent and often life-threatening. The limited duration of the average open heart procedure provides less time for major complications to occur, although a few deserve mention.

A relatively common complication suffered by patients who undergo cardiopulmonary bypass (CPB) is called "postpump syndrome," and is characterized by complement activation, cytokine production, activation of various white blood cell types, and depressed lung function. The depressed lung function infrequently progresses to acute respiratory distress syndrome or ARDS (0.5 to 1.7 percent of CPB patients developed ARDS), but tends to be fatal if such progression occurs (50 to 91.6 percent mortality) (Asimakopoulos et al., 1999). The inflammatory response observed is not attributed solely to blood exposure to the extracorporeal circuit but is likely also due to a combination of operative trauma, reperfusion injury, and exposure to endotoxin during the procedure (Asimakopoulos et al., 1999). Hemorrhagic and thrombotic problems during CPB are of grave concern, and traditionally, CPB support has required the use of high doses of anticoagulant to prevent clotting in the extracorporeal circuit at the expense of a possible increase in bleeding. This bleeding risk is further magnified by the consumption of coagulation factors and platelets by extracorporeal surfaces and activation of fibrinolytic pathways. Investigations into minimizing this phenomenon have led to the development of anticoagulant (heparin) fiber coatings for the oxygenators (Wendel and Ziemer, 1999). The presence of a heparin coating have led some to reduce the amount of systemic heparin provided during CPB in an effort to limit bleeding (Aldea et al., 1996; Aldea et al., 1998). Although there is evidence that bleeding is reduced, the approach is controversial in many circles as clinical markers of blood clotting remain elevated, resulting in lingering thromboembolism concerns (Kuitunen et al., 1997; Kumano et al., 1999). In addition, it is not clear how much benefit can be attributed to the heparinized circuit itself. Retrospective data using identical heparin-bonded circuits with full versus reduced anticoagulation show a significant benefit of the reduced anticoagulation in terms of postoperative bleeding and blood loss, along with reduced ventilation support requirements (Ovrum et al., 2003). Further research is required to elucidate what and how much protective effect is provided by heparin-coated fibers.

The more chronic support provided by ECMO is plagued by complications and poor outcomes. Survival rates for ECMO support range from 88 percent for neonates in respiratory failure to 33 percent for adults in cardiac failure (Bartlett et. al., 2000). Similar to CPB, hemorrhagic and thrombotic complications occur and have led to intense investigation into the long-term neurologic outcomes of these patients (Graziani et al., 1997; Nield et al., 2000), although the exact relationship between ECMO and outcomes remains unclear (Vaucher et al., 1996; Rais-Bahrami et al., 2000). In addition, longer-term support with hollow fiber membrane oxygenators results in the manifestation of a particular phenomenon where plasma from the blood side seeps into the pores of the fibers in a process termed *weeping*. The effect of this phenomenon is to increase the diffusion distance for oxygen and carbon dioxide, thereby reducing mass transfer performance. Originally thought to be due to temperature changes and condensation of water in the fiber interior (Mottaghy et al., 1989), evidence suggests deposition of circulating phospholipid at the fluid-gas interface results in a change in hydrophobicity on the pore surface that mediates penetration of the plasma (Montoya et al., 1992).

3.9.5 Future Trends

Future developments in cardiopulmonary bypass will focus on improving the biocompatibility of the device through minimization of hematologic alterations. One current approach involves coating the oxygenator fibers with a layer of polysiloxane in an effort to limit the postperfusion syndrome (Shimamoto et al., 2000). ECMO, with its higher longevity requirements, will similarly benefit from new coatings and materials. General measures to improve the biocompatibility of the fibers include coatings and additives to limit plasma infiltration into the device (Shimono et al., 1996), limit platelet deposition on the surface (Gu et al., 1998) and platelet activation (Defraigne et al., 2000), and minimize leukocyte and complement activation (Watanabe et al., 1999; Saito et al., 2000). Although not a new concept, novel methods to improve mass transfer through the thinning or disruption of the boundary layer are currently being developed. Some approaches include the use of fibers mounted on a rapidly spinning disc (Borovetz et al., 1997; Reeder et al., 1998), cone (Makarewicz et al., 1994) or cylinder (Svitek et al., 2005), the pulsing and distention of silicone sheets (Fiore et al., 2000), and the pulsation of a balloon mounted inside circumferentially organized fibers designed for placement in the vena cava (Federspiel et al., 1997). Some of these devices offer the opportunity to combine the features of a blood pump and artificial lung, and therefore represent a significant leap over current bypass systems.

ACKNOWLEDGMENTS

The support of the McGowan Institute for Regenerative Medicine at the University of Pittsburgh is acknowledged. Fellowship support was provided to Kenneth Gage during the writing of the first edition of this chapter from the Department of Energy under the Krell Institute's Computational Science Graduate Fellowship (CSGF).

This work was supported by the Department of Energy Computational Science Graduate Fellowship Program of the Office of Science and National Nuclear Security Administration in the Department of Energy under contract DE-FG02-97ER25308.

REFERENCES

(1988). "Comparative evaluation of prosthetic, reversed, and in situ vein bypass grafts in distal popliteal and tibial-peroneal revascularization. Veterans Administration Cooperative Study Group 141." *Arch Surg*, **123**(4):434–8.

Abiomed Inc. (2007). "Heart Replacement." Retrieved Jun 13, 2008, from http: //www.abiomed.com/products/heart replacement.cfm.

Akins, C. W. (1995). "Results with mechanical cardiac valvular prostheses." *Ann Thorac Surg*, **60**(6):1836–44.

Al Suwaidi, J., P. B. Berger, et al. (2000). "Coronary artery stents." *JAMA*, **284**(14):1828–36.

Aldea, G. S., M. Doursounian, et al. (1996). "Heparin-bonded circuits with a reduced anticoagulation protocol in primary CABG: a prospective, randomized study." *Ann Thorac Surg*, **62**(2):410–7; discussion 417–8.

Aldea, G. S., P. O'Gara, et al. (1998). "Effect of anticoagulation protocol on outcome in patients undergoing CABG with heparin-bonded cardiopulmonary bypass circuits." *Ann Thorac Surg*, **65**(2):425–33.

Anderson, H. L., III and R. H. Bartlett (2000). Chapter 123: Extracorporeal life support for respiratory failure and multiple organ failure. *Textbook of Critical Care*. A. Grenvik, S. M. Ayres, P. R. Holbrook and W. C. Shoemaker. Philadelphia, PA. U.S.A., W. B. Saunders.

Anderson, H. V., R. E. Shaw, et al. (2002). "A contemporary overview of percutaneous coronary interventions. The American College of Cardiology-National Cardiovascular Data Registry (ACC-NCDR)." *J Am Coll Cardiol*, **39**(7):1096–103.

Appelgren, P., U. Ransjo, et al. (1996). "Surface heparinization of central venous catheters reduces microbial colonization in vitro and in vivo: results from a prospective, randomized trial." *Crit Care Med*, **24**(9):1482–9.

Arafa, O. E., T. H. Pedersen, et al. (1999). "Vascular complications of the intraaortic balloon pump in patients undergoing open heart operations: 15-year experience." *Ann Thorac Surg*, **67**(3):645–51.

Asimakopoulos, G., P. L. Smith, et al. (1999). "Lung injury and acute respiratory distress syndrome after cardiopulmonary bypass." *Ann Thorac Surg*, **68**(3):1107–15.

Babaliaros, V. and P. Block (2007). "State of the art percutaneous intervention for the treatment of valvular heart disease: a review of the current technologies and ongoing research in the field of percutaneous valve replacement and repair." *Cardiology*, **107**(2):87–96.

Bagshaw, S. M., L. R. Berthiaume, et al. (2008). "Continuous versus intermittent renal replacement therapy for critically ill patients with acute kidney injury: a meta-analysis." *Crit Care Med*, **36**(2):610–7.

Bai, J., H. Lin, et al. (1994). "A study of optimal configuration and control of a multi-chamber balloon for intraaortic balloon pumping." *Ann Biomed Eng*, **22**(5):524–31.

Baldus, S., R. Koster, et al. (2000). "Treatment of aortocoronary vein graft lesions with membrane-covered stents: A multicenter surveillance trial." *Circulation*, **102**(17):2024–7.

Bandyk, D. F. and G. E. Esses (1994). "Prosthetic graft infection." *Surg Clin North Am*, **74**(3):571–90.

Bartlett, R. H., D. W. Roloff, et al. (2000). "Extracorporeal life support: the University of Michigan experience." *JAMA*, **283**(7):904–8.

Berger, K., L. R. Sauvage, et al. (1972). "Healing of arterial prostheses in man: its incompleteness." *Ann Surg*, **175**(1):118–27.

Bernstein, A. D., A. J. Camm, et al. (1993). "North American Society of Pacing and Electrophysiology policy statement. The NASPE/BPEG defibrillator code." *Pacing Clin Electrophysiol*, **16**(9):1776–80.

Bernstein, A. D., A. J. Camm, et al. (1987). "The NASPE/BPEG generic pacemaker code for antibradyarrhythmia and adaptive-rate pacing and antitachyarrhythmia devices." *Pacing Clin Electrophysiol*, **10**(4 Pt 1): 794–9.

Bernstein, A. D., J. C. Daubert, et al. (2002). "The revised NASPE/BPEG generic code for antibradycardia, adaptive-rate, and multisite pacing. North American Society of Pacing and Electrophysiology/British Pacing and Electrophysiology Group." *Pacing Clin Electrophysiol*, **25**(2):260–4.

Bernstein, A. D. and V. Parsonnet (1996a). "The NASPE/BPEG pacemaker-lead code (NBL code)." *Pacing Clin Electrophysiol*, **19**(11 Pt 1):1535–6.

Bernstein, A. D. and V. Parsonnet (1996b). "Survey of cardiac pacing and defibrillation in the United States in 1993." *Am J Cardiol*, **78**(2):187–96.

Bernstein, A. D. and V. Parsonnet (2001). "Survey of cardiac pacing and implanted defibrillator practice patterns in the United States in 1997." *Pacing Clin Electrophysiol*, **24**(5):842–55.

Bertrand, O. F., R. Sipehia, et al. (1998). "Biocompatibility aspects of new stent technology." *J Am Coll, Cardiol*, **32**(3):562–71.

Besarab, A., J. Work, et al. (2006). "Clinical practice guidelines for vascular access." *Am J Kidney Dis*, **48**(l Suppl 1): S176 276.

Biancari, F. and M. Lepantalo (1998). "Extra-anatomic bypass surgery for critical leg ischemia. A review." *J Cardiovasc Surg (Torino)*, **39**(3):295–301.

Bolooki, H. (1998a). Chapter 6: Balloon pump equipment. *Clinical Application of the Intra-Aortic Balloon Pump*. H. Bolooki. Armonk, NY, U.S.A., Futura Pub. Co.:73–85.

Bolooki, H. (1998b). Chapter 7: Balloon pump consoles and catheters. *Clinical Application of the Intra-Aortic Balloon Pump*. H. Bolooki. Armonk, NY, U.S.A., Futura Pub. Co.:87–107.

Bolooki, H. (1998c). Chapter 8: Physiology of balloon pumping. *Clinical Application of the Intra-Aortic Balloon Pump*. H. Bolooki. Armonk, NY, U.S.A., Futura Pub. Co.:109–161.

Bonhoeffer, P., Y. Boudjemline, et al. (2000). "Percutaneous replacement of pulmonary valve in a right-ventricle to pulmonary-artery prosthetic conduit with valve dysfunction." *Lancet*, **356**(9239): 1403–5.

Bonow, R. O., B. Carabello, et al. (1998). "Guidelines for the management of patients with valvular heart disease: executive summary. A report of the American College of Cardiology/American Heart Association Task Force on Practice Guidelines (Committee on Management of Patients with Valvular Heart Disease)." *Circulation*, **98**(18):1949–84.

Bonow, R. O., B. A. Carabello, et al. (2006). "ACC/AHA 2006 guidelines for the management of patients with valvular heart disease: a report of the American College of Cardiology/American Heart Association Task Force on Practice Guidelines (writing Committee to Revise the 1998 guidelines for the management of patients with valvular heart disease) developed in collaboration with the Society of Cardiovascular Anesthesiologists endorsed by the Society for Cardiovascular Angiography and Interventions and the Society of Thoracic Surgeons." *J Am Coll Cardiol*, **48**(3):el-148.

Boriani, G., I. Diemberger, et al. (2007). "How, why, and when may atrial defibrillation find a specific role in implantable devices? A clinical viewpoint." *Pacing Clin Electrophysiol*, **30**(3):422–33.

Borovetz, H. S., P. Litwak, et al. (1997) Membrane apparatus with enhanced mass transfer via active mixing. U.S.A. **Patent 6,106,776.** April 11, 1997.

Brewster, D. C. (2000). Chapter 37: Prosthetic grafts. *Vascular Surgery*. R. B. Rutherford. Philadelphia, PA, U.S.A., W. B. Saunders & Co.:559–584.

Bunt, T. J. (1983). "Synthetic vascular graft infections. I. Graft infections." *Surgery*, **93**(6):733–46.

Busch, T., H. Sirbu, et al. (1997). "Vascular complications related to intraaortic balloon counterpulsation: an analysis of ten years experience." *Thorac Cardiovasc Surg*, **45**(2):55–9.

Butany, J. and M. J. Collins (2005). "Analysis of prosthetic cardiac devices: a guide for the practising pathologist." *J Clin Pathol*, **58**(2):113–24.

Calligaro, K. D. and F. J. Veith (1991). "Diagnosis and management of infected prosthetic aortic grafts." *Surgery*, **110**(5):805–13.

Canaud, B., H. Leray-Moragues, et al. (2000). "Temporary vascular access for extracorporeal therapies." *Ther Apher*, **4**(3):249–55.

Cazeau, S., C. Leclercq, et al. (2001). "Effects of multisite biventricular pacing in patients with heart failure and intraventricular conduction delay." *N Engl J Med*, **344**(12):873–80.

Centers for Medicare and Medicaid Services. (2005, 12/14/2005). "Fistula first breakthrough." Retrieved June 1, 2008, from http://www.cms.hhs.gov/ESRDQualityImproveInit/04 FistulaFirstBreakthrough.asp.

Chenoweth, D. E. (1984). "Complement activation during hemodialysis: clinical observations, proposed mechanisms, and theoretical implications." *Artif Organs*, **8**(3):281–90.

Cimochowski, G. E., E. Worley, et al. (1990). "Superiority of the internal jugular over the subclavian access for temporary dialysis." *Nephron*, **54**(2):154–61.

Clark, W. R. (2000). "Hemodialyzer membranes and configurations: a historical perspective." *Semin Dial*, **13**(5):309–11.

Clowes, G. H., Jr., A. L. Hopkins, et al. (1956). "An artificial lung dependent upon diffusion of oxygen and carbon dioxide through plastic membranes." *J Thorac Surg*, **32**(5):630–7.

Clowes, G. H. A., Jr. and W. E. Neville (1957). "Further development of a blood oxygenator dependent upon the diffusion of gases through plastic membranes." *Trans Am Soc Artif Intern Organs*, **3**:52–58.

Cohen, M., M. S. Dawson, et al. (2000). "Sex and other predictors of intra-aortic balloon counterpulsation-related complications: prospective study of 1119 consecutive patients." *Am Heart J*, **139**(2 Pt 1):282–7.

Cohen, M., J. J. Ferguson, 3rd, et al. (2002). "Comparison of outcomes after 8 vs. 9.5 French size intra-aortic balloon counterpulsation catheters based on 9,332 patients in the prospective Benchmark registry." *Catheter Cardiovasc Interv*, **56**(2):200–6.

Comerota, A. J., F. A. Weaver, et al. (1996). "Results of a prospective, randomized trial of surgery versus thrombolysis for occluded lower extremity bypass grafts." *Am J Surg*, **172**(2):105–12.

Connolly, J. E., J. H. Kwaan, et al. (1984). "Newer developments of extra-anatomic bypass." *Surg Gynecol Obstet*, **158**(5):415–8.

Contreras, M. A., W. C. Quist, et al. (2000). "Effect of porosity on small-diameter vascular graft healing." *Microsurgery*, **20**(1):15–21.

Copeland, J. G., R. G. Smith, et al. (2004). "Cardiac replacement with a total artificial heart as a bridge to transplantation." *N Engl J Med*, **351**(9):859–67.

Crain, M. R., M. W. Mewissen, et al. (1996). "Fibrin sleeve stripping for salvage of failing hemodialysis catheters: technique and initial results." *Radiology*, **198**(1):41–4.

Cribier, A., H. Eltchaninoff, et al. (2002). "Percutaneous transcatheter implantation of an aortic valve prosthesis for calcific aortic stenosis: first human case description." *Circulation*, **106**(24):3006–8.

Crossley, G. H. (2000). "Cardiac pacing leads." *Cardiol Clin*, **18**(1):95–112, viii–ix.

Crump, J. A. and P. J. Collignon (2000). "Intravascular catheter-associated infections." *Eur J Clin Microbiol Infect Dis*, **19**(1):1–8.

Darouiche, R. O., Raad, II, et al. (1999). "A comparison of two antimicrobial-impregnated central venous catheters. Catheter Study Group." *N Engl J Med*, **340**(1):1–8.

David, T. E., D. E. Uden, et al. (1983). "The importance of the mitral apparatus in left ventricular function after correction of mitral regurgitation." *Circulation*, **68**(3 Pt 2):II76–82.

Davids, L., T. Dower, et al. (1999). Chapter 1: The lack of healing in conventional vascular grafts. *Tissue Engineering of Vascular Prosthetic Grafts*. P. Zilla and H. P. Greisler. Austin, TX, U.S.A., R.G. Landes Biosciences Co.:3–44.

De Hart, J., G. Cacciola, et al. (1998). "A three-dimensional analysis of a fibre-reinforced aortic valve prosthesis." *J Biomech*, **31**(7):629–38.

de Voogt, W. G. (1999). "Pacemaker leads: performance and progress." *Am J Cardiol*, **83**(5B):187D–191D.

De Wachter, D. and P. Verdonck (2002). "Numerical calculation of hemolysis levels in peripheral hemodialysis cannulas." *Artif Organs*, **26**(7):576–82.

Defraigne, J. O., J. Pincemail, et al. (2000). "SMA circuits reduce platelet consumption and platelet factor release during cardiac surgery." *Ann Thorac Surg*, **70**(6):2075–81.

DeFrances, C. J., K. A. Cullen, et al. (2007). "Annual summary with detailed diagnosis and procedure data. National Hospital Discharge Survey, 2005." *Vital Health Stat*, **13**(165):1–209.

Denker, B. M., G. M. Chertow, et al. (2000). Chapter 57: Hemodialysis. *The Kidney*. B. M. Brenner. Philadelphia, PA, U.S.A., W.B. Saunders Co.:2373–453.

Deutsch, M., J. Meinhart, et al. (1999). "Clinical autologous in vitro endothelialization of infrainguinal ePTFE grafts in 100 patients: a 9-year experience." *Surgery* **126**(5):847–55.

Devine, C., B. Hons, et al. (2001). "Heparin-bonded Dacron or polytetrafluoroethylene for femoropopliteal bypass grafting: a multicenter trial." *J Vasc Surg*, **33**(3):533–9.

Diethrich, E. B. (2003). "Future potential of endovascular techniques for vascular surgeons." *Semin Vasc Surg*, **16**(4):255–61; discussion 261.

Dohmen, P. M., A. Lembcke, et al. (2007). "Mid-term clinical results using a tissue-engineered pulmonary valve to reconstruct the right ventricular outflow tract during the Ross procedure." *Ann Thorac Surg*, **84**(3):729–36.

Dowling, R. D. and S. W. Etoch (2000). "Clinically available extracorporeal assist devices." *Prog Cardiovasc Dis*, **43**(1):27–36.

Drinker, P. A. and J. L. Lehr (1978). "Engineering aspects of ECMO technology." *Artif Organs*, **2**(1):6–11.

Earnshaw, J. J. (2000), "The current role of rifampicin-impregnated grafts: pragmatism versus science." *Eur J Vasc Endovasc Surg*, **20**(5):409–12.

Eberhart, A., Z. Zhang, et al. (1999). "A new generation of polyurethane vascular prostheses: rara avis or ignis fatuus?" *J Biomed Mater Res*, **48**(4):546–58.

Edmunds, L. H., Jr., R. E. Clark, et al. (1996). "Guidelines for reporting morbidity and mortality after cardiac valvular operations. The American Association for Thoracic Surgery, Ad Hoc Liaison Committee for Standardizing Definitions of Prosthetic Heart Valve Morbidity." *Ann Thorac Surg*, **62**(3):932–5.

Eloot, S., J. Y. De Vos, et al. (2004). "Diffusive clearance of small and middle-sized molecules in combined dialyzer flow configurations." *Int J Artif Organs*, **27**(3):205–13.

Epstein, A. E., J. P. DiMarco, et al. (2008). "ACC/AHA/HRS 2008 Guidelines for Device-Based Therapy of Cardiac Rhythm Abnormalities: A Report of the American College of Cardiology/American Heart Association Task Force on Practice Guidelines (Writing Committee to Revise the ACC/AHA/NASPE 2002 Guideline Update for Implantation of Cardiac Pacemakers and Antiarrhythmia Devices): Developed in Collaboration With the American Association for Thoracic Surgery and Society of Thoracic Surgeons." *Circulation*, **117**(21):e350–408.

Eybl, E., M. Grimm, et al. (1992). "Endothelial ceil lining of bioprosthetic heart valve materials." *J Thorac Cardiovasc Surg*, **104**(3):763–9.

Faries, P. L., F. W. Logerfo, et al. (2000). "A comparative study of alternative conduits for lower extremity revascularization: all-autogenous conduit versus prosthetic grafts." *J Vasc Surg*, **32**(6):1080–90.

Federspiel, W. J., M. S. Hout, et al. (1997). "Development of a low flow resistance intravenous oxygenator." *ASAIO J*, **43**(5):M725–30.

Ferguson, J. J., 3rd, M. Cohen, et al. (2001). "The current practice of intra-aortic balloon counterpulsation: results from the Benchmark Registry." *J Am Coll Cardiol*, **38**(5):1456–62.

Fiore, G. B., M. L. Costantino, et al. (2000). "The pumping oxygenator: design criteria and first in vitro results." *Artif Organs*, **24**(10):797–807.

Fischman, D. L., M. B. Leon, et al. (1994). "A randomized comparison of coronary-stent placement and balloon angioplasty in the treatment of coronary artery disease. Stent Restenosis Study Investigators." *N Engl J Med*, **331**(8):496–501.

Foster, M. C., T. Mikulin, et al. (1986). "A review of 155 extra-anatomic bypass grafts." *Ann R Coll Surg Engl*, **68**(4):216–8.

Gage, K, L. and W. R. Wagner (2002). Cardiovascular Devices. *Standard Handbook of Biomedical Engineering and Design*. M. Kutz. New York NY. U.S.A., McGraw-Hill Professional: 20.1–20.48.

Galletti, P. M. (1993). "Cardiopulmonary bypass: a historical perspective." *Artif Organs*, **17**(8):675–86.

Galletti, P. M. and C. T. Mora (1995). Chapter 1. Cardiopulmonary bypass: The historical foundation, the future promise. *Cardiopulmonary Bypass: Principles and Techniques of Extracorporeal Circulation*. C. T. Mora. New York, NY. U.S.A., Springer-Verlag: 3–18.

Gerber, T. C., R. A. Nishimura, et al. (2001). "Left ventricular and biventricular pacing in congestive heart failure." *Mayo Clin Proc*, **76**(8):803–12.

Golden, M. A., S. R. Hanson, et al. (1990). "Healing of polytetrafluoroethylene arterial grafts is influenced by graft porosity." *J Vasc Surg*, **11**(6):838–44; discussion 845.

Grassmann, A., S. Gioberge, et al. (2005). "ESRD patients in 2004: global overview of patient numbers, treatment modalities and associated trends." *Nephrol Dial Transplant*, **20**(12):2587–93.

Gray, R. J., A. Levitin, et al. (2000). "Percutaneous fibrin sheath stripping versus transcatheter urokinase infusion for malfunctioning well-positioned tunneled central venous dialysis catheters: a prospective, randomized trial." *J Vasc Interv Radiol*, **11**(9):1121–9.

Graziani, L. J., M. Gringtas, et al. (1997). "Cerebrovascular complications and neurodevelopmental sequelae of neonatal ECMO." *Clin Perinatol*, **24**(3):655–75.

Gregoratos, G., M. D. Cheitlin, et al. (1998). "ACC/AHA Guidelines for Implantation of Cardiac Pacemakers and Antiarrhythmia Devices: Executive Summary—a report of the American College of Cardiology/American Heart Association Task Force on Practice Guidelines (Committee on Pacemaker Implantation)." *Circulation*, **97**(13):1325–35.

Greisler, H. P. (1991). *New Biologic and Synthetic Vascular Prostheses*. Austin, TX, U.S.A., R.G. Landes Biosciences Co.

Greisler, H. P. (1996). "Growth factor release from vascular grafts." *J Control Release*, **39**(2–3):287–280.

Grooteman, M. P. and M. J. Nube (1998). "Haemodialysis-related bioincompatibility: fundamental aspects and clinical relevance." *Neth J Med*, **52**(5):169–78.

Grube, E., J. C. Laborde, et al. (2005). "First report on a human percutaneous transluminal implantation of a self-expanding valve prosthesis for interventional treatment of aortic valve stenosis." *Catheter Cardiovasc Interv*, **66**(4):465–9.

Gu, Y. J., P. W. Boonstra, et al. (1998). "Cardiopulmonary bypass circuit treated with surface-modifying additives: a clinical evaluation of blood compatibility." *Ann Thorac Surg*, **65**(5):1342–7.

Gulbins, H., A. Pritisanac, et al. (2006). "Successful endothelialization of porcine glutaraldehyde-fixed aortic valves in a heterotopic sheep model." *Ann Thorac Surg*, **81**(4):1472–9.

Hakim, R. M. and J. M. Lazarus (1995). "Initiation of dialysis." *J Am Soc Nephrol*, **6**(5):1319–28.

Hammermeister, K., G. K. Sethi, et al. (2000). "Outcomes 15 years after valve replacement with a mechanical versus a bioprosthetic valve: final report of the Veterans Affairs randomized trial." *J Am Coll Cardiol*, **36**(4):1152–8.

Harris, L. M. (2005). Chapter 48: The modified biograft. *Vascular Surgery*. R. B. Rutherford, Philadelphia, PA, U.S.A., Elsevier Saunders. **V 1.**

Hasaniya, N. W., M. Angelis, et al. (1996). "Efficacy of subcutaneous silver-impregnated cuffs in preventing central venous catheter infections." *Chest*, **109**(4):1030–2.

Heath, M. J. and M. L. Dickstein (2000). "Perioperative management of the left ventricular assist device recipient." *Prog Cardiovasc Dis*, **43**(1):47–54.

Helmus, M. N. and J. A. Hubbell (1993). "Materials Selection." *Cardiovasc Pathol*, **2**(3 Suppl 1):53–71.

Henry, M., C. Klonaris, et al (2000). "State of the art: which stent for which lesion in peripheral interventions?" *Tex Heart Inst J*, **27**(2):119–26.

Hirsch, A. T., Z. J. Haskal, et al. (2006). "ACC/AHA 2005 Practice Guidelines for the management of patients with peripheral arterial disease (lower extremity, renal, mesenteric, and abdominal aortic): a collaborative report from the American Association for Vascular Surgery/Society for Vascular Surgery, Society for Cardiovascular Angiography and Interventions, Society for Vascular Medicine and Biology, Society of Interventional Radiology, and the ACC/AHA Task Force on Practice Guidelines (Writing Committee to Develop Guidelines for the Management of Patients With Peripheral Arterial Disease): endorsed by the American Association of Cardiovascular and Pulmonary Rehabilitation; National Heart, Lung, and Blood Institute; Society for Vascular Nursing; TransAtlantic Inter-Society Consensus; and Vascular Disease Foundation." *Circulation*, **113**(11):e463–654.

Hoggard, J., T. Saad, et al. (2008). "Guidelines for venous access in patients with chronic kidney disease." *Semin Dial*, **21**(2):186–91.

Holman, W. L., J. L. Skinner, et al. (1999). "Infection during circulatory support with ventricular assist devices." *Ann Thorac Surg*, **68**(2):711–6.

Holmes, D. R., Jr., J. Hirshfeld, Jr., et al. (1998). "ACC Expert Consensus document on coronary artery stents. Document of the American College of Cardiology." *J Am Coll Cardiol*, **32**(5):1471–82.

Horstkotte, D. (1996). "Results with mechanical cardiac valvular prostheses [Letter]." *Ann Thorac Surg*, **62**(5):1565–7.

Hoshal, V. L., Jr., R. G. Ause, et al. (1971). "Fibrin sleeve formation on indwelling subclavian central venous catheters." *Arch Surg*, **102**(4):253–8.

Humes, H. D., W. H. Fissell, et al. (2002a). "The bioartificial kidney in the treatment of acute renal failure." *Kidney Int*, **61**(Suppl 80):S121–5.

Humes, H. D., W. H. Fisseli, et al. (2002b). "Metabolic replacement of kidney function in uremic animals with a bioartificial kidney containing human cells." *Am J Kidney Dis*, **39**(5):1078–87.

Humes, H. D., S. M. MacKay, et al. (1999). "Tissue engineering of a bioartificial renal tubule assist device: in vitro transport and metabolic characteristics." *Kidney Int*, **55**(6):2502–14

Hurle, A., P. Llamas, et al. (1997). "Paraplegia complicating intraaortic balloon pumping." *Ann Thorac Surg*, **63**(4):1217–8.

Jeffrey, K. and V. Parsonnet (1998). "Cardiac pacing, 1960–1985: a quarter century of medical and industrial innovation." *Circulation*, **97**(19):1978–91.

Johnson, R. J. (1994). "Complement activation during extracorporeal therapy: biochemistry, cell biology and clinical relevance." *Nephrol Dial Transplant*, **9** (Suppl 2):36–45.

Jones, C. H. (1998). "Continuous renal replacement therapy in acute renal failure: membranes for CRRT." *Artif Organs*, **22**(1):2–7.

Kannan, R. Y., H. J. Salacinski, et al. (2005). "Current status of prosthetic bypass grafts: a review." *J Biomed Mater Res B Appl Biomater*, **74**(1):570–81.

Kantrowitz, A. (1990). "Origins of intraaortic balloon pumping." *Ann Thorac Surg*, **50**(4):672–4.

Kantrowitz, A., P. S. Freed, et al. (1992). "Initial clinical trial of a closed loop, fully automatic intra-aortic balloon pump." *ASAIO J*, **38** (3):M617–21.

Kantrowitz, A., S. Tjonneland, et al. (1968). "Initial clinical experience with intraaortic balloon pumping in cardiogenic shock." *JAMA*, **203**(2):113–8.

Kapadia, M. R., D. A. Popowich, et al. (2008). "Modified prosthetic vascular conduits." *Circulation*, **117**(14):1873–82.

Kasirajan, V., P. M. McCarthy, et al. (2000). "Clinical experience with long-term use of implantable left ventricular assist devices: indications, implantation, and outcomes." *Semin Thorac Cardiovasc Surg*, **12**(3):229–37.

Kaufman, J. S. (2000). "Antithrombotic agents and the prevention of access thrombosis." *Semin Dial*, **13**(1):40–6.

Kirklin, J. K. and W. L. Holman (2006). "Mechanical circulatory support therapy as a bridge to transplant or recovery (new advances)." *Curr Opin Cardiol*, **21**(2):120–6.

Kleine, P., M. Perthel, et al. (2000). "Downstream turbulence and high intensity transient signals (HITS) following aortic valve replacement with Medtronic Hall or St. Jude Medical valve substitutes." *Eur J Cardiothorac Surg*, **17**(1):20–4.

Klinkmann, H. and J. Vienken (1995). "Membranes for dialysis." *Nephrol Dial Transplant*, **10** (Suppl 3):39–45.

Kohler, T. R., J. R. Stratton, et al. (1992). "Conventional versus high-porosity polytetrafluoroethylene grafts: clinical evaluation." *Surgery*, **112**(5):901–7.

Kolff, W. J., H. T. J. Berk, et al., (1944). "The artificial kidney: A dialyzer with a great area." *Acta Med Scanty*, **117**(2):121–134.

Krafczyk, M., M. Cerrolaza, et al. (1998). "Analysis of 3D transient blood flow passing through an artificial aortic valve by Lattice-Boltzmann methods." *J Biomech*, **31**(5):453–62.

Krajcer, Z. and M. H. Howell (2000). "Update on endovascular treatment of peripheral vascular disease: new tools, techniques, and indications." *Tex Heart Inst J*, **27**(4):369–85.

Kuitunen, A. H., L. J. Heikkila, et al. (1997). "Cardiopulmonary bypass with heparin-coated circuits and reduced systemic anticoagulation." *Ann Thorac Surg*, **63**(2):438–44.

Kumano, H., S. Suehiro, et al. (1999). "Coagulofibrinolysis during heparin-coated cardiopulmonary bypass with reduced heparinization." *Ann Thorac Surg*, **68**(4):1252–6.

Kumbasar, S. D., E. Semiz, et al. (1999). "Mechanical complications of intra-aortic balloon counterpulsation." *Int J Cardiol*, **70**(1):69–73.

Kusumoto, F. M. and N. Goldschlager (1996). "Cardiac pacing." *N Engl J Med*, **334**(2):89–97.

L'Heureux, N., N. Dusserre, et al. (2007a). "Technology insight: the evolution of tissue-engineered vascular grafts—from research to clinical practice." *Nat Clin Pract Cardiovasc Med*, **4**(7):389–95.

L'Heureux, N., T. N. McAllister, et al. (2007b). "Tissue-engineered blood vessel for adult arterial revascularization." *N Engl J Med*, **357**(14):1451–3.

L'Heureux, N., S. Paquet, et al. (1998). "A completely biological tissue-engineered human blood vessel." *Faseb J*, **12**(1):47–56.

Laas, J., P. Kleine, et al. (1999). "Orientation of tilting disc and bileaflet aortic valve substitutes for optimal hemodynamics." *Ann Thorac Surg*, **68**(3):1096–9.

Lazar, H. L., Y. Bao, et al. (1999). "Decreased incidence of arterial thrombosis using heparin-bonded intraaortic balloons." *Ann Thorac Surg*, **67**(2):446–9.

Lehner, G., T. Fischlein, et al. (1997). "Endothelialized biological heart valve prostheses in the non-human primate model." *Eur J Cardiothorac Surg*, **11**(3):498–504.

Leon, M. B., P. S. Teirstein, et al. (2001). "Localized intracoronary gamma-radiation therapy to inhibit the recurrence of restenosis after stenting." *N Engl J Med*, **344**(4):250–6.

Leung, S. K. and C. P. Lau (2000). "Developments in sensor-driven pacing." *Cardiol Clin*, **18**(1):113–55, ix.

Leypoldt, J. K. and A. K. Cheung (1996). "Characterization of molecular transport in artificial kidneys." *Artif Organs*, **20**(5):381–9.

Lim, W. L., Y. T. Chew, et al. (1998). "Steady flow dynamics of prosthetic aortic heart valves: a comparative evaluation with PIV techniques." *J Biomech*, **31**(5):411–21.

Londrey, G. L., D. E. Ramsey, et al. (1991). "Infrapopliteal bypass for severe ischemia: comparison of autogenous vein, composite, and prosthetic grafts." *J Vasc Surg*, **13**(5):631–6.

Mackay, J. and G. A. Mensah. (2004). "The atlas of heart disease and stroke." Retrieved May 1st, 2008, from http://www.who.int/cardiovascular diseases/resources/atlas/en/index.html.

Makarewicz, A. J., L. F. Mockros, et al. (1994). "A pumping artificial lung." *ASAIO J*, **40**(3):M518–21.

Makhijani, V. B., H. Q. Yang, et al. (1997). "Three-dimensional coupled fluid-structure simulation of pericardial bioprosthetic aortic valve function." *ASAIO J*, **43**(5):M387–92.

Maki, D. G., L. Cobb, et al. (1988). "An attachable silver-impregnated cuff for prevention of infection with central venous catheters: a prospective randomized multicenter trial." *Am J Med*, **85**(3):307–14.

Maki, D. G., D. M. Kluger, et al. (2006). "The risk of bloodstream infection in adults with different intravascular devices: a systematic review of 200 published prospective studies." *Mayo Clin Proc* , **81**(9):1159–71.

Maki, D. G. and L. A. Mermel (1998). Infections due to infusion therapy. *Hospital Infections*. J. V. Bennett and P. S. Brachman. Philadelphia, PA, USA, Lippincott-Raven Publishers:689–724.

Maki, D. G., S. M. Stolz, et al. (1997). "Prevention of central venous catheter-related bloodstream infection by use of an antiseptic-impregnated catheter. A randomized, controlled trial." *Ann Intern* Med, **127**(4):257–66.

Mareels, G., D. S. De Wachter, et al. (2004). "Computational fluid dynamics-analysis of the Niagara hemodialysis catheter in a right heart model." *Artif Organs*, **28**(7):639–48.

Mareels, G., R. Kaminsky, et al. (2007). "Particle image velocimetry-validated, computational fluid dynamics-based design to reduce shear stress and residence time in central venous hemodialysis catheters." *ASAIO J*, **53**(4):438–46.

Marin, M. G., J. C. Lee, et al. (2000). "Prevention of nosocomial bloodstream infections: effectiveness of antimicrobial-impregnated and heparin-bonded central venous catheters." *Crit Care Med*, **28**(9):3332–8.

Mathers, C. D. and D. Loncar (2006). "Projections of global mortality and burden of disease from 2002 to 2030." *PLoS Med*, **3**(11):e442.

Mattos, M. A., K. J. Hodgson, et al. (1999). "Vascular stents." *Curr Probl Surg*, **36**(12):909–1053.

McCarthy, P. M. and K. Hoercher (2000). "Clinically available intracorporeal left ventricular assist devices," *Prog Cardiovasc Dis*, **43**(1):37–46.

McGiffin, D. C. and J. K. Kirklin (1995). Chapter 32: Cardiopulmonary bypass for cardiac surgery. *Surgery of the Chest*. D. C. Sabiston Jr. and F. C. Spencer. Philadelphia, PA. U.S.A., W.B. Saunders. **V2**:1256–1271.

Mehlhorn, U., A. Kroner, et al. (1999). "30 years clinical intra-aortic balloon pumping: facts and figures." *Thorac Cardiovasc Surg*., **47** (Suppl 2):298–303.

Mendelson, K. and F. I. Schoen (2006). "Heart valve tissue engineering: concepts, approaches, progress, and challenges." *Ann Biomed Eng*, **34**(12):1799–819.

Mermel, L. A., B. M. Farr, et al. (2001). "Guidelines for the management of intravascular catheter-related infections." *Clin Infect Dis*, **32**(9):1249–72.

Merport, M., T. P. Murphy, et al. (2000). "Fibrin sheath stripping versus catheter exchange for the treatment of failed tunneled hemodialysis catheters: randomized clinical trial." *J Vasc Interv Radiol*, **11**(9)**:**1115–20.

Meyer, M. M. (2000). "Renal replacement therapies." *Crit Care Clin*, **16**(1):29–58.

Mitrani, R. D., J. D. Simmons, et al. (1999). "Cardiac pacemakers: current and future status." *Curr Probl Cardiol*, **24**(6):341–420.

Moller, M. and P. Arnsbo (1996). "Appraisal of pacing lead performance from the Danish Pacemaker Register." *Pacing Clin Electrophysiol*, **19**(9):1327–36.

Mond, H. G., M. Irwin, et al. (2004). "The world survey of cardiac pacing and cardioverter defibrillators: calendar year 2001." *Pacing Clin Electrophysiol*, **27**(7):955–64.

Montoya, J. P., C. J. Shanley, et al. (1992). "Plasma leakage through microporous membranes. Role of phospholipids." *ASAIO J*, **38**(3):M399–405.

Morice, M. C., P. W. Serruys, et al. (2002). "A randomized comparison of a sirolimus-eluting stent with a standard stent for coronary revascularization." *N Engl J Med*, **346**(23):1773–80.

Morley-Davies, A. and S. M. Cobbe (1997). "Cardiac pacing." *Lancet*, **349**(9044):41–6.

Morris, M. M., B. H. KenKnight, et al. (1999). "A preview of implantable cardioverter defibrillator systems in the next millennium: an integrative cardiac rhythm management approach." *Am J Cardiol*, **83**(5B):48D–54D.

Moses, J. W., M. B. Leon, et al. (2003). "Sirolimus-eluting stents versus standard stents in patients with stenosis in a native coronary artery." *N Engl J Med*, **349**(14):1315–23.

Mottaghy, K., B. Oedekoven, et al. (1989). "Technical aspects of plasma leakage prevention in microporous capillary membrane oxygenators." *ASAIO Trans*, **35**(3):640–3.

Mueller, X. M., H. T. Tevaearai, et al. (1999). "Thrombogenicity of deflated intraaortic balloon: impact of heparin coating." *Artif Organs*, **23**(2):195–8.

Namyslowski, J. and N. H. Patel (1999). "Central venous access: A new task for interventional radiologists." *Cardiovasc Intervent Radiol*, **22**(5):355–68.

Nield, T. A., D. Langenbacher, et al. (2000). "Neurodevelopmental outcome at 3.5 years of age in children treated with extracorporeal life support: relationship to primary diagnosis." *J Pediatr*, **136**(3):338–44.

Niklason, L. E., J. Gao, et al. (1999). "Functional arteries grown in vitro." *Science*, **284**(5413):489–93.

Norgren, L., W. R. Hiatt, et al. (2007). "Inter-Society Consensus for the Management of Peripheral Arterial Disease (TASC II)." *J Vasc Surg* **45**(Suppl S):S5–67.

O'Grady, N. P., M. Alexander, et al (2002). "Guidelines for the Prevention of Intravascular Catheter-Related Infections." *Clin Infect Dis*, **35**(11):1281–1307.

Oesterle, S. N., R. Whitbourn, et al. (1998). "The stent decade: 1987 to 1997. Stanford Stent Summit faculty." *Am Heart J*, **136**(4 Pt 1):578–99.

Okabe, T., Y. Asakura, et al. (1999). "Evaluation of scaffolding effects of five different types of stents by intravascular ultrasound analysis." *Am J Cardiol*, **84**(9):981–6.

Ovrum, E., G. Tangen, et al. (2003). "Heparin-coated circuits (Duraflo II) with reduced versus full anticoagulation during coronary artery bypass surgery." *J Card Surg*, **18**(2):140–6.

Owings, M. F. and L. Lawrence (1999). "Detailed diagnoses and procedures, National Hospital Discharge Survey, 1997." *Vital Health Stat*, **13**(145):1–157.

Palder, S. B., R. L. Kirkman, et al. (1985). "Vascular access for hemodialysis. Patency rates and results of revision." *Ann Surg*, **202**(2):235–9.

Park, P. K., B. E. Jarrell, et al. (1990). "Thrombus-free, human endothelial surface in the midregion of a Dacron vascular graft in the splanchnic venous circuit—observations after nine months of implantation." *J Vasc Surg*, **11**(3):468–75.

Pasquinelli, G., A. Freyrie, et al. (1990). "Healing of prosthetic arterial grafts." *Scanning Micros*, **4**(2):351–62.

Pearson, M. L. (1996). "Guideline for prevention of intravascular device-related infections. Part I. Intravascular device-related infections: an overview. The Hospital Infection Control Practices Advisory Committee." *Am J Infect Control*, **24**(4):262–77.

Peek, G. J., F. Clemens, et al. (2006). "CESAR: conventional ventilatory support vs extracorporeal membrane oxygenation for severe adult respiratory failure." *BMC Health Serv Res*, **6**:163.

Pertosa, G., G. Grandaliano, et al. (2000). "Clinical relevance of cytokine production in hemodialysis." *Kidney Int*, **58**(Suppl 76):Sl04–11.

Pinski, S. L. and R. G. Trohman (2000). "Permanent pacing via implantable defibrillators." *Pacing Clin Electrophysiol*, **23**(11 Pt l):1667–82.

Raad, I. (1998). "Intravascular-catheter-related infections." *Lancet*, **351** (9106):893–8.

Raad, I., R. Darouiche, et al. (1997). "Central venous catheters coated with minocycline and rifampin for the prevention of catheter-related colonization and bloodstream infections. A randomized, double-blind trial. The Texas Medical Center Catheter Study Group." *Ann Intern Med*, **127**(4):267–74.

Rais-Bahrami, K., A. E. Wagner, et al. (2000). "Neurodevelopmental outcome in ECMO vs near-miss ECMO patients at 5 years of age." *Clin Pediatr (Phila)*, **39**(3):145–52.

Reeder, G. D., M. J. Gartner, et al. (1998) Membrane apparatus with enhanced mass transfer, heat transfer, and pumping capabilities via active mixing. U.S.A. **Patent 6,217,826**. Sep 21, 1998.

Robinson, D. A., A. Lennox, et al. (1999). "Graft dilatation following abdominal aortic aneurysm resection and grafting." *Aust N Z J Surg*, **69**(12):849–51.

Rockall, A. G., A. Harris, et al. (1997). "Stripping of failing haemodialysis catheters using the Ampitaz gooseneck snare." *Clin Radiol*, **52**(8):616–20.

Rogers, C. and E. R. Edelman (1995). "Endovascular stent design dictates experimental restenosis and thrombosis." *Circulation*, **91**(12):2995–3001.

Ronco, C., M. Ballestri, et al. (2000). "New developments in hemodialyzers." *Blood Purif*, **18**(4): 267–75.

Rosamond, W., K. Flegal, et al. (2008). "Heart Disease and Stroke Statistics—2008 Update: A Report From the American Heart Association Statistics Committee and Stroke Statistics Subcommittee." *Circulation*, **117**(4):e25–146.

Rose, E. A., A. C. Gelijns, et al. (2001). "Long-term mechanical left ventricular assistance for end-stage heart failure." *N Engl J Med*, **345**(20):1435–43.

Rosenthal, M. B. (2007). "Nonpayment for performance? Medicare's new reimbursement rule" *N Engl J Med*, **357**(16):1573–5.

Roy, B. J., P. Rycus, et al. (2000). "The changing demographics of neonatal extracorporeal membrane oxygenation patients reported to the Extracorporeal Life Support Organization (ELSO) Registry." *Pediatrics*, **106**(6):1334–8.

Saito, N., S. Motoyama, et al. (2000). "Effects of new polymer-coated extracorporeal circuits on biocompatibility during cardiopulmonary bypass." *Artif Organs*, **24**(7):547–54.

Salem, D. N., P. D. Stein, et al. (2004). "Antithrombotic therapy in valvular heart disease—native and prosthetic: the Seventh ACCP Conference on Antithrombotic and Thrombolytic Therapy." *Chest*, **126**(3 Suppl):457S–482S.

Sauren, L. D., R. E. Accord, et al. (2007). "Combined Impella and intra-aortic balloon pump support to improve both ventricular unloading and coronary blood flow for myocardial recovery: an experimental study." *Artif Organs*, **31**(11):839–42.

Sauvage, L. R., K. Berger, et al. (1975). "Presence of endothelium in an axillary-femoral graft of knitted Dacron with an external velour surface." *Ann Surg*, **182**(6):749–53.

Sauvage, L. R., K. E. Berger, et al. (1974). "Interspecies healing of porous arterial prostheses: observations, 1960 to 1974." *Arch Surg*, **109**(5):698–705.

Schachinger, V., C. W. Hamm, et al. (2003), "A randomized trial of polytetrafluoroethylene-membrane-covered stents compared with conventional stents in aortocoronary saphenous vein grafts." *J Am Coll Cardiol*, **42**(8):1360–9.

Schetz, M. (1999). "Non-renal indications for continuous renal replacement therapy." *Kidney Int*, **52**(Suppl 72): S88–94.

Schillinger, F., D. Schillinger, et al. (1991). "Post catheterisation vein stenosis in haemodialysis: comparative angiographic study of 50 subclavian and 50 internal jugular accesses." *Nephrol Dial Transplant*, **6**(10):722–4.

Schmidt, J. A. and L. J. Stotts (1998). "Bipolar pacemaker leads: new materials, new technology." *J Invest Surg*, **11**(1):75–81.

Schoen, F. J. and R. J. Levy (1999). "Founder's Award, 25th Annual Meeting of the Society for Biomaterials, perspectives. Providence, RI, April 28-May 2, 1999. Tissue heart valves: current challenges and future research perspectives." *J Biomed Mater Res*, **47**(4):439–65.

Scholz, K. H., S. Ragab, et al. (1998). "Complications of intra-aortic balloon counterpulsation. The role of catheter size and duration of support in a multivariate analysis of risk." *Eur Heart J*, **19**(3):458–65.

Schwab, S. J. and G. Beathard (1999). "The hemodialysis catheter conundrum: hate living with them, but can't live without them." *Kidney Int*, **56**(1):1–17.

Schwartz, R. S., K. C. Huber, et al. (1992). "Restenosis and the proportional neointimal response to coronary artery injury: results in a porcine model." *J Am Coll Cardiol*, **19**(2):267–74.

Seeger, J. M. (2000). "Management of patients with prosthetic vascular graft infection." *Am Surg*, **66**(2):166–77.

Serruys, P. W., P. de Jaegere, et al. (1994). "A comparison of balloon-expandable-stent implantation with balloon angioplasty in patients with coronary artery disease. Benestent Study Group." *N Engl J Med*, **331**(8):489–95.

Serruys, P. W., M. J. Kutryk, et al. (2006). "Coronary-artery stents." *N Engl J Med*, **354**(5):483–95.

Shimamoto, A., S. Kanemitsu, et al. (2000). "Biocompatibility of silicone-coated oxygenator in cardiopulmonary bypass." *Ann Thorac Surg*, **69**(1):115–20.

Shimono, T., Y. Shomura, et al. (1996). "Experimental evaluation of a newly developed ultrathin silicone layer coated hollow fiber oxygenator." *ASAIO J*, **42**(5):M451–4.

Shin'oka, T., G. Matsumura, et al. (2005). "Midterm clinical result of tissue-engineered vascular autografts seeded with autologous bone marrow cells." *J Thorac Cardiovasc Surg*, **l29**(6):1330–8.

Shinoka, T., P. X. Ma, et al. (1996). "Tissue-engineered heart valves. Autologous valve leaflet replacement study in a lamb model." *Circulation*, **94**(9 Suppl):II164–8.

Sitges-Serra, A. (1999). "Strategies for prevention of catheter-related bloodstream infections." *Support Care Cancer*, **7**(6):391–5.

Slaughter, M. S., M. A. Sobieski, et al. (2007a). "Home discharge experience with the Thoratec TLC-II portable driver." *ASAIO J*, **53**(2):132–5.

Slaughter, M. S., S. S. Tsui, et al. (2007b). "Results of a multicenter clinical trial with the Thoratec Implantable Ventricular Assist Device." *J Thorac Cardiovasc Surg*, **133**(6):1573–80.

Smith, S. C., Jr., T. E. Feldman, et al. (2006). "ACC/AHA/SCAI 2005 Guideline Update for Percutaneous Coronary Intervention: A Report of the American College of Cardiology/American Heart Association Task Force on Practice Guidelines (ACC/AHA/SCAI Writing Committee to Update the 2001 Guidelines for Percutaneous Coronary Intervention)." *J Am Coll Cardiol*, **47**(l):el–121.

Sobieski, M. A., T. A. George, et al. (2004). "The Thoratec mobile computer: initial in-hospital and outpatient experience." *ASAIO J*, **50**(4):373–5.

Sodian, R., S. P. Hoerstrup, et al. (2000). "Early in vivo experience with tissue-engineered trileaflet heart valves." *Circulation*, **102**(19 Suppl 3):III22–9.

Stammers, A. H. (1997). "Historical aspects of cardiopulmonary bypass: from antiquity to acceptance." *J Cardiothorac Vasc Anesth*, **11**(3):266–74.

Stankovic, G., A. Colombo, et al. (2003). "Randomized evaluation of polytetrafluoroethylene-covered stent in saphenous vein grafts: the Randomized Evaluation of polytetrafluoroethylene COVERed stent in Saphenous vein grafts (RECOVERS) Trial." *Circulation*, **108**(1)**:**37–42.

Stavarski, D. H. (1996). "Complications of intra-aortic balloon pumping. Preventable or not preventable?" *Crit Care Nurs Clin North Am*, **8**(4):409–21.

Stevenson, L. W., R. L. Kormos, et al. (2001). "Mechanical cardiac support 2000: current applications and future trial design. June 15–16, 2000 Bethesda, Maryland." *J Am Coll Cardiol*, **37**(1):340–70.

Stone, G. W., S. G. Ellis, et al. (2004). "A polymer-based, paclitaxel-eluting stent in patients with coronary artery disease." *N Engl J Med*, **350**(3):221–31.

Sullivan, T. M., S. M. Taylor, et al. (2002). "Has endovascular surgery reduced the number of open vascular operations performed by an established surgical practice?" *J Vasc Surg*, **36**(3):514–9.

Svennevig, J. L. (2000). "Off-pump vs on-pump surgery. A review." *Scand Cardiovasc J*, **34**(1):7–11.

Svitek, R. G., B. J. Frankowski, et al. (2005). "Evaluation of a pumping assist lung that uses a rotating fiber bundle." *ASAIOJ*, **51**(6):773–80.

Thomas, C. L., Ed. (1989), *Taber's Cyclopedic Medical Dictionary*. Philadelphia, PA, U.S.A., F.A. Davis Co.

Thomas, M. R. (2005). "Brachytherapy: here today, gone tomorrow?" *Heart*, **91** (Suppl 3): iii32–4.

TMI Study Group (1985). "The Thrombolysis in Myocardial Infarction (TIMI) trial. Phase I findings." *N Engl J Med*, **312**(14):932–6.

Torchiana, D. F., G. Hirsch, et at. (1997). "Intraaortic balloon pumping for cardiac support: trends in practice and outcome, 1968 to 1995." *J Thorac Cardiovasc Surg*, **113**(4)758–64; discussion 764–9.

Trerotola, S. O. (2000). "Hemodialysis catheter placement and management." Radiology, **215**(3):651–8.

Triolo, P. M. and J. D. Andrade (1983a). "Surface modification and characterization of some commonly used catheter materials. II. Friction characterization." *J Biomed Mater Res*, **17**(1):149–65.

Triolo, P. M. and J. D. Andrade (1983b). "Surface modification and evaluation of some commonly used catheter materials. I. Surface properties." *J Biomed Mater Res*, **17**(1):129–47.

Tumlin, J., R. Wali, et al. (2008). "Efficacy and safety of renal tubule cell therapy for acute renal failure." *J Am Soc Nephrol*, **19**(5):1034–40.

Turco, M. A., M. Buchbinder, et al. (2006). "Pivotal, randomized U.S. study of the Symbiottrade mark covered stent system in patients with saphenous vein graft disease: eight-month angiographic and clinical results from the Symbiot III trial." *Catheter Cardiovasc Interv*, **68**(3):379–88.

Twardowski, Z. J. (1998). "High-dose intradialytic urokinase to restore the patency of permanent central vein hemodialysis catheters." *Am J Kidney Dis*, **31**(5):841–7.

Tyers, G. F., P. Mills, et al. (1997). "Bipolar leads for use with permanently implantable cardiac pacing systems: a review of limitations of traditional and coaxial configurations and the development and testing of new conductor, insulation, and, electrode designs." *J Invest Surg*, **10**(1–2):1–15.

US Renal Data System (2000). USRDS 2000 Annual Data Report: National Institute of Diabetes and Digestive and Kidney Diseases, National Institutes of Health, Bethesda, MD, U.S.A.

US Renal Data System (2007). USRDS 2007 Annual Data Report: Atlas of Chronic Kidney Disease and End-Stage Renal Disease in the United States. National Institute of Diabetes and Digestive and Kidney Diseases, National Institutes of Health, Bethesda, MD, U.S.A.

Valles, J., C. Leon, et al. (1997). "Nosocomial bacteremia in critically ill patients: a multicenter study evaluating epidemiology and prognosis. Spanish Collaborative Group for Infections in Intensive Care Units of Sociedad Espanola de Medicina Intensive y Unidades Coronarias (SEMIUC)." *Clin Infect Dis*, **24**(3):387–95.

Van Belle, E., S. Susen, et al. (2007). "Drug-eluting stents: trading restenosis for thrombosis?" *J Thromb Haemost,* **5** (Suppl 1):238–45.

Vaucher, Y. E., G. G. Dudell, et al. (1996). "Predictors of early childhood outcome in candidates for extracorporeal membrane oxygenation." *J Pediatr*, **128**(1):109–17.

Veith, F. J., S. K. Gupta, et al. (1986). "Six-year prospective multicenter randomized comparison of autologous saphenous vein and expanded polytetrafluoroethylene grafts in infrainguinal arterial reconstructions." *J Vasc Surg*, **3**(1):104–14.

Verin, V., Y. Popowski, et al. (2001). "Endoluminal beta-radiation therapy for the prevention of coronary restenosis after balloon angioplasty. The Dose-Finding Study Group." *N Engl J Med*, **344**(4):243–9.

Virmani, R. and A. Farb (1999). "Pathology of in-stent restenosis." *Curr Opin Lipidol*, **10**(6):499–506.

Vongpatanasin, W., L. D. Hillis, et al. (1996). "Prosthetic heart valves." *N Engl J Med*, **335**(6):407–16.

Wagner, W. R., P. C. Johnson, et al. (1993). "Evaluation of bioprosthetic valve-associated thrombus in ventricular assist device patients." *Circulation*, **88**(5 Pt 1):2023–9.

Waksman, R. (1999). "Intracoronary radiation therapy for restenosis prevention: status of the clinical trials." *Cardiovasc Radiat Med*, **1**(1):20–9.

Watanabe, H., J. Hayashi, et al. (1999). "Biocompatibility of a silicone-coated polypropylene hollow fiber oxygenator in an in vitro model." *Ann Thorac Surg*, **67**(5):1315–9.

Weeks, S. M. (2002). "Unconventional venous access." *Tech Vasc Interv Radiol*, **5**(2):114–20.

Wegner, J. A. (1997). "Oxygenator anatomy and function." *J Cardiothorac Vasc Anesth*, **11**(3):275–81.

Wendel, H. P. and G. Ziemer (1999). "Coating-techniques to improve the hemocompatibility of artificial devices used for extracorporeal circulation." *Eur J Cardiothorac Surg*, **16**(3):342–50.

Wesolowski, S. A., C. C. Fries, et al. (1961). "Porosity: primary determinant of ultimate fate of synthetic vascular grafts." *Surgery*, **50**:91–6.

Williams, S. K., T. Carter, et al. (1992). "Formation of a multilayer cellular lining on a polyurethane vascular graft following endothelial cell sodding." *J Biomed Mater Res*, **26**(1):103–17.

Willman, V. L., J. M. Anderson, et al. (1999). Expert panel review of the NHLBI Total Artificial Heart (TAH) Program June 1998–November 1999. National Heart Lung and Blood Institute, National Institutes of Health, Bethesda, MD, USA: 28pp.

Wilson, W., K. A. Taubert, et al. (2007). "Prevention of infective endocarditis: guidelines from the American Heart Association: a guideline from the American Heart Association Rheumatic Fever, Endocarditis, and Kawasaki Disease Committee, Council on Cardiovascular Disease in the Young, and the Council on Clinical Cardiology, Council on Cardiovascular Surgery and Anesthesia, and the Quality of Care and Outcomes Research Interdisciplinary Working Group." *Circulation*, **116**(15):1736–54.

Windecker, S. (2007). "Percutaneous left ventricular assist devices for treatment of patients with cardiogenic shock." *Curr Opin Crit Care*, **13**(5):521–7.

Windecker, S. and B. Meier (2007). "Late coronary stent thrombosis." *Circulation*, **116**(17):1952–65.

Winters, K. J., S. C. Smith, et al. (1999). "Reduction in ischemic vascular complications with a hydrophilic-coated intra-aortic balloon catheter." *Catheter Cardiovasc Interv*, **46**(3):357–62.

Yun, K. L., C. F. Sintek, et al. (1999). "Randomized trial of partial versus complete chordal preservation methods of mitral valve replacement: A preliminary report." *Circulation*, **100**(19 Suppl):II90–4.

Zapol, W. M., M. T. Snider, et al. (1979). "Extracorporeal membrane oxygenation in severe acute respiratory failure. A randomized prospective study." *JAMA*, **242**(20):2193–6.

Zilla, P., D. Bezuidenhout, et al. (2007). "Prosthetic vascular grafts: Wrong models, wrong questions and no healing." *Biomaterials*, **28**(34):5009–27.

Zilla, P., J. Brink, et al. (2008). "Prosthetic heart valves: catering for the few." *Biomaterials*, **29**(4):385–406.

CHAPTER 4
DESIGN OF RESPIRATORY DEVICES

David M. Shade
Johns Hopkins Hospital, Baltimore, Maryland

Arthur T. Johnson
University of Maryland, College Park, Maryland

4.1 INTRODUCTION

Respiratory medical devices generally fall into categories designed to measure volume, flow, pressure, or gas concentration. Many of these devices have been used in some form for many years, so design is both sophisticated and incremental. A thorough knowledge of pulmonary physiology and existing devices can be very helpful when proposing improvements. Most respiratory devices are composed of one or more simpler components, often linked to a processing unit of some type, such as a standalone personal computer (PC). Remarkably varied and sophisticated diagnostic instruments can be constructed from these basic building blocks combined with values, tubing, pumps, and mouthpieces.

4.2 PULMONARY PHYSIOLOGY

Before delving too deeply into the instrumentation, it will be helpful to review briefly the function of the respiratory system and the parameters most often measured in pulmonary medicine.

The human respiratory system is composed of two lungs contained within the thorax, or chest-cavity. The primary function of the lungs is gas exchange with the blood, providing a continuous source of oxygen for transport to body tissues, and eliminating carbon dioxide produced as a waste product of cellular metabolism. Gas exchange occurs in the alveoli, tiny thin-walled air-filled sacs numbering approximately 300 million in normal adult lungs. The alveoli are connected to the outside environment through a system of conducting airways that ends with the oral and nasal cavities. Alveoli are surrounded by and in close proximity to pulmonary capillaries, the tiny vessels containing blood to participate in gas exchange. The network of alveoli and airways is interdependent, so that the walls of the alveoli are shared among neighboring lung units.

Inspiration of fresh air occurs when respiratory muscles, chiefly the diaphragm, contract, expanding the chest wall and decreasing slightly the pressure surrounding the lungs but within the chest cavity (the *pleural pressure*). This drop in pleural pressure tends to pull outward on the outer lung surfaces, which in turn pull outward on more central lung units due to interdependence, and so on, with the result that the pressure within the alveolar air spaces falls. When alveolar pressure falls below the surrounding atmospheric pressure, air flows down the pressure gradient, filling the alveoli with inspired gas. Because lung tissue is elastic, it will tend to deflate when inspiratory muscle forces are released. In a normal person at rest, expiration is a passive phase and requires no muscular activity.

If all of a person's muscles were paralyzed and the lung was then permitted to empty, the lung volume would decrease to the *functional residual capacity* (FRC). At this volume, lung elasticity tends to favor further emptying, but the chest wall favors expansion. At higher volumes, both structures favor emptying (see Fig. 4.1). FRC, then, represents an equilibrium between the tendency of the lungs to empty further and the tendency of the chest wall to spring outward. In order to decrease the volume of the lung below FRC, expiratory muscles must be used to contract the chest wall and increase the pleural pressure. When the lung is emptied as much as is possible, there remains trapped within the alveoli and airways a volume of gas termed the *residual volume* (RV). The gas becomes trapped when the airways through which gas must travel collapse due to the high pleural pressure surrounding them. The amount of additional gas that may be expired with effort after the lung has reached FRC is termed the *expiratory reserve volume* (ERV). Thus, FRC is the sum of RV and ERV (FRC = RV + ERV).

During quiet breathing, passive expiration ends at FRC as the lung and chest wall reach equilibrium. The subsequent inspiration will increase the lung's volume by an amount termed the *tidal volume* (TV), which is typically about 500 mL for an adult at rest. Of course, the normal resting breath is far smaller than a deep breath; a maximum inspiration occurs when the lung is inflated to the *total lung capacity* (TLC), the largest volume that can be contained within the lung. TLC is determined by the balance between the increasing recoil (or "pull") of the lung and chest wall as they are inflated and the decreasing strength of the muscles as they are stretched. The difference between the TLC and the RV is termed the *vital capacity* (VC) and represents the largest volume of gas that can be

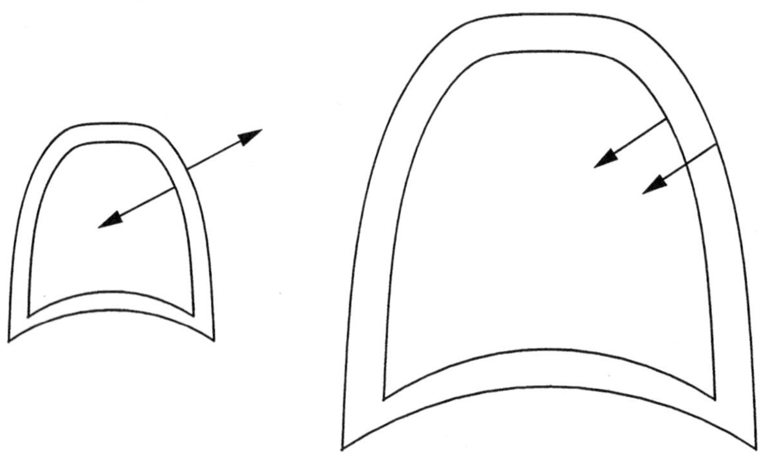

A B

FIGURE 4.1 At lower volumes (*a*), the lung favors emptying but the chest wall favors expansion. At higher volumes (*b*), both the lung and the chest wall favor emptying. The resting volume of the lung is above the residual volume; the resting volume of the chest wall is typically about 60 percent of TLC.

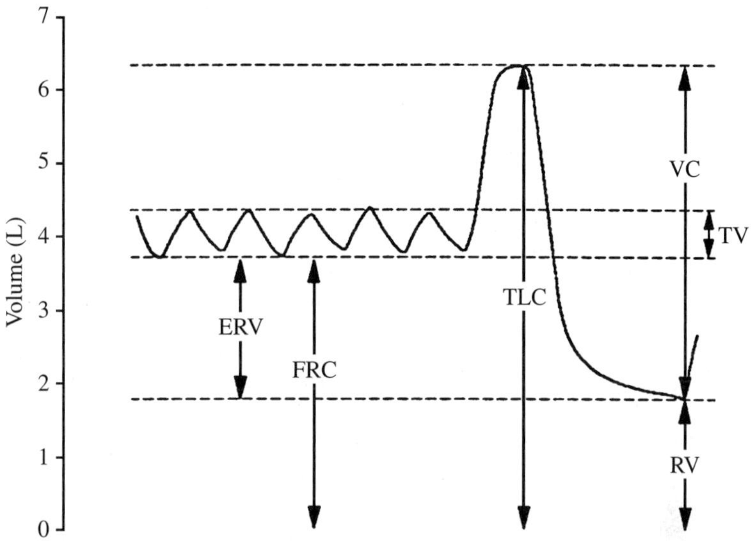

FIGURE 4.2 Spirometer tracings showing the lung volumes. Note that since the zero point of the spirometer may be set arbitrarily, only volumes not depending on zero (VC, TV, and ERV in this figure) may be measured directly.

exhaled, starting from full inflation, in a single breath. Thus, TLC = RV + VC. Figure 4.2 shows a diagram of the various lung volumes and capacities.

Unlike TV, which is determined in large part by effort and ventilatory drive, TLC, RV, and VC are parameters that reflect certain properties of the pulmonary physiology. For example, a condition tending to increase the propensity of the airways to collapse would tend to increase the RV, and thereby decrease the VC, without changing the TLC. Asthmatics, in fact, may exhibit just this propensity during an asthma attack. Likewise, a condition increasing the elasticity (or "stiffness") of the lung would tend to decrease the TLC, and perhaps the VC, as the muscles became unable to supply sufficient force for continued inspiration. One condition causing such a change is asbestosis. Measurement of the various static lung volumes can be helpful both in classifying a lung disease and in tracking its progress or responsiveness to treatment.

During the process of ventilation, gases must travel through the airways linking the alveoli with the nose and mouth. These airways impose a pneumatic resistance to the flow of air, which, similar to an electrical resistance limiting current, reduces the flow for a given pressure gradient. During quiet breathing, most of the resistance to airflow occurs in the upper airway and not in the smaller airways within the lung. The resistance of the airways themselves is affected by the volume of the lung at the time of measurement, because as the lung approaches full inflation, the airways are stretched radially, achieving their greatest diameter and hence their lowest resistance. Another lung parameter affecting both static and dynamic changes is the lung compliance, a measure of tissue elasticity. The compliance is defined as the change in volume divided by the change in pressure across the wall of the lung, has units of volume over pressure, and is typically measured as the slope of a plot of lung volume against transmural pressure. Even in a person having normal muscle strength, it is possible to have marked reductions in the static lung volumes (such as TLC, VC, and RV) because of increases in the stiffness of the lung tissue. Like the resistance, compliance depends on the volume of gas contained within the lung. As the lung volume approaches TLC, it takes considerably greater pressure to continue inflation when compared with similar inflations taken nearer to FRC, representing a reduction in lung compliance at higher lung volumes.

Similar to electrical resistance and capacitance, airway resistance and lung compliance together impose a frequency-dependent impedance to ventilation. Thus, the normal lung emptying passively follows an exponential decay with a single time constant equal to the product of the resistance and the compliance. Because the lung is composed of millions of lung units, potentially having regional differences in impedance, dynamic characteristics of ventilation affect how quickly the lung may inflate or deflate, and may also result in portions of the lung being underventilated, while other portions are either normally ventilated or even overventilated.

In addition to ventilating the alveoli, another important function of the respiratory system is gas exchange, the process of moving oxygen into and carbon dioxide from the blood supply. Gas exchange occurs through the passive diffusion of gases across the alveolar membrane. Diffusive gas exchange is affected by the thickness and permeability of the alveolar membrane, the total surface area available for diffusion, and the availability of blood flow to receive or deliver the diffused gases. One common pulmonary test, the *diffusion capacity*, indirectly assesses the alveolar membrane by measuring the diffusion of carbon monoxide from the lungs into the blood. Of course, gas exchange can occur only with gas that has actually reached the alveoli, which is considerably less than the amount of gas moving through the nose and mouth. In fact, in a normal person at rest, only about two-thirds of the air inspired in a single breath reaches the alveoli. The remaining one-third occupies the *dead space*, portions of the lung, airways, and nasopharynx that do not participate in gas exchange. In certain conditions, alveoli that are ventilated may not participate in gas exchange due to aberrations in diffusion or to alterations in blood flow that reduce or eliminate perfusion. These nonexchanging alveoli increase the *physiologic dead space* (as distinguished from *anatomic dead space*, which comprises the mouth, nasopharynx, trachea, and other conducting airways) and reduce the alveolar ventilation. Dead space ventilation, then, is "wasted" ventilation and must be subtracted from the total ventilation in order to determine the effective alveolar ventilation.

Once the pulmonary circulation has undergone gas exchange with ventilated alveoli, the oxygen-enriched blood circulates to body tissues, which consume the oxygen and replace it with carbon dioxide. The net consumption of oxygen ($\dot{V}_{O_2}$) is not equal to the net respiratory production of carbon dioxide ($\dot{V}_{CO_2}$), owing to the fact that cellular metabolic pathways do not maintain a 1:1 balance between the two, and also to the fact that carbon dioxide may be excreted in the urine as well as through the respiratory system. At rest, the ratio of $\dot{V}_{CO_2}$ to $\dot{V}_{O_2}$, the *respiratory quotient* (RQ), is typically 0.7. During maximum exercise, this value may rise to well above 1.0. Measurements of $\dot{V}_{O_2}$, $\dot{V}_{CO_2}$, and RQ are important in assessing the adequacy of nutrition of a critically ill patient, the diagnosis and treatment of patients with various pulmonary and cardiovascular diseases, and the training of elite athletes.

Most of the physiological parameters related to the respiratory system vary across age groups, gender, and ethnicity, and most are affected significantly by the size of the individual being assessed (large people tend to have large lungs). Therefore, interpreting the meaning of measured parameters often relies on comparing results with those obtained in large population studies of "normal" (disease-free) people of similar characteristics. There are many sources for the equations available to predict these normal values. While many devices attempt to include information about the predicted values, the most useful devices will allow the user to choose from among many sets.

4.3 IMPORTANT PRINCIPLES OF GAS PHYSICS

Most measurements made in the context of the respiratory system assume that the gas or gas mixture involved obeys the *ideal gas law*:

$$PV = nRT \tag{4.1}$$

where P = pressure (atmospheres, atm)
V = volume (liters, L)
n = moles of gas (mol)
T = temperature (kelvin, K)
R = gas constant [= 0.082057 (atm • L)/(mol • K)]

TABLE 4.1 Constituents of Air

	Ambient		Inspired		Alveolar		Expired	
	mmHg	%	mmHg	%	mmHg	%	mmHg	%
Nitrogen (N_2)	584.1	76.86	556.8	73.26	566.2	74.50	583.7	76.80
Oxygen (O_2)	156.6	20.60	149.2	19.64	100.0	13.16	103.1	13.56
Carbon dioxide (CO_2)	0.2	0.03	0.2	0.03	40.0	5.26	41.2	5.43
Water (H_2O)	12.0	1.58	47.0	6.18	47.0	6.18	25.0	3.29
Other	7.1	0.93	6.8	0.89	6.8	0.89	7.0	0.92

Assume ambient temperature of 24°C, ambient relative humidity of 50%, barometric pressure of 760 mmHg, and body temperature of 37°C.

The amount of each gas present in a mixture of gases may be represented conveniently in several ways: by its percentage (or fraction) of the whole, by its absolute volume in a known total volume, or by its partial pressure. The partial pressure of a gas in a mixture is the pressure that would be exerted by that gas on the walls of its container in the absence of all other gases. According to *Dalton's law*, the sum of the partial pressures of all gases present in a mixture is equal to the total pressure exerted by the mixture. For a gas mixture at atmospheric pressure, then,

$$P_B = \sum_{i=1}^{N} P_i \tag{4.2}$$

where P_B = the ambient atmospheric pressure (typically ~760 mmHg at sea level)
P_i = the partial pressure of the ith species
N = the total number of gases present in the mixture

The fractional concentration of a species is simply its partial pressure divided by the total pressure. Typical components of inspired and expired air are shown in Table 4.1.

Special note must be made of the presence of water vapor as it presents an often-overlooked factor. The amount of water a gas mixture is *capable* of containing is limited by the availability of water and the temperature of the mixture. The relative humidity measures the percentage of this upper limit actually achieved. The relationship between temperature and the maximum possible partial pressure of water has been determined empirically; one suitable equation over common temperature ranges is

$$P_{H_2O} = 14.47 - 0.705T + 0.0428T^2 \tag{4.3}$$

where P_{H_2O} is partial pressure of water vap or (mmHg) and T is temperature (degrees Celsius).

At room temperature, the maximum possible P_{H_2O} is approximately 25 mmHg. The maximum possible P_{H_2O} rises to about 47 mmHg as the temperature rises to normal body temperature (37°C). Thus, upon inspiration, a sample of air is warmed and humidified, while expiration leads to cooling and condensation of excess water vapor. This is important for several reasons. First, the concentration of a gas as it exists within the lung differs from that in the air prior to inspiration or following expiration, as it is diluted or concentrated by changes in water vapor concentration. Second, even if a known fixed volume of gas is injected into the lung, such as by a ventilator, the volume of the lung does not increase by that same volume. Lastly, a warm moist gas which is exhaled undergoes cooling and condensation, and even if rewarmed will not reach 100 percent relative humidity and will therefore contain less water than initially, unless a source of water is available as the gas is rewarmed.

The combined effects of changes in temperature, pressure, and water vapor concentration are frequently accounted for by applying an appropriate correction factor, calculated as shown in Table 4.2.

TABLE 4.2 Gas Conversion Factors (Volume and Flow)

To convert from	To	Multiply by: Formula	Multiply by: Typical value
ATPS	BTPS	$\frac{BP - pH_2O}{BP - 47} \cdot \frac{310}{273 + T}$	1.080
	STPD	$\frac{BP - pH_2O}{760} \cdot \frac{273}{273 + T}$	0.892
	ATPD	$\frac{BP - pH_2O}{BP}$	0.971
ATPD	BTPS	$\frac{BP}{BP - 47} \cdot \frac{310}{273 + T}$	1.113
	STPD	$\frac{BP}{760} \cdot \frac{273}{273 + T}$	0.919
	ATPS	$\frac{BP}{BP - pH_2O}$	1.030
BTPS	STPD	$\frac{BP - 47}{760} \cdot \frac{273}{310}$	0.826
	ATPS	$\frac{BP - 47}{BP - pH_2O} \cdot \frac{273 + T}{310}$	0.926
	ATPD	$\frac{BP - 47}{BP} \cdot \frac{273 + T}{310}$	0.899
STPD	BTPS	$\frac{760}{BP - 47} \cdot \frac{310}{273}$	1.210
	ATPS	$\frac{760}{BP - pH_2O} \cdot \frac{273 + T}{273}$	1.121
	ATPD	$\frac{760}{BP} \cdot \frac{273 + T}{273}$	1.088

BP = barometric pressure
T = temperature (°C)
ATPS = ambient temperature and pressure, saturated
ATPD = ambient temperature and pressure, dry
STPD = standard temperature and pressure, dry
BTPS = body temperature and pressure, saturated

The "typical values" assume a barometric pressure of 760 mmHg and a temperature of 24°C.
Standard pressure is 760 mmHg and standard temperature is 0°C (= 273 K).
Body temperature is 37°C (= 310 K).

Under ideal conditions, seldom encountered, gas flowing through a straight tube would exhibit only *laminar flow* (the absence of all turbulence). In laminar flow, every molecule in the gas stream has only axial velocity, and moves only in the direction of the bulk flow. Under conditions of complete turbulence, the gas molecules move in all directions, with no net flow. Flows encountered in practice exhibit some characteristics of both laminarity and turbulence (Fig. 4.3). Factors tending to favor increasing turbulence include decreasing tube radius, increasing gas density, and increasing bulk flow rate. Turbulence is increased by sharp angles and geometric obstructions in the gas stream. Laminar flow is increased by having a straight, smooth-bore tube with a length at least 6 times its diameter prior to flow measurement.

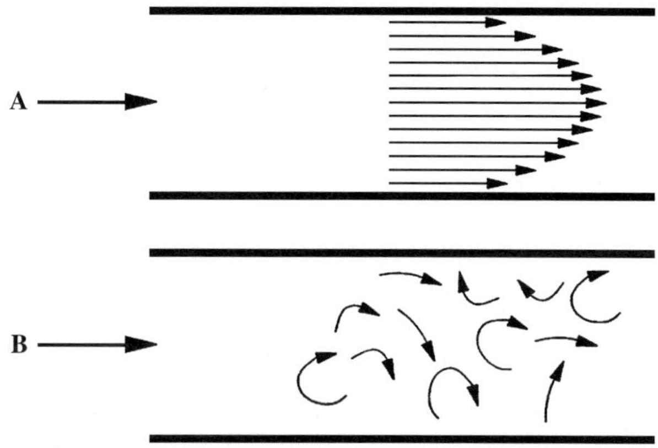

FIGURE 4.3 Representations of laminar (*a*) and turbulent (*b*) flow through a straight tube. With laminar flow, the pressure drop across a length of tube is proportional to the flow. With turbulence, the pressure approaches proportionality with the square of flow. The velocity profile under laminar flow conditions is parabolic, with higher flows near the center of the tube than near the boundary.

The pressure required to move gas along a straight tube under conditions of laminar flow is given by the Poiseuille equation:

$$\Delta P = \frac{\dot{V} 8 \eta l}{\pi r^4} \tag{4.4}$$

where ΔP = pressure drop
$\dot{V}$ = flow
η = gas viscosity
l = length of tube
r = radius of tube

Thus, for a given straight tube, the Poiseuille equation predicts a linear relationship between pressure and flow and gives rise to the pneumatic analog of Ohm's law:

$$\Delta P = \dot{V} R \qquad \text{(compare with } \Delta V = IR\text{)} \tag{4.5}$$

where R is resistance, given by $8\eta l/\pi r^4$.

This Ohm's law representation of the pressure-flow relationship forms the basis for measurements of airways resistance and is the principle on which several flow-measuring devices are based. The pressure required to move gas under conditions of turbulence is always greater than that required to achieve the same flow under laminar conditions, as additional pressure (or energy) is required to accelerate molecules in directions other than the direction of bulk flow. This will be manifested as an upward curve and deviation from linearity on a plot of flow (x axis) versus pressure drop (y axis).

Turbulence in flow through a straight tube may be estimated by calculating the *Reynold's number:*

$$N_R = \frac{2 s r \rho}{\eta} \tag{4.6}$$

where N_R = Reynold's number
s = linear velocity of flow
ρ = gas density

and other variables are as shown above.

Reynold's numbers greater than 2000 are predictive of significant turbulence. It should be noted that while turbulent flow depends on both gas density and viscosity, laminar flow depends only on viscosity.

4.4 DEVICE COMPONENTS

4.4.1 Volume

Gas volumes may be measured directly using one of several volume-displacement *spirometers*. The simplest and oldest design, the water-sealed spirometer, uses a hollow cylinder, or bell, which is inverted and lowered into a bucket of water containing a tube for the movement of gas (Fig. 4.4). The bell rises or lowers as gas moves into or out of the gas space trapped between the bell and the water. In order to prevent excess compression of the gas within the bell, earlier models used a chain and counter-weight, although newer models are designed with lightweight bells in which gas compression is not significant. A pen is often attached to the bell, which may graph the volume-time tracing on an attached *kymograph*, a rotating drum with recording paper. Many spirometers also incorporate a linear potentiometer attached to the bell for easy electrical recording via a simple amplifier. The basic principle of operation is that the height of the bell is related to its volume by the formula for the volume of a cylinder:

$$V = \pi r^2 h \tag{4.7}$$

A similar approach is used in the dry-seal spirometer. In this case, the bell is sealed to its base with a thin layer of latex (or some other thin and flexible material). As gas is introduced into the bell, the latex prevents its escape and forces the bell to move, as with the water-sealed spirometer. Dry-seal spirometers may be mounted horizontally, and may employ a moving piston instead of a moving bell. Manual and electrical recording are achieved as with the water-sealed spirometer. A third type of volume-displacement spirometer, somewhat less common recently, is the bellows, or wedge,

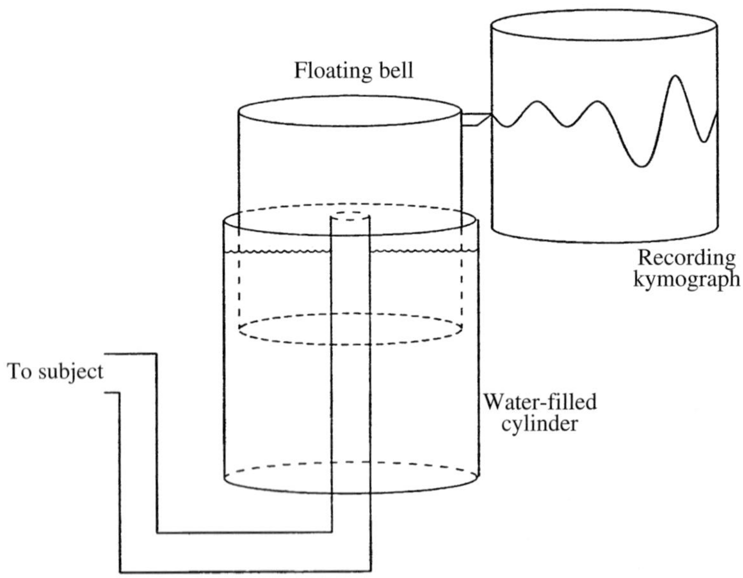

FIGURE 4.4 Schematic drawing of the water-sealed spirometer. The kymograph rotates at a constant speed, allowing for the inscription of a volume (y axis) versus time (x axis) plot as the bell moves up and down in response to gas movement at the outlet.

spirometer. In this device, the gas to be measured is contained within a bellows whose expansion is recorded via a pen or a rotational potentiometer.

Volume-displacement spirometers offer the advantage of simple construction and use. They do not require computers or processors for simple volume and time measurements. Perhaps most importantly, they are easy to calibrate and do not depend on the composition of gases they are used to measure. However, they do suffer from some disadvantages. First, they are bulky. Water-sealed spirometers, in particular, can be heavy when they are filled with water, and they are prone to spillage when tipped. Second, owing to their mechanical action, they have a limited frequency response and are not well suited to rapidly changing signals (although they do have satisfactory frequency response for most common measurements). Last, the maximum volume they can measure is limited by their size. Thus, for an experiment in which tidal volume is measured over a period of 5 minutes, the volume-displacement spirometer would be difficult to employ, without a series of complicated valves, as it would be filled before the experiment was over. Nevertheless, the volume-displacement spirometer remains popular for simple measurements of volume and time.

A completely different approach, applicable only to volumes of gas as inspired or expired from the body, relies on the changes in chest (and sometimes abdominal) geometry that accompany breathing. One design uses two elastic bands, one placed around the chest, the other around the abdomen. The bands contain strain gages that measure the relative expansion of each of the compartments. This device requires calibration with each patient or subject on whom it is to be used. It is affected by movement artifact, changes in patient position, or changes in the relative movements of chest and abdomen during breathing. It is best employed on patients at rest, during quiet breathing, such as during sleep. Its accuracy seldom exceeds ± 20 percent. A similar device uses electrodes placed on the chest wall to measure transthoracic impedance as a means to estimate changes in chest geometry. These devices offer the advantage of easy long-term measurements without the need for mouthpieces or other cumbersome connections, but their relative inaccuracy limits their usefulness.

4.4.2 Flow

Flow is the time-derivative of volume, or

$$\dot{V} = \frac{dV}{dt} \tag{4.8}$$

Thus, any device capable of measuring either volume or flow can also report the other, given an appropriate time measurement and the needed processing. For this reason, and others given below, flow-measuring devices have become popular methods for measuring both volumes and flows (although volume-displacement spirometers also can easily calculate and report flow measurements).

There are three common groups of flow-measuring sensors. The pressure-drop pneumotachometers rely on the Poiseuille equation by imposing a fixed resistance on the gas flow and measuring the pressure drop across the resistance. Assuming laminar flow, the pressure drop will be linearly related to the flow rate. The resistive element may come in several forms, but two of the most common are the Lilly and the Fleisch (Fig. 4.5). The Lilly type uses a fine screen (similar to a window screen) to provide resistance. Often, three screens are used, with the outer screens meant to maintain laminar flow and to prevent debris and exhaled droplets from damaging the middle screen across which the pressure drop is measured. The Fleisch type uses a group of small parallel tubes as its resistive element.

In their simplest designs, both types rely on laminar flow to maintain a linear output. Thus, they may be rated for a maximum flow rate, above which linearity is compromised, as predicted by increases in the Reynold's number. In practice, deviations from linearity may be seen even below the maximum rated flow. Sometimes this may be due to suboptimal geometry between the device and the connecting tubes and valves. Another cause of inaccuracy may be condensation of water from the warm moist exhaled gas as it contacts the colder surfaces of the pneumotachometer. In addition to causing computational difficulties because of changes in gas volume as water vapor is lost, the condensed water that is deposited on the resistive element may change its resistance and diminish its

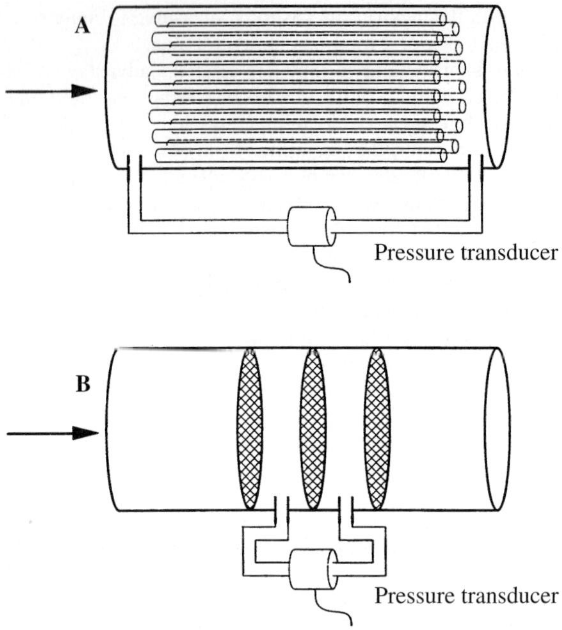

FIGURE 4.5 Schematic representations of the Fleisch (*a*) and Lilly (*b*) types of pneumotachographs for measuring flow. In both types, the small open ports are connected to opposite sides of a differential pressure transducer. The pressure difference between the open ports is related to the flow through the device by an equation that depends in part on the degree of turbulence present.

accuracy. This is often countered by heating the device to body temperature, thus preventing condensation. The reliance on linearity minimized the usefulness of this class of device until sufficient portable processing power was available that linearity no longer was required. Most devices now used no longer assume linearity, but instead characterize the flow versus pressure relationship over the entire useful range. This may be done by measuring the response to a series of known flows, but is more often calculated using an algorithm described by Yeh and colleagues (1982) using a calibration syringe of known volume. Under conditions of laminar flow, where only gas viscosity is important, the specific composition of the gas being measured is usually of little concern, since most gases present in common respiratory measurements are of similar viscosity (see Table 4.3). However, if

TABLE 4.3 Physical Constants of Common Respiratory Gases

Species	Viscosity, μP	Density, g/L	Thermal conductivity, 10^{-6} cal/(s · cm^2 · °C/cm)	Magnetic susceptibility, 10^{-6} cgs units
N_2	178.1	0.625	56.20	–12.0
O_2	201.8	0.714	57.24	3449.0
CO_2	148.0	0.982	33.68	–21.0
He	194.1	0.089	333.50	–1.88
H_2	87.6	0.089	405.00	–3.98
CO	175.3	0.625	53.85	–9.8
Ne	311.1	0.446	107.03	–6.74
CH_4	108.7	0.446	71.08	

All values taken near room temperature (19 to 30°C) from tables in *CRC Handbook of Chemistry and Physics*. Robert C. Weast, 61st edition, 1981.

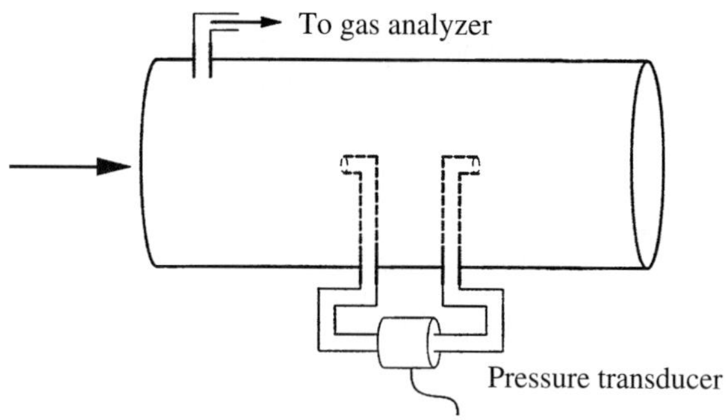

FIGURE 4.6 Schematic representation of a pitot tube. Some designs incorporate elements to better control the degree of turbulence. The gas analyzer is used to measure the density of the gas.

gases with a different viscosity will be used, the device must be carefully calibrated with gases having that same composition.

A different variety of pressure drop flow sensor relies on the Pitot effect instead of Ohm's law. In one design of this type of device, two pressure-sensing "taps" are placed within the gas stream, one pointed directly upstream and the other pointed directly downstream (Fig. 4.6). The pressure difference is no longer described by the Poiseuille equation, but rather is described by Bernoulli's law, which states that the pressure difference between the taps is a function of the density of the gas measured and the square of its velocity. Velocity is related to volumetric flow by the cross-sectional area of the apparatus. Because this device is affected by gas density, it is usually employed in conjunction with analyzers providing precise measurements of the types and concentrations of gases present, allowing for calculation of the mixture's density, but limiting the device's usefulness as a standalone flow sensor.

The second group of flow-measuring sensors, commonly referred to as hot-wire anemometers, is based on the principle that flowing gas will cool a heat source, and that greater flows will cause greater cooling of the heat source. The devices contain a heated wire (some designs incorporate a second heated wire, at a different temperature, as a reference), which is maintained at a constant temperature via feedback circuitry (Fig. 4.7). The current required to maintain the stable temperature is related to the bulk flow through the device. The hot-wire anemometer is affected slightly by the thermal conductivity of the gases present, but is generally less sensitive to changes in gas composition than pressure-drop flow sensors. The accuracy of this type of flow sensor, too, is affected by changing amounts of turbulence.

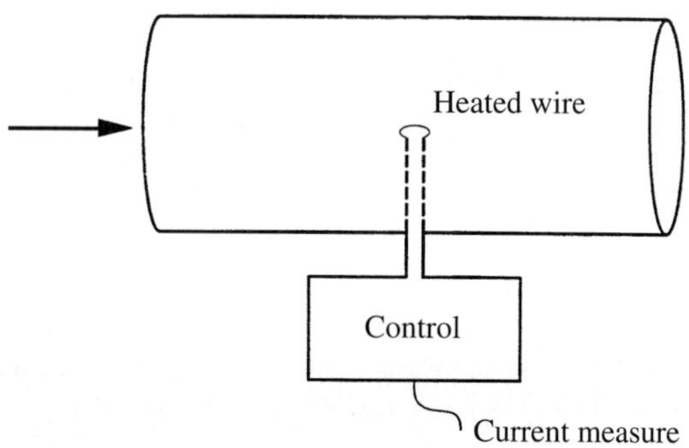

FIGURE 4.7 Schematic representation of a hot-wire anemometer. The flow is related to the current required by the feedback control circuitry to maintain the heated wire at a constant temperature.

The third group of flow sensors are the turbines, devices that are based on a rotating vane placed in the gas stream, much like a wind speed indicator on a simple weather station. The rotation of the vane is proportional to the velocity and density of the gas stream. As with the Pitot-effect devices, gas velocity is related to volumetric flow by the cross-sectional area of the apparatus. Turbine flow sensors can be purely mechanical, with precision gearings and a display dial, making for a very portable device requiring no electricity. Battery-powered models using an LED and a light sensor to count the rotations of the vane are also common. Turbine sensors must overcome several challenges to remain accurate, however. First, the moving parts must be lightweight to reduce the effects of inertia, which tend to impair the frequency response of the device. At the same time, however, the vanes must be made strong enough to withstand the forces of high flow rates.

The chief advantages of flow sensors are their small size and their ability to measure continuously in flow-through designs. They all offer good dynamic range, with frequency responses that exceed that needed for most or all respiratory measurements. They suffer from the need for more complex calibrations and generally require a computer or processor unit. The Pitot-effect device requires simultaneous measurement of gas concentrations. The hot-wire anemometer requires external circuitry capable of heating the wires sufficiently and somewhat sophisticated feedback circuitry. The turbine sensors can be fragile and susceptible to damage.

4.4.3 Pressure

Although there are a variety of pressure transducer types available, for most respiratory applications the newer solid-state pressure transducers offer the most attractive alternative. Variable capacitance transducers generally use the deflection of conductive plates by the input pressure differential to generate an output signal. Similarly, variable inductance transducers use the input pressure differential to create a change in inductance. In both cases, the transducer requires an input AC excitation signal in order to create an output signal. The circuitry used to create the excitation, and to output a usable pressure signal, is often referred to as a carrier-demodulator. These types of transducers are very precise, offer a large variety of input ranges, and maintain stable calibrations. However, they can be somewhat expensive and require dedicated external circuitry.

Solid-state pressure transducers come in a single package, often quite small, and also offer a wide choice of input pressure ranges. Typically, they use the input pressure differential to deform slightly a semiconductor plate separating two chambers exposed to each of the two input pressure levels. Any difference between the two levels will deform the separating plate, changing its conductive properties. Onboard circuitry usually allows the transducer to accept a DC excitation voltage, and provides a linear, temperature-corrected DC output voltage. These transducers are offered by a large number of vendors at affordable pricing.

All of these pressure transducers offer frequency response characteristics acceptable for most or all respiratory applications. In situations requiring the measurement of a single pressure (e.g., the pressure at the mouth during breathing), one of the two input ports to the transducer is left open to atmospheric pressure. In other situations requiring the measurement of a pressure differential (e.g., measuring the output of a pressure-drop flow sensor), the two ports of the transducer are attached to the two taps of the sensor.

4.4.4 Gas Concentration

There are a large number of gas analysis technologies available to measure the concentrations of various species present in a gas mixture. Some of the more common types used in respiratory applications are based on principles of *thermal conductivity*, *infrared absorption*, *zirconium fuel cell technology*, *paramagnetism*, *emission spectroscopy*, *gas chromatography*, and *mass spectrometry*. In many cases, some gases in a mixture interfere with the analysis for other gases and must be removed. Most often, interfering gases to be removed are water vapor and carbon dioxide. Water vapor may

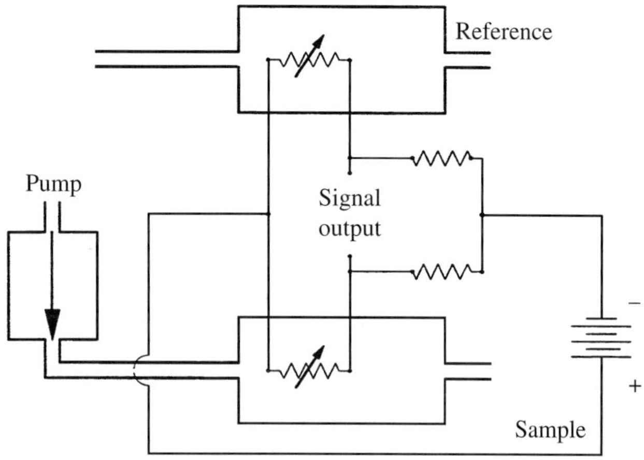

FIGURE 4.8 Schematic drawing of a thermal conductivity meter. The electrical elements are configured in a typical Wheatstone bridge circuit. The variable resistors are usually thermistors.

be removed by passing the gas stream through a canister of calcium sulfate ($CaSO_4$). Alternatively, water vapor may be removed, or equilibrated to a known level, by passing the gas mixture through a length of nafion, tubing with walls that are able to remove water because they are impregnated with a material with a high affinity for water. Placing the nafion within the lumen of larger tubing through which is run dry nitrogen (running in the direction opposite to the gas mixture to be analyzed) will remove all the water vapor from the mixture, whereas leaving the nafion tubing exposed to room air will equilibrate the water vapor concentration with ambient levels. Carbon dioxide is most often removed by passing the gas stream through a canister containing either barium hydroxide [$Ba(OH)_2$] or sodium hydroxide (NaOH). In both cases, the chemical combines with the gaseous CO_2 removing it from the gas mixture. Also, both chemical CO_2 scrubbers produce water as a by-product of the reaction and therefore should be placed upstream to a water removal system, if needed. Usually, any chemical scrubber will be impregnated with an indicator that changes color as the chemical becomes consumed, alerting the user to the need for replacement.

Thermal conductivity meters measure the ability of a gas mixture to conduct heat away from a heat source (Fig. 4.8). They usually employ two thermistors, one exposed to sample gas and the other to a reference sample containing none of the gases to be measured, arranged in a conventional Wheatstone bridge. Thermal conductivity is most commonly used to measure helium concentration, although it can be used to measure carbon dioxide concentrations if used carefully. Both carbon dioxide and water vapor interfere with helium analysis and must be removed from the gas mixture prior to helium analysis. Water vapor, like helium, has a higher thermal conductivity than other gases found in air, and thus will cause false elevation in the helium reading. Carbon dioxide, on the other hand, has a lower thermal conductivity and will cause a lowered helium reading. Thermal conductivity meters tend to be quite linear, making them easy to use, but they have relatively slow response times on the order of 20 to 30 seconds.

Infrared (IR) absorption is a common method of gas analysis and can be used for measurements of carbon dioxide, carbon monoxide, and methane, among others (Fig. 4.9). IR analyzers run the gas mixture through a sample chamber illuminated at one end with an IR light source. At the other end of the chamber is an IR detector. Parallel to the sample chamber is a reference chamber, which is usually filled with room air and uses the same IR source and detector as the sample chamber. The gases to be analyzed absorb some of the IR radiation, decreasing the amount reaching the detector. A motor rotates a "chopper blade" which alternately blocks one of the two chambers from the source. By synchronizing the chopper rotation with the signal at the detector, the analyzer can determine the relative

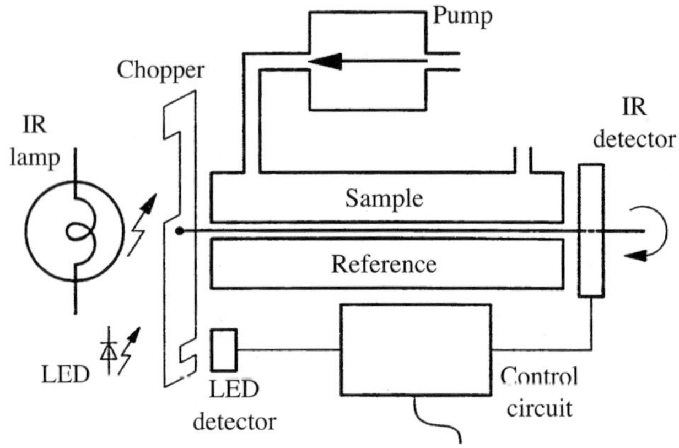

FIGURE 4.9 Schematic showing the function of an infrared (IR) gas analyzer. The chopper rotates, allowing light from the IR lamp to illuminate only one of the two gas-filled chambers (sample and reference) at a time. The IR light passes through the illuminated chamber, where it is differentially absorbed by the gases present. The IR detector measures the amount of IR light transmitted through the whole chamber. The LED and LED detector allow the control circuit to determine which of the two gas-filled chambers is illuminated at any time. The control circuit measures and linearizes the differential IR absorbance of the two chambers, and outputs the usable signal.

absorption in the reference chamber. This synchronization can be achieved by using a standard LED and light detector to determine the position of the chopper opening. The IR analyzer is sensitive to the pressure within the sample chamber, and thus requires either a constant flow through the chamber using a stable pump, or no gas flow after a pump has filled the chamber with the gas to be analyzed. IR analyzers can be designed to have rapid response times. When used as a CO analyzer, CO_2 is an interfering gas and must be removed or subtracted mathematically. H_2O is an interfering gas for almost all other gases and should be removed or equilibrated prior to analysis.

The zirconium fuel cell employs a zirconium substrate coated by platinum to create an electrode sensitive only to oxygen. Oxygen diffuses through the platinum coating on one side, passes through the zirconium, and completes the circuit on the other side of the fuel cell. So long as there is an oxygen concentration difference on the two sides, the movement of oxygen ions creates a current and induces a voltage, which is logarithmically related to the oxygen concentration difference. The zirconium is heated to high temperature (> 700°C), requiring adequate warm-up time (20 to 30 minutes) and power requirements not suited to highly portable applications. The analyzer is sensitive to the pressures within it and thus requires a stable sample flow. It offers a rapid response time and is relatively insensitive to interfering gases.

Paramagnetism refers to the propensity for certain molecules to align themselves when exposed to a magnetic field. Oxygen exhibits very high magnetic susceptibility compared to other common respiratory gases. The paramagnetic oxygen analyzer introduces a gas mixture into a hollow dumbbell-shaped structure suspended in a magnetic field. The greater the oxygen content, the greater the force tending to move the dumbbell toward alignment in the field. The oxygen concentration may be measured either as the deflection of the dumbbell or as the force required to prevent the dumbbell from moving. The analyzer is sensitive to pressure, and thus flow rates must be held steady during measurement. Response times on modern analyzers are quite fast and may be suitable for rapid sampling.

Emission spectroscopy is used to measure nitrogen concentrations. Nitrogen is drawn via a strong vacuum through a needle valve into a *Geisler tube*, a very low pressure chamber where it is exposed to a strong electric field (on the order of 25 kV) (Fig. 4.10). The N_2 ionizes and emits light, which is filtered and picked up by a photodetector, where the signal is amplified and linearized, and output

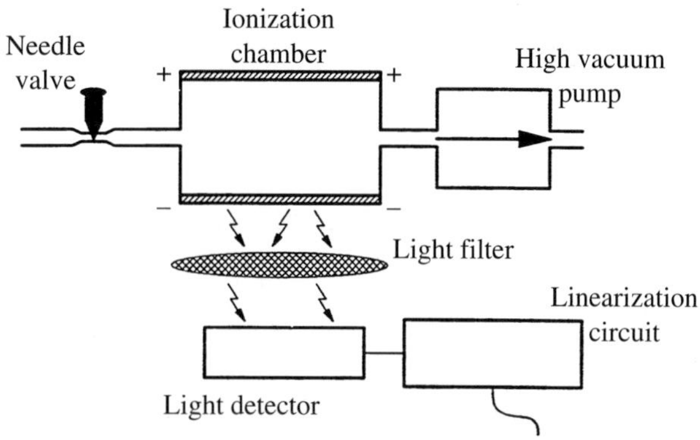

FIGURE 4.10 Schematic drawing of an emission spectroscopy analyzer, typically used to measure nitrogen concentrations. The output varies with the pressure within the ionization chamber, so the needle valve and vacuum pump must carefully regulate that pressure.

to a recorder. The output is quite sensitive to the pressure within the chamber, and thus the vacuum pump and needle valve must both be quite stable. This type of nitrogen analyzer has a rapid response time and is relatively insensitive to interfering gases. However, achieving and maintaining the required vacuum can be challenging to the designer. An alternative approach to the analysis of nitrogen concentration is to measure O_2 and CO_2 concentrations and, if water vapor pressure has been removed, calculate the remainder to be nitrogen (assuming no other gases are present).

Gas chromatography separates a mixture of gases by passing the sample through a column containing a material, which selectively impedes the progress of different species along its length (Fig. 4.11). The gas sample is mixed with a carrier gas (usually helium, which thereby renders the analyzer unable to measure helium concentrations) and run through the column. Species that are less impeded by the column material exit the column first, followed sequentially by other species. The concentrations of the now separated species are measured using another type of detector, frequently a thermal conductivity meter. Water vapor is usually removed prior to passing the gas through the column. The gas chromatograph offers the advantage of being able to measure several different gases with one analyzer, but has relatively slow response times and is unsuitable for continuous sampling with changing inputs.

The mass spectrometer, like the gas chromatograph, is capable of measuring many or all constituents in a gas mixture within a single analyzer. The gas mixture is drawn via a vacuum into a low-pressure

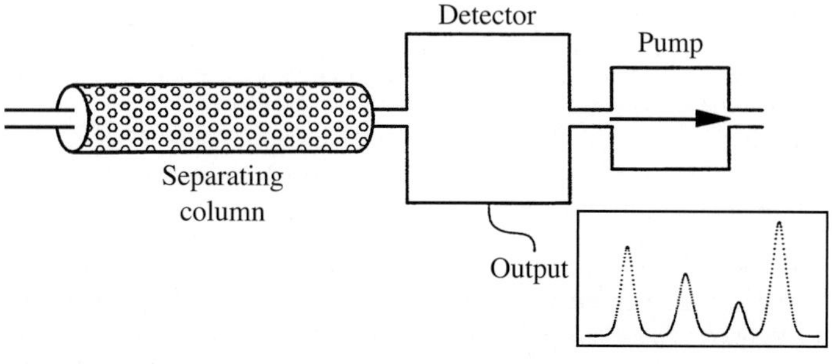

FIGURE 4.11 Schematic diagram of a gas chromatography (GC) analyzer. The gas mixture to be analyzed is drawn through the column where it is separated into its constituent species. The separated gases are then drawn through another gas detector (often a thermal conductivity analyzer), where concentrations are measured.

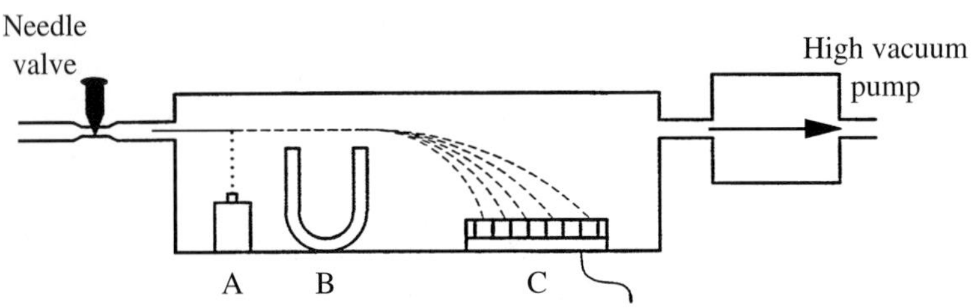

FIGURE 4.12 Schematic drawing of a mass spectrometer. The gas is ionized by an ion gun (A) and then passes through a magnetic field (B). The charged particles follow a circular path with a radius dependent on the mass-to-charge ratio. The collector (C) is composed of a series of particle detectors at various distances along its length. Each detector's output indicates the concentration of a different gas species. The spectrometer collector does not distinguish between ionized particles having the same mass-to-charge ratio, and thus there are certain gases which cannot be analyzed separately.

chamber where its molecules are ionized by an electron gun (Fig. 4.12). The charged ions are accelerated by an electric field down a chamber, and are then exposed to a magnetic field. The ions are deflected along an arc by the magnetic field according to their mass and charge: larger ions exhibit a greater radius of curvature than smaller ions with the same charge. Detectors count the number of ions at various locations within the analyzer. Because the analyzer distinguishes species based on molecular mass, different ions with the same mass and charge cannot be separated. The mass spectrometer has a rapid response time and is well suited to continuous sampling and measurement. It is, however, quite large and expensive. Water vapor is usually removed from the gas stream prior to analysis.

All of the gas analyzers described above have been used successfully in clinical practice, and although they have different advantages and disadvantages, all are well suited to certain types of applications.

4.5 COMMON RESPIRATORY MEASUREMENTS

Putting the preceding discussions into practice is the everyday mission of the *Pulmonary Function Laboratory*, a common clinical unit designed to make respiratory measurements on hospital patients and research subjects. Some of the most common measurements and the devices used to make them will be described below.

4.5.1 Spirometry

Spirometry is the most common respiratory measurement and reports, in a single maneuver, a remarkable range of valuable parameters. In this test, the patient inspires fully to TLC and then expires rapidly and forcefully, blowing hard until the lung volume reaches RV. A tracing of volume versus time is obtained, from which many parameters may be measured, including FVC, FEV_1 (the volume of air exhaled during the first second), and the ratio of FEV_1/FVC (Fig. 4.13). Spirometry also reports the maximum, or peak, expiratory flow, as well as instantaneous flows at specified lung volumes. Spirometry may be performed using a volume-displacement spirometer, with electrical or mathematical differentiation to measure flows, or using a flow sensor with mathematical integration to obtain volumes. Standards for spirometry have been published by numerous medical societies (see references at the end of this chapter). For such a simple-to-perform test, spirometry is remarkably powerful. It is exceedingly reproducible when compared with other medical tests. It is commonly used for a wide variety of medical purposes, including the detection and classification of various forms of lung disease, the responsiveness to various therapeutic interventions, and the progression

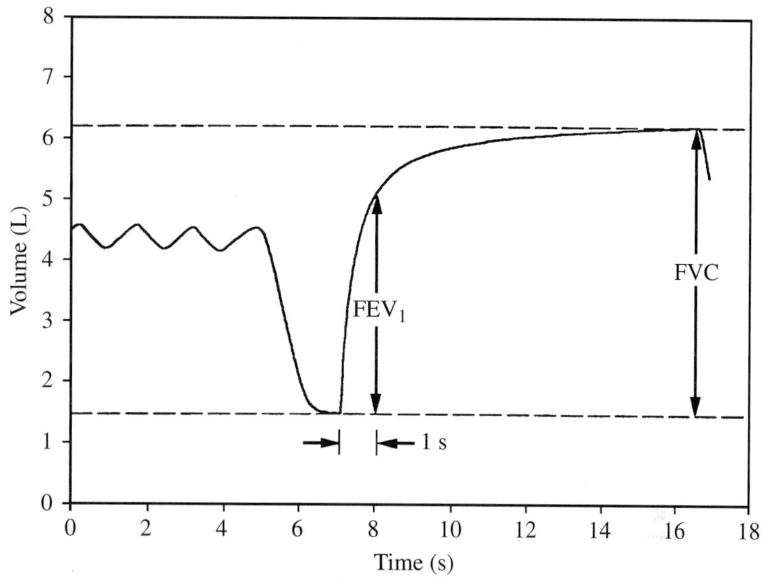

FIGURE 4.13 Spirometer volume-time tracing typical of spirometry during forced expiration. In this representative test, the FEV_1 is 3.64 L and the FVC is 4.73 L.

of pulmonary and nonpulmonary conditions. Indeed, the FEV_1 has been shown in numerous studies to correlate more reliably with mortality than many other common medical tests, for reasons not completely understood. All spirometric parameters are reported at BTPS conditions.

4.5.2 CO Diffusing Capacity

The CO diffusing capacity, DLCO, is calculated by measuring the difference in alveolar CO concentrations at the beginning and end of a period of breath holding. The test begins by having the patient exhale completely to RV and then inspiring rapidly to TLC a breath of gas with a known CO concentration. After a 10-second breath-hold, the patient exhales rapidly (Fig. 4.14). The initial portion of this exhalation is discarded, as it contains gas from the dead space, and a portion of the subsequently exhaled gas, assumed to be well-mixed alveolar gas, is analyzed for CO content. The initial alveolar concentration of CO is not the inspired concentration, as the inspired gas is diluted with gas remaining in the lung prior to inspiration (the RV). In order to assess this dilutional reduction in CO concentration (as contrasted with the later reduction due to diffusion), an inert gas that is readily diluted but does not diffuse or dissolve is added to the inspired gas. Suitable tracer gases for this purpose include helium, methane, and neon. The concentration drop of the tracer gas from beginning to end of breath holding is used to calculate the initial CO alveolar concentration as follows:

$$F_{A\mathrm{CO}} = F_{I\mathrm{CO}} \frac{F_{E\mathrm{TR}}}{F_{I\mathrm{TR}}} \tag{4.9}$$

where F_A = fractional concentration in alveolar gas
F_I = fractional concentration in inspired gas
F_E = fractional concentration in expired gas
CO = carbon monoxide
TR = tracer gas

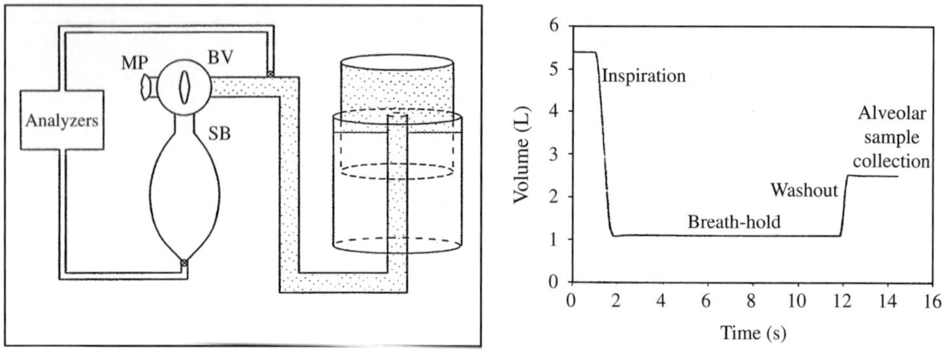

A B

FIGURE 4.14 Illustration of equipment for performing a single-breath diffusing capacity test (*a*). The patient breathes through the mouthpiece (MP). Initially, the breathing valve (BV) is turned so that all breathing is in from and out to the room. After the patient exhales to RV, the breathing valve is turned to attach the patient to the spirometer filled with test gas containing carbon monoxide and helium. The patient inspires rapidly to TLC, breath-holds for 10 seconds, and exhales rapidly. The breathing valve is left connected to the spirometer for the initial portion of this expiration, allowing the spirometer to record the amount of gas washing out the dead space. After the dead space has been flushed, the breathing valve is turned so tht an alveolar sample is collected in the sample bag (SB). Gas analyzers measure the inspired gas concentrations from the spirometer, and the expired gas concentrations from the sample bag. A representative spirometer tracing is shown on the right (*b*).

Over the period of breath holding, the alveolar concentration of CO falls exponentially according to its partial pressure gradient between the gas and blood sides of the alveolar membrane (it is assumed that the blood concentration of CO is zero throughout the short breath-hold). Then, the DLCO is calculated as

$$\text{DLCO} = V_I \frac{F_{I\text{TR}}}{F_{E\text{TR}}} \frac{1}{T} \frac{1}{BP - 47} \ln\left(\frac{F_{A\text{CO}}}{F_{E\text{CO}}}\right) \tag{4.10}$$

where V_I = volume of inspired gas (usually adjusted by an estimate of dead space)
T = duration of breath-hold
BP = ambient barometric pressure

and other parameters are as defined above.

The equipment needed to calculate the DLCO includes either a spirometer or a flow sensor to measure the inspired volume and gas analyzers to measure the concentrations of CO and the tracer gas. In some systems, the sample of expired alveolar gas is collected in a bag for analysis; in other systems with rapidly responding analyzers, the expired gas is sampled continuously for calculation. It is worth noting that using a flow sensor for this test requires that the flow sensor be calibrated with the gases to be used, as described above.

The DLCO is very sensitive for lung abnormalities but is also quite nonspecific. Several conditions can cause marked reductions in DLCO, including emphysema and pulmonary fibrosis. DLCO can be increased in some cases of early heart failure and in cases of pulmonary hemorrhage. DLCO is reported at STPD conditions.

4.5.3 Lung Volumes

There are several different methods available for measuring the TLC, RV, and FRC. These parameters, regardless of how they are measured, are reported at BTPS conditions.

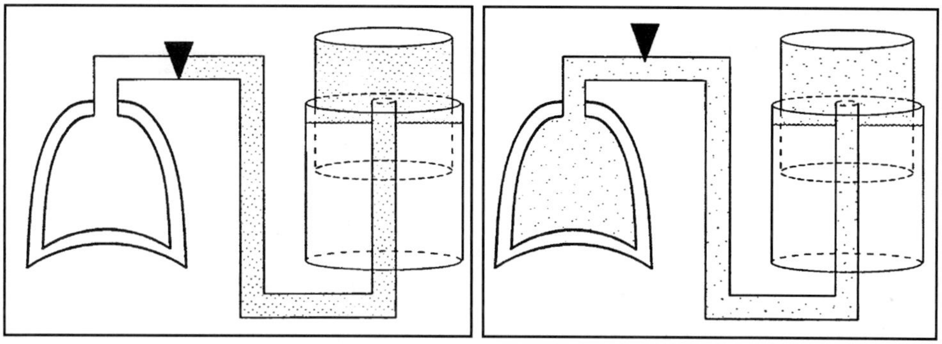

A B

FIGURE 4.15 Diagram illustrating the helium-dilution lung-volume test. Prior to the test (*a*), the spirometer system is filled with a known concentration of helium. When the test is completed (*b*) after the helium has distributed and reached equilibrium with the gas in the lungs, the ratio of final to initial concentration of helium is equal to the ratio of spirometer volume to spirometer plus lung volume. In practice, the spirometer used generally has two ports, not only one as pictured, and allows for better mixing of the gases.

In the *helium-dilution* method, a two-port spirometer is connected with tubes to a breathing valve and a blower motor. The spirometer is filled with a known concentration of helium and the patient, with no helium in the lungs, is attached at FRC by turning the breathing valve. At the beginning of the test, the total amount of helium contained within the system is equal to the initial concentration times the system volume. After 3 to 7 minutes of rebreathing, when the helium has been distributed evenly between the patient's lungs and the system, the final helium concentration is recorded (Fig. 4.15). Then, owing to the fact that helium is inert and does not leave the lung via solution in tissues or diffusion into the blood,

$$\text{FRC} = V_S \frac{F_{\text{IHE}} - F_{\text{FHE}}}{F_{\text{FHE}}} \tag{4.11}$$

where V_S = system volume
F_{IHE} = initial helium concentration
F_{FHE} = final helium concentration

This test requires that some of the gas be circulated through a CO_2-removal canister to prevent exhaled CO_2 from rising to uncomfortable or dangerous levels during the rebreathing period. Oxygen is added periodically to maintain a constant total system volume at end expiration. Once FRC is obtained, TLC and RV may be calculated, after the patient performs one or more VC maneuvers, as described earlier. The helium-dilution system, since it is a closed-system test, is almost always performed using a volume-displacement spirometer. It also requires the use of a helium analyzer.

The *nitrogen-washout* method attempts to "wash out" all of the nitrogen from the lung during a period of 100 percent oxygen breathing (Fig. 4.16). All of the exhaled gas is analyzed for volume and N_2 concentration, which is integrated to give the total volume of nitrogen washed from the lung. By assuming a known initial concentration of nitrogen within the lung, and having measured its volume, the total volume of gas contained within the lung may be calculated as follows:

$$\text{FRC} = \frac{V_{EN_2}}{F_{AN_2}} \tag{4.12}$$

where V_{EN_2} is the total volume of exhaled N_2 and F_{AN_2} is the initial alveolar N_2 concentration (typically taken to be ~0.79).

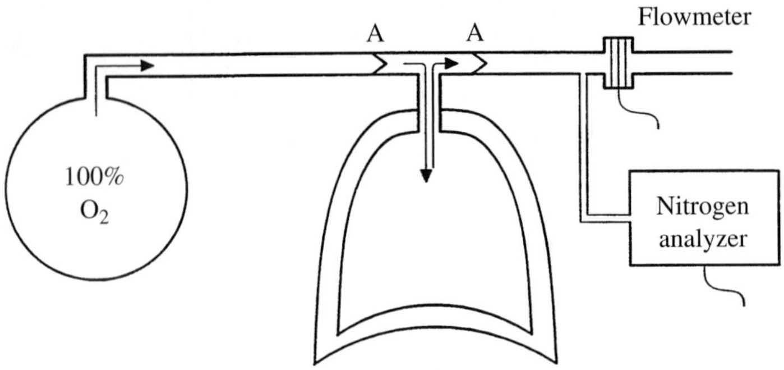

FIGURE 4.16 Equipment setup for a nitrogen-washout lung volume test. The one-way valves (A) keep separate the inspired and expired gas streams, as shown by the directional arrows. The total volume of nitrogen exhaled is calculated by integrating the continuous expired nitrogen concentration over the volume signal, which is in turn generated by integrating the flow signal over time. The nitrogen analyzer is also used to determine when the test is over, as indicated by an expired nitrogen concentration close to zero following the replacement of all lung nitrogen by other gases (oxygen and carbon dioxide).

The total volume of exhaled N_2 may be calculated by collecting all the expired gas in a very large spirometer and making a single measurement of its nitrogen concentration, or the expired gas may be analyzed continuously for N_2 content with simultaneous use of a flow sensor. Even when the expired gas is collected separately, a continuous N_2 signal is helpful to detect leaks in the system that will interfere with accuracy and to determine when the test is completed.

Both the helium-dilution and nitrogen-washout tests also give information about the distribution of gas within the lung, as both will yield a curve closely following exponential decay when the helium concentration or the end-expiratory nitrogen concentration is plotted against time. Although this information may be useful in describing gas mixing within the lung, it has not been widely used in clinical practice.

A third method for measuring lung volumes uses a device known as a *body plethysmograph*, also referred to as a "body box." The body box is a large rigid-walled structure in which the patient is seated, after which the door is closed and sealed completely. In one variety, a small hole in the wall of the cabinet leads to a spirometer or flow sensor. Respiratory efforts within the box causes changes in volume to be recorded on this spirometer as chest wall movement displaces air within the box. In a second variety of body box, there is no hole in the wall of the box and respiratory efforts instead cause pressure swings within the tightly sealed box. At FRC, a valve at the patient's mouth is closed and the patient is instructed to pant. The rhythmic respiratory efforts cause rises and falls in alveolar pressure (measured at the mouth) and opposite pressure or volume swings in the box around the patient (Fig. 4.17). According to Boyle's law, the product of the volume being compressed and its pressure remains constant. Thus

$$\text{FRC} \times P_m = (\text{FRC} - \Delta V)(P_m + \Delta P_m) \tag{4.13}$$

where P_m = pressure measured at the mouth at the beginning of a pant
ΔV = change in lung volume due to compression during a single pant
ΔP_m = change in pressure at the mouth during a single pant

The ΔV is measured either from the change in volume through the port in the side of the box, or by calibrating changes in box pressure to volume changes. The body plethysmograph allows for rapid

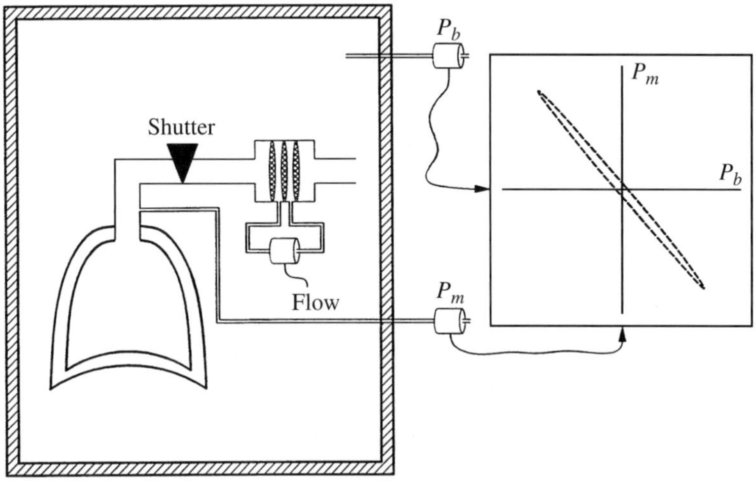

FIGURE 4.17 Illustration of a body plethysmograph, or body box. The patient sits within the sealed rigid-walled box. For measurements of lung volumes, the patient pants against the closed shutter while box pressure (P_b) and mouth pressure (P_m) are recorded as shown. The slope of the relationship between P_b and P_m determines the volume of gas being compressed within the lung. For measurements of airways resistance, the shutter is then opened and an additional recording is made, this time with flow rather than P_m on the *y* axis.

multiple determinations of lung volume. It requires the large rigid box, one or two pressure transducers, and usually a flow sensor or spirometer.

4.5.4 Airways Resistance

Measurements of airways resistance generally assume that Ohm's law applies and therefore that

$$P_A = \dot{V}R_{\text{aw}} \tag{4.14}$$

where P_A = alveolar pressure (measured relative to atmospheric pressure)
$\dot{V}$ = flow
R_{aw} = airways resistance

One method uses a body plethysmograph with a pneumotachograph at the mouth (Fig. 4.17). It repeats the measurements described above in the discussion of lung volumes and adds a series of pants with the mouthpiece valve *open,* allowing for airflow. During open-valve panting, the slope of the relationship between airflow at the mouth and changes in box pressure is recorded. During closed-valve panting, the slope of the relationship between changes in alveolar pressure and changes in box pressure is recorded. The ratio of these two measurements yields the airways resistance as follows:

$$\frac{\text{Closed valve}}{\text{Open valve}} = \frac{P_A/P_{\text{Box}}}{\dot{V}/P_{\text{Box}}} = \frac{P_A}{\dot{V}} = R_{\text{aw}} \tag{4.15}$$

where P_{Box} is pressure within the box and other symbols are as shown above.

4.5.5 Respiratory Resistance

Resistance in the respiratory system is present in the lung tissue and chest wall as well as in the airways. The sum of these three resistances is called *respiratory resistance* (Fig. 4.18).

There are several techniques for measuring respiratory resistance. The first is the forced-oscillation (FO) technique, enabled by placing an audio speaker in the flow pathway to the mouth. The speaker is driven by a low-frequency sine-wave oscillator that imposes flow and pressure oscillations on normal breathing flows and pressures. Flow and pressure oscillations can be somewhat out of phase with each other because of reactive components (compliances and inertances) in the respiratory system. The ratio of the in-phase components gives respiratory resistance, and the ratio of the out-of-phase components gives respiratory reactance. Frequency of the signal can be varied to measure respiratory changes with frequency. Forced random noise (FRN) uses the same technique but uses many different frequency components nearly simultaneously. Impulse oscillometry (IOS) introduces pulses of different frequencies to allow time-dependent changes in the respiratory system to be tracked.

Another technique for measuring respiratory resistance makes use of an airflow perturbation device (APD) (Fig. 4.19). In this approach, the patient breathes through a mouthpiece connected to a flow sensor. A pressure transducer measures the pressure at the mouth. At the outlet of the flow sensor is a rapidly rotating wheel that intermittently creates a *partial* obstruction to airflow. During the time that there is no obstruction, the airflow is described by

$$P_A = \dot{V}_{\text{open}}(R_{\text{resp}} + R_{\text{open}}) \tag{4.16}$$

$$R_{\text{open}} = \frac{P_{m,\text{open}}}{\dot{V}_{\text{open}}} \tag{4.17}$$

where P_A = alveolar pressure (relative to atmospheric)
$\dot{V}_{\text{open}}$ = flow with no obstruction
R_{resp} = respiratory resistance
R_{open} = resistance of the flow sensor and the device with no obstruction
$P_{m,\text{open}}$ = mouth pressure with no obstruction

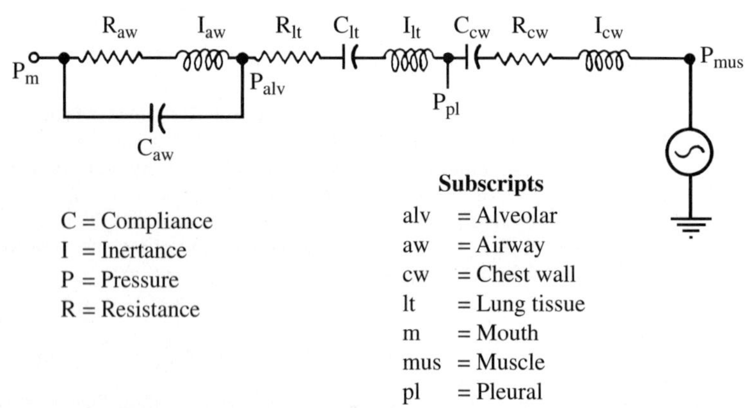

FIGURE 4.18 Lumped-parameter model of the respiratory system considered as three components comprising airways, lung tissue, and chest wall.

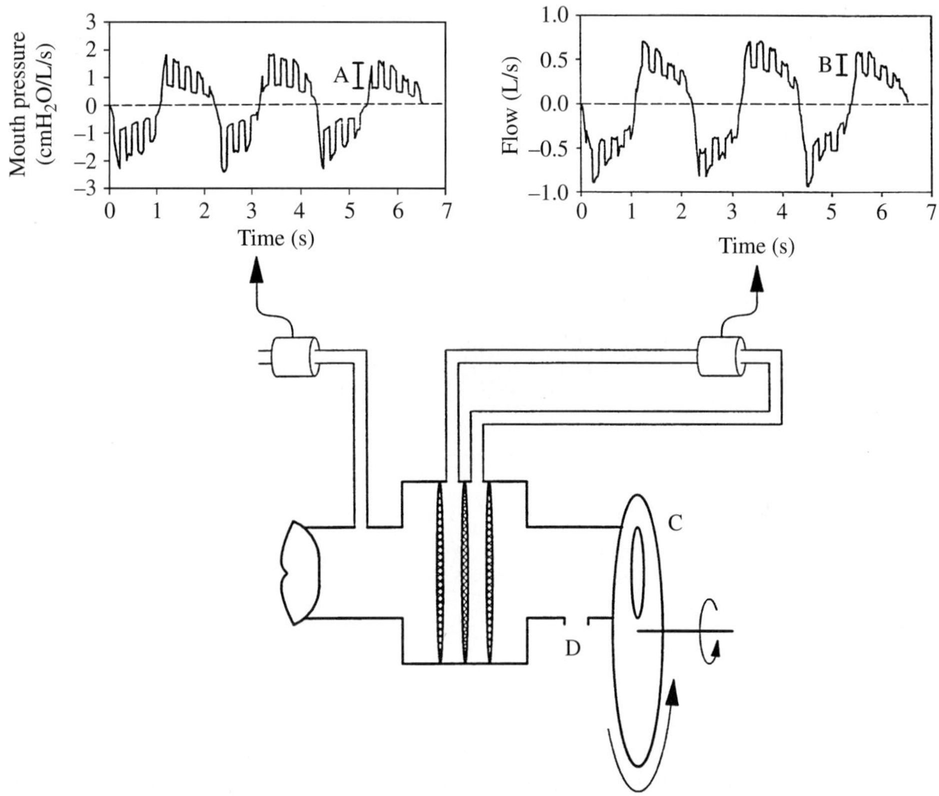

FIGURE 4.19 Diagram of the airflow perturbation device (APD). The rotating disk (C) creates changes in resistance through which the patient breathes. The ratio of delta pressure (A) to delta flow (B) with the partial obstructions is equal to the patient's airways resistance. The side opening (D) provides a flow outlet for periods when the rotating disk obstructs the outlet of the flow sensor.

When there is a partial obstruction, airflow is described by

$$P_A = \dot{V}_{obs}(R_{resp} + R_{obs}) \tag{4.18}$$

$$R_{obs} = \frac{P_{m,obs}}{\dot{V}_{obs}} \tag{4.19}$$

where $\dot{V}_{obs}$ = flow with a partial obstruction
R_{obs} = resistance of the flow sensor and the device with a partial obstruction
$P_{m,obs}$ = mouth pressure with a partial obstruction

If the wheel spins rapidly enough so that each partial obstruction is short, the alveolar pressure is assumed to remain constant. Solving these equations yields

$$R_{resp} = \frac{P_{m,obs} - P_{m,open}}{\dot{V}_{open} - \dot{V}_{obs}} = \frac{\Delta P}{-\Delta \dot{V}} \tag{4.20}$$

The APD has been used to determine respiratory resistance of people from very young to very old, and the results demonstrate the decline of resistance with child age as growth makes airways larger (Fig. 4.20).

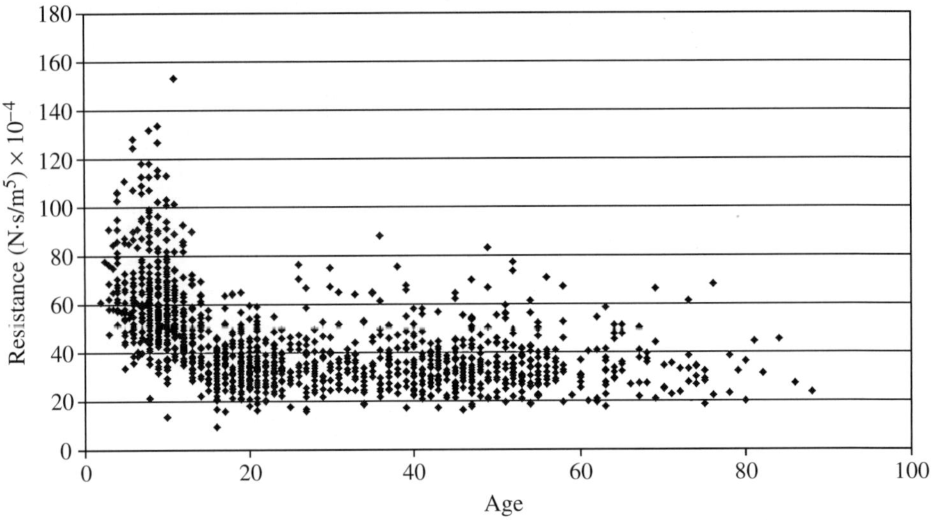

FIGURE 4.20 Respiratory resistance with age as measured by the APD.

4.5.6 Oxygen Consumption and Carbon Dioxide Production

The simplest method for measuring carbon dioxide production ($\dot{V}_{CO_2}$) is to collect a timed sample of expired gas in a balloon or spirometer, measuring the total volume of gas collected and its CO_2 concentration. If the inspired gas is assumed to contain no CO_2 (a reasonable assumption for most measurement purposes), then all of the CO_2 contained within the expired gas came from the $\dot{V}_{CO_2}$ which may be calculated as

$$\dot{V}_{CO_2} = \frac{VF_{ECO_2}}{\text{Time}} \tag{4.21}$$

Unfortunately, a similar equation does not hold for measurements of $\dot{V}_{O_2}$. The reason for this is that the inspired gas does contain oxygen, and thus there must be included a term to account for the fact that the oxygen consumed is the relatively small difference between the large amounts of total oxygen inspired and expired. Thus, an equation for $\dot{V}_{O_2}$ is

$$\dot{V}_{O_2} = \dot{V}_i F_{IO_2} - \dot{V}_e F_{EO_2} \tag{4.22}$$

where $\dot{V}_e$ is average expiratory ventilation in liters per minute and $\dot{V}_i$ is average inspiratory ventilation in liters per minute and F_{IO_2} and F_{EO_2} are the inspired and expired oxygen concentrations, respectively.

Note that, as described earlier, the $\dot{V}_{O_2}$ does not ordinarily equal the $\dot{V}_{CO_2}$, which means as a consequence that $\dot{V}_e$ does not equal $\dot{V}_i$. Some devices do measure separately the $\dot{V}_e$ and the $\dot{V}_i$, either with two flow sensors or a single flow sensor measuring in both directions (inspiration and expiration). However, it is possible to obtain a reasonably accurate calculation of $\dot{V}_{O_2}$ by noting that, in the steady state, there is no net consumption nor production of N_2. Thus, the following equation for N_2 consumption may be set to zero:

$$\dot{V}_{N_2} = \dot{V}_i F_{IN_2} - \dot{V}_e F_{EN_2} = 0 \tag{4.23}$$

Solving this for $\dot{V}_i$ yields

$$\dot{V}_i = \dot{V}_e \frac{F_{EN_2}}{F_{IN_2}} \tag{4.24}$$

Both F_{EN_2} and F_{IN_2} are known, so long as inspired concentrations of oxygen and carbon dioxide are known and no other gases (besides water vapor) are present, as follows:

$$F_{IN_2} = 1 - F_{IO_2} - F_{ICO_2} \tag{4.25}$$

$$F_{EN_2} = 1 - F_{EO_2} - F_{ECO_2} \tag{4.26}$$

Thus, combining these equations, $\dot{V}_{O_2}$ may be calculated as follows:

$$\dot{V}_{O_2} = \dot{V}_e \left[\frac{1 - F_{EO_2} - F_{ECO_2}}{1 - F_{IO_2} - F_{ICO_2}}\right] F_{IO_2} - \dot{V}_e F_{EO_2} \tag{4.27}$$

Measurements of $\dot{V}_{O_2}$ and $\dot{V}_{CO_2}$, while possible with balloons ("Douglas bags") or large spirometers, are more commonly performed with a flow sensor and continuous O_2 and CO_2 sampling.

4.6 OTHER DEVICES

It is not possible in this space to describe all respiratory measurements and devices. However, those that have been described do represent some of those most commonly encountered in routine clinical and research applications. Commercially available systems, complete with software and printers, make easy work of performing these common measurements in the usual manner, and are constructed with components as described above. Often, however, these systems are ill-suited to making measurements that differ, even only slightly, from common practice. Thus, an understanding of their function may benefit both the researcher and the clinician.

4.7 DESIGN OF RESPIRATORY DEVICES

The designer of respiratory devices is, in many ways, faced with the same challenges as with other medical devices. There are many different aspects to consider, with device function being but one of these. In addition to device performance, there are safety, user interface, legal, biocompatibility, marketing, cost, and adaptability issues to face.

4.7.1 Concurrent Engineering

Modern engineering design methods often employ concurrent engineering, wherein designs are the result of teams of people representing various specialties working together toward a common goal. Especially for larger projects, teams may be formed from design engineers, marketing specialists, manufacturing engineers, packaging specialists, legal and regulatory specialists, servicing specialists, and others. Their common goal is to design an acceptable product in the shortest possible time for the smallest cost.

Before the adoption of concurrent engineering practices, each of these functions occurred in sequence: the marketing specialist surveyed past and potential users to determine what people liked and didn't like about prior models from this firm and from the competition; design engineers used computer model methods to create a new basic design; packaging specialists worked to create an attractive instrument that functioned according to user expectations; manufacturing people took this instrument and developed the means to mass-produce it and the quality-assurance tests to be sure that each device met or exceeded minimum standards; the legal and regulatory specialists developed the data to meet government requirements in the country of use; sales personnel found potential users, compared the new device with the competition, and adapted the device to specific user needs; then the servicing specialists responded to customer concerns by developing quick field tests, parts kits, and field manuals to repair defective devices on site.

This procedure was time consuming and expensive. If the manufacturing engineer found that the device could not be produced effectively as designed, then the whole design process had to be revisited. The same holds true for other steps in the process. There are legends about instruments that would not function without failure and that could not be serviced economically. The results were very expensive calamities.

Simultaneously considering all of these design aspects shortens the design process and allows industry to respond much quicker to customer needs or technological breakthroughs. What once took 5 to 10 years to develop can now be done in 1 year or less. Perhaps because of this, attention has turned to regulatory delays for device approval, which are now an unproportionately large amount of time.

Small projects by small companies may not use formal concurrent engineering teams in the way that large projects in large companies require their use. However, the same functions need to be represented in the same parallel way. Because many medical devices are produced by small companies with few employees, the design engineer working for one of these companies must be able to wear many hats.

4.7.2 Technical Design

Design of medical devices employs a combination of fundamental engineering principles and empirical data. Almost all respiratory devices incorporate the need to move air from one place to another. At the least, it is usually desired to reduce airflow resistance and dead volume of the air circuit. There is no substitute for a thorough knowledge of fluid mechanics in order to realize these goals. Minimizing the number of sharp bends, sudden constrictions, and obstructions can reduce resistance; reducing turbulence, tubing length, and compliant members can reduce dead volume. This knowledge comes from engineering principles and can be predicted beforehand.

A field as mature as the field of respiratory devices develops around a great deal of empirical knowledge. This information could, perhaps, be predicted from first principles, but often is determined by experimental measurement on previous devices or on prototypes of newly developed devices. Two devices where empirical knowledge is important are the body plethysmograph and the hospital ventilator. Each of these is a complex device that has undergone many embodiments over the years; each has been required to become more accurate or more versatile; each has been improved through knowledge gained by use.

The design process, then, is to begin a new device from basic engineering considerations and to make improvements based more and more on empirical information. Computer-aided design (CAD) and computer-aided manufacturing (CAM) programs are often constructed to incorporate the state of knowledge in compact and easily used form. This has the advantage of allowing the information base to be constantly accessible without dependence on the memories of any particular individual. This makes these proprietary computer programs some of the most valuable assets of any company, and gives companies that have been manufacturing the same kind of medical device for many iterations an almost insurmountable advantage over younger companies that attempt to improve the same kind of device. Thus, newer companies are usually found developing newer kinds of devices that do not require as much empirical knowledge to produce. When these newer companies develop substantial amounts of their own empirical technical knowledge, they become valuable for their technical information bases, and they become acquisition targets by larger companies wishing to develop their own devices of that type.

4.7.3 Safety

Most respiratory devices are noninvasive, which reduces the safety burden somewhat because there is no direct route for introduction of microbes into the interior of the body as with other types of devices. One of the main causes for safety concern is due to saliva: this fluid could be the pathway for stray electrical currents to enter the body. Even more important is the transmission of respiratory diseases.

Saliva contains a mixture of ionic substances and can conduct electricity. For this reason, there can be no direct electrical pathway from the ac supply to the patient. Thus use of isolation transformers should be seriously considered, especially when young children are to be measured. An alternative is the use of battery-powered units, which are especially attractive because there cannot be a stray path to ac electrical ground as long as the unit is not hooked to an ac electrical outlet. Although most hospitals have grounded ac outlets and ground fault interrupters, respiratory medical devices are being used in homes, clinics, and schools where such safety precautions may not be installed.

Saliva can carry disease organisms. To minimize the transmission of disease, disposable cardboard mouthpieces are used with many respiratory measurement devices. Respiratory devices should, if possible, be designed to include sterilizable parts in the airflow path. This would reduce the possibility that microbes hitchhiking on aerosol particles would be passed from patient to patient. When appropriate, disposable filters may also help prevent microbe transmission.

Some ventilators and pulmonary function equipment connect to cylinders of gas, for example, to supplemental oxygen, carbon monoxide, helium, and others. Connectors for gas cylinders of different gases are different to prevent accidentally connecting to the wrong kind of gas. If a mistake is made, asphyxiation and death may be the result. There have been hospital deaths attributed to this simple mistake. Be sure to use the correct connector.

4.7.4. Costs

The range of costs for pulmonary function equipment is from less than \$300 for simple spirometers to \$50,000 for hospital body plethysmographs. The cost must be appropriate for the use. In general, home-use devices are much less costly than hospital devices. Home devices are usually much simpler and may not be as accurate or reliable as hospital devices. The design engineer must know the market for a new device before investing inordinate amounts of time or before including too many options that lead to inappropriate purchase prices.

Much of the cost of a new medical device is incurred due to governmental regulatory requirements. There is no practical solution to this because approval to manufacture requires amounts of device details and human trials to assure that the device is safe and effective.

4.7.5 Materials

Many of the materials incorporated in respiratory medical devices do not directly contact the person using the device. Therefore, materials are not subject to the same biocompatibility constraints as are implantable or surface contact devices. There is a need, however, to be sure that materials are rugged enough to stand up to repeated use under sometimes frantic circumstances. An endotracheal tube, for instance, must not fail during insertion into the trachea. In addition, materials in the air passage cannot give off toxic gases or undesirable odors or flavors. Finally, parts that are to be disinfected periodically must be able to withstand the disinfection process. This is especially important, given the prevalence of chemical disinfection with fairly corrosive agents.

4.7.6 Legal Liability

All medical devices are possible sources for legal action. Misuse or malfunctioning of the device can bring tort claims against the hospital, the owner of rented equipment, and the company of manufacture.

The designer of respiratory medical devices must design the device to minimize accidental misuse by the user by making the device as foolproof as possible, especially during emergency situations where the attention is on the patient and not the device. If an injury can be attributed to a device, either because of malfunction or faulty design, the manufacturer can face severe penalties.

4.7.7 Optional Functions

There is a tendency on the part of a designer to incorporate many additional functions to give the device additional capabilities. There are cases where this is counterproductive, especially if the complexity of device use increases beyond the point where mistakes can be made. Increasing the number of options often shifts the burden for a measurement from the device to the nurse or technician. Especially if these options are rarely used, they may not be useful even if they are appealing to the designer and marketing specialists. If options are to be included, make them hierarchical: the most important functions should be obtained with little effort by the user. Additional functions can be accessed with extra effort. For instance, the display on a computerized pulmonary function device should not show all possible measurements made with the device; only the one to three most important measurements should be displayed. Additional values, tables, or graphs can be displayed with additional switches, knobs, or touching the screen. Keep it simple.

4.7.8 Calibration

All hospital equipment requires periodic calibration to assure accurate measurements. Automatic calibration features allow for quick calibration at the point of use. If the instrument can self-calibrate, even for just the most important points, then it will be much more useful than if it must be moved to a shop for calibration. Some instruments undergo self-calibration when they are turned on. Other instruments are normally always powered, and can be calibrated either by pressing a button or by a timer (although this may interfere with a measurement). More thorough calibrations still need to be completed in a biomedical maintenance laboratory.

If the device has a linear input-output response, then there are normally only two calibration points, one at the device zero (null input), and the other at the span value (maximum input). It is not uncommon that significant drift occurs in the zero value alone; it is not so common that the span value drifts independent of the zero value. That is fortunate, because a null input is easier to calibrate than a span input. The instrument can be made to measure the output for null input and correct all readings accordingly.

Calibration of the device should be an important consideration when the product is being designed.

4.7.9 Human Factor Issues

Human factor considerations can be easily overlooked in the initial design of a medical instrument, which can result in the need for costly redesigns and delays in testing and approval. In these days when concurrent engineering practices are being applied to designs of everything from light bulbs to automobiles, it is important for the biomedical engineer to understand the medical environment in which the device is to be used. Especially important is to understand the various expectations for the device from personnel involved in its use.

The Patient. There is not one stereotypical patient, but several. One of these is a normal, healthy individual who is undergoing a routine physical examination. This examination might be for school, for personal reasons, or for work. There may be some apprehension exhibited by the patient when confronted by medical surroundings. Especially with a new medical device or test, the patient will wonder what it will do to him or her. The patient will likely exhibit slight hyperventilation, her/his respiratory system may not be entirely normal, and the operation of the device can be viewed with suspicion.

Another patient may enter the hospital with a severe pulmonary condition. She/he may suffer from extreme dyspnea, can be nearly unconscious, and may exhibit symptoms of panic. Movement to standard pulmonary function testing equipment may require too much exertion, and he or she may be too preoccupied to fully cooperate. Special breathing maneuvers may not be within his/her capabilities. The operation of the device must be fast and able to occur where he/she is located, and, unlike the first patient, the instrument offers hope, not a threat.

The Technician. The technician is highly trained, but not in the way an engineer is trained. The technician is oriented toward the patient, and can coax and cajole the best effort and the best measurements from the patient. The technician can also add consistency to the measurement, because he/she often adds a great deal of discrimination when it comes to deciding whether a measurement should be kept or repeated.

The technician does not coax and cajole instruments very well. Operation of the instrument is ideally automatic up to the point where a decision is made whether or not to repeat a test. Too many buttons and choices take too much attention away from the patient, which the technician may not like.

The Physician. The physician shoulders the ultimate responsibility for diagnosis and treatment. She/he is busy, and has little time to devote to undependable instrumentation. The medical device, like the technician, must do what she/he wants instead of the other way round. The physician must have confidence in both the technician and the device in order that she/he may be able to rely on measurement results and make a determination of the problem without wasting unnecessary time. The device should give unequivocal results whenever possible so as not to create confusion or uncertainty. The physician generally prefers new medical devices that are familiar and relate to other devices and methods she/he has used in the past. Once accepted by the physician, the assumption is made that the new medical device gives accurate results. In reality, the device does not always need to be extremely accurate, but it must be consistent.

The Engineer. It is the engineer who knows each flaw in the measurement. She/he wants to be proud of the instrument, and wants it to be perfect. The engineer wishes to be appreciated for all the bits of creativity and insight that have been incorporated into the machine and is disappointed when these are not appreciated. Her/his tendency, in the face of a compromise between machine and patient, is to require more of the patient. This tendency must be resisted. The engineer must have faith in her/his abilities, patience with those in the medical profession, and care in her/his approach. Above all, she/he must realize that the medical world is different from her/his own, and that, while nothing can stand between medicine and a technique that it craves, there is no path more strewn with obstacles than the path toward acceptance of a new medical device.

4.7.10 Physical Characteristics

Aesthetic design is important for device acceptance. Many respiratory devices are relatively small, and compactness is usually a positive attribute. There was a time when the very size and massive appearance of a device connoted robustness, but styles change, and now the appearance of elegance is in vogue. The device must look clean, small, lightweight, and sanitary. Computer displays should have an appearance similar to popular computer programs of the day. The color of the device should be rather neutral instead of gaudy.

Most medical devices are accepted better if they are lightweight. Respiratory devices may be used in the home, and home may be located up several flights of stairs. Even hospital equipment must be moved for cleaning or storage, so lighter devices are appreciated. Portability is beneficial.

Medical devices should be quiet. They should not appear to be contraptions to nurses and technical staff, and they should not cause loss of confidence in patients. They should not add to the din of a hospital environment, especially during emergencies, when communications among healthcare professionals are most critical.

Devices must be rugged. They should be designed not to break if they are to fall on the floor during a medical emergency. They must be able to withstand fluids that are sometimes all around in a medical setting. They must be able to tolerate electrical surges, and they should operate even when placed in unconventional orientations.

If they can be made to work correctly in dusty or dirty environments, or at extreme temperatures, then they can be used under severe field conditions. However, most medical devices are expected to be used in clean conditions at moderate temperatures. Such conditions prevail in most modern hospitals in the developed world. In third-world countries or during combat, however, medical environments are not as well-controlled.

4.7.11 Governmental Regulatory Requirement

The U.S. Food and Drug Administration (FDA) is the main regulatory body for medical device approval in the United States. It is the job of the FDA to determine that a new medical device is both safe and effective. Each medical device must meet both criteria of safety (it can do no harm) and effectiveness (it must do what it purports to do).

Most new medical devices must undergo a process of premarket notification. Certain class I devices (see the FDA Web site at www.fda.gov) are exempt from this requirement. There are certain respiratory-related devices in the list of class I devices, but, in general, they are ancillary to respiratory diagnostic measurement and health care.

If the medical device is intended to be used in a new way or is based on a fundamental scientific technology different from other devices, then the approval process is extremely thorough and is called premarket approval (PMA). If the device can be justified as a minor modification of a device that has received prior FDA approval for manufacture, then it undergoes an abbreviated 501(k) approval process. Neither of these processes is a trivial step, and specialists are often employed just to guide the device through to approval.

Medical device approval processes in other countries may or may not be similar to the process in the U.S. Mutual Recognition Agreements and may be negotiated between different governments to allow judgments by national conformity assessment bodies to be accepted in other countries.

REFERENCES

American Association for Respiratory Care, 1994a, Clinical Practice Guideline: Body Plethysmography. *Respir Care.* **39**(12):1184–1190.

American Association for Respiratory Care, 1994b, Clinical Practice Guideline: Static Lung Volumes. *Respir Care.* **39**(8):830–836.

American Association for Respiratory Care,1996, Clinical Practice Guideline: Spirometry. *Respir Care.* **41**(7):629–636.

American Association for Respiratory Care, 1999, Clinical Practice Guideline: Single-breath Carbon Monoxide Diffusing Capacity. *Respir Care.* **44**(5):539–546.

American Thoracic Society, 1991, Lung Function Testing: Selection of Reference Values and Interpretive Strategies. *Am Rev Respir Dis.* **144**(5):1202–1218.

American Thoracic Society, 1995a, Single Breath Carbon Monoxide Diffusing Capacity (transfer factor). *Am Rev Respir Dis.* **152**:2185–2198.

American Thoracic Society, 1995b, Standardization of Spirometry61994 Update. *Am Rev Respir Dis.* **152**:1107–1136.

Clausen, J. L. (ed), 1982, *Pulmonary Function Testing Guidelines and Controversies: Equipment, Methods, and Normal Values.* Orlando, Grune & Stratton.

CNN, 2000, Oxygen tank mix-up blamed in deaths of Ohio nursing home residents. Dec. 14, 2000; http://www.cnn.com/2000/US/12/14/nursinghome.deaths.ap.

Coates, A. L., R. Peslin, D. Rodenstein, and J. Stocks, 1997, Measurement of Lung Volumes by Plethysmography. *Eur Respir J.* **10**:1415–1427.

Dubois, A. B., S. Y. Botelho, and J. H. Comroe, 1956, A New Method for Measuring Airway Resistance in Man Using a Body Plethysmograph: Values in Normal Subjects and in Patients with Respiratory Disease. *J Clin Invest.* **35**:327–335.

Fessler, H. E., and D. M. Shade, 1998, Measurement of Vascular Pressure. *In* Tobin M. J. (ed): *Principles and Practice of Intensive Care Monitoring*. New York, McGraw-Hill.

Gardner, R. M., J. L. Hankinson, and B. J. West, 1980, Evaluating Commercially Available Spirometers. *Am Rev Respir Dis.* **121**(1):73–82.

Geddes, L. A., and L. E. Baker, 1989, *Principles of Applied Biomedical Instrumentation* (3d ed). New York, J Wiley.

Johnson, A. T., and J. D. Bronzino, 1995, Respiratory System. *In* Bronzino J. D. (ed): *The Biomedical Engineering Handbook*. New York, CRC Press and IEEE Press.

Johnson, A. T., 1986, Conversion Between Plethysmograph and Perturbational Airways Resistance Measurements, *IEEE Trans Biomed BME.* **33**:803–806.

Johnson, A. T., and C. –S. Lin, 1983a, Airflow Perturbation Device for Measuring Airway Resistance of Animals, *Trans ASAE.* **26**:503–506.

Johnson, A. T., and C. –S. Lin, 1983b, Airflow Resistance of Conscious Boars, *Trans ASAE.* **26**:1150–1152.

Johnson, A. T., and J. M. Milano, 1987, Relation Between Limiting Exhalation Flow Rate and Lung Volume, *IEEE Trans Biomed BME.* **34**:257–258.

Johnson, A. T., C. –S. Lin, and J. N. Hochheimer, 1984, Airflow Perturbation Device for Measuring Airways Resistance of Humans and Animals, *IEEE Trans Biomed BME.* **31**:622–626.

Johnson, A. T., H. M. Berlin , and S. A. Purnell, 1974, Perturbation Device for Noninvasive Measurement of Airway Resistance, *Med Instr.* **8**:141.

Johnson, A. T., J. N. Hochheimer, and J. Windle, 1984, Airflow Perturbation Device for Respiratory Research and Medical Screening, *J ISRP.* **2**:338–346.

Lausted, C. G., and A. T. Johnson, 1999, Respiratory Resistance Measured by an Airflow Perturbation Device, *Physiol Meas.* **20**:21–35.

Leff, A. R., and P. T. Schumacker, 1993, *Respiratory Physiology: Basics and Applications*. Philadelphia, WB Saunders.

Lin, C. –S., A. T. Johnson, and N. Yaramanoglu, 1985, Model Analysis of the Airflow Perturbation Device, *Inn Tech Biol Med.* **6**:461–472.

Meneely, G. R., and N. L. Kaltreider, 1949, The Volume of the Lung Determined by Helium Dilution. *J Clin Invest.* **28**:129–139.

Miller, M. R., and A. C. Pincock, 1986, Linearity and Temperature Control of the Fleisch Pneumotachograph. *J Appl Physiol.* **60**(2):710–715.

Morris, A. H., R. E. Kanner, R. O. Crapo, and R. M. Gardner. Clinical Pulmonary Function Testing, 1984, *A Manual of Uniform Laboratory Procedures*, 2d ed. Salt Lake City, Intermoutain Thoracic Society.

Neas, L. M., and J. Schwartz, 1998, Pulmonary Function Levels as Predictors of Mortality in a National Sample of US Adults. *Am J Epidemiol.* **147**(11):1011–1018.

Nelson, S. B., R. M. Gardner, R. O. Crapo, and R. L. Jensen, 1990, Performance Evaluation of Contemporary Spirometers. *Chest.* **97**:288–297.

Ogilvie, C. M., R. E. Forster, W. S. Blakemore, and J. W. Morton, 1957, A Standardized Breath Holding Technique for the Clinical Measurement of the Diffusing Capacity of the Lung for Carbon Monoxide. *J Clin Invest.* **36**:1–17.

Porszasz, J., T. J. Barstow, and K. Wasserman, 1984, Evaluation of a Symmetrically Disposed Pitot Tube Flowmeter for Measuring Gas Flow During Exercise. *J Appl Physiol.* **77**(6):2659–2665.

Punjabi, N. M., D. Shade, and R. A. Wise, 1998, Correction of Single-Breath Helium Lung Volumes in Patients with Airflow Obstruction. *Chest.* **114**:907–918.

Roussos, C., and P. T. Macklem, 1982, The Respiratory Muscles. *New Engl J Med.* **307**:786–797.

Ruppel, G. L., 1997, *Manual of Pulmonary Function Testing*, 7th ed. St. Louis, Mosby Year Book.

Rutala, D. R., W. A. Rutala, D. J. Weber, and C. A. Thomann, 1991, Infection Risks Associated with Spirometry. *Infect Control Hosp Epidemiol.* **12**:89–92.

Turner, M. J., I. M. MacLeod, and A. D. Rothberg, 1989, Effects of Temperature and Composition on the Viscosity of Respiratory Gases. *J Appl Physiol.* **67**(1):472–477.

Wanger, J. (ed), 1998, *Pulmonary Function Laboratory Management and Procedure Manual.* New York, American Thoracic Society.

Wanger, J., 1996, *Pulmonary Function Testing: A Practical Approach*, 2d ed. Baltimore, Williams & Wilkins.

Wilson, A. F. (ed), 1985, *Pulmonary Function Testing Indications and Interpretations*. Orlando, Grune & Stratton.

Yeh, M. P., T. D. Adams, R. M. Gardner, and F. G. Yanowitz FG, 1984, Effect of O_2, N_2, and CO_2 Composition on Nonlinearity of Fleisch Pneumotachograph Characteristics. *J Appl Physiol.* **56**(5):1423–1425.

Yeh, M. P., R. M. Gardner, T. D. Adams, and F. G. Yanowitz, 1982, Computerized Determination of Pneumotachometer Characteristics Using a Calibrated Syringe. *J Appl Physiol.* **53**(1):280–285.

CHAPTER 5
DESIGN OF ARTIFICIAL KIDNEYS

Narender P. Reddy
University of Akron, Akron, Ohio

5.1 INTRODUCTION

The human kidney constitutes one of the most vital and sensitive organs, and represents the most complex mass transfer and excretory mechanisms of the body. In addition to excreting urea and other metabolic waste products, the kidneys regulate the body fluid volume, the ionic content (Na^+, C^-, K^+), and the acid base balance through the excretion of water, excess ions, and elimination of H^+ and HCO_3. Also, the kidney performs several nonexcretory functions, including the production of numerous hormones.[1] Significant failure of the kidney function often results in quick buildup of urea and other metabolic waste, which in turn leads to cessation of vital metabolic reactions. In acute renal failure, complete recovery is expected in few days or weeks. Chronic renal failure, on the other hand, can lead to irrevocable loss of kidney function.[2] Chronic renal failure can result from a number of etiologies, including chronic infection, glomerular nephritis, renal ischemia (inhibition of blood flow), reflex nephropathy, diabetes mellitus, etc. Renal failure leads to uremia, and uremia leads to weakness, lethargy, fuzzy consciousness, vomiting, and may sometimes lead to seizure and coma. The artificial kidney device presents a life-saving opportunity for patients with chronic renal failure.

In the natural kidney, most components of the blood, except blood cells and proteins, are first filtered out using ultrafiltration, and then the essential nutrients (glucose, amino acids, etc.) and the required amounts of electrolytes (Na, K, Cl, HCO_3, Ca, Mg, etc.) and water are reabsorbed through either passive, active, or facilitated transport. The waste products are not reabsorbed and therefore are excreted in the urine. This complex process of filtration and reabsorption may be difficult to duplicate in the artificial kidney device.

The artificial kidney device removes excess waste from the blood using the principle of dialysis. Dialysis represents the movement of solute and water through a semipermeable membrane separating the two solutions. These artificial kidney devices are also called *hemodialyzers*. The word "heme" refers to blood. In the hemodialyzers, blood flows on one side of the semipermeable membrane and dialysate fluid flows on the other side of the membrane. The membrane in these devices is usually chosen such that all species, except proteins and blood cells, can potentially transfer. The dialysate fluid is an aqueous make-up solution consisting of glucose and electrolytes in water, and does not contain any waste products such as urea, creatinine, uric acid, phenols, sulfates, etc.[3] As the blood flows

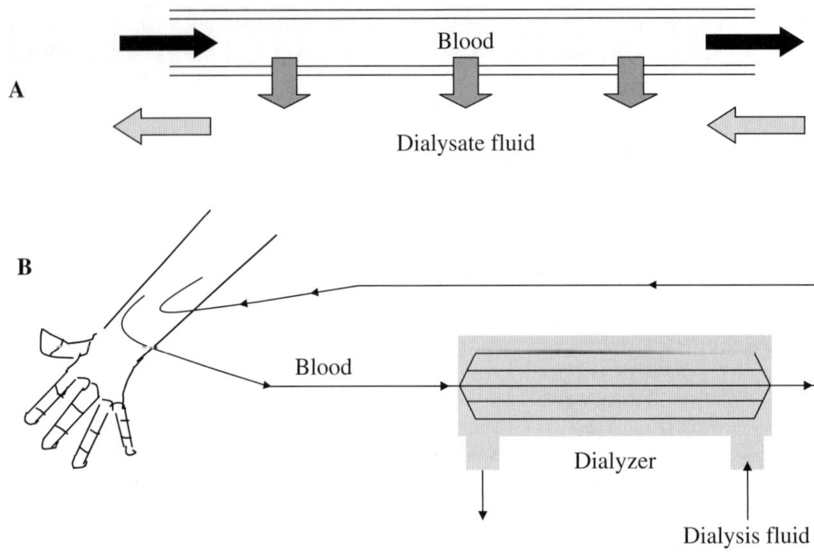

FIGURE 5.1 Hemodialysis. (*a*) The principle of dialysis: blood flows through the inside of the hollow fiber and dialysate fluid flows on the outside of the hollow fiber. The hollow fiber wall acts as a semipermeable membrane. The toxic waste products are removed by either diffusion (low flux dialysis) or by convection (high flux dialysis). (*b*) Blood from the patient's artery flows into the hollow fibers in the dialysis membrane, and the cleaned blood is returned back to the patient's vein.

through the dialyzer, these waste products diffuse, out of the blood, across the membrane into the dialysate fluid. In the patient with chronic renal failure, in addition to the waste product buildup, usually there is a buildup of certain solutes such as NaCl, $NaHCO_3$, etc. The dialysis process should also remove the excess concentration of these solutes. Moreover, excess water must also be removed by the dialyzer. This is achieved by creating a slight pressure gradient across the semipermeable membrane. The removal of middle waste molecules can be effectively achieved by convection and adsorption. High flux dialyzers use membranes with large pores for removal of uremic toxins and fluid.[4] The high flux dialysis is also referred to as high efficiency dialysis.

Most of the artificial kidney devices are hollow-fiber–type devices with blood flowing inside of the hollow fibers and dialysis fluid flowing on the outside of the fibers (Fig. 5.1*a*). Blood from the patient's artery is connected through tubing to the artificial kidney device and is returned to the patient's vein through tubing from the artificial kidney (Fig. 5.1*b*). There are several requirements in the design of a hemodialyzer device.

5.2 REQUIREMENTS OF AN ARTIFICIAL KIDNEY

1. The device should be safe. Safety is the most important consideration in the design of any medical device.

   Biological Safety. The device should have high biocompatibility and blood compatibility.[5] The device should not cause hemolysis. *Hemolysis* is the destruction of red blood cells. The device should not adsorb or filter vital blood components. Also, the device should not introduce any foreign materials or toxic materials into the blood. The device should efficiently remove toxic material. While most toxic substances are in the low molecular weight, certain toxins are in the middle molecular weight. At the same time, the membrane should not remove essential proteins such as blood serum albumin. Accumulation of β_2-microglobulin leads to a clinical condition called amyloidosis.[6] The molecular weight of β_2-microglobulin is around 11,800 Da.[7] The molecular weight of albumin is 66,400 Da. Simply increasing the membrane size to remove the β_2-microglobulin can lead to the removal of essential molecules like the blood serum albumin, which is close in molecular weight to the toxic molecules. Removal of β_2-microglobulin has been shown to reduce morbidity in end-state renal disease (ESRD) patients.[8] In addition, the interaction of blood with the dialyzer membrane often results in human complement activation.[9] This immunological reaction may result in undesirable effects or even in morbidity in ESRD patients.[10] In high flux dialysis, although a positive pressure gradient exists across the hollow fiber tube, the large axial pressure drop may result in lower pressure in certain portion of the distal (venous) end of the fiber. Thus in these regions of the fiber, the pressure could be lesser than that in the dialysate fluid causing back filtration of dialysate fluid in these high flux dialyzers.[11,12] This may result in complement-activating factors (cytokine-inducing substances) to be back transported into the blood, causing significant complement activation and the associated immunological reactions.[11]

Reliable vascular access is essential for repeated hemodialysis.[12] A fistula is constructed by joining a major artery in the wrist (e.g., radial artery) with an adjacent vein such that a portion of the arterial blood takes a shortcut directly into the vein. Woven tubes of synthetic materials such as Dacron, and expanded polyterofluoroethylene (PTFE, Gortex, Impra) as synthetic grafts should be biocompatible and blood compatible and should not cause clotting. Transcutaneous vascular access device should also be blood compatible and biocompatible and should not cause clotting. The transcutaneous access device should allow easy and quick connections. These access devices should not cause infection. The National Kidney Foundation has issued clinical guidelines for vascular access.[13]

Chemical Safety. Water quality, for dialysate fluid, is a major safety concern.[14] The patient's blood is exposed to approximately 20,000 L of dialysate fluid each year. Consequently, impurities which are considered insignificant for drinking water may be potentially harmful for the dialysis patient and can create long-term toxic effects. Substances present in the dialysate fluid, even in low concentrations, can enter the blood stream and cause damage. For example, chloramine can cause hemolytic anemia. Special attention should be paid to substances that bind to the plasma proteins. For example, aluminum in small quantities can cause severe brain and bone damage in long-term dialysis patients. Lead, cadmium, mercury, and selenium, etc., have similar toxic effects. The Association for the Advancement of Medical Instrumentation (AAMI) has set up standards for hemodialyzers and water quality for hemodialysis (Table 5.1). In addition, the water used to makeup the dialysate fluid should not have excess microbial content. Improper water treatment or inadequate design can lead to biofilm growth on various conduits of the artificial kidney machine. Bacteria at these biofilm sites may release pyrogen or cytokine-inducing substances and other endotoxins into the dialysate fluid. Although the microorganisms cannot cross the dialysis membrane, the pyrogen lipids and cytokine-inducing substances produced by these organisms can cross the dialysis membrane and can lead to infection.[15–17]

Proper sterilization of the device (cartridge, etc.) is important. All membranes are not compatible with all types of sterilization. For instance, ethylene oxide (EtO), when conjugated with human blood serum albumin, may lead to anaphylactic reactions observed in some patients on EtO-sterilized hemodialyzers.

Mechanical Safety. The dialysis membrane should have high shear strength (resistance to tearing) and high ultimate strength. The membrane should maintain adequate strength and dimensional stability while wet. The membrane often loses water-soluble components and often adsorbs components of the surrounding medium, which can lead to changes in dimensions and mechanical properties.

The blood side flow resistance should be low enough to maintain adequate blood flow with minimal pumping. Artificial pumping of blood may cause hemolysis (destruction of red blood cells). Therefore, pressure developed by patient's own heart should be able to pump the blood through the dialyzer machine back to the heart. The normal blood pressure in the adult is pulsatile with 120 mmHg systolic (upper peak of the wave) and 70 mmHg diastolic (lower peak of the waveform), with an average pressure of 100 mmHg. Blood pressure in children is even lower. Usually, a roller-type blood pump is used to pump blood. This blood pump is placed in between the arterial access line and the blood inlet manifold of the artificial kidney device.

TABLE 5.1 Allowed Limits for Impurities in ppm

Contaminant	EP	New AAMI (Draft RD-62a)
Aluminum	0.01	0.01
Ammonium	0.2	
Antimony		0.005
Arsenic		0.005
Barium		0.1
Beryllium		0.0004
Cadmium		0.001
Calcium	2 (0.05 mmol/L)	2
Chloramines	0.1	0.1
Total chlorine	0.1	
Free chlorine		0.5
Chlorides	50	
Chromium		0.014
Copper		0.1
Cyanide		0.002
Fluorides	0.2	0.2
Heavy metals	0.1	
Lead		0.005
Magnesium	2 (0.07 mmol/L)	4
Mercury	0.001	0.0002
Nitrates	2	2
Potassium	2 (0.1 mmol/L)	8
Sodium	50 (2.2 mmol/L)	70
Selenium		0.09
Silver		0.005
Sulfates	50	100
Thallium		0.002
Zinc	0.1	0.1
Bacteria	100 CFU/mL	200 CFU/mL (action at 100)
Endotoxin	0.25 EU/mL	2.0 EU/mL (action at 1.0)

Source: Reproduced from Ref. 14 with permission.

Human Factors Safety. The device should be easy to operate and should be fool-proof. The blood inlet and outlet connections and the dialysate inlet and outlet connections should be such that they permit only error-free operation. The part of the device which contains the hollow fibers should be preassembled and prepackaged into a cartridge, and presterilized.

Size and color coding of various connections will ensure safety. For example, the blood inlet manifold should be of the size such that only the inlet tubing bringing the arterial blood should be able to connect. The arterial (access) pressure and the return venous pressure should be monitored. Air leak into the arterial and the venous lines should be detected automatically. Air in the blood causes blood embolism and clotting. In addition, blood leak into the dialysate fluid should be detected automatically. The device should be designed to avoid error-prone stage.

Alarms should be incorporated into the dialysis machine to signal system malfunction. There should be alarms for (1) low arterial pressure, (2) high arterial pressure, (3) low venous pressure, (4) high venous pressure, (5) air leaks (air in the blood lines), (6) transmembrane pressure, and (7) blood pump torque. These alarms should be easily audible (70 dB) and visible from 2 to 3 m distance. The dialyzer should be designed such that system malfunction should be able to automatically shut off the blood pump and clamp the blood lines such that the patient is isolated.

2. The device should be efficient in removing nitrogen, and other waste material and toxic products of metabolism. It should also remove excess ionic species. The device should efficiently remove toxic middle molecules.
3. The device should have small priming volume. The *priming volume* is the volume of the artificial-kidney–occupied blood. This amount of blood is lost in every dialysis session. Therefore, the priming volume should be small. The normal blood volume in adult is approximately 5 L. Therefore, the priming volume should not exceed 250 mL corresponding to 5 percent of the blood volume. It should be noted that the blood volume in children is much lower.
4. The device should be reliable.

5.3 LOW FLUX VERSUS HIGH FLUX DIALYSIS

Hemodialysis involves the transfer of solutes and water from the blood to the dialysate fluid through a semipermeable membrane. In the conventional or low flux dialysis, the solutes are removed by diffusion across the semipermeable membrane, and minute quantity of water is removed by using slight pressure across the membrane. The membrane in low flux dialysis usually has low water permeability such that an ultrafiltration controller is not needed to prevent excess water loss from the patient. On the other hand, membranes used in high flux dialysis have high water permeability, and the solutes are removed by diffusion and convection. While diffusion depends on the concentration gradient and the solute permeability of the membrane, convection depends on the membrane sieving coefficient, water permeability, and the transmural pressure gradient.[7] Solute transfer flux (dW) for a differential length can be expressed as

$$dW = dW \text{ diffusion} + dW \text{ convection}$$

$$dW = k_D \times \Delta C \times dA + S \times k_U \times (\Delta P - \Delta\pi) \times C \times dA \tag{5.1}$$

where dA = the membrane surface area for a differential length along the membrane
C = the concentration of the solute in the blood
ΔC = the concentration difference across the membrane
k_D = the solute permeability for the membrane
k_U = the ultrafiltration coefficient
ΔP = the pressure drop across the membrane
$\Delta\pi$ = the osmotic pressure gradient
S = the sieving coefficient

The ultrafiltration coefficient (k_U) for high flux dialyzers is typically in the range of 20 to 50 mL/h/mmHg. With convective removal of the middle molecules, there is a significant water loss. Saline (make-up solution of water and essential nutrients) is infused into the patient along with the cleaned (dialyzed) blood. Therefore, these high flux dialyzers require precise ultrafiltration control. The ultrafiltration coefficient is generally in the range of 15 to 30 mL/h/mmHg.[18–20] The U.S. FDA defines high flux hemodialyzers as those with an ultrafiltration coefficient k_U greater than 12 mL/h/mmHg.

The sieving coefficient (S) and the solute permeability (k_D) depend on the ratio of solute radius to pore radius. The solute permeability (k_D) drastically decreases with increasing solute radius. The sieving coefficient (S) also decreases with increasing solute diameter (molecular weight).[7,21] Figure 5.2 shows the relationship between sieving coefficient (S) and solute molecular weight for various pore sizes. The removal of middle molecules by diffusion is very limited. Middle molecules are defined as uremic toxins that have intermediate molecular weight between conventional small molecules and serum albumin. In particular, β_2-microglobulins have a molecular weight of 11,800 Da and present a major problem. The diffusion coefficient for β_2-microglobulin is 13.7×10^{-7} cm^2/s, whereas for serum albumin the diffusion

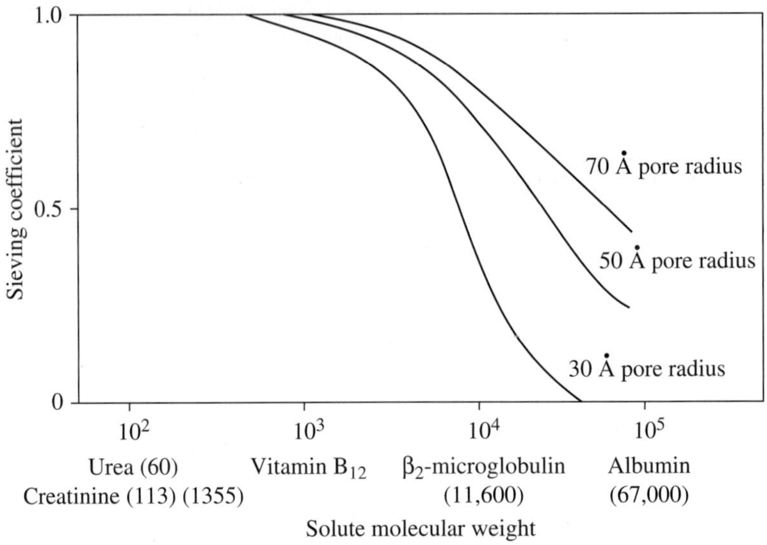

FIGURE 5.2 The relationship between sieving coefficient and solute molecular weight. *(Reproduced from Ref. 7 with permission.)*

coefficient is 6.3×10^{-7} cm^2/s.[7] Moreover, the blood concentration of β_2-microglobulins is 0.06 g/L, whereas the blood concentration of serum albumin is very high 50 g/L. Therefore, it is difficult to separate the β_2-microglobulin from serum albumin using diffusion. The middle molecules are removed by convective transport in high flux dialysis. Although the conventional membranes used in low flux dialysis with 15- to 30-Å pore size will not leak albumin, the extraction of β_2-microglobulin is not sufficient. More than 50-Å pore size is required to achieve a 60 percent removal of β_2-microglobulin. This large pore size leads to significant leakage of albumin. Also, adsorption of blood serum albumin to the dialysis membrane is a major problem.[22] Therefore, the challenge in the design and selection of the membrane is to achieve an effective removal of middle molecules without the loss of serum albumin.

Extraction (E) is a dimension less parameter that can be used to compare the performance of various dialyzers[23]:

$$E = (C_{Bi} - C_{Bo})/(C_{Bi} - C_{Di}) \tag{5.2}$$

Concentration of waste products in the dialysate fluid C_{DI} is zero as the dialysate fluid enters the dialyzer. Therefore,

$$E = (C_{Bi} - C_{Bo})/C_{Bi} \tag{5.3}$$

Although engineers prefer extraction, clinical preference is the use of clearance ($\boldsymbol{K}$) to compare various dialyzers:

$$\text{Clearance } \boldsymbol{K} = Q_B\,(C_{Bi} - C_{Bo})/C_{Bi} \tag{5.4}$$

where Q_B is the blood flow rate to the artificial kidney. For the artificial kidney device, the clearance

$$\boldsymbol{K} = Q_B\,E \tag{5.5}$$

The extraction coefficient for countercurrent flow dialysis without significant ultrafiltration can be expressed as[23]

$$E = (1 - \exp (k_D A (1 - Z)/Q_B)/(Z - \exp (k_D A (1 - Z) Q_B)) \tag{5.6}$$

The term $(k_D A/Q_B)$ is a dimension-less quantity and is referred to as the number of mass transfer units N_T. Therefore,

$$E = (1 - \exp (N_T(1 - Z))/(Z - \exp (N_T(1 - Z))) \tag{5.7}$$

where Z is the ratio of blood flow rate (Q_B) to the dialysate flow rate (Q_D):

$$Z = Q_B/Q_D \tag{5.8}$$

The extraction coefficient E increases with decreasing Z. When $Z = 0$, regardless of the dialyzer (countercurrent, cocurrent, or mixed flow), the extraction coefficient can be expressed as

$$E = 1 - \exp (-N_T) \tag{5.9}$$

The clearance for countercurrent flow low flux dialysis can be expressed as

$$K = Q_B E = Q_B(1 - \exp (N_T (1 - Z))/(Z - \exp (N_T(1 - Z)) \tag{5.10}$$

In the conventional or low flux dialysis, the blood flow rates are in the range of 200 to 250 mL/min. In the high flux dialysis, the blood flow rates are above 400 mL/min. For low flux as well as high flux dialysis, clearance depends on extraction and therefore on k_D and k_U. These parameters in turn depend on the type of membrane used.

5.4 MEMBRANES FOR DIALYSIS

The properties of the semipermeable membrane play a major role in dialysis. The membrane should have high permeability to water and organic metabolites and at the same time should be able to retain plasma proteins. In particular, the membrane should be able to remove middle molecules such as β_2-microglobulins and advanced glycation end products (AGE), and at the same time should not cause any depletion of serum albumin and other proteins.[7,24] In addition, the membrane should be biocompatible and blood compatible. An ideal membrane does not adsorb blood proteins or hormones. C. P. Sharma[25] provides an excellent review of membranes for hemodialysis.

Cellulose, modified cellulose, and synthetic polymers are the three types of membranes used in dialysis. Cellulose membranes were used initially as they have good permeability with uniform pore size and are hydrophilic.[25] Protein adsorption decreases with increasing hydrophilicity. However, cellulose membranes are known for biocompatibility and hemocompatibility problems.[25–27] Cellulose and regenerated cellulose membranes lead to the release of thromboxane, histamine, interleukin-1, and tumor necrosis factor, etc.[26] In addition, significant transient leucopenia has been observed with these membranes. Cellulose is a long-chain molecule containing hydroxyl (OH) groups. The free hydroxyl groups have been associated with the complement activation and leucopenia observed when using cellulose or regenerated cellulose membranes.[27]

Substituted cellulose has been developed to reduce the hemocompatibility problems associated with cellulose.[25] Cellulose acetate (diacetate and triacetate) membranes are formed by bonding acetate to the hydroxyl groups. This modified cellulose membranes have tertiary amino compounds bound to the hydroxyl groups. This modified cellulose is marketed under the trade name Hemophan. While cellulose acetate membranes induce significant platelet activation, platelet activation with Hemophan membranes is not as pronounced.[25,26,28]

Synthetically modified cellulose is produced by replacing some hydroxyl groups with benzyl groups by ether bonds. These membranes offer a combination of hydrophobic (benzyl groups) to reduce complement activation and hydrophilic (hydroxyl groups) to reduce protein adsorption. In another type of synthetic modification, the surface hydroxyl groups are replaced by grafting polyethelene glycol.[29] Although there is an improved compatibility with the modified cellulose membranes, the improvement is far from the desired.

Advantages of cellulose and it's derivatives include uniform pore size, ability to form thin membranes of the order of 5 to 15 μm, high mechanical strength, chemical stability and high tenacity even in the wet state, reduced tendency for protein adsorption, and excellent permeability to small molecules. Disadvantages of the cellulose and modified cellulose membranes include complement activation, leucopenia, and inability to eliminate toxic middle molecules such as β_2-microglobulin. Vitamin E–bonded cellulose available under the trade name Excebrane has improved blood compatibility and microglobulin clearance when compared to cellulose.[30,31] In addition, oxidative DNA damage has been less pronounced when compared to cellulose membranes. However, more pronounced leukopenia was observed with vitamin E–modified cellulose when compared to synthetic polysulfone membranes.[32]

Synthetic membranes offer superior blood compatibility and middle molecule clearance. Synthetic membranes, in general, are more hydrophobic than cellulose-based membranes. Polysulfone is the most widely used synthetic membrane. Polysulfone membranes have high water permeability and significantly improved biocompatibility.[33] Polysulfone is used for both low flux and high flux dialysis. Helixone is a commercially available polysulfone high flux membrane which efficiently removes middle molecules, such as β_2-microglobulin, in a narrow range without the loss of albumin. This is achieved by uniform pore in Helixone membranes, which are produced by nanocontrolled spinning techniques. Polyethersulfone membranes available under the trade name Diapes are thin (30 m) and have higher water permeability with increased middle molecule (β_2-microglobulins and AGE) clearance.[25,34,35]

Polymethylmethacrylate (PMMA) membranes have good middle molecule clearance, and have excellent biocompatibility. Both polysulfone membranes and PMMA membranes effectively eliminate several immunogenic products, including neutrophil elastase. Immunoglobulin light chains are uremic toxins which are effectively eliminated by PMMA membranes.[25,36–38]

Polyacrylonitrile-based membranes have very good biocompatibility and enhanced permeability. AN69 is a commercially available high flux membrane made from copolymer of acrylonitrile and sodium methyl sulfonate.[39] AN69 has excellent blood compatibility due to its negative surface charge, and has high permeability with pores in the range of 25 to 55 Å. AN69 membrane effectively removes β_2-microglobulin AGE peptides by convection (high flux) and adsorption. In addition AN69 eliminates immunogenic substances such as C3a and C5a, and factor D, etc., by adsorption. However, AN69 membranes lead to severe adverse reaction in patients who are on medical treatment with angiotensin-converting enzyme (ACE) inhibitors.[40,41]

In general, high flux synthetic membranes have increased biocompatibility, blood compatibility, and increased middle molecule clearance when compared to membranes made of cellulose and its derivatives. Clinical studies have revealed lower mortality, lower microglobulin and triglyceride values, and lower incidence of amyloid disease in synthetic high flux membranes (polysulfone, AN69, and PMMA, etc.) when compared to cellulose-derived membranes.[25] However, the clearance of these middle molecule toxins, even with the high flux dialysis, using synthetic membranes is much lower when compared to the clearance in the natural kidney.

5.4.1 The Dialysis System

Blood flows through hollow fibers and dialysate fluid flows outside the hollow fibers, and the hollow fiber wall acts as a membrane separating the blood and the dialysate fluid. Therefore, there are three distinct circulation components: the dialysis circuit; the blood circuit, and the hollow fiber which interfaces both. Figure 5.3 describes the dialysis system for low flux dialysis. The basics of hemodialysis machine are well described by Misra.[42] The dialysis fluid forms a major component of

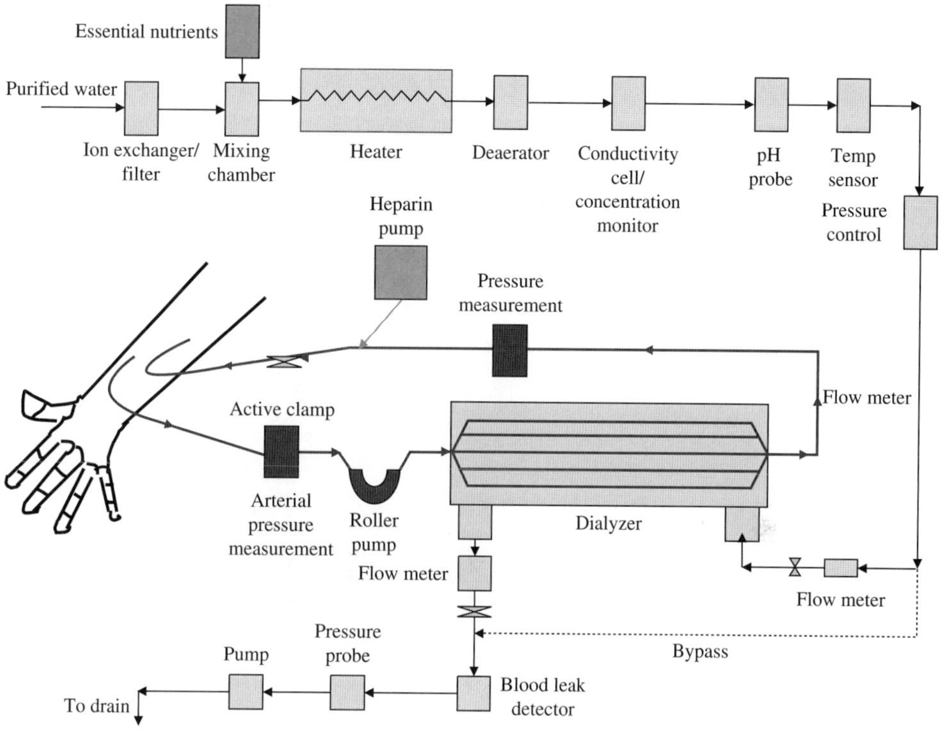

FIGURE 5.3 The dialysis system for low flux dialysis.

the dialysis system. The stringent requirements for the water quality demand several levels of water purification, including ion exchange and distillation. The required nutrients (Na^+, K^+, Cl^-, glucose, etc.) are proportioned and mixed with water. The mixture is then heated to body temperature to avoid heat transfer between the dialysate fluid and the blood. The heated dialysate fluid is now deaerated to trap bubbles. The mixing and heating, etc., are performed in the dialysis machine (Fig. 5.4). The dialysis fluid usually flows counterclockwise outside the hollow fiber (semipermeable membrane) carrying the blood. The hollow fibers are preassembled and prepackaged into a cartridge with blood and dialysis fluid inlet and outlet manifolds. These cartridges come in various sizes having different number of fibers and therefore different surface area (Fig. 5.5). In low flux dialysis, the transmural (transmembrane) pressure gradient across the hollow fiber is negligible; however, a slight negative pressure is used to remove some water. On the other hand, for high flux dialysis, the negative pressure has to be precisely controlled. Since there is a significant rate of fluid removal from the blood, a make-up solution is introduced into the blood stream before it is returned to the vein (Fig. 5.6). This fluid replacement has to be regulated precisely. Other components of the dialysate circuit include a blood leak detector in the dialysate output line (Fig. 5.3). The blood leak detector detects for any blood in the dialysate fluid that might have leaked from the hollow fiber (across the membrane) into the dialysate fluid using a photo detector. While the dialysate fluid does not absorb red or infrared light, the red blood cell absorbs red and infrared light. The dialysate fluid is then pumped into the drain. The pressure in the dialysate fluid is precisely regulated.[42]

There is a roller blood pump in the arterial line between the arterial access and the blood inflow manifold of the artificial kidney machine. Blood pressure is measured in the arterial line between the access and the blood pump. Also, blood pressure is measured in the return venous line. An air leak detector in the return blood line (downstream of the exhaust blood manifold) detects any air in the blood line. In addition, there is a heparin pump placed before the blood enters the venous return

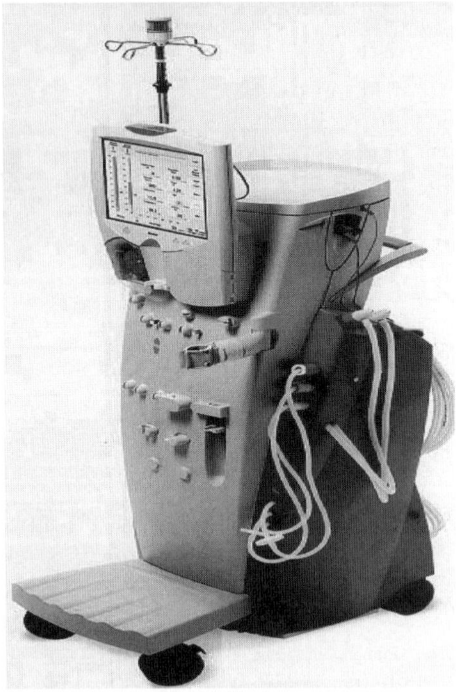

FIGURE 5.4 The Baxter hemodialyzer machine. (*Photograph Courtesy of Baxter Inc., reproduced with permission.*)

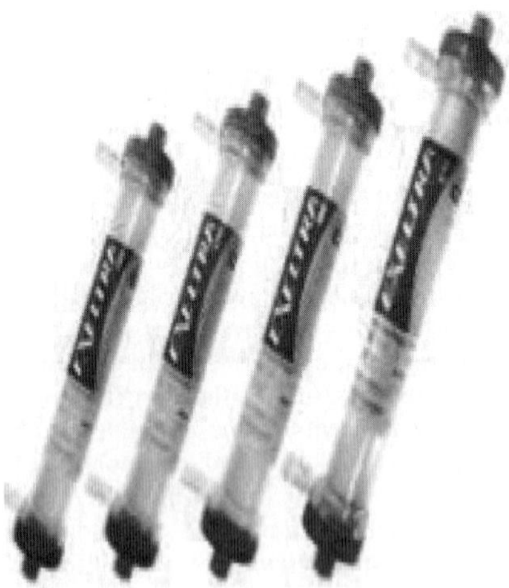

A: BAXTER EXELTRA dialysis catridges for high flox dialysis (CTA membrane) gamma sterilized

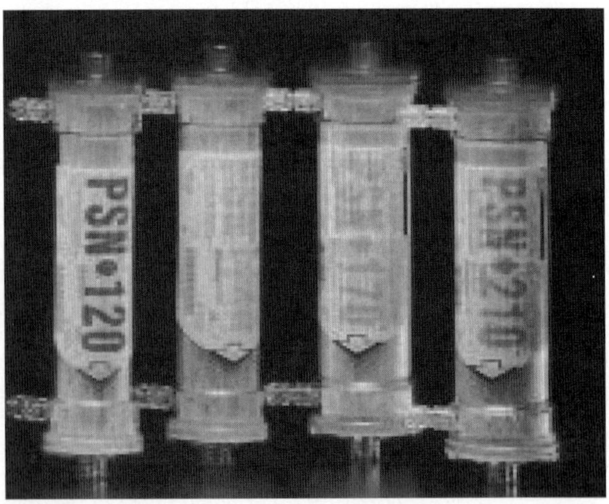

B: BAXTER PSN (poly synthane) Dialysis cartridges for mid flux dialysis (PSN membrane) ETO sterilized

FIGURE 5.5 Hemodialysis cartridges come in various sizes with different surface areas. (*Courtesy of Baxter Inc., reproduced with permission.*)

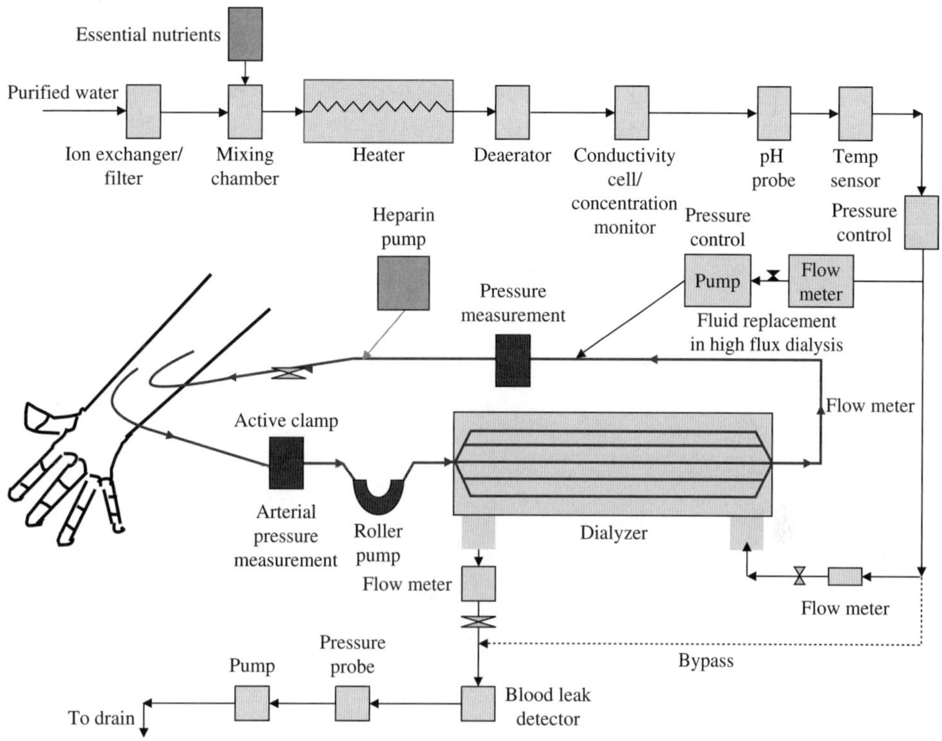

FIGURE 5.6 The hemodialysis system for high flux dialysis. Replacement fluid is added to the blood before returning to the patient's vein.

access to prevent clotting. Heparin is an anticlotting hormone. The treatment regimes vary from clinic to clinic and from patient to patient.

5.5 TREATMENT PROTOCOL AND ADEQUACY OF DIALYSIS

Let us consider a simple one-compartmental model for the prescription of treatment protocols for dialysis using an artificial kidney device (Fig. 5.7). While the blood urea concentration (BUN) in the normal individual is usually 15 mg% (mg% = milligrams of the substance per 100 mL of blood), the BUN in uremic patients could reach 50 mg%. The purpose of the dialysis is to bring the BUN level closer to the normal. During the dialysis, some hormones also diffuse out of the dialyzer membrane along with the urea molecule. Too rapid dialysis often may lead to depression in the individual due to the rapid loss of hormones.[23] On the other hand, too slow dialysis may lead to unreasonable time required at the hospital. Simple modeling can be used to calculate the treatment protocols. Let us consider a one-compartmental model of the tissue where we assume that the blood and tissue are well mixed, and that the concentration of urea is uniform throughout the body.[43] Let C_{Bi} be the concentration of urea at the inlet of the dialyzer in the arterial line which takes blood into the dialyzer, that is, at the outlet of the body. Let C_{Bo} be the concentration of urea at the exit of the dialyzer in the venous line which brings the blood back to the body, that is, at the inlet of the body compartment. Mass balance demands that the rate of change of mass in the body be equal to the net rate of mass coming into the body from the dialyzer, plus the metabolic production rate G:

$$(VdC/dt) = Q_B\,(C_{Bo} - C_{Bi}) + G = -Q_B\,C\,(1 - C_{Bo}/C_{Bi}) + G \qquad (5.11)$$

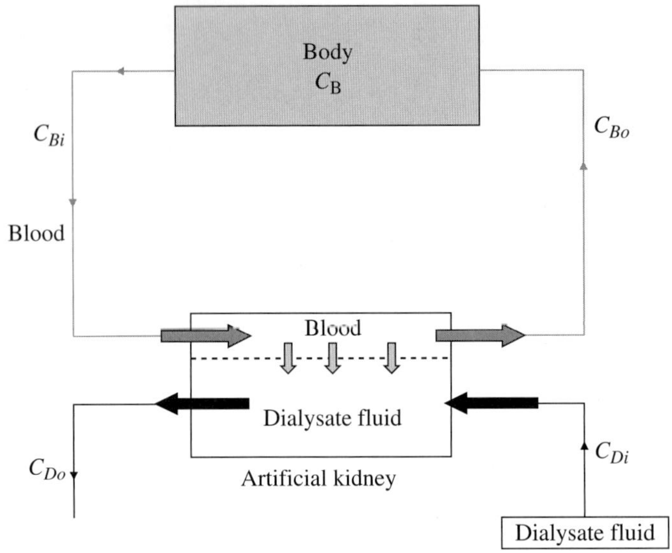

FIGURE 5.7 Patient-dialyzer interaction modeling using one-compartmental model of the body.

where V = the tissue volume plus the blood volume
Q = the blood flow rate to the kidney
G = the metabolic production rate of urea in the body

Extraction ratio for low flux dialysis can be further expressed in terms of the concentrations as follows:

$$E = 1 - (C_{Bo}/C_{Bi}) = 1 - \exp(-kA/Q_B) \tag{5.12}$$

where A is the interfacial membrane surface area for mass transfer and k is the permeability of the membrane for that particular solute (urea in the present context).

Since Q does not change during dialysis, and since k and A are design parameters, extraction ratio E remains a constant for low flux dialysis.

It should be pointed out that C_{Bi} is the concentration at the outlet of the body and therefore at the inlet of the dialyzer, and C_{Bo} is the concentration in the blood coming into the body and therefore going out of the dialyzer (Fig. 5.7). Also, it should be noted that the concentration in the blood going out of the body C_{Bi} is the same as the concentration in the body (C) since we assumed that the entire body (tissue and blood) constitutes a homogeneous well-mixed compartment. Therefore, Eq. (5.11) can be rewritten as follows upon substitution of Eq. (5.12):

$$(VdC/dt) = -Q_B\, C\, E + G \tag{5.13}$$

For low flux dialysis, the volume does not change significantly:

$$V(dC/dt) = -Q_B\, C\, E + G \tag{5.14}$$

When the dialyzer is turned on, metabolic production rate G can be assumed to be negligible when compared to the other term in the equation, and upon integration will result in

$$C = C^0 \exp[-(Q\, E/V)\, t] = C^0 \exp[-(Kt/V)] \tag{5.15}$$

where C^0 is the initial concentration of urea in the tissue and $\mathbf{K}$ is clearance ($\mathbf{K} = Q_B E$).

When the patient is *not* on dialysis, then the blood flow to the dialyzer Q is zero, and therefore,

$$V\,(dC/dt) = G \tag{5.16}$$

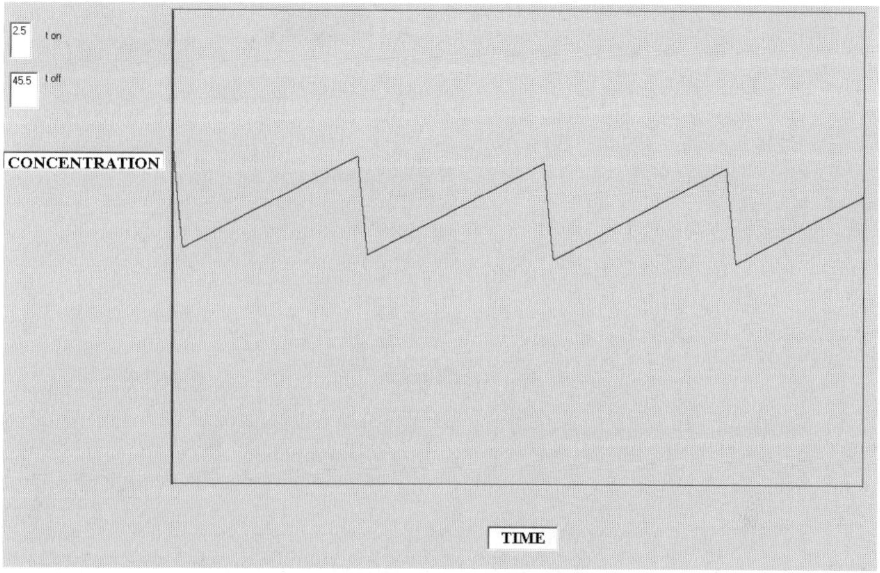

FIGURE 5.8 Concentration of urea as a function of time. Concentration decreases exponentially when the patient is on dialysis during the dialysis session, and slowly rises when the patient is off-dialysis.

When the patient is *not* on dialysis, the concentration of urea would increase linearly if the metabolic production rate is constant or will increase exponentially if the metabolic production rate is a linear function of the concentration (first-order reaction). When the patient is *on* dialysis, the concentration would decrease exponentially. This way, the treatment protocol can be prescribed after simulating different *on* and *off* times (e.g., turn on the dialyzer for $2\frac{1}{2}$ hours every 2 days) to bring the BUN under control (Fig. 5.8).

Now, let us examine the limitations of the one-compartmental model. First, the entire blood and tissue are assumed to be in equilibrium. However, it is well known that intracellular urea concentration may be significantly different from the extracellular compartment. Moreover, urea may be preferentially produced in certain organs like brain, heart, muscle, etc. An accurate treatment requires a multicompartmental model.

Let us consider a two-compartmental model (Fig. 5.9) consisting of an intracellular pool (compartment 1) and an extracellular pool (compartment 2). Urea is produced by intracellular pool and is transported across the cell membrane into the interstitial fluids and then into the blood stream. Mass balance for these two compartments can be expressed as follows:

$$V_1 (dC_1/dt) = G - \mathrm{B} (C_1 - C_2) \tag{5.17}$$

where $\mathrm{B} (C_1 - C_2)$ = the interfacial transfer from compartment 1 to compartment 2 (from intracellular to extracellular pool)

C_1, C_2 = concentrations of urea in compartments 1 and compartment 2

B = constant

The constant B is a product of permeability of the cellular membrane for urea and the interfacial surface area:

$$V_2 (dC_2/dt) = \mathrm{B} (C_1 - C_2) - Q\, C_2\, E \tag{5.18}$$

Blood flow to the dialyzer (Q) is zero when the patient is not on dialysis machine. However, the two-compartmental model may not be sufficient if one wants to find the concentration of urea in the brain tissue. A multicompartmental model involving separate compartments for brain, heart, kidney, lean tissue, etc., may be needed to accurately determine the concentration of urea in critical organs.

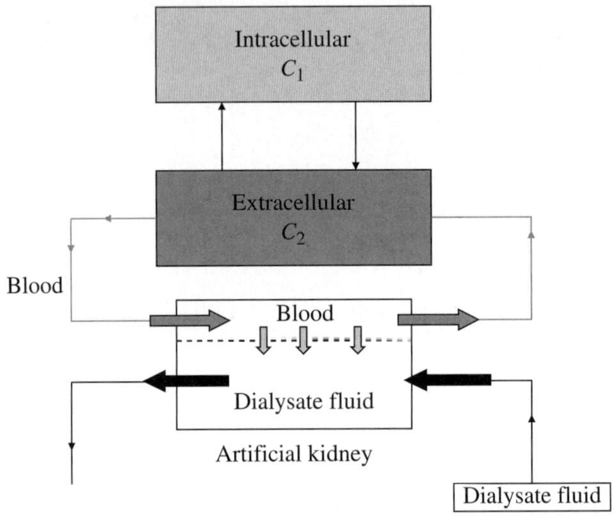

FIGURE 5.9 Patient-dialysis interaction modeling using two-compartmental model of the body consisting of an extracellular compartment (blood and interstitial fluid), and an intracellular compartment.

From the single-compartmental model Eq. (5.15),

$$(C/C^0) = \exp\,[-(\mathbf{K}t/V)] \tag{5.19}$$

The quantity $\mathbf{K}t/V$ provides a measure of the delivered dialysis dose, and has been used in the clinic in the management of dialysis patients.[44–46] As a rough estimation, the quantity $\mathbf{K}t/V$ can be calculated by taking the inverse logarithm of the ratio of postdialysis to predialysis BUN. However, an accurate method would be to solve the multicompartmental model equations taking into account the metabolic production rate of urea G.[44] Computer programs exist for solving the urea kinetic modeling differential equations taking into account the postdialysis urea rebound often observed in patients.[47] The National Kidney Foundation (NKF) has issued guidelines on calculating the $\mathbf{K}t/V$ value.[48] Daugirdas[49] has derived an empirical relationship which takes into account the amount of urea removed via ultrafiltration and urea generated in the tissue:

$$\mathbf{K}t/V = -\ln\,(R - 0.008\,T) + (4 - 3.5\,R)\,U/W \tag{5.20}$$

where R = the ratio of postdialysis to predialysis BUN
T = the time in hours (h)
U = the ultrafiltration volume in liters (L)
W = the patient's postdialysis weight in kilograms (kg)

Equation (5.20) is referred to as Daugirdas II formula and has been endorsed by the NKF as a measure of dialysis adequacy.[44,45] The NKF has established Dialysis Outcome Quality Initiative (DOQI) clinical practice guidelines. For a thrice-a-week-dialysis program, NKF guidelines require a $\mathbf{K}t/V$ value of 1.2 or larger.[44,45] It should be noted that the minimum $\mathbf{K}t/V$ value required for clinically adequate dialysis depends on the frequency of dialysis.

The above guidelines for $\mathbf{K}t/V$ are for urea clearance. There are numerous other uremic toxins that have to be removed.[45,50] Inadequate removal of middle molecules, such as β_2-microglobulin, and a loss of blood serum albumin are major problems. The Clinical Performance Measures Project has set blood serum albumin >4 g/dL as a target for incenter dialysis patients.

In addition to removing the toxic waste materials, the natural kidney reabsorbs many essential nutrients and amino acids from the filtrate. In the natural kidney, the filtrate from the glomerulus in the Bowman's capsule passes through the proximal tubule and the distal tubule before it is rejected as urine. In the proximal tubule, salt, essential ions, glucose, water, amino acids, small protein, peptides, glutathione, and other substances are reabsorbed through active, passive, and facilitated transport mechanisms. The artificial kidney does not reabsorb some of the essential nutrients, such as the amino acids, small protein, and peptides, etc. Activated charcoal microcapsules have been suggested for use in the artificial kidney.[51] However, there are numerous drawbacks with the charcoal kidney. There continues to be a need for replacing the other functions of the natural kidney, such the amino acid and peptide reabsorption. Humes et al.[52] are developing a bioengineered artificial kidney device.

5.6 BIOENGINEERED ARTIFICIAL KIDNEY

Recent advances in tissue engineering and tissue culture have created opportunities for the development of bioengineered artificial kidney devices. Humes et al.[52,53] have successfully developed a bioengineered renal tubule assist device (RAD) by seeding proximal tubule cells on the inner surface of hollow fibers made of polysulfone. The inner luminal surface of polysulfone was first coated with a synthetic protein, Pro-Nectin-L, to promote cellular attachment to the surface. Tubule cells were then seeded onto this surface. For preclinical trials, investigators have extracted tubule cells from pigs. However, for further studies and clinical trials, they have extracted proximal tubule cells from human postmortem kidney specimens and transplant discards. After seeding, the bioreactors (tubule-cell–seeded hollow fibers) were perfused with culture media initially through diffusion and later with convective flow. The bioreactors were then evaluated for reabsorption protein, amino acids, glucose, etc. Initial experiments were conducted with tubule cells seeded onto single hollow fibers and then with tubule cells seeded onto commercially available polysulfone catridges. In preclinical anesthetized dog experiments, a commercial high flux hollow fiber artificial kidney was used to remove waste materials, and the ultrafiltrate from this artificial kidney was then perfused through the RAD bioreactor cartridge as shown in Fig. 5.10.

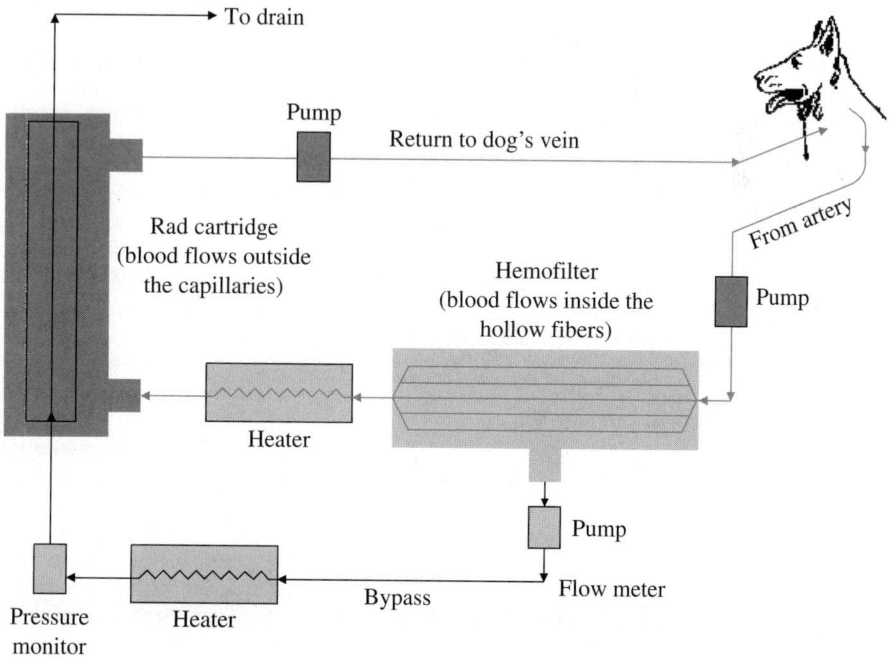

FIGURE 5.10 The bio-artificial kidney being developed by Humes et al. Renal tubule assist device (RAD) is in series with a hemofilter. Renal tubule cells are grown on the inside wall of a synthetic hollow fiber. The renal tubule cells produce and/or reabsorb essential hormones. The RAD cartridge consists of the bio-hollow tubes. The waste from the hemofilter flows through the inside of the bio-hollow tubes and the blood flows on the outside of these tubes in the RAD cartridge, absorbing the essential hormones produced by the renal tubule cells in the wall of the bio-hollow tube.

The investigators have found that the RAD bioreactor was able to reabsorb glucose, glutathione, 1-25 dihydroxy-vitamin D_3, etc. In addition, the RAD bioreactors were able to generate ammonia in a quantity comparable to the natural kidney. Clinical trials are currently ongoing.

The bioengineered artificial kidney with real tubular cells from the kidney seeded onto synthetic polymeric hollow fibers is promising. These RAD bioreactors form the beginning of bioengineered artificial kidney devices and provide a foundation for the development of artificial devices for full restoration of the kidney function. Perhaps, one day, the renal glomerular cells can also be grown on hollow fiber polymer cartridges to form a bioengineered glomerulus and Bowman's capsule, which, together with the RAD, could form a total bioengineered artificial kidney device.

5.7 CONCLUSION

The purpose of the artificial kidney device is to remove urea and other toxic waste molecules. Blood flows on one side of a semipermeable membrane and dialysate solution flows on the other side of the membrane. The toxic waste molecules are removed by either diffusion, or convection, or both. *Diffusion* is the primary mechanism of waste product removal in the conventional low flux dialysis. High flux dialysis involves solute removal by convection and diffusion, but convection is the primary mechanism. Toxic middle molecules (e.g., β_2-microglobulin) are effectively eliminated in the high flux dialysis. However, high flux dialysis may lead to the loss of blood serum albumin, which is closer in molecular weight to the toxic middle molecules. Biocompatibility is a major requirement of hemodialysis membranes. The conventional cellulose base membranes are associated with biocompatibility problems, including complement activation and lucopenia. Substituted cellulose and synthetic membranes have significantly improved biocompatibility. Polyacrylonitrile based and polysulfone membranes have excellent biocompatibility. There are stringent water quality requirements for use in dialysis fluid. Quantitative measures such as $\mathbf{K}t/V$ are clinically useful for the prescription and assessment of adequacy of dialysis. Designing a membrane to effectively remove toxic middle molecules without the loss of blood serum albumin presents continuing challenge. The present artificial kidney systems do not duplicate all the functions of the kidney. The future direction is toward tissue-engineered renal assistive devices in series with hemodialysis cartridges.

REFERENCES

1. Guyton AC: *Text Book of Medical Physiology*. Philadelphia, Pa. Saunders, 7th ed., 1986.
2. Singh AK: *Chronic Kidney Disease*. Philadelphia, Pa. Saunders, 2005.
3. Light PD: Dialysate composition in hemodialysis and peritonial dialysis, in Henrich WL (ed.), *Principles and Practice of Dialysis*. Philadelphia, Pa. Lippincott Williams & Wilkins, 3d ed., 2004, pp. 28–44.
4. Leypoldt JK: Solute fluxes in different treatment modalities. *Nephrology, Dialysis and Transplantation*, **15**(Suppl. 1):3–9, 2000.
5. Cheung AK: Biocompatibility of hemodialysis membranes. *J. Am. Soc. Nephrol.* **1**:155–161, 1990.
6. Jadoul M: Dialysis-related amyloidosis: importance of biocompatibility and age. *Nephrology, Dialysis and Transplantation,* **13**(Suppl. 7):61–64, 1998.
7. Ohmno M, Suzuki M, Miayagi M, Yagi T, Sakurai H., Ukai T: CTA hemodialyis membrane design for β_2-microglobulin removal Cellulosics, in Kennedy JF, Phillips GO, Williams PA (eds.), *Chemical, Biochemical, and Material Aspects*. New York, N.Y. Harwood, 1993, pp. 415–420.
8. Winchester JF, Salsberg JA, Levin NW: Beta-2 microglobulin in ESRD: an in-depth review. *Adv. Renal Repl. Th.*, **10**:279–309, 2003.
9. Canaud B, Kessler M, Pedrini LA, Tattersall J, Wee PM, Vanholder RM, Wanner C: Biochemical reactions subsequent to complement and leukocyte activation. *Nephr. Dialysis Transpl.* **17**-S7:32–34, 2002.
10. Canaud B, Kessler M, Pedrini LA, Tattersall J, Wee PM, Vanholder RM, Wanner C: Clinical morbidity and mortality in response to complement and leukocyte activation. *Nephr. Dialysis Transpl.* **17**-S7:34–37, 2002.

11. Henrich W: *Prinicples and Practice of Dialysis*, Philadelphia, Pa. Lippincott Williams & Wilkins, 3d ed., 2004.
12. Ronco C: Backfiltration: a controversial issue in modern dialysis. *Int. J. Artif. Org.* **11**:69–74, 1988.
13. Ronco C, Levin NW: *Hemodialysis, Vascular Access, and Peritoneal Dialysis Access.* New York, N.Y., Basel, 2004.
14. Cappelli G, Inguaggiato P, Ferramosca E, Albertazzi A: Water treatment for hemodialysis, in Ronco C, Greca L (eds.), *Hemodialysis Technology*. Basel, Karger, 2002, pp. 317–324.
15. Wber V, Linsberger I, Rossmanith E, Weber C, Falkenhagen D: Pyrogen transfer across high and low flux hemodialysis membranes. *Artif. Organs.* **28**:210–217, 2004.
16. Schindler R, Christ-Kohlrausch F, Frei U, Shaldon S: Differences in permeability of high-flux dialyzer membranes for bacterial pyrogens. *Clin. Nephrol.* **59**:447–454, 2003.
17. Schindler R: Causes and therapy of microinflammation in renal failure. *Nephrol. Dial. Transpl.* **19**(Suppl. 5):34–40, 2004.
18. Woods HF, Nandakumar M: Improved outcome for hemodialysis patients treated with high-flux membranes. *Nephrol. Dial. Traspl.* **15**(Suppl. 1):36–42, 2000.
19. Akizawa T, Kinugasa E, Ideura T: Classification of dialysis membranes by performance. *Contrib. Nephrol.* **113**:25–31, 1995.
20. Clark WR, Hamburger RJ, Lysaght MJ: Effect of membrane composition and structure on solute removal and biocompatibility in hemodialysis. *Kidney Int.* **56**:2005–2015, 1999.
21. Leypoldt JK, Cheung AK: Characterization of molecular transport in artificial kidney. *Art. Org.* **20**:381–389, 1996.
22. Clark WR, Macias WL, Molitoris BA, Wang NH: Plasma-protein adsorption to highly permeable hemodialysis membranes. *Kidney Int.* **48**:481–488, 1995.
23. Cooney D: *Biomedical Engineering Principles*. New York, N.Y., M. Dekker, 1976.
24. Vienken J, Bowry S: Quo vadis dialysis membrane? *Artif. Organs.* **26**:152–159, 2002.
25. Sharma CP: Membranes for dialysis, in *Encyclopedia of Surface and Colloid Science*. Dekker, 2004, pp. 1–15.
26. Cases A, Reverter J, Escolar G, Sanz C, Sorribes C, Ordinas A: In-vivo evaluation of platelet activation by different cellulosic membranes. *Art. Organs*, **21**:330–334, 1997.
27. Cheung AK, Parker CJ, Wilcox L, Janatova J: Activation of the alternate pathway of complement by cellulosic membranes. *Kidney Int.* **36**:257–265, 1989.
28. Verbeelen D, Jochmans K, Herman AG, Van der Niepen P, Sennesaei J, De Walele M: Evaluation of platelets and hemostasis during hemodialysis with six different membranes. *Nephron.* **59**:567–572, 1991.
29. Sirolli V, Di Stante S, Stuard S, Stuard S, Di Liberato L, Amoroso L, Cappelli P, Bonomini M: Biocompatibility and functional performance of polythene glycol acid-grafted cellulose: An alternative to synthetic membranes for use in hemodialysis. *Int. J. Art. Organs.* **23**:356–364, 2000.
30. Sasaki M, Hosoya N, Saruhasi, M: Vitamin E modified cellulose membrane. *Art. Organs.* **24**:779–789, 2000.
31. Zaluska WT, Ksiazek A, Rolski J: Effect of vitamin E modified cellulose membrane on human lymphocyte, monocyte, and granulocyte CD11b/CD18 adhesion molecule expression during hemodialysis. *ASAIO J.* **47**:619–622, 2001.
32. Dhondt A, Vanholder R, Florieux G, Waterloos MA, De Smet R, Lesaffer G, Lameire N: Vitamin E-bonded cellulose membrane and hemodialysis bioincompatibility: absence of an acute benefit on expression of leukocyte surface molecules. *Am. J. Kidney Dis.* **36**:1140–1146, 2000.
33. Hakim NA: Influence of hemodialysis membrane on outcome of ESRD patients. *Am. J. Kidney Dis.* **32**:71–75, 1998.
34. Cianciolo G, Stefoni S, Donati G, De Pascalis A, Iannelli S, Manna C, Coli L, et al. Intra- and post-dialytic platelet activation and PDGF-AB release: cellulose diacetate vs polysulfone membranes. *Nephrol. Dial. Transplant.* **16**(6):1222–1229, June 2001.
35. Jaber BL, Fonski JA, Cendorogio M, Balakrishnan VS, Razegi, P, Dinarello, CA, Pereira BJ: New polyether sulfone dialyzers attenuate passage of cytokine-inducing substances from pseudomonas contaminated dialysate. *Blood Purif.* **16**:210–219, 1998.
36. Kanda H, Kubo K, Hamasaki K, Kanda A, Nakao A, Kitamura T, Fujita T, Yamamoto K, Mimura T: Influence of various hemodialysis membranes on the plasma (1–3-D)-glucan level. *Kidney Int.* **60**:319, 2001.
37. Falkenhagen D, Brown GS: Clinical evaluation of three hemodialyzers containing PMMA membranes of different surface area, with special attention to thrombogenicity. *Nephrol. Dial. Transplant.* **6**(Suppl. 2):43–8, 1991.

38. Kato A, Takita T, Furuhashi M, Takahashi T, Watanable T, Maruyama Y, Hishida A: Polymethylmethacrylate efficacy in reduction of renal itching in hemodialysis patients: cross-over study and tumor necrosis factor. *Art. Organs.* **25**:441–447, 2000.

39. Renaux J, Atti M: The AN69 Dialysis membrane, in Ronco C, La Grecca G (eds.), *Hemodialysis Technology.* Basel, Karger, 2002, pp. 111–119.

40. Varresen L, Water M, Vanrenterghem Y, Michielsen P: Angiotensin converting enzyme inhibitors and anaphylactoid reactions to high flux, membrane dialysis. *Lancet.* **336**:1360–1362, 1990.

41. John B, Kannu H, Anjeet I, Ahmad R: Anaphylactic reaction during hemodialysis on AN69 membrane in a patient receiving angiotensin II receptor antagonist. *Nephrol. Dial. Transplant.* **16**:1955–1956, 2001.

42. Misra M: The basics of hemodialysis equipment. *Hemodial. Int.* **9**:30–36, 2005.

43. Reddy NP: Modeling and simulation of biomedical systems, in Kutz M (ed.), *Standard Handbook of Biomedical Engineering and Design,* New York, N.Y., McGraw-Hill, 2003, pp. 1.13–1.17.

44. O'Connor A, Wish B: Hemodialysis adequacy and timing of dialysis initiation, in Henrich WL (ed.), *Principles and Practice of Dialysis.* Philadelphia, Pa. Lippincott Williams & Wilkins, 3d ed., 2004, pp. 111–127.

45. Kumar VA, Depner TA: Approach to hemodialysis kinetic modeling, in Henrich WL (ed.), *Principles and Practice of Dialysis*, Philadelphia, Pa. Lippincott Williams & Wilkins, 3d ed., 2004, pp. 82–102.

46. Leypoldt JK: *The Artificial Kidney: Physiological Modeling and Tissue Engineering*, Austin, Tex, R.G. Landes, 1999.

47. Depner TA: *Multi-Compartment Models: Prescribing Hemodialysis—A Guide to Urea Modeling,* Boston, Mass. Kluwater Academic, 1991, pp. 91–126.

48. National Kidney Foundation: K/DOQI clinical practice guidelines for hemodialysis 2000. *Am. J. Kidney Dis.* **37**:S7–S64, 2001.

49. Daugirdas JT: Second generation logarithmic estimates of single pool variable volume *Kt/V*: an analysis of error. *J. Am Soc. Nephrol.* **4**:1205–1231, 2001.

50. Maduell F: Hemodiafiltration. *Hemodialysis Int.* **9**:47–55, 2005.

51. Chandy T, Sharma C: Activated charcoal microcapsules and their applications. *J. Biomat.* **13**:129–157, 1999.

52. Humes HD, Buffington DA, MacKay SM, Funke AJ, Weitzel WF: Replacement of renal function in uremic animals with a tissue-engineered kidney. *Nature Biotech.* **17**:451–455, 1999.

53. Humes HD, Weitzel WF, Bartlett RH, Swinker FG, Paganni EP, Luderer JR, Sobota J: Initial clinical results of the bioartificial kidney containing human cells in ICU patients with acute renal failure. *Kidney Int.* **66**:1578–1588, 2004.

CHAPTER 6
DESIGN OF CONTROLLED-RELEASE DRUG DELIVERY SYSTEMS

Steve I. Shen, Shilditya Bhattacharya, Bhaskara R. Jasti, and Xiaoling Li
Thomas J. Long School of Pharmacy and Health Science, University of the Pacific, Stockton, California,

With the advances in science and technology, many new chemical molecules are being created and tested for therapeutic uses in a much faster pace. The U.S. Food and Drug Administration (FDA) approved 22 to 53 new molecular entities each year between 1993 and 2006 and slowly decreased to 17 in 2007,[1] the lowest in about 24 years. A major problem is the translation of in vitro activity of new molecules to efficacy in the humans. Creation of these drug molecules is only part of the drug product development. Every drug molecule needs a delivery system to carry the drug to the site of action upon administration to the patient. Delivery of the drugs can be achieved using various types of dosage forms, including tablets, capsules, creams, ointments, liquids, aerosols, injections, and suppositories. Most of these conventional drug delivery systems are known to provide immediate release of the drug with little or no control over delivery rate. To achieve and maintain therapeutically effective plasma concentrations, several doses are needed daily, which may cause significant fluctuations in plasma levels (Fig. 6.1). Because of these fluctuations in drug plasma levels, the drug level could fall below the minimum effective concentration (MEC) or exceed the minimum toxic concentration (MTC). Such fluctuations result in unwanted side effects or lack of intended therapeutic benefit to the patient.

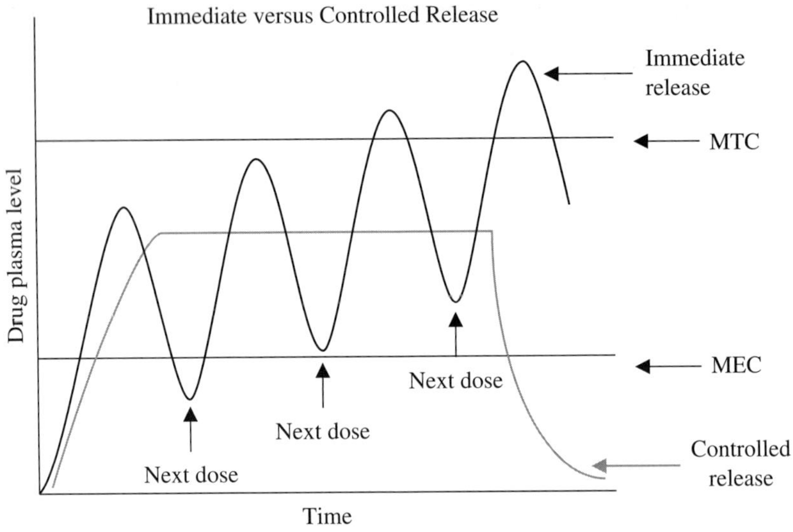

FIGURE 6.1 Schematic representation of therapeutic and toxic levels from immediate versus controlled-release dosage forms.

Sustained-release and controlled-release drug delivery systems can reduce the undesired fluctuations of drug levels, thus diminishing side effects while improving the therapeutic outcome of the drug (Fig. 6.1). The terms, *sustained release* and *controlled release* refer to two different types of drug delivery systems, although they are often used interchangeably. Sustained-release dosage forms are systems that prolong the duration of the action by slowing the release of the drug, usually at the cost of delayed onset and its pharmacological action. Controlled-release drug systems are more sophisticated than just simply delaying the release rate and are designed to deliver the drug at a specific release rate within a predetermined time period. Targeted delivery systems are also considered as a controlled delivery system, since they provide spatial control of drug release to a specific site of the body.

Advantages of controlled-release drug delivery systems include delivery of drug to the required site, maintenance of drug levels within a desired range, reduced side effects, fewer administrations, and improved patient compliance. However, there are potential disadvantages that should not be overlooked. Disadvantages of using such delivery systems include possible toxicity of the materials used, dose dumping, requirement of surgical procedures to implant or remove the system, and higher manufacturing costs. In pharmaceutical industry, design and development of controlled/sustained-release drug delivery systems have been used as a strategic means to prolong the proprietary status of drug products that are reaching the end of their patent life. A typical example is modifying an existing drug product that requires several doses a day to a single daily dosing to maintain the dominance over generic competitions. For some drugs, controlled delivery is necessary, since immediate release dosage forms cannot achieve desired pharmacological action. These include highly water-soluble drugs that need slower release and longer duration of action, highly lipophilic drugs that require enhancement of solubility to achieve therapeutic level, short half-life drugs that require repeated administration, and drugs with nonspecific action that requires the delivery to target sites. Additionally, with the decrease in percentage of successful new molecules, many drug companies are utilizing the controlled-release drug delivery systems as a means to strengthen their drug life cycle management.

An ideal drug delivery system should deliver precise amounts of drug at a preprogrammed rate to achieve a drug level necessary for treatment of the disease. For most drugs that show a clear relationship between concentration and response, the drug concentration will be maintained within the therapeutic range when the drug is released by zero-order rate. In order to design a controlled-release delivery system, many factors such as physicochemical properties of drug, route of drug administration, and pharmacological and biological effects must be considered.

6.1 PHYSICOCHEMICAL PROPERTIES OF DRUG

Physicochemical properties such as solubility, stability, lipophilicity, and molecular interactions play a major role in biological effectiveness of the drug. Solubility is a measure of the amount of solute that can be dissolved in the solvent. For a drug to be absorbed, it must first dissolve in the physiological fluids of the body at a reasonably fast dissolution rate. Drug molecules with very low aqueous solubility often have lower bioavailability because of the limited amount of dissolved drug at the site of absorption. In general, drugs with lower than 10 mg/mL in aqueous solutions are likely to exhibit low and erratic oral bioavailability.

Once the drug is administered, biological fluids that are in direct contact with drug molecule may influence the stability of the drug. Drugs may be susceptible to both chemical and enzymatic degradation, which results in a loss of activity of the drug. Drugs with poor acidic stability, when coated with enteric coating materials, will bypass the acidic stomach and release the drug at lower portion of the gastrointestinal (GI) tract. Drugs can also be protected from enzymatic cleavage by modifying the chemical structure to form prodrugs.

The ability of drug partitioning into lipid phase can be evaluated by the distribution of drug between lipid and water phase at equilibrium. A distribution constant, the partition coefficient K, is commonly used to describe the equilibrium of drug concentrations in two phases.

$$K = \frac{\text{Drug}_{\text{lipid}}}{\text{Drug}_{\text{water}}} \tag{6.1}$$

The partition coefficient of a drug reflects the permeability of a drug through the biological membrane and/or the polymer membrane. Commonly, partition coefficient is determined by equilibrating the drug in a saturated mixture of octanol (lipid phase) and water. Drugs with high partition coefficient can easily penetrate biological membranes as they are made of lipid bilayers, but are unable to proceed further due to higher affinity to the membrane than the aqueous surroundings. Drugs with low partition coefficient can easily move around the aqueous regions of the body, but will not cross the biological membranes easily.

In addition to the inherent properties of drug molecules, molecular interactions such as drug–drug, drug–protein, and drug–metal ion binding are important factors that can significantly change the pharmacokinetic parameters of a drug. These factors should also be taken into consideration when designing controlled drug delivery systems.

6.2 ROUTES OF DRUG ADMINISTRATION

Various routes of administration pose different challenges for product design. As a result of the different barriers and pathways involved, selection of an administration route is an important factor for design of drug delivery system. For example, the oral route is the most widely utilized route because of its ease of administration and large surface area of the GI tract (200 m^2). The presence of microvilli makes this the largest absorptive surface of the body (4500 m^2).[2] The challenges of oral administration are short GI transit time, extreme acidic pH, abundant presence of digestive enzymes, and first-pass metabolism in the liver. Several products were designed to prolong the retention time of the drug in the GI tract. A hydrodynamically balanced drug delivery system (HBS) is designed to achieve bulk density of less than 1 when contacted with gastric fluids rendering the drug formulation to remain buoyant. This dosage form is also called *floating* capsules or tablets because of this characteristic.[3]

Another commonly used route for drug delivery is parenteral administration. The routes used for parenteral therapy include intradermal, subcutaneous, intravenous, intracardiac, intramuscular, intra-arterial, and intrasynovial. Parenteral administrations offer immediate response, in such situations as cardiac arrest or shock, and good bioavailability for drugs that undergo degradation by digestive enzymes in GI tract. The disadvantages of parenteral administrations are difficulty of administration, requirement of sterile conditions, and cost of manufacturing.

In addition, skin with surface area of 2 m^2 is a commonly used route for drug delivery. Advantages of the transdermal route include avoidance of first-pass effect, potential of multiday therapy with a single application, rapid termination of drug effects, and easy identification of medication in an emergency. The limitations are skin irritation and/or sensitization, variation of intra- and interindividual percutaneous absorption, the limited time that a delivery system can remain affixed, and higher cost.[4]

Most of the controlled-release delivery systems available in the market for systemic delivery of drugs utilize oral, parenteral, and transdermal route for their administration. Advances in biotechnology produced many gene, peptide, and protein drugs with specific demands on route of delivery. Thus, other routes such as buccal, nasal, ocular, pulmonary, rectal, and vaginal are gaining more attention.

6.3 PHARMACOLOGICAL AND BIOLOGICAL EFFECTS

It is important to consider the human dimension in the design of the drug delivery systems. Biological factors, such as age, weight, gender, ethnicity, physiological processes, and disease state, will change the pharmacokinetics and pharmacodynamics of a drug. For example, dosing newborn infants requires caution due to their immature hepatic function and higher water content in the body. Geriatric patients may suffer from reduced sensitivity of certain receptors that may lead to insensitivity to certain drugs. It has been found that different ethnic groups respond to drugs differently. Diuretics and calcium channel blockers are recommended as the first-line therapy in hypertensive Black patients, while beta-blockers work better for Caucasian patients. Pathological changes may influence the distribution and bioavailability of the drug by altering the physiological process. Decreased kidney and/or liver functions will affect the clearance of many drugs.

In this chapter, the discussion of the design of drug delivery system is based on various approaches: prodrug approach, diffusion-controlled reservoir and matrix systems, dissolution/coating-controlled systems, osmotically controlled systems, ion-exchange resin systems, gastroretentive systems, and approaches for macromolecular drug delivery. The aim of this chapter is to introduce the basic concepts for the designs of various drug delivery systems. Readers can refer to Refs. 2 to 9 for further details.

6.4 PRODRUG

The molecule with the most potent form does not always have the desired physicochemical properties needed for drug dissolution and/or absorption. In fact, of all the pharmaceutically active ingredients, 43 percent are sparingly soluble or insoluble in water. In the prodrug approach for drug delivery, active ingredients are chemically modified by connecting specialized functional groups that will be removed in the body after administration releasing the parent molecule.[8] These latent groups are used in a transient manner to change the properties of the parent drug to achieve a specific function, for example, alter permeability, solubility, or stability. After the prodrug has achieved its goal, the functional group is removed in the body (enzymatic cleavage or hydrolysis) and the parent compound is released to elicit its pharmacological action (Fig. 6.2).

The prodrug approach has been used for one or more of the following reasons:

To Change Half-Life. Half-life is defined as time required by the biological system for removing 50 percent of administered drug. Drugs with very short half-life may not be therapeutically beneficial

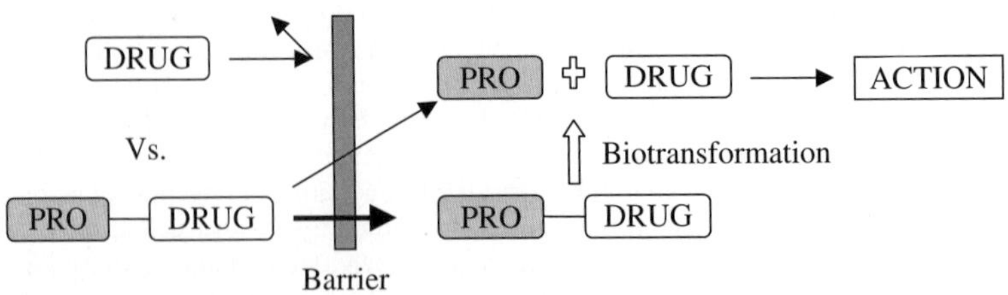

FIGURE 6.2 Schematic design of prodrug principle.

TABLE 6.1 Examples of Marketed Prodrugs

Product Name	Prodrug	Active Drug	Principle for Prodrug Approach
Vasotec® (Merck)	Enalapril	Enalaprilat	
Valtrex® (GSK)	Valaciclovir	Aciclovir	
Sinemet® (BMS)	Levedopa	Dopamine	
Tamiflu® (Roche)	Oseltamivir phosphate	Oseltamivir carboxylate	
Benicar® (Daichi)	Olmesartan	Olmesartan	To cross a biological barrier at the site of absorption
Sankyo (Forest)	medoxomil		
Famvir® (Novartis)	Famciclovir	Penciclovir	
Vantin® (Pfizer)	Cefpodoxime proxetil	Cefpodoxime	
Valcyte® (Roche)	Valganciclovir	Ganciclovir	
Monopril® (BMS)	Fosinopril	Fosinoprilat	
Cerebyx® (Pfizer)	Fosphenytoin	Phenytoin	For ease of intravenous administration

unless this characteristic is improved. Attaching the drug to a polymer as part of a pendent will enhance its half-life. Modification of the drug to protect the site of degradation or metabolism is another method to achieve longer half-life.

To Cross a Biological Barrier. Drugs with unbalanced hydrophilic or hydrophobic properties will not effectively cross the biological barriers. Attachment of labile functional groups can change the properties of the parent drug and allow the prodrug to cross the barrier.

To Increase Retention Time. When intended for a part of the body with high tissue turnover rate, such as intestinal mucosa, a drug linked to a mucoadhesive polymer can increase adhesion to the site and have better bioavailability.

To Target a Specific Site. Connecting specialized functional groups that have site-specific affinity (peptide, antibody, etc.) can allow the parent drug to be delivered to targeted area of the body to produce site-specific therapeutic action. Some of the prodrugs available in the market are listed in Table 6.1.

6.5 DIFFUSION-CONTROLLED DELIVERY SYSTEMS

Diffusion process has been utilized in design of controlled-release drug delivery systems for several decades. This process is a consequence of constant thermal motion of molecules, which results in net movement of molecules from a high-concentration to a low-concentration region. The rate of diffusion is dependent on temperature, size, mass, and viscosity of the environment.

Molecular motion increases as temperature is raised due to a higher average kinetic energy in the system:

$$E = \frac{kT}{2} = \frac{mv^2}{2} \tag{6.2}$$

where E = kinetic energy
k = Boltzmann's constant
T = temperature
m = mass
v = velocity

This equation shows that an increase in temperature is exponentially correlated to velocity (v^2). Size and mass are also significant factors in the diffusion process. At a given temperature, the mass of molecule is inversely proportional to velocity [Eq. (6.2)]. Larger molecules interact more with the surrounding environment, causing them to have slower velocity. Accordingly, large molecules diffuse much slower than light and small particles. Viscosity of the environment is another important parameter in diffusion, since the rate of molecular movement is associated with the viscosity of the environment. Diffusion is fastest in the gas phase, slower in the liquid phase, and slowest in the solid phase.

Mathematically, the rate of drug delivery in diffusion-controlled delivery systems can be described by Fick's laws. Fick's first law of diffusion is expressed as[9]

$$j = -D\frac{dC}{dx} \tag{6.3}$$

where J = flux of diffusion
D = the diffusivity of drug molecule
dC/dx = the concentration gradient of the drug molecule across diffusional barrier with thickness dx

According to the diffusion principle, controlled-release drug delivery systems can be designed as a reservoir system or a matrix system. Drug released from both reservoir- and matrix-type devices follow the principle of diffusion, but they show two different release patterns as shown in Fig. 6.3.

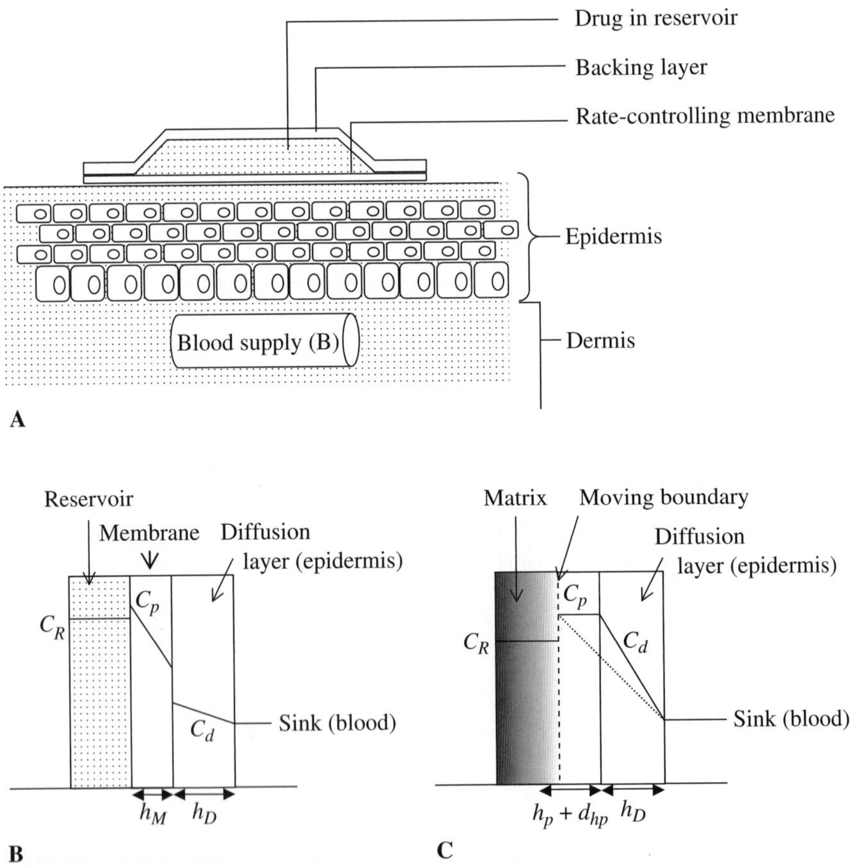

FIGURE 6.3 Schematic illustration of a transdermal drug delivery system in use (*a*), concentration profiles of reservoir (*b*), and matrix type of system (*c*).

In Fig. 6.3, C_R is drug concentration in the reservoir or matrix compartment, C_P is solubility of drug in the polymer phase, C_D is the concentration in diffusion layer, h_m is thickness of the membrane, h_d is thickness of diffusion layer, and $h_P + dh_P$ indicates the changing thickness of the depletion zone of matrix.

In a reservoir system, if the active agent is in a saturated state, the driving force is kept constant until it is no longer saturated. For matrix systems, because of the changing thickness of the depletion zone, release kinetics is a function of the square root of time.[10] A typical reservoir system for transdermal delivery consists of a backing layer, a rate-limiting membrane, protective liner, and a reservoir compartment. The drug is enclosed within the reservoir compartment and released through a rate-controlling polymer membrane (Fig. 6.4).

Membranes used to enclose the device can be made from various types of polymers. The rate of release can be varied by selecting polymer and varying the thickness of the rate-controlling membrane. The drug in reservoir can be in solid, suspension, or liquid form.

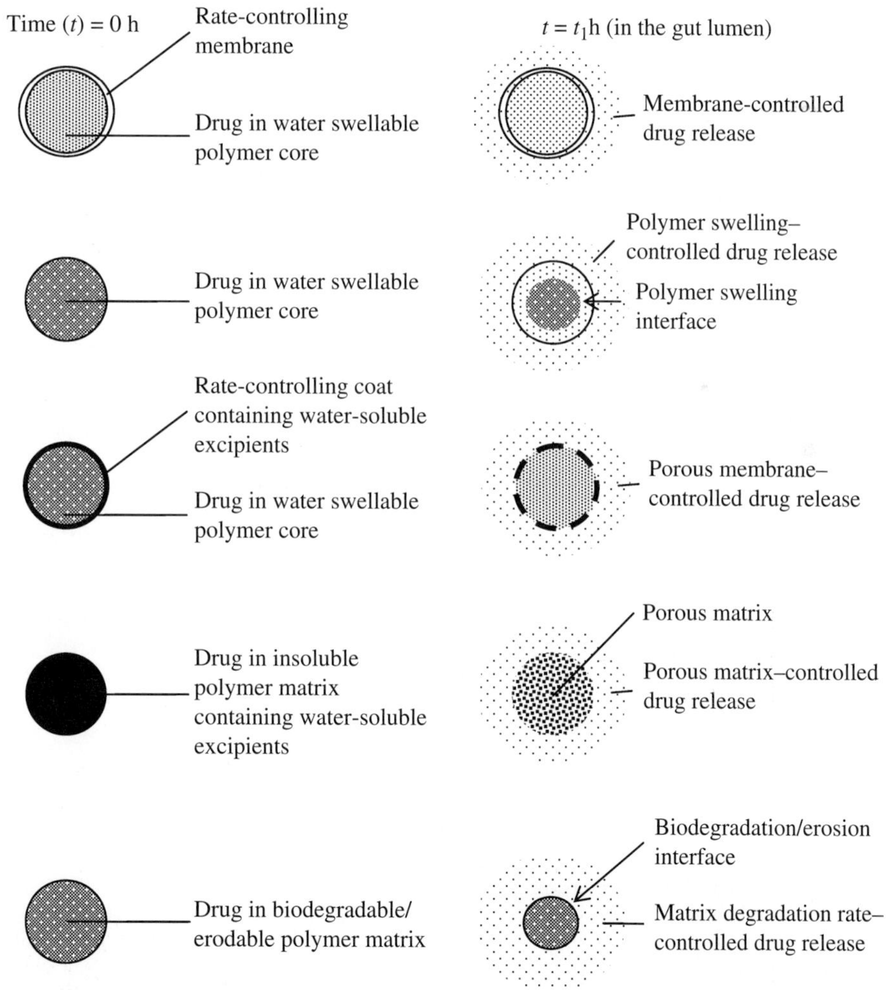

FIGURE 6.4 Schematic illustration of various design principles from controlled-release dosage forms.

Analysis of diffusion-controlled reservoir or matrix drug delivery systems require few assumptions: (1) the diffusion coefficient of a drug molecule in a medium must be constant; (2) the controlled drug release must have a pseudosteady state; (3) dissolution of solid drug must occur prior to the drug release process; and (4) the interfacial partitioning of drug is related to its solubility in polymer and in solution as defined by

$$K = \frac{C_s}{C_p} \tag{6.4}$$

where K = partition coefficient of the drug molecule from polymer to solution
C_s = solubility of drug in the solution phase
C_p = solubility of drug in polymer phase

With the above assumptions, the cumulative amount Q of drug released from a diffusion-controlled reservoir-type drug delivery device with a unit surface area can be described as follows[2]:

$$Q = \frac{C_p K D_d D_m}{K D_d h_m + D_m h_d} t - \frac{D_d D_m}{K D_d h_m + D_m h_d} \int_0^t C_{b(t)} dt \tag{6.5}$$

where D_m = diffusivity of drug in polymer membrane with thickness h_m
D_d = diffusivity of hydrodynamic diffusion layer with thickness h_d
C_b = concentration of drug in reservoir side
t = time

Under sink condition, where $C_{b(t)} \approx 0$ or $C_s \rangle\rangle C_{b(t)}$, Eq. (6.5) is reduced to

$$Q = \frac{C_p K D_d D_m}{K D_d h_m + D_m h_d} t \tag{6.6}$$

This relationship shows that release of drug can be a constant, with rate of drug release being

$$\frac{Q}{t} = \frac{C_p K D_d D_m}{K D_d h_m + D_m h_d} \tag{6.7}$$

In extreme cases, the rate of release may depend mainly on one of the layers, either polymer membrane layer or hydrodynamic diffusion layer. If the polymer membrane is the rate-controlling layer, $K D_d h_m >> D_m h_d$, the equation can be simplified to

$$\frac{Q}{t} = \frac{C_p D_m}{h_m} \tag{6.8}$$

which shows that the release rate is directly proportional to its solubility of the drug in polymer and inversely proportional to thickness of the polymer membrane.

Delivery systems designed on this principle can be administered by different routes: intrauterine such as Progestasert, implants such as Norplant, transdermal such as Transderm-Nitro, and ocular such as Ocusert.

A matrix system, often described as monolithic device, is designed to uniformly distribute the drug within a polymer as a solid block. Matrix devices are favored over other design due to their simplicity, low manufacturing costs, and lack of accidental dose dumping which may occur with reservoir systems when the rate-controlling membrane ruptures.

The release properties of the device depend highly upon the structure of the matrix whether it is porous or nonporous. The rate of drug release is controlled by the concentration or solubility of drug in the polymer and diffusivity of the drug through the polymer for nonporous system. For a porous matrix, the solubility of the drug in the network and the tortuosity of the network add another dimension to affect the rate of release. In addition, drug loading influences the release, since high loading can complicate the release mechanism because of formation of cavities as the drug is leaving the device. These cavities will fill with fluids and increase the rate of release.

The cumulative amount released from a matrix-controlled device is described by[2]

$$Q = \left(C_A - \frac{C_p}{2}\right) h_p \tag{6.9}$$

where C_A is initial amount of drug, C_p is solubility of drug in polymer, and h_p is a time-dependent variable defined by

$$h_p^2 + \frac{2(C_A - C_p)D_p h_d h_p}{\left(C_A - \frac{C_p}{2}\right) D_d \bar{k} K} = \frac{2C_p D_p}{C_A - \frac{C_p}{2}} t \tag{6.10}$$

where $\bar{k}$ = the constant for relative magnitude of the concentration in diffusion layer and depletion zone

D_p = the diffusivity of drug in the polymer devices

and other parameters are the same as described for Eqs. (6.4) to (6.9). At a very early stage of the release process, when there is a very thin depletion zone, the following will be true:

$$h_p^2 << \frac{2(C_A - C_p)D_p h_d h_p}{\left(C_A - \frac{C_p}{2}\right) D_d \bar{k} K}$$

Equation (6.10) can be reduced to

$$h_p \approx \frac{C_p D_d \bar{k} K}{(C_A - C_p) h_d} \tag{6.11}$$

and placing Eq. (6.11) into Eq. (6.9) gives

$$\frac{Q}{t} = \frac{C_p D_d \bar{k} K}{h_d} \qquad \left(\text{if } C_A - C_p \approx C_A - \frac{C_p}{2}\right) \tag{6.12}$$

Since $KC_p = C_s$, Eq. (6.12) becomes

$$\frac{Q}{t} = \frac{C_s D_d \bar{k}}{h_d} \tag{6.13}$$

The $\bar{k}$ term implies that the matrix system is more sensitive to the magnitude of concentration difference between depletion and diffusion layers.

If

$$h_p^2 >> \frac{2(C_A - C_p)D_p h_d h_p}{\left(C_A - \frac{C_p}{2}\right) D_d \bar{k} K}$$

where the depletion zone is much larger and the system has a very thin diffusion layer, Eq. (6.10) becomes

$$h_p \approx \left(\frac{2C_p D_p}{(C_A - \frac{C_p}{2})} t \right)^{1/2} \tag{6.14}$$

and placing Eq. (6.14) into Eq. (6.9) makes

$$\frac{Q}{t^{1/2}} = [(2C_A - C_p)C_p D_p]^{1/2} \tag{6.15}$$

Equation (6.15) indicates that after the depletion zone is large enough, the cumulative amount of drug released (Q) is proportional to the square root of time ($t^{1/2}$).

6.6 DISSOLUTION/COATING-CONTROLLED DELIVERY SYSTEMS

Controlled release of drug can be achieved by utilizing the rate-limiting step in the dissolution process of a solid drug with relatively low aqueous solubility. The dissolution rate can be quantitatively described by Noyes-Whitney equation as follows:

$$\frac{dC}{dt} = \frac{DA}{h}(C_0 - C_t) \tag{6.16}$$

where dC/dt = rate of drug dissolution
D = diffusion coefficient of drug in diffusion layer
h = thickness of diffusion layer
A = surface area of drug particles
C_0 = saturation concentration of the drug in diffusion layer
C_t = concentration of drug in bulk fluids at time t

The surface area A of the drug particle is directly proportional to the rate of dissolution. For a given amount of drug, reducing particle size increases its surface area and dissolution rate. However, small particles tend to agglomerate and form aggregates. Using a specialized milling technique with stabilizer and other excipients, aggregation can be prevented to make microparticles smaller than 400 nm in diameter to improve the dissolution of the drug in the body.

The saturation solubility C_0 can also be manipulated to change the rate of dissolution. Both the physical and chemical properties of a drug can be modified to alter the saturation solubility. For example, salt form of a drug is much more soluble in aqueous environment than the parent drug. The solubility of a drug can also be modified when the drug forms complex with excipients, resulting in a complex with solubility different from the drug itself.

Controlled or sustained release of drug from delivery systems can also be designed by enclosing drug in a polymer shell/coating. After the dissolution or erosion of the coating, drug molecules become available for absorption. Release of drug at a predetermined time is accomplished by controlling the thickness of coating. In Spansule® systems, drug molecules are enclosed in beads of varying thickness to control the time and amount of drug release. The encapsulated particles with thin coatings will dissolve and release the drug first while a thicker coating will take longer to dissolve and will release the drug at later time. Coating-controlled delivery systems can also be designed to prevent the degradation of the drug in the acidic environment of the stomach, which can reach as low as pH 1.0. Such systems are generally referred to as *enteric-coated systems*. In addition, enteric coating also protects stomach from ulceration caused by drug agents. Release of the drug from coating-controlled delivery systems may depend upon the polymer used. A combination of diffusion and dissolution mechanisms may be required to define the drug release from such systems.

6.7 BIODEGRADABLE/ERODIBLE DELIVERY SYSTEMS

Biologically degradable systems contain polymers that degrade into smaller fragments inside the body to release the drug in a controlled manner. Zero-order release can be achieved in these systems as long as the surface area or activity of the labile linkage between the drug and polymeric backbone are kept constant during drug release. Another advantage of biodegradable systems is that, when formulated for depot injection, surgical removal can be avoided. These new delivery systems can protect and stabilize bioactive agents, enable long-term administration, and have potential for delivery of macromolecules.

A summary of different matrix and coating-controlled release mechanisms is illustrated in Fig. 6.4.

6.8 OSMOTIC PUMP

This type of delivery device has a semipermeable membrane that allows controlled amount of water to diffuse into the core of the device filled with a hydrophilic component.[11] A water-sensitive component in the core can either dissolve or expand to create osmotic pressure and push the drug out of device through a small delivery orifice which is drilled to a diameter that correlates to a specific rate. In an elementary osmotic pump, the drug molecule is mixed with osmotic agent in the core of the device (Fig. 6.5). For drugs that are highly or poorly water-soluble, a two-compartment push-pull bilayer system has been developed, in which drug core is separated from the push compartment (Fig. 6.5). The main advantage of osmotic pump system is that constant release rate can be achieved since it relies simply on the passage of water into the system and the human body is made up of 70 percent water. The release rate of the device can be modified by changing the amount of osmotic agent, surface area and thickness of semipermeable membrane, and/or the size of the hole.

The rate of water diffusing into osmotic device is expressed as[12]

$$\frac{dV}{dt} = \left(\frac{AK}{h}\right)(\Delta\pi - \Delta P) \tag{6.17}$$

where dV/dt = change of volume over change in time
A = area
K = permeability
h = thickness of membrane
$\Delta\pi$ = difference in osmotic pressure between drug device and release environment
ΔP = difference in hydrostatic pressure

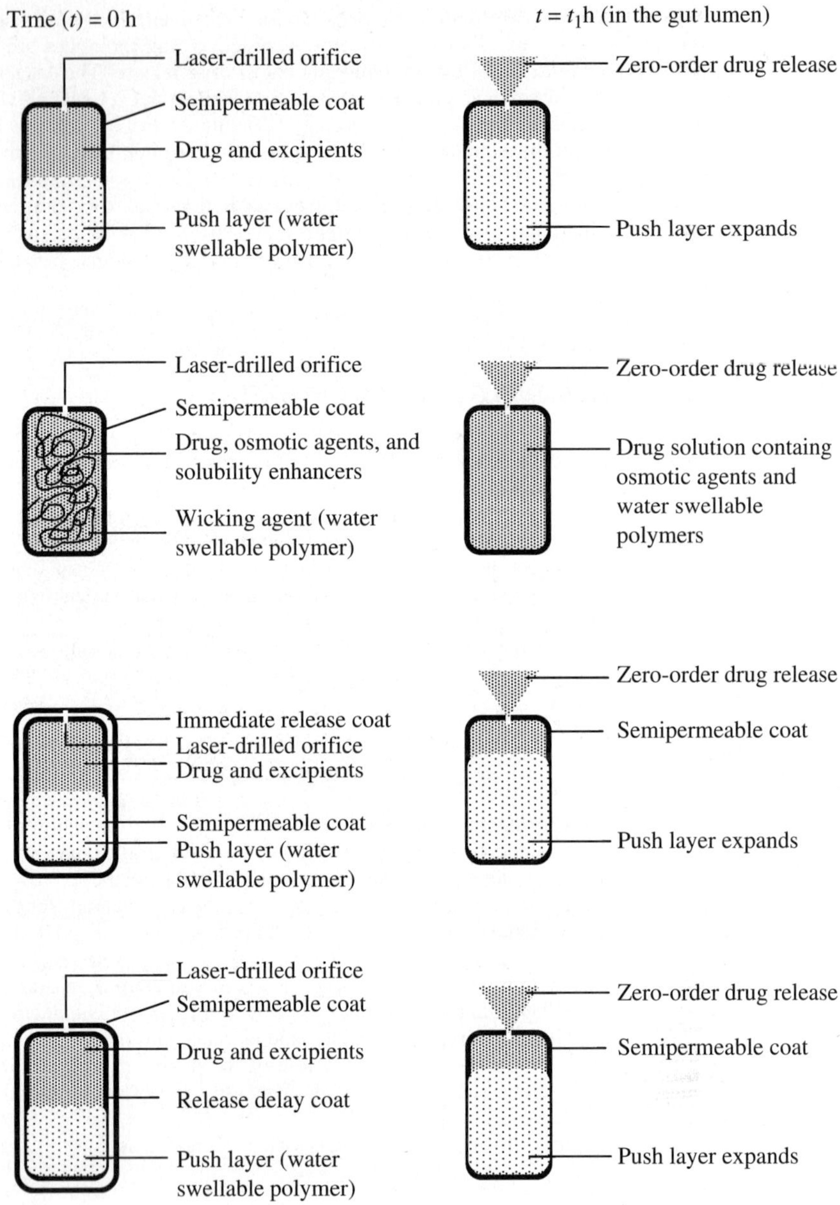

FIGURE 6.5 Schematic illustration of various mechanisms of osmotic-controlled release dosage forms.

If the osmotic pressure difference is much larger than the hydrostatic pressure difference ($\Delta\pi >> \Delta P$), the equation can be simplified to

$$\frac{dV}{dt} = \left(\frac{AK}{h}\right)(\Delta\pi) \tag{6.18}$$

The rate of drug pumped out of the device dM/dt can be expressed as

$$\frac{dM}{dt} = \left(\frac{dV}{dt}\right)C \tag{6.19}$$

where C is the drug concentration. As long as the osmotically active agent provides the constant osmotic pressure, the delivery system will release the drug at a zero-order. The zero-order delivery rate can be expressed as

$$\left(\frac{dM}{dt}\right)_z = \frac{AK}{h}\pi_s C \tag{6.20}$$

where π_s is osmotic pressure generated by saturated solution and all other symbols are the same as described earlier.

6.9 ION-EXCHANGE RESINS

The ion-exchange resin system can be designed by binding drug to the resin. After the formation of drug/resin complex, drug can be released by an ion-exchange reaction with the presence of counter ions. In this type of delivery system, the nature of the ionizable groups attached determines the chemical behavior of an ion-exchange resin (Fig. 6.6).

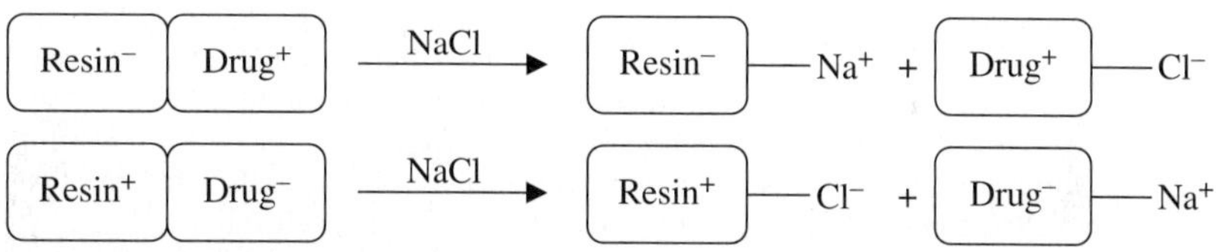

An ion-exchange reaction can be expressed as

$$[A^+] + [R^-][B^+] \longleftrightarrow [B^+] + [R^-][A^+]$$

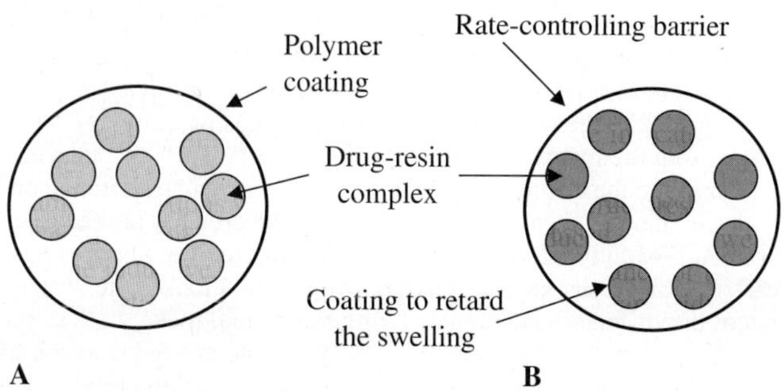

FIGURE 6.6 Schematic illustration of first generation (*a*) and second generation (*b*) ion-exchange drug delivery system.

and the selectivity coefficient (K_B^A) is defined as

$$K_B^A = \frac{[A_R^+][B^+]}{[A^+][B_R^+]} \tag{6.21}$$

where $[A^+]$ = concentration of free counter ion
$[B_R^+]$ = concentration of drug bound of the resin
$[B^+]$ = concentration of drug freed from resin
$[A_R^+]$ = concentration of counter ion bound to the resin

Factors that affect the selectivity coefficient include type of functional groups, valence and nature of exchanging ions, and nature of nonexchanging ions. Although it is known that ionic strength of GI fluid is maintained at a relatively constant level, first generation ion-exchange drug delivery systems had difficulty controlling the drug release rate because of lack of control of exchange ion concentration. The second-generation ion-exchange drug delivery system (Pennkinetic system) made an improvement by treating the drug-resin complex further with an impregnating agent such as polyethylene glycol 4000 to retard the swelling in water (Fig. 6.6*b*). These particles are then coated with a water-permeable polymer such as ethyl cellulose to act as a rate-controlling barrier to regulate the drug release.[13]

6.10 GASTRORETENTIVE DELIVERY SYSTEMS

Gastroretentive delivery systems were initially designed for oral delivery of antibiotics to the stomach to combat *Helicobacter pylori* infections, which are found in the pyloric region of the stomach. But later on, the delivery platform was utilized to deliver drugs with narrow window for absorption and drugs intended for local action in the stomach like antacids. Drugs such as acyclovir, bisphosphonates, captopril, furosemide, metformin, gabapentin, levodopa, baclofen, and ciprofloxacin have narrow absorption window located in the upper intestine, and their absorption would be benefited from a prolonged residence time of the drug at the site of absorption.

There are several approaches for gastroretention of dosage forms. Swelling and expandable dosage forms, mucoadhesive beads, and floating beads are some of the strategies that have been used. Empting of gastric content is controlled by contents in the stomach and size of the object being emptied. A fed stomach empties slower than the fasted stomach. Thus, any dosage form administered with food will be retained in the stomach for a longer period than administered in a fasted state. Objects larger than 20 mm in size tend to be retained in the fed stomach, which provides the basis for expandable and swellable gastroretentive dosage forms. Swelling-type tablets are designed with polymers, which undergo rapid relaxation in aqueous media, forming hydrogels from which the drug slowly diffuses out into the gastric lumen. Expandable systems can be designed in different shapes, such as, films, strips, propellers, and various other geometrical shapes, which form a part of the delivery system or are loaded with drugs themselves. Upon contact with gastric fluids they expand by polymer relaxation to attain a specific shape and render themselves resistant to gastric emptying. Another approach for the gastroretention is mucoadhesion or bioadhesion to the gastric mucosa. Drug-loaded beads with mucoadhesive coating stick to the gastric mucosa even after gastric emptying has taken place and continue to release drugs from the matrix. Certain natural polymers, such as chitosan, possess amine groups that tend to be ionized in the acidic gastric pH. The positively charged amine on chitosan interacts electrostatically with the anionic mucus to provide bioadhesive property to the beads and microparticles of the delivery system. Floating systems have also been explored for gastroretention. In these systems generation of carbon dioxide gas in situ provides swelling and makes the system buoyant in the stomach. But two major disadvantages encountered with the system make it a less-preferred alternative for gastroretention. Firstly, the floating system can only operate in a fed stomach where there is enough fluid held for a considerable amount of time. A fasted stomach has little fluid and drinking water in a fasted state does not simulate a fed state as the gastric contents are emptied almost immediately. Thus, the floating systems cannot operate in the fasted state. Secondly, the patient has to be erect, either standing or sitting, after the administration of a floating device. Supine position of the patient will move the floating device near to the pyloric sphincter from where it can pass into the intestine. Therefore, in addition to drug and system design considerations, the physiological considerations should also be considered when designing a gastroretentive delivery system.

6.11 DELIVERY OF MACROMOLECULES

The advances in biotechnology have introduced many proteins and other macromolecules that have potential therapeutic applications. These macromolecules bring new challenges to formulation scientists, since the digestive system is highly effective in metabolizing these molecules, making oral delivery almost impossible, while parenteral routes are painful and difficult to administer. A potential carrier for oral delivery of macromolecules is polymerized liposomes.[14] *Liposomes* are lipid vesicles that target the drug to selected tissues either by passive or active mechanisms.[15] Advantages of liposomes include increased efficacy and therapeutic index, reduction in toxicity of the encapsulated agent, and increased stability via encapsulation. One major weakness of liposome is the potential leakage of encapsulated drugs because of the stability of liposome. Unlike traditional liposomes, the polymerized liposomes are more rigid due to cross-linking and allow the polymerized liposomes to withstand harsh stomach acids and phospholipase. This carrier is currently being tested for oral delivery of vaccines.

Pulmonary route is also being utilized as a route for delivery of macromolecules. The lung's large absorptive surface area of around 100 m^2 makes this route a promising alternative route for protein administration. Drug particle size is a key parameter to pulmonary drug delivery. To reduce the particle size, a special drying process called *glass stabilization technology* was developed. By using this technology, dried powder particles can be designed at an optimum size of 1 to 5 μm for deep lung delivery. Advantages of powder formulation include higher stability of peptide and protein for longer shelf-life, lower risk of microbial growth, and higher drug loading compared to liquid formulation.[16] Liquid formulations for accurate and reproducible pulmonary delivery are now made possible by technology which converts large or small molecules into fine-particle aerosols and deposits them deep into the lungs. The device has a drug chamber that holds the liquid formulation, and upon activation, the pressure will drive the liquid through fine pores, creating the microsized mist for pulmonary delivery.

Transdermal needleless injection devices are another candidate for protein delivery.[17] The device propels the drug with a supersonic stream of helium gas. When the helium ampule is activated, the gas stream breaks the membrane which holds the drug. The drug particles are picked up by a stream of gas and propelled fast enough to penetrate the stratum corneum (the rate-limiting barrier of the skin). This delivery device is ideal for painless delivery of vaccine through the skin to higher drug loading. Limitations to this device are the upper threshold of approximately 3 mg and temporary permeability change of skin at the site of administration. An alternative way to penetrate the skin barrier has been developed utilizing thin titanium screens with precision microprojections to physically create pathways through the skin and allow for transportation of macromolecules. Another example of macromolecular delivery is an implantable osmotic pump designed to deliver protein drugs in a precise manner for up to 1 year. This implantable device uses osmotic pressure to push the drug formulation out of the device through the delivery orifice.

6.12 CONCLUSION

Controlled-release delivery devices have been developed for almost 40 years. Most of the devices utilize the fundamental principles of diffusion, dissolution, ion exchange, and osmosis (Table 6.2). Optimal design of a drug delivery system will require a detailed understanding of release mechanisms, properties of drugs and carrier materials, barrier characteristics, pharmacological effect of drugs, and pharmacokinetics. With development in the field of biotechnology, there is an increase in the number of protein and other macromolecular drugs. These drugs introduce new challenges and opportunities for the design of drug delivery systems.

TABLE 6.2 Examples of Various Marketed Controlled-Release Drug Delivery Products

Design Principle	Product Name	Active Ingredient	Route of Administration	Developer/ Manufacturer
Diffusion (reservior)	Estraderm	Estradiol	Transdermal	Alza/Novartis
	Norplant	Levonorgestrel	Subdermal implant	Wyeth-Ayerst Laboratory
	Ocusert	Pilocarpine	Ocular	Alza
	Progestasert	Progesterone	Intrauterine	Alza
	Transderm Scop	Scopolamine	Transdermal	Alza/Novartis
Diffusion (matrix)	Nitro-Dur	Nitroglycerine	Transdermal	Key Pharmaceutical
	Nitrodisc	Nitroglycerine	Transdermal	Searle
Mixed (matrix-reservoir)	Catapress-TTS	Clonidine	Transdermal	Alza/Boehinger Ingelheim
	Oxytrol	Oxybutynin	Transdermal	Watson
	Duragesic	Fentanyl	Transdermal	J&J (Ortho McNeil Janssen)
	Deponit	Nitroglycerine	Transdermal	Pharma-Schwarz
Porous matrix	K-Tab	Potassium chloride	Oral tablet	Abbot Labs.
Hydrodynamically balanced system	Medopar DR	Levodopa and benserazide	Oral tablet	Roche
	Glucophage XR	Metformin	Oral tablet	Bristol Myer Squibb
	Xatral OD	Alfuzosin	Oral tablet	Skye Pharma
	Valrelease	Diazepam	Oral tablet	Roche
Ion-exchange	Colestid	Colestipol	Oral tablet or granules	Upjohn
	Questran	Cholestyramine	Oral tablet or powder	Bristol Labs
	Tussionex Pennkinetic	Chlorpheniramine and hydrocodone	Oral suspension	Fisons
Nanocrystal technology	Rapamune	Sirolimus	Oral tablet	Elan/Wyeth-Ayerst Laboratory
Coating	Compazine Spansule	Prochlorperazine	Oral capsules	Glaxo Smith Kline
	Verelam PM	Verapamil	Oral capsules	Schwarz Pharma/ Elan
	Innopran XL	Propranolol	Oral capsules	Reliant
	Dexedrine CR	Dextroamphetamine	Oral capsules	Glaxo Smith Kline
	Fefol-Vit	Ferrous sulfate and vitamins	Oral capsules	Glaxo Smith Kline
	Ecotrin	Aspirin	Oral tablet	Glaxo Smith Kline
	Voltaren	Diclofenac	Oral tablet	Geigy
	Eskalith CR	Lithium carbonate	Oral tablet	Glaxo Smith Kline
	Adalat® CC	Nifedipine	Oral tablet	Bayer
	Ery-Tab®	Erythromycin	Oral tablet	Abbot
	Focalin® XR	Dexmethylphenidate	Oral tablet	Novartis
	Lialda™	5-Aminosalicylic acid	Oral tablet	Shire
	Sular®	Nisoldipine	Oral tablet	Sciele Pharma/ Bayer
	Coreg™ CR	Carvedilol	Oral tablet	Glaxo Smith Kline

(Continued)

TABLE 6.2 Examples of Various Marketed Controlled-Release Drug Delivery Products (*Continued*)

Design Principle	Product Name	Active Ingredient	Route of Administration	Developer/ Manufacturer
Biodegradable/ erodable matrix	Cipro XR	Ciprofloxacin	Oral tablet	Schering Plough
	Paxil CR	Paroxetine	Oral tablet	Glaxo Smith Kline
	Ambien CR	Zolpidem tartarate	Oral tablet	Sanofi Aventis
	Risperidal Consta	Risperidone	Parenteral	J&J (Ortho McNeil)
	Locteron	rAlpha interferon	Parenteral	Biolex
	Sinemet CR	Carbidopa and levedopa	Tablet	Merck
	hGH-OctoDEX	hGrowth hormone	Parenteral	Octoplus
	Naprelan	Naproxen sodium	Tablet	Roche
	Abraxane	Paclitaxel	Parenteral	Abraxis/Astrazeneca
	Gliadel Wafer	Carmustine	Implant	MGI Pharma
	Zoladex	Goserelin	Implant	Astrazeneca
	Remoxy	Oxycodone	Capsule	Durect
Gastroretentive dosage	Valrelease	Levedopa	Oral capsule	Roche
	Topalkan	Al-Mg antacid with alginic acid	Tablet	Pierre Fabre Sante
	Gaviscon	Alginates	Tablet	Glaxo Smith Kline
	Glumetza	Metformin	Tablet	Depomed/King Pharma
	Proquin XR	Ciprofloxacin	Tablet	Depomed
	Gabapentin GR	Depomed	Tablet	Depomed
Osmotic pumps	Calan SR	Verapamil	Oral tablet	Alza/GD Searle
	Cardura XL	Doxazosin	Oral tablet	Alza/Pfizer
	Covera HS	Verapamil	Oral tablet	Alza/ Pfizer
	DUROS	Potential carrier for macromolecules	Implant	Alza
	Ditropan	Oxybutynin	Oral tablet	Alza/UCB Pharma
	Minipress XL	Prazosin	Oral tablet	Alza/Pfizer
	Teczem	Enalapril and diltiazem	Oral tablet	Merck/Aventis
	Glucotrol XL	Glipizide	Oral tablet	Pfizer
	Concerta	Methylphenidate	Oral tablet	J&J (Ortho McNeil)
	Procardia XL	Nifedipine	Oral tablet	Pfizer
	Dyna Circ CR	Isradipine	Oral tablet	Reliant Pharma
	Sudafed 24h	Pseudoephidrine	Oral tablet	Pfizer
	Volmax	Albuterol	Oral tablet	Alza/Muro Pharmaceuticals
Liposome	Ambisome	Amphotericin B	Parenteral	Gilead/Astellas
	Amphotec	Amphotericin B	Parenteral	Sequus Pharmaceuticals
	Doxil	Doxorubicin	Parenteral	Sequus Pharmaceuticals
	DaunoXome	Daunorubicin	Parenteral	Diatos/Gilead
	Liprostin	PGE-1	Parenteral	Endovasc
	Depocyt	Cytarabine	Parenteral	Skye Pharma
	Abelcet	AmphoterecinB	Parenteral	Enzon
	LipoTaxen	Paclitaxel	Parenteral	Lipoxen

(*Continued*)

TABLE 6.2 Examples of Various Marketed Controlled-Release Drug Delivery Products (*Continued*)

Design Principle	Product Name	Active Ingredient	Route of Administration	Developer/ Manufacturer
Thermally triggered release	ThermoDox	Doxorubicin	Parenteral	Celsion
Pegylated systems	Macugen	Pegaptanib sodium	Parenteral	Pfizer/OSI
	Oncaspar	PEG–L-asparginase	L-asparginase	Enzon
	Adagen	PEG–Adenosine Deaminase	Parenteral	Enzon
	PEGIntron	PEG–Interferon α2b	Parenteral	Schering Plough
	PEGASYS	PEG–Interferon α2a	Parenteral	Roche
	Neulasta	Pegfilgastrim	Parenteral	Amgen
Ligand-based targeted delivery	Herceptin	Trastuzumab	Parenteral	Genentech
	Avastin	Bevacizumab	Parenteral	Genentech
	Rituxan	Rituximab	Parenteral	Genentech/Biogen Idec
	Raptiva	Efalizumab	Parenteral	Genentech
	Xolair	Omalizumab	Parenteral (sc)	Genentech/Novartis
	Remicade	IgG1κ (anti-TNFα)	Parenteral	Centocor
	Bexxar	Tositumomab	Parenteral	Glaxo Smith Kline
	Tysabri	Natalizumab	Parenteral	Biogen Idec/Elan
	Soliris	Eculizumab	Parenteral	Alexion
Programmable drug delivery systems	Animas 2020	Insulin	Parenteral	J&J (Animas Corp.)
	MiniMed Paradigm REAL-Time	Insulin	Parenteral	Medtronic
	CozMore Insulin pump system	Insulin	Parenteral	Smiths Medical MD
	Accu-Chek Spirit	Insulin	Parenteral	Roche
	OmniPod	Insulin	Parenteral	Insulet Corp.
	Amigo Nipro	Insulin	Parenteral	Nipro Diabetes Systems

REFERENCES

1. CDER 1999 Report to the Nation. *Improving Public Health Through Human Drugs. US Department of Human Services*, Food and Drug Administration, and Center for Drug Evaluation and Research.
2. Y. E. Chien, *Novel Drug Delivery Systems*, 2d ed., Marcel Dekker, New York, 1992.
3. V. S. Gerogiannis, D. M. Rekkas, and P. P. Dallas, Floating and Swelling Characteristics of Various Excipients Used in Controlled-Release Technology, *Drug Dev. Ind. Pharm.* **19**:1061–1081, 1993.
4. R. O. Potts and G. W. Cleary, Transdermal Drug Delivery: Useful Paradigms, *J. Drug Target*, **3**(4):247–251, 1995.
5. J. R. Robinson and V. H. Lee (eds.), *Controlled Drug Delivery: Fundamentals and Applications,* 2d ed., Marcel Dekker, New York, 1987.
6. S. D. Bruck (ed.), *Controlled Drug Delivery*, vols. 1 and 2, CRC Press, Florida, 1984.
7. S. Cohen and H. Bernstein (eds.), *Microparticulate Systems for Delivery of Proteins and Vaccines*, Marcel Dekker, New York, 1996.
8. H. Bundgaard (eds.), *Design of Prodrugs*, Elsevier Science, New York, 1985.
9. J. Crank, *The Mathematics of Diffusion*, 2d ed., Oxford Press, 1975.

10. R. A. Lipper and W. I. Higuchi, Analysis of Theoretical Behavior of a Proposed Zero-Order Drug Delivery System, *J. Pharm. Sci.*, **66**(2):163–164, 1977.

11. F. Theeuwes, Elementary Osmotic Pump, *J. Pharm. Sci.*, **64**:1987–1991, 1975.

12. C. Kim, *Controlled Release Dosage Form Design*, Technomic, Pennsylvania, 2000.

13. S. Motycha and J. G. Naira, Influence of Wax Coatings on Release Rate of Anions from Ion-Exchange Resin Beads, *J. Pharm. Sci.*, **67**(4):500–503, 1978.

14. J. Okada, S. Cohen, and R. Langer, In vitro Evaluation of Polymerized Liposomes as an Oral Drug Delivery System, *Pharm. Res.*, **12**(4):576–582, 1995.

15. A. D. Bangham, Diffusion of Univalent Ions Across the Lamellae of Swollen Phospholipids, *J. Mol. Biol.*, **13**:238–252, 1965.

16. J. R. White and R. K. Campbell, Inhaled Insulin: An Overview, *Clin. Diab.*, **19**(1):13–16, 2001.

17. T. L. Brukoth, B. J. Bellhouse, G. Hewson, D. J. Longridge, A. G. Muddle, and D. F. Saphie, Transdermal and Transmucosal Powdered Drug Delivery, *Crit. Rev. Ther. Drug Carrier Sys.*, **16**(4):331–384, 1999.

CHAPTER 7
STERILE MEDICAL DEVICE PACKAGE DEVELOPMENT

Patrick J. Nolan
DDL, Inc., Eden Prairie, Minnesota

The objective of this chapter is to provide an overview of the process and techniques of designing and developing a package system for a medical device. An all-inclusive discussion of this subject is beyond the scope of this chapter; however, numerous references are provided for further detail and study of the subject. The information provided in this chapter is a compilation from the references cited as well as from the experiences of the author in developing package systems for medical devices.

7.1 INTRODUCTION

Implementation of a standard for the process of designing and developing a package for terminally sterilized medical devices is essential to the overall effort of marketing a sterile device in the international and domestic communities. It is incumbent upon the medical device manufacturer to ensure that a safe, reliable, and fully functional device arrives at the point of end use. This assurance is complicated by the fact that the sterile barrier system must maintain its barrier integrity throughout its intended shelf life and through the rigors of manufacture and shipping and handling. The total product development effort must include the packaging system design process and encompasses the following functions:

- Package design
- Package prototyping
- Manufacturing process validation
- Sterilization process
- Distribution and environmental effects

The anticipated sterilization method and the intended product application, shelf life, transport, and storage methods all combine to influence the package system design and choice of packaging materials. The process of developing a package system seems straightforward and basic. In actuality, the package design process is complicated by the fact that if products are terminally sterilized in the sterile barrier system, then the device packages must allow effective sterilization of their contents by a wide array of methods, and therefore the materials must be compatible with the sterilization method. Consequently, the sterile barrier system must provide a consistent and continuous barrier to environmental microorganisms and bacteria so as to maintain product sterility. The package system must be designed to prevent product damage and loss of functionality from the dynamic hazards of shock and vibration, which are inherent in the distribution environment. In addition, the medical device manufacturer must have documented evidence that the performance of the package system is not adversely affected, and that it maintains its stability over the claimed shelf life. The interactions of the materials and product, combined with the manufacturing processes required to bring the product to its end use, influence the package design and manufacturing of the finished product.

The importance of packaging in bringing a medical device to market was illustrated in a speech by George Brdlik in 1982. These points are no less true today than they were in 1982. Brdlik stated:

Packaging is too often neglected as an important characteristic of a medical device. When sterile medical devices are involved, deficient packaging can cause the following problems:

- *Increased risk of patient infection if product sterility is compromised by defective seals, pinholes fragile packaging materials, or packaging which shreds, delaminates, or tears upon opening.*
- *Hampering of a surgical procedure because of difficulties in product identification or aseptic transfer, or if a product selected for use must be replaced because the package is either initially defective or damaged upon opening.*
- *Increased hospital costs due to discarded products or excessive storage space requirements.*
- *Increased manufacturing costs for refund/replacement of damaged products and recall of products with potentially compromised sterility or integrity.*

In essence, poor packaging can transform the best, safest, and most economical medical device into an inferior, unsafe, and expensive product.

This chapter provides a systematic and standardized approach to developing a comprehensive package system that meets regulatory hurdles and ensures a high degree of confidence that the sterile medical device product will meet its performance specifications at the point of end use. These elements include

- Selection of materials
- Design of the package
- Package prototyping
- Process validation
- Final package design validation

All of these elements must be combined to produce a package system that meets regulatory, industry, and consumer's requirements.

7.2 REGULATORY HISTORY

The regulatory burden for validating the manufacturing process and package system has become significant and important. It was started in 1938 with the amended Food and Drug Act of 1906 in which medical devices were first regulated, and then progressed to the Quality Systems Regulation (QSR) that specifies the requirements for components, device master record, and environmental controls, just to name a few.

It is appropriate here to present a brief history of how the medical device industry became regulated and how eventually the Food and Drug Administration (FDA) recognized the importance of the package system as an integral part, and in fact a component of the medical device.

As mentioned earlier, the FDA began regulating medical devices in 1938. At that time, the Federal Food, Drug, and Cosmetic Act extended the FDA's legal authority to control foods and drugs and bestowed the agency with new legal powers over cosmetics and medical devices. However, the act was limited in scope in that the regulatory actions could only be taken after a device was introduced into interstate commerce, and only after the device was found to be adulterated or misbranded. Surprisingly, the burden was on the government to provide evidence of violation of the act. In addition, the 1938 act could not prevent the introduction and marketing of "quack" medical devices. However, there was also an explosion of legitimate and sophisticated new devices using postwar biotechnology. These devices not only presented huge potential benefits to patient healthcare, but also caused an increased risk for harm. It became apparent that additional legal controls were necessary in order to harness the potential good from the new technologies. A government committee studied the best approach to new comprehensive device legislation, and, as a result, in 1976 a new law amended the 1938 act and provided the FDA with significant additional authority concerning the regulation of medical devices. The amendments included classification of all devices with graded regulatory requirements, medical device manufacturer registration, device listing, premarket approval (PMA), investigational device exemption (IDE), good manufacturing practices (GMP), records and reporting requirements, preemption of state and local regulations, and performance standards. Two years later in 1978, the FDA published the GMP regulations that provided a series of requirements that prescribed the facilities, methods, and controls to be used in the manufacture, packaging, and storage of medical devices. The law has since been modified with the most substantive action occurring in 1990 with the passage of the Safe Medical Devices Act (SMDA). It broadly expanded FDA's enforcement powers by authorizing the levying of civil penalties and creating a series of postapproval controls for monitoring the performance of medical devices.

Over the past 18 years, the FDA has significantly changed the way medical devices are regulated. The issuance of guidance documents effectively circumvented rulemaking and public comment. Publishing FDA's interpretation of the GMP effectively causes the manufacturer to comply with that interpretation. Legally, guidances are not binding on the public, whereas certain rules are. But for all practical purposes, there is little difference between the two. For example, two of these guidance documents include

- Guideline on General Principles of Process Validation—1987
- Preproduction Quality Assurance Planning: Recommendations for Medical Device Manufacturers

FDA issues dozens of guidances each year on specific products and processes. The last significant piece of legislation for medical devices came with the signing of the Food and Drug Administration Modernization Act of 1997 (FDAMA). This legislation essentially changed FDA's approach to standards-based enforcement and adds a system to recognize national and international standards in product reviews. The FDA will publish the recognized standards in the *Federal Register*, and these standards will then serve as guidance, enabling companies to use them to satisfy premarket submission requirements through a declaration of conformity. The list of recognized standards is provided in the FDA Guidance document entitled "Guidance for Recognition and Use of Consensus Standards: Availability." This legislative change enables companies to submit a one-page 510(k) that simply states that the device complies with a stated list of recognized standards.

Significant legislation affecting medical devices and packaging includes

- 1938—Federal Food, Drug, and Cosmetic Act
- 1976—Medical Device Amendments (MDA)
- 1978—GMP Regulations published in *Federal Register*

- 1990—Safe Medical Device Act (SMDA)
- 1997—Food and Drug Administration Modernization Act (FDAMA)

So, medical device manufacturers are subject to the provisions of the FDAMA and the GMP when doing business in the United States. The regulations are published in 21 CFR (Code of Federal Regulation), Part 820. The section dealing specifically with the requirements for packaging is Section 820.130. FDA approves products for use through the investigational device exemption (IDE), premarket application (PMA), and 510(k) processes. Additional information on the medical device approvals process can be found at the following Web site: http://www.fda.gov/CDRH/devadvice/ide/approval.shtml. There may be additional regulatory burdens when the device is being marketed outside of the United States. Some of these regulations are discussed in Sec. 7.2.1.

7.2.1 International Regulations

International regulations play a significant role in the marketing and use of medical devices. The European Union "Council Directive concerning medical devices" (MDD) is the European equivalent of the FDA regulations. The MDD (93/42/EEC), also known as the "Medical Device Directive," as published in the EEC in 1993, (http://www.translate.com/multilingual_standard/MDD.pdf) lists the essential requirements for devices and packages, and all medical devices sold on the European free market must meet the specifics of this directive, which overrides all national regulations. The "Essential Requirements" section for medical devices and packages is found in Annex I of the MDD. General requirements for ensuring that characteristics of the medical device are not altered or adversely affected during their intended use as a result of transport and storage are found in Sec. 5. There are more specific requirements for infection and microbial contamination as it relates to packaging in Sec. 8. It is incumbent on the medical device manufacturer to conform to all of the sections of the "Essential Requirements," not just the packaging requirements.

ISO 11607. An ISO standard approved in 1997 by the international community, and most recently revised and republished in 2006, has become essential to the development and validation of a package system for a terminally sterilized medical device. Compliance with this standard and other European standards ensures compliance with the packaging provisions of the MDD "Essential Requirements." The two-part ISO 11607 standard is entitled

- *Packaging for terminally sterilized medical devices—Part 1: Requirements for materials, sterile barrier systems, and packaging systems;*
- *Packaging for terminally sterilized medical devices—Part 2: Validation requirements for forming, sealing, and assembly processes.*

ISO 11607 is the foremost standard for validating packaging for terminally sterilized medical devices. Packaging must comply with ISO 11607 to ensure that the enclosed medical device is kept sterile throughout all the elements and hazards generated by the manufacturing, shipping, and storage environments.

What revisions Were Made to the ISO 11607 Standard Since 2004? The ISO 11607 standard was revised to harmonize with the provisions of the EN 868-1 standard as discussed below. As a result, the new ISO 11607-01 comprises two parts:

- Part 1: Materials and designs
- Part 2: Processes

A summary of the changes are as follows:

Terminology Many terms have been added or eliminated from the current standard, including:
The Definition of "medical device." ISO 11607-01 includes some medical devices that were not previously covered by the old standard.

"Primary package" replaced by "sterile barrier system"(SBS). This is defined as the "minimum package that prevents ingress of microorganisms and allows aseptic presentation of the product at the point of end use."

"Final package" replaced by "package system." This is defined as "(the) combination of the sterile barrier system and protective package." This combined package could include the second sterile barrier, or outer package, in a dual pouch or tray; a paperboard carton or shelf box; and the shipping container. These all may combine to form the "package system."

The elimination of "package integrity." This was defined as "unimpaired physical condition of a final package." Now it is implied that package integrity is lost if the sterile barrier system is breached or does not "prevent the ingress of microorganisms to the product."

Test Method Validation Test data will only be accepted from ISO 11607 validated test methods, which may include a precision and bias statement and is based on round-robin testing of the test method itself by several labs. However, a test method validation is not complete until it is actually performed in a specific test lab with standard materials to show that the lab can produce data equal to that shown in the precision and bias statement. This is not to say that a test method developed by an individual company could not be used to test a specific attribute of the material or package. However, the method must be validated by determining its precision and bias against a "standard." The validation must be documented and retained as evidence that the repeatability and reproducibility were determined and are within acceptable tolerance as those shown in the precision and bias statement. In addition, the sensitivity of the method must be determined. This would apply in the case of a package leak test to demonstrate package integrity.

Compliance Responsibilities Compliance responsibilities that were clearly outlined in Sec. 4.4 of the old standard have been omitted from the new ISO 11607-01. Therefore, some confusion may arise over certain areas of responsibility such as

- Who should test the packaging suppliers' seals?
- Who is responsible for validating package sealing equipment?
- Who is responsible for evaluating the biocompatibility or other material characteristics such as microbial barrier properties?

However, members of the Standards Revision Committee from AAMI, TC198, WG7 stated that the rationale for elimination of assignment of responsibilities was that under the old standard when an auditor assessed compliance to the standard, and a device manufacturer handled an aspect that was "assigned" to a package supplier, the auditor would have to determine that compliance with the standard was not achieved. The important point is whether the requirement is met, not who did the work.

Ultimately, the medical device manufacturer must take care up-front with contractors and vendors to determine roles and responsibility in the entire package development and validation process.

Worst-Case Packaging The revised standard places additional emphasis on the concept of testing the "worst-case" package configuration. More on this concept later.

Stability Testing (Accelerated Aging) as a Separate Entity Another significant change was to separate performance testing (distribution and transportation) from stability testing (shelf life) in the final package system validation. Previous studies had combined these effects of aging with extreme environmental conditions and dynamic events inherent in distribution in a sequential test method. The new thinking as stated by the AAMI Committee was "Stability testing and performance testing should be treated as separate entites." More on this concept in later.

The FDA has recognized this standard for product reviews in its 1997 *Guidance for Recognition and Use of Consensus Standards: Availability.* This standard specifies the basic attributes that materials must have for use in packaging for terminally sterile medical devices. In addition, it provides the producer or manufacturer the guidance to conduct a formal qualification and validation of the packaging operations. There must be a documented process validation program that demonstrates the efficacy and reproducibility of all sterilization and packaging processes to ensure the package integrity at the point of end use.

Finally, the new ISO standard provides a series of recommended tests and criteria to evaluate the performance of the complete package under all of the stresses and hazards inherent in the packaging and distribution process. These tests are listed in Annex B of the standard and include, but are not limited to, the following types:

- Internal pressure
- Dye penetration
- Gas sensing
- Vacuum leak
- Seal strength
- Transportation simulation
- Accelerated aging
- Microbial barrier

For more interpretive information regarding the ISO 11607 standard, the AAMI Committee has published a Technical Information Report (TIR) entitled; AAMI TIR-22:2007, Guidance for ANSI/AAMI/ISO 11607, Packaging for terminally sterilized medical devices—Part 1 and Part 2: 2006. The scope of this document is to provide guidance on the application of ANSI/AAMI/ISO 11607 standard within the regulatory framework of the FDA that exists at the time of the publication of the document. The TIR22 is a guidance document and should be used in conjunction with the ANSI/AAMI/ISO 11607 standard. Another guidance document available to help medical device manufacturers become compliant to ISO 11607 includes a publication by DuPont entitled; "DuPont Tyvek Compliance to ISO 11607-1:2006." It can be found at (www.MedicalPackaging.DuPont.com).

EN 868 Part 1. This European standard, entitled *Packaging Materials and Systems for Medical Devices Which Are to Be Sterilized: General Requirements and Test Methods*, provides detailed guidance on meeting the requirements of the MDD. It includes more detail on the selection and validation of packaging materials than does Clause 4 of the ISO 11607 standard. However, there are some differences, and both standards must be considered when evaluating the packaging system for compliance to the FDA and MDD regulations.

Standards within the EN 868 series fall into two distinct categories—horizontal and vertical. The EN 868 Part 1 is a horizontal standard since it specifies the requirements for a broad range of packaging materials, types, and designs. The requirements are essentially the same as ISO 11607, Part 1; however, the ISO document also includes requirements for package forming and final package validation as described in Part 2. If you comply with the ISO 11607 Part 1, you will comply with EN 868, Part 1 since the documents have been harmonized as of the revisions to ISO 11607 in 2006.

Vertical standards within the 868 series include detailed requirements for individual materials or specific package types or medical device products. These standards are designated as Parts 2 through 10. They specify limits for material properties for

- Sterilization wraps (Part 2)
- Paper for use in the manufacture of paper bags, pouches, and reels (Parts 3, 4, 5)
- Paper for the manufacture of packs for medical use for sterilization by ethylene oxide EtO or irradiation (Part 6)
- Adhesive-coated paper for the manufacture of heat-sealable packs for medical use for sterilization by EtO or irradiation (Part 7)
- Reusable sterilization containers for steam sterilization conforming to EN 285 (Part 8)
- Uncoated nonwoven polyolefin materials for use in the manufacture of heat-sealable pouches, reels, and lids (Part 9)

- Adhesive-coated nonwoven polyolefin materials for use in the manufacture of heat-sealable pouches, reels, and lids (Part 10)

The "Essential Requirements" of the MDD can be effectively met by complying with the requirements of the ISO 11607 and EN 868, Part 1 standards.

CE Mark. A CE Mark can be affixed to the medical device when all of the essential requirements of the MDD and other directives, as appropriate, are met. The declaration of conformity that contains the documented evidence that all requirements have been met achieves this.

7.3 FUNCTIONS OF A PACKAGE

The first step in designing and developing a package system for a medical device is obtaining all of the design inputs. This task provides all of the critical attributes and requirements of the device which could have an effect on the package design and performance. The design inputs also influence the selection of materials appropriate for and compatible with the device. Packages are intended to contain the product. However, for medical devices, there are other functions the package serves; it provides protection, identification, process ability, ease of use, and special applications for device use and presentation. A basic knowledge of the product's use, dimensions, shape, special characteristics (e.g., sharp edges, points, and fragility), distribution environment, application, and barrier requirements are essential to selecting appropriate materials and designing the final package.

7.3.1 Protection

Protection of the device by the package may be provided in several different ways. Primarily, the sterile medical device must be protected from the bacteria and microorganisms natural to the environment. The package must provide a protective barrier from the environment but must also allow the product to be terminally sterilized, be opened easily by medical professionals, and maintain integrity until the point of end use. Materials must allow for the most efficient and effective sterilization method but not be degraded by that method. The package must also provide protection to the product from the hardships of the distribution and handling environment. In addition, there cannot be any damage to the package itself from shock or impacts associated with handling in shipment, resulting in loss of seal integrity. Materials must be resistant to impacts and abrasion. The package must be designed so as to prevent sharp objects from piercing the materials or damaging seals, by eliminating movement of the device inside the package. In some applications, the product may be so fragile that the package must have cushioning characteristics that prevent excess shock energy to be transmitted to the device. Protection of the device over an extended shelf life is another function of the package design requiring material stability over time.

Summarizing the protective features of a package for a sterile medical device, the package must have

- Sterilizability: provide the ability to terminally sterilize the device by one or more methods without degrading the material.
- Shelf life: ensure the stability of the material as a barrier throughout the life cycle of the product.
- Environmental: provide barrier to moisture, air, bacteria, oxygen, light.
- Physical: provide dynamic protection, resist impacts and abrasion, and provide structural support.

The materials most commonly used for medical device packages today incorporate the characteristics required for a protective package.

7.3.2 Identification

Packages must not only provide protection to the product, but they must also communicate what the product is, instructions, warnings and safety information, and other pertinent information such as, lot number, sterilization method, and expiration date. Space must be provided on the package for conveying this information either by printing directly on the package or by applying a label. Often, there must be adequate space for the information in two or more languages. The information must be legible at the point of end use; therefore abrasion, water, and the sterilization process must not damage the printing and labels.

Specific information regarding label requirements can be found at the following Web site: http://www.fda.gov/cdrh/devadvice/33.html.

7.3.3 Processability

By *processability* we mean the ability of the packaging material along with its product to be processed through a series of manufacturing operations that includes mechanical stresses in filling and sealing, chemical or physical actions during sterilization, stresses of shipping and handling, and the environmental effects of aging before the product is finally used. This processability requirement is clearly stated in 21 CFR Part 820.130, "Device Packaging":

> *The device package and any shipping container for a device shall be designed and constructed to protect the device from alteration or damage during the customary conditions of processing, storage, handling and distribution.*

This statement forms the basis for which the requirement to perform package validation testing is established and is described in the ISO 11607 standard as "performance testing."

7.3.4 Ease of Use

Parallel with the increase in the use of disposable medical devices is the requirement for easy-to-open packages that can provide an application for the presentation of the product into the sterile field. The package has to be designed such that the materials are strong enough to withstand the rigors of processing but can be opened without tearing or excessive stress on the package or product.

7.3.5 Special Applications

In some cases the package may serve as a tool in the procedure. The obvious application is as a delivery mechanism for the product to the sterile field; for example, heart valve holders for aseptic transfer to the surgery site. However, even more complex applications may be designed into the package to aid in the procedure.

7.4 PACKAGE TYPES

The form the package takes is fundamentally dependent on the characteristics of the device such as size, shape, profile, weight, center of gravity, physical state, irregularities, sharp edges/points, density, application of the device, shelf life, and other design inputs.

The medical device industry uses a limited variety of types but many different materials in each form. Over the past 20 years, the industry has standardized on the following basic medical device package types.

7.4.1 Thermoform Trays (Semirigid)

Thermoform trays are made from a variety of plastics by molding them to the desired shape through the thermoforming process. Trays are particularly suited for devices with irregular shapes and high profiles since the tray can be designed to accommodate these device characteristics. Trays are ideal for procedure kits that contain several devices as they can be molded with special flanges, undercuts, and snap fits or ridges for securing the components. Semirigid trays are self-supporting.

When designing a tray for a medical device, several criteria must be considered in the selection of the material:

- Tensile strength
- Stiffness
- Impact resistance
- Clarity
- Ease of forming and cutting
- Heat stability
- Compatibility with sterilization processes
- Cost, on a yield basis, versus performance
- Product compatibility
- Ability to be sealed with lidding material

When using a tray for a sterile medical device, in order to perform the most basic protection function, the tray must be sealed to prevent loss of sterility. This is accomplished by using a lidding material that is sealed around the flange area of the tray. Until the advent of Tyvek® into the market, it was difficult to provide lidding material that would provide a means for terminal sterilization using the common sterilization methods of the day. However, Tyvek® has allowed widespread use of thermoform trays for many applications.

7.4.2 Flexible Formed Pouches

This type of package is one in which a flexible material is drawn using the thermoform process into a flexible "tray." The package, essentially, is a formed pouch that allows containment of high-profile devices. These packages are generally not self-supporting.

Characteristics of the formed flexible packages are

- Relatively low cost, suitable to high-volume, low-cost devices
- May be made to be heat sealable
- Ease of forming
- Available for form-fill-seal operations
- Suited to relatively simple tray configurations
- Can conform to product
- Good visibility of product
- Cannot be preformed into a package
- Offer little structural protection
- Limited variety of materials available
- Relatively lower heat resistance

Like the semirigid tray, this package type must also be sealed using a lidding material or top web. The top web material must be designed with the particular barrier properties needed to be compatible with bottom web material and the chosen sterilization process. The top web material must therefore be selected on the basis of the following three factors:

- Type of device—environmental or product barrier requirements
- Method of sterilization—gas, radiation, steam
- Method of dispensing—peel, cut, tear, puncture

7.4.3 Flexible Nonformed Pouches

The most common package in this category, and probably for most single-use medical devices, is the two-web peel pouch. The package form is very common for a variety of medical devices, including gloves, catheters, tubing, adhesive bandages, dressings, sutures, and other low-profile and lightweight products. This flat pouch design is suitable for high-volume, low-cost devices as they provide the basic protection for devices. The most popular form of flat pouch is known as the *chevron* pouch. It gets its name from the peak-shaped end of the package where the initial peeling of the seal begins. This design provides ease of peeling as the peel forces are distributed angularly along the seal line rather than across the entire seal end. Other forms of the flat pouch can be achieved by forming seals across the corner of the package, leaving a tab to initiate the peel.

The typical peel pouch used for devices is made from two separate web materials that are heat sealable or adhesive coated. Since these packages usually contain sterile disposable devices that are terminally sterilized inside the primary package, a porous material is required for one of the webs. Either paper or Tyvek® is used as one of the web materials along with a plastic film such as a laminated polyester and polyethylene.

Some of the benefits of the peel pouch are

- Relatively low cost
- Suitable for small-run or high-volume uses
- Can be fabricated from a wide variety of materials
- Can be prefabricated or formed in-line
- Provide a sterile delivery capability
- Product visibility
- Easy opening
- Printable with product information and instructions

Some of the disadvantages are

- Not useful for high-profile devices
- Not suitable for high-mass products
- Low dynamic protection capabilities
- Not suitable for irregularly shaped devices
- Not suitable for kits or multicomponent devices

Another type of peelable pouch is known as the *header* bag. This package is essentially a two-web pouch in which a portion of one web is a peelable Tyvek® or paper vent. The header bag provides high permeability, ease of opening, and convenient product dispensing. An advantage of this package type is that a basic flexible bag can contain a high-profile device.

7.5 PACKAGING MATERIALS

This part provides a basic overview of some of the more common packaging materials used for medical device packages. Since entire books are published describing the chemical characteristics, applications, and performance properties of packaging materials, it is beyond the scope of this chapter to provide all of the necessary information for the selection of materials for the specific medical device. Consult the references for additional information.

7.5.1 Primary Materials

Tyvek®. Tyvek®, a spun-bonded olefin, is used in almost every major form of sterile package, including peelable pouches, header bags, and lid stock of thermoform trays and kits. Tyvek® is a fibrous web material composed entirely of extremely fine, continuous strands of high-density polyethylene. This material has exceptional characteristics that distinguish it from other materials.

The product characteristics of Tyvek® include

- Outstanding porous microbial barrier
- Strength
- Moisture resistance
- Inertness to most chemicals
- Air permeability
- Clean peeling seals
- Low linting due to continuous filaments
- Low fiber tear

It has superior dry and wet strength and dimension stability. Its excellent puncture and tear resistance and toughness allow for a wide range of applications for medical devices, particularly irregularly shaped and bulky products. This material has an unusual fiber structure that allows for rapid gas and vapor transmission but at the same time provides a barrier to the passage of microorganisms. Tyvek® is used most often with ethylene oxide (EtO) sterilization methods because of its unique property of high porosity and microbial barrier. Tyvek® provides several other attributes useful to package integrity and aesthetics:

- Water repellency—repels water but is porous to moisture vapor
- Chemical resistance—resists usual agents of age degradation (e.g., moisture, oxidation, rot, mildew, and many organic chemicals)
- Radiation stability—unaffected by common levels of radiation used for sterilization
- Low-temperature stability—retains strength and flexibility at subzero temperatures
- High-temperature stability—can be used in steam sterilization methods
- Aesthetic qualities—bright, white, clean appearance for printing

Since Tyvek® does not readily adhere to other plastics, except other polyolefins, through the application of heat and pressure, it has been made a more versatile packaging material by applying coatings that enable it to bond with a wide variety of plastics. There are several grades of Tyvek® used for medical packaging applications, including 1059B, 1073B, and 2FS.

The DuPont™ Medical Packaging has published two very useful documents to help in designing a package system that is in compliance with the ISO 11607 standard. They are

- "Technical Reference Guide for Medical Packaging," first published in 2002; reissued in 2007
- "DuPont™ Tyvek® Compliance to ISO 11607-1:2006"
- These documents can be found at: http://www2.DuPont.com/Medical_Packaging/en_US/tech_info/index.html

Another breathable material which may provide an alternative to Tyvek® has been developed by Oliver Medical called Ovantex®. Ovantex/F is a material made of a proprietary blend of synthetic fibers and cellulose-based components. The barrier properties of this material are superior to medical grade papers and are comparable to some grades of spun-bonded olefin. The consistency of the thickness provides less variation in the sealing process; and tear resistance is superior to paper but not as good as spun-bonded olefin. This material may provide an acceptable alternative to Tyvek®.

Paper. For many years, paper was the only choice for package types until the introduction of Tyvek® as a medical packaging material. However, paper still plays a significant role in the medical device industry. Over the years before the introduction of Tyvek®, paper materials compiled a significant performance record of product protection and patient safety. Although Tyvek® has taken a majority share of the medical device package market, the industry is finding ways to utilize paper in combination with plastics and foils to provide the needed performance characteristics with favorable economics.

The significant features of paper materials that enable it to continue as a feasible packaging material alternative are

- Sustainability
- Cost
- Disposability
- Sterilization
- Combination with other materials
- Versatility
- Peelability
- Range of grades

Some of the limitations of paper as a medical device packaging material are

- Strength—low tear and puncture resistance
- Dimensional stability
- Moisture sensitivity
- Aging—limited under certain environmental conditions

Paper can be used as lidding material for semirigid and flexible trays, and for peelable pouches. Adhesive coatings are required to allow sealing.

Films, Laminates, and Coextrusions. Many films are used in medical device packaging applications. Both flexible formed and nonformed pouches, as well as bags, use films for their manufacture. These materials offer a high degree of versatility and are available in a countless variety of forms in monofilms, laminations, and coextrusions. The specific material to be used for a medical device is dependent on the performance properties required for the device application. For example

- Sterilization method (e.g., the material must tolerate high temperature)
- Protection requirements (e.g., high puncture resistance)
- Peel requirements (e.g., easily peelable)
- Package style (e.g., formable vs. nonformable pouch)
- Barrier properties (e.g., moisture or oxygen barrier)
- Packaging process (e.g., in-line sealing vs. form-fill seal)
- Packaging aesthetics (e.g., visibility of product)

The flexible materials used for medical device packages include a plastic film that is usually a lamination or extrusion-coated material. The material most commonly used for flexible packaging applications is oriented polyester (e.g., Mylar™), which is used as a base for properties such as, dimensional stability, heat resistance, and strength with an adhesively laminated seal layer, such as low-density polyethylene, which provides the film structure with heat sealability. The variety of film combinations is virtually unlimited, and the performance properties of the film can be customized to meet the requirements of the package specifications and the medical device. Other examples of film constructions are

- Polyester/Pe/EVA
- Polyester/Surlyn
- Polyester/nylon/Pe
- Polyester/nylon/PP
- Polyester/PVDV/Pe
- Metallized polyester/Pe
- Polyester/foil/Pe
- Polyester/foil/polyester/Surlyn
- Oriented PP/Pe
- Polycarbonate/Pe/EVA

There may be other combinations of film structures as new materials with different properties are continually being developed. Consult with packaging material suppliers to determine the optimum material for your application.

The thermoplastic films used in flexible applications are suited only for sealing to themselves or to chemically related materials. The sealing of like materials produces fused bonds that may not be peelable and thus applicable for single-use medical devices. To overcome the limitations of sealing like materials, adhesives specifically tailored for seal-peel functionality are applied to the film surface, allowing films to remain unaltered and to retain their performance characteristics. The use of uncoated or coextruded materials for medical device packages is limited in their application by allowing only a narrow sealing range, providing limited sealability on high-speed equipment, allowing sealing of chemically similar materials, and Tyvek® materials. On the other hand, materials coated with an adhesive provide versatility and greater benefits, such as a wider sealing range, easy and consistent sealability to porous materials such as Tyvek® and paper, barrier properties, lower cost, and versatility in adhesive properties dependent on the application (e.g., pouch or tray application).

Foils. Foil laminate materials are used in applications where high moisture, gas, and light barriers are essential. Foil can be used in all forms of packaging and for both medical devices and pharmaceuticals. The lamination of the foil with plastic films is required to provide sealability. Foil materials are being used for lidding of thermoform tray packages where high moisture and gas barriers are required and where the sterilization method allows it (e.g., gamma, e-beam, and steam). Wet devices such as dressings, solutions, sponges, swabs, and other saturated products requiring high moisture barrier are particularly suited to foil packages. Foil laminations with high-density polyethylene or polypropylene are common constructions for these package types. For solutions, a form-fill-seal application is ideal, as the pouch is formed and filled in a multiphase operation on a single machine.

The trend in medical device packaging, over the past 10 years has been to flexible packages, as they are less costly, more resistant to shipping damage, easier to handle, and produce less packaging waste. A foil-laminated package offers many benefits such as strength, high environmental barrier, peelability, easy opening, temperature resistance, opacity for light-sensitive products, sterilizer resistance, ease of formability, compatibility with many products, and tamper evidence.

Thermoformable Plastics. Thermoformed plastics are among the most widely used package types due to their aesthetic appeal, medical device delivery applications, and versatility for customized designs to fit contours of medical devices or several components of procedure kits. The selection of a material for a specific medical device is dependent on several factors such as barrier requirements, sterilization method, and cost. There are many thermoformable plastics; however, not all have the ideal properties that lend themselves to medical device packaging applications. For example, an acrylic-based plastic has very low structural flexibility, low impact resistance, poor clarity, but has a very high radiation resistance. The polyethylene terephthalate (PET) plastics (polyesters) have excellent clarity, structural flexibility, impact resistance, sealability, and radiation resistance, but only marginal water vapor barrier and heat resistance. So each material has its favorable and unfavorable properties, and the material that most closely fits the desired packaging application must be selected. The most common packaging materials for thermoform tray applications are discussed in some detail.

Polyethylene Terephthalate (PET). The generic material called PET, or polyethylene terephthalate, is probably the most widely used material for medical packaging applications due to its favorable characteristics as mentioned previously. This material forms easily in thermoforming operations and provides good barrier performance and sealability with various lidding materials. The material imparts excellent clarity, flexibility, and radiation resistance—all important characteristics for packaging medical devices. It is produced in forms for injection or blow molding of rigid containers like bottles and jars, and in sheet form for thermoforming trays, and blisters. When PET is coextruded with other materials such as glycol to make PETG, the barrier performance characteristics of the material are improved. PETG is not heat sealable, so the lidding stock must be adhesive coated to facilitate a functional seal for the package. Table 7.1 provides some specific physical properties for PET materials.

Polycarbonate (PC). Polycarbonate is used for high-performance package applications where high strength and toughness are required due to the size, density, or shape of the product. In some applications PC is used because of its superior clarity and the aesthetic appeal of the product. PC is the most impact resistant of all the plastics but has only average moisture- and gas-barrier properties (Table 7.2). The cost of PC is somewhat prohibitive in a high-volume product application. However, for low-volume, high-priced devices, such as pacemakers, defibrillators, and other implantable devices, it is an excellent material for thermoform trays. Most of the common sterilization methods, such as autoclave, steam, ethylene oxide, gamma, and e-beam, can be used on packages made from polycarbonate. Typically, PC film for thermoform applications is coextruded with a polyolefin heat-seal layer.

Polyvinyl Chloride (PVC) and Polyvinylidene Chloride (PVdC). The material known as PVC polyvinyl chloride is one vinyl-based polymer used commonly in packaging applications. Another material in the same family is PVdC, also known as polyvinylidene chloride (SARAN™). These materials differ from polyethylene in having a chlorine atom that replaces one hydrogen atom in its chemical structure. This is important, since it is this chlorine atom that has caused the material to lose favor for packaging applications due to environmental concerns. The environmental concern is that when incinerated, the material generates a hydrogen chloride gas. Several European countries have banned the use of vinyl-based materials. The criticism is controversial. The perceived environmental threat has caused many PVC applications to be replaced by PET. PVC is used most frequently in

TABLE 7.1 Specific Physical Properties for PET Materials

PET	
Molecular formula	$(C_{10}H_8O_4)_n$
Density	1370 kg/m^3
Young's modulus (E)	2800–3100 MPa
Tensile strength (σ_t)	55–75 MPa
Elastic limit	50–150%
Notch test	3.6 kJ/m^2
Glass temperature	75°C
Melting point	260°C
Vicat B	170°C
Thermal conductivity	0.24 W/(m · K)
Linear expansion coefficient (α)	7×10^{-5}/K
Specific heat (c)	1.0 kJ/(kg · K)
Water absorption (ASTM)	0.16
Refractive index	1.5750

Source: A.K. van der Vegt and L.E. Govaert, *Polymeren*, van keten tot kunstof, ISBN 90-407-2388–5.

TABLE 7.2 Properties of Polycarbonate

Polycarbonate	
Physical Properties	
Density (ρ)	1200–1220 kg/m^3
Abbe number (V)	34.0
Refractive index (n)	1.584–6
Flammability	V0–V2
Limiting oxygen index	25–27%
Water absorption—equilibrium (ASTM)	0.16–0.35%
Water absorption—over 24 h	0.1%
Radiation resistance	Fair
Ultraviolet (1–380 nm) resistance	Fair
Mechanical Properties	
Young's modulus (E)	2–2.4 GPa
Tensile strength (σ_t)	55–75 MPa
Compressive strength (σ_c)	>80 MPa
Elongation (ε) at break	80–150%
Poisson's ratio (ν)	0.37
Hardness—rockwell	M70
Izod impact strength	600–850 J/m
Notch test	20–35 kJ/m^2
Abrasive resistance—ASTM D1044	10–15 mg/1000 cycles
Coefficient of friction (μ)	0.31
Thermal Properties	
Melting temperature (T_m)	267°C
Glass transition temperature (T_g)	150°C
Heat deflection temperature—10 kN (Vicat B)*	145°C
Heat deflection temperature—0.45 MPa	140°C
Heat deflection temperature—1.8 MPa	128–138°C
Upper working temperature	115–130°C
Lower working temperature	–135°C
Linear thermal expansion coefficient (α)	65–70 × 10^{-6}/K
Specific heat capacity (c)	1.2–1.3 kJ/kg · K
Thermal conductivity (k) at 23°C	0.19–0.22 W/(m · K)
Heat transfer coefficient (h)	0.21 W/(m^2 · K)
Electrical Properties	
Dielectric constant (ε_r) at 1 MHz	2.9
Permittivity (ε) at 1 MHz	2.568 × 10^{-11} F/m
Relative permeability (μ_r) at 1 MHz	0.866
Permeability (μ) at 1 MHz	1.089 μN/A^2
Dielectric strength	15–67 kV/mm
Dissipation factor at 1 MHz	0.01
Surface resistivity	10^{15} Ω/sq
Volume resistivity (ρ)	10^{12}–10^{14} Ω · m

*ASTM D1525-07 Standard Test Method for Vicat Softening Temperature of Plastics, ASTM International, West Conshohocken, PA, 2007, **DOI:** 10.1520/D 1525–07.

Source: Wikipedia (http://en.wikipedia.org/wiki/Polycarbonate).

TABLE 7.3 Properties of Polyvinyl Chloride

Polyvinyl Chloride	
Density	1380 kg/m^3
Young's modulus (E)	2900–3300 MPa
Tensile strength (σ_t)	50–80 MPa
Elongation at break	20–40%
Notch test	2–5 kJ/m^2
Glass temperature	87°C
Melting point	80°C
Vicat B*	85°C
Heat transfer coefficient (λ)	0.16 W/(m · K)
Effective heat of combustion	17.95 MJ/kg
Linear expansion coefficient (α)	8 10^{-5}/K
Specific heat (c)	0.9 kJ/(kg · K)
Water absorption (ASTM)	0.04–0.4
Price	0.5–1.25 €/kg

*Deformation temperature at 10 kN needle load.
Source: Wikipedia (http://en.wikipedia.org/wiki/Polycarbonate).

packaging application for blow-molded bottles, blisters, and thermoform trays. PVC is tough and clear and has excellent barrier properties as well as high impact resistance (Table 7.3).

Polystyrene (PS). Polystyrene (PS) is one of the most versatile, easily fabricated, and cost-effective plastic used in the packaging industry. It can be molded, extruded, and foamed. It is probably best known for its use as cushioning materials for electronic products. There are two types of polystyrene available for packaging applications: general purpose and high impact (HIPS). It is the high-impact type that is used for medical device packaging applications. High-impact polystyrene contains a small amount of rubberlike polybutadiene blended in to overcome the brittleness of the general-purpose material. This makes the HIPS tougher but less clear, usually translucent or opaque. The material may be acceptable for applications where visibility of the device is not required. The advantages of the material are its cost, heat resistance, and ease of formability (Table 7.4). However, it may be susceptible to impact damage during shipping and handling. Another styrene-based material is

TABLE 7.4 Properties of Polystyrene

Polystyrene	
Density	1050 kg/m^3
Density of EPS	25–200 kg/m^3
Specific gravity	1.05
Electrical conductivity (s)	10^{-16} S/m
Thermal conductivity (k)	0.08 W/(m · K)
Young's modulus (E)	3000–3600 MPa
Tensile strength (s_t)	46–60 MPa
Elongation at break	3–4%
Notch test	2–5 kJ/m^2
Glass temperature	95°C
Melting point	240°C
Vicat B	90°C
Heat transfer coefficient (Q)	0.17 W/(m^{2}K)
Linear expansion coefficient (a)	8 10^{-5}/K
Specific heat (c)	1.3 kJ/(kg · K)
Water absorption (ASTM)	0.03–0.1
Decomposition	X years, still decaying

Source: Wikipedia (http://en.wikipedia.org/wiki/Polystrene).

TABLE 7.5 Barrier and Mechanical Strength Properties for Thermoformable Plastics

Plastic	WVTR, nmol/m · s	Oxygen, nmol/m · Gpa	Tensile strength, psi	Elongation, %	Impact strength, kg/cm	Tear strength, g/0.001 in
PET	0.45	6–8	25,000–30,000	120–140	25–30	13–80
Polycarbonte	2.8	N.A.	10,000	92–115	100	16–25
PVdC	0.005–0.05	0.02–0.03	8,000	60–100	5–15	4–6
HDPE	0.095	200–400	3,000–7,500	10–500	1–3	15–300
LDPE	0.35	500–700	1,000–3,500	225–600	4–6	50–300
PVC	0.55	10–40	2,000–16,000	5–500	12–20	Varies
PP	0.16	300–500	9,000–25,000	60–100	5–15	4–6
Polystyrene	1.8	500–800	N.A.	N.A.	N.A.	N.A.

Source: Diana Tweede and Ron Goddard, *Packaging Materials*, Pira International, Leatherhead, Surrey, U.K., 1998.

called *styrene butadiene copolymer* (SBC) and is commonly processed into containers, sheet, and film. It is used extensively in medical packaging applications due to its ability to be sterilized by both gamma irradiation and ethylene oxide.

The styrene materials are commonly recycled in communities where economics or legislation is favorable. However, where these materials are incinerated, PS, like PVC, causes unacceptable gaseous emissions and thus have come under intense environmental pressure and outright banning in some communities.

Other Materials and Properties. There is a host of other materials used in thermoform packaging applications. Some are specifically engineered for high barrier applications while others are resistant to high temperature. Although these materials have their greater use for medical device components, some materials are finding use for various types of packages such as tubes, blown containers, molded closures, and, in some cases, thermoform sheet material.

Table 7.5 shows barrier and mechanical strength properties for the most common thermoformable plastics.

7.5.2 Secondary Materials

Secondary packaging is often used with primary packages to provide several functions in the overall distribution system for a medical device. *Secondary packages* are defined as containers that enclose one or more primary packages. One function the secondary package provides is the communication of information about the device. Protection of the device through the rigors of distribution and handling is another function a secondary package provides. In addition, the secondary package allows for storage of primary packages in a neat and orderly manner before use.

Paperboard Cartons. The most common form of secondary package used for primary medical device packages is the paperboard carton. This package is used for all types of primary packages, including the semirigid tray, flexible formed pouch, chevron pouch, and header bag. It is used most often when the primary package requires some additional protection and as a "shelf box" for storage at the point of end use. A paperboard carton is usually inserted into a shipping container (i.e., shipper) that provides more substantial protection for transport. Many paperboard cartons may be consolidated into a single shipper.

Materials used to fabricate paperboard cartons may also be variously known as boxboard, cartonboard, chipboard, containerboard, and solid fiberboard. They are made in the same manner as paper and allow semirigid formability as well as surface strength and printability. Solid bleached boxboard is the highest quality, as it is made from the purest virgin bleached pulp. This grade of paperboard is most often used for medical devices due to its aesthetic good looks and excellent printability for graphics and product information. Various styles of paperboard carton are available to suit a particular product or primary package type or application.

Corrugated Fiberboard Boxes. A corrugated fiberboard box is used to transport the medical device through the distribution environment and to its ultimate user. This package may be known as the shipping container, shipper, shipping box, transport package, or other name that denotes its purpose as the final package to be offered for shipment. This package may contain only primary package types, or single or multiple secondary packages containing primary packages. In this case the package system may be considered to have a primary, secondary, and tertiary package.

Most shippers are made from a material known as corrugated fiberboard. The paper-based material consists of a corrugated medium sandwiched between two kraft paper faces. It is characterized by the thickness and spacing of the medium (fluting), the weight of the facing layers, and the quality of the paper used. Most medical devices are transported in a grade and style of shipper known as a single wall, C-flute, regular slotted container (RSC).

7.6 COMMON TESTING METHODS

This part details some of the testing methods used and accepted within the medical device industry for characterizing the performance of the package. These methods will be used to validate the packaging processes and to establish performance specifications for continuous monitoring of quality. An ASTM international standard, entitled F2097-07 "Standard Guide for Design and Evaluation of Primary Flexible Packaging for Medical Products," provides a compendium of test methods. Specific individual test methods must be selected based on the pertinent characteristics of the specific product to be packaged and the purpose for testing, research and development, or compliance. Not all test methods will be applicable.

7.6.1 Introduction

The package for a medical device plays a key role in safely delivering specialized treatment to the patient for which the device was designed and developed. It must ensure the efficacy of the device from the point of manufacture to the point of final use. Most single-use terminally sterilized medical devices must be delivered with a very high confidence that the device has remained in a sterile condition throughout its storage, handling, and transport environment. In addition, packaging may have a direct function in the application of the treatment, as it may act as a fixture or dispenser to the physician. Thus, mechanical damage to the package may not be tolerated. The design and development of the packaging system has come under closer and closer scrutiny by both the international and domestic regulatory agencies. This scrutiny has placed a great deal of emphasis on standardizing the package-development process. Some standardization of the packaging process has come in the form of the international standard entitled ISO 11607, "Packaging for Terminally Sterilized Medical Devices." Annex B of the ISO 11607 standard provides "informative" knowledge on standardized test methods and procedures that may be used to demonstrate compliance with the requirements of Part 1 ISO 11607. This section specifically presents the current consensus thinking and some industry test methods available for evaluating the integrity and strength of sterile barrier systems and package system performance.

7.6.2 Package Integrity versus Package Strength

First, there seems to be some confusion within the medical device industry regarding the strength versus the integrity of a package. Package strength concerns the force required to separate two components of the package. It could be the force to separate two flexible components of a pouch or a flexible lid and a thermoform tray. These forces may be measured in pounds per inch width, as in the seal/peel test; or in pounds per square inch, as in the burst test method. Alone, these tests of package strength values do not necessarily prove the integrity of the entire package. For example, since the seal/peel test per ASTM F-88 only evaluates a 1-in segment of the package, there may be other areas of the package which are not sealed adequately to prevent contamination of the product. In fact, the seal width that was actually measured may be within the strength specification but may have a channel leak that could breach the package and negate integrity.

Likewise, the ASTM F-1140 burst test method as referenced by ISO 11607 also has its pitfalls. This method evaluates the whole package by applying pressure to all areas of the package; however, the pressure is not applied equally at all points due to package irregularities and distortions. This can lead to a relatively high degree of variability between tests. Further, the burst test may not detect breaches in the package, such as pinholes and channel leaks, even though the burst test values have met the performance specification.

Even though the package strength specifications are confirmed, the package integrity is not necessarily proven. Seal integrity is defined as *condition of the seal, which ensures that it presents a microbial barrier to at least the same extent as the rest of the packaging*. This definition does not refer to the *strength* of the seal. Package integrity is independent of package strength, although a strong package seal is a convincing indicator of a safe package with seal integrity. Further, if the entire seal area is proven to be homogeneous and continuous, then one could say that the package seals provide integrity. However, this says nothing about the package surfaces that may have pinholes or leaks not detected by seal strength tests. Other mechanical tests may be appropriate for determining package seal homogeneity.

Seal strength is important in the overall scheme of developing the package process, but the seal strength performance specification is used most effectively to monitor the process, not to determine ultimate acceptance. Seal strength is also an important determinant for establishing package process parameters. In fact, the ISO 11607 standard requires that the *seal strength shall be determined at the upper and lower limits of the defined critical sealing process variables and shall be demonstrated to be suitable for the intended purpose*. To restate, seal strength is an important performance attribute for the package and provides suitable guidance in establishing statistical process control limits, but is not the absolute determinant of the acceptability of the package for its intended use. Package integrity at the point of final use is the principal acceptance criterion for a sterile medical device package. However, both performance attributes are essential to the package design and development process.

7.6.3 Determining Package Strength

Package seal strength measurements are fundamental indicators of the package formation process. At a minimum the seal strength serves as a gauge that a sealing process is under control and that the process is producing acceptable sterile barrier systems (packages).

The performance specification or benchmark for the package may be based on the seal and burst test values of packages produced on a specific validated production line. These tests are performed using standardized test methods developed by the American Society for Testing and Materials (ASTM-International). The seal strength test procedure is described in ASTM F88, "Seal Strength of Flexible Barrier Materials," and is the industry's definitive method for characterizing seal strength. This test covers the measurement of the strength of a seal of a given width at a specific point of the package. It does not measure the seal continuity. Other methods such as the 180° peel test may be used to determine the seal continuity or peeling characteristics. The seal strength test is performed by cutting a 1-in-wide strip from the seal of the package. The strip is placed in the tensile test machine by clamping each leg of the sample in the grips, aligning the specimen so that the seal is perpendicular to the direction of pull as shown in Fig. 7.1.

The seal is pulled apart at a rate of 10 to 12 in/min. The peak force required to pull the seal completely apart is recorded. It would be appropriate to perform the test at several points of the package, including the manufacturer's seals (produced by the vendor of the package) and the production seals (produced by the manufacturer of the product). Typical seal strength values lie in the range between 1 and 4 lb. The optimum seal strength varies according to the type of package being tested and its specific applications.

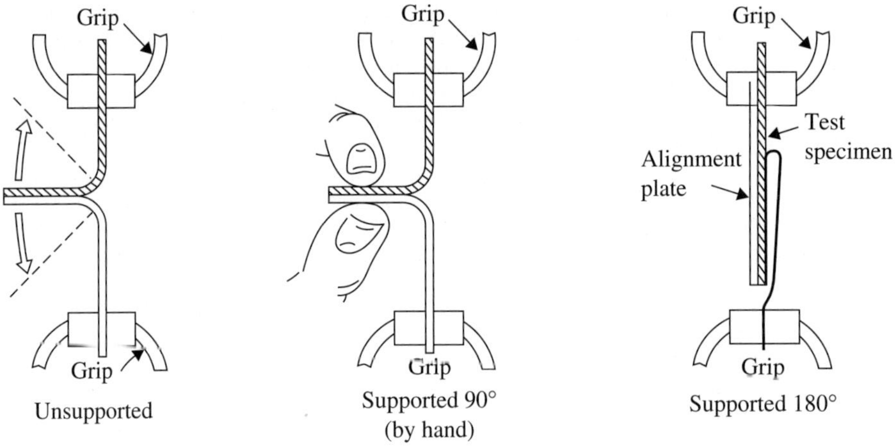

FIGURE 7.1 Techniques for inserting test specimen into the apparatus grips. The technique used to perform the test will provide different results.

The burst test procedure is described in ASTM Standard D-1140, "Failure Resistance of Unrestrained and Nonrigid Packages for Medical Applications" and is a means by which an entire package is tested. This method covers the determination of the ability of package materials or seals to withstand internal pressurization. Since packages may be produced from substandard materials; may be produced with inadequate seals; or combinations thereof, package integrity may be compromised during production, distribution, or storage. Burst testing may provide a rapid means of evaluating overall package quality during production, and overall package integrity after dynamic events associated with shipping and handling.

Two methods of burst testing are provided in the ASTM standard, entitled F1140-07 Standard Test Methods for Internal Pressurization Failure Resistance of Unrestrained Packages. The open-package test is performed in a fixture which clamps the open end but provides a means for pressurizing the package. The pressure is increased in the package at a rate greater than the permeability of the porous package component, until a failure occurs. The type and location of the failure is recorded as well as the maximum pressure at which failure occurred. The open-package test is most useful as a quality assurance procedure on incoming materials to ensure that the supplier of the material is meeting preestablished specifications for seal strength.

The closed-package test is performed on production samples as an internal quality assurance procedure. This method is performed by inserting the pressure source through a component of the package and then increasing the pressure until a failure occurs. The pressure at failure and location and type of failure are recorded. Burst test values typically fall in the range between 0.5 and 3 psi. No correlation has been made between the burst test values and seal strength values.

A recent study has shown that unrestrained pressure testing may lead to inconsistencies in test results while more consistent test results are achieved by restraining the test specimen between parallel plates. In response to these studies a new method was developed to test the package between two parallel restraining plates. The new method is entitled F2054-07 "Standard Test Method for Burst Testing of Flexible Package Seals Using Internal Air Pressurization Within Restraining Plates." Quoting from the scope of the standard:

These test methods cover the procedure for determining the minimum burst strength of a seal placed around the perimeter of a flexible package as it is internally pressurized and enclosed within restraining plates. The test methods described herein are functionally similar to Test Methods F 1140 with the exception of the use of restraining plates. Test Methods F 1140 describes methods of burst testing that do not include the use of restraining plates and are suitable to determine a package's general ability to withstand pressurization stresses. Under Test Methods F 1140 the stresses are not distributed uniformly to all areas of the package seal. Under unrestrained conditions the stress on the package is highest at the middle of the pouch where it inflates to the package's maximum diameter; therefore, Test Methods F 1140 may not reliably detect the weakest area of the seal.

The "Significance and Use" section of the standard describes how and why the standard is used and says:

The burst test internally and increasingly pressurizes a package until an area of the package seal around the perimeter "bursts" open in response to pressurization. By placing the package within restraining plates during pressurization, the dimensional stability of the package is maintained in a manner that results in stresses applied more uniformly along the perimeter of the package, where seals are normally placed. This allows the test to have a higher probability of detecting the weakest area of the seal and provides a measurement of the pressure required to "burst" open the package. This test provides a rapid means of evaluating tendencies for package seal failure when the package is exposed to a pressure differential. Pressure differentials may occur during such processes as sterilization and transportation. This test method provides an indicator of the burst strength of a package, where the burst will normally occur in one or more areas of the seal. An indicator of the minimum burst strength may be of importance to the package manufacturer and end user in ensuring adequate package integrity. This test method cannot provide a measure of package seal uniformity. This test method also cannot provide an evaluation of overall package integrity or the burst strength of areas of the package that contact the surface of the restraining plates used. This test method should be combined with other methods of evaluating overall package integrity, uniformity of the package seal, or opening functionality, if so required.

This test frequently is used to quickly evaluate package seal strength during the manufacturing process and at various stages of the package life cycle.

If correlations between pieces of test equipment are to be made, it is important that all parameters of the test be equivalent. Typical parameters can include, but are not limited to, the package size, material, type and configuration of seal, rate of air flow into the package, pressure detection sensing mechanism and sensitivity (machine response to pressure drop), position of test article, rigidity of restraining plates, and distance between restraining plates.

This test may not necessarily provide correlation with package seal strength as typically measured using Test Methods F 1140 or F 88 (or equivalents).

7.6.4 Package "Conditioning" Tests

When we use the term "conditioning" we are referring to any type of situation that exposes the package to hazards inherent in the life cycle of the package, including shelf life (aging), environmental (temperature and humidity, atmospheric pressure), and dynamics (shock and vibration). These tests do not produce a test result per se, but subject the packages to conditions that may compromise the package system. Consequently, they are not required to be validated, but should represent the best or most realistic simulation of the conditions inherent in the package life cycle. Several guidelines and practices have been developed to provide a standardized means of subjecting packages to conditioning prior to package integrity testing. More detail will be provided in later sections of this chapter; however, the conditioning standards of interest are

- D4169-05 Standard Practice for Performance Testing of Shipping Containers and Systems
- D4332-01(2006) Standard Practice for Conditioning Containers, Packages, or Packaging Components for Testing
- D6653-01(2006) Standard Test Methods for Determining the Effects of High Altitude on Packaging Systems by Vacuum Method
- D7386-08 Standard Practice for Performance Testing of Packages for Single Parcel Delivery Systems
- E171-94(2007) Standard Specification for Standard Atmospheres for Conditioning and Testing Flexible Barrier Materials
- F1980-07 Standard Guide for Accelerated Aging of Sterile Barrier Systems for Medical Devices

7.6.5 Determining Package Integrity

The FDA has recognized ISO 11607 as a consensus standard, which states that, "The manufacturer shall demonstrate the integrity of the package by testing the package. This can be accomplished by physical tests." Examples of physical tests as described in the ISO 11607 standard include internal pressure test, and dye penetration test, gas sensing test, and vacuum leak test. All of these methods have their advantages and disadvantages.

Microbial Challenge/Product Sterility Test Methods. There are really two types of microbial barrier tests: those performed on materials and those performed on whole packages. Microbial barrier tests on materials are performed by packaging manufacturers to ensure that their materials are impervious to microorganisms while allowing sterilant gases to permeate for product sterilization purposes. This is why "breathable" materials are used for sterile barrier systems. These tests are typically performed using ASTM F1608, "Microbial Ranking of Porous Packaging Materials (Exposure Chamber Method)." Microbial barrier testing of materials is significantly less controversial than microbial testing of whole packages since this methodology lends itself to some level of standardization and control. Determining the microbial barrier characteristics of materials is very different from the methods required for a whole package testing. A whole package test is significantly more complex than a single material, and whole package microbial challenge testing has long been discredited as a reliable means of determining package (sterile barrier system) integrity. For this reason the remainder of the package integrity discussion focuses on physical test methods for determining package integrity.

Physical Test Methods. Some of the physical test methods have been available for many years as published ASTM standards. Recently, the industry has taken a closer look at the validity and effectiveness of these methods and has developed new methods for evaluating package integrity.

Visual Inspection. ASTM Subcommittee F2 published standard F1886-98, "Standard Test Method for Determining Integrity of Seals for Medical Packaging by Visual Inspection, to help detail a methodology for visual inspection. This standard describes a method to visually detect channel defects in package seals down to a width of 0.003 in (75 μm) with a 60 to100 percent probability, depending on the package type and size of channel. It provides attribute data (accept/reject) for package integrity of finished, unopened packages. It is generally not effective in detecting pinholes and minute tears in package substrates. In addition, visual inspection cannot be used for packages with two opaque substrates, as transparency of the seal surfaces is essential to the inspection. Its most applicable attribute is for monitoring package quality in production to detect any significant changes in heat-sealing process parameters, which may provide the first indication that the process is out of control. Additional testing using more sensitive methods for leak detection of packages suspicious of having defects may be warranted to confirm whether the channel or void is in fact an unsealed area. Visual inspection is not considered to be the only means by which the manufacturer should evaluate for package integrity.

Internal Pressure Test. The internal pressure or bubble leak test applies an internal pressure to the sterile package while it is submerged in water and notes any escaping air bubbles. The Flexible Packaging Association's (FPA) committee, Sterilization Packaging Manufacturers Council (SPMC), originally published this standard for testing packaging integrity. The standard was entitled FPA/SPMC Standard 005-96, "Standard Test Method for Detection of Leaks in Heat Seal Packages-Internal Pressurization Method," and has since been adopted by ASTM and published as F2096-04, "Standard Test Method for Detecting Gross Leaks in Medical Packaging by Internal Pressurization (Bubble Test)." This has become the industry's definitive method in package validation studies for determining the integrity of the sterile barrier system.

As the standard describes in the "Significance and Use" section:

> *The internal pressurization test method provides a practical way to examine packages for gross leaks, which may render the product nonsterile.*
>
> *This test method is extremely useful in a test laboratory environment where no common package material/size exists.*

This test method may apply to very large or long packages, which do not fit into any other package integrity test method apparatus.

This test method may be used as a means to evaluate package integrity. Package integrity is crucial to consumer safety since heat-sealed packages are designed to provide a contamination free and sterile environment to the product.

The advantages of using this method for determining package integrity are that it is very easy to perform the test, and it is inexpensive to test a large sample size and obtain statistical significance in the test sample set. The equipment costs are low since all that is required is a pressure source and a water bath.

This method has been validated by round-robin testing, and a precision and bias statement has been developed for its repeatability and reproducibility. Its sensitivity for detecting leak size has been found to be 0.010 in (250 μm) with an 81 percent probability. Gross leaks such as 0.010-in pinholes occur most often as a result of handling and distribution hazards that cause tears, gouges, and punctures. Package validations most often fail as a result of the rigors of shipping and distribution. This test is sufficiently sensitive to detect those types of defects caused by the hazards of distribution. Leaks in seals and in material surfaces can be detected using this method. If the method is validated for each package type, it may be possible to consistently detect holes as small as 0.005 in (125 μm).

The method can be used for both porous and nonporous packaging materials. For packages with porous materials, the porous material substrate may be sealed using a label or coating to reduce the porosity of the material. This facilitates the pressurization of the package and reduces the interpretation of what constitutes a leak and where a leak is occurring in the package. The porous material is not evaluated for leakage as the coating may mask or block leaks in that component of the sterile barrier system. However, pinholes, tears, gouges, and channel leaks are readily apparent under a predetermined and validated internal pressure that does not begin to separate the seals.

Validation of the method for the package under investigation must be performed to determine the proper internal pressure and the sensitivity of the method, and to evaluate the ability to detect channel and pinhole leaks over the permeation of any air through the porous substrate.

Vacuum Leak Test. The vacuum leak test is similar in concept to the internal pressure leak test in that the result is a pass/fail for the detection of bubbles emanating from the package while submersed in a water bath. The method is described in ASTM D3078-02, "Standard Test Method for Determination of Leaks in Flexible Packaging by Bubble Emission." The pressure differential is obtained by evacuating the chamber, causing the package to expand due to its internal pressure. This test method covers the determination of gross leaks in flexible packaging containing a headspace gas. Test sensitivity is limited to 1×10^{-5} atm cm^3/s (1×10^{-6} Pa m^3/s) or even less sensitive.

The difficulty in using this method for porous packages is that the pressure differential may not reach a point at which air passes through a channel or material leak before air passes readily through the porous material. Lowering the porosity of the material by coating it with a lacquer or other means could reduce this problem. This test is more suitable for nonporous packages where internal pressure will force air through leaks.

Dye Penetration Test. The ASTM F2 Committee first published a dye penetration test method in 1998, which has become an important method for determining the integrity of sterile barrier system seals. The standard, designated as F1929-98(2004), "Standard Test Method for Detecting Seal Leaks in Porous Medical Packaging by Dye Penetration," provides a standardized method for conducting leak testing of package seals using a low surface tension solution and dye indicator. The "Significance and Use" section of the standard describes the standard's intent as follows:

Harmful biological or particulate contaminants may enter the device through leaks. These leaks are frequently found at seals between package components of the same or dissimilar materials. Leaks may also result from a pinhole in the packaging material.

This dye penetrant procedure is applicable only to individual leaks in a package seal. The presence of a number of small leaks, as found in porous packaging material, which could be detected by other techniques, will not be indicated.

There is no general agreement concerning the level of leakage that is likely to be deleterious to a particular package. However, since these tests are designed to detect leakage, components that exhibit any indication of leakage are normally rejected.

Since leaks may change in size with different ambient conditions, comparisons between test stations are not conclusive. Therefore, this method is usually employed as a go, no-go test.

The dye solution will wick through any porous material over time, but usually not within the maximum time suggested. If wicking does occur, it may be verified by observing the porous side of the subject seal area. The dye will have discolored the surface of the material.

When puncturing the packaging to allow injection of the dye penetrant solution, care should be taken not to puncture other package surfaces. Puncturing of the package is facilitated if it is done adjacent to a dummy device inside the package. The device will provide a tenting effect that will separate the two sides of the package, reducing the chance of accidental puncture of both sides.

The basis of the test method is that when the test solution comes in contact with a channel or breach in the package seal, it will flow through the channel by capillary action. The leak will be indicated by a blue streak visible in the seal and/or a profuse and consistent flow of the dye through the channel.

This test method is generally considered to be more sensitive than the whole package microbial challenge methods discussed earlier in this chapter. It is reported in a study on Tyvek®-to-plastic pouches that seal defects down to 0.0015 in (38 μm) were readily detected with a blue dye solution. The published test standard has verified through round-robin testing that the smallest channel which can be reliably detected is on the order of 0.002 in (50 μm) or larger. In fact, the detection rate for breathable pouches and trays with breathable lids was found to be 98 to 99 percent. It was discovered during the testing that significant reductions in test performance were observed when indicator dyes other than toluidine blue were used. Also, the round robin results are specific for the wetting agent (Triton X-100) used for the solution.

The most effective application for the dye penetration test method is for detecting breaches in the seals of transparent packages since seal defects must be observed easily. It is possible to use this method for opaque packages; however, observation of the seal leak must be made at the seals outside edge and the exact location of the leak may be difficult to ascertain. One attribute of this test methodology is that it is difficult to use for detecting leaks in the surfaces of package components. That is, pinholes, gouges, or abrasions of the materials cannot be detected, since the dye cannot be easily contacted with all of the package surfaces. So, although the dye penetration test is a sensitive leak indicator for seals, it is not a good whole-package integrity test. Other means must be used to detect material leaks, such as the bubble emission leak test. Other attributes of this test method must be considered before incorporating it into a package validation protocol. First the method is difficult to use for packages having a paper component as the dye solution can destroy the material in a very short time—maybe even faster than the dye would travel through a channel. Other porous packages may allow the dye solution to wick through, causing difficulty in detecting a true leak from the permeation or wicking of the solution through the material. Since the dye solution is injected into the package, the method is destructive to the package and, in many instances, also to the product.

Other Package Integrity Test Methods. Several other package integrity test methods have been developed by the ASTM F2 Committee. These include methods using trace gas sensing devices and other mechanical means for determining when a leak exists in a package. Several methods are listed below. These methods are developed around specific types of packages and apparatus:

- F2227-02 (2007), Standard Test Method for Nondestructive Detection of Leaks in Nonsealed and Empty Medical Packaging Trays by CO2 Tracer Gas Method
- F2228-02 (2007), Standard Test Method for Nondestructive Detection of Leaks in Medical Packaging which Incorporates Porous Barrier Material by CO2 Tracer Gas Method
- F2338-07 Standard Test Method for Nondestructive Detection of Leaks in Packages by Vacuum Decay Method
- F2391-05 Standard Test Method for Measuring Package and Seal Integrity Using Helium as the Tracer Gas

All the ASTM test methods are available from ASTM International and are published in the *ASTM Book of Standards*, volume 15.10.

7.6.6 Conclusion

Package seal strength does not necessarily equate to package integrity. These two attributes of a finished medical device package are separate considerations in proving the efficacy of the package. Industry has developed methods for seal strength testing which are used to validate the package process. Although package seal strength is an important performance attribute, the ultimate acceptance of the package is based on its absolute integrity. Some conditioning tests that will subject the package system to events inherent in its life cycle may be performed prior to integrity testing of the sterile barrier system. There are several means available for evaluating the integrity of sterile medical device packages. The application of a particular integrity test depends on many factors, including the type of package, materials of construction, size, desired sensitivity, and objective of the test.

7.7 PACKAGE PROCESS VALIDATION

This part provides an overview of the package manufacturing and the elements that must be considered for validating the package sealing and forming process. The ISO 11607 standard states in the introduction to Part 2:

> *There should be a documented validation program demonstrating the efficacy and reproducibility of all sterilization and packaging processes. Along with the sterilization process, some of the packaging operations that can affect sterile barrier system integrity are forming, sealing, capping or other closure systems, cutting, and process handling.*

7.7.1 Introduction

The product engineering team has developed an exciting new medical device that will improve the quality of life for many patients. The product has been tested and retested. Regulatory questions concerning the product have been defined and answered. Clinical trials to show that the product performs as intended have been completed. The manufacturing process has proven to be consistent and is fully documented. However, the challenge of bringing it to the market is just beginning. Many more questions must be answered before the product can be safely distributed and used by the patient's caregiver. The most basic one is, "How will I get the product to the caregiver in the condition required for safe and proper use?" The most basic answer is "By designing a package system that will combine with the device to create a total product that performs efficiently, safely, and effectively in the hands of the user."

At first glance, the issue of developing a package system seems uncomplicated and elementary. After all, what could be difficult about placing the device into a thermoformed tray, covering it with a Tyvek® lid, inserting it into a paperboard carton, and consolidating the cartons into a shipping unit? In actuality, the process of designing and developing a package for terminally sterilized medical devices is complex and complicated. This is due to all of the interactions of various processes, equipment, materials, and environments that combine to influence the package design and manufacturing of the finished product.

For example, the product engineering team has developed the product as a disposable sterile device that must remain sterile at the point of end use. Therefore, the microbial barrier properties of the packaging materials, along with the suitability of forming and sealing, are crucial for assuring package integrity and product safety. So, the product and package materials must be compatible with the chosen sterilization process. In addition, the product will need to survive the rigors of transportation with its intrinsic hazards of shock, vibration, and environmental conditions. Finally, the manufacturer must have documented evidence that the performance of the package is not adversely affected over time (stability).

Unfortunately, the product engineering team was unaware that there are regulations within the FDA and international community that require a formal package system qualification process and a documented validation program demonstrating the efficacy and reproducibility of all sterilization and packaging processes (i.e., forming, sealing, capping, cutting, and handling). At this point, the engineering staff has realized that the package design and development process should have been an integral part of the product development program and should not have been left to the very end of the development process. Serious delays in distribution of the product have resulted since the package validation process requires significant time and effort to complete. The engineering team now turns to the Regulatory Affairs (RA) department for help in identifying the regulatory requirements for packaging.

Investigation by the RA department for the requirements imposed on packaging reveals an array of documents on the subject. Foremost is the quality systems regulation (QSR) found in Title 21 CFR, Part 820. The requirements for components, device master records, and environmental controls that affect the selection and use of packaging appear throughout the QSR. However, the specific requirements for packaging are in Sec. 820.130.

Further investigation discloses two international documents regulating the design and development of packaging: the International Standards Organization (ISO) 11607 "Packaging for Terminally Sterilized Medical Devices" and European Norm (EN) 868-1, "Packaging Materials Systems for Medical Devices which Are to Be Ssterilized-Part 1: General Requirements and Test Methods." Both of these documents provide an outline of general requirements and test methods for validating the complete package system. RA has reviewed the two international documents and has found that they are very similar, but with a few significant differences. "What standard do we follow?" becomes the next basic question to answer. Since ISO 11607:2000 was published, the new two-part standard has been harmonized the EN 868-1. So, for general requirements of developing a package system, there is only one standard to comply with—ISO 11607.

FDA has helped further answer this question by acknowledging the importance of international consensus standards. The FDA stated in the FDA Modernization Act of 1997: *Guidance for the Recognition and Use of Consensus Standards* that

> *. . . conformance with applicable consensus standards can provide a reasonable assurance of safety and/or effectiveness. Therefore, information submitted on conformance with such standards will have a direct bearing on determination of safety and effectiveness made during the review of IDEs and PMAs. Furthermore, if a premarket submission contains a declaration of conformity to recognized consensus standards, this will in most cases, eliminate the need to review actual test data for those aspects of the device addressed by the standard.*

Consequently, FDA has recognized the ISO 11607 standard as the consensus standard for manufacturing and quality control of packaging processes, materials, product package and design, and sterilization processes. Confusion about the existence of two packaging standards in which to conform is a concern for medical device companies. However, conformance to the EN 868-1 standard has become a moot issue as the ISO 11607 standard has been harmonized by the ISO TC 198 Working Group 7. So now we know what needs to be accomplished in regards to packaging, right? We just need to perform a package process validation. That's simply a matter of following the ISO 11607 standard. Yes, but unfortunately it's not a cookbook recipe to success.

7.7.2 What Is Process Validation (PV)?

The FDA defines validation as "establishing by objective evidence that the process, under anticipated conditions, including worst-case conditions, consistently produces a product which meets all predetermined requirements (and specifications)." Likewise, the ISO 11607 standard, Packaging for Terminally Sterilized Medical Devices, defines validation as a "documented procedure for obtaining and interpreting the results required to establish that a process will consistently yield product complying with predetermined specifications." What these definitions are really saying in a practical sense are that a process validation must address the requirements or application of the package, the interaction of people and equipment used in the manufacture of the package, the consistency with which a package can be made, the effects of processing (e.g., sterilization) on the performance of the package, and the storage and handling of the package. A manufacturer must become intimately involved with how the product is packaged and how to maintain consistency and uniformity. He must have proof that a process performs as it was intended.

The process validation (PV) consists of a series of qualifications of the processes making up the complete package system. These processes include the installation qualification (IQ), operational qualification (OQ), and performance qualification (PQ). Each facet of the packaging system must be challenged and qualified in order to claim validation of the entire system.

ISO 11607 addresses the package system validation in three phases or clauses. Clause 4 specifies the basic attributes required for a wide range of materials as they combine and interact with various medical devices, packaging designs, sterilization methods, and distribution modes. Clause 5 defines the framework of activities to qualify the processes used to make and assemble the final package configuration. Clause 6 is intended to assist in the selection of tests and to provide criteria that can be used to evaluate the performance of the final package.

7.7.3 Why Is Package Validation Important?

The primary objective of a package process validation should be to provide the medical device manufacturer with a high degree of assurance that his product will reach the user in a condition suitable for optimum functionality for its intended purpose, that is, provide a safe and effective medical device.

The specific benefits of the package process validation include not only reducing the manufacturer's risk of product malfunction or the potential of a nonsterile operating condition but also improved customer satisfaction, improved manufacturing efficiencies, reduced costs, reduced development time, and compliance to regulatory requirements. The "Guideline on General Principles of Process Validation" provides valuable understanding on quality systems requirements and may be relied upon with the assurance of its acceptability to FDA.

7.7.4 The Complete Package Validation Process

Prior to beginning any work on a validation, it is essential to write a protocol. The protocol provides a blueprint stating how testing is to be conducted, including the purpose, scope, responsibilities, test parameters, production equipment and settings, and the acceptance criteria for the test. Validation requires careful planning and preparation, and it begins with a well-conceived and well-written protocol.

As was mentioned earlier, the validation process consists of a series of qualifications of unique processes that make up the complete package process system. This total package process system includes the final package design, the materials chosen for the package, and the ability to consistently sterilize the product inside its package. The design of the package and its dynamic interactions with the product, the machinery used to assemble the package, the setup and maintenance of the machine, and consistency of production are other important considerations. If one of these processes is not right, the entire system breaks down and the manufacturer is at risk of malfeasance.

7.7.5 Package Forming and Sealing

While working with a packaging vendor, the package design has been completed. Vendors are usually responsible for validating that the materials are compatible with the sterilization process, and that compliance qualification tests are conducted. This responsibility should be clearly communicated and agreed upon during vendor selection and negotiation. Appropriate materials have been selected and validated for compatibility with the intended product by the manufacturer. But how will we assemble the product into the package using the most efficient and consistent process? The package sealing equipment for the job is identified and purchased; however, it must be properly installed before producing finished packages. Before starting final process development, it must be demonstrated that the process equipment and ancillary systems are capable of consistently operating within the established design and operating limits and tolerances. Part 2 of the ISO standard addresses all of the issues in validation such as equipment qualification, process development, process performance qualification, process control, and process certification and revalidation.

7.7.6 Installation Qualification (IQ)

An equipment installation qualification (IQ) is important because all production facilities have specific requirements for utilities, cleanliness, ambient temperature and humidity, and other variables. For this reason, the equipment should be installed in its intended production location before qualification. In addition, all equipment change parts and accessories are assembled and checked out for proper fit. This phase of the validation includes verifying that the equipment will perform its intended function, establishing calibration and maintenance procedures, and identifying monitoring and control issues. Standard operating procedures (SOPs) must be written for calibration, maintenance, and repair.

Facilities management has confirmed that the equipment has been properly installed, and that it performs in accordance with the manufacturer's specification. We can now begin to produce finished packages on the new equipment.

7.7.7 Operational Qualification (OQ)

In the operational qualification (OQ) the process parameters are challenged to ensure that they will produce sterile barrier systems that meet all defined requirements under all anticipated conditions of manufacturing. This step is designed to show and document that the equipment can run at its operating limits and to determine its performance capabilities relative to the manufacturer's specifications. This is the most critical and time-consuming phase of the validation process. It requires a large amount of performance testing and evaluation. Tests must be chosen that measure relevant performance characteristics of the package for important attributes such as seal strength and integrity. ISO provides examples of tests that may be used for measuring these attributes, including ASTM F88, ASTM D903, and ASTM F1140 for seal strength, and several methods such as internal pressure, dye penetration, gas sensing, and vacuum leak tests for package integrity, which have been discussed previously. These are physical test methods that ISO acknowledges can be used for demonstrating the integrity of the sterile package.

The first step in this phase of the validation is to establish the upper and lower ranges of the process parameters, which produce acceptable package performance. This may be accomplished by testing packages produced from a matrix of process parameter variable combinations, or by a design of experiments (DOE) which will only test packages produced at the extreme range of the process parameters. Where limited quantities of packages are available, one combination of process parameters may be used to produce packages based on historical experience, and then tested for strength and integrity. If these process parameters do not produce packages meeting the prescribed performance specifications, then the process parameters are adjusted until acceptable packages are produced. The flowchart in Fig. 7.2 depicts the process for establishing the machine process parameters.

The packages are produced under standard operating conditions and on the process equipment that has completed an IQ.

Through the rigorous step of OQ, the manufacturing department has now documented the machine process parameters and established the package performance specifications for the package system being developed.

7.7.8 Performance Qualification (PQ)

When the optimum machine process parameters have been established in the OQ, it is essential to determine the effects of sterilization, storage, and shipping and handling on the performance of the critical package attributes. This can be accomplished by measuring the seal strength and integrity after each of the individual processes and the accumulative effects of all these processes. This step

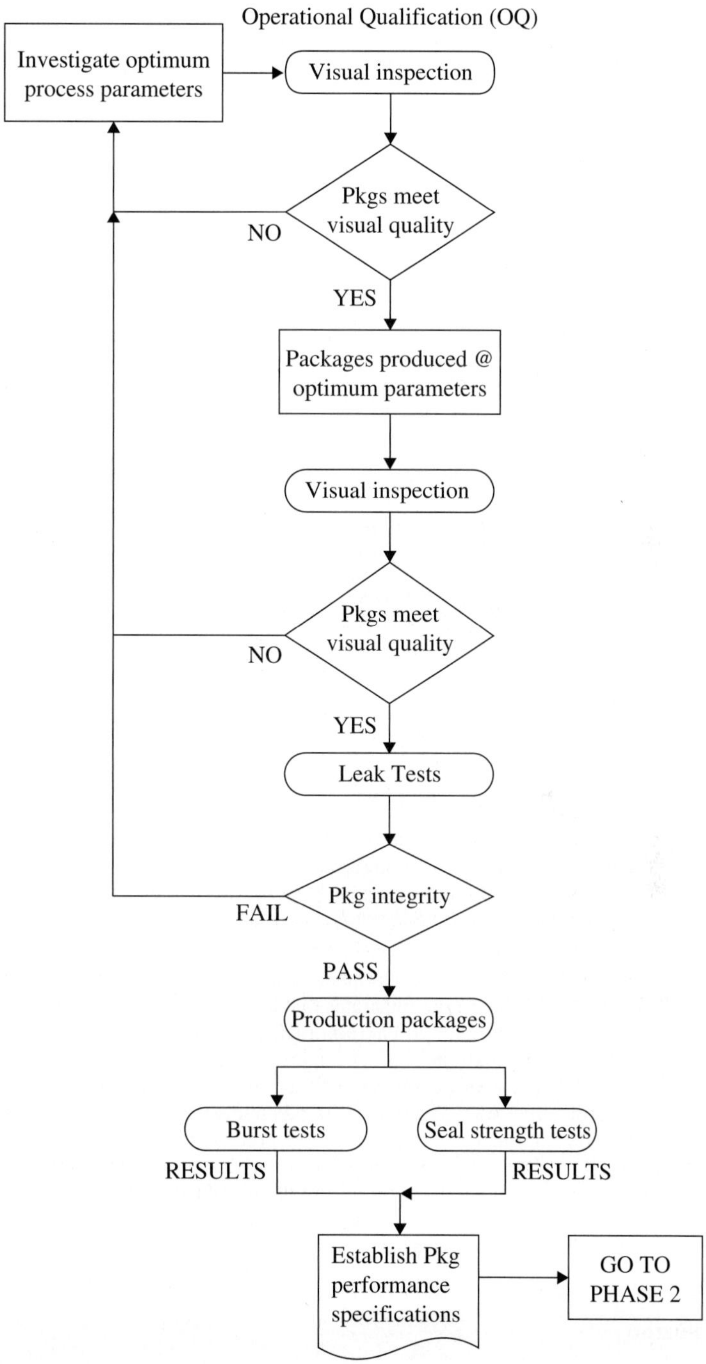

FIGURE 7.2 Operational qualification flowchart example.

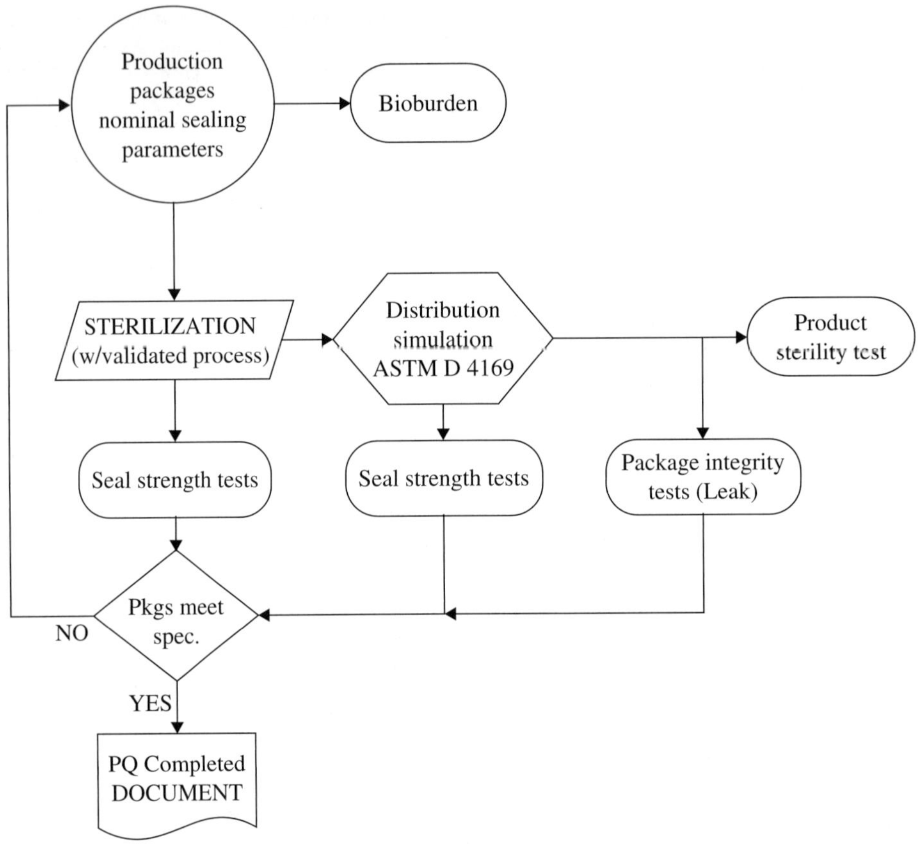

FIGURE 7.3 Performance qualification process flowchart.

in the process validation is to ensure that the process is in control by measuring the consistency with which packages meet the performance specifications. This is done in the process performance qualification (PQ). The PQ demonstrates that the process will consistently produce sterile barrier systems under the specified and optimal (nominal) operating conditions and will also provide a sterile barrier system throughout all the rigors of manufacturing and distribution.

The final phase of the process validation demonstrates that the combined effects of manufacturing, sterilization, storage, and handling do not have an adverse effect on the performance of the package produced under standard operating procedures. The flowchart shown in Fig. 7.3 depicts one protocol for assessing the integrity of the package after exposure to simulated, but realistic, events that the package will encounter during its manufacturing and distribution. These events include, but may not be limited to, the manufacturing process itself, the sterilization process, storage or aging, and handling and shipping hazards.

7.7.9 Conclusion

Medical devices are developed using engineering principles and process qualification techniques to ensure that they perform as intended. So too must the package design and development process be qualified and validated. The complete validation requires a series of qualifications of the entire system (e.g., IQ, OQ, PQ), which ensures that the package will perform in harmony with the product in a consistent and safe manner. This is accomplished by developing a comprehensive plan that cannot be simplified or short-circuited. Product engineering has realized that to accomplish the task of package process validation, the package system must be developed in tandem with the product development. Otherwise, delays of 6 to 12 months could result while the package system is being validated. The ISO 11607 standard provides guidance to assist medical device companies in developing sterile medical device package systems that perform efficiently, safely, and effectively in the hands of the caregiver. Remembering that the standard provides designers and manufacturers of medical devices with a *framework* of laboratory tests and evaluations that can be used to qualify the overall performance of the package, there are many means within this framework to achieve the end result.

7.8 SHELF-LIFE STUDIES

This part provides guidance for conducting accelerated aging or stability studies for medical device packages. A distinction between accelerated aging and environmental challenging should be made here. The ASTM Standard F1327, "Standard Terminology Relating to Barrier Materials for Medical Packaging," defines the two events as follows:

> *Accelerated aging—a technique to simulate the effects of time on a sterile barrier system or packaging system by subjecting the packaging to elevated temperatures under conditions otherwise representative of controlled environment storage conditions. The equivalent time is generally estimated by assuming the degradation of packaging materials following the kinetics described by the Arrhenius reaction rate function.*
>
> *Environmental challenging—the process of subjecting a sterile barrier system or package system to extremes of temperature and/or humidity with the goal of determining sensitivities of the packaging system to environmental stresses. In contrast to accelerated aging, environmental challenging often includes conditions and/or transitions of temperature and humidity that equal or exceed those that can be encountered in a packaging system life cycle.*

This part discusses the techniques used for accelerated aging while the environmental challenging will be discussed in Sec. 7.9. The distinction in these environmental testing techniques is important because for accelerated aging, the key is to choose a test temperature that does not damage the materials from conditions that would not be expected to occur in real time or are outside of the recommended use for the materials, but still "age" the materials in an accelerated manner; the purpose of environmental challenging techniques is to asses package performance at the realistic extreme conditions possible in the package life cycle or to stress the packaging materials near or past its failure point.

Developers of medical device packaging have struggled for years to justify shelf-life claims and establish expiration dating for packaged medical devices. Much has been published over the past decade describing techniques for conducting accelerated aging programs. However, the theory of accelerated aging is complex enough for homogeneous materials, let alone device systems involving several different materials, such as in complete medical device packages. The rapidly changing market place, technological developments, and regulations that govern them demand that the manufacturer be responsive, which places a priority on the ability of the manufacturer to develop products meeting all of the regulatory burdens in a timely and expeditious manner. Establishing shelf-life claims can be a significant bottleneck in the product development timeline. Real-time aging protocols would significantly hamper the product development cycle as well as marketability and are impracticable in today's fast-paced environment.

The adoption of the European Medical Device Directive (MDD) in June 1998 and the mandatory implementation of the CE label on all sterile medical devices marketed in the European Community have resulted in the compulsory use of expiration dates on all medical device packages. In order to obtain the CE label, *all* the "Essential Requirements" of the directive must be met. The MDD states that the label must bear . . . where appropriate, an indication of the date by which the device should be used, in safety, expressed as the year and month.

Compliance to the MDD's "Essential Requirements" is met by using harmonized standards. These standards may be European Norm (EN) or International Standards Organization (ISO) standards that meet the essential requirements of the directive. For the development of medical device package systems, ISO 11607 has been developed and is used to meet essential *packaging* requirements of the directive. Specifically, for meeting the directive requirement as stated above, the revised ISO 11607 provision states (f): "The following properties shall be evaluated: any shelf-life limitations for presterilization and poststerilization storage." Further, under Sec. 6.2.3 (i), "the design and development of the package system shall consider . . . expiry date limitations of the product." And finally in Sec. 6.4, "Stability Testing," "the stability testing shall demonstrate that the sterile barrier system maintains integrity over time."

The net result is that manufacturers must supply documented evidence to support product-expiration claims. This is accomplished by monitoring measurable characteristics before, during, and after the test to determine the effects of time on package performance.

Expiration claims could be documented by real-time shelf-life testing; however, the timelines for product development would be adversely affected. The developers of the ISO 11607 standard recognized this hindrance and therefore have allowed that ". . . stability testing using accelerated aging protocols shall be regarded as sufficient evidence for claimed expiry dates until data from real-time aging studies are available." This provision is beneficial; however, no guidance is provided as to what conditions of adverse severity are permissible or technically reliable. It therefore has become crucial that guidance and standards be provided to help manufacturers establish product shelf-life and expiration claims.

7.8.1 10-Degree Rule

There are no published standard test methods for performing an accelerated aging study. However, guidance on accelerated aging of packages is available from ASTM in the F1980, "Standard Guide for Accelerated Aging of Sterile Medical Device Packages." The ASTM guide was, in part, based on the landmark technical paper by Robert Reich, which introduced the Von't Hoff theory as an appropriate rationale for the accelerated aging of packaging. This theory, based on the Arrhenius rate kinetics theory of materials, states simply "a rise in temperature of 10°C will double the rate of a chemical reaction." The rule is commonly expressed as a Q_{10} value. So, for example, a doubling of the chemical reaction rate makes the Q_{10} value 2.0. The aging factor (AF) is derived from the following equation:

$$\text{AF} = Q_{10}^{(T_H - T_L)/10}$$

where Q_{10} = rate of chemical reaction (usually 2.0)
T_H = high temperature (test temperature)
T_L = low temperature (ambient)

Figure 7.4 indicates the relationship between the aging temperatures versus equivalency to a 1-year room temperature aging using various Q_{10} values. Other authors such as Geoffrey Clark of the Food and Drug Administration (FDA) have used the Q_{10} rule as rationale for accelerated aging protocols. In Clark's guidance document entitled *Shelf Life of Medical Devices*, Clark used test temperatures of 40°C and a Q_{10} value of 1.8 for intraocular and contact lenses. This guidance has been applied by industry to other medical devices and package systems and represents a very conservative estimate for real-time aging equivalents.

Karl Hemmerich described the 10-degree rule (Q_{10}) in his 1998 article entitled "General Aging Theory and Simplified Protocol for Accelerated Aging of Medical Devices." In it, he concludes, "the 10-degree rule will likely be conservative in the prediction of shelf life. However, the technique depends on numerous assumptions that must be verified by real-time validation testing conducted at room temperature." Reich suggested that using this approach for accelerated aging of medical grade packaging *should be used with some reservations, since the rate kinetics of the (packaging) systems are not fully understood*. Further, the Q_{10} values are based on the rate kinetics of a single chemical reaction; however, the concept of accelerated aging of packages involves *assumptions regarding the uniform aging rates of one or more packaging materials, plus any adhesive reactions*. In addition,

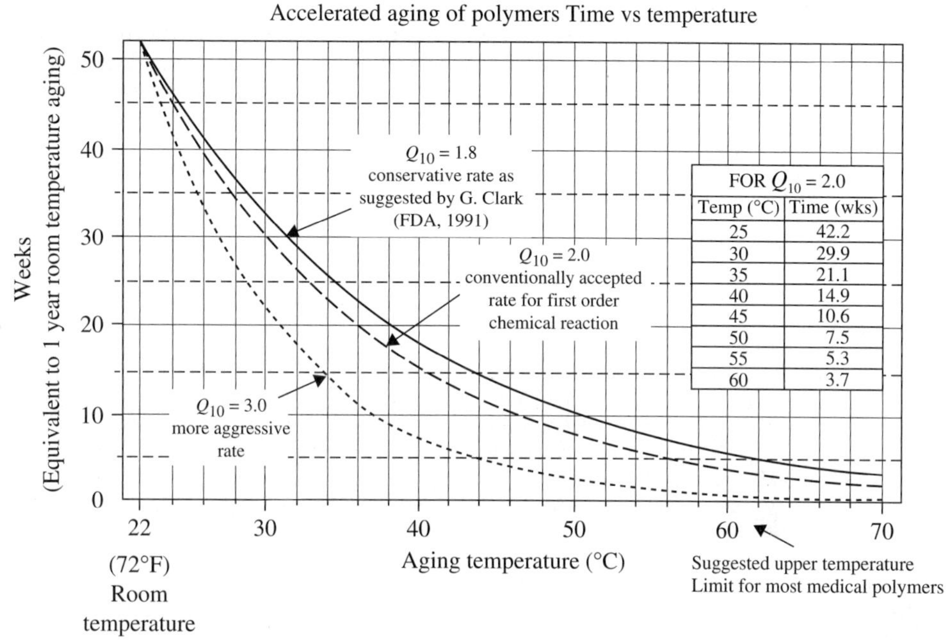

FIGURE 7.4 Accelerated aging of polymers: time versus temperature. The table is calculated for the time (weeks) equivalent to one year room temperature (e.g. 22°C) aging when a polymer is heat aged at a selected temperature (°C). (*From Hemmerich, K., "General Aging Theory and Simplified Protocol for Accelerated Aging of Medical Devices," Medical Plastics and Biomaterials, July/August 1998*, pp. 16–23.) $Q_{10} = \Delta 10°C$ reaction rate constant; $Q_{10} = 1.8$, conservative rate as suggested by G. Clark (FDA, 1991); $Q_{10} = 2.0$, conventionally accepted rate for first order chemical reaction; $Q_{10} = 3.0$, more aggressive rate; 60°C is the suggested upper temperature for most medical polymers.

caution should be exercised that the aging temperatures do not produce unrealistic failure conditions that would never occur under real-time, ambient conditions. A temperature of 60°C is the suggested upper temperature limit for most medical polymers, and a more realistic upper limit should be 55°C.

Reich concludes, however, that the *concept can be useful (as a rationale) for the accelerated aging of packages.* Hemmerich concurs that "this type of conservative relationship is appropriate for a wide range of medical polymers that have been previously characterized." Nevertheless, "the simplified protocol for accelerated shelf-life testing is not a replacement for more complex and advanced accelerated aging (techniques)."

7.8.2 Advanced Aging Techniques

John Donohue and Spiro Apostolou offer more complex and advanced techniques for predicting shelf life of medical devices in their article published in MDDI in June 1998. Their contention is that the Arrhenius and Q_{10} techniques are not reliable predictors of future performance for most medical devices. However, the D&A and variable Q_{10} techniques "are relatively easy to use and have been shown to be more accurate in predicting actual shelf life." The D&A technique assumes nothing and uses only the data to predict the future. The level of damage (LOD) of a physical performance property such as brittleness, number of package seal failures, or color of a plastic at various elevated temperatures and time intervals are some performance parameters used to predict the LOD of the same physical property of real-time aged materials. Short-term (i.e., 1 year) real-time data are required to establish the benchmark performance for comparison to the same property measured at various elevated temperatures, and for subsequently predicting longer-term real-time performance or time to equivalent damage (TED).

The Q_{10} method assumes that the ratio of the times to equivalent damage at low temperatures (usually 10°C apart) has a constant value. In fact, the value of Q_{10} will decrease with increasing temperature. Donohue and Apostolou suggest the use of a modified or variable Q_{10} method in which the ratio of the time to equivalent damage between two temperatures is used as a variable. In this method the TED ratio is equal to the Arrhenius equation, and the Q_{10} is determined with the TED ratio as a variable as follows:

$$Q_{10}^{(T_H - T_L)/10} = \text{TED } T_L/\text{TED } T_H$$

So

$$Q_{10} = (\text{TED } T_L/\text{TED } T_H)^{1/[(T_H - T_L)/10]}$$

Again, it is necessary to acquire performance data for ambient storage conditions as well as for elevated conditions in order to determine the TED ratio, and before this method can be employed for predicting a variable Q_{10}.

Lambert and Tang describe a method of aging using an iterative process that provides an opportunity to refine and validate the initial, conservative aging factor (Q_{10}). The basic concept is to collect a number of parallel real-time aged and accelerated aged data points at early time points such that a correlation between the two can be developed, thereby defining the actual aging factor of the system under investigation. One limitation of this method is that real-time aged package performance data are required in which to compare accelerated aged data and make iterations on the conservative Q_{10}. A basic eight-step concept was flowcharted by Lambert and Tang as shown in Fig. 7.5.

7.8.3 Guidance Documents

The American Society for Testing and Materials (ASTM) Committee F2 on Flexible Barrier Materials published ASTM F-1980, "Standard Guide for Accelerated Aging of Sterile Medical Device Packages." The scope of the guide is *to provide information for developing accelerated aging protocols to rapidly determine the effects due to the passage of time and environmental effects on the sterile integrity of packages and the physical properties of their component packaging materials*. Additional guidance on accelerated aging protocols is provided in the AAMI Technical Information Report 17 (TIR 17). The information obtained from utilizing these guides may be used to support expiration date claims for medical device packages. It is hoped that it will provide the necessary rationale for accelerated aging protocols which satisfies both the FDA's Quality System Regulations (QSR) and the essential requirements for packaging in the MDD.

The ASTM Guide provides referenced documents (many of which are cited in this chapter) which render credibility to the current suggested methodology for aging medical device packages. The guide condones the simplified Q_{10} method as rationale for using accelerated aging for medical device packages. The guide states, "Conservative accelerated aging factors must be used if little information is known about the package under investigation." The ASTM Guide was revised in 2007 to clarify the use of humidity conditions in the accelerated aging protocol. As the Sterilization Packaging Manufacturers Council (SPMC) stated in their whitepaper on "The Role of Humidity on the Accelerated Aging of Sterilizable Medical Packaging," "While the role of temperature is well documented and understood in the aging process, the impact of humidity is not."

The guide simply stated that "The effects of humidity may need to be considered. . . ." For this reason the guide was revised to provide clarity on when to use humidity in the protocol, and how much. So the concept of absolute humidity (water concentration) was included for guidance in selecting a realistic humidity condition for accelerated aging protocols. The chart of "Concentration of Water in Air as Function of Temperature and Relative Humidity," as shown in Fig. 7.6, was added. So if a fixed absolute humidity is established for accelerated aging protocols and the test temperature is varied, the corresponding relative humidity can be determined so that the test equipment can be set up for the study. This conversion is necessary since test chambers are controlled based on the relative humidity in the interior of the chamber.

Although the method provides conservative estimates of product/package shelf life resulting in longer test durations than would be necessary using more complex aging methods, it does not require

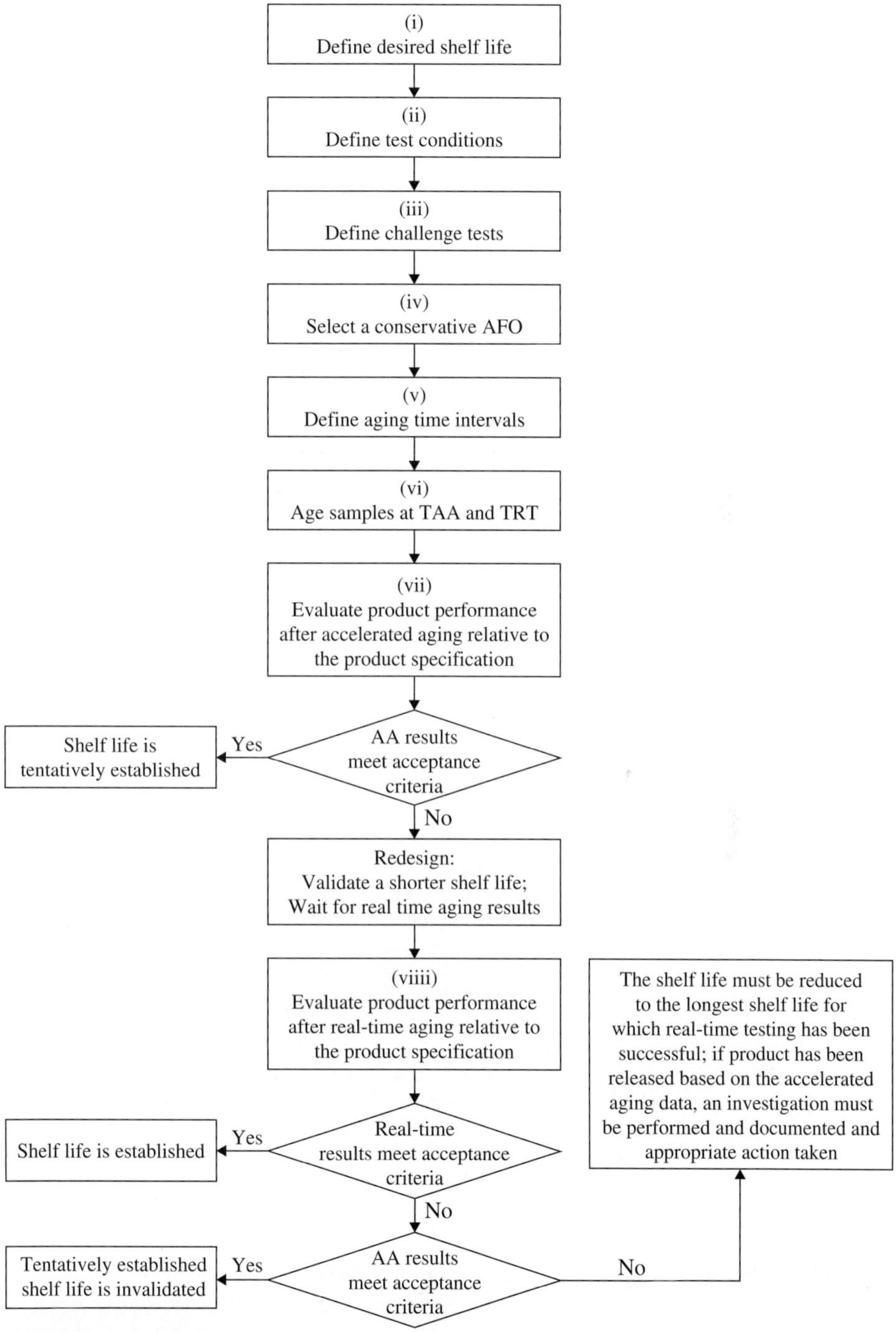

FIGURE 7.5 Eight-step process for accelerated aging.

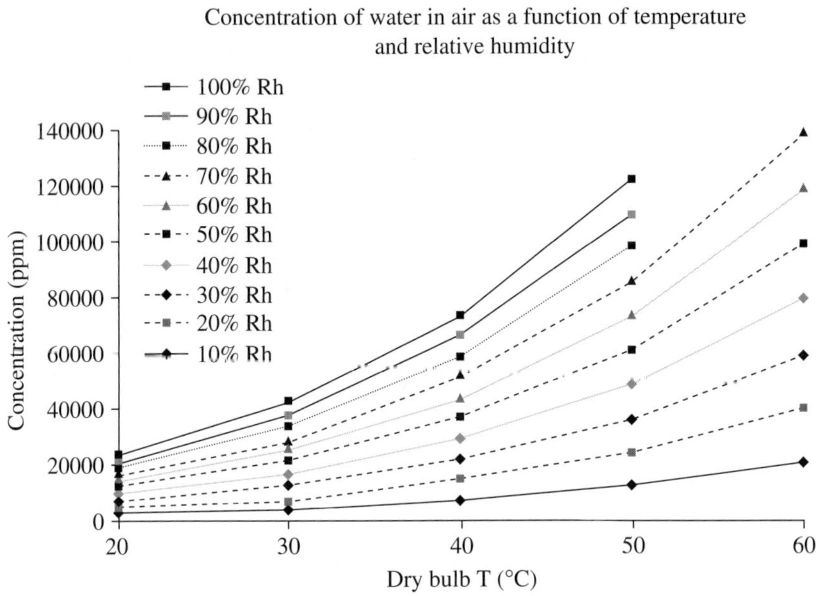

FIGURE 7.6 Chart for determining equivalent absolute and relative humidities at various temperatures.

benchmark real-time data up-front in the development process which could further delay introduction of new products. In addition, it requires fewer samples and conditioning resources. Still, it may be advantageous to refine the aging process in subsequent studies using the more complex techniques summarized in this article. With more information about the system under investigation and with information demonstrating the correlation between real-time performance and accelerated aging performance, more aggressive and accurate aging factors may be defined.

7.8.4 Conclusion

There is no shortage of rationale to support accelerated aging protocols as demonstrated by the published literature. Any manufacturer using techniques described in the literature will be successful in meeting the provisions of national and international regulations. Some techniques require very little information about the system under investigation and make assumptions about material rate kinetics resulting in conservative estimates, while others require real-time performance data in order to define material rate kinetics and predict long-term performance. Which technique to choose for an accelerated aging program will depend upon the manufacturer's resources, expertise, and product development timelines. As the SPMC so aptly stated: "the medical device manufacturer must make the final decision regarding the suitability of a packaging material to ensure efficacy of the sterilized medical device." So the guidance documents and standards are intended to serve in choosing the conditions for testing a package so that informed judgments can be made regarding the performance of the packaging over time.

7.9 FINAL PACKAGE SYSTEM VALIDATION PROTOCOL

The efficacy of sterile medical device packages at the point of end use is of great concern to not only the producer of the product, but also the general public, and foremost the regulatory community. The Food and Drug Administration (FDA) has the regulatory responsibility to ensure that medical devices perform their intended function and pose no undo risk to the patient. Not only must the product itself meet stringent regulatory requirements, but the package must also perform consistently under variable manufacturing conditions, sterilization procedures, and distribution hazards; and perhaps over an extended shelf life.

The development of a final package system validation protocol consists of a documented plan or protocol to evaluate the package design and manufacturing process and ensure that it meets all of the critical parameter and requirements of the standard (ANSI/AAMI/ISO 11607-1:2006, 4.3, 6.3, 6.4). A comprehensive discussion of the final package system validation steps can be found in the AAMI TIR 22:2007. A summary of the steps are

- Develop plan objectives
- Understand the packaging system design configuration
- Group packaging systems for validation
- Determine sample size
- Define acceptance criteria
- Prepare packages for testing
- Define the shipping environment
- Define product/package shelf life
- Document the results

It is generally accepted industry practice to evaluate the integrity of sterile medical device packages by subjecting a fully processed package to extremes in sterilization processes, performing a simulated shelf life or accelerated aging study, conducting a simulated distribution and handling stress test, and then evaluating the efficacy of the package for sterility through physical test methods.

The flowchart in Fig. 7.7 shows one validation plan that has been used to gain compliance with the requirements for the final package system validation. This flowchart should be written into a detailed validation plan that is signed by all the parties. The written protocol will have a thorough description of the package configuration, including a detailed description of the different levels of packaging (e.g., sterile barrier system, carton, shelf pack, shipping container) used in the package system being validated.

In this protocol, the accelerated aging or stability and other distribution and handling requirements for the validation are treated as separate entities. As was discussed in Sec. 7.7, FDA requires documented evidence to support published expiration dates on medical device packages. The European Union has required expiration dates on all medical device packages as specified in the EC Directive 93/42/EEC, which states "the label must bear . . . where appropriate, an indication of the date by which the device should be used, in safety, expressed as the year and month." Consequently, manufacturers are being forced to comply with European directives based on the ISO standards. The new revised ISO 11607 standard has indicated that the shelf-life study should be treated as a separate entity from performance testing. The new thinking, as stated by the AAMI Packaging Committee, is that

> *"Stability testing and performance testing should be treated as separate entities for (some) very important reasons:*
>
> 1. *When a medical device manufacturer is selecting SBS materials for a family of devices, he or she does not want to conduct costly and time consuming repetitions of stability testing when nothing has changed regarding the device materials, SBS materials, or critical process parameters. If stability testing and package performance testing are conducted in parallel, there is always a risk that any failure that occurs cannot be assigned to a specific cause. Did the failure occur as a result of distribution stresses or did aging cause the failure? Exposing package systems to the rogors of simulated distribution testing after long exposure to elevated temperatures usually seen with accelerated aging testing (2 to 16 weeks or more at 40 to 55°C) can result in failures that would not normally be seen during distribution. This can lead to unnecessary, costly, and time-consuming delays in the introduction of new product to the marketplace.*

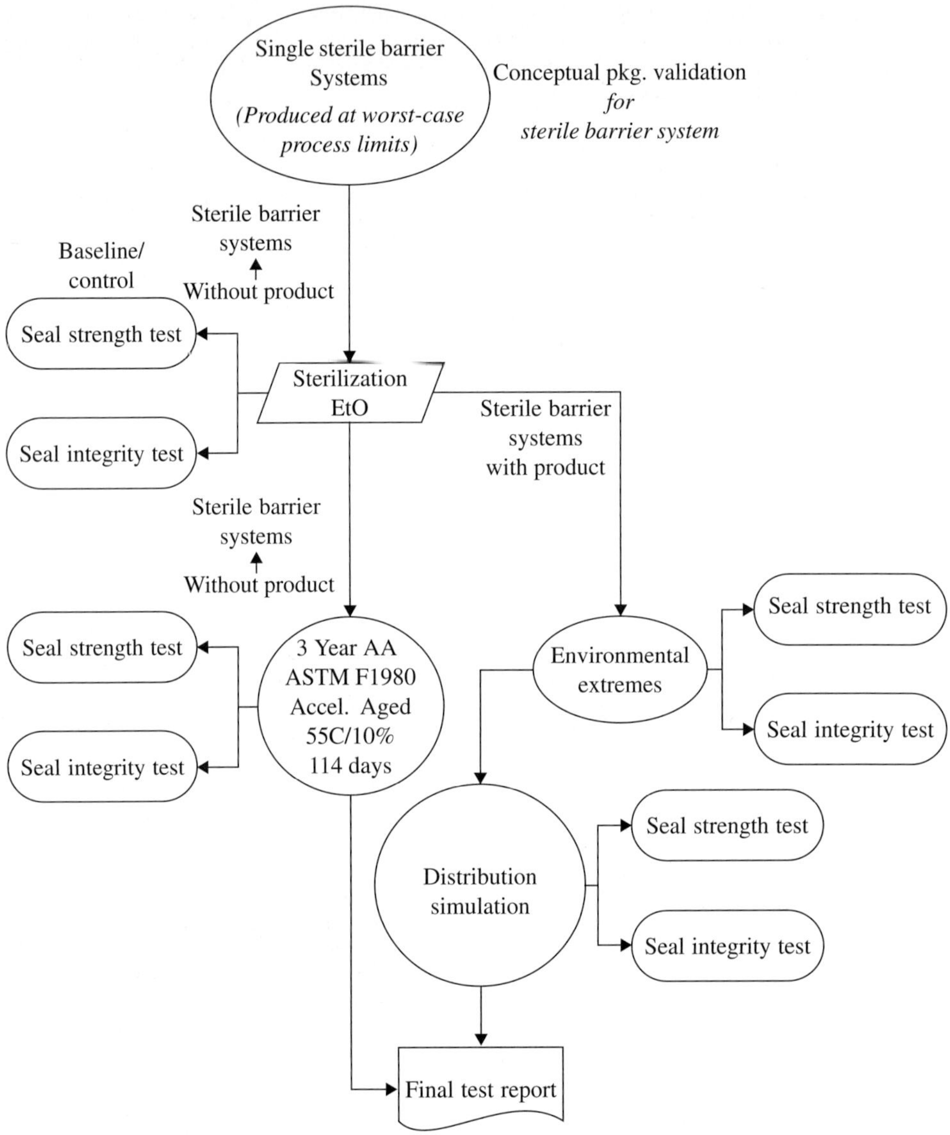

FIGURE 7.7 Conceptual flowchart for completing the requirements for a final package system validation.

2. *The working group's (TC198/WG7) rationale was that when the !10 equation is applied, there is no component for freeze-thaw cycles or humidity. When a package fails a test that incorporates these dynamics, it tells you nothing about shelf life. When treated separately, the packaging engineer can determine whether the failure was related to shelf-life testing or dynamic testing. If cumulative stresses are a concern, the dynamic testing can be after exposure to aging conditions. Of course the ISO 11607 document allows for these to be done together (in sequence)."*

So, in the example protocol, the accelerated aging study is shown as a parallel path to the environmental challenge and distribution and handling segments of the flowchart. Other protocols having the same elements may be designed to comply with the requirements of the standard.

7.9.1 Validating a Package "Family"

In order to reduce the burden of testing, thought should be given to other package system designs and devices that may require validation. Similar medical devices and package designs may constitute a "device family" and may be tested as a group when packaging materials, manufacturing/assembly machinery, sterilization process, and all other aspects of the device and package system are comparable. In this case the worst-case configuration for the device, materials, processes, and logistics for the package must be validated. A rationale for determining the worst-case configuration must be developed to support the technical decision. Another consideration for reducing the burden of testing might be to leverage existing package systems that have been validated in the past. Here the burden will be to demonstrate and document the similarity between the package systems in question.

7.9.2 Worst-Case Package System

When the worst-case scenario is being used to cover multiple package systems and designs, a distinction must be made between the worst-case sterile barrier system and the worst-case package system. This distinction was necessary because the revised standard placed additional emphasis on the concept of testing the "worst-case" package configuration. But it was not clear what was meant by this requirement. The AAMI Packaging Committee helps by clarifying this requirement by stating that "Don't confuse worst-case process parameters with worst-case package configuration. The requirements for a worst-case process is discussed in ISO 11607-2:2006 clauses 5.3 and 5.4. The worst-case may not be (at) the lower limits. The use of worst-case SBS does not necessarily require MDMs to acquire from sterile packaging manufacturers (SPMs) special lots of preformed SBS made at worst-case conditions specifically for design performance qualification. It means that when the MDM is placing a closure seal on a preformed SBS or is sealing a lid to a blister tray, for example, he or she should seek out the process variable that produces the weakest SBS and test samples made under those conditions. When addressing the design configuration worst-case (scenario), one approach is to evaluate the worst-case configuration for the device and package family. Using IV sets as an example, these products can range from simple tubes with fittings to a complex system of tubes, ports, and valves. If you wish to classify IV sets as a family that can be packaged in, for example, a specified header bag, you must identify the family, determine the worst case example (the one with the most tubes, ports, and valves, for instance), and use it for the design qualification performance testing."

7.9.3 Test Sample Size Considerations

This is one of the most confounding aspects of developing the final package system validation plan. The protocol plan must weigh the economics of providing a high level of confidence against the risk associated with producing a package system that will fail and cause harm to the public. Here's how the SPMC answers the question of what sample size to use for package integrity testing:

> *"It is not possible to simply recommend and 'appropriate' test quantity for attribute data (testing) whether in initial, pivotal, or release stages. The subject of sample size determination is not a trivial one, and in the medical device area is directly related to managing risk. Risk varies significantly with the nature of the medical device, particularly for those designed for implantation. Also of significant concern is the reliability and reproducibility of the measurement system, and the degree to which those systems have been validated. These and other considerations are generally considered toward the end for determining an appropriate AQL level, which can then be used to determine sample sizes for testing."*

There are several references to consult to get a better understanding of all the considerations and to determine rational sample sizes for package system validations. These include *The Handbook of Applied Acceptance Sampling: Plans, Procedures, Principle*, and an article published in *MDDI Magazine* "Sample Size Selection Using a Margin of Error Approach," by Nick Fotis and Laura Bix.

The sample size will vary, depending on several characteristics of the validation plan:

- The packaging system being evaluated
- The type of result for the test (e.g., attribute or variable data)
- The risk tolerance of the company

Since the ultimate acceptance of the package system is dependent on the condition of the sterile barrier system, the strength and integrity tests must be performed on a statistically significant sample size based on the confidence interval and reliability.

When considering the sample size of the shipping box (protective package), it must be understood that the unit of test is the shipping box, and one shipping box holding 24 sterile barrier systems is a sample size of one when subjecting it to the performance tests (distribution simulation). Many studies will only require a sample size of one if the shipping box contains enough sterile barrier systems to obtain a statistically significant sample size for integrity testing.

In all cases the sample size will depend upon company risk policy, tester reliability and precision, economics, and regulatory requirements.

7.9.4 Defining the Shelf-Life Study

As the FDA moves toward harmonization with the European standards through revision of its GMP and through adoption of ISO and CEN standards, the need for guidance on the performance of accelerated aging protocols is crucial.

The net result of publishing expiration dates is that there must be some documented evidence which supports the product expiration claims; thus, the need to perform shelf-life studies. However, real-time shelf-life studies are not an alternative in a fast-changing industry which can see two to three generations of products developed over the time it would take to document a 2-year shelf-life claim. So, the need for accelerated aging protocols as an alternative in developing a product and introducing it into the marketplace in a timely fashion is essential. Concurrent real-time studies must be performed to substantiate results of accelerated studies.

Ideally, accelerated aging involves a single measurable characteristic under extreme conditions to simulate, in a short time, the conditions the package would likely be subjected to during its designated shelf life. Some protocols rotate the packages through three environments designed to simulate the aging process. These conditions include high temperature and high humidity, high temperature and low humidity, and freezing conditions. The use of humidity in aging protocols has been discussed earlier, and caution should be taken when using high humidity for aging studies. Low temperature is included since it has been implicated in package failure through cold creep and material embrittlement, and packages may, in fact, be exposed to these temperatures in winter time distribution systems or in the cargo areas of aircraft. However, these conditions represent more of an environmental challenge and do not have any influence on determining the package shelf life.

Current information found in the previously mentioned guidance documents can be reduced to four basic principles for determining shelf-life and consequent expiration dating:

- Determine an acceptable target expiration date based on R&D data, on the likely distribution and storage conditions that the product will encounter prior to its use, and on the company's marketing strategies.
- Select the test temperature parameters that will be tested based on the physical properties of the packaging materials (e.g., glass transition temperature).
- Conduct the testing under consistent procedures.
- Once all the testing has been completed, validate the test data.

Notice that these principles do not explicitly define the test parameters. However, the theory postulated by von't Hoff using the Q_{10} value (which states that a rise in temperature of 10°C will double the rate of chemical reaction) is the most convenient method of estimating the approximate ambient storage time equivalent at a selected accelerated aging temperature, despite the known limitations and concerns for use on complex and dissimilar material structures.

For the aging study shown in the flowchart in Fig. 7.7, using an accelerated aging temperature of 55°C, the equivalent ambient storage time for 1 year is 26 days. Remember, the accelerated aging in this protocol is treated as a separate entity and the combined effects of aging and distribution handling are not determined. Caution must be taken not to accelerate the aging too much, since elevating the temperature of packaging materials could result in a mode of failure that might never be observed in real life (i.e., material/product interaction, creep or deformation).

7.9.5 Defining the Shipping Environment—Environmental Stress Testing

The parallel leg of the package validation protocol shown in Fig. 7.7 is based on the accepted fact that sterile medical device packages do not typically lose their sterility simply by being stored on a shelf. Package failures are a result of environmental extremes and dynamic events which may have occurred during the manufacturing process, during shipping and handling to the sterilization facility, or during distribution or transit to the point of end use. All of these processes may subject the finished package to forces involving handling shocks, vibration, high and low temperature, and humidity extremes. The GMP for Medical Devices Part 820.130 states that "the device package and any shipping container for a device shall be designed and constructed to protect the device from alteration or damage during the customary conditions of processing, storage, handling, and distribution."

There are optional methods available to satisfy this segment of the package validation process. First, the package could be tested by simply shipping it to a destination using the anticipated shipping mode (i.e., overnight parcel, common carrier). This method, although economical, does not lend itself to a high degree of control and repeatability. Alternatively, laboratory simulations provide a means of subjecting packages to the anticipated distribution hazards of shock, vibration, and dynamic compression in a controlled and repeatable manner. Observations of the package performance, as it is subjected to various hazards, can be accomplished in the laboratory, and corrective action can be taken to alleviate any anticipated problems in a timely fashion. Laboratory methods can be performed using standardized laboratory simulations such as ASTM D4169, "Performance Testing of Shipping Containers and Systems" or International Safe Transit (ISTA) procedures like Procedure 1A, 2A, or 3A. More information on the ISTA standards can be found at the ISTA Web site, www.ista.org.

The standardized laboratory procedures sequence a number of distribution "elements" or dynamic tests that use realistic test intensity levels. The ASTM method also allows the user who has significant knowledge of his or her distribution system to design a test sequence which more closely matches a specific shipping environment. This may allow for a laboratory simulation based on actual field measurements, including, vibration, drops, temperature and humidity, and atmospheric pressure.

The most common standardized distribution simulation test used for medical device package validation is the ASTM D4169, Distribution Cycle #13. This method is designed for packages weighing less than 100 lb and being transported by air and motor freight (small parcel distribution system). This test "provides a uniform basis of evaluating in the laboratory, the ability of shipping units to withstand the distribution environment. This is accomplished by subjecting the packages to a test plan consisting of a sequence of anticipated hazard elements encountered in the chosen distribution environment." A new method that has incorporated specific field data from the small parcel delivery system (e.g., UPS, FedEx, DHL) has been published by ASTM and is entitled ASTM D7386-08 "Standard Practice for Performance Testing of Packages for Single Parcel Delivery Systems." This is thought to be a more realistic standardized simulation of the distribution environment to which most medical device packages are subjected.

7.9.6 Defining the Acceptance Criteria—Package Integrity Evaluation

Of course, simply subjecting a medical device package to extremes in temperature and humidity conditions for an extended period of time, and then "shaking, rattling, and rolling" it during transportation simulation and/or subjecting it to environmental extremes, does not indicate the package's ability to maintain its sterile barrier.

Package integrity testing was discussed in an earlier part of this chapter. It uses physical test methods for determining the positive or negative outcome of the package system validation. The acceptance criteria for a sterile barrier system is generally defined to be the ability to deliver the medical device to the end user in an undamaged and sterile condition. Other detailed acceptance criteria may apply to the protective packaging and secondary packaging, but the form and parameters may vary widely. Acceptance criteria could take the form of pass/fail outcomes or be based on a quantitative scoring system or rating of damage levels.

7.9.7 Revalidation of Package Systems

Revalidation of the package system is required when changes have been made to the device, packaging design, packaging materials, and process parameters and/or equipment that will affect the original validation.

7.9.8 Summary

It is now generally recognized that manufacturers must conduct all three types of tests—physical, transportation simulation, and package integrity—to validate packaging materials and processes. The protocol presented here offers the most comprehensive and justifiable methodologies, based on the published literature, for determining the effectiveness of a medical device package design to maintain its sterile condition from the point of sterilization to the point of end use and to comply with regulatory standards.

REFERENCES

21 CFR, Part 820, *Good Manufacturing Practices for Medical Devices: General,* June 1997.

AAMI Technical Information Report (TIR) No. 22-1998, *Guidance for ANSI/AAMI/ISO 11607-1997, Packaging for Terminally Sterilized Medical Devices*, Association for the Advancement of Medical Devices and Instrumentation, Arlington, VA, July 1998.

AAMI TIR 17: 1997, *Radiation Sterilization—Material Characterization*, Association for the Advancement of Medical Instrumentation.

AAMI TIR22, *Guidance for ANSI/AAMI/ISO 11607, Packaging for Terminally Sterilized Medical Devices—Part 1 and Part 2: 2006*, Association for the Advancement of Medical Instrumentation, approved March 20, 2007.

American Society for Testing and Materials, ASTM D 4169, Performance Testing of Shipping Containers and Systems, *ASTM Book of Standards*, Vol. 15.09.

ANSI/AAMI/ISO 11607: 1997, *Packaging for Terminally Sterilized Medical Devices*, Association for the Advancement of Medical Instrumentation, February 24, 1997.

ANSI/AAMI/ISO 11607-1:2006, *Packaging for Terminally Sterilized Medical Devices-Part 1: Requirements for Materials, Sterile Barrier Systems, and Packaging Systems,* American National Standards Institute, 2005.

ANSI/AAMI/ISO 11607-1: 2006, *Packaging for Terminally Sterilized Medical Devices—Part 1: Requirements for Materials, Sterile Barrier Systems, and Packaging Systems,* Association for the Advancement of Medical Instrumentation, Arlington, VA, 2006.

ANSI/AAMI/ISO 11607-2: 2006, *Packaging for Terminally Sterilized Medical Devices—Part 2: Validation Requirements for Forming, Sealing, and Assembly Processes,* Association for the Advancement of Medical Instrumentation, Arlington, VA, 2006.

ASTM *Book of Standards*, Vol. 15.10, ASTM International, West Conshohocken, PA, www.astm.org.

ASTM D7386-08, *Standard Practice for Performance Testing of Packages for Single Parcel Delivery Systems*, ASTM International, West Conshohocken, PA, www.astm.org.

ASTM F1980-07, *Standard Guide for Accelerated Aging of Sterile Barrier Systems for Medical Devices*, ASTM International, West Conshohocken, PA, www.astm.org.

Clark, G., *Shelf Life of Medical Devices*, Rockville, MD, FDA Division of Small Manufacturers Assistance, April 1991.

Code of Federal Regulations 21 CFR Part 820, *Good Manufacturing Practices for Medical Devices: General,* June 1997.

Donohue, J., and Apostolou, S., Predicting Shelf Life from Accelerated Aging Data: The D&A and Variable Q10 Techniques, *Medical Device Diagnostic Industry*, pp. 68–72, June 1998.

Dyke, Denis G., Medical Packaging Validation: Complying with the Quality System Regulation and ISO 11607, *Medical Device and Diagnostic Industry*, August 1998.

EN 868 Part 1, *Packaging Materials and Systems for Medical Devices Which are to be Sterilized: General Requirements and Test Methods*, December 1997.

EN 868-1: 1997, *Packaging Materials and Systems for Medical Devices Which Are to Be Sterilized—Part 1: General Requirements and Test Methods*, February 1997.

FDA Modernization Act of 1997: *Guidance for the Recognition and Use of Consensus Standards: Availability*, Docket No. 98D-0085, www.fda.gov/cdrh/modact/fro225af.html.

FDA Modernization Act of 1997: Guidance for the Recognition and Use of Consensus Standards; Availability, *Federal Register*, February 25, 1998, Vol. 63, No. 37, pp. 9561–69, www.fda.gov/cdrh/modact/fr0225af.html.

Fielding, Paul, Medical Packaging Legislation in Europe, *Medical Device and Diagnostic Industry Magazine*, November 1999.

Fotis, N, et al., Six Myths about ISO 11607, *Medical Device and Diagnostic Industry Magazine*, May 2007.

Fotis, N., and Bix, L., Sample Size Selection Using a Margin of Error Approach, *Medical Device and Diagnostic Industry Magazine*, October 2006.

Freiherr, G., Issues in Medical Packaging: Cost-Consciousness Leads the Way in New World Order, *Medical Device and Diagnostic Industry*, pp. 51–57, August 1994.

Hackett, Earl T., Dye Penetration Effective for Detecting Package Seal Defects, *Packaging Technology and Engineering*, August 1996.

Hemmerich, K., General Aging Theory and Simplified Protocol for Accelerated Aging of Medical Devices, *Medical Plastics and Biomaterials*, pp. 16–23, July/August 1998.

Henke, C., and Reich, R., The Current Status of Microbial-Barrier Testing of Medical Device Packaging, *Medical Device and Diagnostic Industry*, pp. 46–49, 94, August 1992.

Hooten, Fred W., A Brief History of FDA Good Manufacturing Practices, *Medical Device and Diagnostic Industry Magazine*, May 1996.

Hudson, B., and Simmons, L., Streamlining Package Seal Validation, *Medical Device and Diagnostic Industry*, pp. 49–52, 89, October 1992.

International Safe Transit Association, ISTA Project 1A, *Pre-Shipment Test Procedures*, 2009.

Jones, Lois, et al., In Quest of Sterile Packaging: Part 1; Approaches to Package Testing, *Medical Device and Diagnostics Industry*, August 1995.

Jones, Lois, et al., In Quest of Sterile Packaging: Part 2; Physical Package Integrity Test Methods, *Medical Device and Diagnostics Industry*, September 1995.

Lambert, B., and Tang, F., Overview of ANSI/AAMI Material Qualification Guidance; Iterative Accelerated Aging Method, Proceedings 1, Session 108, pp. 55–64, *Medical Design and Manufacturing-West*, Anaheim, CA, 1997.

Medical Device Directive (MDD), Council Directive 93/42/EEC, *Official Journal of European Communities*, **14**(10), 1992.

Nolan, Patrick J., Medical Device Package Design: A Protocol for Sterile Package Integrity Validation, *Medical Device and Diagnostic Industry*, November 1995.

Nolan, Patrick J., Physical Test Methods for Validating Package Integrity, *The Validation Consultant*, **3**(6), July 1996.

Obrien, Joseph P., *Medical Device Packaging Handbook*, Marcel Dekker, NY, 1990.

Reich, R., Sharp, D., and Anderson, H., Accelerated Aging of Packages: Consideration, Suggestions and Use in Expiration Date Verification, *Medical Device Diagnostic Industry*, **10**(3):34–38, 1988.

Reich, R., Sharpe, D., and Anderson, H., Accelerated Aging of Packages: Consideration, Suggestions, and Use in Expiration Date Verification, *Medical Device and Diagnostic Industry*, pp. 34–38, March 1988.

Spitzley, J., A Preview of the HIMA Sterile Packaging Guidance Document, *Medical Device and Diagnostic Industry*, pp. 59–61, December 1991.

Spitzley, J., How Effective is Microbial Challenge Testing for Intact Sterile Packaging?, *Medical Device and Diagnostic Industry*, pp. 44–46, August 1993.

Spitzley, John, How Effective is Microbial Challenge testing for Intact Sterile Packaging?, *Medical Device and Diagnostics Industry*, **15**(8):44–46, 1993.

SPMC, *The Role of Humidity on the Accelerated Aging of Sterilizable Medical Packaging*, www.sterilizationpackaging.org.

Stephens, K., *The Handbook of Applied Acceptance Sampling: Plans, Procedures, Principle*, ASQ Quality Press, Milwaukee, WI, 2001.

The Council of the European Communities, Directive 93/42/EEC, *Medical Device Directive (MDD)*, June 1993.

Tweede, Diana, and Goddard, Ron, *Packaging Materials,* Pira International, Leatherhead, Surrey, UK, 1998.

P · A · R · T · 2

DIAGNOSTIC EQUIPMENT DESIGN

CHAPTER 8
DESIGN OF MAGNETIC RESONANCE SYSTEMS

Daniel J. Schaefer
MR Systems Engineering, Milwaukee, Wisconsin

8.1 INTRODUCTION

Atomic nuclei containing odd numbers of nucleons (i.e., protons and neutrons) have magnetic moments. Hydrogen (^1H) nuclei (protons) have the highest magnetic moment of any nuclei and are the most abundant nuclei in biological materials. To obtain high signal-to-noise ratios, hydrogen nuclei are typically used in magnetic resonance imaging and spectroscopy. Note that many other nuclei (e.g., ^2H, ^{13}C, ^{19}F, ^{23}Na, ^{31}P, and ^{39}K) may also be studied using magnetic resonance.

In the absence of an external static magnetic field, magnetic moments of the various nuclei point in random directions. So, without a static magnetic field, there is no net magnetization vector from the ensemble of all the nuclei. However, in the presence of a static magnetic field, the magnetic moments tend to align. For ^1H nuclei, some nuclei align parallel with the static magnetic field, which is the lowest energy state (and so the most populated state). Other ^1H nuclei align antiparallel with the static magnetic field. The energy of nuclei with a magnetic moment $\vec{m}$ in a static magnetic field $\vec{B}_0$ may be expressed as[1]

$$W_m = \vec{m} \bullet \vec{B}_0 \tag{8.1}$$

The difference in energy between protons aligned with the static magnetic field and those aligned antiparallel is the energy available in magnetic resonance (MR) experiments. This energy is twice that given in Eq. (8.1). Recall that the kinetic energy of the same nuclei at temperature T may be expressed as[2]

$$W_T = \mathrm{K}T \tag{8.2}$$

where K is Boltzmann's constant. The fraction of nuclei aligned with B_0 may be expressed as

$$\eta = 1 - e^{2mB_0/KT} \approx \frac{2mB_0}{KT} \tag{8.3}$$

For protons at 1.5 T at body temperature (37°C), about one proton in 100,000 is aligned with the static magnetic field. Aligned protons provide the MR signal. So, assuming all other parameters equal, higher static magnetic fields provide higher signal levels.

Nuclei with magnetic moments precess in static magnetic fields at frequencies proportional to the local static magnetic field strength. Let B_0 represent the static magnetic field strength, let γ represent a proportionality constant called the magnetogyric ratio, and let the radian precession frequency be ω (= $2\pi f$, where f is the linear frequency of precession). Then the relationships between these quantities may be expressed mathematically as the Larmor[3] equation:

$$\omega = \gamma B_0 \tag{8.4}$$

Properly designed coils may receive signals induced by the time-varying magnetic flux. Ideally, magnetic resonance scanners would produce perfectly homogeneous magnetic fields. In magnetic resonance spectroscopy (MRS), nearby nuclei with magnetic moments may alter the local static magnetic field and the precession frequency so that various chemical components may be identified by the received spectrum.

If small, linear "gradient" magnetic fields are added to the static magnetic field, then received frequency would correlate to physical location. Magnetic resonance imaging uses magnetic field gradients to spatially encode all three dimensions. Note that the most widely used nucleus in MR is the hydrogen nucleus or proton.

For diagnostic purposes, signals from various tissues should differ sufficiently to provide contrast to distinguish them. There are two relaxation processes in magnetic resonance.[4] One mechanism is called spin-lattice or T_1 relaxation. In the absence of a static magnetic field, a collection of nuclei with magnetic moments are randomly oriented and the net macroscopic magnetic moment vector is zero. In the presence of a static magnetic field, the collection of nuclei with magnetic moments has a net macroscopic magnetic moment vector aligned with the static magnetic field. Consider a static magnetic field in which there are nuclei with magnetic moments. When resonant RF pulses excite the nuclei, the macroscopic magnetic moment vector tips by some angle related to the RF waveform. Gradually, the nuclei lose energy to the lattice and the macroscopic magnetic moment vector relaxes back to alignment with the static magnetic field. This type of relaxation is called spin-lattice or longitudinal or T_1 relaxation. Biologically relevant T_1 values are typically in the 100- to 2000-ms range.[5]

The other relaxation mechanism is called spin-spin or T_2 relaxation. The presence of other nuclei with magnetic moments causes changes in the local magnetic field. These changes lead to slightly different precession frequencies for the spins. As the spins get out of phase, signal is lost. This type of relaxation is called spin-spin or transverse or T_2 relaxation. Note that $T_2 \leq T_1$, because T_1 depends on T_2 loss mechanisms as well as others. Typical T_2 values of biological interest are in the 20- to 300-ms range.[5]

Fortunately, various tissues differ in their T_1 and T_2 properties. Different imaging sequences and pulse parameters can be used to optimize contrast between tissues. So, MR pulse sequences are analogous to histological stains; different sequences and parameters can be used to highlight (or obscure) differences.

Magnetic resonance scanners use static magnetic fields to produce conditions for magnetic resonance (see Fig. 8.1). In addition, three coil sets (along with amplifiers and eddy-current correction devices) are needed to spatially encode the patient by producing time-varying gradient magnetic fields. Radio frequency (RF) transmit and receive coils, amplifiers, and receivers are used to excite the nuclei and to receive signals. Computers are useful to control the scanner and to process and display results (i.e., images, spectra, or flow velocities). Other equipment includes patient tables, patient-gating systems, patient-monitoring equipment, and safety systems.

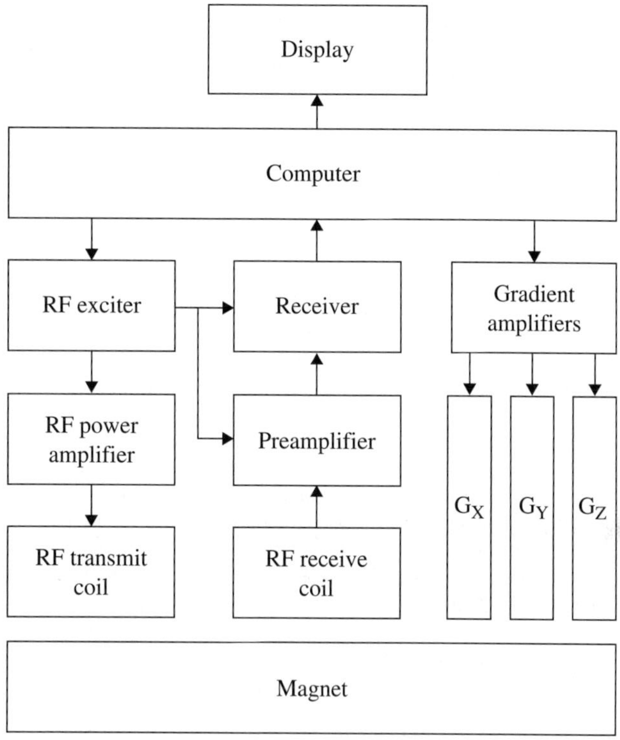

FIGURE 8.1 Components comprising a MR system are illustrated.

8.2 MR MAGNET CHARACTERISTICS

Static magnetic fields of MR scanners are generated either by resistive electromagnets, permanent magnets, or (more commonly) by superconducting magnets. Superconducting magnets are usually the least massive. Superconducting magnets use cryogens. When superconducting magnets quench (i.e., when they warm up and are no longer superconducting), proper venting must prevent asphyxiation hazards for developing. In addition, mechanical design must prevent magnet damage from quenches.

Typically, the static magnetic field is parallel to the floor and aligned with the long (superior/inferior) axis of the patient. However, there are systems where the static magnetic field is along the anterior/posterior axis of the patient and some where the static field is along the left/right patient axis. While patients are typically horizontal, in some magnets the patient may be vertical. Most superconducting magnets have horizontal openings for the patient and at field strengths of 0.5 to 3 T. Most vertical magnets are permanent or resistive, though there are vertical superconducting magnets as well. Vertical magnets currently have field strengths up to 0.7 T.

Magnetic fringe fields from large, strong, unshielded magnets used in MR could require large areas to accommodate siting. To alleviate this problem, passive shielding can be achieved using ferromagnetic materials arranged as numerically determined. Often, magnets are actively shielded (sometimes in addition to some passive shielding). Bucking coils that oppose the static magnetic field are added to increase the rate the static magnetic field diminishes with distance. Actively shielded magnets decrease siting costs.

Many superconducting magnets employ recirculation devices to prevent loss of cryogens. Such systems have lower operating costs.

8.2.1 Field Strength and Signal-to-Noise Ratio (SNR)

As discussed above, the fraction of nuclei that are available for MR interactions increases with static magnetic field strength, B_0. Noise in MR scans depends on the square root of the product of 4 times the bandwidth, temperature, Boltzmann's constant, and the resistance of the object to be imaged. Note that increased bandwidth (leading to a higher noise floor) may be needed as B_0 inhomogeneity becomes worse. As discussed below, B_0 inhomogeneities may also lead to some signal loss.

In magnetic resonance imaging raw data are acquired over some period of time. Raw data are then converted into image data through the use of Fourier transform.[4] Any temporal instability in B_0 will result in "ghosts" typically displaced and propagating from the desired image. Energy (and signal) in the desired image is diminished by the energy used to form the ghosts. So, image signal is lost and the apparent noise floor increases with B_0 temporal instabilities. B_0 fields of resistive magnets change with power line current fluctuations and with temperature. Resistive magnets are not used for imaging until some warm-up period has passed. Permanent-magnet B_0 will drift with temperature variations. Superconducting magnets have the highest temporal B_0 stability a few hours after ramping to field.

Another source of B_0 instability is the movement of nearby objects with large magnetic moments such as trucks and forklifts. Such objects may vary the static magnet field during imaging, resulting in image ghost artifacts propagating from the intended image. This effect depends on the size of the magnetic moment, its orientation, and on its distance from the magnet isocenter. Siting specifications typically are designed to prevent such problems. Note that a common misperception is that actively shielded magnets reduce susceptibility to B_0 instabilities from nearby magnetic moments. Unfortunately, this is not the case.

8.2.2 B_0 Homogeneity

Inhomogeneous static magnetic fields can result in apparent T_2 values called T_{2*}, which are shorter than T_2. Let the inhomogeneity be ΔB_0, then T_{2*} may be expressed as[6]

$$\frac{1}{T_{2*}} = \frac{1}{T_2} + \frac{\gamma \Delta B_0}{2} \tag{8.5}$$

Spin echo pulse sequences use a 90° RF pulse followed after half an echo time (TE) by a 180° RF pulse. Spin-echo signals s decay as[7]

$$s \propto e^{(-T_E/T_2)} \tag{8.6}$$

Shorter T_2 results in less signal. The static field of MR scanners must be very uniform to prevent signal loss and image artifacts. Typically, B_0 inhomogeneity of MR scanners is about 10 parts per million (ppm) over perhaps a 40-cm-diameter spherical volume (dsv) for imaging.[8] In spectroscopy, measurements of small frequency shifts must be accurately made, and B_0 inhomogeneity is typically limited to perhaps 0.1 ppm over a 10-cm dsv.[8]

Clearly, MR magnets demand high homogeneity of the static magnetic field. In solenoidal magnets, geometry and relative coil currents determine homogeneity. A perfectly uniform current density flowing orthogonal to the desired B_0 vector on a spherical surface will produce a perfectly uniform B_0 field in the sphere.[8] Patient access needs render such a design impractical. A Helmholtz pair (two coils of the same radius spaced half a radius apart with the same current flowing in the same direction) is a first approximation to the uniform spherical current density. Typically four or six primary (not counting active shield coils) coils are used. Higher degrees of homogeneity are possible as more coils are used.

No matter how clever the magnet design, the local environment may perturb the desired static magnetic field. Field "shims," either in the form of coils (which may be resistive or superconducting) and/or well-placed bits of ferromagnetic material, are used to achieve the desired magnet homogeneity.

The static magnetic field is sampled at numerous points on a spherical or cylindrical surface. Then field errors are expanded in terms of, for example, spherical harmonics. Shim coils typically are designed[9] to produce fields that approximate the desired harmonic (or other expansion). The current appropriate for correcting each term is then set for each coil shim. Alternatively, the correct size and position of each shim is calculated. The lowest-order shims can usually be achieved by placing constant currents on the three gradient coil axes.

8.2.3 Forces

Forces on ferrous objects near magnets may be of concern. The acceleration a (normalized to that of gravity g) of objects experiencing magnetic forces depends on the permeability of free space μ_0, susceptibility χ, density ρ, and on the magnetic field B and its spatial gradient[10]:

$$a = \frac{\chi}{\mu_0 \rho g} B \frac{\partial B}{\partial z} \tag{8.7}$$

From Eq. (8.7) it is clear that the greatest forces on ferromagnetic objects are where the product of field strength and spatial gradient is the largest. For superconducting magnets, this position is normally close to the coil windings.

8.3 GRADIENT CHARACTERISTICS

A computer commonly generates digital waveforms for the three gradient axes and for the radiofrequency coils. These waveforms (which for gradients may include corrections for eddy currents) are converted into analog signals, amplified, and sent to the appropriate coils. Received signals are converted into digital signals and reconstructed into images using Fourier transforms.[4] The reconstructed images are then electronically displayed. The computer system may also monitor MR scanner subsystems, including those associated with patient safety.

In MR, the static magnetic field is usually taken as the z direction. Linear variations of the static magnetic field (i.e., $\partial Bz/\partial x$, $\partial Bz/\partial y$, and $\partial Bz/\partial z$) are produced by separate gradient coil sets for the three (x, y, and z) coordinates. Only gradient field components in the z direction matter for MR imaging physics. However, magnetic fields form closed loops. So, other non-z components are produced as well. These other components may produce unwanted imaging artifacts and may influence patient physiological responses to switched gradients.

Considerations in gradient coil design include gradient linearity, gradient slew rate (i.e., how quickly the gradient amplitude can change), gradient power dissipation, eddy currents, and gradient-induced nerve stimulation. For simplicity in discussing these issues, consider the Maxwell pair (see Fig. 8.2).[11] If two filamentary, circular loops carry current I in opposing directions, have radii a, and are spaced a distance $2d$ apart, then the magnetic induction B may be expressed as

$$\begin{aligned} B &= \frac{\mu_0 I a^2}{2(a^2+(z-d)^2)^{3/2}} - \frac{\mu_0 I a^2}{2(a^2+(z+d)^2)^{3/2}} \\ &\approx \left(\frac{3\mu I a^2 d}{(a^2+d^2)^{5/2}}\right) z - \left(\frac{5\mu I a^2 d(3a^2-4d^2)}{(a^2+d^2)^{9/2}}\right) z^3 + \left(\frac{21\mu I a^2 d(5a^4-20a^2d^2+8d^4)}{8(a^2+d^2)^{13/2}}\right) z^5 + \text{higher orders} \end{aligned} \tag{8.8}$$

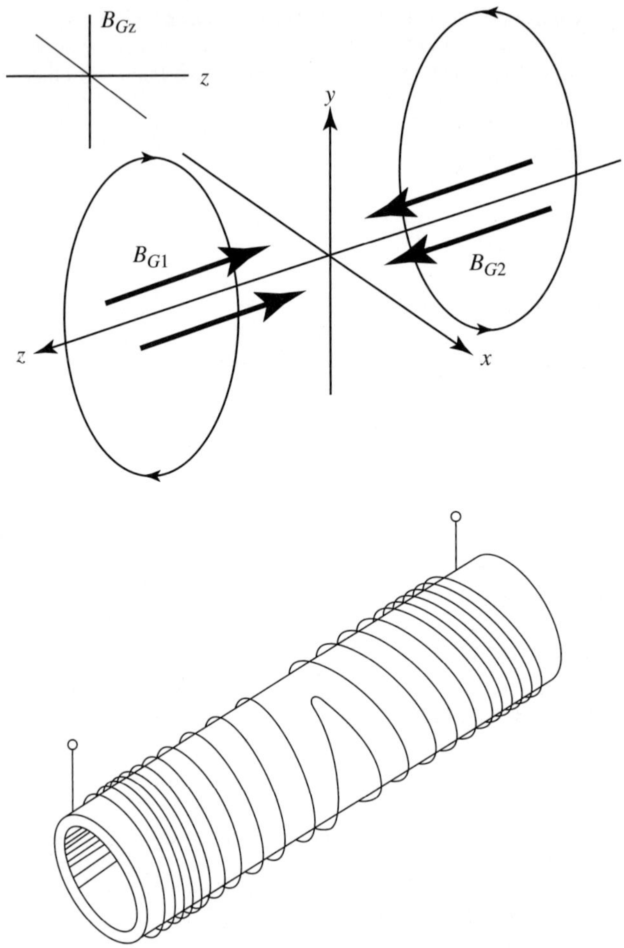

FIGURE 8.2 A filamentary, single turn Maxwell coil pair z gradient coil is illustrated. In addition, a typical unshielded z gradient coil is shown.

The portion of Eq. (8.8) following the approximation sign is a Taylor series expansion about $z = 0$. Note that if the factor of z^3 were zero, gradient error would be reduced to terms dependent on z^5. Selecting $d = 0.5\sqrt{3}$ makes the z^3 factor vanish. The remaining relative error from the ideal gradient may be approximated by dividing the fifth-order z factor by the first-order z factor:

$$\text{Error} \approx \frac{176z^4}{343a^4} \tag{8.9}$$

Equation (8.9) predicts that, for Maxwell coils, the gradient deviates 10 percent from the ideal linearity at $z/a = 0.66$. For $a = 0.3$ m, this deviation takes place at $z = 0.2$ m (e.g., the field of view would be 40 cm if 10 percent deviation from linearity was the maximum desired).

The first term in z of the expansion of Eq. (8.8) is the gradient amplitude G for a Maxwell pair. So from Eq. (8.7), the current needed to produce a gradient G may be expressed as

$$I = \frac{49Ga^2\sqrt{21}}{144\mu_0} \tag{8.10}$$

Let R_L be the resistance per unit length of the coil. The total resistance of a Maxwell pair then is $4\pi a R_L$. The power P dissipated in the gradient coil depends on the product of the total resistance and the square of the current:

$$P = 4\pi a R_L \left(\frac{49Ga^2\sqrt{21}}{144\mu} \right)^2 = \frac{16{,}807\pi R_L G^2 a^5}{1728\mu^2} \tag{8.11}$$

Equation (8.11) illustrates that gradient dissipation goes with the fifth power of coil diameter and with the square of gradient strength. So, a Maxwell head gradient coil with half the diameter of a whole-body Maxwell gradient coil dissipates only 3 percent as much power (assuming gradient strength is unchanged).

Axial gradient coil sets of commercial MR scanners typically use more than the two coils that make up a Maxwell pair. Normally, gradient field series expansions are made and coil location, radius, and current are selected to obtain high linearity or low inductance.[12,13] One such axial coil[12] is shown in Fig. 8.1. Often an outer bucking gradient coil is combined with the inner coil to cancel gradient-induced fields on nearby conductive structures.[14] Undesirable magnetic fields (and resulting image artifacts) associated with eddy currents can then be considerably reduced.

Typical transverse (x and y) gradient coils for superconducting systems include four planar coil sets bent around a cylinder. One very simplified configuration is shown in Fig. 8.3. The pair of coils at one end of the cylinder produces a magnetic vector that for a y gradient, for example, points up. The pair at the other end of the cylinder produces a magnetic field that points down. Near isocenter, magnetic vectors of transverse gradient coils point along z and produce the desired gradient field. Magnetic induction from these coils will be highest near coil conductors where fields point up or down. For transverse coils the largest gradient magnetic field components near patients is not along z. A "thumbprint" transverse coil[13] is also shown in Fig. 8.3.

Switched gradient coils with inductance L will experience a voltage V, which depends on the time (t) rate of change of gradient current:

$$V = L\frac{dI}{dt} \tag{8.12}$$

Gradient coils must be designed to avoid electrical breakdown for the highest desired dI/dt levels.

8.3.1 Gradient-Induced Eddy Currents

Gradient-induced eddy currents produce unwanted distortions to the desired magnetic field. Eddy currents can cause signal loss, ghosting, and incomplete cancellation of static material in angiographic imaging. Eddy currents may be considerably reduced by using actively shielded gradient coils to null fields on conductive surfaces.[14] The addition of such "bucking" coils reduces gradient strength per unit current for the coils.

It is also possible to reduce eddy current effects by predistorting gradient waveforms. Eddy currents combined with predistorted waveforms result in intended gradient waveforms.[15–17] Predistortion cannot correct for spatially dependent eddy current effects.

8.3.2 Gradient-Induced Stimulation

As MR imaging has evolved, so has the demand for higher gradient slew rates. Higher slew rates translate to shorter echo times, higher signal, less distortion artifact, and the possibility of imaging faster biological events. Lossy inductances have associated time constants of inductance/resistance. So, higher gradient slew rates imply lower gradient coil inductances and typically larger, faster gradient amplifiers. High gradient slew rates will induce electric fields in patients. It is imperative that these gradient-induced electric fields be limited to values incapable of harming patients. Safety standards[18–20] are designed to protect patients from cardiac stimulation by a significant margin through avoiding gradient-induced patient discomfort from peripheral nerve stimulation.[21–47]

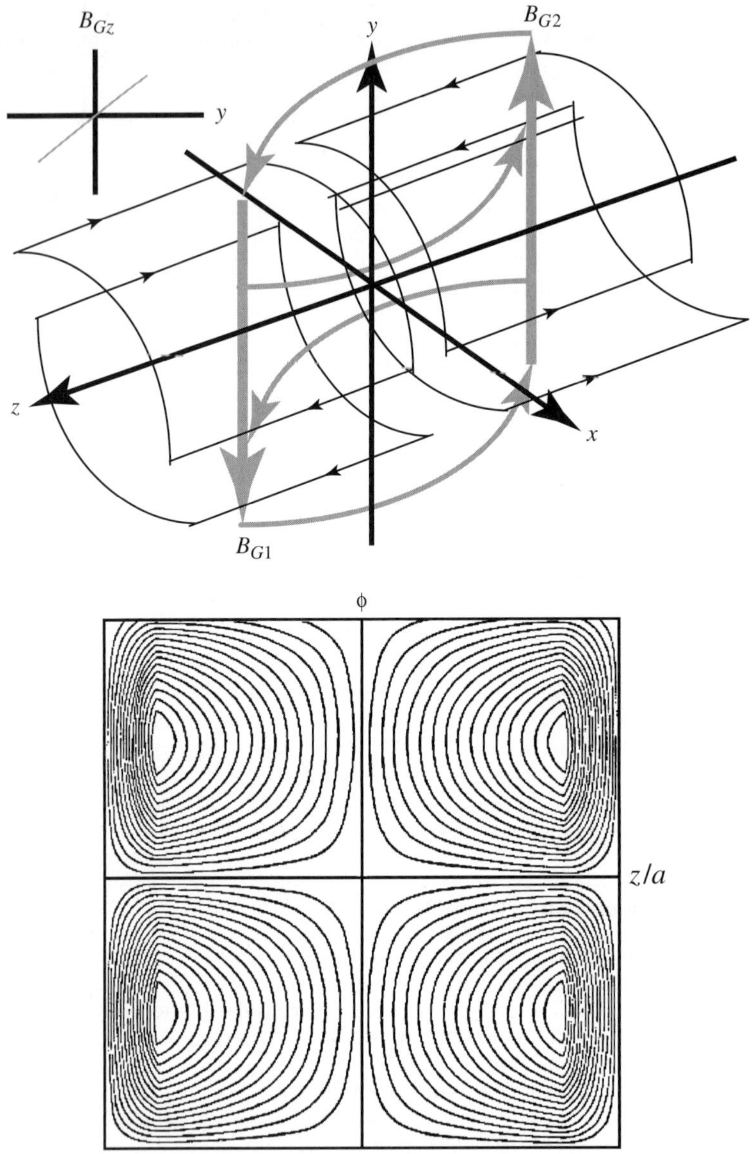

FIGURE 8.3 A filamentary, single turn, saddle transverse gradient coil set is illustrated. In addition, patterns for a typical unshielded transverse gradient coil is shown.

8.3.3 Acoustic Noise

Time-varying magnetic field gradients spatially encode the anatomy of the patient in MR imaging. Switched gradients may also produce acoustic noise. There are two sources of gradient-generated acoustic noise. A conductor of length $\vec{l}$ carrying current I in a static magnetic field $\vec{B}_0$ will experience a force $\vec{F}_m$ due to the magnet[48,49]:

$$\vec{F}_m = I\vec{l} \times \vec{B}_0 \tag{8.13}$$

There is also a force on the coil that is independent of the static magnetic field. Consider the potential energy U_b of a gradient coil with inductance L[49]:

$$U_b = \tfrac{1}{2}\, LI^2 = \int F_c\, dq \tag{8.14}$$

F_c is the force on the coil due to a displacement and q is an arbitrary coordinate. Note that the force on the coil will be in a direction that increases inductance. Hence, the force will try to increase the radius or compress the turns axially. From the derivative of the above equation, an expression for the force may be obtained[49]:

$$F_c = \frac{I}{2\left(\dfrac{dL}{dq}\right)} \tag{8.15}$$

The acoustic noise produced by forces on gradient coils must be limited to appropriate levels to avoid hearing loss.[18–20,50–55] Various schemes to reduce gradient-produced acoustic noise have been reported.[56–58]

8.4 RADIO-FREQUENCY MAGNETIC FIELD AND COILS

Resonant radio-frequency (RF) magnetic fields, orthogonal to the static magnetic field, are used in magnetic resonance (MR) to interrogate (excite) a region of interest for imaging or for spectroscopy.[3,4] The patient may absorb some portion of the transmitted RF energy.[59–63] Heating is the potential safety concern with absorbed RF energy.[64] It is essential for patient safety to limit whole-body and localized heating to appropriate levels.[18–20,59–84]

Resonant frequency scales with static field strength and nuclei of interest. For protons the resonant RF frequency is 42.57 MHz/T[3]. Adjusting tip angle maximizes received signals in MR. Tip angles are proportional to area under the envelope of RF waveforms. For a given waveform, RF energy is proportional to the square of tip angle. Only the magnetic component of the RF field is useful in MR. Efforts are made by manufacturers to reduce electric field coupling to patients. The distribution of RF power deposition in MR tends to be peripheral due to magnetic induction.[59–61] Note that plane wave exposures (in non-MR applications) may lead to greater heating at depth.[63,64]

RF pules are typically transmitted by resonant RF coils. Transmit RF coils may be whole-body coils or local coils. Safety concerns with whole-body RF transmit coils are primarily to limit whole-body temperature elevation to appropriate levels. As shall be explored later, elevation of core body temperatures to sufficiently high levels may be life-threatening.[59–84] With local transmit coils, the primary safety concern is to limit local heating to prevent localized burns.[85–87]

Average RF power is proportional to the number of images per unit time. Patient geometry, RF waveform, tip angle, and whether the system is quadrature during transmit determine peak power. Quadrature excitation lowers RF power requirements by a factor of 2 and stirs any field inhomogeneities.[60,63] Both mechanisms lower the local specific absorption rate (SAR).

8.4.1 Transmit Birdcage Coils

One means of achieving rather homogeneous radiofrequency magnetic fields in MR is through the use of birdcage transmit coils[88] (see Fig. 8.4). Birdcage coils ideally would produce uniform $\vec{B}_1$ fields. Let $\vec{\mathbf{A}}$ be the magnetic vector potential. Components of $\vec{\mathbf{A}}$ (and thus the electric field as well) must be parallel to the current density on the conductors that produced them. Perfectly uniform $\vec{B}_1$ requires an infinitely long birdcage coil (or a spherical current density). The $\vec{B}_1$ field is related to magnetic vector potential:

$$\vec{B}_1 = \nabla \times \vec{\mathbf{A}} = \hat{a}_x\left[\frac{\partial A_z}{\partial y} - \frac{\partial A_y}{\partial z}\right] + \hat{a}_y\left[\frac{\partial A_x}{\partial z} - \frac{\partial A_z}{\partial x}\right] + \hat{a}_z\left[\frac{\partial A_y}{\partial x} - \frac{\partial A_x}{\partial y}\right] \tag{8.16}$$

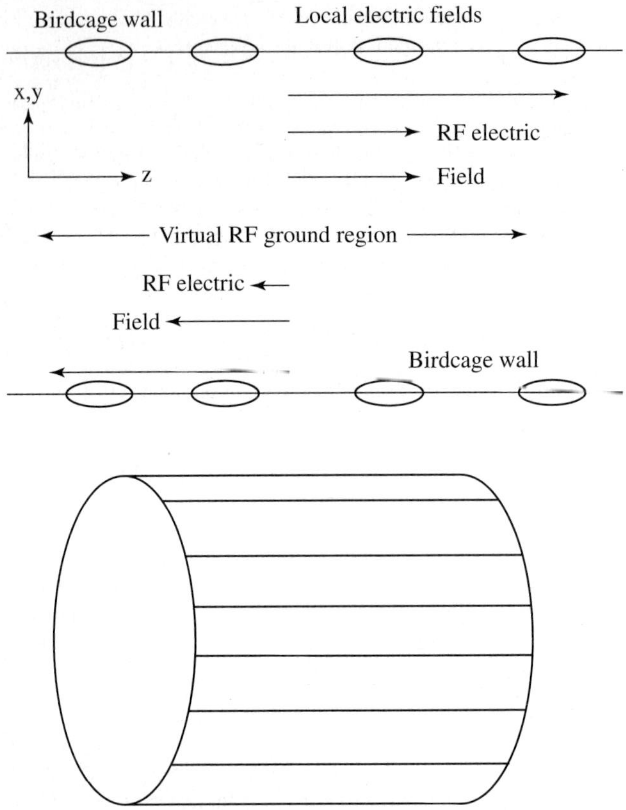

FIGURE 8.4 Electric fields inside a low-pass, RF birdcage coil are presented. Note that electric fields reach their maximum magnitude at the coil and fall to zero along the coil axis. Capacitors along the coil wall may also give rise to locally high electric fields. Any conductors should be routed along regions of low electric field or orthogonal to the electric field. Below is an illustration of a birdcage coil.

Let a be the radius of the birdcage coil. Assume that (at the moment of time we look) $B_1 = B_{1x}$ ($B_{1y} = B_{1z} = 0$). Assume conductors of the RF coil lie only parallel to the z direction, then $A_y = A_x = 0$. Let θ be the angle between the conductor, the center of the cylinder, and the x axis. Then it is possible to find B_{1x} and A_z (remember that B_1 is constant, independent of z):

$$B_{1x} = \frac{\partial A_z}{\partial z} \quad \rightarrow A_z = B_1 y = B_1 a \sin\theta \tag{8.17}$$

So, an infinitely long coil with infinite conductors parallel to z, lying on the surface of a cylinder, will produce a uniform B_1 field, provided current varies with $\sin\theta$.

Of course, real birdcage coils are not infinitely long. Current is returned through end rings at the ends of the finite, cylindrical coil. End rings sum (or integrate) current from the straight coil conductors (which I will call *legs*). So, if coil leg current varies as $\sin\theta$, then current in the end rings varies as $\cos\theta$. Let N be the number of legs in the birdcage coil. Schenck[89,90] showed that peak end ring current amplitude is a factor $1/[2 \sin(\pi/N)]$ larger than the peak current in the coil legs. Let D be the length-to-diameter ratio of the birdcage coil, a be the coil radius, and I be the

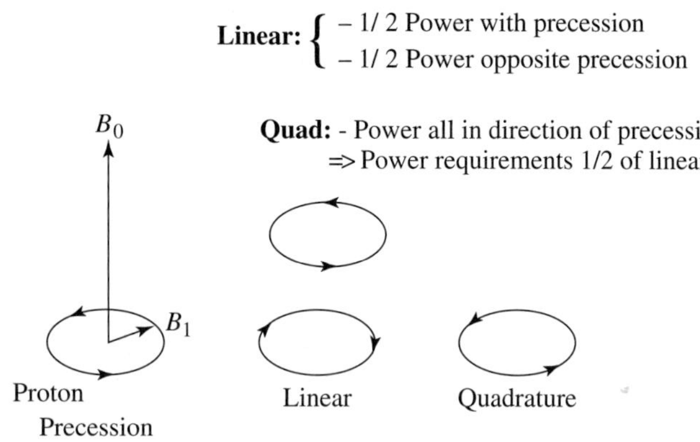

FIGURE 8.5 Comparisons of quadrature and linear RF excitation of spins are shown. Note that linear excitation wastes half the applied power.

maximum current in the legs of the birdcage coil. Schenck also showed that the radiofrequecy magnetic induction B_1 at the center of a birdcage coil is given by

$$B_1 = \frac{\mu_0 I N \sin\left(\frac{\pi}{N}\right)}{2\pi a} \frac{D(D^2+2)}{(1+D^2)^{3/2}} \tag{8.18}$$

B_1, as expressed in Eq. (8.18), is maximum when $D = \sqrt{2}$. However, Eq. (8.18) is within 95 percent of its maximum value for $D > 0.9$. Longer birdcage coils result in higher radiofrequency deposition in patients. Shorter birdcage coils are desirable. Typically, birdcage coils are designed with $D \approx 1$.

In MR, the nuclear spins of interest precess about the static magnetic field. Consider a transmit B_1 field in which the B_1 vector constantly points parallel or antiparallel to, for example, the y axis. This linear polarization with respect to the B_1 component may be considered to consist of two counterrotating components of equal magnitude (see Fig. 8.5). One of the rotating components will be in the same direction as the nuclear precession and so will contribute to MR physics. The other component will participate in MR physics. Instead, that component will only waste energy by unnecessarily depositing RF energy in patients. Quadrature coils are driven electrically and physically 90° apart. Quadrature transmit coils are designed to excite only the B_1 component which rotates in the same direction as the precessing nuclei. Peak power requirements are reduced by a factor of 2 using quadrature coils.

Quadrature receive coils receive correlated signals but uncorrelated noise from the two receive channels. The result is a $\sqrt{2}$ improvement in signal-to-noise ratio over linear coils. In addition, quadrature imaging reduces diagonal shading in images.

8.4.2 Shielding

To prevent undesirable interactions with surrounding conductive structures, transmit coils are often shielded. Shielding reduces coil losses and in receive-coils reduces noise as well. The coil quality factor is the ratio of the inductive reactance of the coil to the resistance of the coil. Let the radian frequency be ω, coil inductance be L, coil losses be R, BW be the bandwidth, and f_c be the center frequency of the coil; then the coil quality factor Q may be expressed as[89]

$$Q = \frac{f_c}{BW} = \frac{\omega L}{R} \tag{8.19}$$

High quality factors improve signal-to-noise ratios for receive coils. Note that extremely high Q may result in *making* precise coil tuning more critical.

8.4.3 Receive Coils

RF receive coils receive signal and noise from the matter in the coil. If only a small region were to be imaged, then signal may be generated only from the region of interest while noise is received from the entire sample in the coil.[86,87,91] To reduce noise in the image, it is sensible to receive with the smallest coil capable of spanning the region of interest. This concept is referred to as *fill factor*.

Transmit coils may also double as receive coils. Frequently, a larger, relatively homogeneous coil such as a birdcage body coil will be used to transmit the excitation pulses. Then, a smaller, less homogeneous receive-only coil called a *surface coil*[86,87,91] will be used to receive the signal. The smaller coil generally has a better fill factor and so produces higher signal-to-noise ratios (SNR) than would have been possible with the larger coil.

Large surface coil currents may result if receive-only surface coils were resonant while RF transmit pulses are generated on the body coil. Such currents can produce opposing B_1 fields which may destroy transmit homogeneity. In addition, these large currents could result in locally high RF deposition near the coils. Boesiger[85] has shown conditions where the surface coil amplified normal body coil heating 47-fold. To prevent such problems, blocking networks[86,87] are used (see Fig. 8.6). These blocking networks present high impedances to surface coil currents during body coil transmit. The required blocking impedance depends on coil area, magnet frequency, and how large an opposing field is to be allowed. Typical blocking impedances are a few hundred ohms. Poorly designed surface coil blocking networks may become warm. IEC 60601-1 sets a surface temperature limit of 41°C for objects that may touch people.[92]

The high blocking impedance is switched out during receive. During receive, the surface coil is made resonant. The transmit body coil normally would couple noise from the rest of the body into surface coils during receive, degrading images. To prevent this sort of coupling, body coils are detuned during the receive phase.

Further increases in SNR might be obtained using phased-array surface coils.[93] Phased-array coils are designed to be orthogonal (received noise is uncorrelated). If data from each coil are separately received and reconstructed, then SNR can be significantly increased over levels possible with individual coils that are not orthogonal. The coils are made orthogonal by slightly overlapping them until their mutual inductance approaches zero.

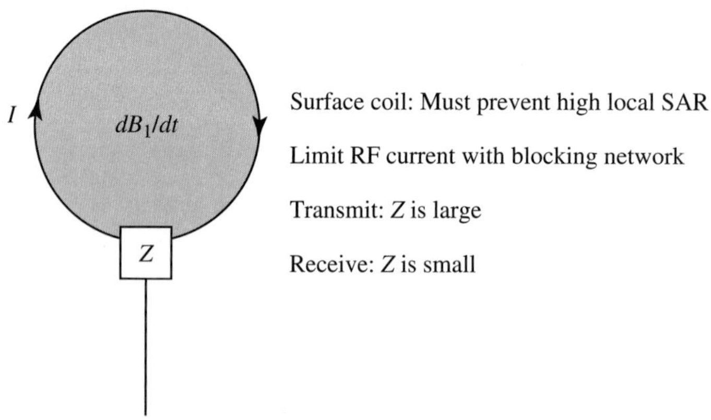

FIGURE 8.6 A receive-only surface coil with a blocking network is shown. During body coil transmit the blocking network, Z, becomes a high impedance to prevent high induced currents from flowing on the coil. Such currents could lead to very high local SAR levels. During surface coil receive, the blocking network becomes a very low impedance to improve the image signal-to-noise ratio.

At higher field strengths, most of the RF losses are due to patients. However, for low field systems, patient losses are much smaller than coil losses. One approach for reducing the SNR impact of such low field coil losses is to use superconducting surface coils.[94] These coils are typically limited in size and require attached cryostats. In addition, very high Q translates to very narrow bandwidths and tight tolerances on tuning.

Receiver Coil Arrays. Signal-to-noise ratio may be improved by replacing a single, large field of view coil with an array of smaller coils that combine for a field of view similar to the larger coil. Each smaller coil receives less noise than the larger coil. Since noise is not correlated, while signals are (due to coil design) signal to noise is typically higher when receiver coil arrays are used. Typically, noise from adjacent coil elements is designed to be uncorrelated by appropriate overlap or circuit design.

Parallel Imaging. Magnetic resonance parallel imaging techniques use multiple receiver coils (with different spatial sensitivities). These receiver coils are used to supply some portion of the spatial encoding information to reduce the total number of gradient phase encodings.[95–101] The techniques typically are used to obtain shorter scan times and may shorten readout times. Some image artifacts can be reduced using parallel imaging.

Typically, in parallel imaging receiver coil spatial sensitivity is determined from low-resolution reference images. Then aliased data sets can be generated for each individual coil. Receiver coil spatial sensitivity information may then be used with either image-domain or frequency (k-space)-domain reconstruction techniques to generate full field of view (nonaliased) images.

Signal to noise in parallel imaging is reduced by the shorter imaging time and by nonideal coil geometry. Nonideal coil geometry finds expression in the g factor. The g factor refers to the pixel-by-pixel signal-to-noise ratio obtained with parallel imaging divided by the signal-to-noise ratio using equivalent conventional techniques with the same receive coils. The g factor is only defined in regions where signal to noise is above a threshold and technically applies only to image-based parallel imaging methods.

The reduction of the number of phase-codings needed due to multiple receiver coils in parallel imaging is called the *acceleration factor*. Maximum acceleration factors are somewhat less than the number of parallel imaging receiver coils.

8.4.4 Preamplifiers

Low-noise figure preamplifiers with noise impedances matched and relatively near the receiver coils are required to avoid degrading SNR. Quadrature systems with preamplifiers on each channel have small SNR advantages over quadrature systems employing low loss combiners and a single preamplifier.

8.4.5 SAR

During MR scans below 3 T or so, RF power deposition in patients can be approximated from quasistatic analysis, assuming electric field coupling to patients can be neglected.[10,34] Let R be the radius, σ the conductivity, and ρ the density of a homogeneous, sphere of tissue (Fig. 8.1). Assume that this sphere is placed in a uniform RF magnetic field of strength B_1 and frequency ω. Let the radiofrequency duty cycle be η. Then average specific absorption rate (SAR), SAR_{ave}, may be expressed as[63]

$$\mathrm{SAR}_{\mathrm{ave}} = \frac{\sigma\eta\omega^2 B_1^2 R^2}{20\rho} \tag{8.20}$$

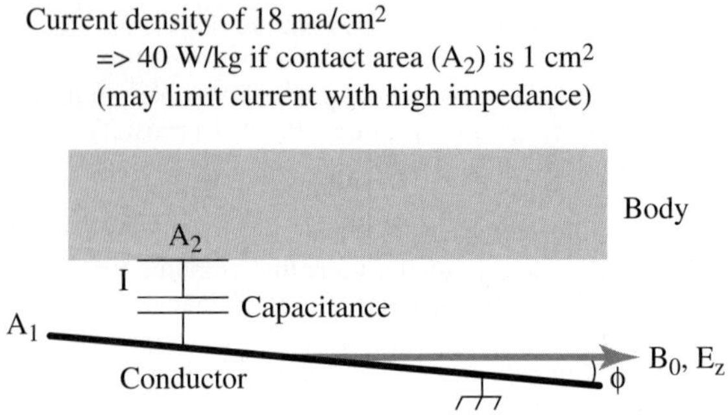

FIGURE 8.7 The effect of conductors on local power deposition is illustrated. A straight conductor experiences a gradient-induced electrical potential related to the vector component of the electric field over the conductor length. The conductor contacts a patient over some cross sectional area. Local SAR is 40 W/kg (well beyond the 8 W/kg guideline) if the local current density is as little as 18 ma/cm^2. Local SAR may be limited by increasing conductor impedance, or by increasing contact area, or by orienting the conductor orthogonal to the electric field, or by making the conductor shorter.

For homogeneous spheres, it turns out that the maximum peak SAR at a point is located on the outer radius of the sphere and is 2.5 times the average for the sphere.

RF heating during MR is by magnetic induction. Power deposition in homogeneous spheres immersed in uniform RF magnetic fields increases with the fifth power of the radius. Heating is largely peripheral with little deep body heating.[63]

As discussed above, RF body coils induce electric fields in the body of patients. The induced electric fields are largest near the RF coil conductors (Fig. 8.4). RF coils may have high electric fields near capacitors on the coil as well. Ensuring patients are kept well away from coil conductors (using pads, for example), especially during high SAR exams, may reduce local heating concerns. Note that in low-pass birdcage coils, the centerline of the coil is nearly a virtual ground. Any conductors that must be introduced into the bore will minimally affect local SAR if they are placed along this virtual ground.

If conductive loops (e.g., monitoring equipment or even coiled transmission line) are introduced into the scanner, high local SAR levels may result (Fig. 8.6). Even straight conductors may increase local SAR significantly (Fig. 8.7). For patient safety, fiber optic devices should be used instead of conductors, when possible.

8.5 OTHER MR SYSTEMS

8.5.1 Computer Systems

Typically, MR pulse sequences (including radiofrequency and gradient waveforms) are computer generated and computer controlled. The computer also generates eddy current compensation for the gradients and perhaps other types of compensation for imperfections. Patient tables are typically under computer control. RF receivers interface with computers that convert the raw received data into images. Computers typically display and possibly monitor patient comfort and patient safety parameters. Computers typically monitor system hardware as well.

8.5.2 Gating

Often MR scans need to be synchronized with (gated by) a physiological input such as the electrocardiogram or peripheral pulse or possibly respiration. Many MR systems provide the ability to gate the scanner from these waveforms. It is imperative that the gating waveforms be sufficiently free of artifacts induced by the MR system (gradient or RF interference or B_0 enhanced "T" waves appearing to be "R" waves) to permit accurate gating. It is also imperative that gating hardware should not increase the chances of local power deposition in patients. Elimination of conductors (e.g., by using fiber optic devices) in the scanner greatly reduces local power deposition concerns. Finally, the gating equipment must not introduce signals that interfere with the scanner and show up as image artifacts.

8.5.3 Other MR Hardware

Other essential MR hardware may include patient tables, patient comfort systems (pads, lights, airflow, or headphones), and venting systems for magnets with cryogens. Patient tables may be used to transport patients, to move the region of interest into the center of the magnet for the examination, and to permit rapid removal of patients from scanners during emergencies. Pads may add to patient comfort and may be essential in reducing concerns of localized RF power deposition. Lighting and airflow may reduce patient anxiety.

8.6 SAFETY STANDARDS

MR is a rapidly evolving technology. It is imperative that MR safety standards protect patient safety during exams, while not preventing safe development of future diagnostic techniques. While many safety standards govern various aspects of MR hardware development, two that are unique to MR are listed in Table 8.1. The Food and Drug Administration (FDA) published "Non-Significant Risk Criteria" for magnetic resonance devices.[19] These criteria state under what conditions MR patient studies need investigational device exemption (IDE). The International Electrotechnical Commission (IEC)[20] developed a widely used MR safety standard. The IEC MR safety standard is three-tiered. The *normal operating mode* is for routine scanning of patients. The operator must take a deliberate action (usually an ACCEPT button) to enter the *first controlled operating mode*. This mode provides higher scanner performance, but requires more operator monitoring of the patient. Finally, there is a *second controlled operating mode* used only for research purposes under limits controlled by an Investigational Review Board (IRB). In Table 8.1, values from the new, recently approved, second edition of the IEC MR Safety Standard are presented along with FDA criteria.

Another IEC safety standard[92] also establishes safety criteria for electrical safety and limits surface contact temperatures to 41°C. Note that during high SAR scans, skin temperature approaches 37°C (a 4°C margin for temperature rise). During very low SAR scans, skin temperature is typically 33°C (an 8°C margin).

8.7 NEMA MR MEASUREMENT STANDARDS

The National Electrical Manufacturers Association (NEMA) has developed a number of useful standards for measurement of MR parameters. The current list of NEMA MR standards is given in Table 8.2. Note that these standards are now freely available. For more information see http://www.nema.org/.

TABLE 8.1 MR Safety Standards

Safety parameter	FDA significant risk criteria (http://www.fda.gov/cdrh/ode/magdev.html)	IEC 60601-2-33 normal mode	IEC 60601-2-33 controlled mode (operator takes deliberate action to enter)	IEC 60601-2-33 second controlled mode (needs IRB approval)
B_0	$B_0 > 4$ T	$B_0 \leq 2.0$ T	2 T < $B_0 \leq 4$ T	$B_0 > 4$ T
WB SAR	Whole-body ave. SAR ≥ 4 W/kg with 15 min ave.	Whole-body ave. SAR ≤ 2 W/kg with 6 min ave.	Whole-body ave. SAR ≤ 4 W/kg with 6 min ave.	Whole-body ave SAR > 4 W/kg with 6 min ave.
Head SAR	Ave. head SAR > 3 W/kg with 10 min ave.	Ave. head SAR ≤ 3.2 W/kg with 6 min ave.	Ave. head SAR ≤ 3.2 W/kg with 6 min ave.	Ave. head SAR > 3.2 W/kg with 6 min ave.
Local SAR	Local SAR > 8 W/kg in any gram (head or torso)	Local SAR ≤ 10 W/kg in head or trunk, ≤ 20 W/kg in extremities with 6 min ave.	Local SAR ≤ 10 W/kg in head or trunk, ≤ 20 W/kg in extremities with 6 min ave.	Local SAR > 10 W/kg in head or trunk, > 20 W/kg in extremities with 6 min ave.
Partial body SAR	N/A	SAR ≤ 10–8 W/kg (exposed mass/total mass limits between 2 and 10 W/kg): 6 min ave.	Partial SAR ≤ 10–6 W/kg (exposed mass/total mass limits between 4 and 10 W/kg): 6 min ave.	Partial SAR > first controlled mode
Short-term SAR	N/A	SAR over any 10 s period may be up to 3 times appropriate long-term SAR level	SAR over any 10 s period may be up to 3 times appropriate long-term SAR level	SAR > first controlled mode
dB/dt	Sufficient for severe discomfort	$dB/dt \leq 80\%$ of peripheral nerve mean	$dB/dt \leq 100\%$ of peripheral nerve mean	dB/dt > first controlled mode

TABLE 8.2 NEMA Standards*

Standard (as listed in NEMA catalog)	Title
MS 1-2001	Determination of Signal-to-Noise Ratio (SNR) in Diagnostic Magnetic Resonance Images
MS 2-1989 (R-1996)	Determination of Two-Dimensional Geometric Distortion in Diagnostic Magnetic Resonance Images
MS 3-1989 (R-1994)	Determination of Image Uniformity in Diagnostic Magnetic Resonance Images
MS 4-1989 (Revision 1998)	Acoustic Noise Measurement Procedure for Diagnostic Magnetic Resonance Images
MS 5-1991 (R-1996)	Determination of Slice Thickness in Diagnostic Magnetic Resonance Imaging
MS 6-1991 (Revision 2000)	Characterization of Special Purpose Coils for Diagnostic Magnetic Resonance Images
MS 7-1993 (Revision 1998)	Measurement Procedure for Time-Varying Gradient Fields (dB/dt) for Diagnostic Magnetic Resonance Imaging Devices
MS 8-1993 (R-2000)	Characterization of the Specific Absorption Rate for Magnetic Resonance Imaging Systems
MS 9-2001*	Characterization of Phased Array Coils for Diagnostic Magnetic Resonance Imaging Systems
MS 10-2001*	Determination of Local Specific Absorption Rate for Magnetic Resonance Imaging Systems
MS 11-2001*	Alternate Measurement Procedure for Time-Varying Gradient Fields (dB/dt) by Measuring Electric Field Gradients for Magnetic Resonance Imaging Systems

*Not finished at publication time.

REFERENCES

1. Halliday, D. and R. Resnick, 1966, *Physics*, New York: John Wiley, p. 826.
2. Moore, W. J., 1972, *Physical Chemistry*, Englewood Cliffs, New Jersey: Prentice Hall, pp. 140–143.
3. Mansfield, P. and P. G. Morris, 1982, "NMR imaging in biomedicine," In: *Advances in Magnetic Resonance*, Suppl. 2, J. S. Waugh, ed., New York: Academic Press, p. 32.
4. Keller, P. J., 1990, *Basic Principles of Magnetic Resonance Imaging*, General Electric Company, Milwaukee, pp. 16–37.
5. Bottomley, P. A., T. H. Foster, R. E. Argersinger, and L. M. Pfiefer, 1984, "A review of normal tissue hydrogen NMR relaxation times and relaxation mechanisms from 1-100 MHz: Dependence on tissue type, NMR frequency, temperature, species, excision, and age," *Med. Phys.*, **11**:425.
6. Glover, G. H., 1993, "Gradient Echo Imaging," In: The American Association of Physicists in Medicine (AAPM) Monograph No. 21: *The Physics of MRI*, P. Sprawls and M. Bronskill, eds., American Institute of Physics, New York, pp. 188–205.
7. McVeigh, E. and E. Atalar, 1993, "Balancing contrast, Resolution, and signal-to-noise ratio in magnetic resonance imaging," In: The American Association of Physicists in Medicine (AAPM) Monograph No. 21: *The Physics of MRI*, P. Sprawls and M. Bronskill, eds., American Institute of Physics, New York, pp. 234–267.
8. Thomas, S. R., 1993, "Magnets and gradient coils: types and characteristics," In: The American Association of Physicists in Medicine (AAPM) Monograph No. 21: *The Physics of MRI*, P. Sprawls and M. Bronskill, eds., American Institute of Physics, New York, pp. 56–97.
9. Golay, M. J., 1968, "Field homogenizing coils for nuclear spin resonance instrumentation," *Rev. Sci. Inst.*, **29**:313–315.
10. Schenck, J. F., 2000, "Safety of strong, static magnetic fields (invited)," *J. Magn. Reson. Imaging*, **12**:2–19.
11. Mansfield, P. and P. G. Morris, 1982, "NMR imaging in biomedicine," In: *Advances in Magnetic Resonance*, Suppl. 2, J. S. Waugh, ed., New York: Academic Press, p. 271.

12. Schenck, J. F., 1986, "Axial magnetic field gradient coil suitable for use with NMR apparatus," U. S. Patent No. 4617516.

13. Schenck, J. F., M. A. Hussain, and W. A. Edelstein, 1987, "Transverse gradient coils for nuclear magnetic resonance imaging," U. S. Patent No. 4646024.

14. Roemer, P. B. and J. S. Hickey, 1986, "Self-shielded gradient coils for nuclear magnetic resonance imaging," U. S. Patent No. 4737716.

15. Hughes, D. G., S. Robertson, and P. S. Allen, 1992, "Intensity artifacts in MRI caused by gradient-switching in an animal-size NMR magnet," *Magn. Reson. Med.,* **25**:167–179.

16. Henkelman, R. M. and M. J. Bronskill, 1987, "Artifacts in magnetic resonance imaging," *Rev. Magn. Reson. Med.,* **2**(1):121–126.

17. Jehenson, P., M. Westphal, and N. Schuff, 1990, "Analytical method for the compensation of eddy-current effects induced by pulsed magnetic field gradients in NMR systems," *J. Magn. Reson. Imaging*, **90**:264–278.

18. FDA, 1988, (August 2), "Guidance for content and review of a magnetic resonance diagnostic device 510 (k) application: safety parameter action levels," Center for Devices and Radiological Health Report (Rockville, Maryland).

19. FDA, 1997, "Magnetic resonance diagnostic devices criteria for significant risk investigations" at http://www. fda. gov/cdrh/ode/magdev. html.

20. IEC 60601-2-33, 1995 (2d ed., approved October 2001), Medical Electrical Equipment—Part 2: "Particular requirements for the safety of magnetic resonance equipment for medical diagnosis," International Electrotechnical Commission (IEC)*, 3, rue de Varembé, P. O. Box 131, CH-1211 Geneva 20, Switzerland. (In the United States, copies of this standard can be obtained from the American National Standards Institute (ANSI), 11 West 42nd Street, New York, NY 10036).

21. Nyenhuis, J. A., J. D. Bourland, A. V. Kildishev, and D. J. Schaefer, 2001, "Health effects and safety of intense gradient fields," In: *Magnetic Resonance Procedures: Health Effects and Safety*, F. G. Shellock, ed., New York: CRC Press, pp. 31–54.

22. Schaefer, D. J., J. D. Bourland, and J. A. Nyenhuis, 2000, "Review of patient safety in time-varying gradient fields (invited)," *J. Magn. Reson. Imaging*, **12**(1):20–29.

23. Bourland, J. D., J. A. Nyenhuis, and D. J. Schaefer, 1999, "Physiologic effects of intense MRI gradient fields," *Neuroimaging Clin. N. Am.,* **9**(2):363–377.

24. Schaefer, D. J., 1998, "Safety aspects of switched gradient fields," E. Kanal, ed., *MRI Clin. N. Am.,* **6**(4):731–747.

25. Reilly, J. P., 1989, "Cardiac sensitivity to electrical stimulation," U. S. Food and Drug Administration Report, MT 89–101.

26. Cohen, M. S., R. Weisskoff, and H. Kantor, 1990, "Sensory stimulation by time varying magnetic fields," *Magn. Reson.,* **14**:409–414.

27. Bourland, J. D., J. A. Nyenhuis, G. A. Mouchawar, L. A. Geddes, D. J. Schaefer, and M. E. Riehl, 1990, *Human Peripheral Nerve Stimulation from z-Gradients,* Abstracts of the Society of Magnetic Resonance in Medicine. Works in Progress, p. 1157.

28. Budinger, T. F., H. Fischer, D. Hentshel, H. E. Reinflder, and F. Schmitt, 1991, "Physiological effects of fast oscillating magnetic field gradients," *J. Comput. Assist. Tomogr.,* **15**:609–614.

29. Bourland, J. D., J. A. Nyenhuis, G. A. Mouchawar, T. Z. Elabbady, L. A. Geddes, D. J. Schaefer, and M. E. Riehl, 1991, *Physiologic Indicators of High MRI Gradient-Induced Fields*, Book of Abstracts, Works in Progress, Society of Magnetic Resonance in Medicine, 10th Annual Meeting, San Francisco, p. 1276.

30. Nyenhuis, J. A., J. D. Bourland, G. A. Mouchawar, T. Z. Elabbady, L. A. Geddes, D. J. Schaefer, and M. E. Riehl, 1991, *Comparison of Stimulation Effects of Longitudinal and Transverse MRI Gradient Coils*, Abstract in Works in Progress, Society of Magnetic Resonance in Medicine, p. 1275.

31. Bourland, J. D., J. A. Nyenhuis, G. A. Mouchawar, L. A. Geddes, D. J. Schaefer, and M. E. Riehl, 1991, *z-Gradient Coil Eddy-Current Stimulation of Skeletal and Cardiac Muscle in the Dog*, Book of Abstracts, Society of Magnetic Resonance in Medicine, 10th Annual Meeting, San Francisco, p. 969.

32. Reilly, J. P., 1992, "Principles of nerve and heart excitation by time-varying magnetic fields," *Ann. N. Y. Acad. Sci.,* **649**:96–117.

33. Nyenhuis, J. A., J. D. Bourland, D. J. Schaefer, K. S. Foster, W. E. Schoelein, G. A. Mouchawar, T. Z. Elabbady, L. A. Geddes, and M. E. Riehl, 1992, *Measurement of Cardiac Stimulation Thresholds for Pulsed z-Gradient Fields in a 1. 5 T Magnet*, Abstract in 11th Annual SMRM (Berlin), p. 586.

34. Bourland, J. D., J. A. Nyenhuis, D. J. Schaefer, K. S. Foster, W. E. Schoelein, G. A. Mouchawar, T. Z. Elabbady, L. A. Geddes, and M. E. Riehl, 1992, *Gated, Gradient-Induced Cardiac Stimulation in the Dog: Absence of Ventricular Fibrillation*, Abstract in Works in Progress of 11th Annual SMRM (Berlin), p. 4808.

35. Mansfield, P. and P. R. Harvey, 1993, "Limits to neural stimulation in echo-planar imaging," *Magn. Reson. Med.*, **29**:746–758.

36. Irnich, W. and F. Schmitt, 1995, "Magnetostimulation in MRI," *Magn. Reson. Med.*, **33**:619–623.

37. Mouchawar, G. A., J. A. Nyenhuis, J. D. Bourland, L. A. Geddes, D. J. Schaefer, and M. E. Riehl, 1993, "Magnetic stimulation of excitable tissue: calculation of induced eddy-currents with a three-dimensional finite element model," *IEEE Trans. Magn.*, **29**(6):3355–3357.

38. Schaefer, D. J., J. D. Bourland, J. A. Nyenhuis, K. S. Foster, W. F. Wirth, L. A. Geddes, and M. E. Riehl, 1994, *Determination of Gradient-Induced, Human Peripheral Nerve Stimulation Thresholds for Trapezoidal Pulse Trains*, Abstract published by the Society of Magnetic Resonance, 2nd Meeting, San Francisco, p. 101.

39. Ehrhardt, J. C., C. S. Lin, V. A. Magnotta, S. M. Baker, D. J. Fisher, and W. T. C. Yuh, 1993, *Neural Stimulation in a Whole-Body Echo-Planar Imaging System*, Abstract in 12th Annual SMRM (New York), vol. 3, p. 1372.

40. Rohan, M. L. and R. R. Rzedzian, 1992, "Stimulation by time-varying magnetic fields," *Ann. N. Y. Acad. Sci.*, **649:**118–128.

41. Schaefer, D. J., J. D. Bourland, J. A. Nyenhuis, K. S. Foster, P. E. Licato, and L. A. Geddes, 1995, *Effects of Simultaneous Gradient Combinations on Human Peripheral Nerve Stimulation Thresholds*, Society of Magnetic Resonance, 3rd Meeting, Nice, France, p. 1220.

42. Bourland, J. D., J. A. Nyenhuis, W. A. Noe, D. J. Schaefer, K. S. Foster, and L. A. Geddes, 1996, *Motor and Sensory Strength-Duration Curves for MRI Gradient Fields*, Abstracts of the Society of Magnetic Resonance, 4th Meeting, New York City, p. 1724.

43. Nyenhuis, J. A., J. D. Bourland, and D. J. Schaefer, 1996, *Analysis from a Stimulation Perspective of Magnetic Field Patterns of MR Gradient Coils*, Abstracts of the Magnetism and Magnetic Materials Conference.

44. Bourland, J. D., J. A. Nyenhuis, K. S. Foster, G. P. Graber, D. J. Schaefer, and L. A. Geddes, 1997, *Threshold and Pain Strength-Duration Curves for MRI Gradient Fields*, Abstracts of the International Society of Magnetic Resonance in Medicine, Vancouver, Canada, p. 1974.

45. Havel, W., J. Nyenhuis, J. Bourland, K. Foster, L. Geddes, G. Graber, M. Waninger, and D. Schaefer, Jan. 6–9, 1998, *Comparison of Rectangular and Damped Sinusoidal dB/dt Waveforms in Magnetic Stimulation*, Abstracts of the 7th Joint MMM-INTERMAG Conference, San Francisco.

46. Abart, J., K. Eberhardt, H. Fischer, W. Huk, E. Richer, F. Schmitt, T. Storch, and E. Zeitler, 1997, "Peripheral nerve stimulation by time-varying magnetic fields," *J. Comput. Assist. Tomogr.*, **21**(4):532–538.

47. Ham, C. L. G., J. M. L. Engels, G. T. van de Weil, and A. Machielsen, 1997, "Peripheral nerve stimulation during MRI: effects of high gradient amplitudes and switching rates," *J. Magn. Reson. Imaging*, **7**(5):933–937.

48. Halliday, D. and R. Resnick, 1966, *Physics*, New York: John Wiley, pp. 819–820.

49. Schaefer, D. J., 1993, "Bioeffects of MRI and patient safety," In: The American Association of Physicists in Medicine (AAPM) Monograph No. 21: *The Physics of MR Imaging,* American Institute of Physics, New York, pp. 607–646.

50. Hedeen, R. A. and W. A. Edelstein, 1997, "Characteristics and prediction of gradient acoustic noise in MR imagers," *Magn. Reson. Med.* **37**:7–10.

51. McJury, M., "Acoustic noise and magnetic resonance procedures," 2001, In: *Magnetic Resonance Procedures: Health Effects and Safety*, F. G. Shellock, ed., New York: CRC Press, pp. 115–138.

52. McJury, M. and F. G. Shellock, 2000, "Auditory noise associated with MR procedures: a review (invited)," *J. Med. Reson. Imaging*, **12**:37–45.

53. Melnick, W., "Hearing loss from noise exposure," In: *Handbook of Noise Control,* C. M. Harris, ed., New York: McGraw-Hill, p. 2.

54. Robinson, D. W. "Characteristics of occupational Noise-Induced Hearing Loss," In: *Effects of Noise on Hearing*, D. Henderson, R. P. Hamernik, D. S. Dosjanjh, J. H. Mills, eds., New York: Raven Press, 1976, pp. 383–405.
55. Brummett, R. E., J. M. Talbot, and P. Charuhas, 1988, "Potential hearing loss resulting from MR imaging," *Radiology*, **169**:539–540.
56. Mansfield, P. M., P. M. Glover, and R. W. Bowtell, 1994, "Active acoustic screening: design principles for quiet gradient coils in MRI," *Meas. Sci. Technol.,* **5**:1021–1025.
57. Cho, Z. H., S. T. Chung, J. Y. Chung, et al., 1998, "A new silent magnetic resonance imaging using a rotating DC gradient," *Magn. Reson. Med.,* **39**:317–321.
58. Chen, C. K., T. D. Chiueh, and J. H. Chen, 1999, "Active cancellation system of acoustic noise in MR imaging," *IEEE Trans. Biomed. Eng.,* **46**:186–190.
59. Shellock, F. G., 2000, "Radiofrequency energy-induced heating during MR procedures: A review," *J. Med. Reson. Imaging*, **12**:30–36.
60. Schaefer, D. J., 2001, "Health effects and safety of radiofrequency power deposition associated with magnetic resonance procedures," In: *Magnetic Resonance Procedures: Health Effects and Safety*, F. G. Shellock, ed., New York: CRC Press, pp. 55–74.
61. Shellock, F. G. and D. J. Schaefer, 2001, "Radiofrequency energy-induced current density distributions for radiofrequency and gradient magnetic fields used for magnetic resonance procedures," In: *Magnetic Resonance Procedures: Health Effects and Safety*, F. G. Shellock, ed., New York: CRC Press, pp. 75–97.
62. Smith, C. D., J. A. Nyenhuis, and A. V. Kildishev, 2001, "Health effects of induced electric fields: implications for metallic implants," In: *Magnetic Resonance Procedures: Health Effects and Safety*, F. G. Shellock, ed., New York: CRC Press, pp. 393–414.
63. Schaefer, D. J., 1998, "Safety aspects of radio frequency power deposition in magnetic resonance," E. Kanal, ed., *MRI Clin. N. Am.,* **6**(4):775–789.
64. Elder, J. E., 1984, "Special senses," In: *Biological Effects of Radio-Frequency Radiation*, J. E. Elder and D. F. Cahill, eds., EPA-600/8-83-026F, U. S. Environment Protection Agency, Res. Tri. Pk., North Carolina, Sec. 5, pp. 64–78.
65. Bottomley, P. A. and E. R. Andrew, 1978, "RF penetration, phase-shift, and power dissipation in biological tissue: implications for NMR imaging," *Phys. Med. Biol.,* **23**:630–643.
66. Abart, J., G. Brinker, W. Irlbacher, and J. Grebmeir, 1989, "Temperature and heart rate changes in MRI at SAR levels up to 3 W/kg," Poster Presentation, *SMRM Book of Abstracts*, p. 998.
67. Adair, E. R. and L. G. Berglund, 1986, "On the thermoregulatory consequences of NMR imaging," *Magn. Reson. Imaging,* (4):321–333.
68. Adair, E. R. and L. G. Berglund, 1989, "Thermoregulatory consequences of cardiovascular impairment during NMR imaging in warm/humid environments," *Magn. Reson. Imag,* (7):25.
69. Athey, T. W., 1989, "A model of the temperature rise in the head due to magnetic resonance imaging procedures," *Magn. Reson. Med.,* **9**:177–184.
70. Athey, T. W., 1992, "Current FDA guidance for MR patient exposure and considerations for the future," *Ann. N. Y. Acad. Sci.,* **649**:242–257.
71. Barber, B. J., D. J. Schaefer, C. J. Gordon, D. C. Zawieja, and J. Hecker, 1990, "Thermal effects of MR imaging: worst-case studies on sheep," *AJR*, **155**:1105–1110.
72. Benjamin, F. B., 1952, "Pain reaction to locally applied heat," *J. Appl. Physiol*., (52):250–263.
73. Bernhardt, J. H., 1992, "Non-ionizing radiation safety: radio-frequency radiation, electric and magnetic fields," *Phys. Med. Biol.,* **4**:807–844.
74. Budinger, T. F. and C. Cullander, 1984, "Health effects of in-vivo nuclear magnetic resonance," In: *Clinical Magnetic Resonance Imaging*, A. R. Margulis, C. B. Higgins, L. Kaufman, L. E. Crooks, eds., San Francisco: Radiology Research and Education Foundation, Chap. 27.
75. Carlson, L. D. and A. C. L. Hsieh, 1982, *Control of Energy Exchange*, London: Macmillan, pp. 56, 73, 85.
76. Goldman, R. F., E. B. Green, and P. F. Iampietro, 1965, "Tolerance of hot wet environments by resting men," *J. Appl. Physiol.,* **20**(2):271–277.
77. Guy, A. W., J. C. Lin, P. O. Kramer, and A. F. Emery, 1975, "Effect of 2450 MHz Radiation on the Rabbit Eye," *IEEE Trans. Microwave Theory Tech.,* MTT-23:492–498.
78. Kanal, E., 1992, "An overview of electromagnetic safety considerations associated with magnetic resonance imaging," *Ann. N. Y. Acad. Sci.,* **649**:204–224.

79. Saunders, R. D. and H. Smith, 1984, "Safety aspects of NMR clinical imaging," *Br. Med. Bull.*, **40**(2):148–154.

80. Shellock, F. G., D. J. Schaefer, W. Grunfest, and J. V. Crues, 1987, "Thermal effects of high-field (1. 5 Tesla) magnetic resonance imaging of the spine: clinical experience above a specific absorption rate of 0. 4 W/kg," *Acta Radiol.*, **369**:514–516.

81. Shellock, F. G. and J. V. Crues, 1987, "Temperature, heart rate, and blood pressure changes associated with clinical magnetic resonance imaging at 1. 5 Tesla," *Radiology*, **163**:259–262.

82. Shellock, F. G., 1989, "Biological effects and safety aspects of magnetic resonance imaging," *Magn. Reson. Q.*, **5**(4):243–261.

83. Shellock, F. G., D. J. Schaefer, and J. V. Crues, 1990, "Alterations in body and skin temperatures caused by MR imaging: is the recommended exposure for radiofrequency radiation too conservative," *Br. J. Radiol.*, **62**:904–909.

84. Smith, D. A., S. K. Clarren, and M. A. S. Harvey, 1978, "Hyperthermia as a possible teratogenic agent," *Pediatrics*, **92**(6):878–883.

85. Boesigner, P., R. Buchli, M. Saner, and D. Meier, 1992, "An overview of electromagnetic safety considerations associated with magnetic resonance imaging," *Ann. N. Y. Acad. Sci.*, **649**:160–165.

86. Edelstein, W. A., C. J. Hardy, and O. M. Mueller, 1986, "Electronic decoupling of surface-coil receivers for NMR imaging and spectroscopy," *J. Magn. Reson.*, **67**:156–161.

87. Haase, A., 1985, "A new method for the decoupling of multiple NMR probes," *J. Magn. Reson.*, **61**:130–136.

88. Hayes, C. E., W. A. Edelstein, J. F. Schenck, O. M. Mueller, and M. Eash, 1985, "An efficient, highly homogeneous radiofrequency coil for whole-body NMR imaging at 1. 5 T," *J. Magn. Reson.*, **63**:622–628.

89. Schenck, J. F., 1993, "Radiofrequency Coils: Types and Characteristics," In: The American Association of Physicists in Medicine (AAPM) Monograph No. 21: *The Physics of MRI*, P. Sprawls and M. Bronskill, eds., American Institute of Physics, New York, pp. 98–134.

90. Schenck, J. F., E. B. Boskamp, D. J. Schaefer, W. D. Barber, and R. H. Vander Heiden, 1998, *Estimating Local SAR Produced by RF Transmitter Coils: Examples Using the Birdcage Coil,* Abstracts of the International Society of Magnetic Resonance in Medicine, 6th Meeting, Sydney, Australia, p. 649.

91. Edelstein, W. A., T. H. Foster, and J. F. Schenck, 1985, *The Relative Sensitivity of Surface Coils to Deep Lying Tissues*, Abstracts of the Society of Magnetic Resonance in Medicine, Berkeley, pp. 964–965.

92. IEC 60601-1-1, Medical Electrical Equipment—Part 1: General Requirements for Safety; Safety Requirements for Medical Electrical Systems, 1992-06, Amendment 1, 1995-11 (General), International Electrotechnical Commission (IEC)*, 3, rue de Varembé, P. O. Box 131, CH-1211 Geneva 20, Switzerland, (in the United States, copies of this standard can be obtained from the American National Standards Institute (ANSI), 11 West 42 nd Street, New York, NY 10036).

93. Roemer, P. B., W. A. Edelstein, C. E. Hayes, S. P. Souza, and O. M. Muller, 1990, "The NMR phased-array," *Magn. Reson. Med.*, **16**:192–225.

94. Ginefri, J. C., L. Darrasse, and P. Crozat, 2001, "High-temperature superconducting surface coil for in vivo microimaging of the human skin," *Magn. Reson. Med.*, **45**(3):376–382.

95. Carlson, J. W., 1987, "An algorithm for NMR imaging reconstruction based on multiple RF receiver coils," *J. Magn. Reson.*, **74**:376–380.

96. Hutchinson, M. and U. Raff, 1988, "Fast MRI data acquisition using multiple detectors," *Magn. Reson. Med.*, **6**(1):87–91.

97. Kwiat, D., S. Einav, and G. Navon, 1991, "A decoupled coil detector array for fast image acquisition in magnetic resonance imaging," *Med. Phys.*, **18**(2):251–265.

98. Kelton, J. R., R. L. Magin, and S. M. Wright, 1989, "An algorithm for rapid image acquisition using multiple receiver coils," *Eighth Annual Meeting of the Society for Magnetic Resonance in Medicine*, Amsterdam, Netherlands, p. 1172.

99. Ra, J. B. and C. Y. Rim, 1993, "Fast imaging using subencoding data sets from multiple detectors," *Magn. Reson. Med.*, **30**(1):142–145.

100. Sodickson, D. K. and W. J. Manning, 1997, "Simultaneous acquisition of spatial harmonics (SMASH): fast imaging with radiofrequency coil arrays," *Magn. Reson. Med.*, **38**(4):591–603.

101. Pruessmann, K. P., M. Weiger, M. B. Scheidegger, and P. Boesiger, 1999, "SENSE: Sensitivity encoding for fast MRI," *Magn. Reson. Med.*, **42**(5):952–962.

CHAPTER 9
INSTRUMENTATION DESIGN FOR ULTRASONIC IMAGING

Kai E. Thomenius
GE Corporate Research and Development
Schenectady, New York

9.1 INTRODUCTION

The purpose of this chapter is to show how piezoelectric transduction, sound wave propagation, and interaction with scattering targets are taken advantage of in image formation with an ultrasound instrument. These instruments have evolved over the last 40 years from relatively simple hand-moved scanners built around an off-the-shelf oscilloscope to rather sophisticated imaging computers. Much technology has been perfected during this evolution. For example, transducers have grown from circular single-element probes to precision arrays with more than 1000 elements. With better front-end electronics, the operating frequencies have increased as weaker echoes can be handled. As the gate counts of VLSI ASICs (very large-scale integration application-specific integrated circuits) have increased, the numbers of processing channels in array-based systems have risen. With the introduction of reasonably low-cost high-speed (20 to 60 MHz) 8- to 14-bit analog-to-digital (A/D) converters, digital beam formation has become the standard. Further, we are witnessing today the beginning of a shift to completely software-based beam formation that has the potential of elimination of the very high development costs of ASICs. Along with these developments is a shift to more and more compact systems. Throughout its history, medical ultrasound has been a very dynamic field; it appears that this will not change in the near future. The organization of this chapter is based on the discussion of a block diagram of a generalized ultrasound system. Each component of the block diagram will be reviewed in considerable detail. Different design approaches for the various blocks will be reviewed and their advantages and disadvantages discussed. Those areas of the block diagram which are targets of significant current research are summarized along with the major industry trends.

9.2 BASIC CONCEPTS

9.2.1 Image Formation

Image formation in medical ultrasound is accomplished by a pulse-echo mechanism in which a thin ultrasound beam is transmitted and echoes generated by the interaction of that beam with scattering targets are received by a transducer or a set of transducer elements. The transmit and receive processing used to create this beam is referred to as *beam formation*. Due to its central role in ultrasonic imaging, beam formation will be discussed in detail later on.

The strength of the received echoes is usually displayed as increased brightness on the screen (hence the name for the basic ultrasonic imaging mode, B-mode, with B for brightness). A two-dimensional data set is acquired as the transmitted beam is steered or its point of origin is moved to different locations on the transducer face. The data set that is acquired in this manner will have some set of orientations of the acoustic rays. The process of interpolating this data set to form a TV raster image is usually referred to as scan conversion. With Doppler signal processing, mean Doppler shifts (which correspond to velocities of the scatterers such as red blood cells) at each position in the image can be determined from as few as 4 to 12 repeated transmissions. The magnitudes of these mean frequencies can be displayed in color superimposed on the B-mode image and can be used to show areas with significant blood flow.

9.2.2 Physical Constants and Typical System Operating Parameters

It may be useful to consider typical system operating parameters. The following table lists some physical constants that help define the operating parameters of today's systems:

Typical attenuation in tissue	0.5 dB/cm · MHz for one-way travel
Speed of sound in tissue	1540 m/s (or roughly 13 μs/cm for round-trip travel)

One of the challenges of ultrasonic imaging relates to that very high attenuation. To put this in numerical terms, a typical 5-MHz transducer is expected to penetrate approximately 10 cm. Thus, the signal leaving the transmitting transducer will undergo attenuation in the order of 25 dB before it reaches a scattering site. At that point, a small fraction of the energy will be reflected, let us say the reflected echo will be another 30 dB down; and the return will bring about another 25 dB of attenuation. Thus, the entire attenuation has been about 80 dB. A typical ultrasound image will contain some 40 to 50 dB of dynamic range; hence, needless to say, there is a strong need for careful low-noise designs for ultrasound front ends.

The following table gives some system design parameters commonly used for B-mode imaging:

Transducer frequencies	2–15 MHz
Transducer bandwidth	50–90% fractional bandwidth
Typical depths of penetration	18 cm (abdominal imaging)
	16 cm (cardiac imaging)
	5 cm (small parts and peripheral vascular imaging)
Time to acquire one 20-cm acoustic ray	~260 μs
Pulse repetition frequency (PRF)	4 kHz
Typical number of rays in an image	128–400
Data acquisition frame rates	10–80 frames/s

Due to frequency-dependent attenuation, applications with greater penetration requirements use the lower transducer frequencies. The instrument parameters have been selected or have evolved to their current values as manufacturers have optimized their instruments to the needs of the various clinical applications. Given compromises that have to be made, resolution of scanners is been limited to roughly 0.4 mm with 7- to 12-MHz transducers to approximately 2 to 4 mm with the 2.5- to 3.5-MHz transducers. The penetration at which these resolutions can be achieved is approximately 4 cm for the higher frequencies and 15 cm or more for the lower frequencies. Whether or not this performance can be achieved on any given patient is dependent on factors such as uniformity of speed of sound, which is highly patient dependent (O'Donnell, 1988). The degree of and correction for sound speed variations in ultrasound systems continues to receive much attention (Fink, 1992; Flax, 1988; Li, 1995; Nock, 1988; O'Donnell, 1988; Trahey, 1988; Zhu, 1993a, 1993b; Krishnan, 1996; Rigby, 2000; Silverstein, 2001).

9.2.3 Clinical Applications

B-mode imaging has found numerous uses in today's clinic (Goldberg, 1990; Sarti, 1987). Some of these are

Abdominal imaging	Identification of tumors, cysts in liver, kidneys
Cardiology	Valvular insufficiency (flail leaflet), myocardial dyskinesis, septal defects, congenital malformations

Obstetrics	Fetal growth, congenital malformations
Peripheral vasculature	Extent of plaque, blood vessel tortuosity

Many of these diagnoses are based on relatively gross anatomical information that is available from the ultrasound image. In addition there is a large amount of additional information imparted to the echoes by the scattering process. Some of this information is displayed on B-mode images and is of major value to the clinician. This information is critical to diagnoses such as diffuse disease processes, the identification of tumors, quality of myocardial dynamics, and so forth. It is for these reasons the signal integrity and retention of maximum dynamic range is of key value in the image formation process.

Sales of ultrasound instruments are divided among the four areas listed above roughly as follows (source: Klein Biomedical Consultants):

Radiology	39%
Cardiology	35%
Obstetrics/gynecology	16%
Peripheral vasculature	5%

This gives a rough idea of the level of utilization in the several areas; however, it also should be noted that the marketplace is currently undergoing significant changes with the health-care reform activity. Also, there is much overlap between the segments. For example, many radiologists do perform obstetric or peripheral vascular examinations and echocardiologists perform increasing amounts of peripheral vascular work. In terms of instrumentation sales, these are believed to be approximately $4.0 billion in year 2008. The growth of the total revenues has flattened of the last decade; however, there are areas such as highly miniaturized systems that are experiencing double digit growth rates as new markets are opening up. Ultrasound is also seen as a likely beneficiary of the reduced spending in the very high-end of imagers such as CT, PET, SPECT, and MRI scanners.

9.2.4 Classifications of Ultrasound Instruments

Ultrasonic instruments can be classified in many of different ways (Christensen, 1988). Among these are

Types of electronic beam steering	Phased arrays versus steering by element selection
Clinical applications	See Sec. 9.2.3
Nature of beam formation	Analog versus digital
Portability	Console-based systems versus handhelds

With respect to steering methods, the huge majority of instruments (perhaps more than 99 percent) sold today are electronically (as opposed to mechanically) steered. Phased-array systems are dominant in echocardiographic applications where aperture size is limited by rib spacings, while the other beam-steering methods are more often used in radiologic and obstetric and gynecological examinations. The latter grouping is sometimes referred to as *general imaging ultrasound*. The shift to digital beam formation is accelerating, and it is likely that today nearly all instruments sold will have digital beam formers. This is true even for the lower-price points.

9.3 TYPICAL SYSTEM BLOCK DIAGRAM

The block diagram in Fig. 9.1 shows the signal-processing steps required for B-mode image formation. The actual implementations vary considerably among manufacturers and the types of systems. For example, the grouping of functions might be different from one system to the next, depending

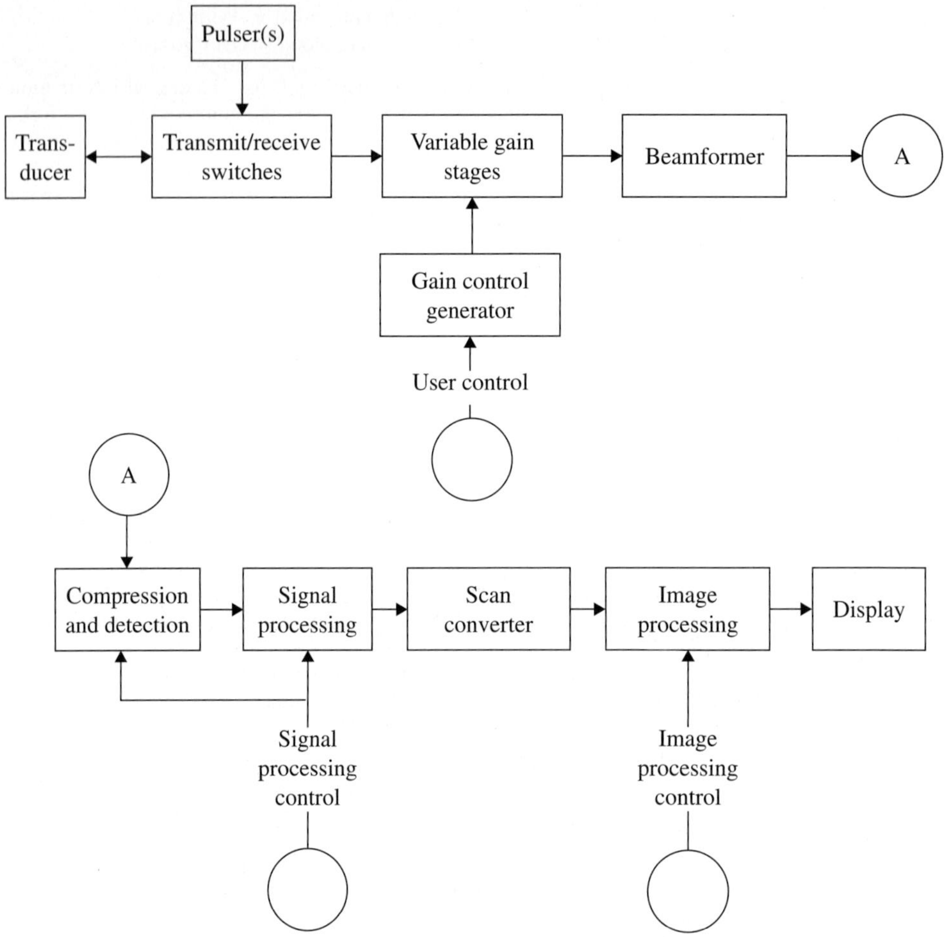

FIGURE 9.1 Block diagram of a typical ultrasound system. The blank circles represent points of at which user control is introduced.

on the choices made by the system designers; however, the basic functionality shown by each block has to be there.

One point that the block diagram may not convey adequately is the degree of duplication of functions in today's systems. For example, in systems with 128 processing channels, there will usually be 128 pulsers, 128 transmit/receive switches (T/R switches), and so forth. In such systems the use of large-scale integration and application specific integrated circuits (ASICs) is highly important for cost and space reduction. For the most part, the block diagram for digital and analog beam formers is quite similar, although there will usually be a large number of additional support circuitry required for synchronization, interpolation, and decimation of the sampled waveforms, and so forth.

Depending on the particular system implementation, the full RF bandwidth will be retained through the top part of the block diagram. The class of heterodyned systems performs frequency mixing at the beam former level, and the signal spectrum is shifted to either an intermediate frequency or all the way to the baseband. With digital beam formers, A/D conversion occurs after the variable gain stages. The digital beam former systems can be designed with similar heterodyning approaches, although there are many different approaches to delay generation. In addition to the digital and analog forms of beam formers, it is also possible to use charge-coupled devices for this purpose and these, in fact, are receiving increased attention at the present time.

The following paragraphs introduce and describe briefly the functions of the most important blocks in Fig. 9.1. The most important of these will receive greater attention in the remainder of the chapter.

9.3.1 B-Mode Transducers

As has been noted in the previous chapter, the mode of transduction in ultrasound systems takes advantage of the piezoelectric characteristic of certain ceramics. There are several types of transducers currently in use, and the nature of processing of acoustic data is different among them. These differences are highlighted in later sections as appropriate.

The piezoceramics can be fabricated in a number of ways to perform B-mode imaging. In its simplest form, the B-mode transducer is a circular *single-element transducer* with a fixed geometric focus. This type of a transducer has been replaced today by more sophisticated multielement transducers, although some extremely low-cost systems based on mechanically driven single-element probes are available. The next more complicated designs are *annular arrays* that are also circular but, as the name implies, are composed of several (4 to 12) rings. These transducers can be used with mechanically steered systems, although very few, if any, are currently available. Both the single-element and annular-array transducers usually have concave-curved transmitting surface or an acoustic lens to focus the acoustic energy at a given location. The next broad transducer category is that of *linear arrays* which are built by dividing a piezoceramic strip into a large number of line-source-like elements. The number of elements in such arrays can exceed 200, although 128 is a typical number. A variation of the linear array is the *curvilinear array* that is built on a curved surface. With linear arrays the acquired image is rectangular in shape, while with curvilinear arrays (and single element, annular arrays, and certain linear arrays) it is sector shaped. Both linear and curvilinear arrays have either a lens or are curved to focus the ultrasound in the plane perpendicular to the imaging plane. With both of these types of arrays, focusing in the image plane is done electronically. Finally, in order to improve on slice thickness, some form of electronic elevation focusing is being introduced into today's systems. This is realized by the use of multiple rows of elements that form a two-dimensional array of elements (Wildes, 1997). Arrays which are connected to form a symmetrical aperture about the center line are sometimes referred to either as 1.25-D or 1.5-D arrays, depending on whether improved slice thickness in the elevation direction is achieved by increasing the aperture size or by performing electronic focusing with those rows of elements. Finally, in the last 5 years, two-dimensional (or 2D) arrays, which are capable of steering the acoustic beam in two dimensions, have become commercially available. These are aimed largely at the echocardiology market.

The transducer or transduction itself has received considerable attention from researchers due to its critical position in the signal-processing sequence (Hunt, 1983; Szabo, 2004). Much progress has been made in the areas of sensitivity, bandwidth, and the use of composite materials. Bandwidths of today's transducers can exceed 80 percent of the center frequency. This gives the system designer additional flexibility with the available imaging frequencies and allows the optimization of image quality among the various imaging modes as well as over a larger cross section of patients. There is some potential of increasing the transmitted signal bandwidths to more than 100 percent with a new class of transducers referred to as *single-crystal relaxors*. Also, the Khuri-Yakub Ultrasound Group at Stanford University has shown that silicon-based MEMS (microelectromechanical systems) devices can be made to perform transduction for ultrasound purposes (Johnson, 2002).

9.3.2 Pulser, T/R Switch, Variable Gain Stage (or TGC Amplification)

This group of blocks is among the most critical from the analog signal-to-noise ratio point of view (Analog Devices, 1999; Schafer, 1985; Wells, 1983). The piezoceramic array elements are energized with the pulser and the transduction occurs as has been described. With the newer generation of instruments, the excitation waveform is typically a short burst of one- to three-cycle duration. Earlier generations (pre-Doppler) of instruments tended to use shock excitation with very wide bandwidths. The transducer element, with its limited bandwidth, filters this signal both during transmission and reception to a typical burst. The pulser voltages used vary considerably but values around 150 V are common. Use of a short burst (say with a bandwidth in the 30 to 50 percent range) can give the system designer the ability to move the frequency centroid within the limits of the transducer bandwidth. In some imaging modes such as B-mode, the spatial-peak temporal-average intensity (I_{spta}, an FDA-regulated acoustic power output parameter) value tends to be low; however, the peak pressures tend to be high. This situation has suggested the use of coded excitation, or transmission of longer codes that can be detected without loss of axial resolution (Chiao, 2005). In this manner the average acoustic power output can be increased and greater penetration depth realized.

The T/R switches are used to isolate the high voltages associated with pulsing from the very sensitive amplification stage(s) associated with the variable gain stage (or TGC amplifier for time gain compensation). Given the bandwidths available from today's transducers (80 percent and more in some cases), the noise floor assuming a 50-Ω source impedance is in the area of few microvolts rms. With narrower bandwidths this can be lowered, but some imaging performance will be lost. If the T/R switch can handle signals in the order of 1 V, the dynamic range in the neighborhood of more than 100 dB may be achieved. It is a significant implementation challenge to have the noise floor reach the thermal noise levels associated with a source impedance; in practice there are a good number of interfering sources that compromise this. In addition, some processing steps such as the T/R switching cause additional losses in the SNR.

The TGC stages supply the gain required to compensate for the attenuation brought about by the propagation of sound in tissue. During the echo reception time that ranges from 40 to 240 μs, the gain of these amplifiers is swept over a range approaching 60 to 70 dB, depending on the clinical examination and the number of A/D converter bits available. The value of this gain at any depth is under user control with a set of slide pots often referred to as the TGC slide pots. The dynamic range available from typical TGC amplifiers is in the order of 60 dB. One can think of the TGC amplifiers as providing a dynamic range window into the total range available at the transducer. This is illustrated in Fig. 9.2.

It is interesting to note that the commercial impact of multichannel ultrasound instruments is such that special purpose TGC amplifier ICs have been developed for this function by major integrated circuit manufacturers (Analog Devices, 1999; Texas Instruments, 2006).

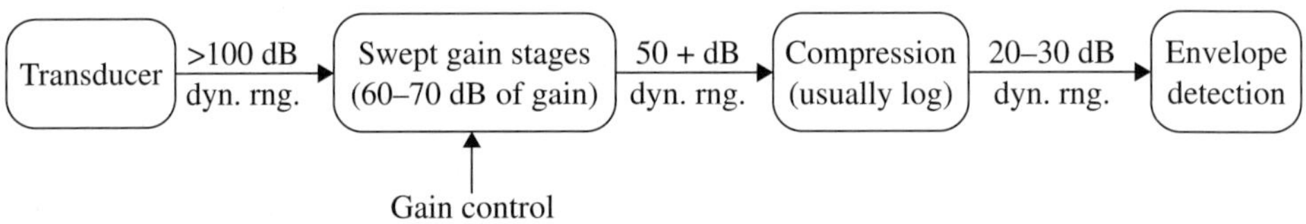

FIGURE 9.2 Front-end block diagram with signal-processing steps and corresponding dynamic ranges.

9.4 BEAM FORMATION

Beam formation can be considered to be composed of two separate processes: beam steering and focusing (Macovski, 1983; Hedrick, 1996). The implementation of these two functions may or may not be separated, depending on the system design. Focusing will be discussed first.

9.4.1 Focusing

Analogously to optics, the spatial variation in system sensitivity can be modified by the action of focusing on the transmitted acoustic beam and, during reception, on its echoes. One can view focusing as the modification of the localized phases (or, more correctly for wideband systems, time shifts)

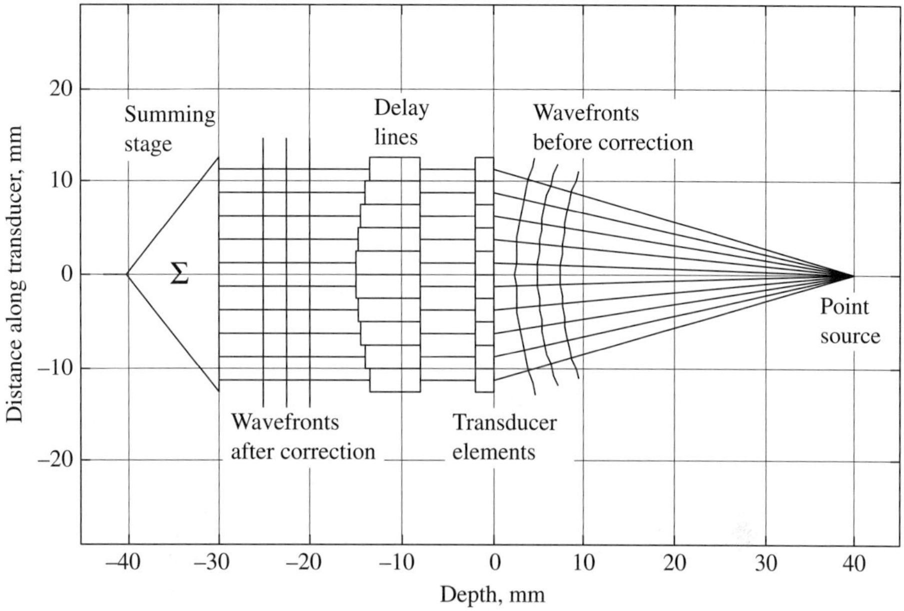

FIGURE 9.3 Schematic of focusing during reception. The echoes from a point source (at 40 mm) are shown impinging on a transducer array. The difference in the reception times is corrected by the delay lines. As an example, the echo will be received first by the center elements. Hence, their delays are the longest.

of the acoustic beam so as to cause constructive interference at desired locations. One simple way to accomplish focusing is by curving the transducer element so as to form a phase front that, after traveling a defined distance, will cause the beam to add constructively at a desired focal point. With transducer arrays the formation of the desired phase front during transmission can be accomplished by electronically altering the sequence of excitation of the individual elements. Similarly, during reception, the signals from the array elements can be routed through delay lines of appropriate lengths so that echoes from specific locations will have constructive interference (Thurstone, 1973). These processes are shown schematically in Fig. 9.3.

As suggested by Fig. 9.3, the echoes from a point source will have a spherical wavefront. The center elements of the array will receive these echoes at first, while the outer elements will receive them last. To compensate for this and to achieve constructive interference at the summer, the center elements will be given the longest delays as suggested by the length dimension of the delay lines. The calculations to determine the differential delays among the received echoes are straightforward.

An attractive formalism for expressing the array-based focusing in mathematical terms is due to Trahey (1988). The total transmitted pressure wave $T(t)$ at a point p can be expressed as a sum of the contributions from N array elements as follows:

$$T(t) = \sum_{n=1}^{N} \frac{A_T(n)}{r(n)} S\left[t - t_T(n) + \frac{r(n)}{c}\right] \tag{9.1}$$

where $A_T(n)$ = the pressure amplitude contribution of the nth element of the array at point p
$r(n)$ = the distance from the nth element to the focus
$S(t)$ = the waveshape of the pressure pulse generated by any given element of the array
$t_T(n)$ = the focusing time delay for element n shown as the length of delay lines in Fig. 3
c = the speed of sound in the medium

Assuming that at location p there is a point target with reflectivity W_p, then the signal after the summer in Fig. 9.3 can be described by

$$R(t) = W_p \sum_{n=1}^{N} \frac{A_R(n)}{r(n)} T\left[t - t_R(n) + \frac{r(n)}{c}\right] \tag{9.2}$$

where $A_T(n)$ = the pressure amplitude contribution of the nth element to echoes from point p
$T(t)$ = given by Eq. (9.1)
$t_R(n)$ = the receive focusing delay for element n

The remaining parameters of Eq. (9.2) were defined in Eq. (9.1). It should be noted that the $A_T(n)$ and $A_R(n)$ terms in Eqs. (9.1) and (9.2) will, in general, be different since the transmit and receive operation need not be symmetric. The terms include tissue attenuation, element sensitivity variation, and transmit or receive apodizations.

It might be useful at this point to discuss several methods by which the receive delays for either focusing or beam steering are implemented. The previous paragraph refers to the use of delay lines for this purpose. Analog delay lines are an older, albeit a very cost-effective method. However, lumped-constant delay lines do suffer from several limitations. Among these is the limited bandwidth associated with longer delay lines. Delays needed for focusing for most apertures are less than 0.5 μs; however, for phased-array beam steering (see below) they may be as long as 8 μs for larger apertures required for 2.5- to 3.5-MHz operation or up to 5 μs required for 5- to 7-MHz operation. Delay lines suitable for the latter case are relatively expensive. In addition, there are concerns about the amplitude variations with tapped delay lines as different taps are selected, delay uniformity over a production lot, and delay variations with temperature. In response to these difficulties, there has been a major migration to digital beam formation over the last 15 years (Thomenius, 1996).

An alternate method of introducing focusing delays for both analog and digital beam formers is by heterodyning (Maslak, 1979). This is usually done in conjunction with mixing the received signal with a lower local oscillator frequency with the goal of moving the received energy to a different location on the frequency spectrum. If the phase of the local oscillator is varied appropriately for each of the array signals, the location of constructive interference can be placed at a desired location. The limitations of this are associated with the reduced bandwidth over which the delay correction will be accurate and the reduced range of phase correction that is possible. Finally, as noted above, focusing (and beam steering) can be accomplished by relatively straightforward digital techniques in a digital beam former. A number of different methods of digital beam former implementation have been published in the sonar and ultrasound literature (Mucci, 1984; Steinberg, 1992).

Figure 9.4 shows the formation of the focal region for a 20-mm aperture circular transducer with a geometric focal distance of 100 mm and being excited with a CW signal of 3.0 MHz. At the left-hand side of the pressure profile, the rectangular section from –10 to 10 mm corresponds to the pressure at the transducer aperture. In the near field, there are numerous peaks and valleys corresponding to areas where there is partial constructive and destructive interference. As one looks closer to the focal region, these peaks and valleys grow in size as the areas of constructive and destructive interference become larger. Finally, at the focal point the entire aperture contributes to the formation of the main beam.

One way of assessing the quality of a beam is to look at its beamwidth along the transducer axis. The 6- and 20-dB beamwidths are plotted in Fig. 9.5. It is important to recognize that the beamwidths shown are those for a circular aperture. Due to the axial symmetry, the beamwidths shown will be achieved in all the planes, that is, in the imaging plane as well as the plane perpendicular to it (this plane is often referred to as the *elevation plane* from radar literature). This will not be the case with rectangular transducers. With rectangular transducers, the focusing in the image plane is done electronically, that is, in a manner similar to annular arrays. However, in the elevation plane, the focusing in today's systems is done either by a lens or by the curvature of the elements. In such cases, the focal location will be fixed and cannot be changed electronically. Remedying this limitation of rectangular transducers is currently an active area of study. The introduction of the so-called *elevation focusing* will be discussed in greater detail in a later chapter.

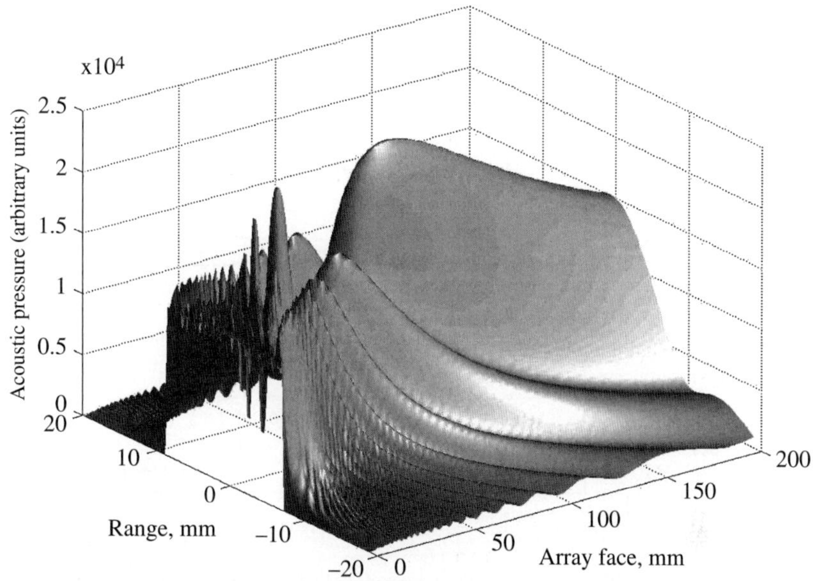

FIGURE 9.4 Spatial cross-sectional pressure distribution due to a circular transducer with a diameter of 20 mm, frequency of 3.0 MHz, and a radius of curvature of 100 mm. The left-hand side corresponds to the transducer aperture. All spatial dimensions are in millimeters, the *x* and *y* axes are not to scale. This pressure distribution was determined by the use of angular spectrum techniques (Schafer, 1989).

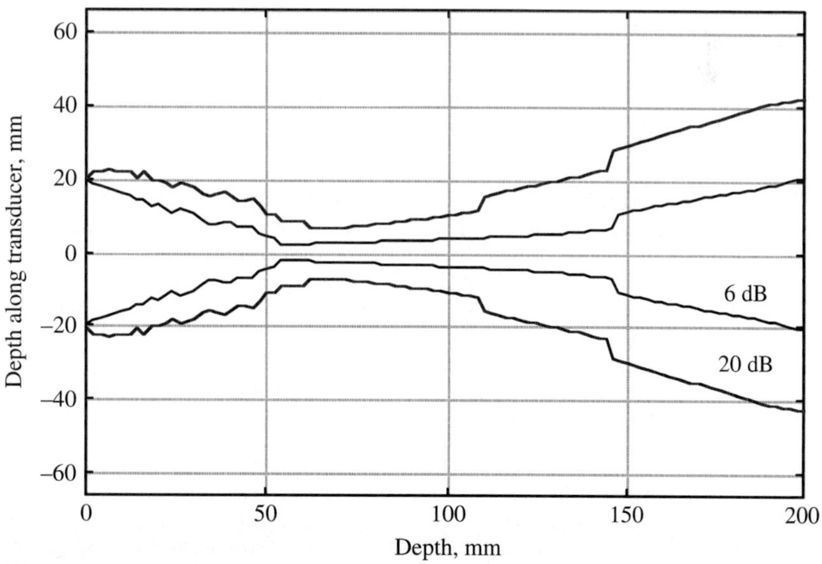

FIGURE 9.5 A 6- and 20-dB beam contours for the beam generated by a 3.0-MHz, 19-mm aperture, 100-mm focus transducer undergoing CW excitation. The *x* and *y* axes are to scale so that one can get a sense of the beam dimensions with respect to the depth of penetration.

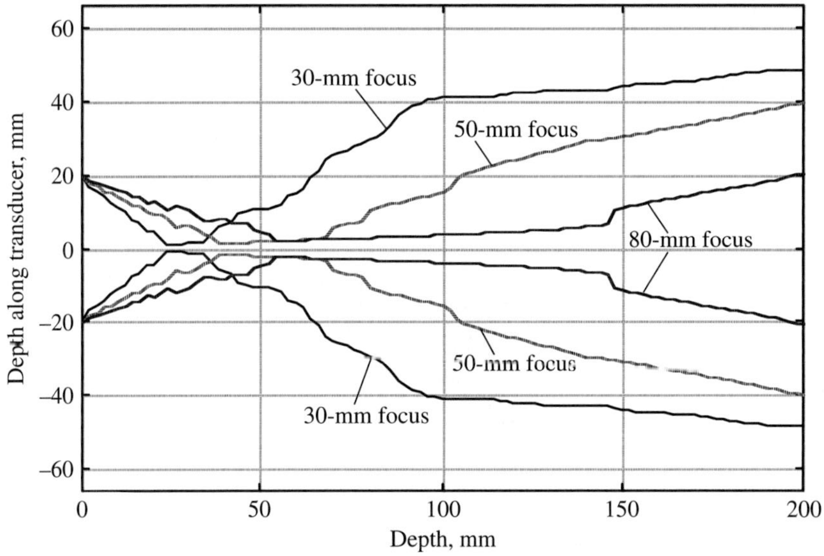

FIGURE 9.6 Three 6-dB beam profiles for the above transducer. The radius of curvature for the three cases are 30, 50, and 80 mm. The graph with a solid line corresponds to the 30-mm focus, the dot-dash (.-) to the 50-mm focus, and the dash-dash (--) to the 80-mm focus.

There is considerable diagnostic importance that has to be attached to the 20-dB and higher beamwidths. Sometimes the performance at such levels is discussed as the *contrast resolution* of a system. The wider the beam is, say at 40 dB below the peak value at a given depth, the more unwanted echoes will be brought in by these sidelobes. Small cysts and blood vessels may be completely filled in by such echoes. Also, if a pathological condition alters the backscatter strength of a small region by a modest amount, this variation may become imperceptible due to the acoustic energy introduced by the sidelobes.

With array-type transducers, the timing of the excitation or the delays during reception can be varied, thereby causing a change in the focal location. This is demonstrated in Fig. 9.6 where three different 6-dB profiles are shown. During transmission, the user can select the focal location as dictated by the clinical study being performed. There are operating modes sometimes referred to as *composite imaging modes,* in which the final image is a composite of the data acquired during transmission and reception from several distributed focal locations. Not only can one change the transmit focal location but also the aperture size and transmit frequency between the transmissions. With this approach, one can achieve superior image uniformity at the expense of frame rate that will be decreased by the number of transmissions along a single look angle.

During reception there is yet another possibility to improve the performance of the system. As the transmitted wavefront travels away from the transducer, the delays introduced by the focusing can be varied, thereby changing the receive focus with the location of the wavefront. At the same time, the size of the receive aperture can be continuously increased to try to maintain beamwidth as long as possible. This approach is referred to as *dynamic focusing* and is now a standard feature in all systems. In a typical implementation, dynamic focusing is introduced via course delays that may correspond to increments of the A/D converter sampling clock. A fine delay can be introduced via interpolation filtering. Such a system may have a sampling clock that samples data at 40 MHz, or in 25-ns increments. With 4:1 interpolation, this timing increment can be reduced to 6.25 ns. Thus, digital beam formation offers excellent time delay accuracy.

9.4.2 Beam Steering

There are a number of different methods of steering an acoustic beam currently in use. These can be grouped into three categories:

1. Mechanical
2. Element selection
3. Phased array

The major implication of the selection of the beam-steering approach is in the cost of the instrument. Mechanically steered systems tend to be the simplest and hence the least expensive while the phased arrays the most expensive. The great majority of recent vintage scanners have the latter two types of beam steering. The following paragraphs will discuss the relevant features of each of the three types.

Mechanical Steering. The simplest method of beam steering is to use a mechanism to reorient a transducer (usually a circular aperture) to a predetermined set of orientations so as to capture the required two-dimensional data set. This approach was dominant during the 1970s; however, in the last 15 years electronically steered systems have become, by far, the most popular and driven the mechanical systems to near extinction. Mechanically systems usually use either a single-element transducer or an annular array transducer. The former will have a fixed focus, while the latter does allow the focal point to be moved electronically. A very interesting application for mechanical scanners today is that of extremely low-cost systems (Richard, 2008) and the use in the acquisition of 3D data sets. In the latter case, a conventional linear or curvilinear array is mechanically oscillated rapidly and a real-time 3D volume is acquired. The resulting surface-rendered images are sometimes referred to as 4D images, time being the fourth dimension (GE, 2008).

There are a number of very attractive aspects to mechanical systems with their circular transducers. Among these are low cost and the ability to focus the sound beam electronically in all planes, in other words, axisymmetrically. The low cost arises from the relatively low cost associated with the mechanisms used to move the transducer in comparison to the multielement transducer arrays and supporting electronics needed with electronic beam-steering. The ability to focus the acoustic energy in all planes is a unique advantage since most mechanically steered systems use either single element–or annular array–type transducers. With the annular arrays, one has the capability to move the focus electronically in all planes as opposed to the electronically steered arrays that are usually rectangular in shape and will have electronic focusing only in one plane. The number of transducer elements in an annular array is usually less than 12, typically 6 or 8. With electronically steered arrays, the element count can go as high as 192 or more. As a consequence, the costs tend to be higher. Today, mechanical scanners exist in niche markets such as intravascular imaging or in extremely low-cost systems, or with 3D/4D scanners.

Some of the drawbacks associated with mechanical steering involve the inertia associated with the transducer, the mechanism, and the fluid within the nosepiece of the transducer. The inertia introduces limitations to the frame rate and clearly does not permit random access to look angles as needed (the electronically steered approaches supply this capability). The ability to steer the beam at will is important in several situations but most importantly in Doppler applications. Further, electronic beam formation affords numerous advanced features to be implemented such as the acquisition of multiple lines simultaneously and elimination of the effects due to variations in speed of sound in tissue.

Steering by Element Selection. Another relatively low-cost beam-steering approach involves steering of the beam by element selection. In this approach one doesn't strictly steer the beam but rather changes the location of its origin, thereby achieving coverage over a 2D tomographic slice. This method is applied with both linear and curvilinear arrays. Figure 9.7 shows the application in the case of curvilinear arrays. For this particular case, the 2D image will be sector shaped; with linear arrays it will, of course, be rectangular. This is a relatively low-cost approach since aside from the multiplexing

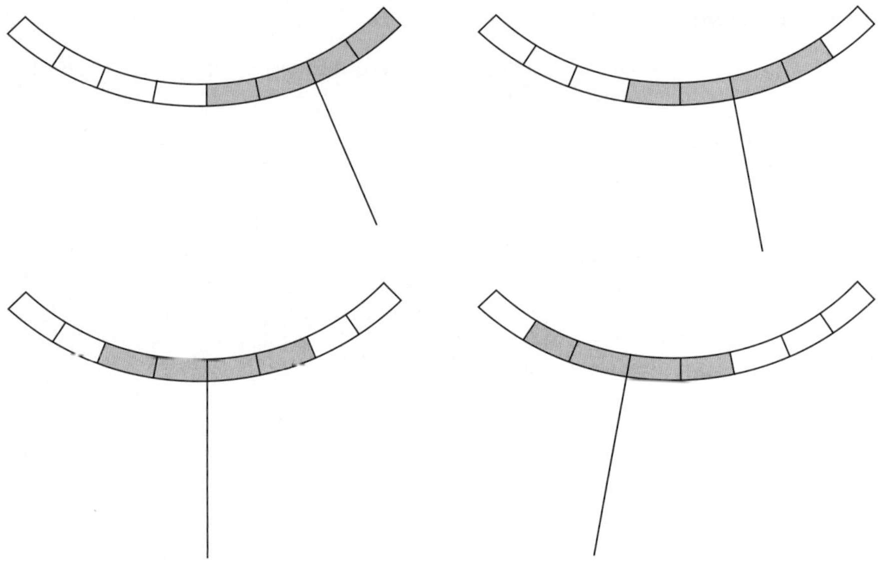

FIGURE 9.7 Steering by element selection for a curvilinear array. The beam will shift to a new location as the center of the active aperture is shifter over the entire array.

required for element selection, the electronics required to accomplish beam formation are merely the focusing circuitry.

The line densities achievable with this mode of beam steering are not as variable as with mechanical steering since they will be dependent on element center-to-center spacing. There are methods by which one can increase the achieved line density. Figure 9.7 shows an acquisition approach, sometimes referred to as *full stepping*. The line density with full stepping will equal to the element density since the beam center will always be at the junction between two elements. It is possible to change the sizes of the transmit and receive apertures, and thereby change the transmit and receive beam centers. This changes the effective location of the resultant beam and introduces the possibility of an increased line density. Half and even quarter stepping schemes exist, although care has to be taken that the resulting beam travels along the expected path.

Steering with Phased Arrays. The most complicated form of beam steering involves the use of phased-array concepts derived from radar (Steinberg, 1976; Thurstone, 1973; Thomenius, 1996). Most ultrasonic phased-array transducers have between 64 and 256 elements. Transmit beam steering in phased-array system is achieved by adding an incremental delay to the firing time of each of the array elements that is linearly related to the position of that element in the array. Similarly, during reception the delay that is applied to each of the echoes received by the array elements is incremented or decremented by a position-dependent factor. This differential time delay Δt is given by

$$\Delta t = \frac{x_n}{c}\tan(\theta) \tag{9.3}$$

where x_n = the location of the array element n
θ = the desired beam-steering angle

The application of such a delay increment during reception is illustrated in Fig. 9.8. Since the beam-steering angle is such that the echoes will reach the array elements toward the bottom of the figure first, the longest delays will be imposed on the echoes from those elements. Since the

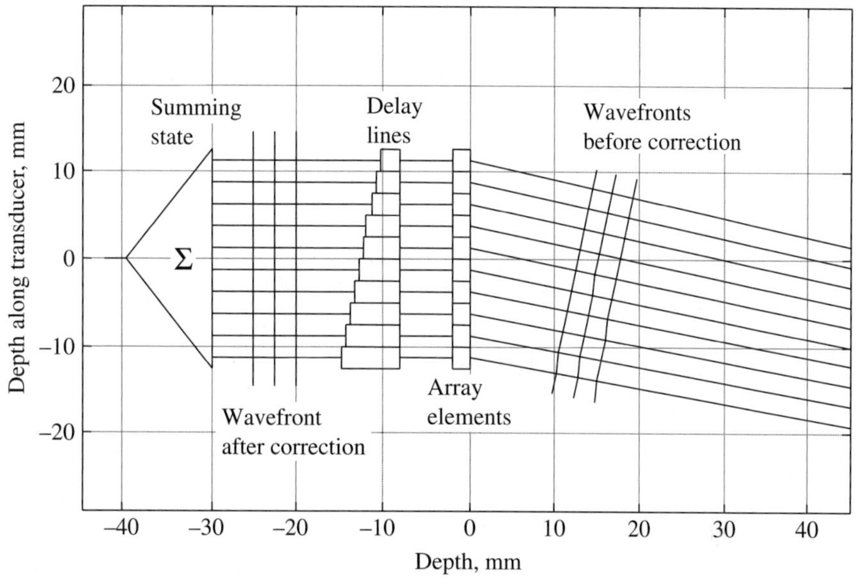

FIGURE 9.8 Beam steering in a phased array system during reception. A linearly increasing time delay differential is introduced for each of the delay lines to correct for the linear time difference in the arrival times.

wavefront is linear, the arrival times of the remaining echoes have a linear relationship; hence the linear decrement on the delays from one element to the next.

In addition to beam steering, one can combine focusing and beam-steering delays in the same process. This is illustrated in Fig. 9.9. Echoes from a near field point source (at 40 mm) are shown arriving at the array elements. The arrival times of the echoes have a nonlinear component so the

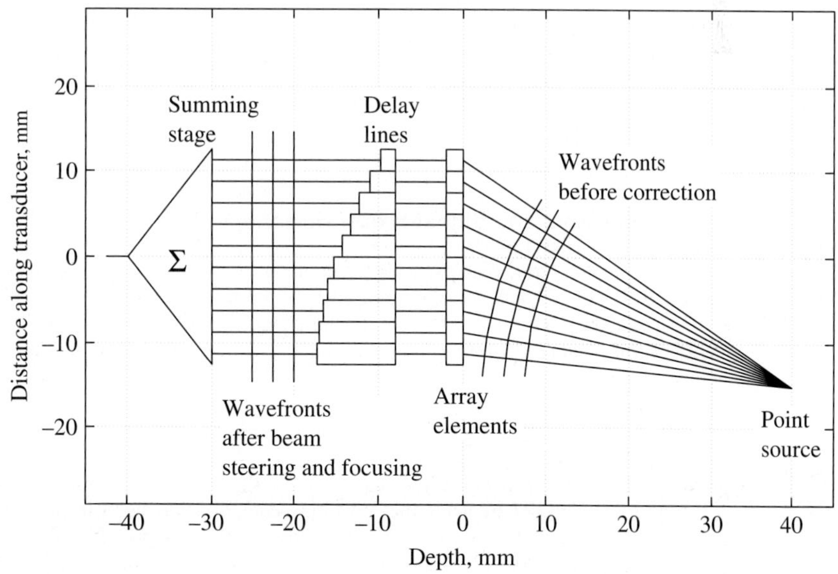

FIGURE 9.9 Schematic of beam steering and focusing during reception in a phased array type system. In addition to the focusing correction (also shown in Figure 3), phased array systems add a linearly increasing time shift to the receive delay lines to achieve constructive interference in the desired direction.

delay lines cannot compensate with a simple linear increment as in Fig. 9.8. It can be shown easily that the differential time delay between channels can be determined from the law of cosines.

As the process of steering and focusing is repeated for a sequence of look angles, a sector-shaped image data set is acquired. The line density available from phased array scanners is not as restricted as with curvilinear arrays, but some limitations exist in certain systems due to the relatively large size of delay increments available in tapped delay lines. Heterodyned systems and digital beam formers have less limitations in this area.

All linear and curvilinear array systems have limitations or design constraints associated with the existence of *grating lobes* that are due to leakage of acoustic energy in unwanted angles. It turns out that for certain larger center-to-center array element spacings, there will be constructive interference at look angles other than the main beam. This difficulty is particularly serious for the case of phased-array systems due to the need for beam steering. It turns out that the grating lobes move with the steering angle and can be brought into the visible region by the simple act of beam steering.

Grating lobes can be completely avoided by keeping the center-to-center spacing at one-half of the wavelength at the highest contemplated operating frequency. (It turns out this is completely analogous to the familiar sampling theorem which states the temporal sampling has to occur at a frequency that is twice that of the highest spectral component of the signal being processed (Steinberg, 1976). This has the drawback of forcing the use of a larger number of array elements and their processing channels. This, and the expensive processing required for each channel, causes the phased-array systems to be more expensive than the other types.

9.4.3 Harmonic Imaging

A recent development in the area of B-mode imaging is that of imaging of the harmonics generated during propagation of acoustic waves in tissue (Averkiou, 1997; Jiang, 1998; Wells, 2006; Kollmann, 2007). While all the discussion so far has assumed that the propagation of these waves is linear, this is actually not the case. There is a difference in the speed of sound in the compressional and rarefactional parts of the acoustic pressure wave. As a consequence, the positive half of a propagating sine wave will move faster than the negative half; this results in the formation of harmonic energy. An image formed from such harmonics will be superior to that from the fundamental part of the spectrum due to reduced reverberant energy and narrower main beam. The acceptance of this form of imaging has been so rapid that in certain clinical applications (e.g., echocardiology), harmonic imaging is the default operating mode. From the point of view of beam former design, there is relatively little that needs to be done differently other than developing the ability to transmit at a lower frequency while receiving at twice the transmit frequency.

9.4.4 Compression, Detection, and Signal-Processing Steps

The sequence of the processing steps between the beam former and scan conversion is different among the various commercial systems, but the goals of the steps remain the same. The beam former output will be a wideband RF, an IF, or a complex baseband signal, which will usually be bandpass filtered to reduce out-of-band noise contributions. In systems with very wideband processing, frequency diversity techniques (e.g., split spectrum processing) can be brought into play to try to reduce the impact of coherent interference or speckle.

With most of today's systems, there is a logarithmic compression of the amplified signal after beam formation amplification. The goal of this is to emphasize the subtle gray level differences between the scatterers from the various types of tissues and from diffuse disease conditions.

There are a number of ways that envelope detection has been implemented. In purely analog approaches, simple full wave-rectification followed by a low-pass filtering has been shown to work quite well. It is also possible to digitize the RF signals earlier in the processing chain, perform the compression and detection processes digitally, and use quadrature detection to determine the signal envelope.

9.5 SIGNAL PROCESSING AND SCAN CONVERSION

As has been noted earlier, the image data is acquired on a polar coordinate grid for sector scanners (e.g., mechanically steered, curvilinear arrays, and phased-array systems) and in a rectangular grid for linear arrays. It is clearly necessary to convert this image data into one of the standard TV raster formats for easier viewing, recording, computer capture, and so on. This is performed in a module in most systems referred to as the *scan converter*. The major function of the scan converter is that of interpolation from, say, a polar data grid to that of the video pixel space. Given the data rates required, it is a challenging task but one that most commercial systems appear to have well under control.

The early scan converters used several clever schemes to accomplish the required function. For example, with sector scanners, certain systems would modulate the A/D converter sampling rate by the look angle of the beam former in such a way that every sample would fall onto a raster line. Once the acoustic frame was completed, and the data along each horizontal raster line was read out, simple one-dimensional interpolation was performed (Park, 1984). The need for more sophisticated processing brought about two-dimensional interpolation methods. Among the first in this area were Larsen et al. (1980) whose approach involved the use of bilinear interpolation. With the Larsen et al. (1980) approach, the sampling rate along each scan line was held at a uniform value that was high enough to meet the sampling theorem requirements. With two axial samples along two adjacent acoustic lines, the echo strength values at each of the pixels enclosed by the acoustic samples were determined. This could be done by either (1) interpolating angularly new axial sample values along a synthetic acoustic ray that traversed through the pixel in question and then performing an axial interpolation along the synthetic ray or (2) by interpolating a new axial sample along both real acoustic rays and then performing the angular interpolation. This basic approach has become the most widely used scan-conversion method among the various manufacturers and seems to have stood the test of time.

More recently, researchers have continued to study the scan conversion problem with different approaches. For example, Berkhoff et al. (1994) have evaluated "fast algorithms" for scan conversion, that is, algorithms that might be executed by software as opposed to dedicated hardware. Given the rapid trend to faster, more powerful, and cost-effective computers and their integration with ultrasound systems, it is likely that more of the scan conversion function will be done in software. Berkhoff et al. (1994) recommend two new algorithms that they compare with several conventional interpolators. With the speed of computers improving at a steady pace, these approaches are increasingly attractive (Chiang, 1997). In other words, with the cost of some of the hardware components such as A/D converters coming down, oversampling the acoustic line data may permit the replacement of bilinear interpolation with simple linear interpolation. Oversampling by a factor of two along with linear interpolation was found to be superior to bilinear interpolation under certain specific circumstances. It is clear there is additional work in this area yet.

9.6 CURRENT TRENDS IN MEDICAL ULTRASOUND SCANNERS

In comparison to the other major imaging modalities such as CT, MRI, or PET, ultrasound is blessed with a relatively simple image data transduction method. The arrays described earlier are all handheld; this is in direct contrast with the other modalities that require room-sized gantries with rapidly rotating 64-slice or higher banks of detectors or superconductive magnetic field sources with rapidly changing gradient fields. The remainder of an ultrasound scanner is largely digital signal processing. The activities of the microelectronics and personal computer industries have brought about major size, cost, and power requirement reductions in the circuitry used by ultrasound scanners. This became apparent with the rapid migration of key parts of the scanner from hardware to software, usually PC-based software. Key among these were transmit beam formation, the scan converter function, and pled with the continuous reduction in feature size of semiconductors along the lines of Moore's law, have enabled the introduction of laptop-sized ultrasound scanners. This particular market segment is the fastest growing for ultrasound scanners (Klein Biomedical Consultants). It is likely that this miniaturization trend will continue even though Moore's law is showing signs of slowing down.

Perhaps the most exciting miniaturization-related aspect of the current miniaturization trend is the introduction of software-based beam formers. As noted in the previous paragraph, much of the back end of a scanner has already migrated to software, usually on a conventional PC. For several years, this migration appeared to be stalled at the receive beam former. However, the last several years have seen the beam former yielding to DSP (digital signal processor) and even PC-based operation (Napolitano, 2003; Verasonics, 2007). Based on these developments, ultrasound scanners have a data acquisition front end with the array, front-end signal processing (e.g., TGC amplifiers) up to the A/D converters, and a processor-based back end. If Moore's law can muster even mild reduction in size for PCs, tomorrow's ultrasound scanner is likely to be a small handheld unit.

9.7 SUMMARY

This chapter has reviewed the fundamentals of the design of ultrasound scanners with a particular focus on the beam formation process. Different types of image data acquisition methods are described along with a historical view of the developments. The entire process from transduction to scan conversion has been discussed, including the relevant numerical specifications of the various parameters. Finally, the current dominant trends that will define the future of these scanners have been discussed. Unlike most of the other imaging modalities, it appears that ultrasound will continue to remain highly dynamic with large shifts in applications away from the radiology and cardiology departments in hospitals to far closer to the offices of the general practitioners and the patient.

REFERENCES

Analog Devices, http://www.analog.com/library/analogDialogue/archives/33-05/ultrasound/.

Averkiou, M. A., Roundhill, D. N., and Powers, J. E., (1997), "A new imaging technique based on the nonlinear properties of tissues." *IEEE Ultrasonics Symposium Proceedings*, pp. 1561–1566.

Berkhoff, A. P., Huisman, H. J., Thijssen, J. M., Jacobs, E. M. G. P., and Homan, R. J. F., (1994), "Fast scan conversion algorithms for displaying ultrasound sector images," *Ultrasonic Imaging*, **16**:87–108.

Chiang, A. M. and Broadstone, S. R., (1997), "Portable ultrasound imaging system," U. S. Patent No. 5,590,658, issued Jan. 7, 1997.

Chiao, R. Y., and Hao, X., (2005), "Coded excitation for diagnostic ultrasound: a system developer's perspective," *IEEE Trans UFFC*, **52**:160–170.

Christensen, D. A., (1988), *Ultrasonic Bioinstrumentation*, Chap. 6, John Wiley & Sons, New York.

Fink, M., (1992), "Time reversal of ultrasonic fields: Part I—basic principles," *IEEE Transactions on Ultrasonics, Ferroelectrics, and Frequency Control.* **39**:555–566.

Flax, S. W., and O'Donnell, M., (1988), "Phase aberration correction using signals from point reflectors and diffuse scatterers: Basic principles," *IEEE Transactions on Ultrasonics, Ferroelectrics, and Frequency Control.* **35**:758–767.

GE, http://www.gehealthcare.com/usen/ultrasound/4d/virtual_4d_mini.html.

Goldberg, B. B., and Kurtz, A. B., (1990), *Atlas of Ultrasound Measurements*, Year Book Medical Publishers, Chicago.

Hedrick, W. R. and Hykes, D. L., (1996), "Beam steering and focusing with linear phased arrays," *Journal of Diagnostic Medical Sonography*, **12**:211–215.

Hunt, J. W., Arditi, M., and Foster, F. S., (1983), "Ultrasound transducers for pulse-echo medical imaging," *IEEE Transactions on Biomedical Engineering,* **30:**453–481.

Jiang, P., Mao, Z., and Lazenby, J., (1998), "A new tissue harmonic imaging scheme with better fundamental frequency cancellation and higher signal-to-noise ratio," *Proceedings of the 1998 IEEE Ultrasonics Symposium.*

Johnson, J., et al., (2002), "Medical imaging using capacitive micromachined ultrasonic transducer arrays," *Ultrasonics*, **40**(1–8):471–476.

Kollmann, C., (2007), "New sonographic techniques for harmonic imaging—underlying physical principles," *European Journal of Radiology*, **64**(2):164–172.

Krishnan, S., Li, and P. C., O'Donnell, M., (1996), "Adaptive compensation of phase and magnitude aberrations," *IEEE Transactions on Ultrasonics, Ferroelectrics, and Frequency Control*, **43**:44–55, January.

Larsen, H. G. and Leavitt, S. C., (1980), "An image display algorithm for use in real-time sector scanners with digital scan conversion," *1980 IEEE Ultrasonics Symposium Proceedings*, pp. 763–765.

Li, P. C. and O'Donnell, M., (1995), "Phase aberration correction on two-dimensional conformal arrays," *IEEE Transactions on Ultrasonics, Ferroelectrics, and Frequency Control*, **42**:73–82.

Macovski, A., (1983), *Medical Imaging Systems*, Chap. 10, Prentice-Hall, Englewood Cliffs, N.J.

Maslak, S. H., (1979), "Acoustic imaging apparatus," U.S. Patent No. 4,140,022, issued Feb. 20, 1979.

Mucci, R. A., (1984), "A comparison of efficient beamforming algorithms," *IEEE Transactions on Acoustic Speech and Signal Processing*, **32**:548–558.

Napolitano, D., et al., (2003), "Zone-based B-mode imaging," *IEEE 2003Ultrasonics Symposium Proceedings*, pp. 25–28.

Nock, L., Trahey, G. E., and Smith, S. W., (1988), "Phase aberration correction in medical ultrasound using speckle brightness as a quality factor," *Journal of Acoustic Society of America*, **85**:1819–1833.

O'Donnell, M. O. and Flax, S. W., (1988), "Phase aberration measurements in medical ultrasound: human studies," *Ultrasonic Imaging*, **10:**1–11.

Park, S. B. and Lee, M. H., (1984), "A new scan conversion algorithm for real-time sector scanner," *1984 IEEE Ultrasonics Symposium Proceedings*, pp. 723–727.

Richard, W. D., et al., (2008), "A low-cost B-mode USB ultrasound probe," *Ultrasonic Imaging*, **30**:21–28.

Rigby, K. W., (2000), "Real-time correction of beamforming time delay errors in abdominal ultrasound imaging," *Proc. SPIE*, **3982**:342–353.

Sarti, D. A., (1987), *Diagnostic Ultrasound—Text and Cases*, Year Book Medical Publishers, Chicago.

Schafer, M. E. and Lewin, P. A., (1984), "The influence of front-end hardware on digital ultrasonic imaging," *IEEE Transactions on Ultrasonics. Ferroelectrics. and Frequency Control,* **31**:295–306.

Schafer, M. E. and Lewin, P. A., (1989), "Transducer characterization using the angular spectrum method," *Journal of Acoustic Society of America,* **85**:2202–2214.

Silverstein, S. D., (2001), "A robust auto-focusing algorithm for medical ultrasound: consistent phase references from scaled cross-correlation functions," *IEEE Signal Processing Letters*, **8**(6):177–179.

Steinberg, B. D., (1976), *Principles of Aperture and Array System Design,* John Wiley & Sons, New York.

Steinberg, B. D., (1992), "Digital beamforming in ultrasound," *IEEE Transactions on Ultrasonics, Ferroelectrics, and Frequency Control*, **39**(6):716–721, November.

Szabo, T. L., (2004), *Diagnostic Ultrasound Imaging: Inside Out,* Elsevier Science:549 pages

Texas Instruments, http://focus.ti.com.cn/cn/lit/an/slaa320/slaa320.pdf.

Thomenius, K. E., (1996), "Evolution of ultrasound beamforming," *Proceedings of IEEE Ultrasonics Symposium,* IEEE Cat. No. 96CH35993, pp. 1615–1622.

Thurstone, F. L. and von Ramm, O. T., (1973), "A new ultrasound imaging technique employing two-dimensional electronic beam steering," In: *Acoustical Holography*, Booth Newell, vol 5, pp. 249–259, Plenum Press, New York.

Trahey, G. E. and Smith, S. W., (1988), "Properties of acoustical speckle in the presence of phase aberration. Part I: First order statistics," *Ultrasonic Imaging*, **10**:12–28.

Verasonics, http://www.verasonics.com/pdf/verasonics_ultrasound_eng.pdf.

Wells, P. N., (2006), "Ultrasound imaging," *Physics in Medicine and Biology*, **51**(13):R83–R98.

Wildes, D. G., et al., (1997), "Elevation performance of 1.25D and 1.5D transducer arrays," *IEEE Transactions on Ultrasonics, Ferroelectrics, and Frequency Control,* **44**:1027–1037.

Zhu, Q. and Steinberg, B. D., (1993a), "Wavefront amplitude distortion and image sidelobe levels: Part I—Theory and computer simulations," *IEEE Transactions on Ultrasonics, Ferroelectrics, and Frequency Control,* **40**:747–753.

Zhu, Q. and Steinberg, B. D., (1993b), "Wavefront amplitude distortion and image sidelobe levels: Part II—In vivo experiments," *IEEE Transactions on Ultrasonics, Ferroelectrics, and Frequency Control,* **40**:754–762.

CHAPTER 10
THE PRINCIPLES OF X-RAY COMPUTED TOMOGRAPHY

Peter Rockett
Oxford University, Oxfordshire, England

Ge Wang
University of Iowa, Iowa City, Iowa

10.1 INTRODUCTION

The object of x-ray computed tomography is to reproduce, in the form of digital data, the internal structure of three-dimensional bodies with as little distortion as possible. This is achieved by the mathematical reconstruction of a series of two-dimensional images produced by the projection of an x-ray beam through the body in question. In this respect the form and functioning of x-ray computed tomography systems are closely linked to the physics of the interaction of x-ray photons with the material body and to the principles that govern the mathematical process of image reconstruction. In depth these are complex matters, but the fundamentals can be simply explained to provide a sound basis for further study.[1–4]

The relative values of absorption and transmission of adjacent elemental ray paths in an x-ray beam provide the contrast in a projected image. The associated interaction of the x-rays with the material body can be defined in terms of collision cross sections that describe the probability of particular events occurring along the ray path.[5] Here, the principal effects, for x-ray energies below 1 MeV, are identified in Sec. 10.2 as the photoelectron event and the Compton scattering event.[6,7] These effects are combined to define a linear attenuation coefficient $\mu(x)$ that describes the variation of photon intensity Φ along the ray path x according to the exponential relation $\Phi = \Phi_0 \exp(-\int_l \mu(x)\, dl)$, where Φ_0 is the initial intensity of the ray and l is the path length.

Taking account of the role of attenuation in the formation of image contrast, the method by which the material features along the ray path are reconstructed can be mathematically formulated in detail. In this process it is recognized that the two-dimensional object function $f(x, y)$ is represented by the attenuation coefficient $\mu(x, y)$. A key assumption in this process is that x-ray photons travel in straight lines and that diffraction effects may be ignored. Given the energetic nature of x-ray photons, this is a reasonable approach and enables considerable simplification of the underlying principles that are discussed in Sec. 10.3. It also permits the observation that from a mathematical view, a perfect representation of the body is theoretically possible, provided the requisite type and number of projected images are available.

An important feature in the formulation of the tomographic reconstruction process is the assumption of linearity attached to the various operations involved. This leads to the concept of a spatially invariant point-spread function that is a measure of the performance of a given operation. In practice the transformation associated with an operation involves the convolution of the input with the point-spread function in the spatial domain to provide the output. This is recognized as a cumbersome mathematical process and leads to an alternative representation that describes the input in terms of sinusoidal functions. The associated transformation is now conducted in the frequency domain and with the transfer function described by the Fourier integral. In discussing these principles, the functions in the spatial domain and the frequency domain are considered to be continuous in their respective independent variables. However, for practical applications the relevant processes involve discrete and finite data sampling. This has a significant effect on the accuracy of the reconstruction, and in this respect certain conditions are imposed on the type and amount of data in order to improve the result.

In Sec. 10.3 the mathematical principles of computed tomography are developed by considering the formation of images by the relative attenuation of a series of parallel ray paths. The fundamental quantity in this process is the line integral $\int_{AB} f(x, y)\, ds$ of the object function $f(x, y)$, which is the radon transform, or projection, of the object along the ray path AB. This leads to the concept that a parallel projection of an object, taken at an angle θ in physical space, is equivalent to a slice of the two-dimensional Fourier transform of the object function $f(x, y)$, inclined at an angle θ in frequency space. According to a process known as the filtered back-projection, the object can be reconstructed by taking the Fourier transform of the radon transform, applying a weighting to represent the effect of discrete steps in projection angle θ, and back-projecting the result through the reconstruction volume.

A natural progression is to consider the advantages that divergent ray-path scanning provides and the increased complexity that this introduces. It should be appreciated that the cardinal measure for developments in computed tomography is, according to the mathematical view, increased computational efficiency with enhanced modeling accuracy, and from the systems view is faster data capture with improved image contrast and higher spatial resolution. These two aspects are inextricably linked, though it is reasonable to conclude that the extensive and continuous development in reconstruction algorithms has tended to be the catalyst for advancement.

The question of absolute accuracy will depend on considerations of what is practically achievable and directly relates to the type and extent of measured data and the configuration of the associated system. The components of a basic laboratory system will comprise a source of x-rays, a specimen stage, one or more imaging detector/camera devices, and a data acquisition system. The type of x-ray source employed will depend on the permissible exposure period and on the degree of resolution required. Large-area sources, measured in square millimeters, with high x-ray flux will be used where the object is liable to movement and the length of exposure is important, as is usually the case in medical imaging. However, small-area sources, measured in square micrometers, with relatively low x-ray flux will be used where resolution is important. This is usually the case for biological research where the application is generally referred to as microtomography, as discussed in Sec. 10.4. This activity is properly classed as microscopy, where the physical layout of the related system can provide high geometric magnification at the detector input plane of about 100 times and high spatial resolution of about 1 μm or better.

With provision for projected high magnification, the beam-line area is relatively extensive and can accommodate a range of ancillary equipment. This attribute makes the laboratory microtomography facility a very versatile instrument. It can operate in a variety of modes and support scanning strategies that are tailored to particular subject shapes, sizes, and material content. With large-area detectors, magnified images can be recorded with divergent cone-beam projection and provide information of the internal structure with a combination of specimen rotation and translation motion. With small-area detectors, images can be recorded with a collimated pencil-beam and transverse raster scanning of the specimen in the manner of a conventional light microscope. These detectors can be energy sensitive and provide information of the chemical composition in addition to structural morphology. Further, by optically collimating the primary x-ray beam to a secondary focus, it is possible to form images by the x-ray fluorescence emission process and hence provide a map of the atomic composition.

A further indication of the versatility of the projection x-ray microscope is the possibility of splitting the beam path in various ways to provide enhanced imaging detail by phase contrast. Although the assumption that diffraction effects may be neglected has proved to be an acceptable approximation for most attenuation contrast imaging applications, they can nevertheless be manipulated to reveal additional information. A medium of varying density will, by virtue of the associated changes in refractive index, create phase differences in the propagating waves of adjacent ray-paths.[8] Under normal circumstances these effects are small and would not be seen in the image. However, if the difference in phase is converted into spatial displacement, very fine detail emerge as phase contrast in the image. This method is currently receiving a great deal of attention as means of providing improved contrast.[9]

10.2 THE INTERACTION OF X-RAYS WITH MATTER

10.2.1 The Collision Model

X-rays are located at the high-energy end of the electromagnetic spectrum and obey the same laws and possess the same wave-particle duality characteristics attributed to visible light (Fig. 10.1). Their location in the energy E (J) distribution is measured by either the wavelength λ (m) value or the frequency ν (Hz) value of the radiation. As the energy of the radiation increases, the wavelength decreases, frequency increases, and the particle description becomes more appropriate. Since x-rays are to be found at the high-energy end, roughly covering the region 10^{18} to 10^{17} Hz, or 0.1 to 10 nm, we may usefully consider them to be photon particles with energy given by $E = h\nu = hc/\lambda$, where Plank's constant $h = 6.6 \times 10^{-34}$ J · s and the speed of light $c = 3.0 \times 10^8$ m/s. Our description of the interaction of x-rays with matter may thus follow the concept of photon particle encounters with material particles such as atoms and free electrons.

We may regard each encounter as a single identifiable process, involving an isolated absorbing or scattering center that acts independently of the surroundings. This is a classical approach to collision processes and leads to the perception of a measured cross section σ^τ (m^2) as representing the area, with reference to a particular collision event τ, occluded by a single absorbing or scattering center. With this representation, the probability P_τ of absorption, or scattering, for a monoenergetic beam of intensity Φ, passing through a thin homogeneous layer of thickness dx and unit cross section, can be

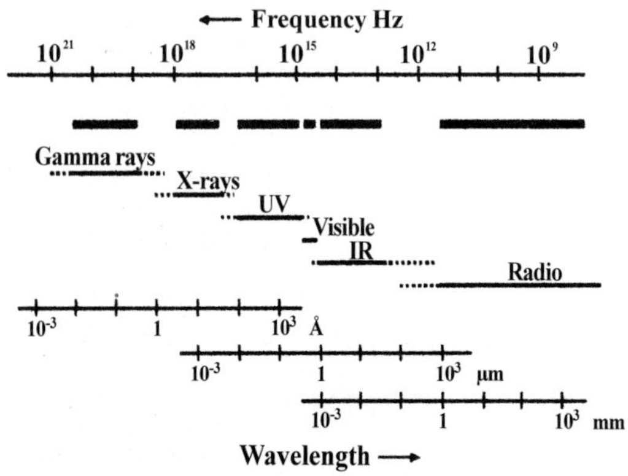

FIGURE 10.1 Electromagnetic spectrum.

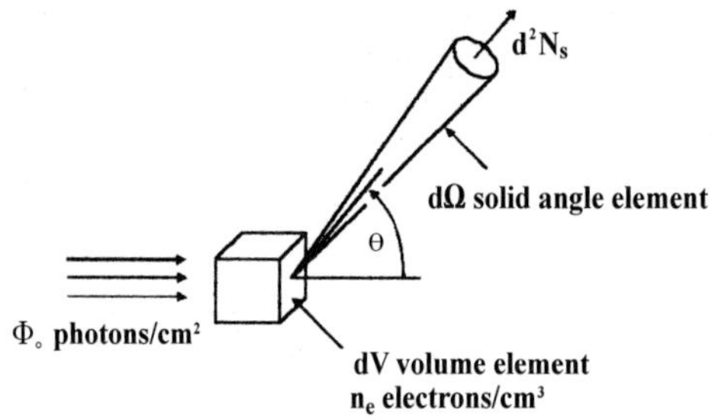

FIGURE 10.2 Photons scattered into solid angle $d\Omega$.

written as $P_\tau = d\Phi/\Phi = n_p\sigma^\tau\, dx$, where n_p is the number density of material atomic or electron particles. Hence, the number of photons dN_s/dV removed per unit volume for event τ is given by

$$\frac{dN_s}{dV} = -\frac{d\Phi}{dx} = \Phi n_p \sigma^\tau \tag{10.1}$$

The angular distribution of photons for scattering events is determined by considering the number of photons scattered at an angle θ into an elemental solid angle $d\Omega$. This leads to the concept of the differential collision cross section $(d\sigma/d\Omega)_\theta$, which can be defined by differentiating Eq. (10.1) with respect to $d\Omega$ to give

$$\frac{d^2N_s}{dV\, d\Omega} = \Phi n_p \left(\frac{d\sigma^\tau}{d\Omega}\right)_\theta \tag{10.2}$$

Here, $d\sigma$ is the probability that the incident photon will be deflected into the elemental solid angle $d\Omega$, so that d^2N_s is the number of photons scattered into $d\Omega$ from volume element dV, for incidence flux Φ (Fig. 10.2).

If the radiation is unpolarized, the differential collision cross section depends only on the angle of deflection θ, so the cross section σ can be determined by integrating $(d\sigma/d\Omega)_\theta$ over a hemisphere, according to

$$\sigma = \int_0^\pi \left(\frac{d\sigma}{d\Omega}\right)_\theta 2\pi \sin\theta\, d\theta \tag{10.3}$$

Since we may interpret the cross section σ^τ as the probability that a photon will be removed from the primary beam, for a single τ event collision site per unit area, the total cross section σ^T for all events can be expressed as

$$\sigma^T = \sum_\tau \sigma^\tau \tag{10.4}$$

where the σ^τ are now considered as components to the overall attenuation process.

10.2.2 Principal Photon Interactions

The principal collision processes observed for x-rays, in the low- to medium-energy range 0 to 200 keV, are photoelectric absorption and Compton scattering. *Absorption losses* refer to events that remove the incident photon from the primary beam by the complete conversion of its energy. *Scattering losses* refer to events that remove the incident photon from the primary beam by a fractional exchange of energy and the redirection of the path of propagation. The relative proportion of either process to the primary beam attenuation varies with x-ray energy. Another scattering process is Thompson scattering, which occurs at low energy and imparts very little energy to the absorber. This involves the interaction of the photon wave and an electron, with the electron-emitting electromagnetic radiation. Encounters of this type cause phase shifts in the incident photon wave and are the basis of phase contrast imaging. However, for attenuation contrast imaging, the effect of phase shift is assumed to be negligible.

For the photoelectric effect, a photon with energy $h\nu_0$ encounters an atom, is completely annihilated, and in the process ejects a bound electron from the atom with kinetic energy E_k. The vacant atomic bound state is repopulated from an adjacent level with the emission of a fluorescent x-ray photon. For Compton scattering, a photon with energy $h\nu_0$ encounters a free electron, is redirected though an angle θ with changed energy $h\nu'$, and the free electron recoils though an angle ϕ with received energy E_k. Both collision processes continuously remove photons from the x-ray beam as it progresses through a material body.

The Photoelectric Effect. The K, L, and M shell electrons of the colliding atom are the principle participants in the photoelectric interaction. When the incident photon possesses an energy $h\nu_0$ greater than the binding, or ionization energy I, the shell electron will be ejected with a kinetic energy E_k according to the conservation of energy relation:

$$h\nu_0 = E_k + I \tag{10.5}$$

The value of the absorption cross section increases with increasing binding energy I, so that a K-shell interaction is roughly 5 times more probable than an L-shell interaction. The event will most readily occur if the photon energy is comparable to the binding energy, in a manner somewhat like a resonance process. This behavior is borne out in practice where the photoelectric cross section σ^{pe} is seen to vary with the inverse cube of the photon energy $h\nu_0$, according to

$$\sigma^{pe} = k\frac{Z^4}{(h\nu_0)^3} \tag{10.6}$$

where the variation with atomic weight Z is a function of the penetration of the incident photon into the Coulomb field presented by the electron shell and k is a constant for that particular shell.

The momentum of the incident photons is mostly imparted to the atomic nucleus with the direction ϕ of the emitted photoelectrons predominantly toward larger angles (Fig. 10.3). The angle is determined by the direction of the electric field associated with the incident radiation. If it is linearly polarized, the photoelectron has a large component of velocity parallel to the electric field. However, at higher energies the photoelectron acquires a forward component of velocity from the incident radiation, as required from conservation of momentum.

The Compton Effect. The Compton effect refers to the scattering of incident photons by the interaction with free electrons. Here, an incident photon of energy $h\nu_0$ is scattered into the angle θ, with

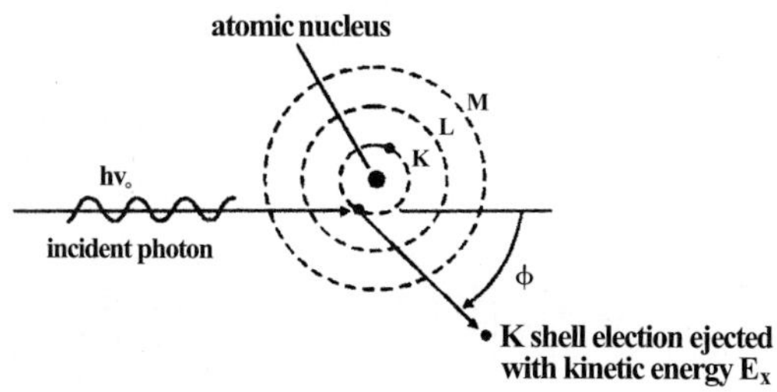

FIGURE 10.3 Photoelectric absorption with energy transfer to ionization and photoelectron motion.

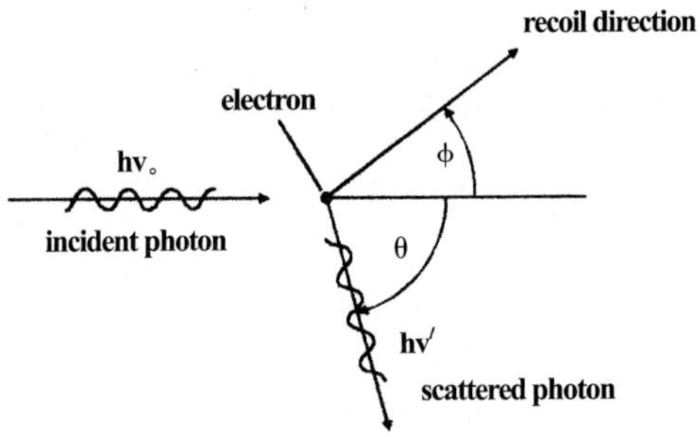

FIGURE 10.4 Geometry of Compton scattering.

reduced energy $h\nu'$, and the electron recoils through the angle ϕ, with increased kinetic energy E_k (Fig. 10.4). The fact that the electrons are free and not bound to an atom reduces the complexity of the problem. As a consequence, the principles of conservation of momentum can be invoked to determine the division of energy between the colliding particles. For the conservation of energy we have $h\nu_0 - h\nu' = E_k$. For conservation of momentum we have in the horizontal direction

$$\frac{h\nu_0}{c} = \frac{h\nu'}{c}\cos\phi + \sqrt{2m_0E_k}\cos\theta \tag{10.7a}$$

and in the vertical direction

$$0 = \frac{h\nu'}{c}\sin\phi + \sqrt{2m_0E_k}\sin\theta \tag{10.7b}$$

where m_0 is the rest mass of the electron. Combining these relations, we obtain an expression for the energy of the scattered photon in terms of the scattering angle:

$$h\nu' = \frac{h\nu_0}{1+\alpha(1-\cos\theta)} \tag{10.8}$$

and the angle of the scattered photon in terms of the electron recoil angle:

$$\cot\phi = (1+\alpha)\tan\left(\frac{\theta}{2}\right) \tag{10.9}$$

where $\alpha = h\nu_0/m_0c^2$ and $m_0c^2 = 0.511$ MeV. It is convenient to rewrite Eq. (10.8) in terms of wavelength, so that

$$\frac{c}{\nu'} - \frac{c}{\nu_0} = \lambda' - \lambda = \frac{h}{m_0c^2}(1-\cos\theta) \tag{10.10}$$

where $h/m_0c^2 = 2.246 \times 10^{-12}$ m is the Compton wavelength. This expression indicates that the change in wavelength, for a given angle of scattering θ, is independent of the incident photon energy.

The collision differential cross section is given by the Klein-Nishina relation:

$$d\sigma = \frac{r_e^2}{2}\left[\left\{1+\frac{\alpha^2(1-\cos\theta)^2}{(1+\cos^2\theta)[1+\alpha(1-\cos\theta)]}\right\}\frac{1+\cos^2\theta}{[1+\alpha(1-\cos\theta)]^2}\right]d\Omega \tag{10.11}$$

where the classical electron radius $r_e = (1/4\pi\epsilon_0)(e^2/mc^2)$. The scattered radiation is strongly peaked in the forward direction, where the cross section falls with increasing angle θ and falls off more

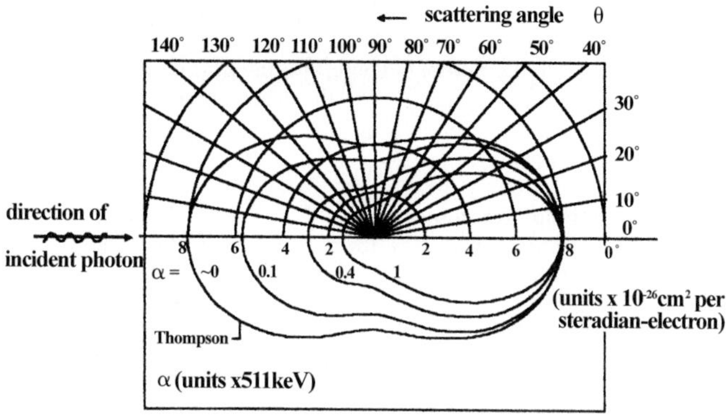

FIGURE 10.5 Compton collision differential cross section.

rapidly for higher values of α (Fig. 10.5). The cross section σ^c for the Compton interaction is found by integrating Eq. (10.11) over a hemisphere, to give

$$\sigma^c = \frac{3}{4}\sigma_o\left[\frac{2(1+\alpha)^2}{\alpha^2(1+2\alpha)} + \frac{\ln(1+2\alpha)}{\alpha}\left(\frac{1}{2} - \frac{1+\alpha}{\alpha^2}\right) - \frac{1+3\alpha}{(1+2\alpha)^2}\right] \tag{10.12}$$

where $\sigma_0 = 8\pi r_e^{2/3}$ is the cross section for Thomson scattering $\alpha \approx 0$.

With reference to Eq. (10.1), the energy ϵ lost from the primary beam per unit volume is given by

$$\in = -\frac{d(\Phi h v_0)}{dx} = \Phi h v_0 n_e \sigma^c \tag{10.13}$$

This can be resolved into the energy that appears as scattered radiation ϵ_s and the energy imparted to the recoil electron ϵ_e, so that $\epsilon = \epsilon_s + \epsilon_e$. With this interpretation we can define a scattering cross section according to $\epsilon_s = \Phi h v_0 n_e \sigma_s^c$ and where

$$\sigma_s^c = \frac{3}{8}\sigma_0\left[\frac{2(2\alpha^3 - 3\alpha - 1)}{\alpha(1+2\alpha)^2} + \frac{8\alpha^2}{3(1+2\alpha)^3} + \frac{\ln(1+2\alpha)}{\alpha^3}\right] \tag{10.14}$$

Similarly, we can define an absorption cross section $\epsilon_e = \Phi h v_0 n_e \sigma_e^c$, that is related to the total cross section according to

$$\sigma_e^c = \sigma^c - \sigma_s^c \tag{10.15}$$

The energy dependencies σ^c, σ_s^c, and σ_e^c can be evaluated from Eqs. (10.12) to (10.15) (Fig. 10.6).

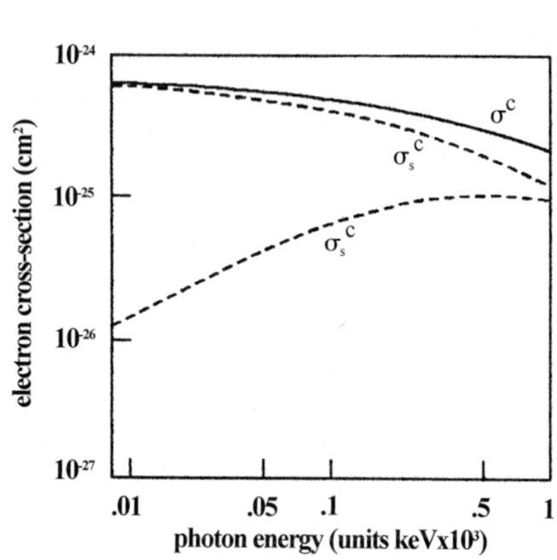

FIGURE 10.6 Compton interaction cross sections.

10.2.3 X-Ray Path Attenuation

For x-rays with energies in the range 0 to 200 keV, the principal mechanisms for attenuating the photon flux are those due to photoelectric absorption with n_a atoms/cm^3 and cross section σ^{pe} cm^2 and Compton collisions with n_e electrons/cm^3 and cross section σ^c cm^2. Therefore, according to Eq. (10.4), we can write the total atomic cross section as

$$\sigma^T = \sigma^{pe} + Z\sigma^c \qquad (10.16)$$

where Z is the atomic number. Therefore, integrating Eq. (10.1) for the removal of photons from a narrow x-ray beam of initial flux/m^2 Φ_0, over a path of length x, gives

$$\Phi = \Phi_0 \exp(-\sigma^T n_a x) \qquad (10.17)$$

This relation holds for monochromatic x-rays propagating through a homogeneous medium. The quantity $\sigma^T n_a$ is known as the linear attenuation coefficient μ, with photoelectric and Compton components

$$\begin{aligned} \mu^{pe} &= n_a \sigma^{pe} \\ \mu^c &= n_e \sigma^c \end{aligned} \qquad (10.18)$$

so that the overall attenuation coefficient is given by

$$\mu = \sigma^T n_a = \mu^{pe} + \mu^c \qquad (10.19)$$

According to Eq. (10.15), the linear attenuation coefficient for the Compton event can be separated into that due to absorption and that due to scattered radiation, so that

$$\mu^c = \mu_e^c + \mu_s^c \qquad (10.20)$$

This means that for a given material substance we have the linear attenuation coefficients grouped as follows:

- Total attenuation $\mu^{pe} + \mu^c$
- Total absorption $\mu^{pe} + \mu_e^c$
- Photoelectric absorption μ^{pe}
- Compton absorption μ_e^c
- Compton scattering μ_s^c

The variation of these terms with x-ray energy is usefully demonstrated for water (Fig. 10.7). With reference to the overall attenuation coefficient [Eq. (10.19)], and to the associated cross section [Eq. (10.16)], for each element there is a photon energy for which $\mu^{pe} = \mu^c$. Values of these energies can be used to indicate the region in which either process is dominant (Fig. 10.8).

The linear attenuation coefficient can be written as $\mu = \sigma^T N_A \rho / A$, where Avagadro's number $N_A = 6.02 \times 10^{23}$ mol^{-1}, A is the atomic weight, and ρ is the density. Given that the interaction cross section σ^T is not a function of the density of the medium, a mass absorption coefficient $\mu/\rho = \sigma^T N_A / A$ can be defined. This is related to the mass of a material required to attenuate an x-ray beam by a given amount. It is the form most often quoted for x-ray attenuation in tables of physical constants.

According to Eq. (10.17), the beam photon flux Φ can be written as

$$\Phi = \Phi_0 \exp(-\mu x) \qquad (10.21)$$

which is the familiar Beer-Lambert law for the attenuation of an x-ray beam passing through matter. When the medium is nonhomogeneous, the attenuation must be integrated along the ray-path length l according to $\Phi = \Phi_0 \exp(-\int_r \mu(x)\, dl)$. For the location $\mathbf{r}$ in two- or three-dimensional space, this becomes

$$\Phi = \Phi_0 \exp\left(-\int_l \mu(\mathbf{r})\, dl\right) \qquad (10.22)$$

If the x-ray source is polychromatic, the attenuation must be integrated over the wavelength λ as well, to give

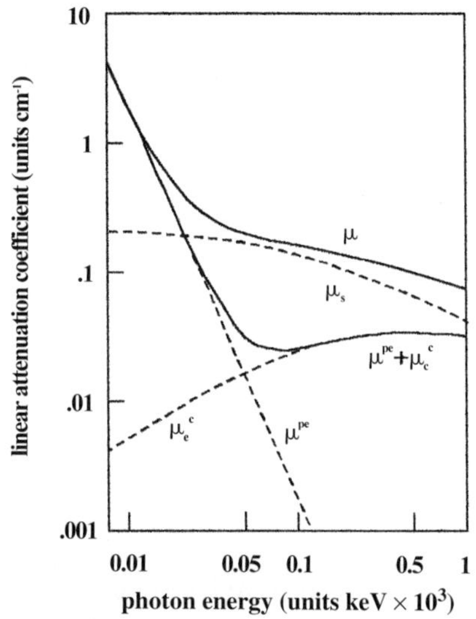

FIGURE 10.7 Linear attenuation coefficients for H_2O.

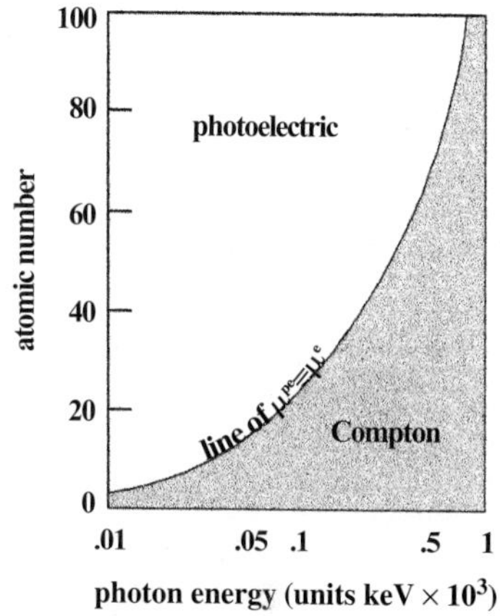

FIGURE 10.8 Region of dominant attenuation process.

$$\Phi = \Phi_0 \exp\left(-\int_\lambda \int_l \mu(\mathbf{r},\lambda)\, dl\, d\lambda\right) \tag{10.23}$$

The presence of water in biological substances, such as soft tissue, has lead to the creation of a unit of attenuation coefficient for tomographic imaging. This is the Hounsfield unit (HU), defined as

$$\mathrm{HU} = \frac{\mu(\text{substance}) - \mu(\text{water})}{\mu(\text{water})} \times 1000 \tag{10.24}$$

The usefulness of this unit for biological imaging is evident by comparing the values in HU for the widely disparate attenuating substances, such as air and bone. Here, air has a value of about −1000 HU and bone about +1000 HU.

10.3 THE MATHEMATICAL MODEL

10.3.1 Linear Systems and the Point-Spread Function

In dealing with the processes that are involved in tomographic reconstruction, the fundamental assumption is made that the individual systems perform linear operations. This ensures that simple relations exist between the input signals and the responding outputs. These systems may be treated schematically as black boxes, with an input $g_{\text{in}}(u)$, producing a corresponding output $g_{\text{out}}(u)$, where the independent variable u may be a one-dimensional time t, or displacement x, a two-dimensional position upon an x, y plane, or a three-dimensional position within an x, y, z volume (Fig. 10.9).

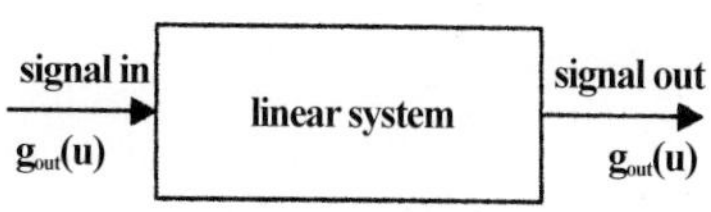

FIGURE 10.9 Black box representation of a linear system.

The principle of linearity prescribes that the weighted input $ag_{\text{in}}(u)$ will produce the output $ag_{\text{out}}(u)$, and the sum of two weighted inputs $ag_{\text{in}}^{(1)}(u) + bg_{\text{in}}^{(2)}(u)$ will produce the output $ag_{\text{out}}^{(1)}(u) + bg_{\text{out}}^{(2)}(u)$, for any real numbers a and b. We can further propose that the linear system be space invariant so that changing the position of the input merely changes the location of the output without altering its functional form. Hence, the image forming system can be treated as a linear superposition of the outputs arising from each of the individual points on the object. An estimate of the effect of the operation of the linear system on the contribution from each point will provide a measure of the performance.

If the operation of the linear system is symbolically represented as $L\{\}$, the relation between the input and output for independent variable u can be written as

$$g_{\text{out}}(u) = L\{g_{\text{in}}(u)\} \tag{10.25}$$

From the properties of the Dirac δ function, which represents a unit area impulse, defined as

$$\delta(u) = \begin{cases} \infty & u = 0 \\ 0 & \text{otherwise} \end{cases} \qquad \text{and} \qquad \int_{-\infty}^{\infty} \delta(u)\, du = 1$$

we have the sifting property $\int_{-\infty}^{\infty} g(u)\delta(u - u_0)\, du = g(u_0)$. Applying this property to Eq. (10.25) gives

$$g_{\text{out}}(u) = L\left\{\int_{-\infty}^{\infty} g_{\text{in}}(u')\,\delta(u' - u)\, du'\right\} \tag{10.26}$$

which expresses $g_{\text{out}}(u)$ as a linear combination of elementary δ functions, each weighted by a number $g_{\text{in}}(u')$. From the linearity principle, the system operator $L\{\}$ can be applied to each of the elementary functions so that Eq. (10.26) can be written as

$$g_{\text{out}}(u) = \int_{-\infty}^{\infty} g_{\text{in}}(u')L\{\delta(u' - u)\}\, du' \tag{10.27}$$

The quantity $L\{\delta(u' - u)\}$ is the response of the system, measured at point u in the output space, to a δ function located at the point u' in the input space, and is called the *impulse response.*

For image forming systems the impulse response is usually referred to as the *point-spread function* (PSF). In this case we consider the response at vector point $\mathbf{r}$ in the image space, to an irradiance distribution $\Phi_0(\mathbf{r}')$ located in object space. An element $d\mathbf{r}'$ located at $\mathbf{r}'$ will emit a radiant flux of $\Phi_0(\mathbf{r}')\, d\mathbf{r}'$, which will be spread by the linear operation $L\{\}$ over a blurred spot defined by the function $p(\mathbf{r}'; \mathbf{r})$. The flux density at the image point $\mathbf{r}$, from the object point $\mathbf{r}'$, will be given by $d\Phi_i(\mathbf{r}) = p(r'; \mathbf{r})\Phi_0(\mathbf{r})\, dr'$, so that the contribution from all points in the object space becomes

$$\Phi_i(\mathbf{r}) = \int_{-\infty}^{\infty} \Phi_0(\mathbf{r}')p(\mathbf{r}';\mathbf{r})\, d\mathbf{r}' \tag{10.28}$$

where $p(\mathbf{r}'; \mathbf{r})$ is the point-spread function. If the system is space invariant, a point source moved over the object space $\mathbf{r}'$ will produce the same blurred spot at the corresponding locations $\vec{\mathbf{r}}$ in the image space. In this case the value of $p(\mathbf{r}'; \mathbf{r})$ depends only on the difference between the location in the object space and the image space, namely $(\mathbf{r}' - \mathbf{r})$, so that $p(\mathbf{r}'; \mathbf{r}) = p(\mathbf{r}' - \mathbf{r})$ and Eq. (10.28) becomes

$$\Phi_i(\mathbf{r}) = \int_{-\infty}^{\infty} \Phi_0(\mathbf{r}')p(\mathbf{r}' - \mathbf{r})\, d\mathbf{r}' \tag{10.29}$$

Equation (10.29) is known as the two-dimensional [i.e., $\vec{\mathbf{r}} = (x, y)$] *convolution integral,* written as

$$g(x, y) = \int_{-\infty}^{\infty}\int_{-\infty}^{\infty} f(x', y')h(x - x', y - y')\, dx'\, dy' \tag{10.30}$$

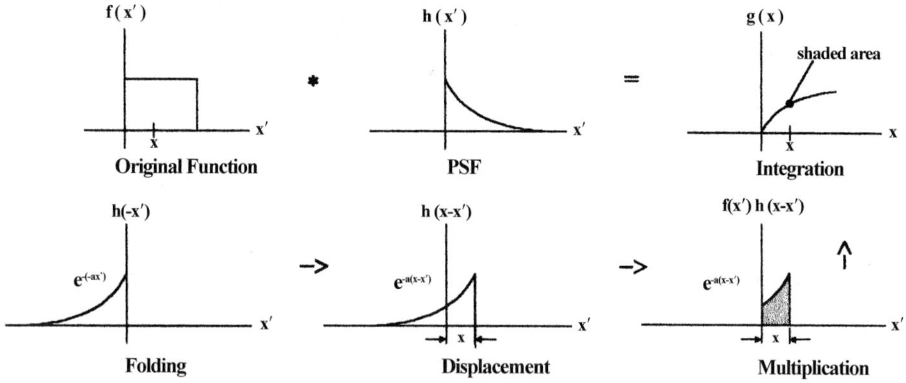

FIGURE 10.10 The convolution process.

This has the shorthand notation $f{**}h = h{**}f$, where ** denotes convolution with double integration. Similarly, $f{*}h = h{*}f$ denotes convolution with single integration.

A physical description of convolution can be expressed in terms of graphical manipulation of the one-dimensional function $f(x')$ (Fig. 10.10). Here, the function $h(x')$ is *folded* by taking the mirror image about the ordinate axis, a *displacement* $h(-x')$ is applied along the abscissa axis, followed by a *multiplication* of the shifted function $h(x - x')$ by $f(x')$. The convolution at location x is then determined by *integration* along the abscissa axis, by finding the area under the product of $h(x - x')$ and $f(x')$. The result of convolution will be the same if the role of the two functions is reversed, that is whether $h(x')$ or $f(x')$ is folded and shifted.

10.3.2 Frequency Domain

The method of resolving the input into a linear combination of δ functions presents a framework for the analysis of linear shift-invariant systems in cartesian space. However, solutions involve the multiple integration of the product of functions and are cumbersome to carry out in practice. Since δ functions are not the only form of input signal decomposition, it is expedient to examine the superposition of complex exponential functions as a possible alternative. In this case the input $g_{in}(\mathbf{u}) = \exp(i2\pi\mathbf{k}\cdot\mathbf{u})$, so that Eq. (10.29) becomes

$$g_{out}(\mathbf{u}) = \int_{-\infty}^{\infty} p(\mathbf{u}' - \mathbf{u}) \exp(+i2\pi\mathbf{k}\cdot\mathbf{u}')\, d\mathbf{u}' \tag{10.31}$$

where $\mathbf{u}$ is the independent variable vector and $\mathbf{k}$ is a given real number vector.

Changing the variables according to $\mathbf{u}'' = \mathbf{u} - \mathbf{u}'$, we have

$$g_{out}(\mathbf{u}) = \exp(i2\pi\mathbf{k}\cdot\mathbf{u}) \int_{-\infty}^{\infty} p(\mathbf{u}'') \exp(-i2\pi\mathbf{k}\cdot\mathbf{u}'')\, d\mathbf{u}'' \tag{10.32}$$

Since the integrand is independent of $\mathbf{u}$, this reduces to

$$g_{out}(\mathbf{u}) = \text{constant} \times g_{in}(\mathbf{u}) \tag{10.33}$$

This indicates that passing a complex exponential through a linear shift-invariant system is equivalent to multiplying it by a complex factor depending on $\mathbf{k}$, which in effect is the transfer function of the system.

The result [Eq. (10.32)] allows us to consider each image to be constructed from a series of sinusoidal functions. This leads to the concept that a function $f(x)$, having a spatial period λ, can be synthesized

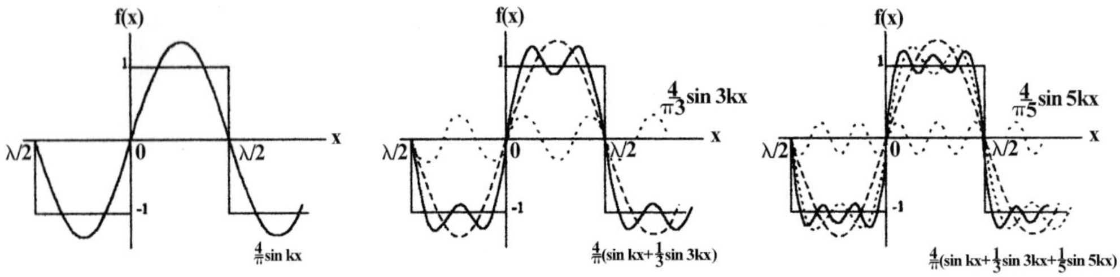

FIGURE 10.11 Synthesis of a periodic square wave.

by a sum of harmonic (sinusoidal) functions whose wavelengths are integral submultiples of λ (i.e., λ, $\lambda/2$, $\lambda/3$). The Fourier series represents this process, according to

$$f(x) = \frac{A_0}{2} + \sum_{m=1}^{\infty} A_m \cos mkx + \sum_{m=1}^{\infty} B_m \sin mkx \tag{10.34}$$

For given $f(x)$, the coefficients are found as

$$A_m = \frac{2}{\lambda}\int_0^{\lambda} f(x') \cos mkx'\, dx' \qquad B_m = \frac{2}{\lambda}\int_0^{\lambda} f(x') \sin mkx'\, dx'$$

where the angular spatial frequency $k = 2\pi/\lambda$.[10]

We make the observation that purely sinusoidal waves have no actual physical reality and that we are invariably dealing with anharmonic features in practice. The synthesis of a periodic square wave into harmonic components provides a good demonstration of the principle (Fig. 10.11).

The effect of reducing the width of the wave is to introduce higher-order harmonics with smaller wavelengths. Consequently, the dimensions of the smallest feature being reproduced determine the total number of terms in the series. If we let the wavelength increase without limit and keep the width of the square-wave peaks constant, they become isolated pulses. This is in the character of nonperiodic functions, where it is no longer meaningful to speak of a fundamental frequency and associated harmonics. We are in effect now considering a series of terms of size approaching zero as the number of the terms approaches infinity. Hence, as we allow $\lambda \to \infty$, the Fourier series is replaced by the Fourier integral, according to

$$f(x) = \frac{1}{\pi}\left[\int_0^{\infty} A(k) \cos kx\, dx + \int_0^{\infty} B(k) \sin kx\, dx\right] \tag{10.35}$$

with the coefficients derived from the given function $f(x)$ written as

$$A(k) = \int_0^{\infty} f(x') \cos kx'\, dx' \qquad B(k) = \int_0^{\infty} f(x') \sin kx'\, dx'$$

The quantities $A(k)$ and $B(k)$ are interpreted as the amplitudes of the *sine* and *cosine* contributions in the range of angular spatial frequency between k and $k + dk$, and are referred to as the *Fourier cosine* and *sine* transforms. If we consolidate the *sine* and *cosine* transforms into a single complex exponential expression, we arrive at the complex form of the Fourier integral. This is the integral in Eq. (10.32), known as the *Fourier transform*, which for the one-dimensional function $f(x)$ is

$$F(\nu) = \Im\{f(x)\} = \int_{-\infty}^{\infty} \exp(-i2\pi\nu x) f(x)\, dx \tag{10.36}$$

where the function $\exp(-i2\pi\nu x)$ is periodic in x with frequency $\nu = k/2\pi$.[11] Hence, to continue with the square-wave example, using Eq. (10.36) we can synthesize an isolated pulse in the *frequency domain* (Fig. 10.12).

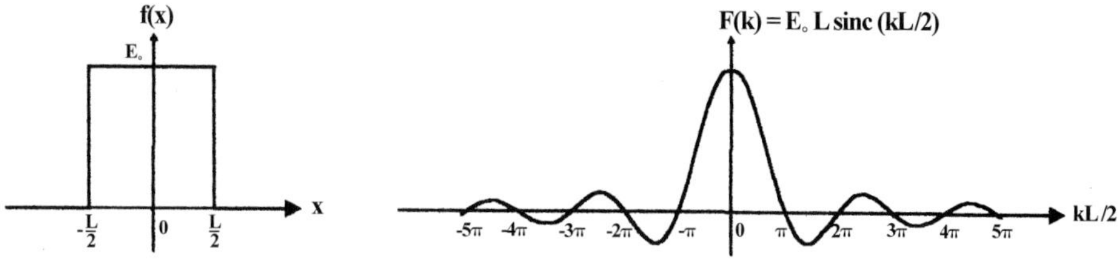

FIGURE 10.12 Fourier transform of a square pulse.

For the two-dimensional or three-dimensional function $f(\mathbf{r})$, the Fourier transform is

$$F(\boldsymbol{\rho}) = \Im\{f(\mathbf{r})\} = \int_{-\infty}^{\infty} \exp(-i2\pi\boldsymbol{\rho}\cdot\mathbf{r}) f(\mathbf{r})\, d\mathbf{r} \tag{10.37}$$

We are particularly interested in two-dimensional space where the function $f(\mathbf{r}) = f(x, y)$. The exponential term $\exp(-i2\pi\boldsymbol{\rho}\cdot\mathbf{r}) = \exp\{-i2\pi(ux + vy)\}$ is periodic in $\mathbf{r} = (x, y)$ with frequency $\boldsymbol{\rho} = (u, v)$. Thus the function $F(\boldsymbol{\rho})$ resides in the spatial *frequency domain*, whereas the function $f(\mathbf{r})$ resides in the physical *space domain.* The usual form of the inverse of the one-dimensional transform is written as

$$f(x) = \Im^{-1}\{F(v)\} = \int_{-\infty}^{\infty} \exp(+i2\pi vx)\, F(v)\, dv \tag{10.38}$$

and that for the two- or three-dimensional transform is written as

$$f(\mathbf{r}) = \Im^{-1}\{F(\boldsymbol{\rho})\} = \int_{-\infty}^{\infty} \exp(+i2\pi\boldsymbol{\rho}\cdot\mathbf{r})\, F(\boldsymbol{\rho})\, d\boldsymbol{\rho} \tag{10.39}$$

The two-dimensional Fourier transform $\Im\{f(x, y)\} = F(u, v)$ has the linearity property

$$\begin{aligned} F\{af_1(x, y) + bf_2(x, y)\} &= aF\{f_1(x, y)\} + bF\{f_2(x, y)\} \\ &= aF_1(u, v) + bF_2(u, v) \end{aligned} \tag{10.40}$$

the scaling property

$$F\{f(\alpha x, \beta y)\} = \frac{1}{|\alpha\beta|} F\left(\frac{u}{\alpha}, \frac{v}{\beta}\right) \tag{10.41}$$

and the shift property

$$F\{f(x-\alpha, y-\beta)\} = F(u, v)\ \exp[-i2\pi(u\alpha + v\beta)] \tag{10.42}$$

The Fourier transform of the two-dimensional convolution [Eq. (10.30)] is

$$\begin{aligned} \Im\{g(x, y)\} &= F\left\{\int_{-\infty}^{\infty}\int_{-\infty}^{\infty} f_1(x', y') f_2(x - x', y - y')\, dx'\, dy'\right\} \\ &= F\{f_1(x, y)\}F\{f_2(x, y)\} = F_1(u, v)F_2(u, v) \end{aligned} \tag{10.43}$$

This shows that the convolution of two functions in the space domain is equivalent to multiplication in the frequency domain. It is this simplifying property that demonstrates the advantage of conducting signal processing in the frequency domain rather than the space domain.

10.3.3 Discrete and Finite Data Sampling

The data contained in a digitally recorded image is an ordered *finite* array of *discrete* values of intensity (grayscale). To manipulate this data, the continuous integrals defining the Fourier transform and convolution must be expressed as approximating summations. For a series of discrete samples $x(n\tau)$ of a continuous function $x(t)$, a representation in the frequency domain can be written as

$$X(w) = \sum_{-\infty}^{\infty} x(n\tau)\exp(-iwn\tau) \tag{10.44}$$

where τ is the sample interval. For a discrete function $x(0), x(2\tau), \ldots, x((N-1)\tau)$ of N elements, Eq. (10.44) becomes

$$X\left(u\frac{1}{N\tau}\right) = \frac{1}{N}\sum_{n=0}^{N-1} x(n\tau)\exp\left\{-i2\pi\left[u\left(\frac{1}{N\tau}\right)\right](n\tau)\right\} \tag{10.45}$$

where the substitution $w = u(1/N\tau)$ has been made, with $u = 0, 1, 2, \ldots, N-1$.

This in effect provides samples $X_0, X_1, \ldots, X_{N-1}$ of the continuous function $X(w)$ at intervals $1/N\tau$ of the frequency w. Hence, for the discrete function $x_0, x_1, \ldots, x_{N-1}$, we can express the Fourier transform as

$$X_u = \frac{1}{N}\sum_{n=0}^{N-1} x_n \exp\left\{-i\left(\frac{2\pi}{N}\right)un\right\} \tag{10.46}$$

for $u = 0, 1, 2, \ldots, N-1$. Hence, a sampling interval of τ in the t domain is equivalent to a sampling interval of $1/N\tau$ in the frequency domain. The inverse of Eq. (10.46) is given by

$$X_n = \sum_{n=0}^{N-1} X_u \exp\left\{i\left(\frac{2\pi}{N}\right)un\right\} \tag{10.47}$$

for $n = 0, 1, 2, \ldots, N-1$. The finite Fourier transform Eq. (10.46) and its inverse Eq. (10.47) define sequences that are periodically replicated, according to the expressions $X_{N,m+k} = X_k$, $x_{N,m+k} = x_k$, for all integer values of m.

To determine the convolution for a discrete sample we follow Eq. (10.43) and find the product of two finite Fourier transforms $Z_u = X_u Y_u$ and take the inverse of the result, according to

$$z_n = \sum_{n=0}^{N-1} \exp\left\{i\left(\frac{2\pi}{N}\right)un\right\}X_u Y_u \tag{10.48}$$

Substituting from Eq. (10.46) and rearranging the order of summation gives

$$Z_n = \frac{1}{N^2}\sum_{p=0}^{N-1}\sum_{q=0}^{N-1} x_p y_q \sum_{u=0}^{N-1} \exp\left\{-i\left(\frac{2\pi}{N}\right)un - up - uq\right\} \tag{10.49}$$

Because of the replication of sequences, the convolution [Eq. (10.49)] can be simplified to

$$z_n = \frac{1}{N}\sum_{q=0}^{N-1} x_{n-q} y_q \tag{10.50}$$

for $n = 0, 1, 2, \ldots, N-1$.

With discrete data sampling, the interval τ between data points determines how well the original signal is modeled. The choice of τ is referred to the Nyquist criterion, which states that a signal must be sampled at least twice during each cycle of the highest signal frequency. This means that if a signal $x(t)$ has a Fourier transform such that

$$X(w) = 0 \qquad \text{for} \qquad w \geq \frac{w_N}{2} \tag{10.51}$$

samples of x must be taken at a rate greater than w_N, so that we require $2\pi/\tau \geq w_N$.

We can illustrate the effect of the sampling interval τ by considering the band-limited transform $X(w)$ of the continuous function $x(t)$. Here, $X(w)$ is zero for values of w outside the interval $(-W, W)$ (Fig. 10.13*a*). If we multiply $x(t)$ by a sampling function $y(t)$, which is a train of impulses with interval τ (Fig. 10.13*b*), we obtain the sampled version $x(n\tau) = y(t)x(t)$ (Fig. 10.13*c*). The transform $F\{y(t)x(t)\} = F\{y(t)\}*F\{x(t)\} = Y(w)*X(w)$ is periodic with interval $1/\tau$. The repetitions of $X(w)$ can

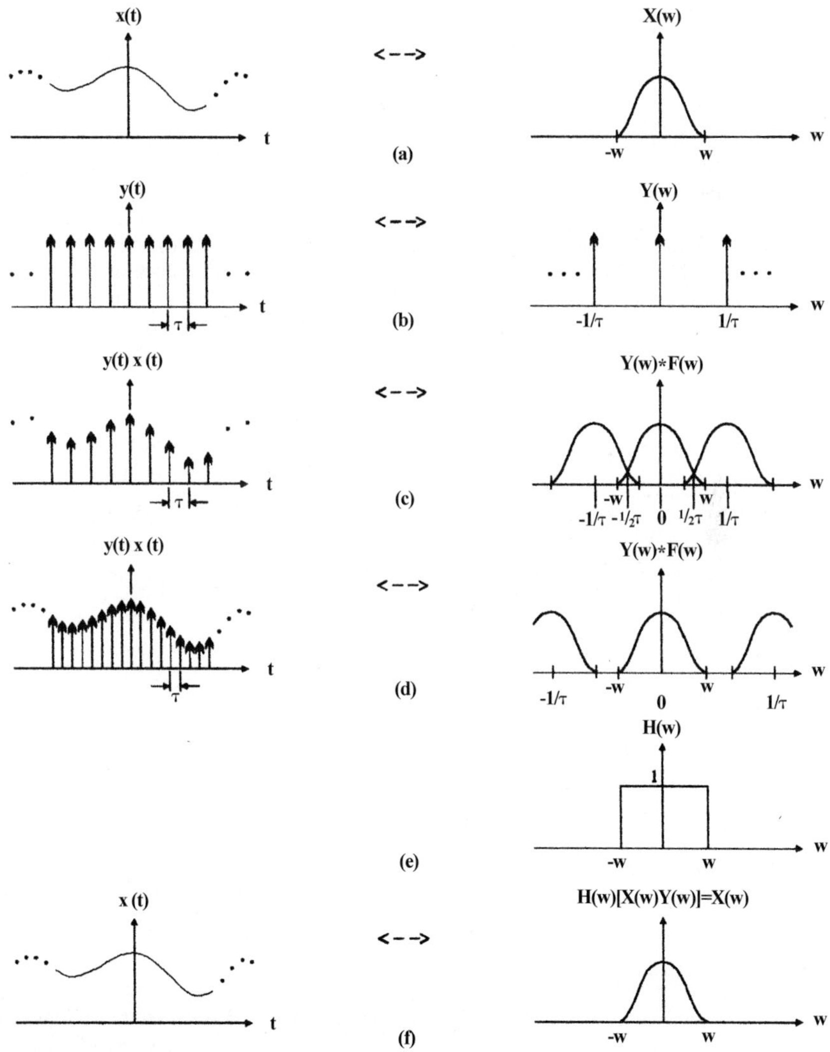

FIGURE 10.13 The effects of sampling interval on a band-limited function.

overlap, with the nearest centers of the overlapped region occurring at $w = \pm 1/2\tau$, providing $1/2\tau < W$. Therefore, to avoid overlapping we require

$$\tau \leq \frac{1}{2W} \tag{10.52}$$

Hence, by decreasing the sampling interval τ, we can separate the transformed functions (Fig. 10.13*d*). This means that we can multiply the transform by the function

$$H(w) = \begin{cases} 1 & -W \leq w \leq W \\ 0 & \text{elsewhere} \end{cases} \tag{10.53}$$

to isolate $X(w)$ (Fig. 10.13*e*). The inverse Fourier transform $F^{-1}\{X(w)\}$ of the isolated function will yield the original *continuous* function $x(t)$ (Fig. 10.13*f*). The complete recovery of a band-limited function, from samples whose spacing satisfies Eq. (10.51), has been formulated as the *Whittaker-Shannon sampling theorem*. If the condition of Eq. (10.51) is not met, the transform in the interval $(-W, W)$ is corrupted by contributions from adjacent periods. This leads to a phenomenon known as *aliasing* and prevents the complete recovery of an undersampled function.[12]

Shannon's sampling theorem is closely related to the Nyquist criterion. With respect to telegraph transmission theory, Nyquist proposed the basic idea that the minimum signal rate must contain the bandwidth of the message. For sampled signals, the bandwidth really ranges from $-f_s/2$ to $f_s/2$, where f_s is the sampling rate. So the minimum sampling rate f_s (known as the Nyquist rate), does contain the signal bandwidth, whose highest frequency is limited to the Nyquist frequency f_s. Shannon gives credit to Nyquist for pointing out the fundamental importance of the time interval $1/2W$ in telegraphy. However, he further established that if a function $f(t)$ contains no frequencies higher than W, it is completely determined by samples at a series of points spaced $W/2$ apart.

10.3.4 Line Integrals and Projections

To describe the process of tomographic reconstruction, we need to formulate a description of the geometry of x-ray paths and the process of absorption along the paths that result in the projected two-dimensional image. This will provide the basic framework from which to develop the method for building up a digital representation of the solid object. We define a single ray path as the straight line joining the x-ray source to a detector cell and passing through the absorbing object (Fig. 10.14). The object is represented by the function $f(x, y)$. The location r and angle θ of ray AB with respect to the (x, y) coordinates is defined by

$$x\cos\theta + y\sin\theta = r \tag{10.54}$$

The level of input signal to the detector cell is determined by the integrated absorption of photons along the ray path according to Eq. (10.22). For the path defined by the (θ, r) coordinates, the photon attenuation, over length l of ray AB in the s direction, is written as

$$\Phi_\theta(r) = \Phi_0 \exp\left(-\int_{AB} f(x, y)\, ds\right) \tag{10.55}$$

This indicates that the object function $f(x, y)$ is the linear attenuation coefficient $\mu(x, y)$ in the plane of the projected rays. Taking the natural logarithm of Eq. (10.55) gives the linear relation

$$P_\theta(r) = -\ln\frac{\Phi_\theta(r)}{\Phi_0} = \int_{AB} f(x, y)\, ds \tag{10.56}$$

This is a line integral of $f(x, y)$ and the quantity $P_\theta(r)$ is called the *radon transform* or the *projection* of $f(x, y)$ along the ray path. It is important to note that the process of reconstructing slices of objects from their projections is simply that of inverting Eq. (10.56). A projection is formed by combining a set of line integrals $P_\theta(r)$, the simplest one being a collection of parallel ray paths with constant θ. This is known as a *parallel projection* (Fig. 10.15).

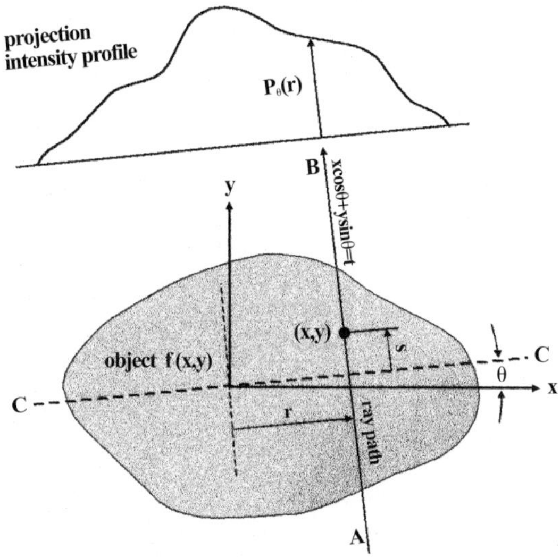

FIGURE 10.14 Projection of object $f(x, y)$ for angle θ.

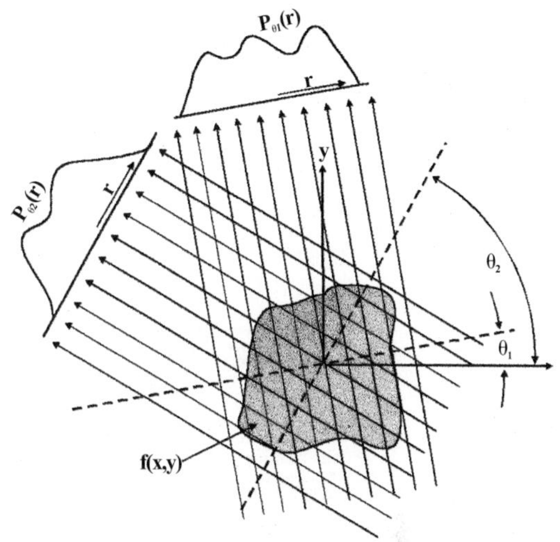

FIGURE 10.15 Parallel projections with varying angle.

The Fourier Slice Theorem. The two-dimensional Fourier transform of the object function, according to Eq. (10.37), is given by

$$F(u, v) = \int_{-\infty}^{\infty} f(x, y) \exp[-i2\pi(ux + vy)]\, dx\, dy \tag{10.57}$$

where (u, v) is the Fourier space, or frequency domain variables, conjugate to the physical space variables (x, y). For a parallel projection at an angle θ, we have the Fourier transform of the line integral [Eq. (10.56)], written as

$$S_\theta(w) = \int_{-\infty}^{\infty} P_\theta(r) \exp(-i2\pi wr)\, dr \tag{10.58}$$

The relationship between the rotated (r, s) coordinate system and the fixed (x, y) coordinate system is given by the matrix equation

$$\begin{bmatrix} r \\ s \end{bmatrix} = \begin{bmatrix} \cos\theta \sin\theta \\ -\sin\theta \cos\theta \end{bmatrix} \begin{bmatrix} x \\ y \end{bmatrix} \tag{10.59}$$

Defining the object function in terms of the rotated coordinate system, for the projection along lines of constant r, we have

$$P_\theta(r) = \int_{-\infty}^{\infty} f(r, s)\, ds \tag{10.60}$$

Substituting this into Eq. (10.58) gives

$$S_\theta(w) = \int_{-\infty}^{\infty} \left[\int_{-\infty}^{\infty} f(r, s) \right] \exp(-i2\pi wr)\, dr \tag{10.61}$$

This can be transformed into the (x, y) coordinate system using Eq. (10.59), to give

$$S_\theta(w) = \int_{-\infty}^{\infty}\int_{-\infty}^{\infty} f(x, y) \exp[-i2\pi w(x\cos\theta + y\sin\theta)]\, dx\, dy \tag{10.62}$$

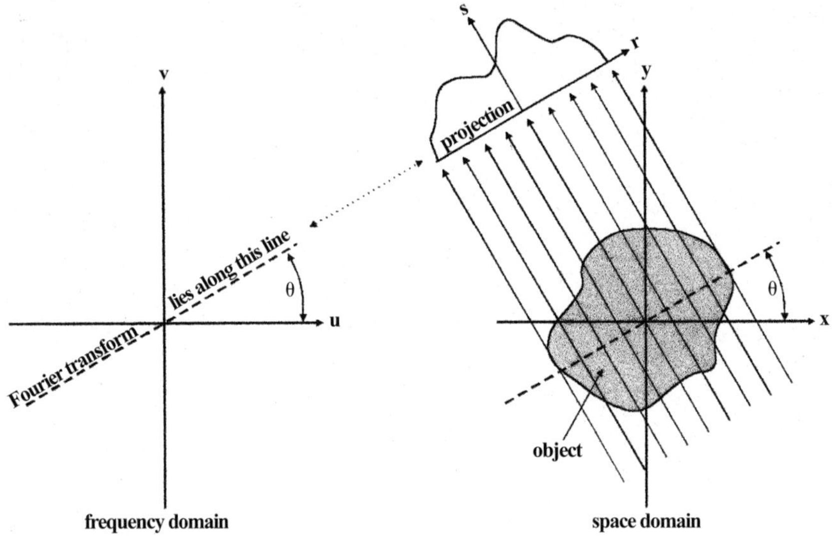

FIGURE 10.16 The Fourier transform of a projection relates to the Fourier transform of the object along a radial line.

The right-hand side of this expression is the two-dimensional Fourier transform at the spatial frequency ($u = w \cos \theta$, $v = w \sin \theta$). Hence, we have the relationship between the projection at angle θ and the two-dimensional transform of the object function, written as

$$S_\theta(w) = F(w, \theta) = F(w\cos\theta, w\sin\theta) \tag{10.63}$$

This is the Fourier slice theorem, which states that the Fourier transform of a parallel projection of an object taken at angle θ to the x axis in physical space is equivalent to a slice of the two-dimensional transform $F(u, v)$ of the object function $f(x, y)$, inclined at an angle θ to the u axis in frequency space (Fig. 10.16).

If an infinite number of projections were taken, $F(u, v)$ would be known at all points in the u, v plane. This means that the object function could be recovered by using the two-dimensional inverse Fourier transform (10.39), written as

$$f(x, y) = \int_{-\infty}^{\infty}\int_{-\infty}^{\infty} F(u, v) \exp[+i2\pi(ux + vy)]\, du\, dv \tag{10.64}$$

In practice, the sampling in each projection is limited, so that $f(x, y)$ is bounded according to $-A/2 < x < A/2$ and $-A/2 < y < A/2$. Also, physical limitations ensure that only a finite number of Fourier components are known, so that $F(u, v)$ is bounded according to $-N/2 < u < N/2$ and $-N/2 < v < N/2$. With reference to the discrete inverse Fourier transform [Eq. (10.47)], and in view of the limiting bounds, Eq. (10.64) becomes

$$f(x, y) = \frac{1}{A^2} \sum_{m=-N/2}^{N/2} \sum_{n=-N/2}^{N/2} F\left(\frac{m}{A}, \frac{n}{A}\right) \exp\left[+i2\pi\left(\frac{m}{A}x + \frac{n}{A}y\right)\right] \tag{10.65}$$

Similarly for the discrete form of the Fourier transform [Eq. (10.46)], we have

$$F(u, v) = \frac{1}{M} \sum_{m=0}^{M-1} \left\{ \frac{1}{N} \sum_{n=0}^{N-1} f(m, n) \exp\left[-i\frac{2\pi}{N}nv\right] \right\} \exp\left[-i\frac{2\pi}{M}mu\right] \tag{10.66}$$

for $u = 0, \ldots, M - 1$; $v = 0, \ldots, N - 1$. The expression within the curly brackets { } is the one-dimensional finite Fourier transform of the mth row of the projected image and can be computed using the fast Fourier transform (FFT) algorithm. To compute $F(u, v)$, each row in the image is replaced by its one-dimensional FFT, followed by the one-dimensional FFT of each column. The spatial resolution of the reconstructed $f(x, y)$, in the plane of the projection, is determined by the range N of Fourier components used.

The proposition of an infinite number of projections is not realistic in practice so that the function $F(u, v)$ is known only along a finite number of radial lines (Fig. 10.17). To implement Eq. (10.65), points on a square grid are interpolated from the values of $F(u, v)$ at the given radial points. However, because the density of the radial points becomes progressively sparser the farther away from the center, the interpolation error increases. This implies that there is greater error in the calculation for higher-frequency components in an image.

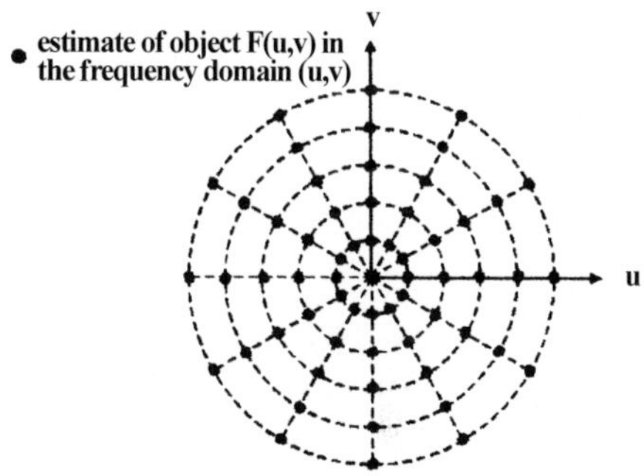

FIGURE 10.17 Finite number of projections provide estimates of Fourier transforms $F(u, v)$ along radial lines.

While the Fourier slice theorem implies that given a sufficient number of projections, an estimate of the two-dimensional transform of the object could be assembled and by inversion an estimate of the object obtained, this simple conceptual model of tomography is not implemented in practice. The approach that is usually adopted for straight ray tomography is that known as the *filtered back-projection algorithm*. This method has the advantage that the reconstruction can be started as soon as the first projection has been taken. Also, if numerical interpolation is necessary to compute the contribution of each projection to an image point, it is usually more accurate to conduct this in physical space rather than in frequency space.

The Filtered Back-Projection. The Fourier slice theorem indicates that each projection is almost an independent operation, a fact that is not immediately obvious from considerations in the space domain. The cautionary "almost" is because the only common information in the Fourier transforms of projections at different angles is the constant [also referred to as "direct current" (dc)] term. Using the argument of independence in the frequency domain, we consider the inverse Fourier transform of each radial line as representing the object with contributions from all other projections reduced to zero. The conception is that the single-projection reconstruction so formed is equivalent to the Fourier transform of the original object multiplied by a simple narrow bandwidth filter (Fig. 10.18*a*). However, because of the angular segmentation, the desired contribution to the summation of projections is that of a pie-wedge filter (Fig. 10.18*c*).

To achieve an estimation of the pie wedge, a simple weighting is taken in the frequency domain, such as multiplying the Fourier transform of the projection $S_\theta(w)$ by the width of the wedge at that frequency. Thus, if there are K projections over 180°, for frequency w, each wedge has width $|w|(2\pi/K)$

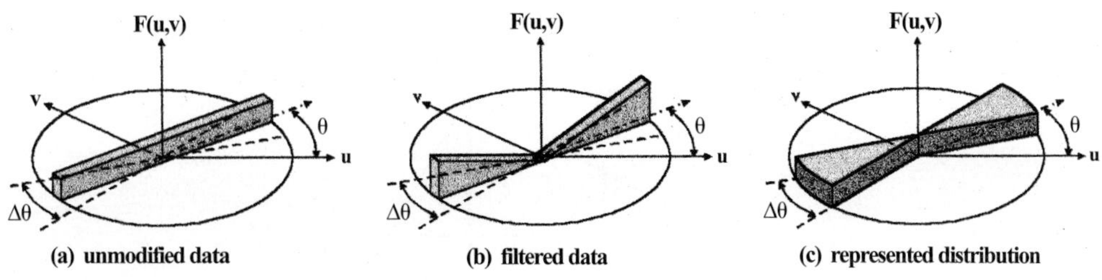

FIGURE 10.18 Frequency domain data from one projection.

and the estimate is a vertical wedge (Fig. 10.18*b*) with the same mass as the pie wedge. The approximation can be made increasingly accurate the greater the number of projections taken.

A formal description of the filtered back-projection process is best served by expressing the object function $f(x, y)$ defined in Eq. (10.64), in an alternative coordinate system. Here, the rectangular coordinate system in the frequency domain (u, v) is exchanged for the polar coordinate system (w, θ), so that

$$f(x, y) = \int_0^{2\pi} \int_0^{\infty} F(w, \theta) \exp[+i2\pi w(x\cos\theta + y\sin\theta)] w\, dw\, d\theta \tag{10.67}$$

given that $u = \cos\theta$ and $v = w \sin\theta$. Splitting the integral into two parts, in the ranges 0 to π and π to 2π, using the property $F(w, \theta + \pi) = F(-w, \theta)$, and substituting from Eqs. (10.59) and (10.62), we get

$$f(x, y) = \int_0^{\pi} \left[\int_{-\infty}^{\infty} S_{\theta}(w) |w| \exp(+i2\pi wr)\, dw \right] d\theta \tag{10.68}$$

If we write the integral inside the straight brackets [] as

$$Q_{\theta}(r) = \int_{-\infty}^{\infty} S_{\theta}(w) |w| \exp(+i2\pi wr)\, dw \tag{10.69}$$

the object function, for projections over 180°, becomes

$$f(x, y) = \int_0^{\pi} Q_{\theta}(x\cos\theta + y\sin\theta)\, d\theta \tag{10.70}$$

The function $Q_{\theta}(r)$ is a filtered projection so that Eq. (10.70) represents a summation of back-projections from the filtered projections. This means that a particular $Q_{\theta}(r)$ will contribute the same value at every point (x, y) in the reconstructed image plane that lies on the line defined by (r, θ) according to Eq. (10.59). This is equivalent to smearing the filtered back-projection along the line *GH* in the reconstructed image plane (Fig. 10.19).

When the highest frequency in the projection is finite, we can express the filtered projection [Eq. (10.69)] as

$$Q_{\theta}(r) = \int_{-\infty}^{\infty} S_{\theta}(w) H(w) \exp(+i2\pi wr)\, du \tag{10.71}$$

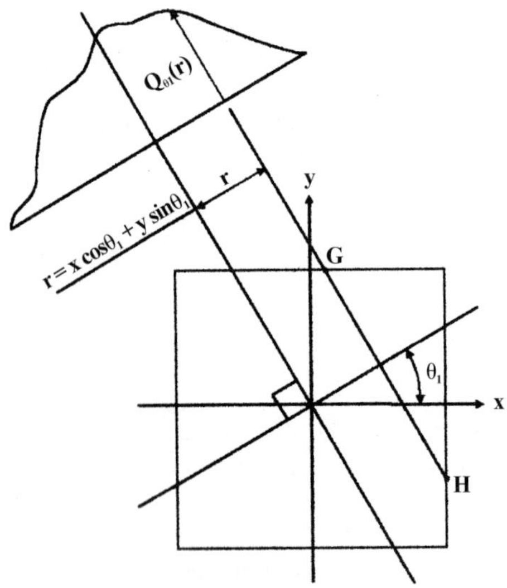

FIGURE 10.19 Filtered back-projection along line *GH*.

where

$$H(w) = |w|\, b_w(w) \qquad \text{and} \qquad b_w(w) = \begin{cases} 1 < |w| < W \\ 0 \text{ otherwise} \end{cases}$$

The filter transfer function $H(w)$ is a ramp in frequency space with a high-frequency cutoff $W = 1/2\tau$ Hz (Fig. 10.20). In the physical space $H(w)$ has the impulse response $h(r) = \int_{-\infty}^{\infty} H(w) \exp(+i2\pi wr)\, dw$, so that, according to Eq. (10.43), the product $S_\theta(w)H(w)$ can be written as $F\{\int_{-\infty}^{\infty} P_\theta(r')h(r - r')\, dr'\}$. Hence the filtered projection [Eq. (10.71)] becomes

$$Q_\theta(r) = F^{-1}\{S_\theta(w)H(w)\} = \int_{-\infty}^{\infty} P_\theta(r')h(r-r')\, dr' \qquad (10.72)$$

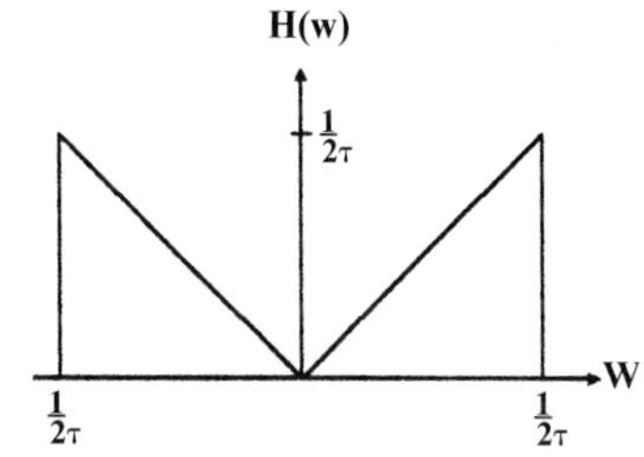

FIGURE 10.20 Ramp filter with high-frequency cutoff.

which is the convolution of the line integral with the filter function in physical space. For a finite number of parallel projections, where $P_\theta = 0$ for $|r| > r_m$, Eq. (10.72) becomes

$$Q_\theta(r) = \int_{-\infty}^{\infty} P_\theta(r)h(x\cos\theta + y\sin\theta - r)\, dr \qquad (10.73)$$

It is instructive to observe that for an unfiltered back-projection, the response to a point object, where $f(x, y) = f(r, s) = (\delta r)\ \delta(s)$, gives the point-spread function $PSF \approx 1/\pi R$, where R is the radial direction from the center. This is generally considered an unfavorable response, and the aim of the filtering is to make the PSF as close to a two-dimensional delta function as possible.

The process of producing a series of parallel ray paths in order to form a one-dimensional projection image involves a linear scanning action across the object. This slow process has to be repeated at each angular step in the rotation of the system. This results in lengthy data collection periods that have proved unacceptable in many cases. These shortcomings can be overcome by generating the line integrals simultaneously for a single projection by using a fan beam source of x-rays in conjunction with a one-dimensional array of detector cells (Fig. 10.21).

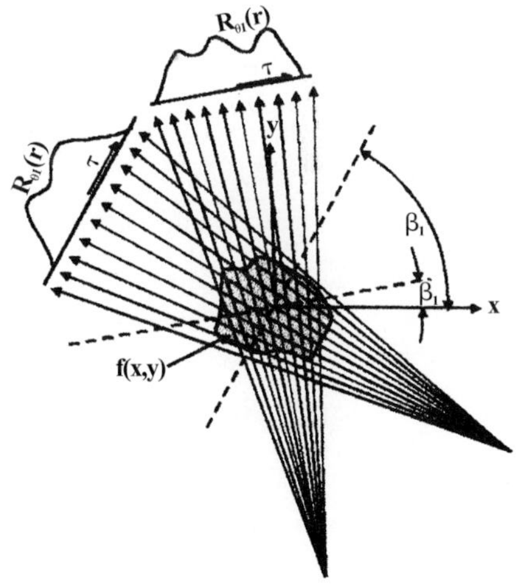

FIGURE 10.21 Fan beam projection with varying angle.

The Fan Beam Reconstruction. With a slit collimated fan beam of x-rays, a projection is formed by the illumination of a fixed line of detector cells. A common detector structure in this respect is the equally spaced collinear array. The projection data for this geometry is represented by the function $R_\beta(p)$, where β is the projection angle of a typical ray path SB and p is the distance along the detector line D_1D_2 to a point at B (Fig. 10.22). To simplify the algebra, the fan beam projection $R_\beta(p)$ is referred to the detector plane moved to D_1'/D_2'. The ray path integral along SB is now associated with the point A on this imaginary detector line at $p = OA$ (Fig. 10.23).

If a parallel projection were impressed upon this geometry, the ray SA defined by (r, θ) would belong to the one-dimensional image $P_\theta(r)$. The relationship between the parallel-beam and fan-beam cases is given by

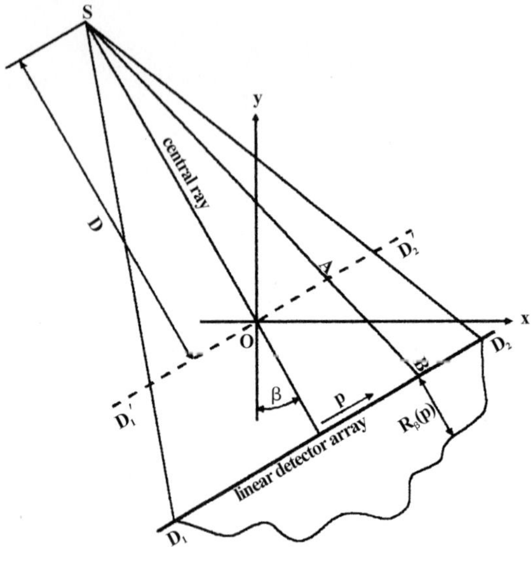

FIGURE 10.22 Linear array of evenly spaced detector cells.

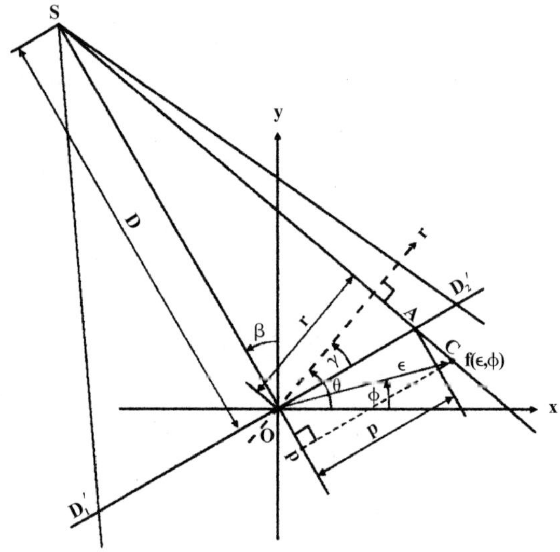

FIGURE 10.23 Fan beam ray-path geometry.

$$r = p\cos\gamma \qquad \theta = \beta + \gamma$$
$$r = \frac{pD}{\sqrt{D^2 + s^2}} \qquad \theta = \beta + \tan^{-1}\frac{p}{D} \tag{10.74}$$

The reconstruction $f(x, y)$ at a point C is given by the substitution of the filtered projection [Eq. (10.73)] into the projection summation [Eq. (10.70)], written as

$$f(x, y) = \frac{1}{2}\int_0^{2\pi}\int_{-t_m}^{t_m} P_\theta(r)h(x\cos\theta + y\sin\theta - r)\,dr\,d\theta \tag{10.75}$$

where the projections are taken over 360°. For the fan beam geometry it is convenient to work in polar coordinates (ϵ, ϕ), so that for $f(x, y) = f(\epsilon, \phi)$ we have

$$f(\epsilon, \phi) = \frac{1}{2}\int_0^{2\pi}\int_{-t_m}^{t_m} P_\theta(r)h[\epsilon\cos(\theta - \phi) - r]\,dr\,d\theta \tag{10.76}$$

Using the geometric relations [Eq. (10.74)], the reconstruction [Eq. (10.76)] can be expressed in terms of the fan beam projection $R_\beta(p)$, to give

$$f(\epsilon, \phi) = \frac{1}{2}\int_0^{2\pi}\frac{1}{U^2}\int_{-\infty}^{\infty} R_\beta(p)h(p' - p)\frac{D}{\sqrt{D^2 + p^2}}\,dp\,d\beta \tag{10.77}$$

where $U(\epsilon, \phi, \beta) = (SO + OP)/D = [D + \epsilon\sin(\beta - \phi)]/D$. Here, $h(p)$ is the inverse Fourier transform of the filter transfer function in Eq. (10.71) and the variable p' is the location p of the pixel along the detector for the object point (ϵ,ϕ) given by $p' = D\{\epsilon\cos(\beta - \phi)/[D + \epsilon\sin(\beta - \phi)]\}$.

Although the fan beam geometry has definite advantages, it is nevertheless a two-dimensional reconstruction method. Like the parallel beam method, it relies on the stacking of sections, with interpolation, to reconstruct the three-dimensional object. Given the advent of large-area-format x-ray detectors, a more efficient technique is to completely illuminate the object with a cone beam

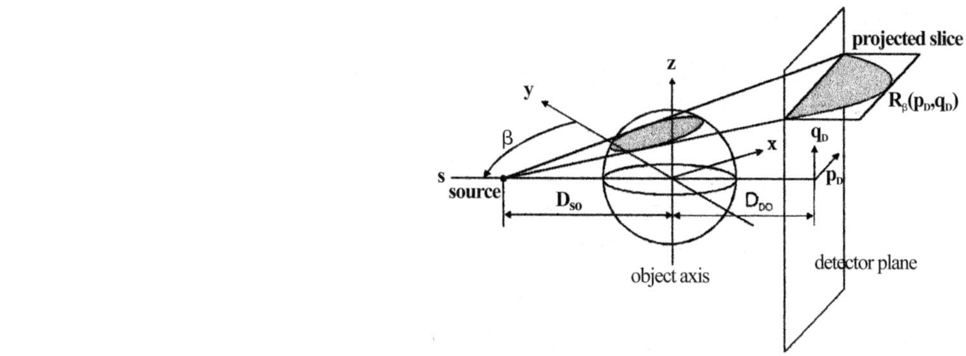

FIGURE 10.24 Cone-beam projection.

and perform the reconstruction as a volume operation rather than an independent slice operation. Consequently, the ray integrals are measured through every point in the object in a comparable time to that taken in measuring a single slice.

The Cone-Beam Reconstruction. With a cone beam of x-rays, a projection is formed by the illumination of a fixed area of detector cells (Fig. 10.24). A common detector structure in this respect is the equally spaced collinear cell array. The projection data for this geometry is represented by the function $R_\beta(p_D, q_D)$, where β is the source angle, p_D the horizontal position, and q_D the vertical position, on the detector plane.

It is convenient to imagine the detector be moved along the detector-source axis to the origin, with an appropriately scaled detector cell location (p, q), according to

$$p = \frac{p_D D_{SO}}{D_{SO} + D_{DO}} \qquad q = \frac{q_D D_{SO}}{D_{SO} + D_{DO}} \tag{10.78}$$

where D_{SO} is the distance from the source to the origin and D_{DO} is the distance from the origin to the detector. Each cone-beam ray terminating at the relocated detector cell (p, q) is contained in a tilted fan specified by the angle of tilt $\bar{\gamma}$ of the central ray and the value of the normal $t = \bar{t}$ to the central ray, given by

$$\bar{t} = q\frac{D_{SO}}{\sqrt{D_{SO}^2 + q^2}} \qquad \bar{\gamma} = \tan^{-1}\frac{q}{D_{SO}} \tag{10.79}$$

The idea is that an object function can be approximately reconstructed by summing the contributions from all the tilted fans. This means that the back-projection is applied within a volume rather than across a plane. The volume elemental cell is a voxel and has the same implication for resolution that the pixel has in the planar representation.

To develop the related analysis, first consider a two-dimensional fan beam rotated about the z axis by β and lying in the x, y plane. If the location of a point (ϵ, ϕ) in polar coordinates for the x, y plane is defined in terms of the rotated coordinate system (r, s), we have the coordinate conversion in the r, s plane, given by

$$\begin{aligned} r &= x\cos\beta + y\sin\beta \qquad & s &= -x\sin\beta + y\cos\beta \\ x &= \epsilon\cos\phi & y &= \epsilon\sin\phi \end{aligned} \tag{10.80}$$

so that

$$p' = \frac{D_{SO}r}{D_{SO} - s} \quad U(x, y, \beta) = \frac{D_{SO} - s}{D_{SO}} \tag{10.81}$$

Hence, the reconstructed object function according to Eq. (10.77) may be written as

$$f(r,s) = \frac{1}{2}\int_0^{2\pi} \frac{D_{SO}^2}{(D_{SO}-s)^2}\int_{-\infty}^{\infty} R_\beta(p)h\left(\frac{D_{SO}r}{D_{SO}-s} - p\right)\frac{D_{SO}}{\sqrt{D_{SO}^2+p^2}}\,dp\,d\beta \tag{10.82}$$

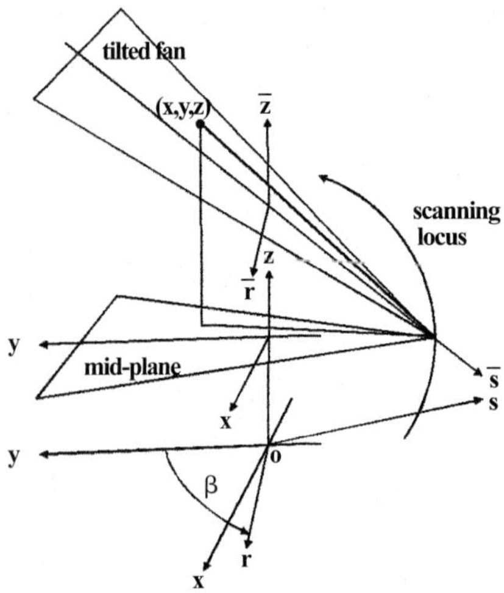

FIGURE 10.25 Tilted fan coordinate geometry.

To contribute to a voxel (r, s, z) for $z \neq 0$ in the cone-beam geometry, the fan beams must be tilted out of the r, s plane to intersect the particular voxel (r, s, z) from various x-ray source orientations. As a result, the location of the reconstruction point in the tilted system is now determined by a new coordinate system $(\bar{r}, \bar{s})$ (Fig. 10.25). Consequently, the fan beam geometry in these new coordinates will change. Specifically, the new source distance is defined by

$$\bar{D}_{SO} = \sqrt{D_{SO}^2 + q^2} \tag{10.83}$$

where q is a detector cell row and represents the height of the z axis intersection of the plane of the fan beam. The incremental angular rotation $d\beta$ will also change according to

$$\bar{D}_{SO}\bar{d}\bar{\beta} = D_{SO}\bar{d}\bar{\beta} \qquad \bar{d}\bar{\beta} = \frac{d\beta D_{SO}}{\sqrt{D_{SO}^2+q^2}} \tag{10.84}$$

Substituting these changes in Eq. (10.82), we have

$$f(\bar{r},\bar{s}) = \frac{1}{2}\int_0^{2\pi} \frac{\bar{D}_{SO}^2}{(\bar{D}_{SO}-\bar{s})^2}\int_{-P_m}^{P_m} R_\beta(p,q)h\left(\frac{\bar{D}_{SO}\bar{r}}{D_{SO}-\bar{s}} - P\right)\frac{\bar{D}_{SO}}{\sqrt{\bar{D}_{SO}^2+p^2}}\,dp\,\bar{d}\bar{\beta} \tag{10.85}$$

In order to work in the original (r, s, z) coordinate system we make the following substitutions in Eq. (10.85):

$$\bar{r} = r \qquad \frac{\bar{s}}{\bar{D}_{SO}} = \frac{s}{D_{SO}} \qquad \frac{q}{D_{SO}} = \frac{z}{D_{SO}-s} \tag{10.86}$$

to give the well-known Feldkamp reconstruction formula[13]

$$f(r,s) = \frac{1}{2}\int_0^{2\pi} \frac{D_{SO}^2}{(D_{SO}-s)^2}\int_{-P_m}^{P_m} R_\beta(p,q)h\left(\frac{D_{SO}r}{D_{SO}-s} - p\right)\frac{D_{SO}}{\sqrt{D_{SO}^2+p^2}}\,dp\,d\beta \tag{10.87}$$

To apply these relations in practice the cone-beam reconstruction algorithm would involve the following arithmetic operations:

1. Multiplication of the projection data $R_\beta(p, q)$ by the ratio of D_{SO} to the source-detector cell distance:

$$\bar{R}_\beta(p,q) = \frac{D_{SO}}{\sqrt{D_{SO}^2+q^2+p^2}}R_\beta(p,q)$$

2. Convolution of the weighted projection $R_\beta(p, q)$ with 1/2 $h(p)$ by multiplying their Fourier transforms with respect to p for each elevation q:

$$Q_\beta(p,q) = \bar{R}_\beta(p,q) * \tfrac{1}{2}h(p)$$

3. Back-projection of each weighted projection over the three-dimensional reconstruction grid:

$$f(r,s,z) = \int_0^{2\pi} \frac{D_{SO}}{(D_{SO}-s)^2} Q_\beta \left(\frac{D_{SO}r}{D_{SO}-s}, \frac{D_{SO}z}{D_{SO}-s} \right) d\beta$$

The inaccuracies resulting from the approximation associated with this type of reconstruction can be made diminishingly small with decreasing cone angle, which is typically ~10° for microtomography.

Algorithms that are based upon the Feldkamp principles have found favor in practice because of their good image quality and fast computational speed. However, the circular path that the source follows lies in a single plane and consequently projects a limited view of the object. Hence, intuitively it is observed that the greater the number of planes containing a source point, the more accurate the reconstruction of the object. To this effect it is possible to state a sufficient condition on the nature of source paths for exact cone-beam reconstruction after the formulation of Smith[14]: "If on every plane that intersects the object there exists at least one cone-beam source point, then the object can be reconstructed precisely." The equivalent statement for a fan-beam reconstruction is "If there exists at least a fan-beam source on any straight line intersecting an object, an exact reconstruction is possible."

The scanning schemes that have been adapted to the above principle may involve the spiral/helical motion that requires lateral displacement with rotation.[15] Extensions of the Feldkamp algorithm, for quite general three-dimensional scanning loci, have been developed by Wang et al.[16] For further discussions on the approximate and accurate cone-beam reconstruction the reader is referred to Ref. 17.

10.4 THE MICROTOMOGRAPHY SYSTEM

10.4.1 The X-Ray Source

The spatial resolution is the principal factor that distinguishes microtomography from conventional medical tomography. In practice, medical systems must provide very high x-ray fluence in order to minimize the exposure times. This means that the x-ray source has a relatively large extended emission area of ~5 mm × 5 mm. The source of x-rays for medical/laboratory systems is created by the bombardment of a solid metal target (tungsten-rhenium) with a directed high-energy electron beam. The conventional design produces electrons from a tungsten spiral wire filament (cathode) held at high voltage. This is heated to a very high temperature, and electrons are extracted in a high voltage field ΔV_{CA} formed between the filament housing and the grounded x-ray target (anode) housing (Fig. 10.26).

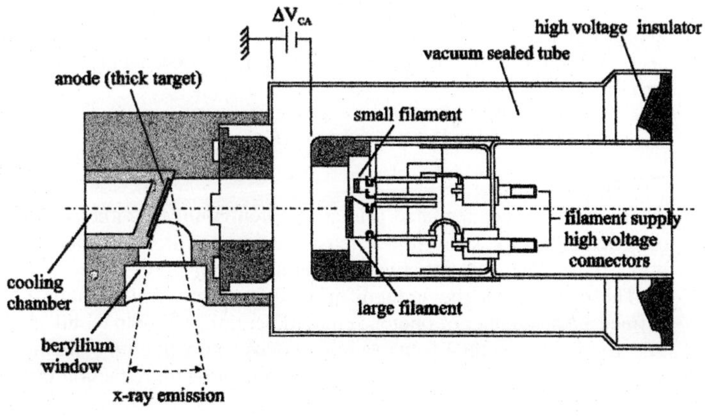

FIGURE 10.26 Medical x-ray tube.

The associated geometry acts as an electrostatic lens and focuses the electron beam onto the target. There is provision for a reduced focal spot size of ~2.5 mm × 2.5 mm from a smaller auxiliary filament with a corresponding reduction in x-ray emission.

The result of the extended source is a geometric unsharpness in the image that can be interpreted as that due to a continuous distribution of point sources representing the x-ray emission area. The extent of the unsharpness U, or blurring, at the edges of the image depends on the extent of the source, according to

$$U = F\left(\frac{D_{SD}}{D_{SO} - 1}\right) \tag{10.88}$$

where F = source size
D_{SO} = source to object distance
D_{SD} = source-to-detector (or image) distance

Hence, if the source size is reduced indefinitely, we have as $F \to 0$ the unsharpness $U \to 0$, and the magnification M is given by

$$M = \frac{D_{SD}}{D_{SO}} \tag{10.89}$$

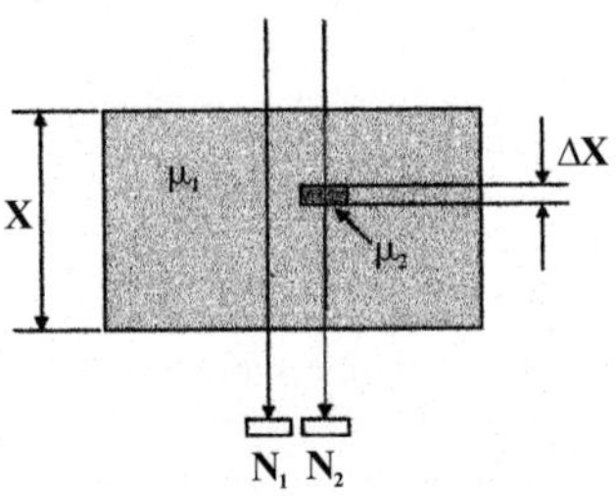

FIGURE 10.27 Threshold of detection for small contrasting object.

To achieve high-resolution $\Delta x \approx 1\ \mu$m, it is necessary to produce a source size $F \approx 1\ \mu$m. However, the penalty for a reduction in source size is a corresponding reduction in photon emission. In order to provide a level of contrast that will support the spatial resolution, consideration must be given to the photon flux. In this respect, a signal-to-noise ratio (SNR) of ~5 is usually chosen as a suitable threshold, for a contrasting feature of relative scale $\Delta x/x$ along a ray path of length x (Fig. 10.27). Here we consider a small contrasting object of thickness Δx and linear attenuation coefficient μ_2, within a larger object of thickness x and attenuation coefficient μ_1. The signal-to-noise ratio for the photon count in adjacent detector cells can be expressed approximately as

$$SNR = \frac{S}{\sigma_s} = \frac{N_1 - N_2}{\sqrt{N_1 + N_2}} \tag{10.90}$$

where the signal S is the difference $N_1 - N_2$ in the number of primary photons counted in the two identical detectors and σ_s is the standard deviation in S.[18] The presence of scattered radiation has been neglected in this derivation. For small contrast, where $|\mu_2 - \mu_1|\Delta x \ll 1$, Eq. (10.90) can be written as

$$SNR = \sqrt{\frac{N_0}{2}\exp(-\mu_1 x)}(\mu_2 - \mu_1)\Delta x \tag{10.91}$$

where N_0 is the unattenuated primary photon count for either detector cell. Hence, to observe the presence of Δx, the x-ray source must provide a sufficiently intense photon flux $\geq N_0$ as a function of μ_1, μ_2, Δx, and x, to satisfy a minimum $SNR \approx 5$.

The measure for the strength of x-ray emission from a point-like source is the brightness β, defined as the number of photons emitted per unit steradian (solid angle), per unit area of the source. The aim is to provide a value as high as possible while recognizing that there are practical limitations to the amount of x-ray emission obtainable with reduction in x-ray source size. For example, if a medical system is overcollimated to achieve a reduction in effective source size, the brightness is insufficient to satisfy the photon flux requirements at the high resolutions in the microdomain.

Therefore, a departure from conventional medical x-ray source design is necessary to achieve the performance required for microtomography applications.

10.4.2 The Microfocal X-Ray Source

The formation of the electron beam is the key to resolution and to the level of photon flux from the x-ray source.[19] In this respect, the electron source brightness β_E and focal quality are functions of the electron energy and the electron current.[20] The principal components that perform this task are the electron gun and the electron lens. The electron gun consists of an electron emitter, or cathode, and two beam-forming electrodes. The electron lens can be either electrostatic or electromagnetic. The latter is usually preferred because the associated focal aberrations are less.

Cathode Condition and Electron Optics. The principal conditions sought for an electron emitter are high brightness, stable geometry, and long life. To achieve a high-quality focus it is important to produce a well-defined virtual source at the electron gun. Here, efficient use is made of the peak cathode brightness of the emitted beam if a single round crossover disk, of effective diameter d_{CO}, is produced by the electron trajectories close to the cathode. Following electron microscopy practice, the choice of cathode structure generally relates to those based on a refractory metal, usually tungsten, or a hexaboride compound, usually lanthanum or cerium. In this respect, a 100-μm wire tungsten (W) hairpin and a lanthanum hexaboride (LaB_6) crystal with 16-μm flat tip, both mounted on a standard Philips base, offer alternative commercial solutions (Fig. 10.28). The tungsten hairpin is low cost, is structurally robust, has a high brightness, and can operate in fairly poor vacuum. However, it suffers from limited lifetime and poor mechanical stability at its high working temperature. The lanthanum hexaboride crystal has a very high brightness, good mechanical stability at its relatively low working temperature, and a very long lifetime (Fig. 10.29). However, it is high in cost, prone to poison unless operated in ultrahigh vacuum, and is structurally delicate.

The shape of the crossover diameter d_{CO}, which is the virtual electron source, is controlled by the geometry of the electrodes that compose the electron gun and the associated voltages (Fig. 10.30). The size, shape, and location of the electrodes, namely the Wehnelt (grid) and the first anode (extractor), relate to the diameter d_W of the Wehnelt aperture, the diameter d_A of the first anode aperture, and to

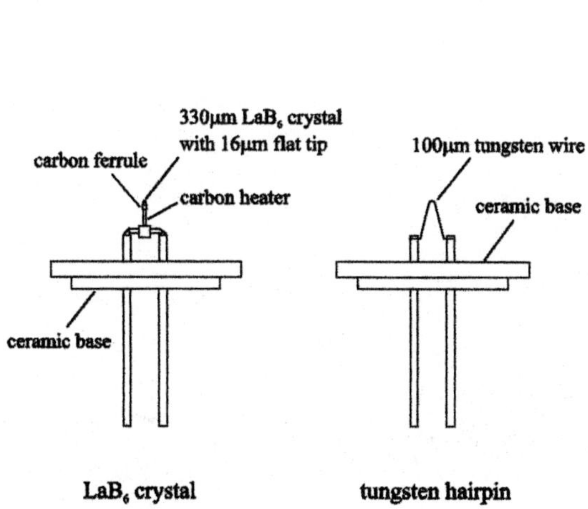

FIGURE 10.28 Electron emission cathodes.

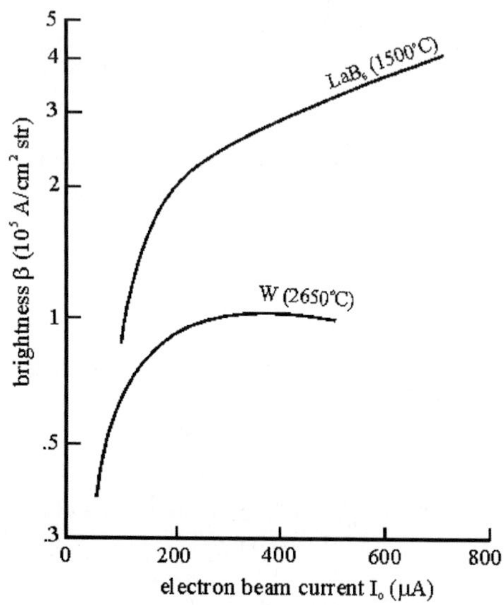

FIGURE 10.29 Electron emission LaB_6 and W cathodes.

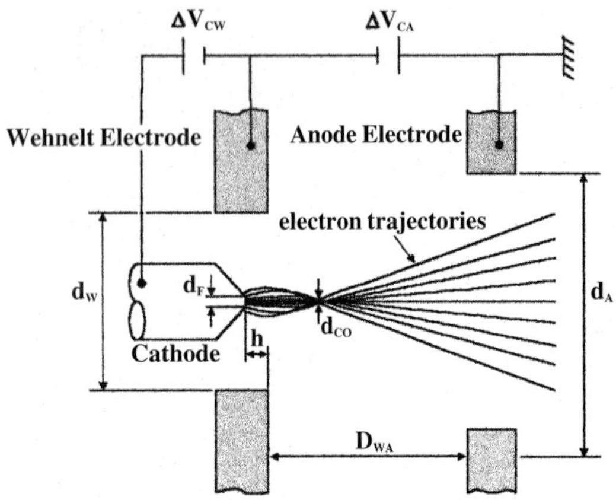

FIGURE 10.30 Electron gun cathode-electrode geometry.

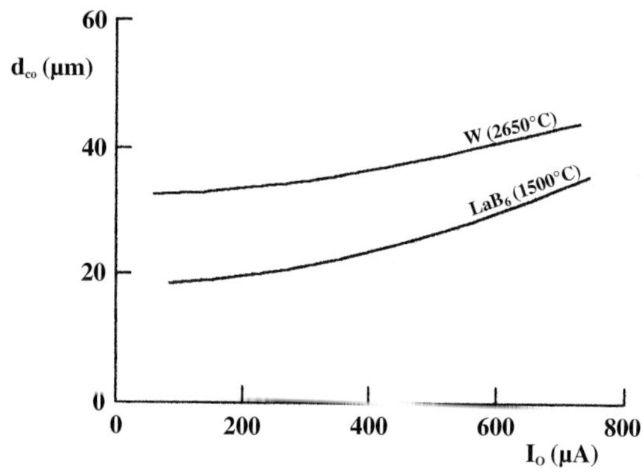

FIGURE 10.31 Crossover diameter, LaB_6 and W.

the spacing D_{WA} between them. The brightness of the electron source is also determined by the ratio d_W/h, where h is the distance of the cathode tip from the Wehnelt face. The voltage difference ΔV_{WA} between the Wehnelt and first anode produces the electron extraction-accelerating field, and the voltage difference ΔV_{CW} between the cathode and Wehnelt produces the electron emission control–retarding field. The size of the crossover diameter d_{CO} is dependent on the type of cathode and varies with the beam current I_0 extracted (Fig. 10.31). The electric fields provided by ΔV_{WA} and ΔV_{CW} are prone to interact at high electron beam currents I_0, causing distortion of the crossover d_{CO}.

With the location of the virtual electron source at the crossover confirmed, the image formation at the x-ray generating target (second anode) is determined according to the principles of electron optics. To achieve high x-ray flux Φ, the electron beam current I_0 must be commensurately high. Therefore, the electron beam shaping apertures are made as large as possible without compromising the focal spot size. A significant source of focal spot aberration arises from off-axis astigmatism caused by axial misalignment of the various optical elements. To minimize this effect, a combination of a single electromagnetic lens with a single defining electron beam aperture is a suitable configuration for high electron beam current and small focal spot.

According to Eq. (10.89) the object must be placed close to the x-ray source in order to work at high x-ray magnification M. Consequently the lens must provide a focus at z_i that is well clear of the base of the electron beam column. In this respect, a suitable shape for the lens can be found by numerically computing the magnetic vector potential A distribution and the flux density **B** distribution throughout the magnetic circuit and coil windings.[21] The calculation involves minimizing the functional:

$$F = \int\int\int_{\text{volume}} \left\{ \frac{1}{2\mu} (\nabla \times \mathbf{A}) \cdot (\nabla \times \mathbf{A}) - \mathbf{J} \cdot \mathbf{A} \right\} dv \tag{10.92}$$

where $\mathbf{A}$ = vector potential, defined by $\mathbf{B} = \nabla \times \mathbf{A}$
∇ = gradient del operator
μ = permeability
$\mathbf{J}$ = current density at any point

The optical properties of the lens are computed numerically from the paraxial electron trajectories $r(z)$, given by

$$\frac{d^2r}{dz^2} + \frac{\eta}{8V_r} B^2(z) r = 0 \tag{10.93}$$

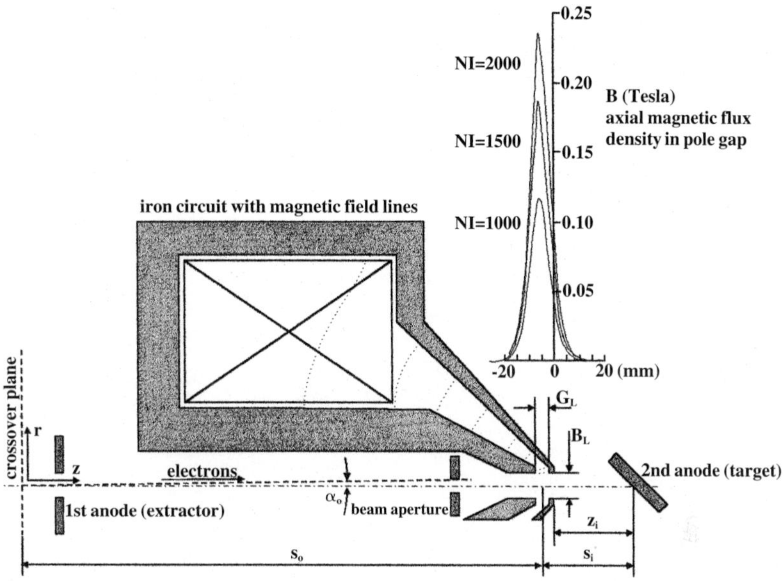

FIGURE 10.32 Electromagnetic lens.

where $B(z)$ = axial magnetic flux density distribution
η = electron charge/rest-mass ratio
V_r = relativistically corrected beam voltage (Fig. 10.32)

There are three components to the focal spot size d_f that strongly influence the design of the electron column, namely, the geometric focus d_m of the crossover d_{CO}, the spherical aberration d_s and the chromatic aberration d_c. The geometric focus of the crossover is controlled by the demagnification M_L of the electron lens and is given by

$$d_m = M_L d_{CO} \tag{10.94}$$

An approximate value of M_L can be calculated from the simple optical relation

$$M_L \approx \frac{S_i}{S_o} \tag{10.95}$$

where s_0 and s_i are the respective distances from the center of the lens pole gap to the crossover and the focus. Hence, the choice of s_0 and s_i, to achieve a desired value of d_m, is the first step in an iterative process that will evaluate M_L from the numerical analysis, Eqs. (10.92) and (10.93). The spherical aberration caustic is given by

$$d_s = \frac{1}{2}C_{so}(\alpha_0)^3 = \frac{1}{2}C_{si}(\alpha_i)^3 \tag{10.96}$$

The spherical aberration coefficients C_{so} and C_{si} are referred to the object side and to the image side, respectively, and the beam semiangles α_o and α_i are referred to in a similar manner. The chromatic aberration caustic is given by

$$d_c = 2C_{co}\alpha_o \frac{\delta V_0}{V_0} = 2C_{ci}\alpha_i \frac{\delta V_0}{V_0} \tag{10.97}$$

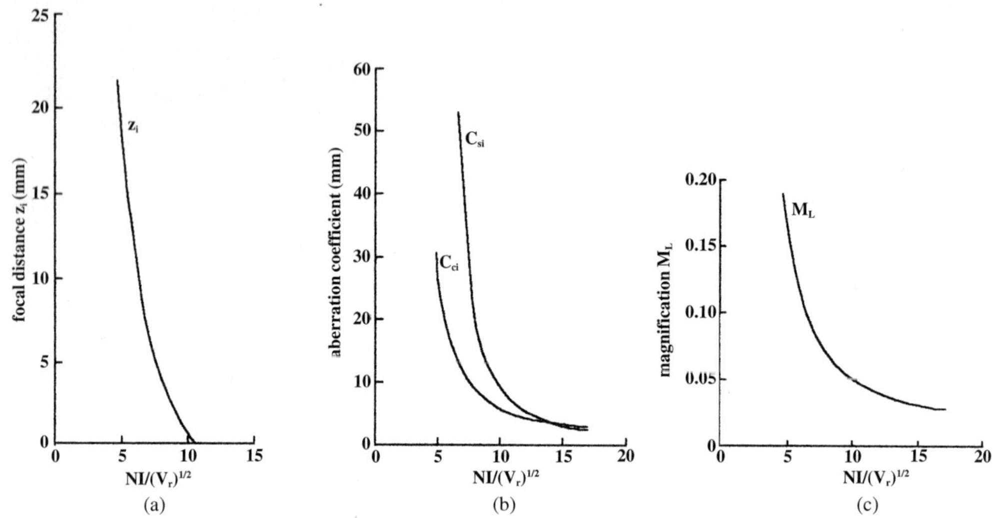

FIGURE 10.33 Electromagnetic lens performance.

The chromatic aberration coefficients C_{co} and C_{ci} are referred to the object side and to the image side respectively and $\pm\delta V_0$ is the variation about the beam voltage V_0. The focal spot size d_f is found by adding the components d_m, d_s, and d_c in quadrature according to

$$d_f = \sqrt{d_m^2 + d_s^2 + d_c^2} \tag{10.98}$$

For good focal quality, low values of C_{si}, C_{ci}, and M_L are sought. For weak lenses, these parameters are dependent on the excitation parameter NI/V_r, where NI is the ampere-turns (excitation) of the lens. In this respect, they are seen to decrease with increasing excitation parameter (Fig. 10.33*b* and *c*). However, to seek a high value of z_i will result in a low value of excitation parameter, which is not the desired outcome (Fig. 10.33*a*). Consequently, a balance must be struck between the need for close access to the x-ray source and the need for a small focal spot size. An important lens parameter in this respect is the pole bore-to-gap ratio B_L/G_L. If this is chosen for optimum performance, a large value of B_L will allow an increase in z_i, without a corresponding increase in aberrations. However, for a given excitation NI, a larger lens bore leads to a reduction in the value of the axial flux density. To compensate, the size of the lens must be increased. A further compromise must be made in the choice of the diameter d_B of the beam-defining aperture. This determines the value of beam current I_0 and also fixes the beam semiangle α_0 referred to the object side, where $I_0 \propto d_B^2$ and $\alpha_o \propto d_B$. An increase in d_B produces a corresponding increase in x-ray flux Φ at the cost of an increase in focal spot size d_f.

A Practical Design. The technology involved in the development of the electron beam column conforms to the principles and practices associated with electron microscopes (Fig. 10.34). To provide versatility with optimum performance, the electron gun accommodates lanthanum hexaboride cathodes, as well as the more conventional tungsten hairpin cathodes. Therefore, the construction complies with standard ultrahigh vacuum (UHV) practice to avoid cathode poisoning. In this respect, the interior vacuum envelope is fabricated from UHV-grade stainless steel, the vacuum seals are flat copper rings (conflat), moving components are sealed with stainless steel bellows, and electrical insulators are metal-ceramic. To maintain the required vacuum $< 10^{-9}$ mbar, the system is turbopumped and all resins, rubber o rings, greases, etc., are rigorously excluded.

The electron chamber has a demountable triode electron gun with a very compact metal-ceramic insulator profile that can support voltages up to 100 kV. Cathode replacement is a routine bench

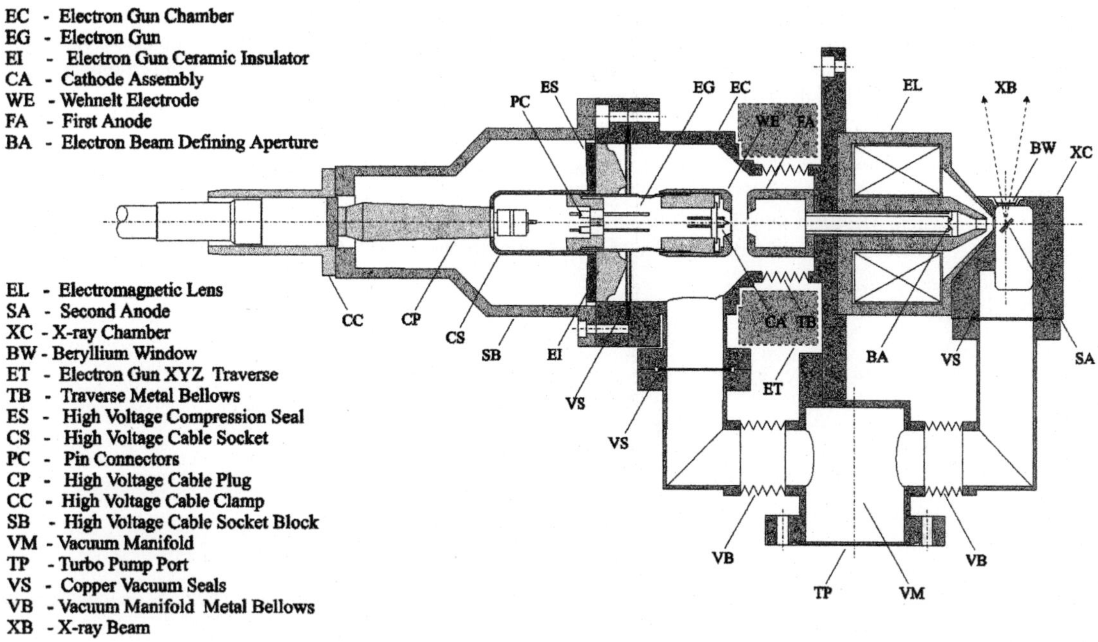

FIGURE 10.34 Microfocal x-ray source.

operation with adjustments for concentricity and axial spacing relative to the Wehnelt electrode for optimum ΔV_{CW}. The electron gun is mounted on a three-axis traverse for alignment with the first anode and for adjustment in the extraction gap to provide optimum ΔV_{WA} over the energy range 0 to 100 keV.

The electromagnetic lens iron circuit is external to the vacuum envelope and provides continuous focus according to $NI \propto \sqrt{V_r}$. The coil windings are cast with high-thermal-conductivity resin to avoid the need for forced cooling. The special geometry permits access to the x-ray source to within 17 mm for large objects and 10 mm for small objects.

The x-ray chamber has a relatively thin (~0.5 mm) beryllium window and houses magnification standards within the vacuum envelope to monitor the electron beam focus. The second anode stage is mounted on a two-axis traverse with a selection of five different target materials for x-ray generation. The individual targets are 6 mm × 8 mm in extent to provide fresh material in the case of damage due to electron beam pitting of the surface.

The high-voltage cable and connector geometry, for the electron gun supply, are based upon a Philips standard cable plug for 100-kV insulation. A silicon seal prevents high-voltage tracking on the atmosphere side of the electron gun insulator. A resin filled cable block has a slightly raised conical face to expel trapped air pockets while compressing the silicon seal. The electrical connections are made with a cable socket in the core of the cable block.

Measured Performance. Under the conditions of space invariance and incoherence, an image can be expressed as the convolution of the object irradiance and the point-spread function, Eq. (10.15). The corresponding statement in the spatial frequency domain, Eq. (10.28), is obtained by taking the Fourier transform of Eq. (10.15). This states that the frequency spectrum of the image irradiance equals the product of the frequency spectrum of the object irradiance distribution and the transform of the point-spread function. In this manner, optical elements functioning as linear operators transform a sinusoidal input into an undistorted sinusoidal output [Eq. (10.33)]. Hence the function that performs this service is the transform of the point-spread function $\Im\{h(x, y)\}$, known as the *optical* *transfer function* $O[u, v]$ (OTF).[22] This is a spatial frequency-dependent complex function with a modulus component called the *modulation transfer function* $M[u, v]$ (MTF) and a phase component called the *phase transfer function* $\Phi[u, v]$ (PTF). The *MTF* is the ratio of the image-to-object modulation, while the *PTF* is a measure of the relative positional shift from object to image.

Taking a one-dimensional distribution for simplicity, we have

$$\Im\{h(x)\} \equiv O[v] = M[v]e^{i\Phi(v)} \tag{10.99}$$

where $M[v]$ and $\Phi(v)$ are *MTF* and *PTF,* respectively. It is customary to define a set of normalized transfer functions by dividing by its zero spatial frequency value

$$O[0] = \int_{-\infty}^{+\infty} h(x)\, dx$$

according to

$$O_n[v] = \frac{\Im\{h(x)\}}{\int_{-\infty}^{+\infty} h(x)\, dx} = \Im\{h_n(x)\} = M_n[v]e^{i\Phi(v)} \tag{10.100}$$

where

$$h_n(x) = \frac{h(x)}{\int_{-\infty}^{+\infty} h(x)\, dx}$$

is the normalized line-spread function and

$$M_n[v] = \frac{M[v]}{O[0]}$$

is the normalized modulation transfer function. If the line-spread function is symmetrical, there is no phase shift so that $\mathrm{Im}\, O_n[v] = 0$, $M_n[v] = \mathrm{Re}\, O_n[v]$, and $\Phi(v) = 0$. A useful parameter in evaluating the performance of a system is the contrast or modulation, defined by

$$\Gamma[v] = \frac{I(v)_{\max} - I(v)_{\min}}{I(v)_{\max} + I(v)_{\min}} \tag{10.101}$$

where $I(v)_{\max}$ is the peak of the profile and $I(v)_{\min}$ is the trough of the profile. Since the *MTF* is the ratio of the image-to-object modulation, we may write, for sinusoids of period λ and corresponding frequency $v = 1/\lambda$ the expression

$$M_n[v] = \frac{\Gamma(v)_{\text{image}}}{\Gamma(v)_{\text{object}}} \tag{10.102}$$

It is a common practice to use the *MTF* to quantify the resolution capability of linear systems associated with image processing. This is because if the individual *MTF*s are known for the components of a system, the overall *MTF* is often simply their product. A natural *resolution standard* would comprise a continuous series of parallel lines with sine wave intensity profiles of increasing frequency. However, this is difficult to produce in practice and it is usual to adopt a simpler pattern known as the *Sayce chart*, which has a parallel line, or rectangular, wave grating with a decreasing spatial period δ and hence increasing spatial frequency $\sigma = 1/\delta$.[23] The rectangular pattern profile $L(x)$ may be expressed in terms of its Fourier series components [Eq. (10.34)], according to

$$L(x) = L_0\left\{1 + \frac{4}{\pi}\Gamma_0(\sigma)_r \sum_{k=1}^{\infty} \frac{(-1)^{k+1}}{2k-1} \cos 2\pi(2k-1)\sigma\right\} \tag{10.103}$$

where the object contrast [Eq. (10.101)], or modulation, is

$$\Gamma_0(\sigma)_r = \frac{L(\sigma)_{\max} - L(\sigma)_{\min}}{L(\sigma)_{\max} + L(\sigma)_{\min}} \tag{10.104}$$

and

$$L_0 = \frac{L(\sigma)_{\max} + L(\sigma)_{\min}}{2}$$

For the object contrast we have the condition $\Gamma_0(\sigma)_r = 1$ for $L(\sigma)_{\min} = 0$.

In seeking a relationship for the value of the *MTF* for a system, we consider the contribution from a single component and offer the output as the input for the next component in the system chain. Hence, the incoherent image $I(x)$ of the rectangular wave grating, formed by convolution of the object $L(x)$ with the line-spread function $h(x)$ of the first component, is given by

$$I(x) = \int_{-\infty}^{\infty} h(x')L(x - x')\,dx' \tag{10.105}$$

If $h(x)$ possesses symmetry, the modulation transfer function value $M_n[(2k - 1)\sigma]$, for the spatial frequencies $(2k - 1)\sigma$, according to Eq. (10.100) may be written as

$$M_n[(2k-1)\sigma] = \frac{\int_{-\infty}^{+\infty} h(x')\cos[2\pi(2k-1)\sigma x]\,dx'}{\int_{-\infty}^{+\infty} h(x')\,dx'}$$

Substituting the expression for the object function Eq. (10.103) into Eq. (10.105), we obtain

$$I(x) = L_0 H_0 \times \left\{1 + \frac{4}{\pi}\Gamma_0(\sigma)_r \sum_{k=1}^{\infty} \frac{(-1)^{k+1} M_n[(2k-1)\sigma]}{2k-1}\cos[2\pi(2k-1)\sigma x]\right\} \tag{10.106}$$

where

$$H_0 = \int_{-\infty}^{+\infty} h(x')\,dx' = O[0]$$

The image contrast $\Gamma_i(v)_r$ can be written in a similar manner to the object contrast [Eq. (10.104)], so that an overall rectangular-wave response, at the spatial frequency $\sigma = 1/\delta$ may be written as

$$M(\sigma)_r = \frac{\Gamma_i(\sigma)_r}{\Gamma_0(\sigma)_r} \tag{10.107}$$

where

$$\Gamma_i(\sigma)_r = \frac{I(\sigma)_{\max} - I(\sigma)_{\min}}{I(\sigma)_{\max} + I(\sigma)_{\min}}$$

Substituting for $L(x)_{\min}$, $L(x)_{\max}$ from Eq. (10.103) and $I(x)_{\min}$, $I(x)_{\max}$ from Eq. (10.106), we find the overall response [Eq. (10.107)] becomes

$$\begin{aligned} M(\sigma)_r &= \frac{4}{\pi}\sum_{k=1}^{\infty}\frac{(-1)^{k+1}}{2k-1}M_n[(2k-1)\sigma] \\ &= \frac{4}{\pi}\left[M_n[\sigma] - \frac{1}{3}M_n[3\sigma] + \frac{1}{5}M_n[5\sigma] - \cdots\right] \end{aligned} \tag{10.108}$$

Solving for the $M_n[\sigma]$ by successively subtracting series for $M_n[k\sigma]/k$, with k chosen to eliminate progressively higher terms in $M_n[k\sigma]$, gives the expression

$$M_n[\sigma] = \frac{\pi}{4}\left[M(\sigma)_r + \frac{1}{3}M(3\sigma)_r - \frac{1}{5}M(5\sigma)_r + \frac{1}{7}M(7\sigma)_r + B_k\frac{1}{k}M(k\sigma)_r \cdots\right] \tag{10.109}$$

where k takes on the odd values 1, 3, 5, etc., and B_k is 1, 0, or −1 according to

$$B_k = (-1)^m(-1)\frac{k-1}{2} \qquad \text{if } r = m$$

$$B_k = 0 \qquad \text{if } r < m$$

Here, m is the total number of primes into which k can be factored and r is the number of different prime factors in k. According to Eq. (10.109) the modulation transfer function can be evaluated in terms of the measured modulation, or contrast values $M(\sigma)_r$. However, since a value of $M(0)_r = 1$ from Eq. (10.108) gives a corresponding value $M_n[\sigma] = 0.9538$ from Eq. (10.109), we must apply a normalizing factor of 1.0484 to the calculated result. We note that the values of M_n are compounded according to the product of the individual MTFs of the imaging components. For the simple x-ray source and detector combination, we have $M_n = M_n^s M_n^D$, where M_n^s is the x-ray source *MTF* and M_n^D is the detector MTF. If the detector is a film emulsion, the *MTF* for the digital scanning device should be included in the product.

It is difficult to construct a suitable resolution standard of the Sayce type for x-ray imaging. Typically the lines would be etched in a gold layer to provide good absorption, but as the line space decreases the lithography process would require the layer to become progressively thinner to maintain the line discrimination. A limited alternative can be constructed from electron microscopy standard 8-μm-thick gold square grid structures. If two of these are superposed and skewed ~8°, the tapered grid intersections will create a continuously varying spatial frequency. A suitable scale is provided by a standard electron microscopy grid of spatial period of $\delta = 24$ μm with a 6-μm bar and 18-μm gap. To stabilize the structure, the grid assembly is sandwiched between standard 8-μm-thick gold disks with suitably sized apertures. This arrangement provides useful contrast values for varying spatial frequency σ but it is not a simple one-dimensional function as discussed in the foregoing analysis. Also, the x-ray source is not a line source with a line-spread function as assumed. Hence, the calculated values of the *MTF* will have a limited accuracy.

The values of $M(\sigma)_r$ and $M_n[\sigma]$ for the microfocal x-ray source are determined from a radiographic film image of the fabricated resolution standard at ×240 magnification (Fig. 10.35). Here, the

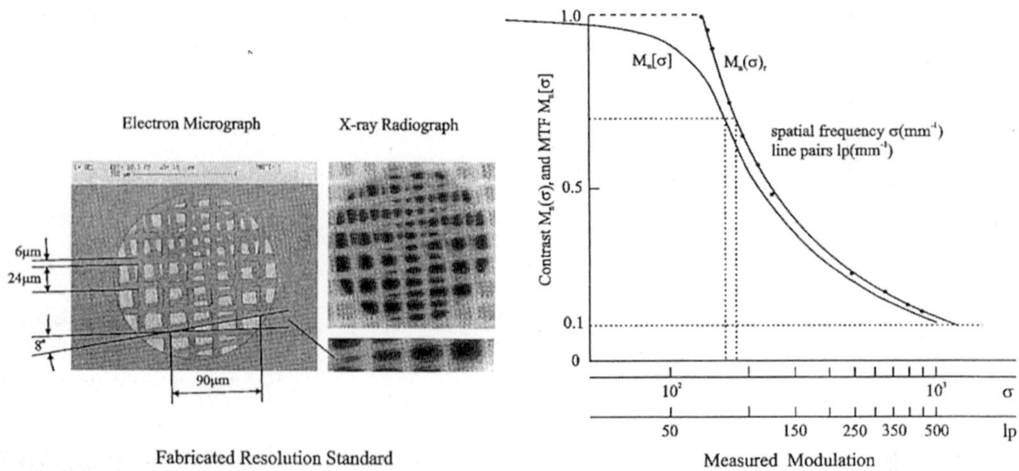

FIGURE 10.35 X-ray source measured resolution.

modulation of intensity profiles is measured at steps along the grid taper, to provide the variation of the contrast with frequency σ. A spatial calibration and modulation reference is provided by an electron micrograph of the resolution standard. The measurements indicate that the resolving power of the x-ray source has a bandwidth of 90 line-pairs/mm (i.e., for $M_r = 0.7071$). At a frequency of 1000 cycles/mm the modulation $M_r = 0.1$, which indicates that features of ~1 μm are resolvable.

X-Ray Generation. We are principally concerned with the deposition of electron beam energy in thick, or electron-opaque, targets. For this type of target the energy is mainly converted internally with the remainder backscattered externally. The x-ray emission is created by deceleration of the incident electrons through the Coulomb interaction with the nuclei of the target and by the removal of bound atomic electrons with the subsequent repopulation of the vacant orbits from adjacent-electron orbits. The former process relates to a broadband continuous spectrum and the latter to a process that produces narrowband discrete line spectra (Fig. 10.36).

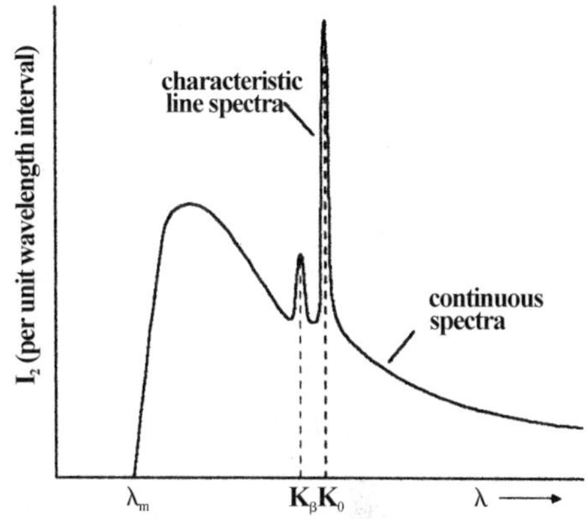

FIGURE 10.36 Spectral distribution of x-ray intensity.

In general, the electrons undergo several collisions before coming to rest so that the continuous spectrum is fairly broadband.[24] The shape of the distribution is dependent on the electron beam energy V_0, so that the envelope $\Phi(\lambda)$ is given by

$$\Phi(\lambda) = \frac{C_1 c Z}{\lambda^2}\left\{\frac{c(\lambda - \lambda_m)}{\lambda\lambda_m} + C_2 Z\right\} \tag{10.110}$$

where the short-wavelength cutoff $\lambda_m = hc/V_0$, C_1 and C_2 are constants, and Z is the atomic number of the target material.[25] Hence, the wavelength of maximum intensity is roughly $3\lambda_m/2$. To reduce the effects of beam hardening, the radiation distribution can be altered by varying the value of V_0 to change the short-wavelength cutoff and by inserting low atomic number material filters such as aluminum, to suppress the long-wave tail.

The intensity of the characteristic spectrum is proportional to Z and the energy depends on the atomic level K, L, M of the interaction. Usually only the higher-energy K series is considered to contribute significantly to the overall radiation. Below 70 keV this is considered negligible and is less than 10 percent for energies in the range 80 to 150 keV. However, for monochromatic applications, such as phase contrast imaging, the presence of characteristic spectra is an important factor.

Historically, the angular distribution of emitted radiation from a thin target has been thoroughly researched. Similar information for electron opaque targets is very limited. From measurements of radiation in the forward hemisphere, the degree of anisotropy for electron opaque targets, expressed as the angle of deviation from the incident electron beam, was found to be ~60°.[26] However, a measurement in the backward hemisphere of a conventional x-ray tube indicated that the radiation distribution was isotropic.[27]

The relation for efficiency η_p of x-ray production of the continuous spectrum, defined as the ratio of x-ray power to that of incident electron beam power, is expressed as

$$\eta_p = KZV_0 \tag{10.111}$$

where $K \approx 10^{-9}$ for V_0 in electron volts. Since the beam power $W_0 = V_0 I_0$ for beam current I_0, the continuous spectrum x-ray power W_c is given by

$$W_c = KZV_0^2 I_0 \tag{10.112}$$

This is a very inefficient process with most of the energy appearing as heat. As a consequence, the temperature of the target material can reach melting point. The liquid metal is subsequently removed by electron beam pressure, resulting in the excavation of a pit or groove. This degradation of the target material creates an enlarged focal spot. Therefore, it is important to determine the maximum power density that a target material can safely accommodate in order to produce maximum x-ray flux to satisfy the threshold of detection condition [Eq. (10.91)].

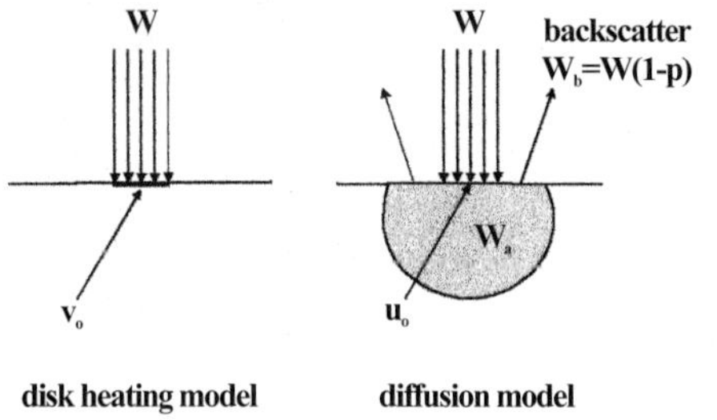

FIGURE 10.37 Heat transfer models.

For the large-focal-diameter electron beams associated with medical x-ray sources, the heat dissipation is considered to occur at the surface and the analytical geometry is that of a disk-heating model.[28] However, this model is inaccurate for focal diameters of small extent where the volume dissipation of heat is an important factor. In this respect the penetration of the beam electrons into the target material must be taken into account (Fig. 10.37). Furthermore, the extent of the electron distribution will contribute to the enlargement of the focal spot, since it represents the volume of x-ray generation within the bulk of the material. For example, at 50 keV the electron penetration depth is ~10 μm which is a significant amount in comparison with a typical microfocal electron beam focal diameter of ~5 μm.

A simple model for the electron motion in the target is to assume that the electrons travel in straight lines to a *depth of complete diffusion*, after which they diffuse evenly in all directions, to cover a total distance called the *range*.[29] Along the *range* an electron is assumed to loose energy according to the Thomson-Whiddington law, written as

$$V_0^2 - V^2 = kx \tag{10.113}$$

where V is the energy after the electron travels a distance x and the constant k is given by

$$k = \frac{b\rho Z}{A} \tag{10.114}$$

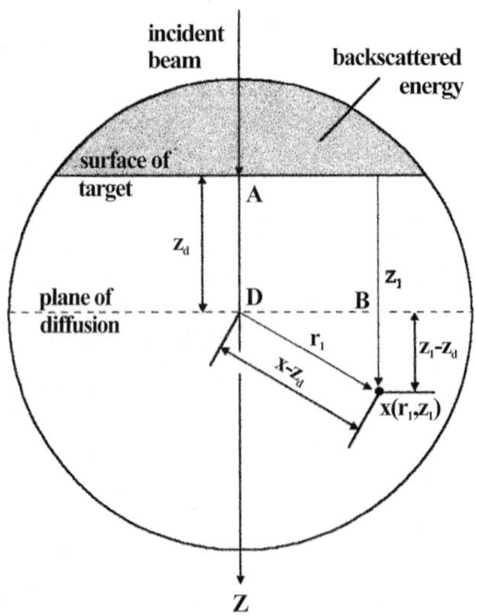

FIGURE 10.38 Model of electron penetration.

where ρ, Z, and A are density, atomic number, and atomic weight, respectively. The parameter b varies slightly with the type of target material but may be assumed to have the constant value $b = 7.75 \times 10^{10}$ eV$^2 \cdot$ m^2/kg. From Eq. (10.113), the electron *range* x_0 is given by

$$x_0 = \frac{V_0^2}{k} \tag{10.115}$$

and the depth of diffusion[29] may be taken to be

$$z_d = \frac{40x_0}{7Z} \tag{10.116}$$

Hence, the diffusion center is nearer to the surface the larger the atomic number of the target material (Fig. 10.38).

The volume in which heat is dissipated is the sphere of radius $x_0 - z_d$ centered at D, which is the center of complete diffusion. The shaded region contains the backscattered beam power. For a small element of the surface, the initial electron beam current dI will be redistributed to a current density dJ at $x(r_1, z_1)$. The corresponding volume density of power dissipated, dW, will be given by

$$dW = -dJ\frac{dV}{dx} \tag{10.117}$$

For uniform diffusion from D, the current density dJ is given by

$$dJ = \frac{dI}{4\pi(x - z_d)^2} \tag{10.118}$$

where it is assumed that $z_1 > z_d$. Substituting Eq. (10.118) into Eq. (10.117) gives

$$dW = \frac{k\,dI}{8\pi(x - z_d)^2(V_0^2 - kx)^{1/2}} \tag{10.119}$$

The total power density dissipation at $x(r_1, z_1)$ is determined by integrating over the beam elements dI. To do this, we consider a gaussian beam current density profile written as

$$J(r) = \frac{I}{1.44\pi a^2}\exp\left(-\frac{r^2}{1.44a^2}\right) \tag{10.120}$$

where I = total beam current
r = radial distance at the surface
a = beam radius at which the current density is $J_{(r=0)}/2$

Hence, the current element dI is given by $J\,dS$. The region of beam cross section that is within the range of $x(r_1, z_1)$ is bounded by a circle on the surface with radius $[(x_0 - z_d)^2 - (z_1 - z_d)^2]^{1/2}$ and center at $x(r_1, 0)$. If $z_1 < z_d$ then $x(r_1, z_1)$ lies between the surface and the depth of diffusion. In this case there is an additional contribution to dW from the incoming beam at $r = r_1$. This is found by replacing dJ in Eq. (10.117) by J at $r = r_1$ from Eq. (10.120), to give

$$dW_0 = \frac{I}{1.44\pi a^2}\exp\left(-\frac{r_1^2}{1.44a^2}\right)\frac{k}{2\left(V_0^2 - kx\right)^{1/2}} \tag{10.121}$$

The steady-state temperature u, in the presence of a volume distributed heat input $W(r, z)$, is determined by the Poisson equation, which for axisymmetric geometry is written as

$$\frac{\partial^2 u}{\partial r^2} + \frac{1}{r}\frac{\partial u}{\partial r} + \frac{\partial^2 u}{\partial z^2} = -\frac{W(r, z)}{\kappa} \tag{10.122}$$

where κ is the thermal conductivity. With the appropriate boundary conditions, solutions to Eq. (10.122) can be computed numerically. In this process it is convenient to normalize the temperature u by the disk-heating model temperature v_0 at the beam center, so that

$$\bar{u} = \frac{u}{v_0} \quad \text{and} \quad v_0 = \frac{0.099W_0}{\pi^{1/2}\kappa a} \tag{10.123}$$

If the power that is absorbed in the target is W_a and the backscattered power in the shaded area (Fig. 10.37) is W_b, the total beam power $W_0 = W_a + W_b = V_0 I_0$. The power retention factor $p = W_d/W_0 = 1 - W_b/W_0$, which is a function of atomic number Z and is independent of voltage V (Fig. 10.39). According to Eqs. (10.115) and (10.116), scaling the electron beam voltage by f will increase the *range* and the *depth of diffusion* by f^2, thus altering the power distribution by $1/f^2$, which in effect is

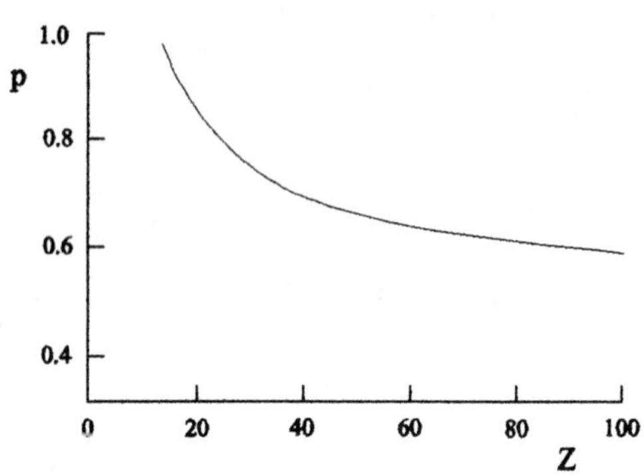

FIGURE 10.39 Fraction of power absorbed by the target.

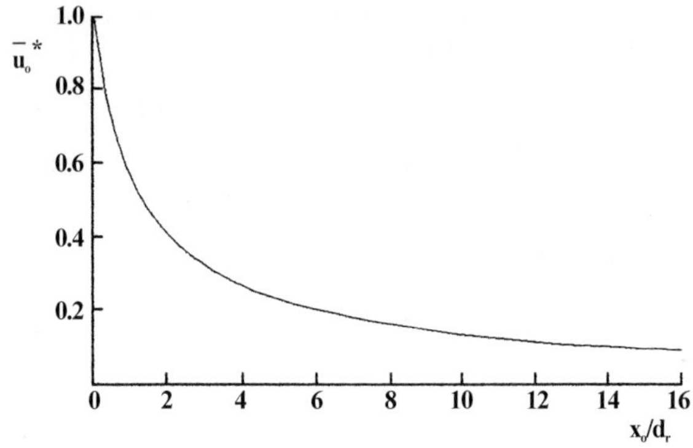

FIGURE 10.40 Temperature rise at the focal spot center.

equivalent to changing the beam diameter d_f by the same amount. Hence, changes in beam voltage and beam diameter result in the same outcome. Therefore, it is sensible to measure *range* in beam diameters as x_0/d_f, noting that for large diameter sources $x_0/d_f \rightarrow 0$ and $\bar{u} \rightarrow p$. This suggests an additional normalization by the power retention factor p to remove the effect of backscatter according to $\bar{u}^* = \bar{u}/p = u/(pv_0)$, which results in a temperature variation with electron range in beam diameters x_0/d_f, based upon absorbed power and independent of the material Z (Fig. 10.40).

If the beam power W_0 is absorbed at the target surface, the temperature rise v_0 is given by Eq. (10.123). This must be corrected for the effects of backscatter and source dispersal to give u_0. In this process, the power retention factor p is taken from Fig. 10.39 for a given material Z, and the temperature rise $\bar{u}^*_0$ is taken from Fig. 10.40 for x_0 calculated from Eqs. (10.114) and (10.115). With the values of v_0, p, and $\bar{u}^*_0$, the true temperature rise u_0 at the beam center is found from $\bar{u}_0 = \bar{u}_0^* p v_0$ (Fig. 10.41).

A high-speed rotating anode is used in conventional x-ray tubes to overcome the heat loading.[28] However, the choice of cooling method is problematical for microfocal applications because of the need to place the specimen close to the x-ray source to achieve high magnification, according to

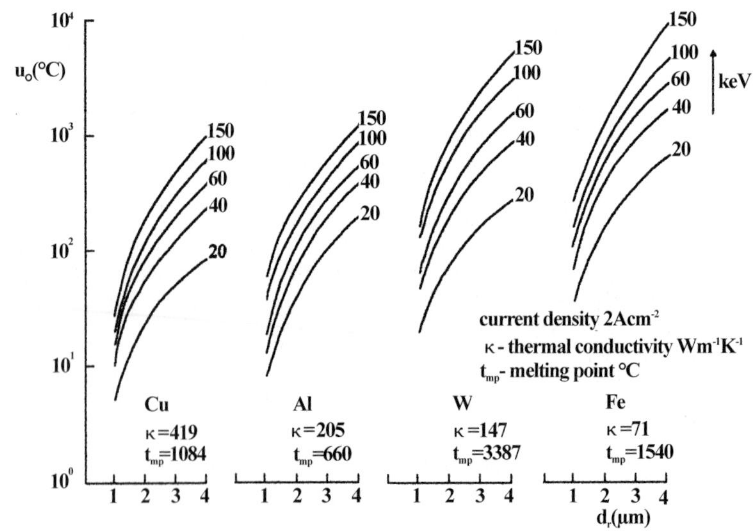

FIGURE 10.41 Heating of a semi-infinite block by a gaussian beam.

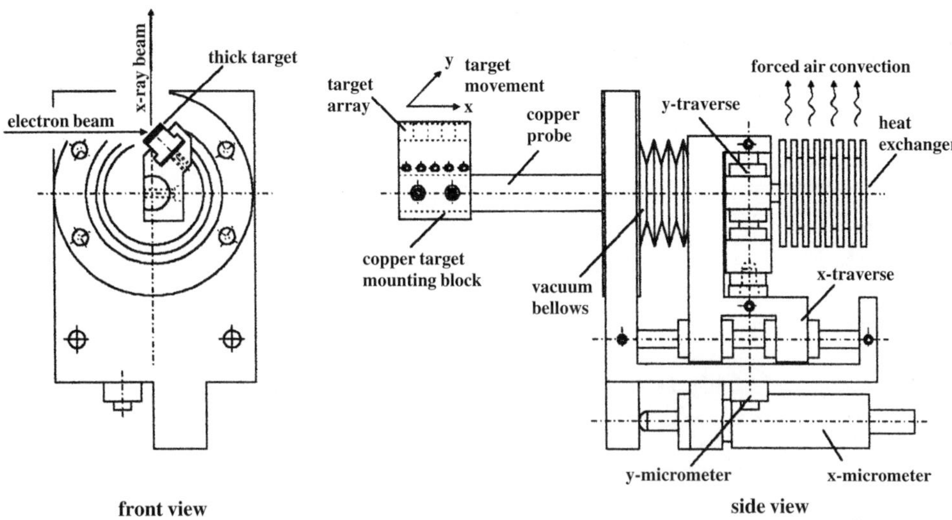

FIGURE 10.42 Microfocal target assembly.

Eq. (10.89). In this respect, rotating anodes are bulky and are difficult to install in a confined space. Furthermore, a range of target (anode) materials should be available within the vacuum envelope to provide the versatility required for research purposes. Since the power dissipation is quite small, ~10 W, it can be argued that thermal conduction in copper, plus forced air convection, should be sufficient to maintain the temperature of the target at an acceptable level. The target assembly installed in the x-ray chamber (Fig. 10.34) adopts this principle with a copper probe supporting several material targets and an external cylindrical heat exchanger receiving forced cooling air (Fig. 10.42). The copper probe is supported on a two-dimensional traverse to select different materials and move fresh material under the electron beam.

10.4.3 Detectors and the Mode of Operation

The high brightness of the microfocal x-ray source enables the microtomography system to operate in two basic modes. These two modes are distinguished by whether the beam is collimated or not and lead to different data acquisition procedures. Also, with the installation of a monochromator, it is possible to perform phase contrast imaging that has a greater sensitivity to density variation than conventional contrast imaging.

Small-Area Detector. In the collimated beam mode the detector is a small-area single-cell device and the specimen is pointwise scanned, in the manner of conventional light microscopy, to record a single frame for each projection (Fig. 10.43). The advantage is that single-cell Si(Li), or HPGe, crystal detectors are available as energy-discriminating devices.[30] These are highly sensitive and possess good energy resolution. They respond to the characteristic spectra and are used in a photon pulse counting mode. This function can provide information on atomic composition of the specimen. A disadvantage is that the data acquisition is a relatively slow process. Also, the magnification is a function of the area raster scanned. The accuracy depends on the specimen scanning stage and detector collimation.

Large-Area Detector. In the uncollimated beam mode, the detector is a large-area multicell device that can record a single frame for each projection without pixel scanning (Fig. 10.44). Consequently data acquisition can be based on the rapid techniques associated with commercially available frame-grabbing hardware/software. However, the device is energy integrating and cannot determine atomic

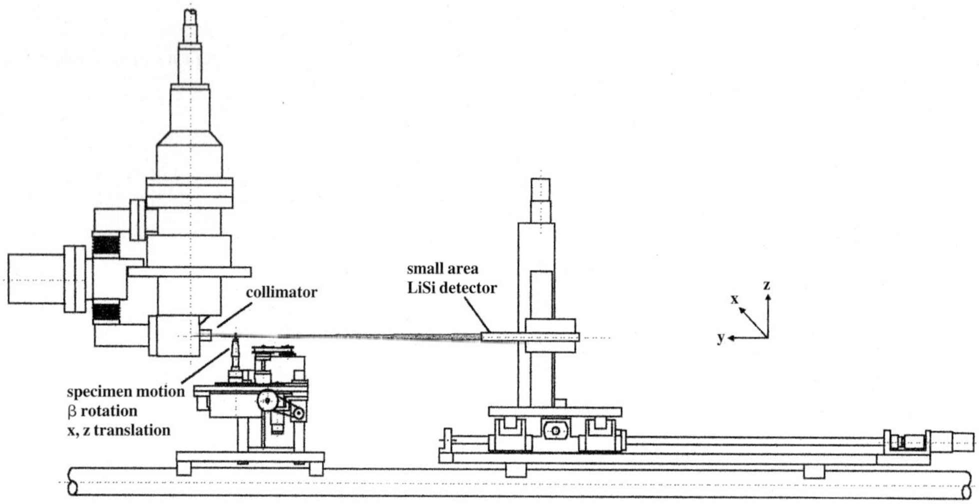

FIGURE 10.43 Raster scan imaging with small-area detector.

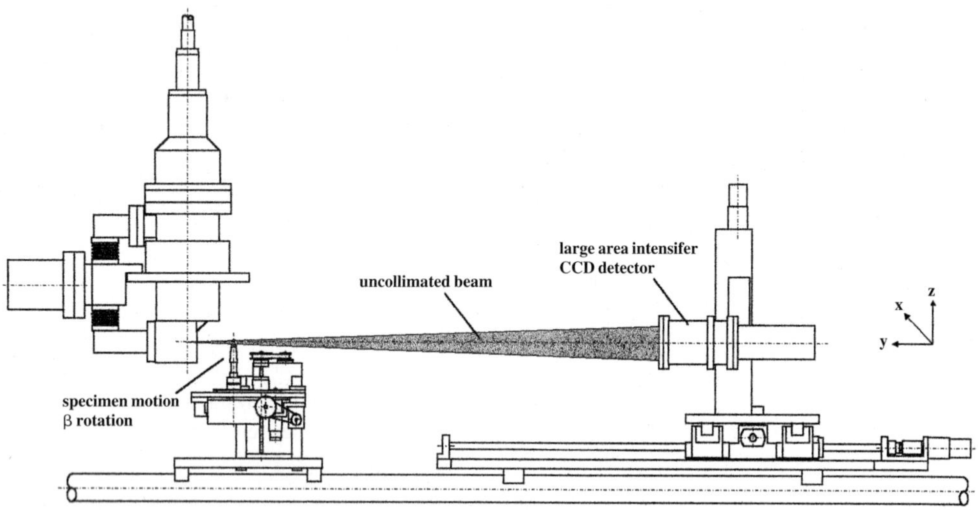

FIGURE 10.44 Direct magnification imaging with large-area detector.

composition. Also, scattering may compromise the image quality, though at the higher magnifications the effect would be reduced because of the larger source to detector distance D_{SD}.

The relative separation of the source, specimen and detector provides direct magnification according to Eq. (10.89). Here, the magnification can be chosen so that the resolution limit of the detector does not compromise the resolution of the x-ray source. For a given detector pixel size d_p at the input plane, the corresponding voxel element size $d_v = d_p/M$. This also determines the size of the specimen to be imaged, since the frame size (height $H_F = d_pN_H$, width $W_F = d_pN_W$) relates to the size of the reconstruction volume (height $H_V = H_F/M$, width $W_V = W_F/M$, depth $D_V = W_F/M$), where $N_H \times N_W$ is the number of frame pixels.

If a wide range of specimen sizes is to be accommodated, the detector/camera input plane needs be of adequate extent, >50 mm. However, the charged coupled device (CCD) that is the actual detector is

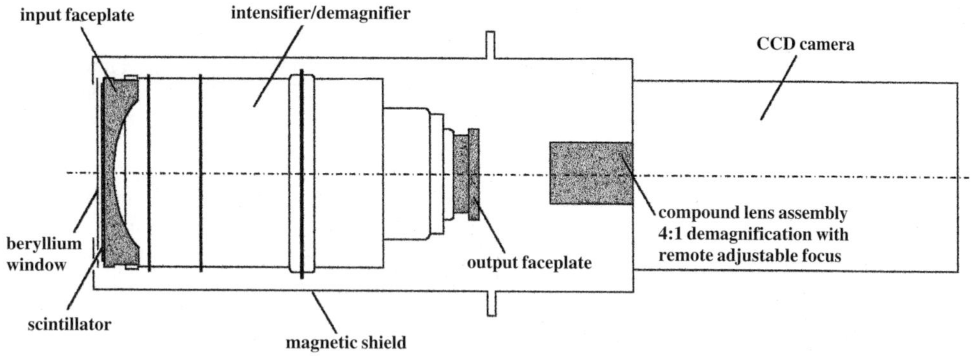

FIGURE 10.45 80-mm intensifier/demagnifier CCD digital x-ray camera.

small in size, ~7 mm × 7 mm. Also, this device is principally sensitive to light and not to x-rays. Hence, the x-ray photons must be down shifted in frequency at the input plane and the image must be reduced to match the CCD. If the image demagnification m is provided by a simple lens system, with an f-number $f/\#$, the light-gathering power will be $\propto 1/(f/\#)^2$. Therefore, $f/\#$ needs to be kept as small as possible which can be achieved by a reduction in m. If a demagnifying intensifier is used, then a portion of the demagnification is provided without loss (Fig. 10.45). Furthermore, if the photon conversion scintillator is coated directly onto the intensifier, rather than onto a conventional fiber-optic faceplate, additional losses are avoided. The aim is to provide as high a *detective quantum efficiency* (DQE) as possible, where DQE = $(\mathrm{snr/SNR})^2$ and *snr*, *SNR* are the signal-to-noise ratios at input and output, respectively.[31]

Phase Contrast Imaging. In conventional x-ray imaging, the contrast is dependent on the photoelectric and Compton scattering processes with sensitivity to density variations $\Delta\rho/\rho$, depending on the relative absorption of adjacent rays. In phase contrast imaging, the contrast is dependent on the elastic Thompson scattering process with sensitivity to density variation $\Delta\rho/\rho$ determined by the refraction of adjacent rays at the boundaries of the structured density variation. The differences in refraction create a slight deviation in the x-ray wavefront so that a phase delay occurs. The small phase differences are separated in a crystal analyzer to form the image. The advantage over absorption contrast is that the phase delay remains significant even when the detail becomes very small. To distinguish the phase delay, the x-rays must be monochromatic and parallel. With a sufficiently coherent source this can be achieved with crystal monochromator (Fig. 10.46).

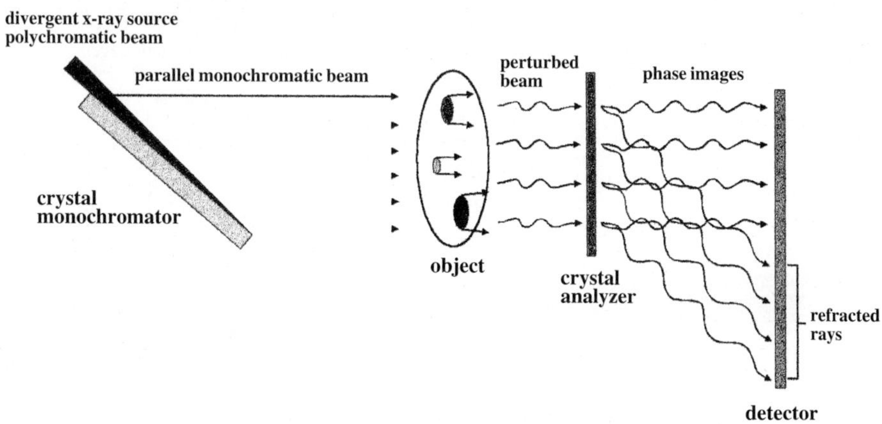

FIGURE 10.46 Phase contrast imaging.

10.4.4 Motion Systems

The specimen motion required for cone-beam reconstruction is a lateral axes (x, z) translation and a vertical axis β rotation. The scanning cycle needs to be under computer control in order to synchronize mechanical movement with data acquisition. Further, the control must provide a level of accuracy that, at the very least, matches the measured resolution of the x-ray source. In practice, an encoded accuracy in lateral translation of 10,000 counts per mm and a rotational accuracy of 2000 counts per degree of revolution can be achieved with commercial components.

The system shown in Fig. 10.47 has a vertical z movement of ~100 mm to facilitate specimen mounting and spiral scanning and a lateral x movement of ~40 mm for specimen alignment. It has an RS232 interface with a PC through a three-axis servo control that uses incremental encoder feedback to monitor position, speed, and direction. The level of proportional, integral, and differential (PID) feedback can be set for the optimum response and accuracy. Motion commands in ASCII format can be executed in immediate real time or loaded for programmed operation (Fig. 10.48). The camera three-axis traverse is servo controlled with a similar RS232 interface (Fig. 10.49). The motion control interfaces are daisy-chain-linked to the controlling PC (Fig. 10.50).

System Alignment. In a basic setting where the detector quarter-shift scheme is not considered, the back-projection function of the cone-beam reconstruction algorithm assumes that the central ray, which passes through the origin of the coordinate system, intersects the center point of the camera input plane. It also assumes that the z axis, which is the rotation axis, is aligned with the detector cell columns of the camera input plane. Hence, the camera must be correctly located with respect to the

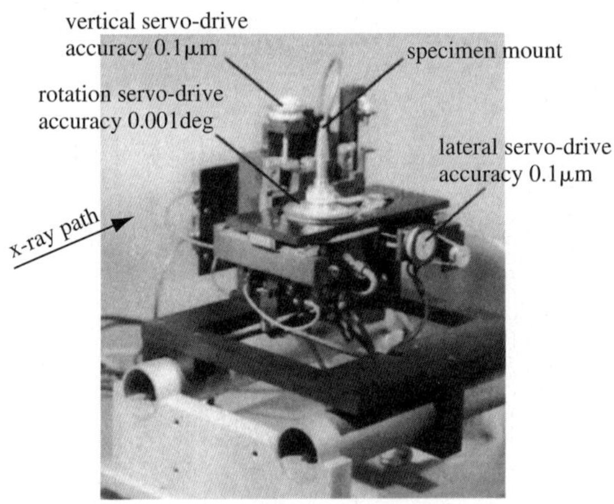

FIGURE 10.47 Servo-controlled specimen motion stage.

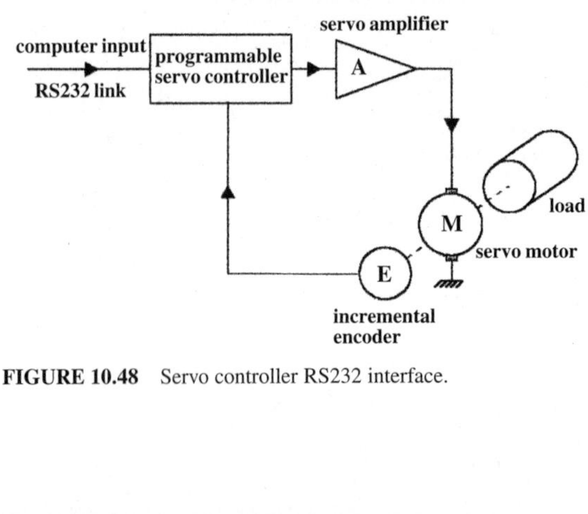

FIGURE 10.48 Servo controller RS232 interface.

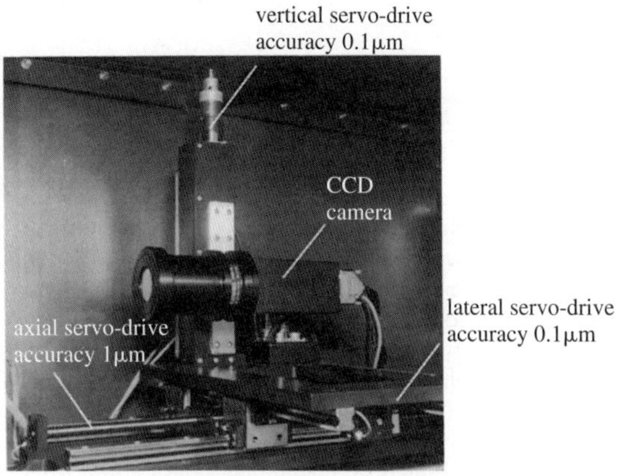

FIGURE 10.49 Servo-controlled camera traverse.

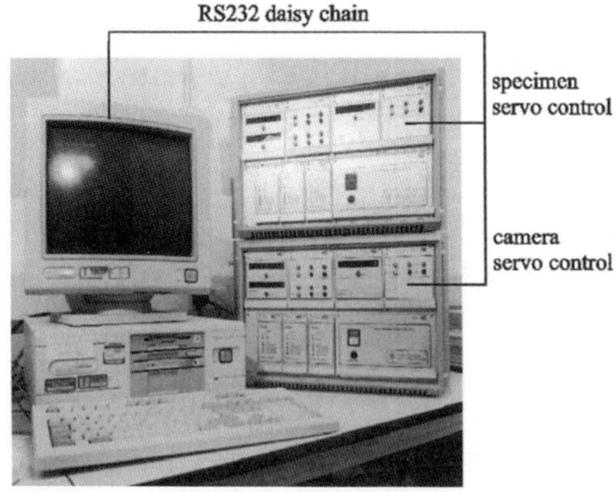

FIGURE 10.50 Motion systems PC interface racks.

x-ray source central ray and the specimen stage rotation axis must be correctly located and aligned with the camera.

In order to center the camera on the central ray, a double-aperture collimator is located over the x-ray chamber window. The aperture size and spacing is selected to provide a 2° cone beam at the first aperture, which is subsequently stopped down to a 1° cone beam by the second aperture. The double aperture ensures that the central ray is orthogonal to the electron beam column and parallel to the instrumentation support rails. The location of the aperture axis can be adjusted to coincide with the x-ray focal spot. The geometry of this arrangement provides a projected image of the collimator aperture for alignment with the camera center point (Fig. 10.51). The camera is translated in x, z until the center of the image, given by $(a + b)/2$ and $(c + d)/2$, is located at the pixel coordinates (511.5, 511.5) that define the frame center.

A small 1.5-mm-diameter precision-machined spindle is mounted on the specimen motion stage to provide an image for alignment of the camera vertical axis with the specimen rotation axis. The camera can be rotated about its longitudinal axis for this purpose. Two images are recorded, at 0° and 180°, to take account of any eccentricity, or tilt of the spindle with respect to the rotational center (Fig. 10.52). The camera is rotated in θ until the average of the coordinates of two locations along the spindle images have the same lateral pixel location.

To align the specimen rotation axis with the camera center point, two images are recorded at 0° and 180° to take account of any eccentricity of the spindle with respect to the rotational center. The spindle is translated in x until the average of the coordinates of the location a, b or c, d is equal to the pixel value 511.5 at the center of the frame (Fig. 10.53).

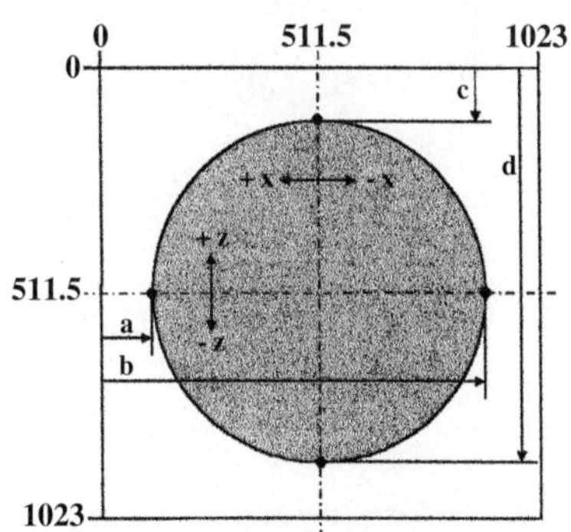

FIGURE 10.51 Camera center point alignment.

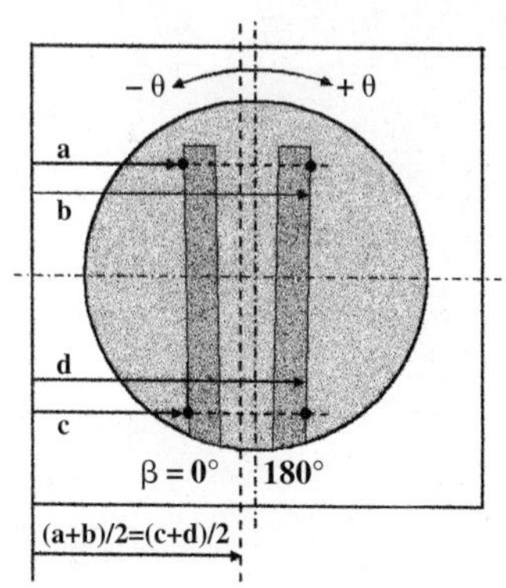

FIGURE 10.52 Camera θ rotation alignment.

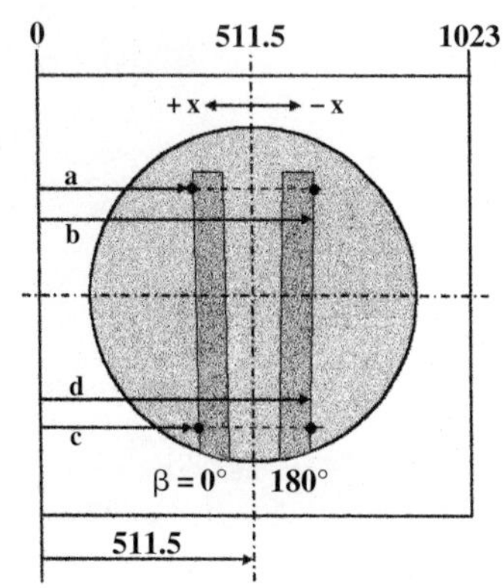

FIGURE 10.53 Specimen rotation axis alignment.

10.4.5 Ancillary Instrumentation

Data Acquisition. The broad interpretation of data acquisition relates to the various operations that are executed in a sequential fashion to secure a complete data set for subsequent computational reconstruction. In a narrower sense, this principally involves specimen motion, frame grabbing, and storing. For an efficient operation, these functions must be carried out automatically with provision for programming operational parameters such as the motion step value and total number of steps/frames, and the camera integration period. The system described in this section has an NT PC with an installed programmable PCI board and a fiber-optic link to control the camera and also communicates with a programmable servo controller for specimen motion via the RS232 port.

The organization of frame grabbing and specimen motion is performed by a programmable interface written in Python, which is an interpreted, interactive, object-oriented language. This provides the handshaking function that is essential for error-free sequential operation. The interface will pick up configuration files that set the camera parameters and servo control parameters. Run-specific details are entered in proffered dialog boxes at the outset of a data acquisition sequence. The image frames are temporarily stored on the PC hard disk and subsequently downloaded onto a Sun Micro Systems SCSI multiple-disk drive.

To provide an example of data quality, a sample of hollow glass spheres (ballotini), size ranging roughly from 10 to 100 μm, is reconstructed using a 2-mm-bore beryllium tube specimen holder (Fig. 10.54). The rotation step interval is 0.5° over 360° to give 720 projected frames of 1024 × 1024 pixel size. The volume is reconstructed using the cone-beam algorithm with a voxel size of 2.5 μm for a projection magnification of ×18. The illustrated tomograph is quarter-size child volume extracted from the full reconstruction. A reference standard was provided by two-dimensional electron micrograph images of a similar sample.

Specimen Stage. The delicate labile nature of biological materials presents a particularly stringent set of conditions for the design of the specimen stage, especially since controlled variations in temperature are often required. The difficulties are compounded by the need to move the specimen in a precisely controlled and accurate manner during the acquisition of projection data for tomographic reconstruction. To illustrate these points, a particular example of a design solution, one that has a proved successful performance, is described as follows.

The requirement is for (1) very accurate linear motion along the lateral x, z axes and very accurate β rotation motion about the vertical z axis, (2) very accurate temperature control, and

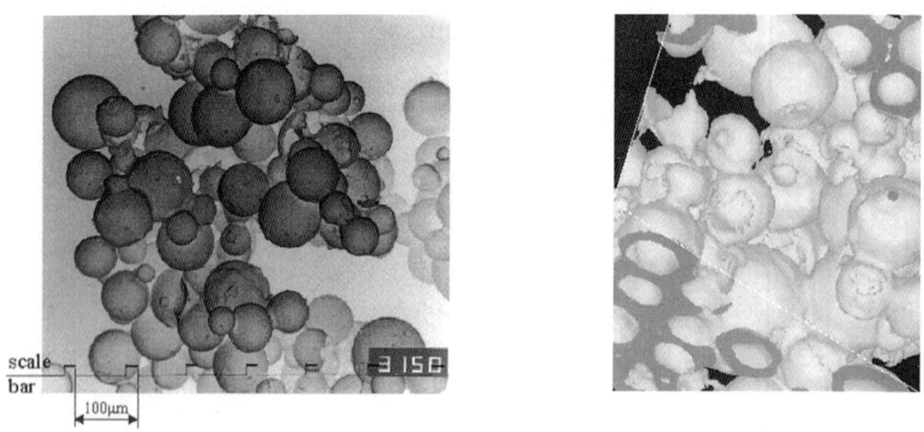

(a) (b)

FIGURE 10.54 Tomographic reconstruction of hollow glass spheres (ballotini). (*a*) Electron micrograph (two-dimensional); (*b*) x-ray tomograph (three-dimensional).

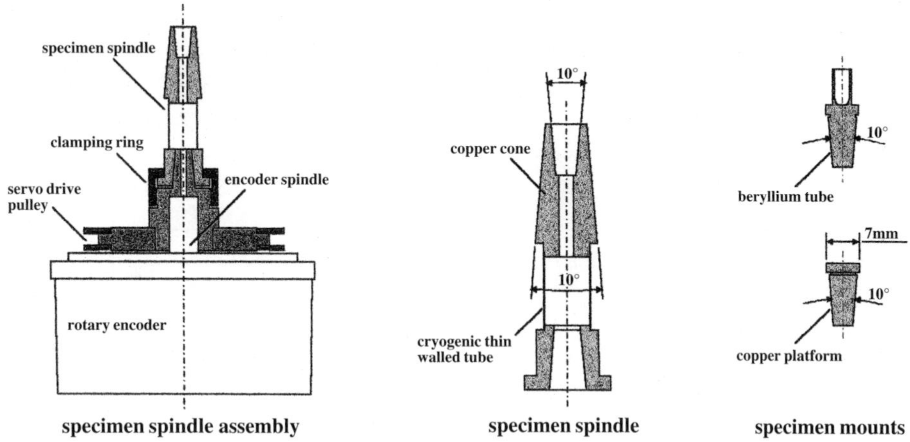

FIGURE 10.55 Specimen rotary stage.

(3) versatile specimen mounting. An important step is to uncouple the motion control system from the thermal control system so that requirements (1) and (2) can function independently. The solution is to let the motion system engage mechanically with the thermal system but allow the latter to passively follow the movement of the specimen. This means that the thermal system must apply only the weakest of constraint to three-dimensional displacement and offer minimal resistance to rotation in the vertical axis.

A cone-on-cone contact is a suitable geometry for mechanical engagement, provided that the cone angle and material are correctly chosen. Since good thermal contact is required, copper is a natural choice, and a 10° cone will provide solid location while keeping the mechanical contact stiction and friction to within acceptable bounds. To minimize shaft bearing inaccuracies, the specimen spindle is built directly onto the highly accurate rotary encoder shaft (Fig. 10.55). Here, a thin-walled stainless steel tube thermally isolates the specimen mount receptacle from the spindle-clamping assembly. The specimen mount also has a conical surface for good thermal contact and alignment. Typical mounting arrangements consist of a copper platform to which stable specimens can be lightly bonded and a thin-walled beryllium tube into which unstable specimens can be inserted.

The contacting component of the thermal system, namely, the copper cold-stage block, is required to float with a small downward force in order to engage positively with the specimen spindle of the motion system. The cold-stage block has a conical bore to receive the specimen spindle and controls the temperature of the specimen mount through thermal conduction across the conical contact surface. Primary heat transfer through thermoelectric coolers maintains the base temperature variation, and secondary heat transfer from buried cartridge heaters maintains temperature control. Solutions to Eq. (10.122) were computed numerically to confirm that a uniform temperature distribution could be maintained with the specific shape and size of the cold-stage block for given values of heat input and heat output. On the basis of these calculations, two 70-W thermoelectric coolers were located at the outer surfaces of the block and four 16-W cartridge heaters were inserted in one surface of the block (Fig. 10.56).

The cold-stage block is counterbalanced through a sprocket-and-chain mechanism to offset the weight and is attached to an unrestrained three-axis miniature slide to permit motion within a 40-mm cubic space (Fig. 10.57). The complete assembly is supported on a micrometer-adjustable pitch/roll plate for alignment of the conical engagement bore with the rotational axis of the motion stage. An environmental chamber, with thin beryllium x-ray path windows, encloses the cold stage and a controlled dry gas bleed prevents water droplet condensation.

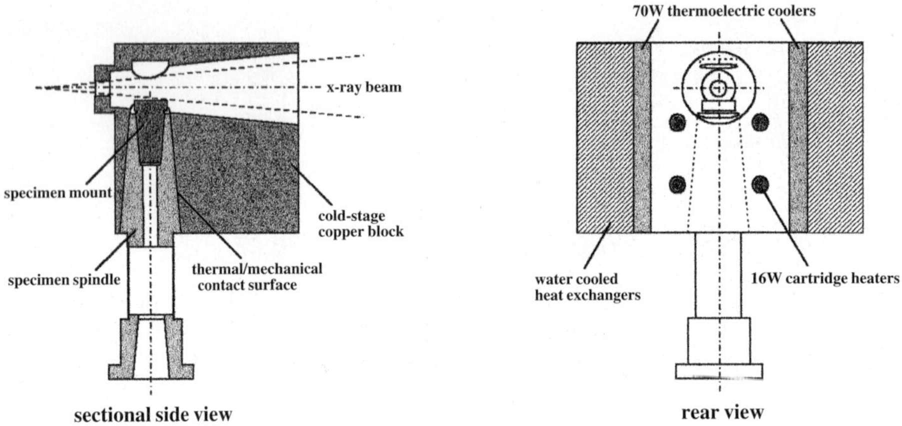

FIGURE 10.56 Cold-stage block assembly.

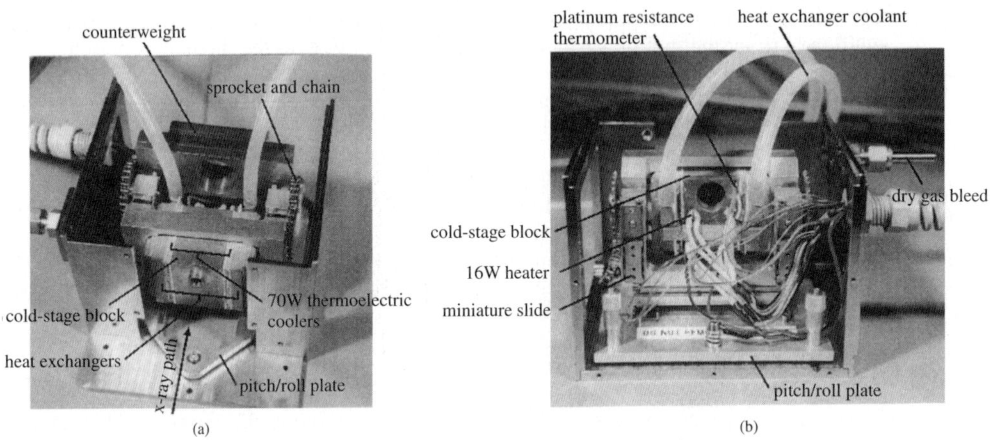

FIGURE 10.57 Thermal control stage assembly. (*a*) Top view; (*b*) rear view with counter weight removed.

Platinum resistance thermometers monitor the temperature, and a three-term tunable PID controller, which is RS232-linked to a PC, stabilizes the value at the set point to an accuracy of at least 0.1°C by regulating the secondary heat transfer. The set point temperature can be programmed, so that precise thermal cycling is available, or manually entered for step variation. The working temperature range is ±50°C with a thermal response ~0.2°C/s.

The system is ideal for examining the rearrangement of microstructural composition of soft-solid materials with variation in temperature. An example of a material that is practically impossible to image in the natural state by conventional optical microscopy is shown in (Fig. 10.58*a*). The volumes depicted are child volumes, containing a region of interest (ROI), extracted from the reconstruction of a frozen four-phase soft-solid structure. The reconstructed volume is derived from 720 filtered and

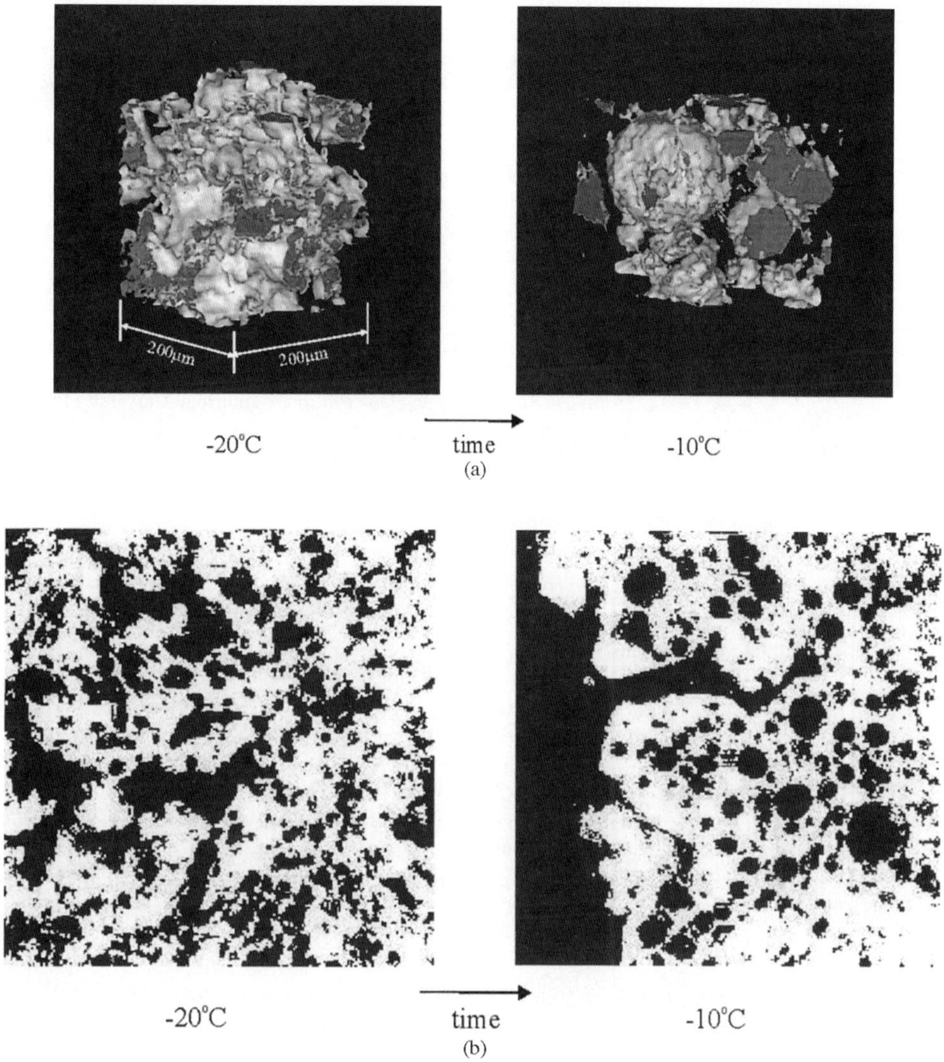

FIGURE 10.58 Soft-solid four-phase composite material. (*a*) Three-dimensional reconstruction; (*b*) two-dimensional slice.

back-projected frames using the Feldkamp cone-beam algorithm, with a resolution of 512 × 512 pixels per frame.

The material was initially chilled to −20°C and subsequently warmed to −10°C. The alteration in the air cell network (black) and the structural rearrangement of the ice plus matrix phase (white) with temperature rise is clearly defined. To provide quantitative measurement of microstructural detail, the volume is sliced across a region of interest (Fig. 10.58*b*). Here, the slice pixel size is 5 μm for a projection magnification of ×18.

REFERENCES

1. G. T. Herman, *Image Reconstruction from Projections—The Fundamentals of Computerized Tomography,* Academic Press, New York, 1980.
2. F. Natterer, *The Mathematics of Computerized Tomography,* John Wiley and Sons, New York, 1986.
3. A. C. Kak and M. Slaney, *Principles of Computerized Tomographic Imaging,* IEEE Press, New York, 1988.
4. H. H. Barrett and W. Swindell, *Radiological Imaging—The Theory of Image Formation, Detection, and Processing,* Academic Press, New York, 1981.
5. N. F. Mott and H. S. W. Massey, *The Theory of Atomic Collisions,* Oxford University Press, London, 1965.
6. A. H. Compton and S. K. Allison, *X-Rays in Theory and Experiment,* D. Van Nostrand, New York, 1935.
7. N. A. Dyson, *X-Rays in Atomic and Nuclear Physics,* Cambridge University Press, Cambridge, 1973.
8. V. Kohn, *Selected Topics in the Theory of Coherent Scattering of X-Rays—Hamburg Lectures,* Kurchatov Institute, Moscow, 1998.
9. J. Baruchel, J.-Y. Buffiere, E. Maire, P. Merl, and G. Peix, *X-Ray Tomography in Material Science,* Hermes Science Publications, Paris, 2000.
10. E. Kreyszig, *Advanced Engineering Mathematics,* John Wiley and Sons, New York, 1988.
11. R. N. Bracewell, *The Fourier Transform and Its Applications,* McGraw-Hill, New York, 1978.
12. R. C. Gonzalez and R. E. Woods, *Digital Image Processing,* Addison-Wesley, New York, 1992.
13. L. A. Feldkamp, L. C. Davis, and J. W. Kress, "Practical Cone-Beam Algorithm," *J. Opt. Soc. Am.,* A **1**(6), June 1984.
14. B. D. Smith, "Image Reconstruction From Cone-Beam Projections—Necessary and Sufficient Conditions and Reconstruction Methods," *IEEE Trans. Med. Imag.,* **4**(1), March 1985.
15. Ge Wang, C. R. Crawford, and W. A. Kalender, "Multirow Detector and Cone-Beam Spiral/Helical CT," *IEEE. Med. Imag*., **19**(9), September 2000.
16. Ge Wang, S. Zhao, and P. Cheng, "Exact and Approximate Cone-Beam X-Ray Microtomography, Modern Microscopies (I)—Instrumentation and Image Processing," *World Scientific,* Singapore, 1998.
17. Ge Wang and M. W. Vannier, "Computerized Tomography," *Encyclopedia of Electrical and Electronics Engineering,* John Wiley and Sons, New York, 1998.
18. C. A. Carlsson, G. Matscheko, and P. Spanne, "Prospects for Microcomputerized-Tomography Using Synchrotron Radiation," *Biological Trace Element Research,* **13**, 1987.
19. P. Rockett and R. W. Parish, "A Wide-Energy Range, High-Resolution Microfocal X-Ray Source," *British Journal of NDT,* March 1986.
20. V. E. Cosslett and W. C. Nixon, *X-Ray Microscopy,* Cambridge Monographs in Physics, N. Feather and D. Shoenberg (eds.), Cambridge University Press, London, 1960.
21. E. Munro, "Computer-Aided Design of Electron Lenses by the Finite Element Method," *Image Processing and Computer Aided Design in Electron Optics,* P. W. Hawkes (ed.), Academic Press, London, 1973.
22. E. Hecht and A. Zajac, *Optics,* Addison-Wesley, London, 1979.
23. J. C. Dainty and R. Shaw, *Image Science,* Academic Press, London, 1974.
24. S. T. Stephenson, "The Continuous X-Ray Spectrum," *Handbuch der Physik,* S. Flugge (ed.), Springer, Berlin, 1957.
25. B. K. Agarwal, *X-ray Spectroscopy,* Springer Series in Optical Sciences, vol. **15**, Berlin, 1979.
26. N. A. Dyson, "The Continuous Spectrum from Electron-Opaque Targets," *Proc. Phys. Soc,* **73**(6), December 1958.

27. A. Bouwers and P. Diepenhorst, *X-Ray Research and Development,* Philips, Eindhoven, 1933.

28. W. J. Oosterkamp, "The Heat Dissipation in the Anode of an X-Ray Tube," *Philips Res. Rep.* **3**, 1948.

29. J. Vine and P. A. Einstein, "Heating Effect of an Electron Beam Impinging on a Solid Surface, Allowing for Penetration," *Proc. IEE,* 1964.

30. J. C. Elliott, P. Anderson, G. R. Davis, F. S. L. Wong, and S. D. Dover, "Computed Tomography, Part II: The Practical Use of a Single Source and Detector," *Journal of Microscopy,* March 1994.

31. J. D. Vincent, *Fundamentals of Infrared Detector Operation and Testing,* John Wiley and Sons, 1990.

CHAPTER 11

NUCLEAR MEDICINE IMAGING INSTRUMENTATION

Mark Madsen
University of Iowa, Iowa City, Iowa

11.1 INTRODUCTION

Nuclear medicine is a diagnostic imaging modality that can be used to obtain clinical information about most of the major tissues and organs of the body. Diagnostic information is obtained from the way the tissues and organs process radiolabeled compounds (radiopharmaceuticals). The radiopharmaceutical is typically administered to the patient through an intravenous injection. The radiopharmaceutical is carried throughout the body by the circulation where it localizes in tissues and organs. Images of these distributions are acquired with a scintillation camera. Ideally, the radiopharmaceutical would only go to abnormal areas. Unfortunately, this is never the case and the abnormal concentration of the radiotracer is often obscured by normal uptake of the radiopharmaceutical in the surrounding tissues. Images of higher contrast and better localization can be obtained with tomographic systems designed for nuclear medicine studies: single photon emission computed tomography (SPECT) and positron emission tomography (PET). These are described in detail below.

Gamma rays are high-energy photons that are emitted as a consequence of radioactive decay. In conventional nuclear medicine, the most commonly used radionuclide is ^{99m}Tc which emits a 140-keV gamma ray. Other radionuclides used in conventional nuclear medicine are given in Table 11.1. With conventional nuclear medicine imaging, the emitted gamma rays that reach the detector are counted individually. This is often referred to as *single photon detection*. One particular type of radioactive decay, beta plus or positron emission, results in the emission of a positron which is the antiparticle of the electron. The positron very quickly annihilates with an electron, producing 2, approximately colinear 511-keV annihilation photons. The simultaneous detection of the 2 annihilation photons by opposed detectors (coincidence detection) provides the basis for PET imaging.

Although radionuclides are nearly ideal tracers, the imaging of radiotracers in the body presents special challenges that are unique. The flux of gamma rays available for imaging is orders of magnitude less than that used in x-ray radiography or CT. In addition, the high energy of the

TABLE 11.1 Common Nuclear Medicine Radionuclides

Radionuclide	Decay	Half-life	Gamma ray energy
^{99m}Tc	IT	6 h	140 keV
^{111}In	EC	67 h	172, 247 keV
^{131}I	β−	8 d	364 keV
^{123}I	EC	13 h	159 keV
^{67}Ga	EC	78 h	93, 185, 300 keV
^{201}Tl	EC	73 h	60–80 keV (x-rays)
^{81m}Kr	IT	13 s	190 keV
^{133}Xe	β−	5.3 d	80 keV

gamma rays makes detection more difficult. This is especially true for the 511-keV annihilation photons associated with PET. As a result, the images produced in nuclear medicine studies are much noisier and have worse spatial resolution than those generated from computed tomography (CT) or magnetic resonance imaging (MRI). In order to appreciate these problems and how they affect the design of nuclear medicine imaging devices, we will briefly review the physics of gamma ray interactions.

The intensity of gamma rays traveling through material is gradually reduced by absorption or scattering. This loss of gamma rays is referred to as *attenuation* and is described by the exponential equation shown below:

$$I(x) = Io \exp(-\mu x) \tag{11.1}$$

where Io = the initial intensity
$I(x)$ = the intensity after traveling a distance x through the material
μ = the linear attenuation coefficient of the material.

Over the range of gamma ray energies used in radionuclide imaging, the two primary interactions that contribute to the attenuation coefficient are photoelectric absorption and Compton scattering. Photoelectric absorption refers to the total absorption of the gamma ray by an inner-shell atomic electron and is the primary interaction in high atomic number (Z) materials such as sodium iodide (the detector material used in the scintillation camera) and lead. In low Z materials such as body tissues, its contribution to attenuation is relatively small. Compton scattering occurs when the incoming gamma ray interacts with a loosely bound outer shell electron. A portion of the gamma ray energy is imparted to the electron and the remaining energy is left with the scattered photon. The amount of energy lost in the event depends on the angle between the gamma ray and scattered photon. Compton scattering is the dominant interaction in body tissues.

High attenuation is desirable in detecting and shielding materials. Ideally, materials used for these purposes would absorb every gamma ray. In the body, attenuation is very undesirable since it reduces the number of events that can be acquired and scattered radiation that reaches the detector causes a significant loss of image contrast.

11.2 CONVENTIONAL GAMMA RAY IMAGING: SCINTILLATION CAMERA

The scintillation camera is the primary imaging instrument used in conventional nuclear medicine and is often referred to as a *gamma camera*. The scintillation camera is a position-sensitive gamma ray imager. Although the entire field of view is available for detection, it processes one event at a time. The spatial resolution is approximately 10 mm and it yields a count rate of 200 to 300 cpm/μCi in the field of view. The field of view covers a large portion of the body and is typically 40 × 50 cm, although other sizes are available. The first scintillation camera was developed by Hal O Anger in 1958.[1] Although this system was very crude, it contained the fundamental components of all future designs: thallium-activated sodium iodide [NaI(T1)] as the primary detector, weighted signals from an array of photomultiplier tubes to determine the location of detected events, and lead collimation as the imaging aperture.

The gamma ray detector of the scintillation camera is a large, thin piece of NaI(T1). Although the crystals originally had a circular cross section, most scintillation cameras now use a rectangular crystal with dimensions as large as 40 × 55 cm. The thickness of NaI(Tl) in most conventional cameras is 9.5 mm, but in systems that are used for coincidence detection, the crystal may be twice as thick. Sodium iodide is a scintillator that converts gamma ray energy into visible light with a relatively high efficiency. The amount of light generated is directly proportional to the absorbed energy and the absorption of one 140-keV gamma ray will yield approximately 5000 visible light photons. There are a number of advantages associated with NaI(Tl) in addition to its high light output. It efficiently absorbs the 140-keV gamma rays of ^{99m}Tc with a photopeak efficiency of 85 percent, and it has a moderate energy resolution. Energy resolution is an important property since it provides the means to discriminate against scattered radiation. Gamma rays that undergo scattering within the patient degrade the quality of images. However, scattered gamma rays necessarily have less energy than unscattered gamma rays and can be selectively eliminated on that basis. Another positive feature of NaI(Tl) is that it can be manufactured in many shapes and sizes. There are disadvantages though. Sodium iodide is hygroscopic and actively absorbs water vapor from the air, resulting in a loss of transparency of the crystal to the scintillation. The detector must be hermetically sealed, and loss of this seal results in irreparable damage. Another disadvantage is that the persistence of the scintillation is long enough that it limits the count rate that the detector can accurately handle. Because conventional nuclear medicine imaging requires very low sensitivity collimators, high count rate is rarely an issue. However, count rate limitations are a very real problem for PET imaging systems where coincidence detection replaces collimation.

Converting the gamma ray energy to visible light is only the first step in the detection process. In order for the information from the scintillation to be useful it has to be converted into an electronic signal with a photomultiplier tube (PMT). The PMT is a vacuum tube with a photoemissive surface called the *photocathode*. Visible light hitting this surface knocks off electrons. These electrons are accelerated to an electric terminal called a *dynode*. The first dynode has a potential of approximately 100 V higher than the photocathode, and the electrons hit it with enough force to knock off about 4 more new electrons. The next dynode is another 100 V higher so the process is repeated. The same process occurs over a total series of 9 dynodes, resulting in a signal amplification of 1,000,000. Proportionality is maintained throughout this amplification so that the size of the resulting electronic pulse is directly proportional to the energy deposited by the gamma ray.

A scintillation camera needs to be able to record the location of gamma ray events over the large area of the NaI(Tl) crystal. This requires uniform sampling by an array of photomultiplier tubes. The PMTs are arranged in a close-packed array that covers the entire surface of the NaI(Tl) crystal (Fig. 11.1). The PMTs used in scintillation cameras are usually 2 or 3 in across, so that as many as 120 PMTs may be used. PMTs have been manufactured in variety of different cross sections in order to maximize their areal coverage. Circular, hexagonal, and square tubes have all been used for this purpose. The signals obtained from the PMTs are used to determine two important properties about the gamma ray interaction: the event location and the energy deposited in the detector from the interaction. The energy information is crucial for normalizing the position signals and for discriminating against scattered radiation.

While the energy of the interaction can be inferred by directly summing the PMT signals in the proximity of the event, the estimation of the event location requires that the PMT signals have spatial weighting factors that are determined by the physical location of each PMT within the array. Separate weighting factors are used for the x and y coordinates, and the location of the event is determined by summing the weighted PMT signals. This process is referred to as Anger logic, since it is the scheme developed by Hal Anger in the first scintillation camera. In the initial designs, all the PMTs in the array participated in the energy and position signal summations. It was subsequently found that the signals from PMTs located far from the event had a poor signal-to-noise

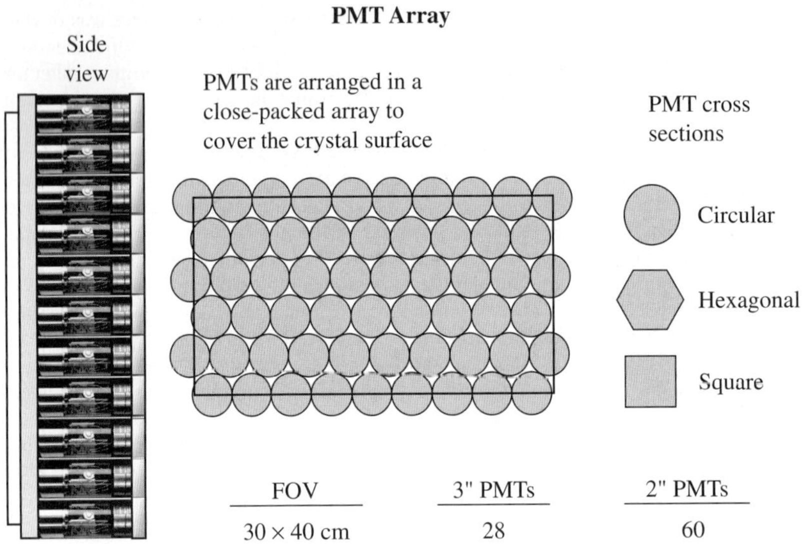

FOV	3" PMTs	2" PMTs
30 × 40 cm	28	60
40 × 55 cm	55	120

FIGURE 11.1 Photomultiplier tube array. The photomultiplier tubes are arranged in a close-packed array to cover the back surface of the single, large NaI(Tl) crystal.

ratio. In modern designs, the PMT signal must exceed a threshold before it is included in the sum. All the processing is performed on each detected event and the decision to include the event as a valid count is not made until the end of the processing when the pulse height analysis is done. Only those events that fall within the selected energy window are recorded (Fig. 11.2).

The position signals determined from summing the weighted PMT signals vary with the brightness of the scintillation which itself depends on the energy absorbed in the crystal. This

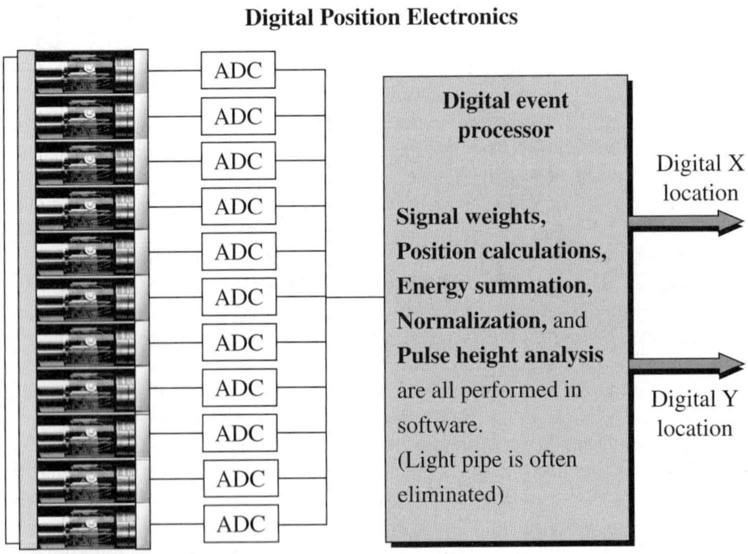

FIGURE 11.2 Scintillation camera signal processing. The output signals from each photomultiplier tube are digitized, allowing them to be processed with a computer algorithm to determine the energy and location of the detected event.

means that an object imaged with a high-energy gamma ray like ^{131}I (364 keV) will be magnified when compared to the same object imaged with ^{99m}Tc (140 keV). This magnification is a concern even when only one gamma ray energy is imaged because of the finite energy resolution of the scintillation camera system. The pulse heights from the absorptions of identical gamma rays vary enough to cause slight minification and magnification ultimately degrading spatial resolution. This problem is avoided by normalizing the position signals with the measured energy signal. Energy normalization removes the image size dependence with signal variations, thereby improving spatial resolution and allowing the simultaneous imaging of more than one radionuclide without distortion.

As has been previously noted, gamma rays that are scattered within the patient have distorted spatial information and degraded image contrast. Because scattered gamma rays necessarily lose energy, they can be selectively avoided by only accepting events that have pulse heights corresponding to the primary gamma ray energy. The pulse height analyzer provides this capability. A "window" is centered to cover 15 to 20 percent of the photopeak. All energy pulses that meet this criterion generate a logic pulse that indicates to the system that a valid event has occurred and these events are recorded.

Once there is an x and y coordinate that locates a valid event, this information has to be stored as image data. Although it is possible on some scintillation camera systems to store the individual coordinates sequentially (referred to as *list mode acquisition*), most systems store the information directly in histogram or matrix mode. With this method, an array of computer memory, typically 128 × 128 or 256 × 256, is reserved for each image frame. The count value of each matrix element or pixel is initially set to 0. The x and y coordinates for each valid event point to a specific pixel, and this pixel is incremented by 1. When the acquisition-stopping criteria are met (e.g., acquisition time or total acquired counts), the image is complete. The information in the matrix is either gray scale or color encoded to display the image data. The entire process is shown schematically in Fig. 11.3. A gamma

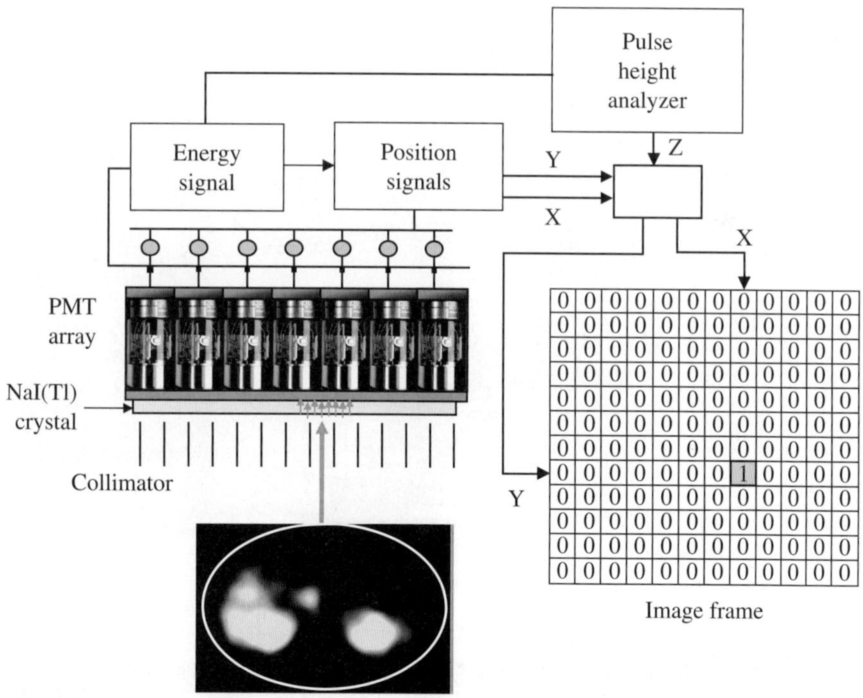

FIGURE 11.3 Scintillation camera image acquisition. The scintillation camera processes each detected event to determine energy and the x and y locations. If an event falls within the selected energy window, the memory location pointed to by the x and y coordinates is incremented. The process continues until a preselected time or count limit is achieved.

ray originating in the patient is absorbed in the NaI(Tl) crystal. The light from the scintillation is sampled by the PMT array which determines both the *x* and *y* coordinates of the event and its energy. If the energy signal falls within the window of the pulse height analyzer, the *x* and *y* coordinates are used to increment the appropriate pixel. This process is repeated for every detected event.

In order to form images with a scintillation camera, a collimator must be mounted in front of the NaI(Tl) crystal. The collimator is the image-forming aperture of the camera system, and it is necessary for the imaging process.[2] The collimator projects the gamma ray pattern originating in the patient onto the NaI(Tl) crystal by selectively absorbing diverging gamma rays. The collimator is a close-packed array of holes with lead walls. Most often the holes have a parallel orientation, but collimators with a fan or cone beam geometry are available. Pinhole collimators are also used for some clinical imaging and are the mainstay of small animal systems. Gamma rays whose trajectory takes them through a hole get to interact with the NaI(Tl), while all the others are absorbed. The design of collimators depends on the gamma ray energy and the ever-present trade-off between count sensitivity and spatial resolution. Collimators used for imaging ^{99m}Tc typically have holes that are 1 to 1.5 mm across and are 20 to 40 mm thick.

Although collimators are necessary for the formation of images, they are the limiting factor in both the count sensitivity and spatial resolution of the scintillation camera. Less than 1 in 5000 gamma rays that hit the front surface of the collimator get through to the crystal. To improve the count sensitivity, the collimator hole size could be increased and the hole length shortened. Unfortunately, these changes degrade the spatial resolution. The spatial resolution of the collimator is constrained by the geometry of the holes and is typically in the range of 6 to 8 mm at 10 cm when used with ^{99m}Tc. This is the dominant factor in determining the overall system resolution since the intrinsic spatial resolution is in the range of 3 to 4 mm. One very important property to remember about collimators is that the spatial resolution gets worse as the source to collimator distance increases. This is illustrated in the set of phantom images that were acquired from 5 to 30 cm from the collimator surface (Fig. 11.4). To obtain the best quality images, it is crucial to keep the collimator as close to the patient as possible.

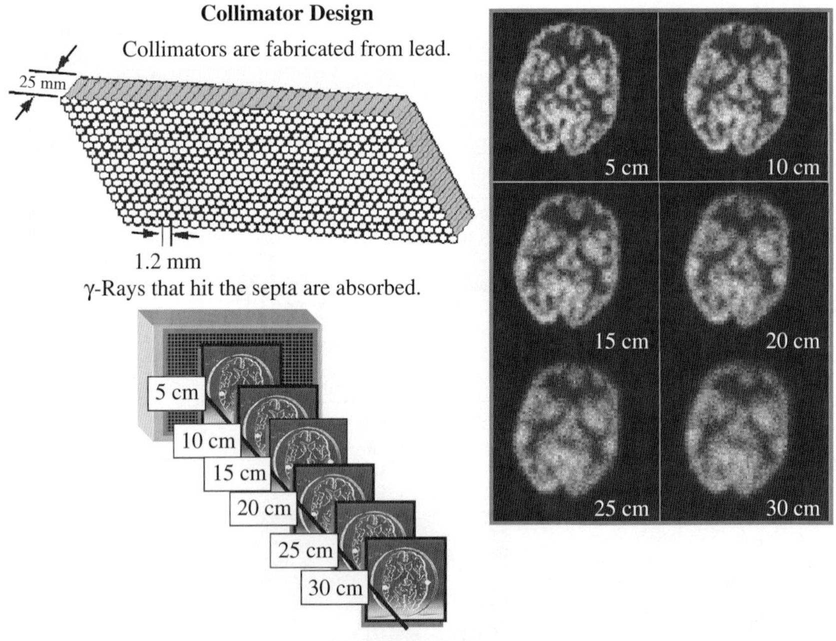

FIGURE 11.4 Collimation. The collimator is the image-forming aperture of the scintillation camera. It projects an image of the radionuclide distribution onto the detector by selectively absorbing diverging gamma rays and passing those gamma rays with a trajectory passing through a hole. Collimators are the limiting factor of both spatial resolution and count sensitivity. Spatial resolution degrades as the source to collimator distance increases.

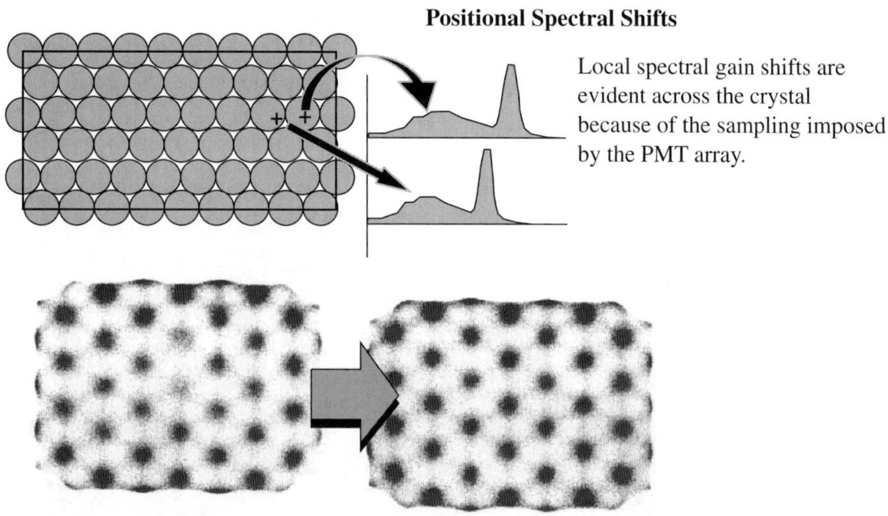

FIGURE 11.5 Energy correction. The magnitude of the energy signals are position dependent, which degrades the overall energy resolution of the camera. This problem is corrected by setting multiple local energy windows across the field of view. While energy correction does not improve uniformity, it makes the camera more stable to scatter conditions.

The modern scintillation camera has improved performance because of improvements in the components and electronics.[3] The availability of digital electronics has allowed the elimination of the light pipe which improves both energy and spatial resolution. However, this requires additional corrections because of the nonlinear response of the PMT array to the scintillations. If a collimated point source were focused on a portion of the NaI(Tl) crystal located exactly on a PMT center, the energy spectrum would be distinctly different than one that was acquired from a point in between two tubes, reflecting the differences in light collection efficiency. This position-dependent shift in the energy spectrum causes an overall loss in energy resolution and also results in regional variations in scatter fraction. The solution to this problem is to locally sample the energy spectra and regionally adjust the energy window for each area. Typically, the camera field of view is divided into a 64 × 64 matrix, and energy window adjustments are made for each of the 4096 regions.

Figure 11.5 shows the effect of energy correction. The images show the response of the scintillation camera to a uniform flux of gamma rays. First, it should be noted that both the corrected and uncorrected images are highly nonuniform and are not adequate for imaging. The energy correction simply makes sure that each region of the crystal is contributing valid photopeak events to the image. This results in only a subtle improvement in uniformity at this stage. However, it makes the subsequent corrections more robust since there will be much less dependence on the effects of scattered radiation, which can vary over a large range depending on the imaging situation.

Because of the nonlinear response of the PMTs, detected events are not correctly positioned using Anger logic alone. The parameter that quantifies how well-detected events are positioned is called *spatial linearity*. The optimization of spatial linearity requires the acquisition of an image from a well-defined distribution. Typically this is accomplished with a highly precise rectangular hole pattern machined in lead that is placed directly on the NaI(Tl) crystal. A distant point source of radioactivity is used to project the image of the hole pattern onto to the scintillation camera. The image of this pattern appears similar to that on the left portion of Fig. 11.6 with distortions caused by spatial nonlinearity. Because the actual and measured location of the holes is known, regional displacements to the x and y coordinates can be calculated for each hole.

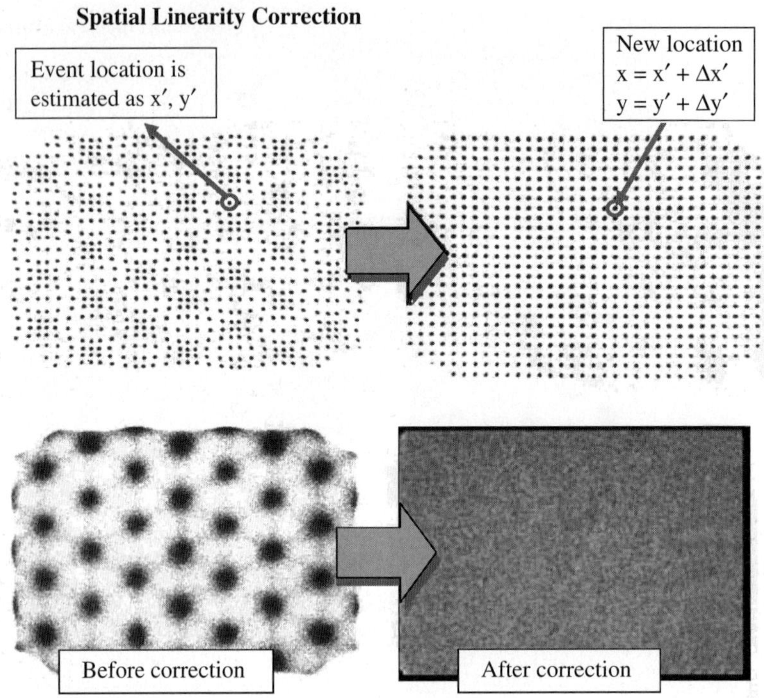

FIGURE 11.6 Spatial linearity correction. Residual positioning errors are corrected by creating a correction map from the image of a precision hole phantom. A lookup table of the position-dependent correction factors allows on the fly repositioning of the detected events that dramatically improves image uniformity.

Displacements for regions in between holes that are not directly sampled are interpolated at a very-high sampling frequency and stored as a lookup table. When a valid event is detected, the initial *x* and *y* coordinates are modified by the appropriated displacements read from the lookup table. Using this approach, events can be accurately positioned to better than 0.5 mm. The improvement in spatial linearity has a profound effect on field uniformity. Both images show the response of the scintillation camera to a uniform flux of gamma rays. With spatial linearity correction, the field becomes uniform to within ±10 percent of the mean image counts. Although this level of uniformity may be adequate for conventional planar imaging, tomographic imaging requires better uniformity.

There are still some residual nonuniformities that exist in the scintillation camera even after energy and spatial linearity correction have been applied. These are further reduced by applying uniformity correction. Typically, a high count flood is acquired and a map of the nonuniformities is stored in a memory buffer. During acquisition, the number of valid events that are acquired is modulated by this reference uniformity map to ensure uniformity. With this additional correction, the field uniformity can be reduced to within ±3 percent of the mean image counts.

Photomultiplier tubes are relatively unstable components. Their performance drifts as they age and the tubes are also sensitive to variations in temperature and humidity. In order for the energy, spatial linearity, and uniformity corrections to remain valid, there must be some way of maintaining the PMTs at a constant operating point. Most scintillation camera systems have PMT stabilization firmware that dynamically adjusts the PMTs in response to a known reference signal. Some vendors use a constant output light-emitting diode inside the detector housing that flashes at a rate of 10 times per second. The individual PMT signals from these calibration flashes are monitored to compare the

TABLE 11.2 Scintillation Camera Specifications (Typical Values)

Parameter	Specification
Crystal size	40 × 50 cm
Crystal thickness	9.5 mm
Efficiency at 140 keV	0.86 (photopeak)
Energy resolution	10%
Intrinsic spatial resolution	3.8 mm
System count sensitivity (general purpose collimator)	135 counts/s/MBq (300 counts/min/μCi)
System spatial resolution at 10 cm	9.5 mm
Intrinsic uniformity	3.5%

measured output to the desired value, and appropriate adjustments are automatically made to maintain the operating point. Another approach uses the ratio between the count rates in a photopeak and scatter window to maintain constant PMT response. Photomultiplier tubes are also very sensitive to magnetic fields, and changes in the orientation of the camera with respect to the earth's magnetic field are enough to cause measurable changes in field uniformity. To reduce this effect, each PMT is individually surrounded with mu-metal shielding.

A number of parameters are used to specify the performance of a scintillation camera.[4] These are listed in Table 11.2 along with representative values. Many of these parameters such as uniformity and spatial resolution are common to many imaging modalities. Others like system dead time and multiwindow spatial registration are specifically related to imaging gamma rays. For example, scintillation cameras have the capability of simultaneously imaging different energy gamma rays. Most scintillation cameras handle at least three and many can handle six or more energy windows. Because it is important that there be no significant distortion of the images obtained at the different energies, the correspondence between images acquired at different energies is monitored by the multiwindow spatial registration (MWSR).

Although the scintillation camera is used for the vast majority of nuclear medicine imaging, a number of special-purpose devices have been developed that deviate from the Anger design.[5,6] These imaging systems either use arrays of individual pixilated scintillators with position-sensitive photon transducers or semiconductor detectors. In every case this has occurred for small field of view devices designed for either a small organ like the heart or breast, or for the imaging of small animals like rats or mice. The pixilated approach has several advantages over the Anger camera.[7] The positioning of events is determined directly by the detector location, and the size of the detector determines the intrinsic resolution. In addition, pixilated detectors do not suffer from edge effects like Anger cameras so that the entire field defined by the detector array is useful. For the pixilated scintillators, several different photon transducers have been used instead of conventional PMTs, including position-sensitive photomultiplier tubes (PSPMTs) and avalanche photodiodes (APDs). An example of the former is a commercially available scintimammography device for diagnosing breast cancer made from 3000 individual 3-mm NaI(Tl) detectors and 48 PSPMTs. Another device in current use in heart imaging uses pixilated cesium iodide [CsI(Tl)] with an array of APDs.[8]

Solid-state semiconductor detectors directly convert the absorbed gamma ray energy into collection of electric charge, obviating the need for photon transducers. Cadmium zinc telluride (CZT) is an attractive solid-state detector that has been manufactured in a pixilated array and has comparable gamma ray detection efficiency to NaI(Tl) at 140 keV. The energy resolution with CZT is nearly a factor of 2 better than that of NaI(Tl). Because of its cost, no large field of view gamma ray imaging devices have been marketed with CZT, but several smaller devices have. These include scintimammography imaging systems and a cardiac SPECT system (see Sec. 11.3.3). There is also a novel SPECT system that has been developed for tomographic mammography that is based on CZT detectors.[9]

11.3 SINGLE PHOTON EMISSION COMPUTED TOMOGRAPHY

SPECT (single photon emission computed tomography) produces tomographic images of the internal distribution of radiopharmaceuticals.[10] It is most commonly used in the diagnosis of coronary artery disease and in tumor detection. Projection images collected by one or more scintillation cameras are mathematically reconstructed to obtain the tomographic slices. SPECT studies are performed for a wide variety of clinical indications and are often used in the diagnosing and monitoring of malignancies. However, myocardial perfusion studies evaluating the heart for coronary artery disease are by far the most common SPECT procedures. Quantitative SPECT yielding absolute radioactivity concentrations requires corrections for attenuation, scatter, and spatial resolution.

A SPECT system typically consists of one or more scintillation cameras mounted to a gantry that can revolve about a fixed horizontal axis (the axis of rotation) (Fig. 11.7*a*). The projection images in a SPECT study usually span a full 360° arc, although myocardial perfusion studies are typically acquired over the 180° arc that minimizes tissue attenuation. SPECT acquisitions are performed with the scintillation camera located at preselected angular locations (step-and-shoot mode), or in a continuous rotation mode. In the step-and-shoot mode, the detector rotates to each angular position and collects data for a preselected frame duration while the detector is motionless. In the continuous rotation mode, the study duration is selected and the rotation speed is adjusted to complete the orbit during this time. Projections are collected as the detector rotates and are binned into a 60 to 120 frames over 360° or 30 to 60 frames over 180° for cardiac studies. It is crucial to maintain close proximity to the body as the detector rotates about the patient to achieve the best possible spatial resolution. Although

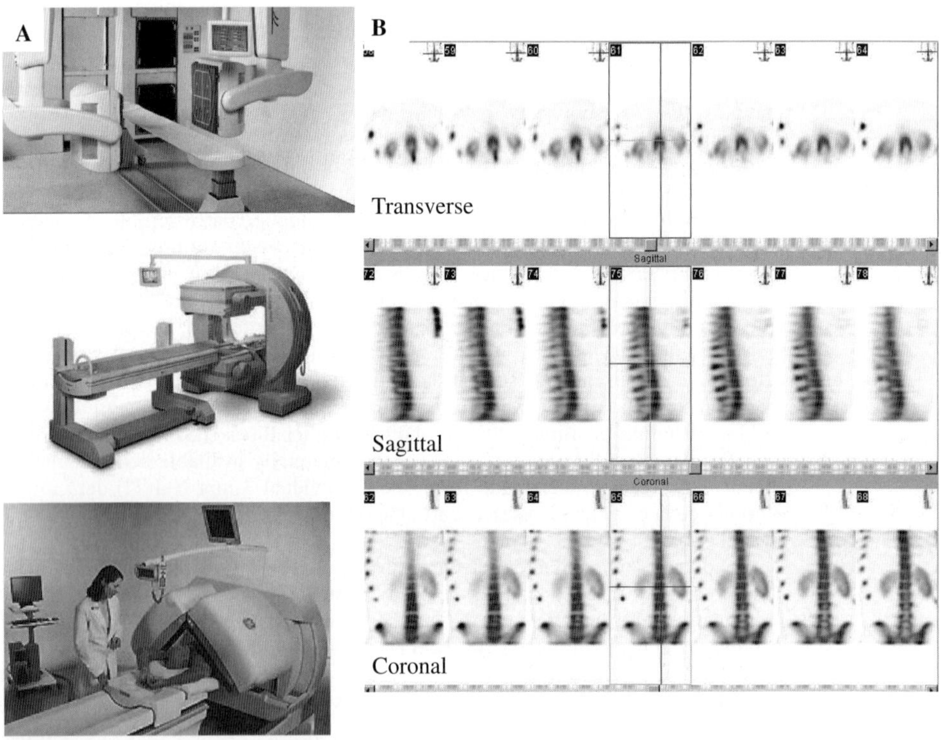

FIGURE 11.7 (*a*) Commercial SPECT systems. Typically two scintillation cameras are mounted on a gantry that can rotate about a patient lying on the table. (*b*) Typical ^{99m}Tc bone SPECT study.

a number of different approaches have been used to accomplish this, the most common method moves the detectors radially in and out as a function of rotation angle. An example bone SPECT study is shown in Fig. 11.7*b*.

The projection images acquired from a SPECT study do not reflect the line integrals of activity within the patient. The primary reason for this is the attenuation of the internally emitted gamma rays by body tissues. If projection images are reconstructed without correcting for tissue attenuation, the resulting images will have artifacts. This is a significant problem with myocardial perfusion since the attenuation artifacts can be mistaken for coronary artery disease. Accurate SPECT attenuation correction requires an independent measurement of the tomographic attenuation coefficients for the volume being imaged. One solution for obtaining this information is to collect transmission data through the patient from an external radioactive source using the gamma camera as a crude CT scanner.[11] Because of the multiple energy imaging capability of the scintillation camera, this transmission information can be collected simultaneously as part of the SPECT acquisition so long as the transmission source and the radiotracer have different gamma ray energies. Typically the radiotracer is labeled with ^{99m}Tc with a 140-keV gamma ray, while the transmission source is ^{153}Gd with a 100-keV gamma ray (Fig. 11.8). Although the quality of the attenuation maps obtained for this approach are poor, there is sufficient information to diminish the attenuation artifacts. An improved attenuation correction can be obtained with a combined SPECT and CT device which will be discussed later. Attenuation compensation requires the use of an iterative reconstruction algorithm that can incorporate the attenuation maps.[12]

Despite the energy discrimination available on all SPECT systems, Compton scattered radiation still accounts for about 30 to 40 percent of the acquired counts in SPECT imaging. Scattered radiation not only decreases contrast, it also impacts other corrections. For example, when attenuation correction is applied without also correcting for scattered radiation, the count density in the heart walls near the liver may be overenhanced. Scatter correction has been performed in several different ways,[13]

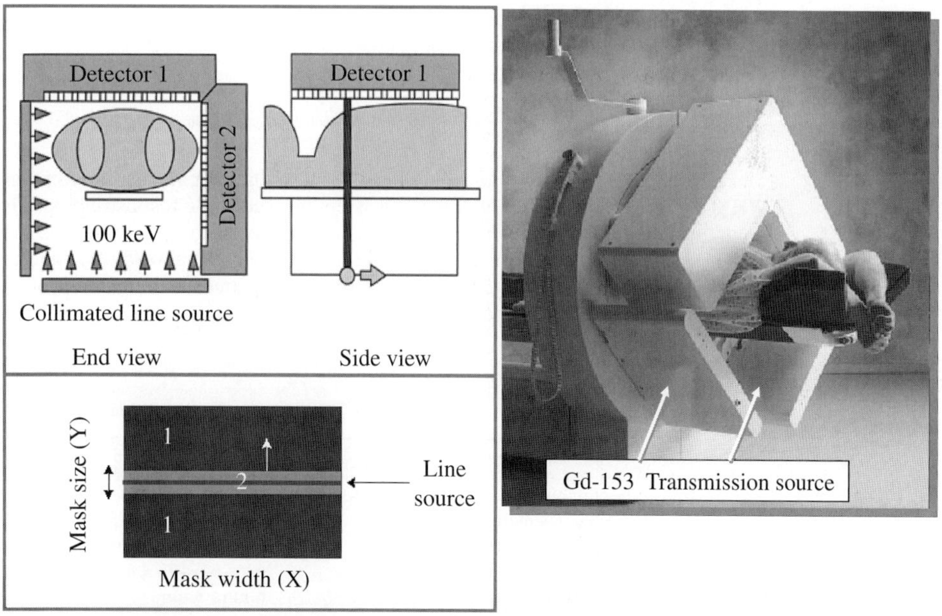

FIGURE 11.8 Transmission imaging with a radionuclide source. Attenuation correction is required for accurate SPECT. In the thorax, this requires the acquisition of a transmission study. This shows one possible configuration where scanning line sources of ^{153}Gd are translated across the field of view using the gamma camera as a crude CT scanner. This information is used to correct myocardial perfusion studies for tissue attenuation. (*Courtesy of GE Medical Systems.*)

but the easiest to implement is the subtraction method where information is simultaneously acquired into a second energy window centered below the photopeak in Compton scatter region of the energy spectrum. After establishing an appropriate normalization factor, the counts from the scatter window are subtracted from the photopeak window and the corrected projections are then used in the reconstruction algorithm.

One other correction that has been implemented with SPECT studies is the compensation for spatial resolution.[14] As discussed in the section on scintillation cameras, the spatial resolution depends on the source to collimator distance. As a result this correction cannot be made with the analytic reconstruction methods (i.e., filtered backprojection) but has been implemented with iterative reconstruction algorithms.

11.3.1 SPECT Image Reconstruction

The details of SPECT image reconstruction are beyond the scope of this article, but the interested reader can see the details in the cited literature.[15,16] Because SPECT image sets are relatively small compared to other medical imaging modalities, the computational and display requirements can be met by personal computers. However, the integration of SPECT studies with CT and MRI put increased demands on memory and storage.

11.3.2 SPECT System Performance

Typical performance specifications for SPECT imaging systems[4] are summarized in Table 11.3. As with conventional planar imaging, the scintillation cameras and the associated collimation are the primary factors affecting the performance. SPECT spatial resolution is nearly isotropic with a FWHM of 8 to 10 mm for brain imaging where the detectors can get close to the radioactive source. The spatial resolution degrades to 12 to 18 mm for body imaging because the detectors cannot be positioned as close. The components of SPECT spatial resolution and their relative importance can be identified from the equation shown below:

$$R_{\text{SPECT}} = \sqrt{R_{\text{col}}^2 + R_{\text{filter}}^2 + R_{\text{int}}^2}$$

As before, R_{int} and R_{col} represent the intrinsic and collimator resolution components. R_{filter} is the FWHM of the smoothing kernel required to yield an acceptable reconstruction. The intrinsic spatial resolution is the least important factor in this calculation since it is usually a factor of 2 or more smaller than the other components. The trade-off between spatial resolution and count sensitivity is explicit in this equation. Decreasing R_{col} to improve spatial resolution will often require R_{filter} to become larger to compensate for increased noise.

TABLE 11.3 SPECT System Performance (Typical Values)

Parameter	Specification
Number of scintillation cameras	1, 2, or 3
Count sensitivity per camera	90 cps/MBq per detector
(High-resolution collimator)	(200 cpm/μCi per detector)
Matrix size	64 × 64; 128 × 128
Pixel size	6 mm; 3 mm
Spatial resolution (brain studies)	8 mm
Spatial resolution (heart studies)	12 mm
SPECT uniformity	15%

11.3.3 SPECT Cardiac Devices

With myocardial perfusion studies, patients are injected with a radioactive tracer that distributes throughout the body, but its distribution in the heart reflects myocardial blood flow. Areas of low tracer uptake indicate coronary artery disease. Two SPECT studies are performed in the evaluation of myocardial perfusion, one where the tracer is administered under normal conditions and the other where it is administered when the patient has had a physical or pharmacologic stress that requires increased cardiac blood flow. Because the heart is located in the left anterior portion of the thorax, gamma rays originating in the heart are highly attenuated for views collected from the right lateral and right posterior portions of the arc. For this reason, SPECT studies of the heart are usually collected using the 180° arc that extends from the left posterior oblique to the right anterior oblique view.[14] This results in reconstructed images with the best contrast, although distortions are often somewhat more pronounced than when 360° data are used.[15] Because of the widespread use of myocardial perfusion imaging, many SPECT systems have been optimized for 180° acquisition by using two detectors arranged at ~ 90°. This reduces the acquisition time by a factor of 2 over single detectors and is approximately 30 percent more efficient than triple-detector SPECT systems. Positioning the detectors at 90° poses some challenges for maintaining close proximity. Most systems rely on the motion of both the detectors and the SPECT table to accomplish this.

The heart is continually moving during the SPECT acquisition, and this further compromises spatial resolution. Because the heart beats many times per minute, it is impossible to directly acquire a stop-action SPECT study. However, since the heart motion is periodic, it is possible to obtain this information by gating the SPECT acquisition.[16] In a gated SPECT acquisition, the cardiac cycle is subdivided and a set of eight images spanning the ECG R-R interval is acquired for each angular view. These images are acquired into predetermined time bins based on the patient's heart rate, which is monitored by the ECG R wave interfaced to the SPECT system. As added benefits of gating, the motion of the heart walls can be observed and ventricular volumes and ejection fractions can be determined.[17]

As previously noted, myocardial perfusion SPECT is easily the most common nuclear medicine procedure and more than 15 million of these are performed each year. It is not surprising then that special-purpose imaging systems have evolved to serve this need. These instruments can be put into three categories: (1) general-purpose SPECT systems that can accommodate both myocardial perfusion as well as other SPECT studies, (2) convention-based systems that have been specifically modified to only perform myocardial perfusion studies, and (3) newly designed devices that are departures from the scintillation-camera–based systems. The devices in the first category look and operate like general-purpose SPECT systems. Typically they have two separate scintillation camera heads that can be configured by the operator to be directly opposed for noncardiac studies or oriented at 90° for myocardial perfusion imaging. The second category features systems with small field of view scintillation cameras that are fixed in a 90° orientation. Instead of having a horizontal table where the patient lies, some of the systems are designed to rotate about a reclining chair. At least one system simplifies the mechanics even further by leaving the detectors stationary and rotating the patient. Because of the overall reduction in size, these systems can fit into relatively small rooms and are substantially cheaper than the category (1) systems. However, in terms of the time it takes to acquire the studies and the methodology, these are very similar. Figure 11.9 shows examples of cardiac SPECT systems along with an example of perfusion images.

The third group currently has two different devices that having different acquisition strategies that reportedly lead to much faster acquisition times and improved spatial resolution.[17] The first device is called the CardiArc and is based on the SPRINT II design. The image receptor is a set of NaI(Tl) bars arranged in an arc. The projections are sampled by a slit-slat combination. Axial slicing is obtained from a horizontal stack of evenly spaced lead plates (the slats), while the transaxial sampling is obtained by six vertical slits in a lead plate. The combination of the slits and slats approximates pinhole sampling and by moving the slit plate, angular samples are acquired. The slit plate is the only moving component of the system. Patients sit in a chair that forms the support for the CardiArc. Because of the six fold sampling and the high resolution of the pinhole geometry, myocardial perfusion studies can be acquired in less than half the time of a conventional SPECT system.

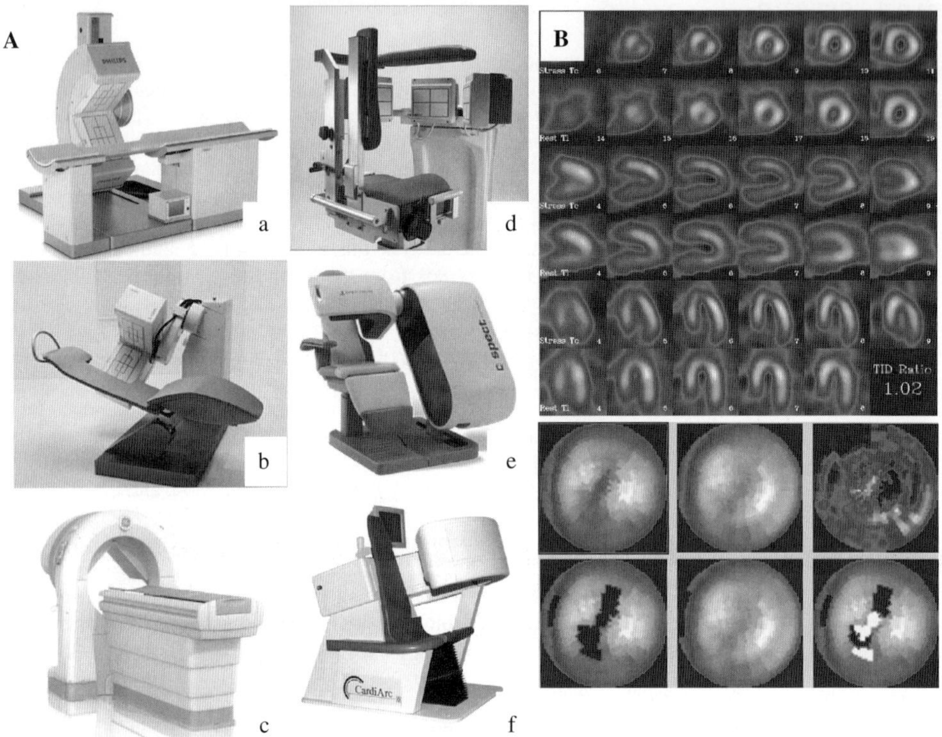

FIGURE 11.9 (*a*) Specialized systems for cardiac SPECT studies. The images on the left are based on conventional SPECT systems (a, b, c). System (d) uses APDs and a pixilated CsI(Tl) detector. The patient rotates while the detectors remain stationary. Systems (e, f) represent new cardiac systems that are fundamentally different than conventional SPECT systems. (*b*) Example of SPECT myocardial perfusion images.

The DSPECT is the other device in the third category.[17] It has a stationary (i.e., nonrotating) right angle gantry with nine individual collimated pixilated CZT modules. Each of the modules can be directed toward an area of interest, and projection samples are acquired as the modules independently rock back and forth. To acquire a myocardial perfusion study, the patient reclines on a chair with the right angle gantry positioned over the chest. A fast scout scan is performed to determine the location of the heart so that the CZT detector modules can be oriented appropriately. This system is reported to have substantially higher count sensitivity than a conventional SPECT system with a twofold improvement in spatial resolution.[18]

11.3.4 SPECT CT

There are several limitations associated with SPECT imaging. Accurate and artifact-free SPECT images require correction for attenuation, and as noted above, that requires obtaining attenuation maps of the image volume. Another problem with SPECT is its poor spatial limitation and lack of anatomical landmarks for unambiguously locating abnormal areas. Combining SPECT imaging with CT imaging addresses both of these concerns.[19] The combination of SPECT and CT in a single device was first investigated by Hasegawa et al.,[20] but the recent introduction of commercial SPECT CT systems is likely mostly the result of the success of PET CT. There are at least three different SPECT CT systems that are available today and a sample SPECT CT study (Fig. 11.10).

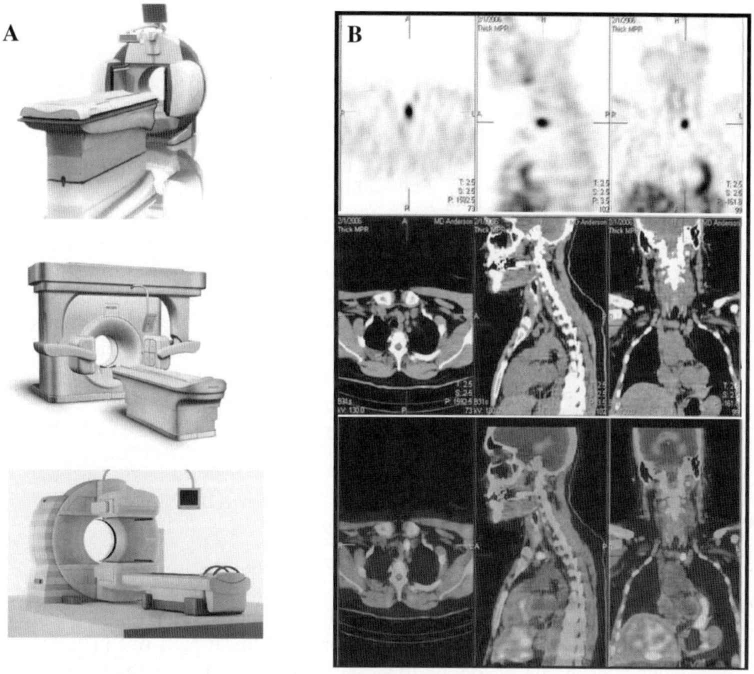

FIGURE 11.10 (*a*) Commercial SPECT CT systems: General Electric Infinia Hawkeye, Philips Precedence, and Siemens Symbia. (*b*) SPECT CT parathyroid study. The combination of the SPECT and CT images allows precise localization of the abnormality. (*Image courtesy of University of Texas, M. D. Anderson Cancer Center.*)

General Electric Healthcare provides a SPECT CT that features a low-power, fixed anode x-ray tube and detector assembly mounted directly onto a dual detector SPECT gantry. Because the SPECT gantry has slip-ring technology, the CT system is capable of helical scanning. Although the CT images from this device are not of diagnostic quality and require several minutes to acquire, they are vastly superior to the images obtained from radionuclide transmission studies and provide more than adequate attenuation correction. Philips Medical System has a dual-detector SPECT system that is suspended by moving arms mounted on the ceiling of the room. This system has been modified so that it is mounted as a bonnet on top of a high-performance CT scanner. The device is available in 6 and 16 slice models with CT slice thickness as fine as 0.65 mm and capable of acquiring whole body CT studies in less than 60 seconds. Additional room shielding is required for the precedence, and the size of the room to house this device is larger than that of a conventional SPECT system. A third system available from Siemens Molecular Imaging fits a diagnostic quality CT scanner within the SPECT gantry ring. It is available with either a 2, 6, or 16 slice CT scanner, and like the Philips product it can produce thin slices while rapidly scanning the whole body. It also requires a larger room and more lead shielding than a conventional SPECT system.

SPECT CT systems are capable of producing high-quality coregistered images that display both functional and anatomic detail. Applications where SPECT CT is expected to add clinical value include myocardial perfusion, bone, and a wide variety of tumor-imaging studies. Although the SPECT CT systems are selling well at this time, it has not yet been established whether they are economically viable. The purchase price of the systems with the diagnostic CT scanners is more than a factor of 2 higher than a conventional SPECT system, and the room renovation costs that potentially need to include extra space, a CT control room, additional room shielding, and special electrical requirements can exceed several hundred thousand dollars. No additional reimbursement money has been provided for SPECT CT studies.

11.3.5 Compton Cameras

Collimators are very inefficient and are the limiting factor in conventional scintillation cameras. One device that eliminates the need for lead collimation is the Compton camera which was investigated during the 1980s and has resurfaced in the past 5 years.[21–23] Instead of restricting the gamma ray trajectories, the Compton camera uses scattering information from two position-sensitive detectors to infer the source location. The gamma ray is Compton scattered from the first detector, and the scattered photon is totally absorbed in the second detector. The energy of the scattered photon is also determined by the second detector and that information allows the calculation of the scattering angle between the incoming gamma ray and the known path between the two detectors. The information from a single event restricts the source to the surface of a cone, and reconstruction algorithms can provide tomographic images of the source distributions. Compton cameras are estimated to improve count sensitivity by a factor of 100; however, useful devices have not yet been developed for clinical imaging. Compton cameras appear to work best with isolated point source distributions and are challenged with the three-dimensional distribution volumes associated with most nuclear medicine studies. As a result, the best application for this approach may be small animal imaging. Preclinical imaging systems designed for small animals utilizing SPECT and PET are reviewed in Sec. 11.5.

11.4 POSITRON EMISSION TOMOGRAPHY

Positron emission tomography (PET) is another approach to nuclear medicine imaging that has several advantages over SPECT. As noted in the introduction to this chapter, PET uses positron-emitting radionuclides that result in the emission of collinear pairs of 511-keV annihilation photons. The coincidence detection of the annihilation photons obviates the need for collimation and makes PET far more efficient than SPECT for detecting radioactivity. Even more importantly, there are positron-emitting radionuclides for oxygen, carbon, nitrogen, and fluorine (Table 11.4), which allows a wide range of molecules to be labeled as diagnostic agents. Many of these radionuclides have short half-lives and require an on-site cyclotron. However, ^{18}F has a sufficiently long half-life that it can be (and is) regionally provided, and there is no populated area of the United States where it is unavailable. Several others such as ^{82}Rb and ^{68}Ga are available from radionuclide generators that provide the radionuclides on demand despite their short half-lives.

Coincidence detection provides spatial resolution without the need for lead collimation by taking advantage of the fact that the annihilation photons resulting from positron emission are approximately colinear. Events are only counted if they are simultaneously detected by two opposed detectors. The sensitive volume defined by the coincidence detectors is called a *line of response* (LOR). As illustrated

TABLE 11.4 PET Radionuclides

Radionuclide	Half-Life	Decay Mode	Positron Energy (MeV)	Photon Energy (keV)	Photons per Decay
^{11}C	20.4 m	β+	0.96	511	2
^{13}N	10.0 m	β+	1.19	511	2
^{15}O	2.0 m	β+	1.72	511	2
^{18}F	109.8 m	β+, EC	0.63	511	1.93
^{82}Rb	76 s	β+, EC	3.35	511	1.9
				776	0.13
^{68}Ga	68.3 m	β+, EC	1.9	511	1.84
^{64}Cu	12.7 h	β–, β+, EC	0.65	511	0.38
				1346	0.005
^{124}I	4.2 d	β+, EC	1.54, 2.17	511	0.5
				603	0.62
				1693	0.3

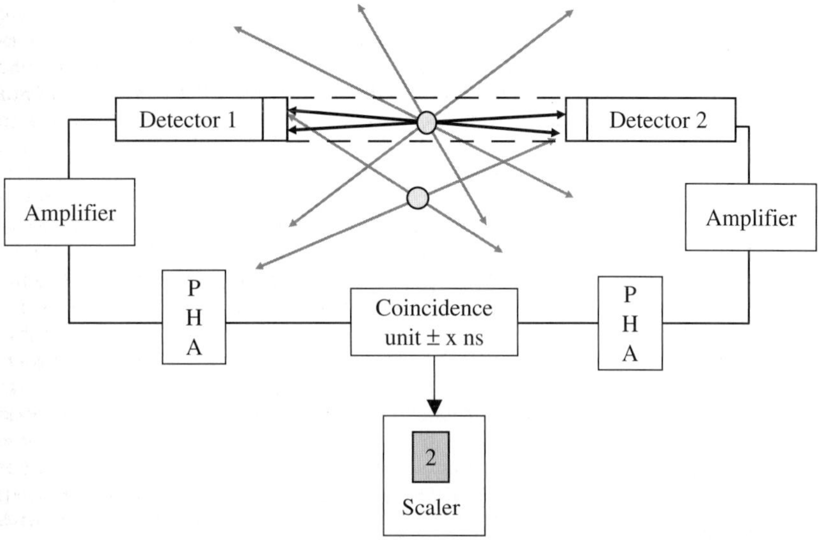

FIGURE 11.11 Coincidence detection. Events are counted only if both detectors are hit simultaneously. Coincidence detection allows source localization without resorting to lead collimation.

in Fig. 11.11, two single detection systems are used with an additional coincidence module. Each individual system will generate a logic pulse when they detect an event that falls in the selected energy window. If the two logic pulses overlap in time at the coincidence module, a coincidence event is recorded. PET systems use a large number (>10,000) of detectors arranged as multiple rings to form a cylinder. Since any one detector can be in coincidence with other detectors in the cylinder, the resulting LORs provide sufficient sampling to collect the projection information required for tomography. The important issues associated with coincidence detection are discussed below.

The intrinsic detection efficiency for a singles detector depends on the atomic number, density, and thickness of the detector. Ideally, the intrinsic detection efficiency should be 1, but at 511 keV that is difficult to achieve, although intrinsic efficiency for some of the detectors is greater than 0.8. Coincidence detection requires that both detectors register an event. Since the interactions at the two detectors are independent, the coincidence intrinsic efficiency depends on the product of the intrinsic efficiency at each detector. As a result, coincidence detection efficiency is always less than that for a single detector, and that difference gets magnified for low-efficiency detectors. Because of the need for high intrinsic efficiency, scintillators are virtually the only materials currently used as detectors in PET imaging systems. A list of the scintillators that are used in PET tomographs along with their properties is given in Table 11.5.

A coincidence event is recorded when there is an overlap of the singles logic outputs at the coincidence modules. The time width of the overlap depends on the scintillation characteristics of the detectors. For current PET scanners, that width ranges from 6 to 12 ns. Although that is a very short

TABLE 11.5 Summary of PET Scintillator Properties

Property	BGO	LSO, LYSO	GSO
Atomic number	73	65	58
Density (g/cm^3)	7.1	7.4	6.7
Intrinsic efficiency (20 mm)	0.85	0.82	0.75
Coincidence efficiency (20 mm)	0.72	0.67	0.56
Energy resolution	15%	10%	8.50%
Decay time (ns)	300	40	60

time compared to most human activities, it is fairly long compared to distances covered by photons traveling at the speed of light. Light travels approximately 30 cm/ns so that a 6 ns duration corresponds to a distance uncertainty of about 90 cm, which is the approximate detector ring diameter. As a result, the differential distance of the source between detectors has no observable effect on the timing of the coincidence events in conventional PET systems.

The arrival time of the annihilation photons is truly simultaneous only when the source is located precisely midway between the two opposed coincidence detectors. If the source is displaced from the midpoint, there will be a corresponding arrival time interval since one annihilation photon will have a shorter distance to travel than the other. As discussed above, this time differential is too small to be useful in conventionally designed PET systems. However, several of the scintillators used in PET tomographs (e.g., LSO, LYSO) are capable of faster response than the 6 to 12 ns timing discussed above. With appropriate electronics, the coincidence timing window has been reduced to 600 ps for these detectors, yielding a source localization uncertainty of 9 cm.[24,25] Even with that reduction, time-of-flight localization cannot be used to directly generate tomographic images, but it can be used to regionally restrict the backprojection operation to areas where the sources are approximately located. In current implementations, the inclusion of time-of-flight information reduces noise in the reconstructed images by a factor of 2. Time-of-flight PET tomographs were actually commercially available for a short time in the 1980s. These systems used BaF_2 detectors which are very fast, but unfortunately have very low detection efficiency. As a result, these devices did not compete well with the conventional PET tomographs based on BGO. In 2006, a time-of-flight machine based on LYSO detectors was reintroduced and is now commercially available.[26]

The only criterion for recording a coincidence event is the overlap of output pulses at the coincidence module. True coincidences occur when a source lies on the LOR defined by two detectors. It is possible that events detected at the two coincidence detectors from sources not on the line of response could happen by chance (Fig. 11.12*a*). As the count rate at each of the singles detectors increases, the likelihood of false coincidences occurring from uncorrelated events increases. These events are called *random* or *accidental coincidences*. The random coincidence rate (R) is directly proportional to the width of the coincidence time window (τ) and the product of the singles rate at the two detectors (S_1 and S_2):

$$R = 2\tau S_1 S_2$$

It is easy to see that while the true coincidence event rate is linear with the source activity, the random coincidence rate increases proportional to the square of the activity. Thus, at high count rates,

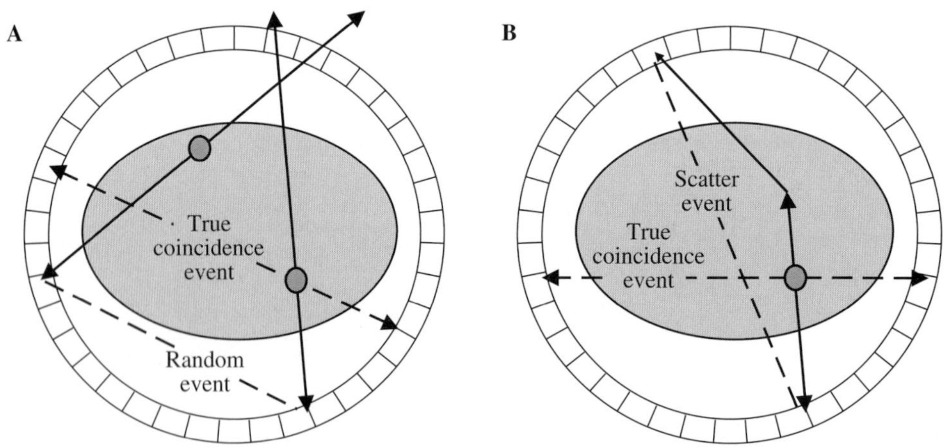

FIGURE 11.12 (*a*) Random coincidence. A true coincidence event occurs when the annihilation photons from a single decay are simultaneously detected by opposed detectors. When annihilation photons from multiple decays are detected, false information is registered. (*b*) If one or more of the annihilation photons is scattered, the apparent LOR does not localize the source. Random and scattered coincidences must be subtracted from the acquisition.

the random coincidence rate can exceed the true coincidence rate. The random coincidences provide false information and need to be removed from the acquired data prior to image reconstruction. It is also obvious that random coincidence rate can be reduced with a smaller coincidence time window. That requires detectors with a fast response time like LSO, LYOS, and GSO.

For sources in air, it is only possible to get a true coincidence event when the source lies in the defining volume between the two coincidence detectors. However, if the sources are distributed in some material, like human tissue, it is possible for one or both of the annihilation photons to be scattered into detectors that don't encompass the LOR of the source (Fig. 11.12*b*). Like the random coincidence event, this provides false information that requires correction. The number of scattered events can be reduced by energy discrimination, but this does not eliminate it all and additional scatter correction techniques are required for PET imaging.

11.4.1 PET Scanner Design

PET imaging systems are based on coincidence detection, and it is possible to use scintillation camera technology to create PET tomographs and for awhile, SPECT/PET hybrid systems were widely available. The low intrinsic efficiency of the gamma cameras made these systems inferior to dedicated PET systems and reimbursement for clinical imaging studies performed with SPECT/PET systems was discontinued, sealing its doom as a commercial product. One dedicated PET system that uses the gamma camera approach is still available. In this design, there are six individual scintillation cameras with 25-mm-thick NaI(Tl) detectors. The detectors are curved so that when they are combined, they form a complete cylinder with a diameter of 90 cm and an axial length of 25 cm. The C-PET operates as a three-dimensional PET system and is less expensive than the ring systems with individual detectors. It has spatial resolution that is comparable to the ring detector systems and much better energy resolution. However, its count sensitivity is about half that of the ring systems.

The best performing whole body PET systems have a large array of scintillation detectors that form a cylinder that the patient passes through.[27] If a single ring of this system is considered, each detector within the ring can form a coincidence event with any of the opposing detectors as shown in Fig. 11.13. The associated lines of response provide all the necessary sampling to generate a tomographic image for one plane. To increase the number of planes, additional rings are combined together to form a large cylinder covering 16 to 18 cm. The number of detectors used in commercial whole body PET systems ranges from 9000 to greater than 20,000. Table 11.6 has a summary of PET system performance specifications.

Four scintillators are currently being used for whole body PET systems[28]: bismuth germanate (BGO), lutetium oxyorthosilicate (LSO), yttrium-doped lutetium oxyorthosilicate (LYSO), and gadolinium oxyorthosilicate (GSO) (Table 11.5). BGO has the best intrinsic efficiency, but its light output is very low and the scintillation decay time is quite long. As would be expected, this results in poor energy resolution and diminished count rate capability. The coincidence intrinsic efficiency of LSO and LYSO is 7 percent below that of BGO, but they have very high light output and the scintillation decay time is almost a factor of 10 shorter. One problem LSO and LYSO have that the other detectors do not share is that they are radioactive so that the detectors have a continual background detection rate. Fortunately, this is not a significant problem in the coincidence mode. GSO intrinsic efficiency is 22 percent less than BGO, but it also has a much higher light output and short decay time.

As stated above, whole body PET systems can have more than 20,000 individual detectors. In the early PET scanners, each detector was coupled directly to a single photomultiplier tube (PMT). The size of the PMT was at that time the limiting factor to detector size and therefore the limiting factor to PET resolution. In the 1980s, the concept of the detector block was developed (Fig. 11.14). In this scheme, an 8 × 8 array of detectors is coupled to four PMTs. Each detector in the array is accurately identified from the ratios of the difference and sums of the PMT signals. This innovation was very important since it provided an economical solution to reducing the detector size while preserving count sensitivity. Block detectors are still in use by two of the commercial vendors. The other major vendor uses an approach similar to the Anger logic used on a scintillation camera. In their design, an array of PMTs views the detector matrix. When an event occurs, the involved detector is determined from summing the position

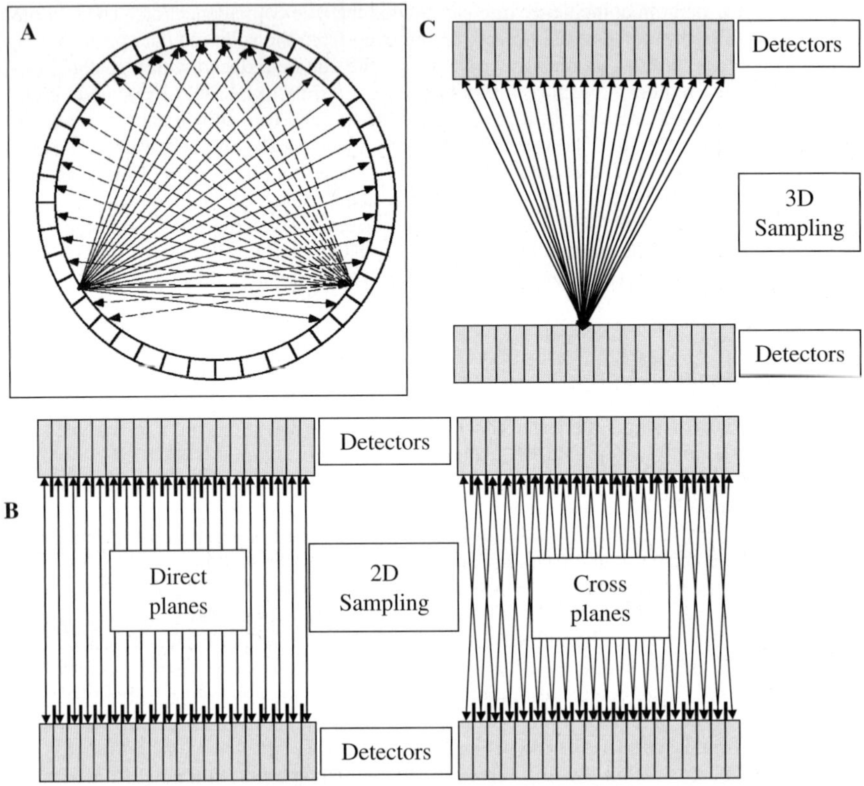

FIGURE 11.13 (*a*) In-plane sampling by the detector ring. Each detector on the ring can potentially be in coincidence with any of the opposed detectors. This provides the sampling required for tomography. (*b*) PET scanners consist of multiple rings (shown in cross section). 2D PET has lead shields to isolate LORs to either direct planes or cross planes. (*c*) 3D PET does not use shields and coincidences can occur between all the rings.

weighted signals of the PMTs in the event proximity. Both of these approaches permit the use of very small detectors. In PET whole body systems, the detector face size ranges from 4 to 6 mm. For small animal PET systems, the detector face size is approaching 1 × 1 mm.

Commercial PET systems were originally designed for two-dimensional (2D) sampling with lead septae (shields) inserted between the rings to restrict the lines of response. This allows coincidence events to be collected within a ring (direct planes) and coincidence events between adjacent rings (cross planes) as shown in Fig. 11.13. Because of the shallow angle that is associated with the cross plane events, these are treated as if they came from a parallel plane midway between the two direct planes. This sampling allows the use of conventional reconstruction algorithms.

TABLE 11.6 Typical 3D PET Performance Values

Parameter	Specification
Axial FOV	16 cm
Sensitivity	7500 cps/MBq
Transverse resolution (FWHM)	5 mm
Axial resolution (FWHM)	5 mm
Peak noise equivalent count rate	70–165 kcps
Scatter fraction	35%

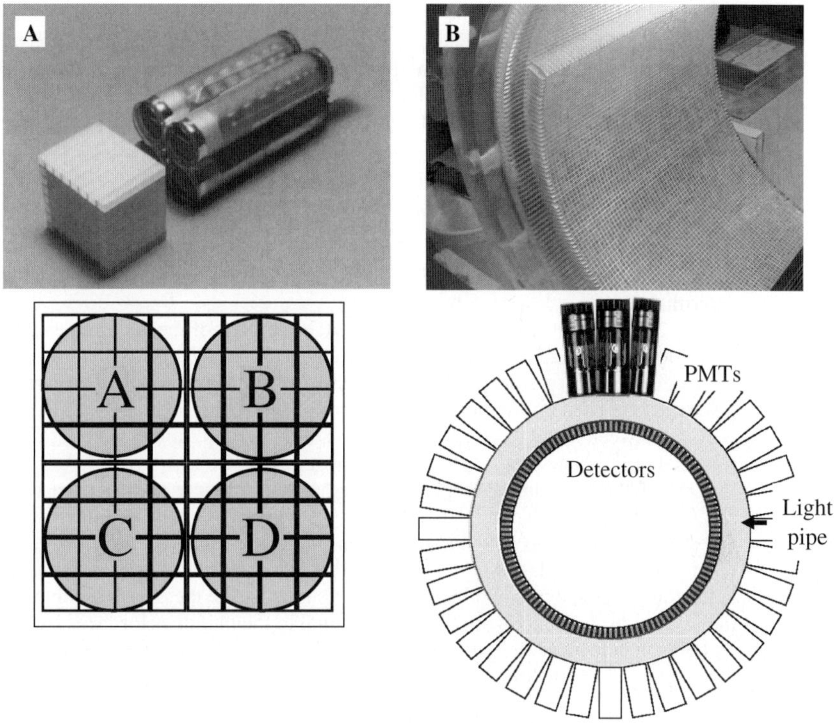

FIGURE 11.14 Sufficient light is emitted to allow the identification of the detector absorbing the annihilation photon. (*a*) Block detector. (*b*) An alternate configuration (Pixelar), using array of detectors with a light pipe and photomultiplier tube array.

In addition to restricting the lines of response, the shields have several other beneficial aspects. Because the overall event rates (both singles and coincidence) are reduced, the electronics can be simplified. The reduction in the singles count rate automatically means that the random coincidence rate is less, and count rate losses due to dead time are also less of a concern. Scattered radiation is also reduced in the 2D mode with the scatter fraction being about 15 percent of the true coincidence data. As a result, corrections for scatter don't need to be extremely accurate, and approximate routines that are fast can be used. Imaging in the 2D mode places a high premium on intrinsic efficiency and BGO is clearly the preferred detector material.

3D PET offers the advantage of much higher count rate when the lead shields are removed and coincidences are allowed between all the rings (Fig. 11.13). The higher count rate allows higher patient throughput and potentially lower radiation dose to the patients. However, the random coincidence and scatter events increase dramatically. The scatter fraction approaches 50 percent of the true coincidence rate with a similar ratio for the randoms. In addition, count rate losses resulting from detector dead time also become a concern. While BGO is the clear choice for 2D PET, its poor energy resolution and large dead time make it less attractive in 3D. LSO and GSO on the other hand make up for their diminished intrinsic efficiency with improved energy resolution and higher count rate capabilities.

Although the overall sensitivity increases in 3D PET, there is a position dependence that is not an issue in 2D PET. A source located in the center of the cylinder interacts with all the rings. As the source moves toward either end, the number of rings decreases along with the sensitivity. The sensitivity profile in 3D has a triangular shape. To compensate for this characteristic, there is a 30 to 50 percent overlap of the bed translation during whole body scans.

Fair comparisons of 2D and 3D PET modes cannot be made solely on the basis of the measured count rates, since the increase in count rate in 3D PET is accompanied by increases in the magnitude of corrections for both randoms and scatter. To effect meaningful comparisons, the concept of the noise equivalent count rate (NECR) is used. The *noise equivalent count rate* is a way of comparing the actual gain associated with an increased sensitivity that also requires increased corrections. The NECR is expressed in terms of the true coincidence count rate (the good data, usually represented by T), the scatter count rate (S), and the random coincidence rate (R):

$$\text{NECR} = T^2/(T + S + cR)$$

where c is a constant that is equal to either 1 or 2 depending on how the random coincidence rate is determined.

For 2D PET, the scatter fraction is about 10 percent of the acquired events and a typical random coincidence rate is 25 percent of the acquired events. In 3D PET both the scatter fraction and the random coincidence rate are close to 50 percent of the true coincidence rate. So even though the observed rate goes up by more than a factor of 6 in going from 2D to 3D PET, the improvement in NEC is between 3 and 4. The NEC is also useful in comparing the count rate performance of the different 3D PET systems.

One of the advantages of PET imaging is its relatively good spatial resolution compared with SPECT. The primary factors that influence spatial resolution include the face size of the detectors, the detector thickness, the detector separation, data smoothing during or after reconstruction, and the pixel size of the displayed images.[27] PET tomographs achieve spatial resolution through coincidence detection. Since the two annihilation photons must strike the opposed coincidence detectors, the spatial resolution associated with the LOR is equal to the half detector face size. This, of course, depends on being able to accurately identify individual detector elements. Because of the uncertainty involved in selecting the correct detector with each event, the spatial resolution is approximately equal to the detector face size.

To achieve high intrinsic efficiency, the detectors used in PET tomographs are typically 20 to 30 mm thick. When an annihilation photon strikes the detector, it can be absorbed anywhere along the detector length. Annihilation photons arriving from the center of the tomograph field of view are likely to travel along the axis of a detector and this presents no problem. However, annihilation photons coming from the edge of the field of view have trajectories that cross many detectors. Because the exact location of the interaction along the detector is unknown, the LOR is essentially broadened, leading to a significant loss of spatial resolution that increases as the source location is displaced from the center of the ring. This parallax effect is often referred to as the *depth of interaction problem* and is illustrated in Fig. 11.15. A variety of techniques have been proposed to measure the depth that the interaction occurs. These include using layers of detectors with identifiable differences in their scintillation properties or by treating the surface of the crystals so that the light yield is depth dependent.[29]

One way of reducing the loss of resolution due to this depth of interaction problem is to use thinner detectors. This is not an option with the current detectors since the detection efficiency would be seriously reduced with any reduction in thickness. Another way to reduce the depth of interaction problem is to increase the ring diameter. There are two drawbacks associated with that approach. The geometric efficiency of the detectors decreases with the square of the source to detector distance. Thus, a larger ring diameter results in a significant drop in count sensitivity. The other reason opposing a larger ring diameter is the loss of spatial resolution associated with the angular dispersion of the annihilation photons. If the positron annihilates at rest, the angle between the 2 annihilation photons is exactly 180°. However, at room (and body) temperature, thermal motion adds about 0.5° (± 0.25) variation in the annihilation angle. This variation produces a loss in spatial resolution that increases with the ring diameter and is approximately 2 mm for whole body PET tomographs (ring diameter approximately 90 cm). The spatial resolution components discussed above can be described as intrinsic because they are fixed by the design configuration of the PET tomograph. The other factors that influence spatial resolution, smoothing, and pixel size vary, depending on reconstruction parameter selections.

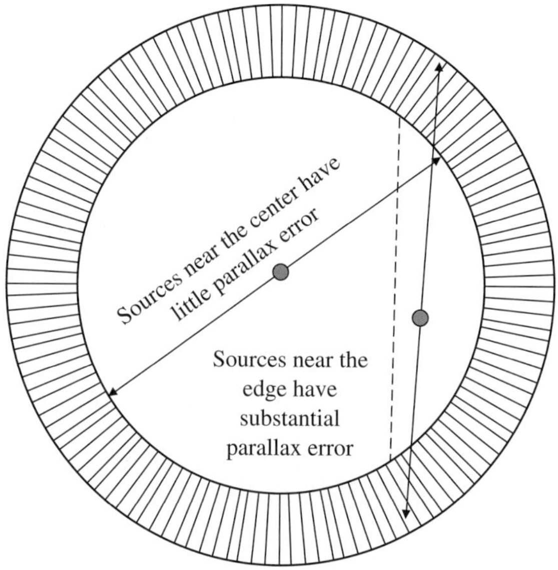

FIGURE 11.15 Depth of interaction effect. The thick detectors used in PET are susceptible to parallax errors because the portion of the detector that absorbs the annihilation photon is unknown. The depth of interaction effect causes spatial resolution to degrade as the source moves toward the edge of the field of view.

A final consideration with PET spatial resolution is the range of the positron in tissue before annihilation. Low-energy positrons such as those emitted by ^{18}F do not travel far and have a negligible effect on spatial resolution. The positrons emitted by ^{82}Rb are very energetic, and the degradation in spatial resolution is very apparent even in whole body PET scanners. The range of the positron is likely to be the ultimate limiting factor in small animal PET imaging.

There are a number of corrections that have to be made to the acquired PET data before it can be reconstructed. These include corrections for sensitivity variations, random coincidences, scatter, and attenuation. The reconstruction algorithm requires a set of measurements that provides projections of the radionuclide distribution from a large number of angles. Changes in the measured count rate should only depend on the in vivo radioactivity distribution and not on variations in the detectors. It is not possible to have all 10,000 plus detectors with uniform sensitivity, so there is some variation that exist from detector to detector. However, even if the detector response was 100 percent uniform, there would still be a need to do a sensitivity correction. This is because both the geometric and intrinsic efficiency vary with the angle of the line of response. A coincidence event that occurs across a ring diameter has a significantly higher chance of being recorded than one that takes place between detectors that are closer together. To compensate for both this angular dependence and for other variations in the detectors, sensitivity scans are acquired as part of the daily quality control. These scans are acquired either using a transmission source or with a uniform cylinder of radioactivity.

As discussed above, the random coincidence rate increases with the square of the singles count rate so it can be a substantial fraction of the acquired counts, especially in 3D PET. Unlike scatter, the distribution of random coincidences is not strongly source dependent, and they tend to be dispersed over the entire imaging field. Random coincidences can be estimated from the singles rate or measured by introducing a time delay into the coincidence circuit. A time window set on this delayed signal will only sample the random coincidences. The estimated random events are usually subtracted from each line of response prior to reconstruction, although some iterative algorithms include this step as part of the reconstruction process.

The annihilation photons traveling through the patient are attenuated largely through Compton scatter interactions. The scattered photon resulting from this interaction loses energy and changes its direction and the inclusion of the scattered event causes a loss of spatial resolution and image contrast. Scattered radiation is fairly easily handled in 2D PET studies because the scatter contribution is about 10 to 15 percent of the acquired events. The scatter component is estimated by fitting the recorded counts that extend beyond the patient boundary to a parabolic or Gaussian function in each projection, which is subtracted from the projection. While this approach is not rigorous, it is sufficiently accurate to correct for scatter in the 2D mode.

Because scatter is a major component of the detected counts in 3D PET, a more sophisticated approach is required. Scatter is estimated from an algorithm that models the transport of photons through the patient.[13] The amount of scatter contaminating any given line of response depends on the activity distribution as well as the tissue density in the patient. So, in order to compute the scatter using this method, both the transmission data and the scatter-contaminated PET data have to be reconstructed. The resultant images are used to estimate the amount of scatter that contributes to each line of response. The scatter component is subtracted and the corrected projection data are presented to the reconstruction algorithm. Although this approach appears to work well and has been adapted on the commercial PET systems, there is still room for improvement. This approach only corrects for activity within the field of view of the tomograph. In many cases, there is significant scatter that originates outside the field of view. Also, the current approach assumes that the annihilation radiation has only one scatter interaction. More sophisticated algorithms are being explored that will expand the range of the correction to include the aforementioned cases. However, the ideal solution is to have better energy resolution so that scatter can be eliminated during the acquisition.

Annihilation radiation like x-rays and gamma rays become less intense as they travel through material objects. The loss of photons from the beam is referred to as *attenuation*. Attenuation is exponential and as a result we can define a quantity called the half value layer (HVL). The *half value layer* is the thickness of material that reduces the intensity of the radiation by half. For soft tissue (water) the HVL for annihilation radiation is 7.2 cm. In order for a coincidence event to be recorded, the 2 annihilation photons have to hit opposing detectors. The amount of attenuation along any specific LOR therefore depends on the total path length through the patient irrespective of where the source is located. For the line of response shown in Fig. 11.16*a*, the coincidence attenuation reduction is the same for all three sources. Trajectories that just graze the edge of the patient have essentially no

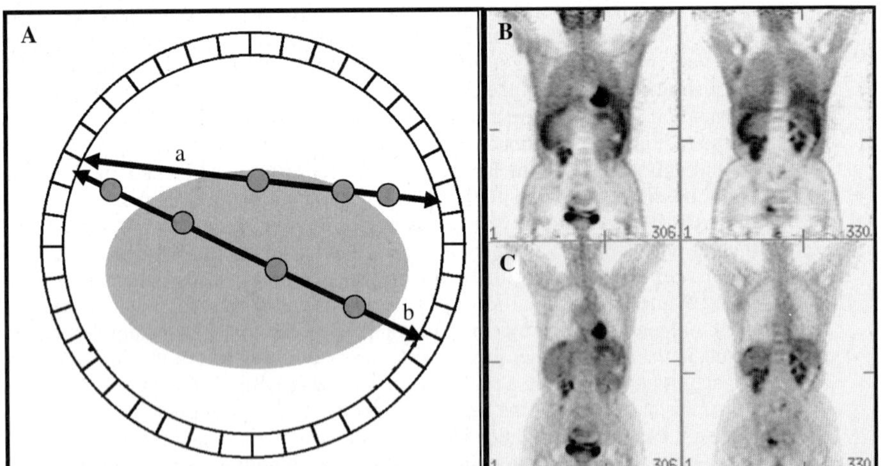

FIGURE 11.16 Attenuation in PET. (*a*) For a given LOR, the attenuation depends only on the path length through the patient and not on the location of the source. Thus, the attenuation factor is the same for each source shown along LOR a. The attenuation factor for LOR b is different than for LOR a, but is the same for each source along b. (*b*) Reconstructed PET images without attenuation correction and the corresponding images (*c*), with attenuation correction. Large artifacts are apparent when attenuation correction is not performed.

attenuation, while those that traverse the thickest portion of the patient can have path lengths of greater than 50 cm in large patients, leading to reductions in the coincidence detection rate of more than a factor of 100. This causes a nonlinear relationship between the detected counts and the source activity. Thus, reconstruction of the acquired data without attenuation correction leads to the characteristic artifacts, including enhanced count density at the skin and in the lung fields and decreased count density in the central portions of the patient (Fig. 11.16*b*).

The amount of attenuation depends only on the trajectory of the annihilation photons through the patient, not on the actual location of the source. Measurement of the transmission factors can be performed using radionuclide sources that revolve about the patient using the PET tomograph as a crude CT scanner.[11,30] Radionuclide sources that have been used for that application include ^{68}Ge and ^{137}Cs. However, collecting the transmission information this way is slow (1 to 3 minutes per bed position) and produces low-resolution, noisy corrections. These problems have been largely solved by using CT tomographic images from the combined PET CT imaging systems (Fig. 11.17).

The CT scanner provides whole body transmission data in less than 1 minute. In addition to the reduction in transmission time, the level of noise in the CT images is much less than that of the radionuclide transmission data. Because the average energy of the x-rays used in the CT scan is 60 to 80 keV, the CT attenuation coefficients have to be mapped to the appropriate values at 511 keV. Although this is a nonlinear process, the mapping has been successfully implemented.[31] However, there are several potential problems that occur when using CT data for attenuation correction.

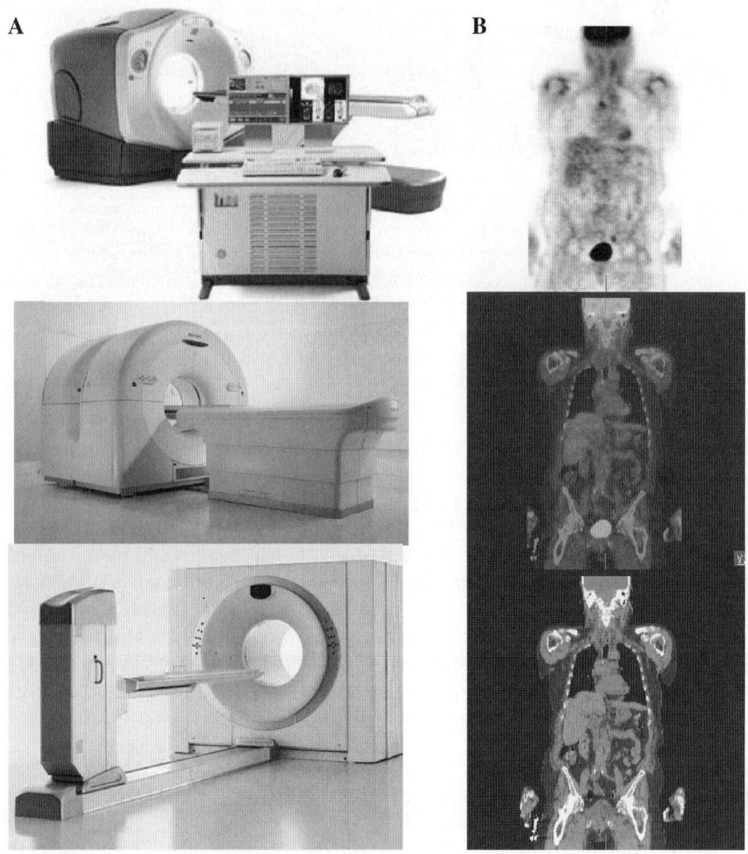

FIGURE 11.17 (*a*) PET CT scanners from General Electric, Philips, and Siemens. (*b*) An example ^{18}F FDG whole body PET CT clinical study.

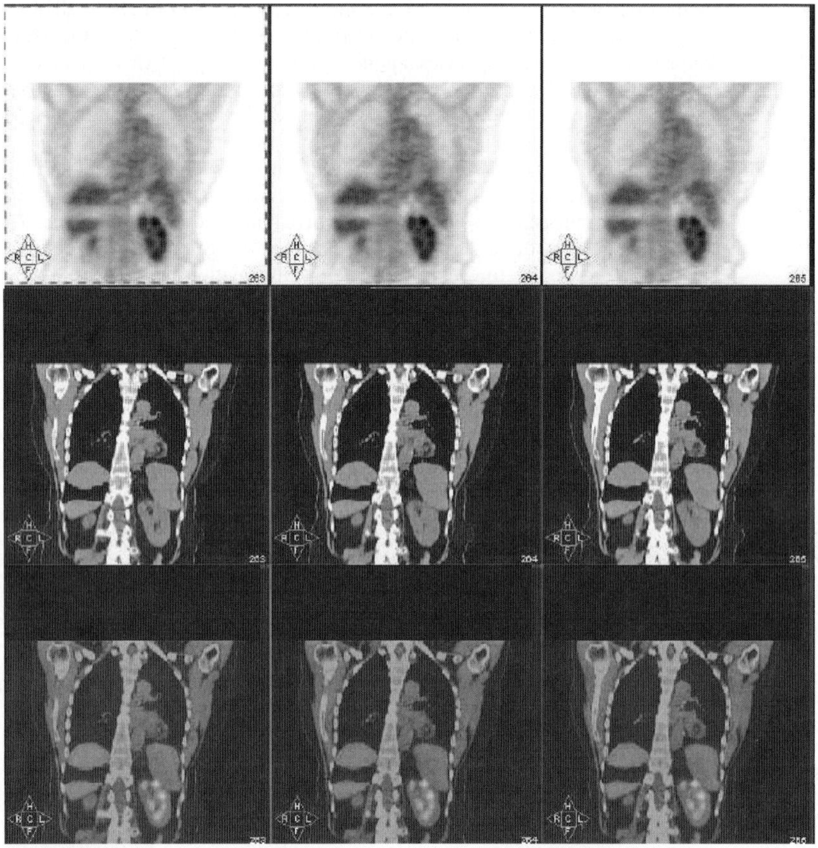

FIGURE 11.18 Breathing artifact on PET CT study. The CT study is acquired in the helical mode. If the patient takes a deep breath during the CT study, a "floating liver" artifact often occurs. Because the CT is used for attenuation correction, the artifact is also evident on the PET images.

The PET portion of the study is acquired over several minutes for each bed position with the patient breathing normally. The CT is acquired as a spiral scan in less than a minute, and ideally the patient should take shallow breaths during the acquisition. Deep breathing during the spiral CT scan creates artifacts in both the CT and the attenuation corrected PET studies[32,33] as shown in Fig. 11.18.

Metal causes rather severe artifacts on CT images and therefore artifacts on PET studies.[34] The problem is fairly widespread, particularly in the mouth, since so many people have heavy metal dental fillings. Another area of concern is artificial joint replacements. A potential solution to this problem is the use of more sophisticated CT reconstruction algorithms that reduce or eliminate metal artifacts. However, these are not widely available on the commercial CT units used in PET/CT. As a result, many clinics are routinely reconstructing and viewing uncorrected (i.e., no attenuation correction) as well as corrected studies to overcome the problems associated with metal artifacts.

11.4.2 PET/CT

The combined PET/CT systems were developed at the University of Pittsburgh by Townsend et al. and were initially introduced as commercial devices in 2001.[35–37] These devices quickly caught on and have virtually replaced all the stand-alone PET tomographs. The PET/CT systems combine a dedicated whole body PET scanner with a diagnostic multislice CT scanner. PET/CT systems offer a number of advantages. The quality of the PET images is significantly improved by the CT transmission correction. The CT transmission study is much faster than the radionuclide transmission so that studies are completed in about half the time of the PET-only systems. This shortened scan time not only provides for higher patient throughput, it also decreases the artifacts associated with patient motion. The other obvious advantage to PET/CT systems is the availability of accurately coregistered images (Fig. 11.17b). All the vendors have convenient viewing software that allows the simultaneous review of the PET, CT, and fused coregistered image sets. The viewing physician can localize an area of concern on any one of the displays and immediately see the corresponding location on the other views. Several groups have shown that information displayed in this manner provides gains in sensitivity, specificity, and confidence of interpretation, especially for the less than experienced reader. Although coregistration of PET and CT is possible with data sets acquired on different systems, the practical implementation is often difficult. Problems include different body orientations (e.g., arms up on one scan, arms down on another), breath-hold conditions, and access to both data sets.

There are issues with the PET/CT systems that have to be considered. The cost of a PET/CT system is at least 50 percent higher than a PET-only system. A much larger room is required so that the patient can be fully translated through both devices. The effective radiation dose to the patient from the CT acquisition adds 500 to 1200 mrem to the study. Also additional technologist training is required for operating the CT scanner. Other issues related to technologist training and health-care personnel include the use of contrast agents for the CT portion of the study.

11.4.3 PET MRI

The combination of PET and CT proved to be very successful and has kindled the desire to combine PET with MRI. There are several challenges posed by performing PET imaging in the vicinity of an MRI system. The photomultiplier tubes still used in all commercial PET systems are very sensitive to magnetic fields. There is sufficient light output from LSO that will allow that the PMTs can be replaced with solid-state avalanche photodiodes.[38] Another problem that needs to be addressed is attenuation correction. The attenuation values found in CT images can be used to accurately estimate attenuation values for the 511-keV annihilation photons. However, the information obtained from an MRI scanner cannot be transformed directly into attenuation coefficients. In some areas like the head that are fairly homogeneous, this may not be difficult to accomplish, but in the thorax the determination of lung attenuation will be very challenging. These problems have not stopped the research and development of PET MRI devices, and prototypes exist for both small animal and human imaging. Human devices include a brain PET MRI system at the Eberhard-Karls University, Tuebingen, Germany, and a whole body PET MRI system at the University of Cambridge, England. An operational small animal PET MRI device has been described by Catana et al.[39]

11.5 SMALL ANIMAL IMAGING

Imaging studies with small animals, especially with mice and rats, provide valuable information in the development of new drugs and treatments for human diseases. There is widespread interest in small animal imaging and it continues to grow. Investigations with rats and mice are indispensable for evaluating pathophysiology, radiopharmaceutical development, and genetic research.[40,41] Targeted research with knock-out and knock-in mice strains is especially important, and all this attention has stimulated the development of imaging systems from many modalities optimized for these animals. Because of the high sensitivity associated with the radiotracers and their ability to deliver crucial information about physiological function, it is natural that both PET and SPECT are major players in small animal imaging. However, small animal imaging presents many challenges because of the small volumes and low radioactivity concentrations that have to be accurately imaged.

The reconstructed spatial resolution is approximately 8 to 15 mm in a PET or SPECT clinical study. To achieve similar sampling of the anatomy of the rat and mouse, the spatial resolution would have to be 1.7 and 0.75 mm, respectively. Unfortunately, spatial resolution is not the sole factor in determining image quality. Adequate count density levels have to be achieved so that the statistical fluctuations do not overwhelm the information content. Count density comparisons of the associated resolution volumes (0.75 mm vs. 8 mm) suggests that the sensitivity of a small animal scanner needs to be more than 2000 times higher than of a human scanner. This is currently far out of reach, but the small size of the animals has one big advantage. In humans, attenuation reduces the coincidence event rate by more than a factor of 50 and in SPECT image by at least a factor of 10. In the rat and mouse, the attenuation reduction factors are less than 2. When attenuation is also considered, the required sensitivity increase is approximately 5 for rat imaging and 55 for mouse imaging. Another gain comes improving the geometric efficiency of the detecting systems by making them just large enough to accommodate rats. Because other compromises required to improve spatial resolution are employed such as small pinholes for SPECT or thinner detectors for PET, the overall sensitivity gain is less than a factor of 5. Thus, we approach the sampling and signal-to-noise limits in animals smaller than rats. To some degree, further gains can be realized by increasing the amount of activity administered to the animals. That also has constraints associated with the count rate capability of the scanner and the volume of injectate tolerated by the animal.

Concerns about the limited anatomical information associated with SPECT and PET are also associated with small animal imaging. As a result, most SPECT and PET small animal imaging systems also include high-resolution CT imaging systems, with some of them capable of spatial resolution better than 10 μm.

11.5.1 Small Animal PET

Many investigators have described small animal PET systems and there are currently more than four commercial systems available. By and large, small animal PET systems are scaled-down versions of clinical PET scanners. These are based on multiple rings of discrete scintillators with LSO, LYSO, or GSO being the most commonly used detectors. To achieve good spatial resolution, the face size of the crystal is small, ranging from less than 1 × 1 mm in some experimental systems up to 2 × 2 mm. The detectors are 10 to 15 mm thick to limit depth of interaction losses. The spatial resolution in these systems ranges from 1.2-to 2.2-mm FWHM. The ring diameter is 15 to 20 cm and the overall detection efficiency is on the order of 2 to 5 percent. Typical small animal PET images are shown in Fig. 11.19*a*.

11.5.2 Small Animal SPECT

Because the spatial resolution of SPECT systems designed for human imaging is fairly coarse, it would seem unlikely that SPECT could ever serve for imaging small animals. What makes small animal SPECT possible is pinhole collimation. Although pinhole imaging has low-count sensitivity for imaging large distributed sources, pinholes become advantageous when imaging localized distributions. Through magnification, pinhole imaging reduces the apparent intrinsic spatial resolution of the detector, resulting in an overall spatial resolution that is predominantly determined by the diameter of the pinhole aperture. Spatial resolution below 2-mm FWHM is routinely achieved with both investigational and commercial devices (see example images in Fig. 11.20), and submillimeter resolution can be achieved by concentrating on small-source distributions within the animal. The accurate modeling of the pinhole aperture is a crucial factor in both the design of the collimators and the reconstruction algorithms and has lead to a number of papers reanalyzing the physics of pinhole imaging.[42–45]

Although spectacular spatial resolution can be achieved through magnification with pinhole collimation, it comes with the very real price of either very large detectors or limited field of view. The need for magnification is reduced for detectors with good intrinsic spatial resolution. While most of the currently available detectors have intrinsic spatial resolution in the range of 2.5 to 3.5 mm, it

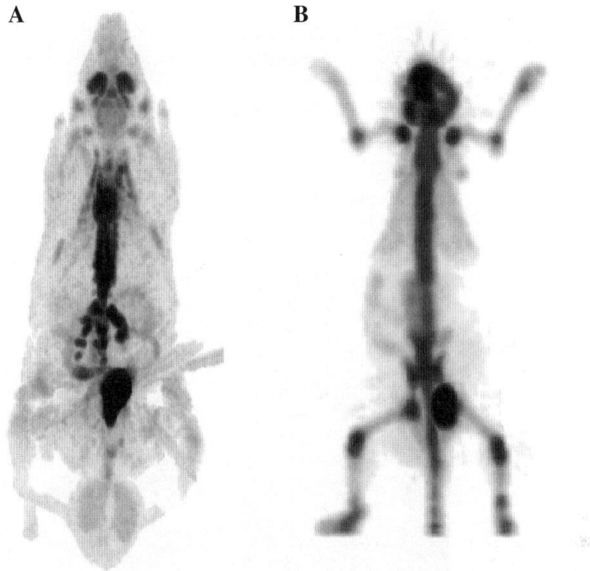

FIGURE 11.19 Small animal PET images. (*a*) Rat images with ^{18}F FDG. (*b*) Mouse imaged with ^{18}F fluoride.

is possible to achieve performance that is nearly a factor of 10 better by using very small pixilated detectors.

The count sensitivity for pinhole-based SPECT system is about 2 orders of magnitude lower than that of the small animal PET systems. One way that can be improved is by adding pinholes. The best performance is achieved when there is minimal overlapping of the images projected onto the detector surface, and that limits the number of pinholes to approximately 10 per detector for systems that image the entire mouse or rat.[46] When the imaging volume is constrained to a smaller region, a much larger number of pinholes can be accommodated.

The investigational and commercial small animal SPECT systems involve a wide range of instrumentation.[5,47–49] Many of the investigational devices use retired clinical SPECT systems that have been fitted with one or more high-resolution pinholes.[50] Other devices have been designed around multiple small field of view gamma cameras with good intrinsic spatial resolution. These devices also use a wide variety of detection instrumentation, including conventional scintillation cameras, pixilated detectors with PSPMTs or APDs, and semiconductor gamma cameras.

11.5.3 Other High-Resolution Devices

Gamma emitters with energies less than 50 keV are not used in human imaging studies because tissue attenuation limits the number of gamma rays that escape the body. Loss of signal from attenuation is not a major consideration with small animal imaging, and that allows a wider range of radionuclides that can be considered as tracers. These low-energy gammas also ease the need for high *Z* and high-density detectors. Position-sensitive devices with very high spatial resolution (< 100 μm) include the silicon strip detector and charge-coupled devices (CCDs).[51,52] Because of their low atomic number, density, and material thickness, they are not useful for imaging with medium- to high-energy gamma rays associated with clinical nuclear medicine studies. However, these detectors have adequate efficiency for very low-energy gamma and x-ray emitters like ^{125}I, and several small animal imaging systems based on these technologies have been proposed.

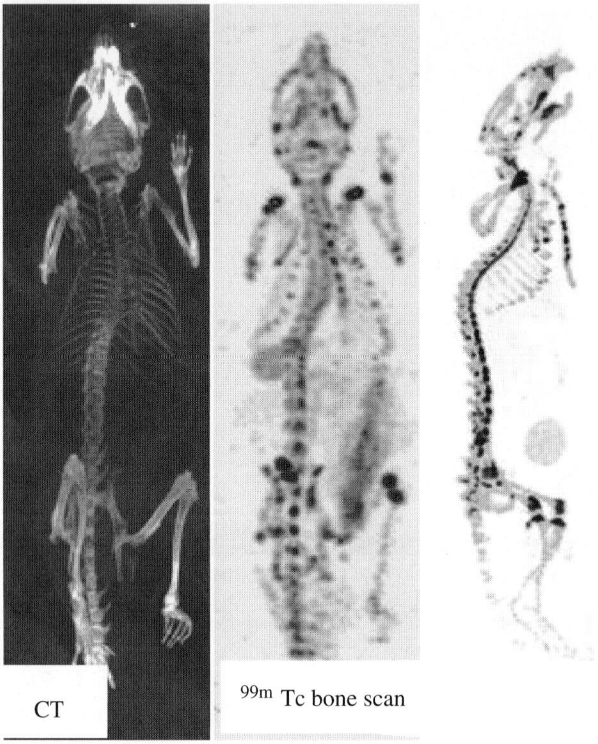

FIGURE 11.20 Example of a small animal SPECT study with co-registered CT. (a) Whole body CT image of a mouse. (b) Co-registered ^{99m}Tc whole body bone scan. (c) Maximum pixel projection image of the ^{99m}Tc bone scan. *Images courtesy of Bioscan, Inc.*

11.6 SUMMARY

Nuclear medicine, including both SPECT and PET, has been on the leading edge of the molecular imaging revolution. Because of the incredibly high sensitivity offered by the radiotracer approach, it is expected that SPECT and PET will remain as valuable clinical modalities and irreplaceable for targeted research with small animals. There will be continued research and development directed toward new radiotracers as well as improved imaging instrumentation.

REFERENCES

1. H. O. Anger, Scintillation camera with multichannel collimators, *J Nucl Med*, **5:**515–31, 1964.
2. D. Gunter, in *Nuclear Medicine*; *Vol. 1*, 2d ed., edited by R. E. Henkin (Mosby, Philadelphia, 2006), p. 107–126.
3. G. Muehllehner, The impact of digital technology on the scintillation camera, *J Nucl Med*, **22**(4):389–91, 1981.
4. H. Hines, R. Kayayan, J. Colsher, D. Hashimoto, R. Schubert, J. Fernando, V. Simcic, P. Vernon, and R. L. Sinclair, National Electrical Manufacturers Association recommendations for implementing SPECT instrumentation quality control, *J Nucl Med*, **41**(2):383–9, 2000.

5. M. Lecchi, L. Ottobrini, C. Martelli, A. Del Sole, and G. Lucignani, Instrumentation and probes for molecular and cellular imaging, *Q J Nucl Med Mol Imaging*, **51**(2):111–26, 2007.
6. H. Zaidi, Recent developments and future trends in nuclear medicine instrumentation, *Z Med Phys*, **16**(1): 5–17, 2006.
7. C. S. Levin, in *Emission Tomography: The Fundamentals of SPECT and PET,* edited by M. N. Wernick and J. N. Aarsvold (Elsevier, San Diego, 2004), pp. 293–334.
8. C. B. Hruska, M. K. O'Connor, and D. A. Collins, Comparison of small field of view gamma camera systems for scintimammography, *Nucl Med Commun*, **26**(5):441–5, 2005.
9. C. N. Brzymialkiewicz, M. P. Tornai, R. L. McKinley, and J. E. Bowsher, Evaluation of fully 3-D emission mammotomography with a compact cadmium zinc telluride detector, *IEEE Trans Med Imaging*, **24**(7): 868–77, 2005.
10. R. J. Jaszczak, The early years of single photon emission computed tomography (SPECT): an anthology of selected reminiscences, *Phys Med Biol*, **51**(13):R99–115, 2006.
11. H. Zaidi and B. Hasegawa, Determination of the attenuation map in emission tomography, *J Nucl Med*, **44**(2):291–315, 2003.
12. D. A. Lalush and M. N. Wernick, in *Emission Tomography: The Fundamentals of SPECT and PET,* edited by M. N. Wernick and J. N. Aarsvold (Elsevier, San Diego, 2004), pp. 44–472.
13. H. Zaidi and K. F. Koral, Scatter modelling and compensation in emission tomography, *Eur J Nucl Med Mol Imaging*, **31**(5):761–82, 2004.
14. M. A. King, S. J. Glick, P. H. Pretorius, R. G. Wells, H. C. Gifford, M. V. Narayanan, and T. Farncombe, in *Emission Tomography: The Fundamentals of SPECT and PET,* edited by M. N. Wernick and J. N. Aarsvold (Elsevier, San Diego, 2004), pp. 473–98.
15. J. Qi and R. M. Leahy, Iterative reconstruction techniques in emission computed tomography, *Phys Med Biol*, **51**(15):R541–78, 2006.
16. M. Defrise and G. T. Gullberg, Image reconstruction, *Phys Med Biol*, **51**(13):R139–54, 2006.
17. J. A. Patton, P. J. Slomka, G. Germano, and D. S. Berman, Recent technologic advances in nuclear cardiology, *J Nucl Cardiol*, **14**(4):501–13, 2007.
18. J. A. Patton, M. P. Sandler, and D. Berman, D-SPECT: A new solid state camera for high speed molecular imaging, *J Nucl Med*, **47(Supplement 1)**: 189P, 2006.
19. M. K. O'Connor and B. J. Kemp, Single-photon emission computed tomography/computed tomography: Basic instrumentation and innovations, *Semin Nucl Med*, **36**(4):258–66, 2006.
20. B. H. Hasegawa, K. Iwata, K. H. Wong, M. C. Wu, A. J. Da Silva, H. R. Tang, W. C. Barber, A. H. Hwang, and A. E. Sakdinawat, Dual-modality imaging of function and physiology, *Acad Radiol*, **9**(11):1305–21, 2002.
21. M. Singh, An electronically collimated gamma camera for single photon emission computed tomography. Part I: Theoretical considerations and design criteria, *Med Phys*, **10**(4):421–7, 1983.
22. A. S. Hoover, J. P. Sullivan, B. Baird, S. P. Brumby, R. M. Kippen, C. W. McCluskey, M. W. Rawool-Sullivan, and E. B. Sorensen, Gamma-ray imaging with a Si/CsI(Tl) Compton detector, *Appl Radiat Isot*, 2006.
23. W. L. Rogers, N. H. Clinthorne, and A. Bolozdynya, in *Emission Tomography: The Fundamentals of SPECT and PET,* edited by M. N. Wernick and J. N. Aarsvold (Elsevier, San Diego, 2004), pp. 383–420.
24. T. K. Lewellen, Time-of-flight PET, *Semin Nucl Med*, **28**(3):268–75, 1998.
25. S. Surti, J. S. Karp, L. M. Popescu, M. E. Daube-Witherspoon, and M. Werner, Investigation of time-of-flight benefit for fully 3-D PET, *IEEE Trans Med Imaging*, **25**(5):529–38, 2006.
26. S. Surti, A. Kuhn, M. E. Werner, A. E. Perkins, J. Kolthammer, and J. S. Karp, Performance of Philips Gemini TF PET/CT scanner with special consideration for its time-of-flight imaging capabilities, *J Nucl Med*, **48**(3):471–80, 2007.
27. G. Muehllehner and J. S. Karp, Positron emission tomography, *Phys Med Biol*, **51**(13):R117–37, 2006.
28. C. L. Melcher, Perspectives on the future development of new scintillators, *Nucl Instrum Methods Phys Res Sec A*, **537**:6–14, 2005.
29. T. Ling, T. K. Lewellen, and R. S. Miyaoka, Depth of interaction decoding of a continuous crystal detector module, *Phys Med Biol*, **52**(8):2213–28, 2007.

30. D. L. Bailey, Transmission scanning in emission tomography, *Eur J Nucl Med*, **25**(7):774–87, 1998.

31. P. E. Kinahan, B. H. Hasegawa, and T. Beyer, X-ray-based attenuation correction for positron emission tomography/computed tomography scanners, *Semin Nucl Med*, **33**(3):166–79, 2003.

32. T. Beyer, S. Rosenbaum, P. Veit, J. Stattaus, S. P. Muller, F. P. Difilippo, H. Schoder, O. Mawlawi, F. Roberts, A. Bockisch, and H. Kuhl, Respiration artifacts in whole-body (18)F-FDG PET/CT studies with combined PET/CT tomographs employing spiral CT technology with 1 to 16 detector rows, *Eur J Nucl Med Mol Imaging*, **32**(12):1429–39, 2005.

33. A. Bockisch, T. Beyer, G. Antoch, L. S. Freudenberg, H. Kuhl, J. F. Debatin, and S. P. Muller, Positron emission tomography/computed tomography—imaging protocols, artifacts, and pitfalls, *Mol Imaging Biol*, **6**(4):188–99, 2004.

34. K. P. Schafers, R. Raupach, and T. Beyer, Combined 18F-FDG-PET/CT imaging of the head and neck. An approach to metal artifact correction, *Nuklearmedizin*, **45**(5):219–22, 2006.

35. T. Beyer and D. W. Townsend, Putting "clear" into nuclear medicine: a decade of PET/CT development, *Eur J Nucl Med Mol Imaging*, **33**(8):857–61, 2006.

36. D. W. Townsend and T. Beyer, A combined PET/CT scanner: The path to true image fusion, *Br J Radiol*, **75 Spec No** S24–30, 2002.

37. D. W. Townsend, T. Beyer, and T. M. Blodgett, PET/CT scanners: a hardware approach to image fusion, *Semin Nucl Med*, **33**(3):193–204, 2003.

38. B. J. Pichler, M. S. Judenhofer, C. Catana, J. H. Walton, M. Kneilling, R. E. Nutt, S. B. Siegel, C. D. Claussen, and S. R. Cherry, Performance test of an LSO-APD detector in a 7-T MRI scanner for simultaneous PET/MRI, *J Nucl Med*, **47**(4):639–47, 2006.

39. C. Catana, Y. Wu, M. S. Judenhofer, J. Qi, B. J. Pichler, and S. R. Cherry, Simultaneous acquisition of multislice PET and MR images: Initial results with a MR-compatible PET scanner, *J Nucl Med*, **47**(12):1968–76, 2006.

40. C. Nanni, D. Rubello, S. Khan, A. Al-Nahhas, and S. Fanti, Role of small animal PET in stimulating the development of new radiopharmaceuticals in oncology, *Nucl Med Commun*, **28**(6):427–9, 2007.

41. D. J. Yang, E. E. Kim, and T. Inoue, Targeted molecular imaging in oncology, *Ann Nucl Med*, **20**(1):1–11, 2006.

42. F. Beekman and F. van der Have, The pinhole: Gateway to ultra-high-resolution three-dimensional radionuclide imaging, *Eur J Nucl Med Mol Imaging*, **34**(2):151–61, 2007.

43. A. Seret and F. Bleeser, Intrinsic uniformity requirements for pinhole SPECT, *J Nucl Med Technol*, **34**(1):43–7, 2006.

44. S. D. Metzler and R. Accorsi, Resolution versus sensitivity-effective diameter in pinhole collimation: Experimental verification, *Phys Med Biol*, **50**(21):5005–17, 2005.

45. R. Accorsi and S. D. Metzler, Resolution-effective diameters for asymmetric-knife-edge pinhole collimators, *IEEE Trans Med Imaging*, **24**(12):1637–46, 2005.

46. Z. Cao, G. Bal, R. Accorsi, and P. D. Acton, Optimal number of pinholes in multi-pinhole SPECT for mouse brain imaging—A simulation study, *Phys Med Biol*, **50**(19):4609–24, 2005.

47. T. Zeniya, H. Watabe, T. Aoi, K. M. Kim, N. Teramoto, T. Takeno, Y. Ohta, T. Hayashi, H. Mashino, T. Ota, S. Yamamoto, and H. Iida, Use of a compact pixellated gamma camera for small animal pinhole SPECT imaging, *Ann Nucl Med*, **20**(6):409–16, 2006.

48. S. R. Meikle, P. Kench, M. Kassiou, and R. B. Banati, Small animal SPECT and its place in the matrix of molecular imaging technologies, *Phys Med Biol*, **50**(22):R45–61, 2005.

49. C. S. Levin, Primer on molecular imaging technology, *Eur J Nucl Med Mol Imaging*, **32(Supplement 2):** S325–45, 2005.

50. B. Vastenhouw and F. Beekman, Submillimeter total-body murine imaging with U-SPECT-I, *J Nucl Med*, **48**(3):487–93, 2007.

51. F. J. Beekman and G. A. de Vree, Photon-counting versus an integrating CCD-based gamma camera: Important consequences for spatial resolution, *Phys Med Biol*, **50**(12):N109–19, 2005.

52. V. V. Nagarkar, I. Shestakova, V. Gaysinskiy, S. V. Tipnis, B. Singh, W. Barber, B. Hasegawa, and G. Entine, in *A CCD-based Detector for SPECT*, Rome, Italy, 2004 (IEEE).

CHAPTER 12
BREAST IMAGING SYSTEMS: DESIGN CHALLENGES FOR ENGINEERS

Mark B. Williams
University of Virginia, Charlottesville, Virginia

Laurie L. Fajardo
University of Iowa, Iowa City, Iowa

12.1 INTRODUCTION

Breast cancer is the second greatest cause (after lung cancer) of cancer-related death among American women, accounting for approximately 40,000 deaths each year. At the present time, early detection and characterization of breast cancers is our most effective weapon, since local disease is in most cases curable. Breast imaging systems can thus be potentially useful if they either are (1) useful for *detection* of cancers or (2) useful for *characterization* of suspicious lesions that may or may not be cancerous. Similarly, from a clinical perspective, methodologies used for breast cancer diagnosis (as opposed to therapy) fall into one of two broad categories: screening or diagnostic. Screening pertains to the population of women exhibiting no symptoms. Diagnostic imaging (otherwise known as problem-solving imaging) is used when there is some suspicion of disease, as a result of the manifestation of some physical symptom, of a physical exam, or of a screening study. The relative effectiveness of a given imaging modality at the tasks of detection and characterization determines whether it will be employed primarily in a screening or diagnostic context. At the present time, x-ray mammography is the only FDA-approved modality for screening, and is by far the most effective modality because of its ability to detect small cancers when they are most treatable (i.e., prior to metastasis). The sensitivity (fraction of all cancers that are detected) by screen-film mammography is approximately 85 percent. Ultrasound, MRI, breast specific gamma imaging, positron emission mammography, and electrical impedance scanning are FDA approved as diagnostic procedures following detection of an abnormality via x-ray mammography.

When designing a system for either screening or diagnostic imaging of the breast, several characteristics of the breast itself present unique engineering challenges. First, unlike parts of the body supported by bone, the breast is a malleable organ. Thus obtaining the exact same configuration for successive imaging studies is difficult, if not impossible. This complicates correlation between follow-up images of a given modality, or between concurrently obtained images from two different modalities. A second challenge arises from the fact that cancers can arise in areas of the breast very close to the chest wall. For example, the focal spot in x-ray mammography must be positioned directly above the chest wall edge of the image receptor in order to assure that x-rays passing through tissue adjacent to the chest wall are imaged. The proximity of the chest and shoulders also presents geometric hindrance affecting MRI coil design and nuclear medicine scanning. A third challenging aspect of breast cancer imaging is the similarity of many of the physical attributes of cancerous material and normal breast tissue. For example, the x-ray attenuation and acoustic impedance of cancerous masses are very similar to those of healthy fibroglandular breast tissue. Thus the imaging process must result in a sufficiently high signal-to-noise ratio that such subtle differences can be ascertained.

12.2 BREAST ANATOMY

The breast is composed primarily of fat and glandular tissue. The glandular tissue is sandwiched between layers of fat and lies above the pectoralis muscle and chest wall. The combination of the adipose and glandular tissue provides the radiographic contrast detected on x-ray mammography. When the ratio of adipose tissue to glandular tissue in the breast is greater, greater radiographic contrast is achieved. Breast tissue composed of only fibroglandular tissue results in a mammogram with lesser radiographic contrast that is more difficult for radiologists to evaluate.

The breast is considered a modified sweat gland and the milk it produces is a modification of sweat. Breast lobules, which produce milk during lactation, are connected by the breast ducts. The breast lobules and ducts are supported by the surrounding connective tissue. Deep and superficial facial layers envelop the stromal, epithelial, and glandular breast elements. Cooper's ligaments, a criss-crossing network of fibrous supporting structures, course between the deep and superficial layers of fascia. Surrounding the cone of glandular tissue is a layer of subcutaneous fat.

The nipple and areola contain erectile smooth muscle as well as sebaceous glands. Between five and nine separate ductal systems intertwine throughout the breast and have separate openings at the nipple. Each major lactiferous duct extends from the nipple-areolar complex into the breast in a branching network of smaller ducts. The area drained by each duct network is called a *lobe*, or *segment* of the breast. The duct network is lined by two types of cells, an inner epithelial layer surrounded by a thinner layer of myoepithelial cells. The final branch from a segmental duct is called the *extralobular terminal duct* and terminates in several acini. The anatomic unit comprising the extralobular duct and its lobule of acini is histologically designated as the terminal ductal lobular unit. It is postulated that most cancers arise in the extralobular terminal ducts, just proximal to the lobule.

Figure 12.1 is a schematic drawing depicting the anatomy of a healthy breast.

12.3 CURRENT CLINICAL BREAST IMAGING

12.3.1 Screening and Diagnostic Mammography

X-ray mammography is a projection onto two dimensions of the three-dimensional x-ray attenuation distribution of the breast. By federal regulation (the Mammography Quality Standards Act), dedicated and specialized radiographic equipment must be used for mammography. Mammographic systems utilize x-ray tubes with small focal spot size (0.1 and 0.3 mm nominal diameters), high-resolution x-ray receptors, and scatter reduction grids between the breast and the receptor. The x-ray focal spot is positioned directly above the edge of the image receptor closest to the patient, so that structures immediately adjacent to the chest wall may be visualized. A typical screening mammogram consists of two views of each breast. The two views are separated by

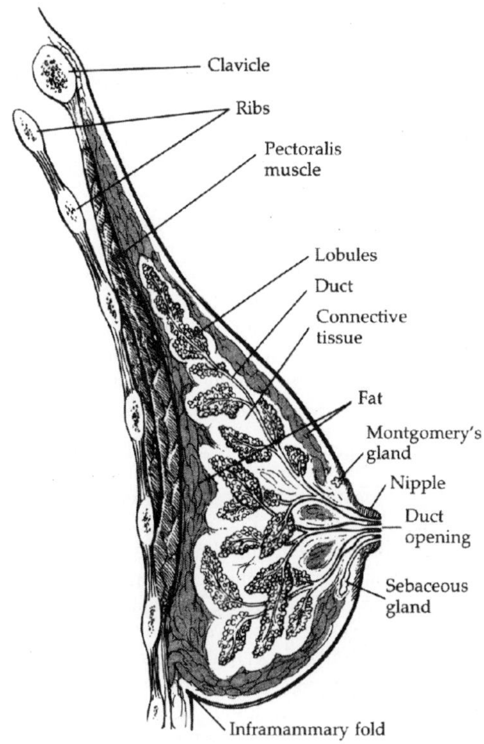

FIGURE 12.1 Schematic diagram showing the anatomy of the human breast.

approximately 45 to 60° in order to help resolve ambiguities produced by overlapping breast structure in a given projection. In addition, one view maximizes visualization of the structures near the lateral portion of the breast, such as the axillary lymph nodes. Both are obtained with the breast under compression using a flat acrylic paddle with low x-ray attenuation. Compression reduces the amount of scatter radiation reaching the detector by reducing the breast thickness, and also spreads out the tissue, thereby reducing the amount of structural overlap in the projection image.

Follow-up diagnostic procedures include additional x-ray views (magnification views, spot views, or unusual projections such as lateral views), ultrasound, and more recently MRI and nuclear medicine imaging (positron emission mammography or single gamma emission scintigraphy). We first present an overview of some of the technical aspects of screening mammography, then describe challenges associated with current and upcoming diagnostic imaging techniques.

X-ray Mammography Image Considerations. X-ray mammography is perhaps the most exacting of all x-ray–based imaging tasks. The main reasons for this are (1) the small difference in x-ray attenuation properties between various breast structures, and between normal and cancerous tissue and (2) the requirement that physically small objects such as microcalcifications be imaged with enough clarity to be detected by the radiologist (microcalcifications are calcium-containing deposits that are associated with early breast cancers, although many calcifications are merely benign). Clinically significant microcalcifications may be 0.2 mm or less in size. They often appear in clusters, and their individual shapes and relative orientations can be a clue as to the likelihood of an associated malignancy. The simultaneous requirements of high contrast resolution and high spatial resolution, along with the desire to minimize radiation dose to the breast, dictate that the image sensor have high sensitivity, low noise, and a narrow point response function. In addition, depending on the size and composition of the breast, the range of x-ray fluence incident on the sensor surface in a given mammogram can be 400:1 or more (Johns and Yaffe, 1987; Nishikawa et al., 1987). Thus the sensitivity and resolution must be maintained over an appreciable dynamic range.

Film-Based Imaging. Most mammography is currently performed using screen-film systems; that is, systems that employ image receptors consisting of film placed in direct contact with an x-ray-to-light converting screen. The screen-film combination, housed in a light-tight cassette, is placed below the breast, with a rotating anode x-ray tube placed 60 to 65 cm above the cassette. A major technical challenge in screen-film mammography arises from the fact that the film is used both as an acquisition and display medium. That means that system parameters such as film speed, detection and light conversion efficiency of the screen, and x-ray spectrum must be chosen not only to maximize the efficiency of the image acquisition process, but also to result in the optimum film darkening to maximize the visual contrast between structures when the film is viewed on a light box. Furthermore, as with other film-based imaging procedures, there is an inescapable trade-off between image contrast and dynamic range. One motivation for the development of digital detectors to replace screen-film receptors in mammography is the desire to increase dynamic range without a concomitant loss of image contrast.

Digital Mammography

Current Technologies for Image Acquisition. The principal motivations for the development of electronic receptors to replace film-based receptors are (1) the limited dynamic range of x-ray intensities over which the sensitivity of film-based systems is appreciable, (2) the inherent noise properties of film due to the random distribution of the grains on the film substrate (Nishikawa and Yaffe, 1985), and (3) the desire to decouple image acquisition and image display, which are inherently coupled in film-based imaging. The desire to overcome these limitations, combined with the advantages inherent in having images in digital form (e.g., computer-aided diagnosis, enhancement through image processing, easier image storage, remote transmission of images, and the possibility for more advanced acquisition approaches such as tomosynthesis, computed tomography, and dual energy imaging), has led to the development of several technical solutions to digital mammographic image acquisition during the past two decades. Leading large area technologies for full-field digital mammography (FFDM) currently include: (1) CsI(Tl) converters optically coupled to arrays of amorphous silicon (a-Si) photodiodes that are read out using a-Si thin-film transistor (TFT) arrays, (2) amorphous selenium (a-Se) converters electrically coupled to a-Si TFT arrays, and (3) storage phosphor plates (typically europium-doped barium fluorobromide) that retain a metastable latent image during x-ray exposure that can be de-excited and quantified using a raster-scanned laser beam. Technologies (1) and (2) are examples of indirect and direct flat-panel technologies, respectively. Indirect flat-panel detectors use an intermediate stage to convert x-rays to visible photons after which a photodetector generates charge. In direct conversion detectors, electron-hole pairs are generated in the x-ray absorber itself without the generation of visible photons. Technology (3) is often called *computed radiography* (CR). In each of the above digital mammography detectors, the detector area is equal to the imaged area. An alternative is to use a narrow, slot-shaped detector that spans the imaged area in one dimension (the chest wall-to-nipple direction), and is scanned from left to right during image acquisition. The x-ray beam, collimated to a similar slot shape, is scanned in synchrony with the detector. Commercial FFDM systems using a CsI-fiber optic taper-CCD combination have been developed (Tesic et al., 1999), and more recently systems employing gas-filled detectors have been introduced (Thunberg et al., 2004). With the full area detector technologies, x-ray tube target materials (molybdenum, rhodium, or tungsten) and external filtration (molybdenum or rhodium) combinations similar to those used in screen-film mammography are employed. For the scanned devices, a tungsten target is typically used, and the tube voltage is often somewhat higher than that used with Mo or Rh targets.

Figure 12.2 compares analog (screen-film) and digital cranial-caudal images of a spiculated mass (1.2-cm invasive ductal carcinoma) located in the upper inner quadrant of the right breast. The mass is seen best in the posterior aspect of the breast on the MLO view. As of this writing, five manufacturers have received approval from the U.S. Food and Drug Administration (FDA) to market full-field digital mammography (FFDM) systems in the United States (some of these manufacturers have more than one FDA-approved FFDM system), including indirect flat-panel systems, direct flat-panel systems, one

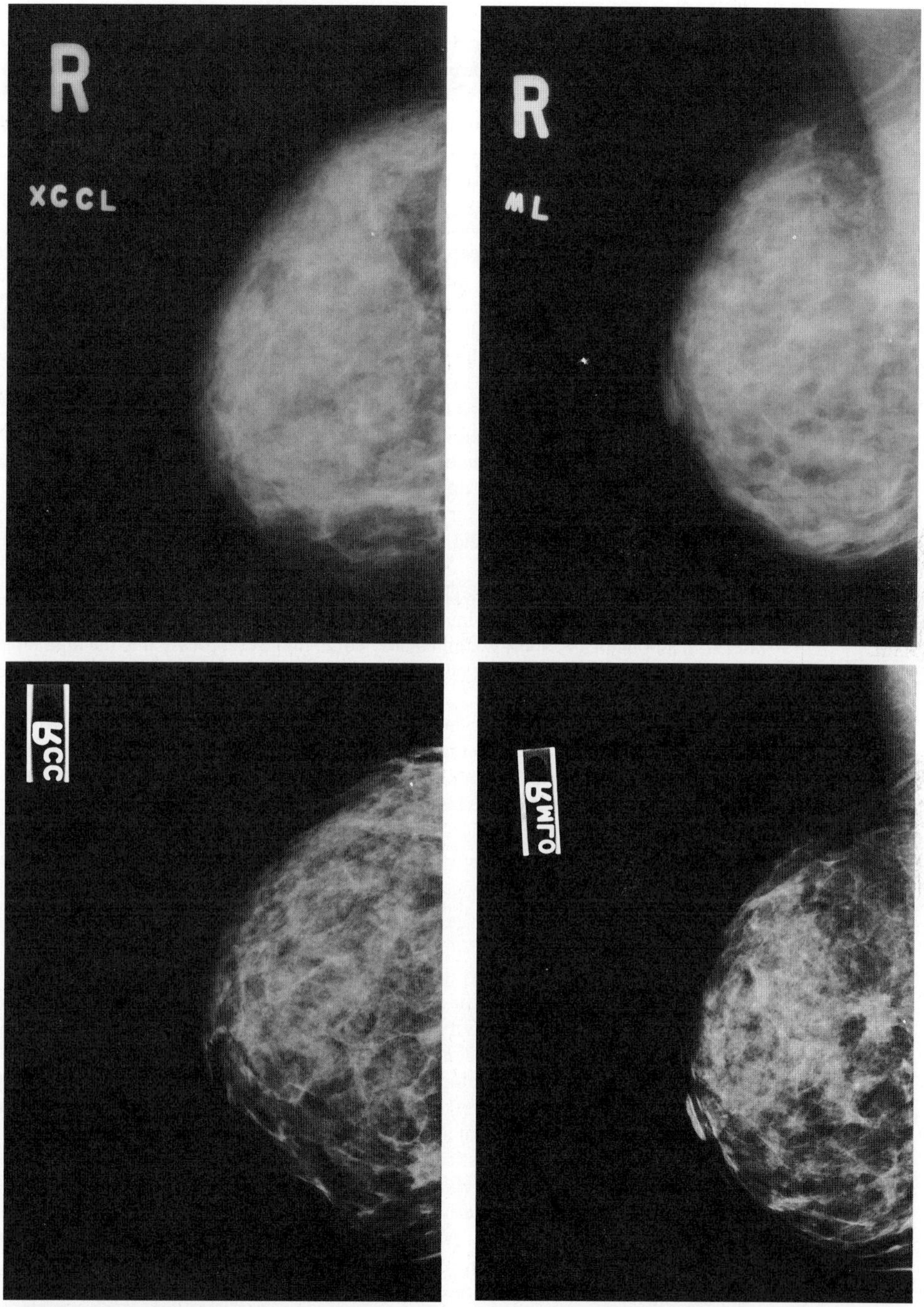

FIGURE 12.2 Analog (top row) and digital (bottom row) images of the right breast of a woman with moderately radio-dense breast tissue and an irregularly shaped mass with spiculated margins (1.2 cm invasive ductal carcinoma) located in the upper inner quadrant of the breast. The mass is seen best in the posterior aspect of the breast on the MLO view (lower right). The improved contrast, enhanced depiction of the suspicious mass, and better visualization of peripheral tissue and skin line in the right image are a result of the larger dynamic range of the digital receptor.

storage phosphor system, and a scanned CCD-based system that is no longer being manufactured. Several other manufacturers are in the process of gathering data for submission to the FDA for approval.

Challenges Facing Digital Mammography. The clinical presence of FFDM is increasing at a high rate. According to the American College of Radiology, as of May 2007, 20 percent of accredited facilities have at least one digital mammography system versus only 16 percent as of January 2007. The current rapid growth is attributed both to the overall trend in radiology toward digital imaging, and to the results of the Digital Mammographic Imaging Screening Trial (DMIST). DMIST enrolled 49,500 asymptomatic women in the United States and Canada, each of whom had both a digital and screen-film mammographic study at the time of enrollment and again a year later. The study concluded that, compared to film-based mammography, FFDM was significantly better for screening women who fell into any of the following categories: (1) under 50 years of age, (2) of any age with heterogeneously or extremely dense breasts, or (3) pre- or perimenopausal women of any age. Although adoption of FFDM into clinical practice is well under way, there are still major challenges that must be addressed. Perhaps the most immediate obstacles have to do with image display. The very large size of the digital images (up to 30 megapixels, with 12 to 16 bits per pixel) far exceeds the matrix size (up to 2000 × 2500 or 5 megapixels) and grayscale depth (typically 8 bits) of current commercially available high-resolution displays. Furthermore, a typical screening study involves simultaneous viewing of four current views (two per breast) alongside the corresponding four views from the previous screening study. Partially for this reason, many early practitioners of FFDM used laser film printers to produce hard copies of the digitally obtained mammograms, so that they could be viewed on a conventional light box, alongside the previous (analog) study.

Another area of ongoing research is the development of image-processing techniques for both laser film and grayscale monitor viewing. In the former case (hard copy display), the characteristics of the laser film automatically apply a nonlinear dynamic range compression to the digital pixel values. In the case of workstation viewing (soft copy display), it is desirable to limit the amount of time that the radiologist must spend adjusting the image display (i.e., adjusting the range of pixel values mapped into the available grayscale levels of the display), so some means of reducing the dynamic range in the mammogram without compromising image quality is needed. One approach is *thickness compensation* (Bick et al., 1996; Byng et al., 1997). This is a software technique that compensates for the decrease in attenuating thickness near the breast periphery by locating region between the area of uniform thickness (where the breast is in contact with the flat compression paddle) and the skin line. Pixel values corresponding to that region are scaled downward to make their values more similar to those in the region of uniform thickness.

12.3.2 Diagnostic Ultrasound

Ultrasound (US) is used as a diagnostic (as opposed to screening) breast imaging modality, in part because it lacks the sensitivity of x-ray mammography for microcalcifications, and its specificity for small masses varies considerably among operators. However, US is recommended by the American College of Radiology as the initial imaging technique for evaluation of masses in women under 30 and in lactating and pregnant women—populations for whom mammography is less sensitive and for whom radiation dose should be minimized. In the majority of breast imaging cases, the primary diagnostic use of ultrasound is the differentiation of solid masses from fluid-filled cysts (Fig. 12.3). Regarding solid mass, there has been a general lack of confidence, in the ability of US to characterize solid masses as benign versus malignant without obtaining histopathology for many cases. Although at least one study has reported that benign and malignant solid breast masses could be differentiated based on US alone (Stavros et al., 1995), subsequent studies have not confirmed this hypothesis, and it is now generally believed that at the present time there are no ultrasound features that, by themselves, are sufficient evidence to forgo biopsy. Recently, the American College of Radiology Imaging Network published its trial evaluating breast ultrasound as a breast cancer screening tool. The study enrolled over 2,800 patients with radiodense breast tissue, of which 2,637 were fully evaluable by either gold standard pathology or follow up imaging. In this study, the investigators found the diagnostic yield

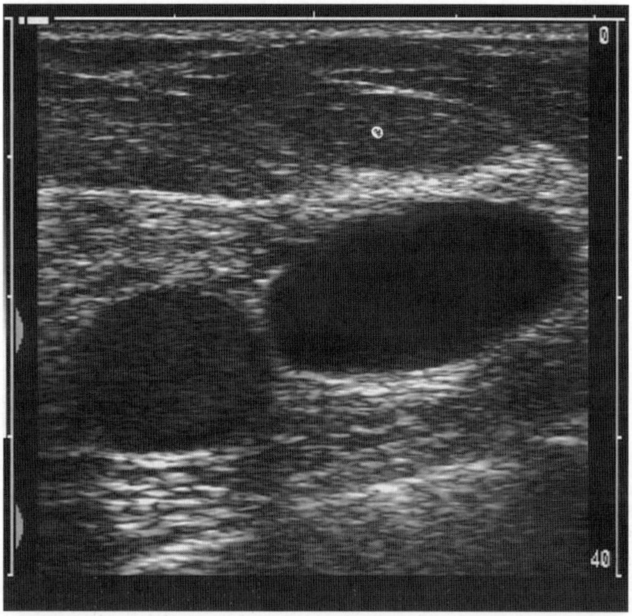

FIGURE 12.3 Ultrasound image demonstrating a mass and a cyst. The round lesion on the left demonstrates homogenous internal echoes consistent with a solid mass (fibroadenoma on biopsy). The oval lesion on the right has no internal echoes (anechoic), consistent with a benign cyst (confirmed by cyst aspiration).

for mammography was 7.6 cancers per 1000 women screened; this increased to 11.8 cancers per 1000 women screened when the data for combined mammography plus ultrasound were evaluated. The supplemental yield of ultrasound was calculated to be 4.2 cancers per 1000 women screened. In a sensitivity predication model, the authors suggested that adding a single screening ultrasound to mammography would yield an additional 1.1 to 7.2 cancers per 1000 high-risk women screened but would substantially increase the number of false positive diagnoses and biopsies performed due to the lower specificity of screening breast ultrasound and the associated operator dependence of this particular examination. The expected value of screening breast ultrasound in the average screening population (which would include radiodense and non-radiodense breast tissue) with respect to sensitivity, specificity, accuracy and cost-effectiveness would be poorer. Newer techniques being explored to improve the ability of US to differentiate benign and malignant masses include intensity histogram analysis (Kitaoka et al., 2001) and disparity processing, in which the sonographer slightly varies the pressure of the probe on the breast surface, and the apparent displacement of the tissue is measured by analysis of the correlation between images obtained at different parts of this compression cycle (Steinberg et al., 2001). This measurement of the elastic properties of the lesion is similar to that employed in breast elastography (briefly described below). In addition to these diagnostic tasks, US also plays a major role in biopsy guidance.

One technical issue affecting US is that its results tend to be more operator-dependent than the other modalities because of variations in positioning of handheld transducers. Automated transducers are much less operator-dependent than handheld transducers. However, handheld transducers permit a more rapid exam, and are better suited for biopsy guidance. In addition to diagnostic tasks, US also plays a major role in biopsy guidance.

12.4 NEW AND DEVELOPING BREAST IMAGING MODALITIES

12.4.1 Introduction

While x-ray mammography is unquestionably the leading currently available modality for early detection of small cancers, it suffers from a relatively low positive predictive value (the fraction of lesions identified as positive that ultimately turn out to be positive). As a result, 65 to 85 percent of all breast biopsies are negative (Kerlikowske et al., 1993; Kopans, 1992). Therefore, adjunct modalities that can differentiate benign and malignant lesions detected by mammography are considered highly desirable. In a report issued by the National Research Council in 2000, the Committee on Technologies for the Early Detection of Breast Cancer identified the breast imaging technologies and their current status (Mammography and Beyond, 2001). A summary, updated to 2007, is shown in Table 12.1.

The first two x-ray imaging modalities have been discussed above. Below, we discuss some of the more advanced (i.e., they have been described in the scientific literature, and have undergone at least preliminary clinical evaluation) and most promising developing breast imaging modalities: tomosynthesis, breast CT, breast MRI, scintimammography, breast PET, and electrical impedance imaging. We also briefly discuss optical imaging and elastography.

12.4.2 Tomosynthesis and Breast CT

Tomosynthesis. In projection radiography, the images of anatomy throughout the imaged volume are superimposed, potentially masking the presence of disease. Three-dimensional (3D) imaging

TABLE 12.1 Status of Developing Breast Imaging Technologies

Technology	Screening	Diagnosis	FDA approved?
Screen-film mammography	+++	+++	Yes
Full-field digital mammography	+++	+++	Yes
Tomosynthesis	+	+	No
Breast CT	0	0	
Computer-assisted detection	++	0	Yes
Ultrasound (US)	+	+++	Yes
Novel US methods	0	0	No
Elastography (MR and US)	0	0	No
Magnetic resonance imaging (MRI)	++	+++	Yes
Magnetic resonance spectroscopy (MRS)	–/0	+/0	Yes
Breast specific gamma imaging	+/0	++	Yes
Positron emission mammography	+/0	++	Yes
Optical imaging	0	+	No
Optical spectroscopy	–	0	No
Thermography	0	+	Yes
Electrical potential measurements	0	+	No
Electrical impedance imaging	0	+	Yes
Electronic palpation	0	NA	No
Thermoacoustic-computed tomography, microwave imaging, Hall effect imaging, magnetomammography	NA	NA	No

Status Description
- – Technology is not useful for the given application.
- NA No data are available regarding use of the technology for given application.
- 0 Preclinical data are suggestive that the technology might be useful for breast cancer detection, but clinical data are absent or very sparse for the given application.
- \+ Clinical data suggest that the technology could play a role in breast cancer detection, but more study is needed to define a role in relation to existing technologies.
- ++ Data suggest that the technology could be useful in selected situations because it adds (or is equivalent) to existing technologies, but not currently recommended for routine use.
- +++ The technology is routinely used to make clinical decisions for the given application.

modalities acquire volumetric rather than planar image data, permitting thin slices of image data to be extracted and viewed individually without superposition of structure from other anatomy outside that slice. X-ray tomosynthesis, whether applied to imaging the breast or other parts of the anatomy, uses multiple views obtained over a range of viewing angles to produce a 3D image. Unlike x-ray CT in which views are obtained over 240 to 360°, a range sufficient to form a mathematically complete projection data set for 3D image reconstruction, the angular range in tomosynthesis is much less, typically 40 to 50°. Tomosynthesis has evolved out of x-ray tomography, which has been practiced since the early 1900s. Early tomographic imaging was performed by linear translation of the x-ray tube and screen-film cassette in opposite directions on either side of the patient. This has the effect of blurring out the images of structures outside of a plane passing through the fulcrum of the tube-receptor motion. The availability within the past decade of large area digital detectors capable of rapid readout has given birth to digital tomosynthesis, in which a series of low-dose digital images is obtained, permitting reconstruction of an arbitrary number of image planes via digital shifting and summation of the images of the series. Figure 12.4 shows planar full field digital mammography images of heterogeneously dense breasts (cranio-caudal (CC) views in 12.4*a* and mediolateral oblique (MLO) views in 12.4*b*). Figures 12.4*c* and 12.4*d* are digital tomosynthesis slices through a suspicious lesion in the right breast. The lesion shape is much more clearly defined in the

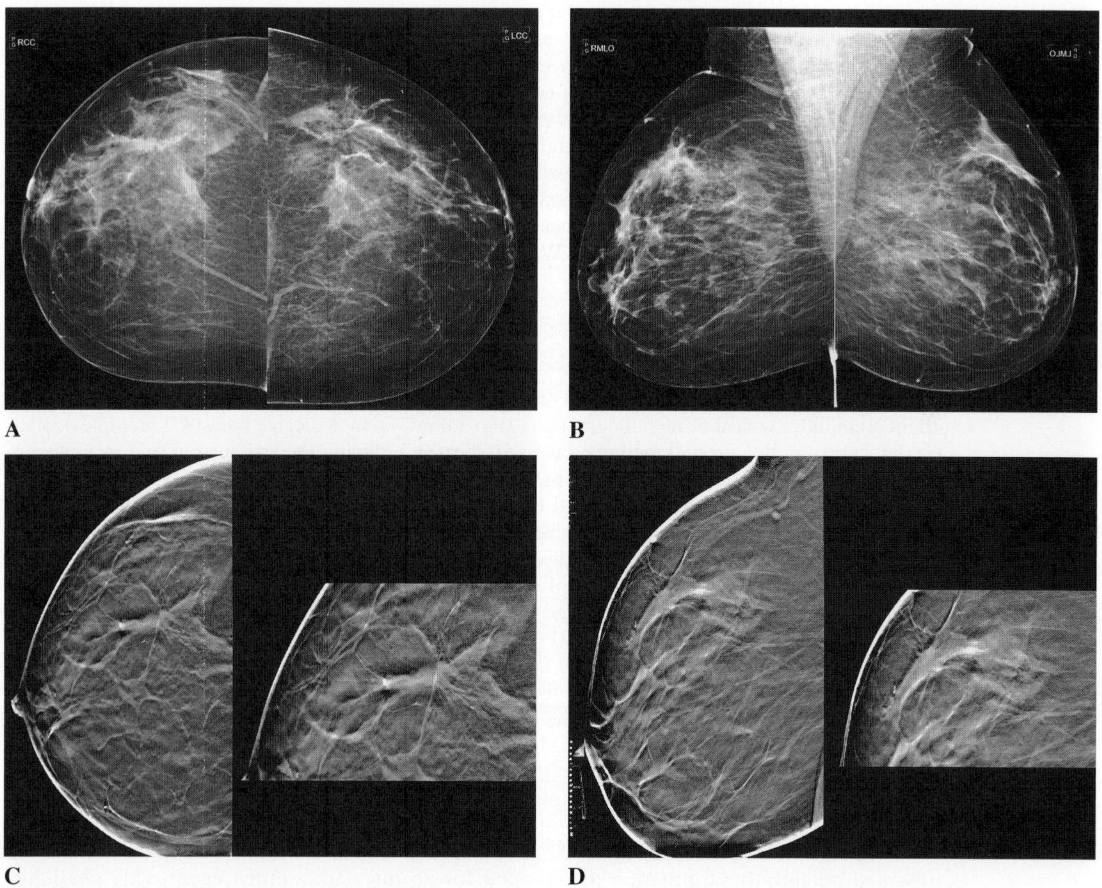

FIGURE 12.4 (a) Cranio-caudal (CC) planar digital mammography images (right and left breasts). (b) Medio-lateral oblique (MLO) planar digital mammography images (right and left breasts). (c) Tomosynthesis slice through a suspicious lesion in the CC view of the right breast (indicated by arrow). Note the clearer depiction of the lesion compared to the planar image in which superimposed structures clutter the region near the lesion. (d) Tomosynthesis slice through the lesion in the MLO view of the right breast (indicated by the arrow).

tomosynthesis images because of the elimination of the superimposed dense breast tissue present in the planar images. Dobbins and Godfrey have written an excellent review of tomographic imaging and tomosynthesis, including descriptions of the several image reconstruction and deblurring strategies (Dobbins and Godfrey, 2003). Among the many clinical applications of digital tomosynthesis are breast imaging (Mainprize et al., 2006; Niklason et al., 1997; Sechopoulos et al., 2007; Wu et al., 2003), chest radiography (Godfrey et al., 2006; McAdams et al., 2006; Pineda et al., 2006), dental imaging (Nair et al., 2003; Webber et al., 1997; Webber et al., 2002; Ziegler et al., 2003), and patient positioning and brachytherapy seed localization in radiation therapy (Godfrey et al., 2007; Reddy and Mendelson, 2005). At the present time a number of mammography equipment manufacturers are actively developing digital tomosynthesis systems for breast imaging. Using an early commercial tomosynthesis unit, researchers at Dartmouth have recently published the results of a study designed to measure the impact of tomosynthesis on recall rates (the fraction of screening mammography patients who are subsequently referred for further workup due to an abnormal mammogram). They reported a reduction of 40 percent in the recall rate among 98 women, when digital screening mammography was supplemented with tomosynthesis (Poplack et al., 2007). Contrast-enhanced tomosynthesis, in which an iodine-based contrast agent is injected intravenously and patients are imaged before and after administration of contrast, is also being investigated as an adjunct to digital mammography (Chen et al., 2007).

A major technical challenge facing breast tomosynthesis is identification of the best acquisition strategy (number of breast compressions, and for each compression the number of views, angular range of views, angular distribution of views, and distribution of x-ray dose among views). The asymmetrical shape of the compressed breast results in preferential radiographic properties for views along directions at small angles relative to the direction of compression, for which the thickness of breast that must be penetrated is less. However, clustering the viewing directions near the compression direction results in incomplete sampling of frequency space and relatively poorer spatial resolution in the direction of compression compared to the other two coordinate directions. This incomplete sampling also results in image artifacts, especially if simple backprojection via shifting and summing is used for reconstruction. The optimum acquisition strategy is thus dependent on the reconstruction technique utilized, and possibly on breast type (Suryanarayanan et al., 2000; Wu et al., 2003; Wu et al., 2004; Zhang et al., 2006).

Breast CT. In recent years, several academic groups have begun the development of dedicated breast CT scanners (Boone et al., 2001; Crotty et al., 2007; Ning et al., 2003). Relative to using a conventional whole-body CT scanner to image the breasts, the primary advantage of a dedicated scanner is the potential reduction of radiation dose from the levels typical of whole-body CT (10 to 20 mGy) to those typical of mammography (1.0 to 3.0 mGy). In dedicated breast CT, complete angular (helical) sampling around the breast is used, thereby reducing the artifacts present in tomosynthesis and producing more isotropic spatial resolution. In virtually all prototype systems, the woman is prone with the uncompressed breast pendant though a hole in the table. A flat-panel detector whose edge is aligned with the chest wall provides cone beam geometry, and in most cases the entire breast is imaged in a single helical acquisition and x-ray exposure. Boone et al. have developed a prototype scanner capable of obtaining 500 views over 360° in 17 s, while delivering a total radiation dose to an average-sized breast equal to that of a conventional two-view planar mammographic study (Boone et al., 2001; Boone et al., 2005). An industrial x-ray tube with a stationary tungsten target is operated at 80 kVp, a tube voltage significantly higher than that used in mammography (25 to 35 kVp). Compared to two-dimensional (2D) FFDM, the system has modest spatial resolution; in the coronal plane the MTF falls to 0.10 at 0.7 to 1.7 cycles/mm, depending on the location within the field of view. This is in part because of a relatively large focal spot size (0.4 mm) and effective detector element size (0.388 mm), and the thickness of the CsI converter (600 μm) (Kwan et al., 2007). Nevertheless, images demonstrate high contrast depiction of anatomical structures in the breast, and a second prototype system is now being tested in a pilot clinical trial.

Compared to breast MRI, breast CT may have advantages in terms of shorter acquisition time and potentially elimination of the need for an injected contrast agent. One challenge facing breast CT is improving the spatial resolution without unacceptable dose increase. Higher spatial resolution is an important goal not just because of the importance of microcalcification detection, but also because microcalcifications indicative of malignant processes are often differentiated from those due to benign processes by their shape. Accurate shape depiction requires resolution superior to that necessary for simple detection. In a similar fashion, malignant and benign masses are often distinguished by the appearance of their borders (margins), with spiculated margins having a much higher correlation with malignancy than smooth margins. To overcome this limitation, developers of breast CT imaging systems are working with x-ray tube developers to build special low kVp and smaller focal spot x-ray tubes for breast CT imaging. A second challenge for breast CT is imaging breast tissue lying adjacent to the chest wall. This problem arises because of the nonzero thickness of the table upon which the patient lies prone, and the difficulty of positioning the x-ray focal spot and active portion of the detector very close to the bottom surface of the table. In terms of promoting clinical acceptance of breast CT, an advancement that would add to its clinical utility is the development of techniques for image-guided biopsy, such as those currently available using stereotactic x-ray imaging. Accurate needle placement is likely to be more difficult for the uncompressed and unrestrained breast than for a compressed breast. However, this technical challenge can likely be overcome using image-guided biopsy approaches similar to those used for MRI-guided breast biopsy.

12.4.3 MRI

At present, mammography is the primary imaging modality used to detect early clinically occult breast cancer. Despite advances in mammographic technique, there are limitations in sensitivity and specificity that remain. These limitations have stimulated exploration into alternative or adjunctive imaging techniques. MRI of the breast provides higher soft tissue contrast than conventional mammography. This provides the potential for improved lesion detection and characterization. Studies have already demonstrated the potential for breast MRI to distinguish benign from malignant breast lesions and to detect mammographically and clinically occult cancer (Dash et al., 1986; El Yousef et al., 1984; Stelling et al., 1985). The first studies using MRI to detect both benign and malignant breast lesions concluded that it was not possible to detect and characterize lesions on the basis of signal intensities on T1-and T2-weighted images (Dash et al., 1986; El Yousef et al., 1984; Stelling et al., 1985). However, reports on the use of gadolinium-enhanced breast MRI were more encouraging. Cancers enhance relative to other breast tissues following the administration of intravenous Gd-DTPA (Kaiser and Zeitler, 1989). Indeed, in one study, 20 percent of cancers were seen only after the administration of Gd-DTPA (Heywang et al., 1989). In addition, several studies reported on MRI detection of breast cancer not visible on mammography (Harms et al., 1993; Heywang et al., 1989). The detection of mammographically occult multifocal cancer in up to 30 percent of patients has led to the recommendations that MRI can be successfully used to stage patients who are potential candidates for breast conservation therapy (Harms et al., 1993). Figure 12.5 shows an example of mammographically occult ductal carcinoma in situ (DCIS) identified via gadolinium-enhanced MRI.

However, the presence of contrast enhancement alone is not specific for distinguishing malignant from benign breast lesions. Benign lesions frequently enhance after Gd injection on MRI, including fibroadenomas, benign proliferative change, and inflammatory change. To improve specificity, some investigators recommend dynamic imaging of breast lesions to evaluate the kinetics of enhancement (Heywang et al., 1989; Kaiser and Zeitler, 1989; Stack et al., 1990). Using this technique, cancers have been found to enhance intensely in the early phases of the contrast injection. Benign lesions enhance variably but in a more delayed fashion than malignant lesions. Recently, the American College of Radiology has published its reporting lexicon for breast MRI, which incorporates both lesion morphology and kinetic information to diagnose MR-depicted breast lesions (American College of Radiology, 2003).

Because x-ray mammography is limited by its relatively low specificity, MRI has been suggested as an adjunct imaging study to evaluate patients with abnormal mammograms. One application of breast MRI may be to reduce the number of benign biopsies performed as a result of screening and diagnostic mammography work-up. To distinguish benign from malignant breast lesions using MRI scanning, most investigators rely on studying the time course of signal intensity changes of a breast lesion after contrast injection. However, among reported studies, the scan protocols varied widely

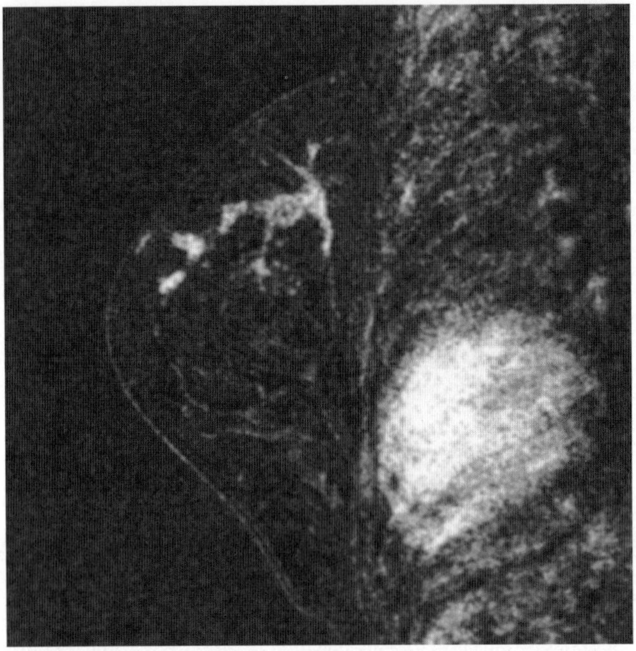

FIGURE 12.5 Post Gd contrast enhanced Ts subtraction image in a 40-year-old high-risk female demonstrates nonmass-like enhancement in the upper out quadrant of the left breast that was confirmed histologically to be segmental involvement with DCIS. Mammogram was normal.

and differ with respect to emphasis on information acquired. For example, Boetes et al. (Boetes et al., 1994) used a protocol consisting of a single-slice non-fat-suppressed gradient echo imaging sequence with 2.6- × 1.3-mm in-plane spatial resolution (10-mm slice) at 2.3-s time intervals. They used the criterion that any lesion with visible enhancement in less than 11.5 s after arterial enhancement was considered suspicious for cancer. These criteria resulted in 95 percent sensitivity and 86 percent specificity for the diagnosis of cancer. Similar sequences have been reported by others using protocols with the time resolution varying from 6 to 60 s. However, problems locating a lesion on the precontrast images in order to perform a single-slice dynamic enhanced examination and the need to detect and evaluate other lesions within the breast have resulted in recommendations that a multislice technique that captures dynamic data from the entire breast after injection of contrast is necessary (Gilles et al., 1994; Hickman et al., 1994; Perman et al., 1994). These investigators advocate using multislice 2D gradient echo, 3D gradient echo, and echo planar techniques, with time resolution varying from 12 s to 1 min, varying special resolution, and varying section thickness. Keyhole imaging techniques that dynamically sample the center of k-space after contrast administration have been suggested as a technique to obtain dynamic high-resolution 3D images of the entire breast (Van Vaals et al., 1993). However, the spatial resolution of enhanced tissue is limited with keyhole techniques because only part of the breast is sampled after contrast is injected. Keyhole imaging is criticized as being suboptimal for assessing lesion architecture. Research to clarify optimal acquisition protocols for breast MRI is needed. Recent work in breast MRI in 3-T magnets is very exciting and holds promise for even higher spatial and temporal resolution and further improvements in image quality. In the future, novel contrast agents may provide more sensitive and more specific discrimination of benign from malignant lesions. In vivo functional measurements of tumor biology using contrast-enhanced MRI, diffusion-weighted MRI, or MR spectroscopy may yield markers that can be used to predict response to treatment more accurately and earlier in treatment.

Also widely varying among investigators are their criteria used for differentiating benign from malignant lesions. Criteria vary from simplistic models that report the percent of lesion enhancement at 2 min following contrast injection to more sophisticated physiologic models that take into account the initial T1 characteristics of a lesion and calculate Gd concentration as a function of time in order to extract pharmacokinetic parameters. Thus, wide variability in the accuracy cited by these investigators for differentiating benign from malignant lesions has been reported (66 to 93 percent) (Daniel et al., 1998; Esserman et al., 1999; Gilles et al., 1994; Hickman et al., 1994; Hylton, 1999; Orel et al., 1994; Perman et al., 1994; Van Vaals et al., 1993). Despite the many differing techniques, it is clear that there is a tendency for cancer to enhance more rapidly than benign lesions after bolus injection of Gd chelate. However, it is also clear that overlap exists in dynamic curves between cancerous and noncancerous lesions, resulting in false-negative diagnosis in all reported series and false-positive diagnosis in many. The development and availability of Breast MRI CAD Systems has improved the interpretation of BMRI tremendously. These software tools perform automated subtraction of contrast enhanced scans obtained at sequential time points during the MRI examination from the initial precontrast scan. The resulting images depict any portion of the breast or a lesions that enhanced and removes all non-enhancing (normal) structures; the data from the sequential images are then used to calculate the temporal time intensity curves that numerically demonstrate the inflow and egress of contract media into/out of breast lesions. In addition, MIP images and other 3-dimensional image reconstructions are easily accomplished to assist the interpreting physician.

Alternative approaches to characterizing enhancing lesions on breast MRI include extracting architectural features that describe breast lesions. The superior soft tissue contrast of MRI and use of higher spatial resolution techniques have prompted investigations in this area and the development of a lexicon for interpreting and reporting breast MRI scans (Gilles et al., 1994; Nunes et al., 1997; Orel et al., 1994; Schnall et al., 2001; American College of Radiology, 2003). Such an advancement would improve the widespread general reliability and comparability among breast MRI examinations performed from one institution to another. Clearly, the relative importance of spatial and temporal resolution in this regard requires further evaluation.

Other reported investigations of breast MRI suggest that MRI demonstrates more extensive cancer than indicated by mammography or predicted by clinical breast examination. Several investigators have now demonstrated that MRI can detect breast cancer that is mammographically occult (Harms et al., 1993; Heywang et al., 1989; Sardanelli et al., 2007a; Sardanelli et al., 2007b; Port et al., 2007; Lehman et al., 2005; Leach et al., 2005; Kuhl et al., 2005; Kriege et al., 2004; Warner et al., 2004) and suggest that MRI may have a role as a screening examination for patients with a high genetic predisposition to breast cancer and in those populations of women having extremely radiodense breast tissue on x-ray mammography. The American Cancer Society recently published its guidelines for breast screening with MRI as an adjunct to mammography, wherein they defined their specific recommendations, the lifetime risk of populations comprising their specific recommendations, and the strength of the evidence on which they based their recommendations (Saslow et al., 2007). An annual MRI screening study along with an annual screening mammogram for women having a BRCA mutation that have not been tested themselves for the BRCA mutation, and women having a lifetime risk of 20 to 25 percent or greater for developing breast cancer as defined by the BRCAPRO (Parmigiani et al., 1998; Berry et al., 1997) or other breast cancer estimation models that are dependent on family history. This recommendation is based on evidence from nonrandomized screening trials and observational studies (Sardanelli et al., 2007a; Sardanelli et al., 2007b; Port et al., 2007; Lehman et al., 2005; Leach et al., 2005; Kuhl et al., 2005; Kriege et al., 2004; Warner et al., 2004).

The recommendations for annual MRI breast screening along with annual mammography for other populations is based on expert concensus opinion regarding the lifetime risk for breast cancer. These populations include women who underwent radiation to the chest between the age of 10 and 30 years and those diagnosed with having Li-Fraumeni syndrome, Cowden syndrome, and Bannayan-Riley-Ruvalcaba syndrome, and individuals with first-degree relatives diagnosed with these syndromes. The panel found insufficient evidence to recommend for or against MRI screening in women whose lifetime risk for developing breast cancer is 15 to 20 percent as defined by BRCAPRO or other models largely dependent on family history, women with a prior pathologic diagnosis of lobular carcinoma in situ, atypical lobular hyperplasia, or in situ or invasive breast cancer.

Likewise, there was insufficient evidence to recommend for or against MRI screening as an adjunct to mammography in women having heterogeneously or extremely radiodense breast parenchyma on mammography. The expert concensus opinion of the panel was that there was no evidence to support MRI screening in women having a less than 15 percent lifetime risk of developing breast carcinoma (Saslow et al., 2007).

12.4.4 Nuclear Imaging Methods

Nuclear imaging involves the injection of pharmaceutical compounds that have been labeled with radioisotopes. The compounds are selected such that they couple to some sort of biological process such as blood flow, metabolic activity, or enzyme production, or such that they tend to accumulate at specific locations in the body, for example, binding to certain cell receptor sites. Thus the relative concentration of these radiotracers in various areas of the body gives information about the relative degree to which these biological activities are occurring. Measurement of this concentration distribution therefore provides *functional* information very different from the *structural* information supplied by modalities such as x-ray mammography and ultrasound. For this reason, nuclear medicine techniques are being explored as adjunct imaging approaches to the structurally oriented x-ray mammography.

Nuclear medicine tracers being considered for breast imaging can conveniently be divided into two groups: those emitting single gamma rays and those emitting positrons. In both cases, the concentration distribution in the breast is mapped by one or more imaging gamma detectors placed in proximity to the patient. In the case of single gamma emitters, the gamma detectors are equipped with some type of physical collimators whose function is to create a unique correlation between a point on the detector surface and a line through the spatially distributed radioactivity source (e.g., the breast). Physical collimation is not necessary in the case of positron-emitting isotopes because of the near colinearity of the gamma ray pair produced by annihilation of the emitted positron with a nearby electron. However, opposing gamma detectors and timing circuitry must be used to detect the two gamma rays of a pair in coincidence. Below we discuss some of the unique challenges presented by nuclear imaging of the breast, and describe some technical solutions currently being explored.

Scintimammography

Conventional Scintimammography. Nuclear medicine imaging of the breast using a tracer emitting single gamma rays and an imaging gamma detector fitted with a collimator is referred to as *breast scintigraphy*, *scintimammography*, or more contemporarily with the advent of dedicated imaging systems, *molecular breast imaging* or breast specific gamma imaging. These terms are typically applied to planar imaging of the breast rather than tomographic imaging, known as single photon emission computed tomography, or SPECT. Early scintimammography studies used conventional, large gamma cameras and imaged the prone patient whose breasts hung pendant through holes in the table. Prone positioning was favored over supine positioning because gravity acts to pull the breast tissue away from the chest wall. Typically two lateral views were obtained, and one anterior-posterior view to aid in medial-lateral tumor localization. The majority of clinical trials to date have employed one of two ^{99m}Tc-labeled pharmaceuticals; sestamibi or tetrafosmin. Reported values for sensitivity and specificity for planar scintimammography performed under these conditions vary according to several factors, a principle one being the distribution of lesion sizes represented in the particular study. In a three-center European trial, sensitivities of 26, 56, 95, and 97 percent were reported for category pT1a (<0.5 cm), pT1b (0.5 to 1.0 cm), pT1c (1.0 to 2.0 cm), and pT2 (>2 cm) cancers, respectively (Scopinaro et al., 1997). A clinical trial (134 women scheduled for open breast biopsy were enrolled) investigating the use of prone ^{99m}Tc-sestamibi scintimammography for pT1 tumors (4.7 percent pT1a, 46.7 percent pT1b, and 48.6 percent pT1c) reported sensitivity, positive predictive value, negative predictive value and accuracy of 81.3, 97.6, 55.6, and 83.6 percent, respectively (Lumachi et al., 2001). The corresponding values for x-ray mammography were 83.2, 89.9, 48.6, and 79.1 percent. In a recent meta-analysis, Hussain et al. reported scintimammography sensitivity and specificity of 85 and 84 percent, respectively for 2424 single-site participants, and 85 and 83 percent, respectively for 3049 multicenter study participants (Hussain et al., 2006). These and other studies demonstrated that scintimammography provides diagnostic information complimentary to that of x-ray mammography (Allen et al., 2000; Buscombe et al., 2001; Palmedo et al., 1998; Scopinaro et al., 1997).

Studies have been made comparing the performance of scintimammography to that of contrast-enhanced MRI as adjuncts to x-ray mammography. In a study of 49 patients comparing contrast MRI with conventional, large-camera scintimammography, Imbriaco et al. found no statistically significant difference in either sensitivity or specificity (Imbriaco et al., 2001). However, comparing contrast MRI with scintimammography using a dedicated breast gamma camera (see the section "Dedicated Cameras") imaging 33 indeterminate lesions, Brem et al. found comparable sensitivity, but significantly greater specificity (71 percent) for scintimammography relative to MRI (25 percent) (Brem et al., 2007). Like MRI, scintimammography is particularly useful for women with radiodense breasts, for whom mammographic interpretation can be difficult.

Technical challenges associated with scintimammography are (1) positioning the camera close to the breast, (2) dealing with the significant scatter radiation arising from gamma rays emitted from regions of the heart and liver, and (3) correcting for contrast degradation due to partial volume averaging and attenuation of gamma rays emitted from the lesion. The first of these issues is driven by the fact that the spatial resolution of cameras with parallel hole collimators is approximately a linear function of the distance between source and collimator. The difficulty of positioning general-purpose gamma cameras close to the breast has led to the fact that while scintimammography using large gamma cameras has excellent sensitivity for tumors larger than about 1 cm, sensitivity is generally poor for smaller, nonpalpable, or medially located lesions. This has been a primary incentive for the development of dedicated gamma cameras for breast imaging.

Dedicated Cameras. One reason for the low sensitivity of conventional scintimammography for small lesions is that it is difficult to position the conventional Anger cameras close to the breast. This is due to their large size, and their appreciable inactive borders. The result is that the lesion-to-collimator distance can often exceed 20 cm. At this distance, the spatial resolution of conventional gamma cameras with high-resolution parallel hole collimators can be 15 to 20 mm. Thus counts originating from the lesion are smeared out over a large area of the image, and small lesions, providing few counts, are lost. One potential method for improving sensitivity is the development of smaller gamma cameras with narrow inactive borders, permitting camera placement adjacent to the chest wall, and near the breast. Several groups have developed such dedicated breast gamma cameras (Cinti et al., 2003; Hruska and O'Connor, 2006; Majewski et al., 2001; More et al., 2006; Pani et al., 1998; Pani et al., 2004; Stebel et al., 2005). Early clinical evaluation of these dedicated systems have shown promising results (Brem et al., 2007; Brem et al., 2005; Scopinaro et al., 1999).

Positron Emission Mammography. In positron emission mammography (PEM), positron-emitting radiotracers are utilized, rather than single gamma ray emitters. Radiotracer location within the breast is determined by detection of the pair of simultaneously emitted 511-keV gamma rays, resulting when the positron annihilates with an electron in the breast. Timing coincidence circuitry is used to identify gamma rays originating from a single annihilation event. To date, breast PET has been based primarily on assessment of either glucose metabolic rate via 2-[^{18}F]fluoro-2-deoxyglucose (FDG) or of estrogen or progestin receptor density using 16α-[^{18}F]fluoroestradiol (FES). Primarily because of its limited sensitivity for small lesions, whole-body PET has limited application in tumor detection (Mankoff and Eubank, 2006). The primary clinical breast cancer applications for whole-body FDG-PET are loco-regional staging (determination of the extent of cancer spreading), and monitoring of loco-regional recurrence following therapy (Avril and Adler, 2007; Eubank, 2007). A European multicenter trial evaluating whole-body FDG-PET for staging recurrent breast cancer demonstrated an overall sensitivity and specificity for both palpable and nonpalpable breast lesions of 80 and 73 percent, respectively (Bender et al., 1997). In a prospective study of 144 patients (185 breast lesions), Avril et al. tested the diagnostic ability of FDG-PET using whole-body PET scanners in patients with masses suggestive of breast cancer (Avril et al., 2000). Histological evaluation of 185 tumors showed a sensitivity of 68.2 and 91.9 percent for pT1 and pT2 tumors, respectively. The overall specificity was only 75.5 percent. However, the positive predictive value (fraction of cases positive on PET that were shown by histology to be malignant) was 96.6 percent. The authors cited partial volume effects (which worsen as the tumor-to-voxel size decreases) and variation of metabolic activity among tumor types as the primary limitations. A retrospective study by Santiago et al. of 133 consecutive breast cancer patients between 1996 and 2000 showed that FDG-PET was 69 percent sensitive and 80 percent specific in predicting clinical status 6 months later, and that in 74 percent of cases, the PET scan affected treatment decisions (Santiago et al., 2006). Yutani et al. compared FDG-PET and sestamibi SPECT in the detection of breast cancer and axillary node metastases (Yutani et al., 2000). The study concluded that MIBI-SPECT is comparable with FDG-PET in detecting breast cancer (overall sensitivities of 76.3 and 78.9 percent, respectively), but that neither whole-body FDG-PET nor whole-body MIBI-SPECT is sufficiently sensitive to rule out axillary lymph node metastasis.

As in the case of single gamma breast imaging dedicated small field of view gamma cameras are being developed (Baghaei et al., 2000; Doshi et al., 2000; Doshi et al., 2001; Jin et al., 2007; Jinyi et al., 2002; Nan et al., 2003; Raylman et al., 2000; Smith et al., 2004; Thompson et al., 1994; Wang et al., 2006; Weinberg et al., 2005; Yuan-Chuan et al., 2006). Most implementations use two-head systems with planar, opposing detectors, rather than the typical ring structure used in whole-body PET scanners. Mild breast compression is typically employed. A four-center study enrolling 94 women with known breast cancer or suspicious lesions compared histopathology results with the assessments of readers using the combination of clinical histories, mammography, and dedicated camera FDG-PET. The overall sensitivity and specificity for dedicated PET alone was 90 and 86 percent, respectively, and these figures improved to 91 and 93 percent when PET was combined with clinical history and mammography (Berg et al., 2006). Raylman et al. are developing dedicated breast PET detectors mounted on a stereotactic biopsy table to perform PET-guided breast biopsy (Raylman et al., 2001).

Spatial resolution in PET is limited by the range of the positron prior to annihilation (which can range from less than 1 mm to several millimeters, depending on the isotope), and noncolinearity of the two gamma rays emitted from the site of annihilation. The latter effect can be somewhat mitigated by reducing the distance between the patient and the detectors. Depth-of-interaction (DOI) effects (uncertainty in the knowledge of the depth within the scintillator crystal of the point of gamma ray absorption) can also degrade resolution by broadening the lines of gamma ray coincidence. A number of design approaches to minimize DOI blurring have been implemented (Huesman et al., 2000; Jinyi et al., 2002; Shao et al., 2002; Wang et al., 2006). In addition, because scattered gamma rays and random coincidences (arising from two different annihilation events) add to the true coincidences to give the total number of counted coincidences, the counting rates encountered in PET are significantly higher than those in single gamma breast imaging, placing more stringent requirements on the readout electronics.

12.4.5 Electrical Impedance Scanning

Electrical impedance scanning (EIS) relies on the differences in conductance and capacitance (dielectric constant) between healthy tissue and malignant tissue. Studies have reported both conductivity and capacitance values 10 to 50 times higher in malignant tissue than in the surrounding healthy tissue (Jossinet, 1996; Morimoto et al., 1993). A commercial EIS scanner called T-scan, developed by Siemens Medical, was approved by the FDA in 1999 to be used as an adjunct tool to mammography (Assenheimer et al., 2001). That device uses a patient-held metallic wand and a scanning probe that is placed against the skin of the breast to complete the electrical circuit using 1.0 to 2.5 V AC. Conductive gel is used to improve conductivity between the skin of the breast and the scanning probe. The scanning probe is moved over the breast and its sensors (256 sensors in high-resolution mode and 64 sensors in normal-resolution mode) measures the current signal at the skin level.

In a prospective study of young (30 to 45 years old) high-risk women, Stojadinovic et al. reported a sensitivity of 38 percent and specificity of 95 percent for EIS using a T-Scan 2000ED system (Stojadinovic et al., 2006). Malich et al. report 88 percent sensitivity and 66 percent specificity in a study of 240 histologically proven breast lesions (Malich et al., 2001b). A 3D electrical impedance scanner has also been constructed and tested clinically (Cherepenin et al., 2001).

Many physical factors affect the performance of EIS, including operator experience, lesion shape, size, and location within the breast (Malich et al., 2003). Sensitivity is low for lesions located more than ~3 cm from the EIS probe on the breast surface. In addition to the expected difficulty of measuring perturbations in the local conductance produced by small lesions, large lesions (with size greater than that of the probe) can also be missed since the conductance and capacitance of the imaged region can then appear uniform. For these reasons, it has been recommended that ultrasound be performed prior to EIS (Malich and Fuchsjager, 2003). In a study comparing ultrasound, MRI, and EIS, Malich et al. obtained 81 percent and 63 percent sensitivity and specificity for EIS in 100 mammographically suspicious lesions. The authors attributed the high false-positive rate to artifacts produced when imaging superficial skin lesions, and resulting from poor contact or air bubbles (Malich et al., 2001a).

12.4.6 Other Techniques

Techniques for using optical radiation for breast imaging (sometimes referred to as optical mammography) have been under development for decades. Due to the fact that the optical absorption coefficient of water drops by nearly 2 orders of magnitude in the frequency range between 600 and 1000 nm relative to either longer or shorter wavelengths, and in this range the absorption coefficient of oxy hemoglobin and deoxy hemoglobin are both about one-tenth of their values in the visible or infrared (Nioka and Chance, 2005), biologic tissue is significantly more translucent for near-infrared (NIR) light than for shorter wavelength visible light. However, within this spectral band, known as the NIR window, elastic scattering of photons dominates absorption [in the breast, the mean free path for absorption is approximately 25 cm, while that for scattering is ~0.001 cm (Nioka and Chance, 2005)]. Optical transport of NIR radiation in the breast is therefore modeled as a diffusion process, and this type of imaging is referred to as *diffuse optical imaging* (DOI) or *diffuse optical tomography* (DOT), if 3D images are reconstructed.

It was also realized, however, that the hemoglobin signals provide information regarding the source of oxygen in the tissue, while the *cyt c ox* signals indicate the intracellular availability of oxygen for oxidative phosphorylation. This ability of recognizing the source/sink relationship greatly enhances the value of NIR spectrophotometry (NIRS) for research and clinical purposes.

NIR breast imaging can be described as either endogenous or exogenous. Endogenous imaging relies on the differences in the IR absorption of oxy hemoglobin and deoxy hemoglobin and on the differences in vasculature between normal and malignant tissues (associated with angiogenesis). Exogenous imaging utilizes injected NIR-excitable fluorescent dyes (such as indocyanine green) to increase contrast between tumors and surrounding healthy tissue.

Photoacoustic tomography is a type of optical imaging that relies on the fact that the absorption of pulsed NIR radiation by tissue leads to heating, followed by rapid thermoelastic expansion and the subsequent generation of broadband thermoelastic waves. Photoacoustic imaging uses short NIR pulses to deposit energy in the breast, but instead of imaging the transmitted NIR radiation, the photoacoustic waves that are emitted by the irradiated tissue and propagate to the surface are detected, typically by an array of ultrasound transducers (Ku et al., 2005; Manohar et al., 2004; Wang et al., 2002). The image is formed by differences in the NIR absorption characteristics of different tissues. As in transmission optical imaging, photoacoustic imaging can be enhanced by the use of optical contrast agents (Alacam et al., 2008; Kim et al., 2007; Ku and Wang, 2005).

Optical mammography offers the potential advantages of being a low-cost, nonionizing diagnostic adjunct to x-ray mammography. There is, however, evidence that laser irradiation can produce long-term physical changes in biological tissue that result in a reduction of optical absorption (Gondek et al., 2006). The principle obstacles to both structural and functional optical breast imaging are the significant levels of scattering of optical photons in biological tissue, rendering the image reconstruction task mathematically ill-posed. It is now generally acknowledged that optical mammography will probably never achieve the submillimeter spatial resolution of other breast imaging modalities such as x-ray, ultrasound, or MRI. Thus most current efforts are geared toward the detection of the presence of particular physiologic states (e.g., hypoxia, angiogenesis, hypermetabolism) rather than the acquisition of a high-resolution structural map. In particular, multiwavelength NIR imaging (Srinivasan et al., 2007) and dynamic DOT imaging (Alacam et al., 2008; Boverman et al., 2007; Nioka et al., 2005) are being developed by a number of investigators.

Elastography is a technique whose goal is to characterize breast masses by measuring their elastic properties under compression. Studies of excised breast specimens have demonstrated that while fat tissue has an elastic modulus that is essentially independent of the strain level (the amount of compression), normal fibroglandular tissue has a modulus that increases by 1 to 2 orders of magnitude with increasing strain (Krouskop et al., 1998). Furthermore, carcinomas are stiffer than normal breast tissue at high strain level, with infiltrating ductal carcinomas being the stiffest type of carcinoma tested (Krouskop et al., 1998). Using a specially constructed device containing a motor-driven cylindrical specimen "indenter" and a load cell, Samani et al. measured the stress-strain curves of 169 ex vivo breast tissue samples. They found that under conditions of small deformation, the elastic modulus of normal breast fat and fibroglandular tissues are similar, while fibroadenomas were approximately twice as stiff. Fibrocystic disease (a benign condition) and malignant tumours exhibited a three- to sixfold increased stiffness, with high-grade invasive ductal carcinoma exhibiting up to a 13-fold increase in stiffness compared to fibroglandular tissue (Samani et al., 2007).

Breast elastography can be performed with ultrasound (UE) or MRI (MRE). Hui et al. compared the performance of UE, mammography, and B-mode ultrasound alone in differentiating benign and malignant breast lesions. They found that the three modalities had approximately equal sensitivity, but that the specificities of mammography (87 percent) and UE (96 percent) were significantly better than that of US alone (73 percent) (Zhi et al., 2007). Other investigators have measured increased specificity for UE compared to B-mode US, but with reduced sensitivity (Thomas et al., 2006).

12.5 FUTURE DIRECTIONS

12.5.1 Multimodality imaging

There is a general consensus in the breast imaging community that no single imaging modality is likely to be able to detect and classify early breast cancers, and that the most complete solution for diagnostic breast imaging is likely to be some combination of complementary modalities. However, again the unique properties of the breast create challenges for successfully merging the information. In particular, the mechanically pliant nature of the breast permits optimization of breast shape for the particular modality used (compressed for x-ray mammography, coil-shaped for breast MRI, pendant for breast scintigraphy, etc.). The result is that multimodality image fusion is extremely difficult. One approach to overcoming this problem is to engineer systems permitting multimodality imaging of the breast in a single configuration. Toward this end, dedicated breast scanners are being developed that integrate digital mammography and ultrasound (Sinha et al., 2007; Surry et al., 2007), digital tomosynthesis and optical imaging (Boverman et al., 2007), NIR spectroscopy and MRI (Carpenter et al., 2007), digital tomosynthesis and limited angle SPECT (More et al., 2007), and breast CT and breast SPECT (Tornai et al., 2003). Figures 12.5 and 12.6 show corresponding structural and functional slices extracted from a dual modality data set. The images were obtained on a dual modality tomographic (DMT) breast scanner developed at the University of Virginia. The DMT scanner uses an upright mammography-style gantry arm, with breast support and compression mechanisms that are independent of the gantry arm and support the breast near the arm's axis of rotation (AOR). This design permits multiple-view, tomographic image acquisition for both modalities (x-ray transmission tomosynthesis and gamma emission tomosynthesis). The DMT scanner employs full isocentric motion in which the tube and x-ray and gamma ray detectors rotate around a common AOR. Figure 12.6 shows a series of slices from a dual modality tomographic scan of a 7.9 cm compressed breast. The slices shown are 1 mm thick and consecutive slices are spaced by 10 mm. The top row contains the x-ray tomosynthesis images; the middle row contains the gamma emission tomosynthesis slices; and the bottom row contains the merged slices. Biopsy indicated poorly differentiated carcinoma. The radiotracer was ^{99m}Tc-sestamibi. This example illustrates both heterogeneous radiographic density and heterogeneous radiotracer uptake.

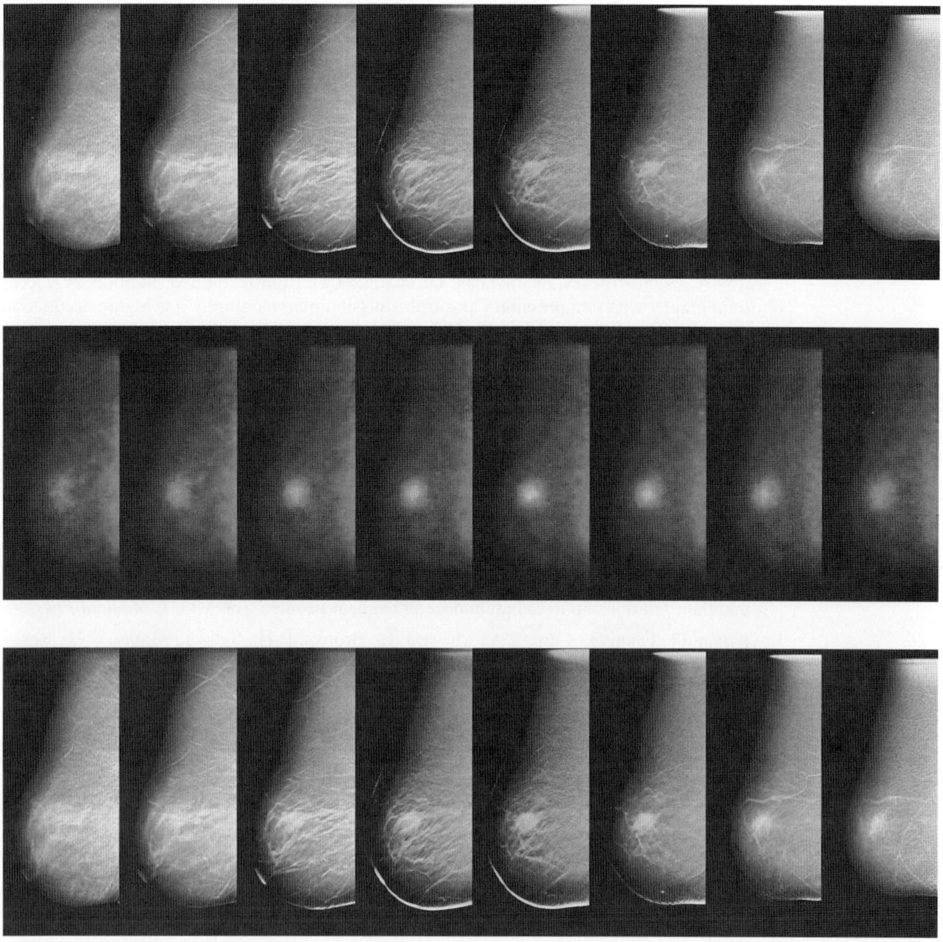

FIGURE 12.6 Slices from a dual modality tomographic scan of a breast with 7.9 cm compressed thickness. The slices are 1 mm thick and consecutive slices are spaced by 10 mm. The top row contains the x-ray tomosynthesis images; the middle row contains the gamma emission tomosynthesis slices; and the bottom row contains the merged slices. The large region of poorly differentiated carcinoma is clearly visible in a number of slices.

REFERENCES

Alacam, B., Yazici, B., Intes, X., Nioka, S., and Chance, B. (2008). Pharmacokinetic-rate images of indocyanine green for breast tumors using near-infrared optical methods. *Physics in Medicine and Biology.* **53**, 837–859.

Allen, M.W., Hendi, P., Schwimmer, J., Bassett, L., and Gambhir, S.S. (2000). Decision analysis for the cost effectiveness of sestamibi scintimammography in minimizing unnecessary biopsies. *Quarterly Journal of Nuclear Medicine.* **44**(2), 168–185.

American College of Radiology (ACR) BIRADS breast imaging and reporting system (2003). *Breast Imaging Atlas*, Reston, VA: American College of Radiology.

Assenheimer, M., Laver-Moskovitz, O., Malonek, D., Manor, D., Nahaliel, U., Nitzan, R., and Saad, A. (2001). The T-SCAN technology: electrical impedance as a diagnostic tool for breast cancer detection. *Physiological Measurement.* **22,** 1–8.

Avril, N., Rose, C.A., Schelling, M., Dose, J., Kuhn, W., Bense, S., Weber, W., Ziegler, S., Graeff, H., and Schwaiger, M. (2000). Breast imaging with positron emission tomography and fluorine-18 fluorodeoxyglucose: use and limitations. *Journal of Clinical Oncology.* **18,** 3495–3502.

Avril, N. and Adler, L.P. (2007). F-18 fluorodeoxyglucose-positron emission tomography imaging for primary breast cancer and loco-regional staging. [Review] [53 refs]. *Radiologic Clinics of North America.* **45,** 645–657.

Baghaei, H., Wai-Hoi, W., Uribe, J., Hongdi, L., Nan, Z., and Yu, W. (2000). Breast cancer imaging studies with a variable field of view PET camera. *IEEE Transactions on Nuclear Science., IEEE Transactions on* **47,** 1080–1084.

Bender, H., Kerst, J., Palmedo, H., Schomburg, A., Wagner, U., Ruhlmann, J., and Biersack, H.J. (1997). Value of (18)fluoro-deoxyglucose positron emission tomography in the staging of recurrent breast carcinoma. *Anticancer Research.* **17,** 1687–1692.

Berg, W.A., Weinberg, I.N., Narayanan, D., et al. (2006). High-resolution fluorodeoxyglucose positron emission tomography with compression ("positron emission mammography") is highly accurate in depicting primary breast cancer. *Breast Journal.* **12,** 309–323.

Berry, D.A., Parmigiani, G., Sanchez, J., et al. (1997). Probability of carrying a mutation of breast-ovarian cancer gene BRCA1 based on family history. *Journal of National Cancer Institute.* **89,** 227–238.

Bick, U., Giger, M., Schmidt, R., Nishikawa, R.M., and Doi, K. (1996). Density correction of peripheral breast tissue on digital mammograms. *Radiographics.* **16,** 1403–1411.

Boetes, C., Barentsz, J., Mus, R., et al. (1994). MRI characterization of suspicious breast lesions with a gadolinium-enhanced turbo FLASH subtraction technique. *Radiology.* **193,** 777–781.

Boone, J.M., Nelson, T.R., Lindfors, K.K., and Seibert, J.A. (2001). Dedicated breast CT: radiation dose and image quality evaluation. *Radiology.* **221,** 657–667.

Boone, J.M., Kwan, A.L.C., Seibert, J.A., Shah, N., Lindfors, K.K., and Nelson, T.R. (2005). Technique factors and their relationship to radiation dose in pendant geometry breast CT. *Medical Physics.* **32,** 3767–3776.

Boverman, G., Fang, Q., Carp, S.A., Miller, E.L., Brooks, D.H., Selb, J., Moore, R.H., Kopans, D.B., and Boas, D.A. (2007). Spatio-temporal imaging of the hemoglobin in the compressed breast with diffuse optical tomography. *Physics in Medicine & Biology.* **52,** 3619–3641.

Brem, R. F., Petrovitch, I., Rapelyea, J. A., et al. (2007). Breast-specific gamma imaging with ^{99m}Tc-Sestamibi and magnetic resonance imaging in the diagnosis of breast cancer—a comparative study. *Breast Journal,* **13**(5): 465–469.

Brem, R.F., Petrovitch, I., Rapelyea, J.A., Young, H., Teal, C., and Kelly, T. (2007). Breast-specific gamma imaging with 99mTc-Sestamibi and magnetic resonance imaging in the diagnosis of breast cancer—a comparative study. *Breast Journal.* **13,** 465–469.

Brem, R.F., Rapelyea, J.A., Zisman, G., Mohtashemi, K., Raub, J., Teal, C.B., Majewski, S., and Welch, B.L. (2005). Occult breast cancer: scintimammography with high-resolution breast-specific gamma camera in women at high risk for breast cancer. *Radiology.* **237,** 274–280.

Buscombe, J.R., Cwikla, J.B., Holloway, B., and Hilson, A.J. (2001). Prediction of the usefulness of combined mammography and scintimammography in suspected primary breast cancer using ROC curves. *Journal of Nuclear Medicine 2001.* **42**(1), 3–8.

Byng, J., Critten, J., and Yaffe, M. (1997). Thickness-equalization processing for mammographic images. *Radiology.* **203,** 568.

Carpenter, C.M., Pogue, B.W., Jiang, S., et al. (2007). Image-guided optical spectroscopy provides molecular-specific information in vivo: MRI-guided spectroscopy of breast cancer hemoglobin, water, and scatterer size. *Optics Letters.* **32,** 933–935.

Chen, S.C., Carton, A.K., Albert, M., Conant, E.F., Schnall, M.D., and Maidment, A.D.A. (2007). Initial clinical experience with contrast-enhanced digital breast tomosynthesis. *Academic Radiology.* **14,** 229–238.

Cherepenin, V., Karpov, A., Korjenevsky, A., Kornienko, V., Mazaletskaya, A., Mazourov, D., and Meister, D. (2001). A 3D electrical impedance tomography (EIT) system for breast cancer detection. *Physiological Measurement.* **22,** 9–18.

Cinti, M.N., Pani, R., Pellegrini, R., et al. (2003). Tumor SNR analysis in scintimammography by dedicated high contrast imager. *IEEE Transactions on Nuclear Science., IEEE Transactions on* **50,** 1618–1623.

Crotty, D.J., McKinley, R.L., and Tornai, M.P. (2007). Experimental spectral measurements of heavy K-edge filtered beams for x-ray computed mammotomography. *Physics in Medicine & Biology.* **52,** 603–616.

Daniel, B., Yen, Y., Glover, G., Ikeda, D., Birdwell, R., Sawyer-Glover, A., Black, J., Plevritis, S., Jeffrey, S., and Herfkens, R. (1998). Breast disease: dynamic spiral MR imaging. *Radiology.* **209,** 499–509.

Dash, N., Lupetin, A., and Daffner, R. (1986). Magnetic resonance imaging in the diagnosis of breast disease. AJR *American Journal of Roentgenology.* **146,** 119–125.

Dobbins, J.T. and Godfrey, D.J. (2003). Digital x-ray tomosynthesis: current state of the art and clinical potential. [Review] [110 refs]. *Physics in Medicine & Biology.* **48,** R65–106.

Doshi, N.K., Shao, Y., Silverman, R.W., and Cherry, S.R. (2000). Design and evaluation of an LSO PET detector for breast cancer imaging. *Medical Physics*. 2000. **27**(7), 1535–1543.

Doshi, N.K., Silverman, R.W., Shao, Y., and Cherry, S.R. (2001). maxPET, a dedicated mammary and axillary region PET imaging system for breast cancer. *IEEE Transactions on Nuclear Science., IEEE Transactions on* **48,** 811–815.

El Yousef, S., Duchesneau, R., and Alfidi, R. (1984). Magnetic resonance imaging of the breast. *Radiology.* **150,** 761–766.

Esserman, L., Hylton, N., George, T., and Weidner, N. (1999). Contrast-enhanced magnetic resonance imaging to assess tumor histopathology and angiogenesis in breast carcinoma. *The Breast Journal.* **5,** 13–21.

Eubank, W.B. (2007). Diagnosis of recurrent and metastatic disease using f-18 fluorodeoxyglucose-positron emission tomography in breast cancer. [Review] [64 refs]. *Radiologic Clinics of North America.* **45,** 659–667.

Gilles, R., Guinebretiere, J., Lucidarme, O., et al. (1994). Nonpalpable breast tumors: diagnosis with contrast-enhanced subtraction dynamic MRI imaging. *Radiology.* **191,** 625–631.

Godfrey, D.J., McAdams, H.P., and Dobbins, J.T. (2006). Optimization of the matrix inversion tomosynthesis (MITS) impulse response and modulation transfer function characteristics for chest imaging. *Medical Physics.* **33,** 655–667.

Godfrey, D.J., Ren, L., Yan, H., Wu, Q., Yoo, S., Oldham, M., and Yin, F.F. (2007). Evaluation of three types of reference image data for external beam radiotherapy target localization using digital tomosynthesis (DTS). *Medical Physics.* **34,** 3374–3384.

Gondek, G., Li, T., Lynch, R.J.M., and Dewhurst, R.J. (2006). Decay of photoacoustic signals from biological tissue irradiated by near infrared laser pulses. *Journal of Biomedical Optics.* **11,** 054036–054Oct.

Harms, S., Flaming, D., Hesley, K.L., et al. (1993). MRI imaging of the breast with rotating delivery of excitation off resonance. *Radiology.* **187,** 493–501.

Heywang, S., Wolf, A., and Pruss, E. (1989). MRI imaging of the breast with Gd-DTPA: use and limitations. *Radiology.* **171,** 95–103.

Hickman, P., Moore, N., and Shepstone, B. (1994). The indeterminate breast mass: assessment using contrast enhanced magnetic resonance imaging. *The British Journal of Radiology.* **67,** 14–20.

Hruska, C.B. and O'Connor, M.K. (2006). Effect of collimator selection on tumor detection for dedicated nuclear breast imaging systems. *IEEE Transactions on Nuclear Science., IEEE Transactions on* **53,** 2680–2689.

Huesman, R.H., Klein, G.J., Moses, W.W., Jinyi, Q., Reutter, B.W., and Virador, P.R.G. (2000). List-mode maximum-likelihood reconstruction applied to positron emission mammography (PEM) with irregular sampling. *IEEE Transactions on Medical Imaging., IEEE Transactions on* **19,** 532–537.

Hussain, R., Buscombe, J.R., Hussain, R., and Buscombe, J.R. (2006). A meta-analysis of scintimammography: an evidence-based approach to its clinical utility. [Review] [42 refs]. *Nuclear Medicine Communications.* **27,** 589–594.

Hylton, N. (1999). Vascularity assessment of breast lesions with gadolinium-enhanced MR imaging. *MRI Clinics of North America.* **7,** 411–420.

Imbriaco, M., Del Vecchio, S., Riccardi, A., Pace, L., Di Salle, F., Di Gennaro, F., Salvatore, M., and Sodano, A. (2001). Scintimammography with 99mTc-MIBI versus dynamic MRI for non-invasive characterization of breast masses. *European Journal of Nuclear Medicine.* **28**(1), 56–63.

Jin, Z., Foudray, A.M.K., Olcott, P.D., Farrell, R., Shah, K., and Levin, C.S. (2007). Performance characterization of a novel thin position-sensitive avalanche photodiode for 1 mm resolution positron emission tomography. *IEEE Transactions on Nuclear Science., IEEE Transactions on* **54,** 415–421.

Jinyi, Q., Kuo, C., Huesman, R.H., Klein, G.J., Moses, W.W., and Reutter, B.W. (2002). Comparison of rectangular and dual-planar positron emission mammography scanners. *IEEE Transactions on Nuclear Science., IEEE Transactions on* **49,** 2089–2096.

Johns, P.C. and Yaffe, M.J. (1987). X-ray characterization of normal and neoplastic breast tissue. *Physics in Medicine & Biology.* **32,** 675–695.

Jossinet, J. (1996). Variability of impedivity in normal and pathological breast tissue. *Medical & Biological Engineering & Computing.* **34,** 346–350.

Kaiser, W. and Zeitler, E. (1989). MRI imaging of the breast: fast imaging sequences with and without Gd-DTPA. *Radiology.* **170,** 681–686.

Kerlikowske, K., Grady, D., Barclay, J., Sickles, E., Eaton, A., and Ernster, V. (1993). Positive predictive value of screening mammography by age and family history of breast cancer. *Journal of American Medical Association.* **270,** 2444–2450.

Kim, G., Huang, S.W., Day, K.C., O'Donnell, M., Agayan, R.R., Day, M.A., Kopelman, R., and Ashkenazi, S. (2007). Indocyanine-green-embedded PEBBLEs as a contrast agent for photoacoustic imaging. *Journal of Biomedical Optics.* **12,** 044020–044Aug.

Kitaoka, F., Sakai, H., Kuroda, Y., Kurata, S., Nakayasu, K., Hongo, H., Iwata, T., and Kanematsu, T. (2001). Internal echo histogram examination has a role in distinguishing malignant tumors from benign masses in the breast. *Clinical Imaging.* **25,** 151–153.

Kopans, D.B. (1992). The positive predictive value of mammography. *American Journal of Roentgenology.* **158,** 521–526.

Kriege, M., Brekelmans, C.T., Boetes, C., et al. (2004). Efficacy of MRI and mammography for breast cancer screening in women with a familial or genetic predisposition. *New England Journal of Medicine.* **351,** 427–437.

Krouskop, T., Wheeler, T., Kallel, F., Garra, B., and Hall, T. (1998). Elastic moduli of breast and prostate tissues under compression. *Ultrasonic Imaging.* **20,** 260–274.

Ku, G., Fornage, B.D., Jin, X., Xu, M., Hunt, K.K., and Wang, L.V. (2005). Thermoacoustic and photoacoustic tomography of thick biological tissues toward breast imaging. *Technology in Cancer Research & Treatment.* **4,** 559–566.

Ku, G. and Wang, L.V. (2005). Deeply penetrating photoacoustic tomography in biological tissues enhanced with an optical contrast agent. *Optics Letters.* **30,** 507–509.

Kuhl, C.S., Schrading, S., Leutner, C.C., et al. (2005). Mammography, breast ultrasound and magnetic resonance imaging for surveillance of women at high familial risk for breast cancer. *Journal of Clinical Oncology.* **23,** 8469–8476.

Kwan, A.L.C., Boone, J.M., Yang, K., and Huang, S.Y. (2007). Evaluation of the spatial resolution characteristics of a cone-beam breast CT scanner. *Medical Physics.* **34,** 275–281.

Leach, M.O., Boggis, C.R., Dixon, A.K., et al. (2005). Screening with magnetic resonance imaging and mammography of a UK population with high familial risk of breast cancer: a prospective multicentre cohort study (MARIBS). *Lancet.* **365,** 1769–1778.

Lehman, C.D., Blume, J.D., Weatherall, P., et al. (2005). Screening women at high risk for breast cancer with mammography and magnetic resonance imaging. *Cancer.* **103,** 1898–1905.

Lumachi, F., Ferretti, G., Povolato, M., Marzola, M.C., Zucchetta, P., Geatti, O., Bui, F., and Brandes, A.A. (2001). Sestamibi scintimammography in pT1 breast cancer: alternative or complementary to X-ray mammography? *Anticancer Research.* **21,** 2201–2205.

Mainprize, J.G., Bloomquist, A.K., Kempston, M.P., Yaffe, M.J., Mainprize, J.G., Bloomquist, A.K., Kempston, M.P., and Yaffe, M.J. (2006). Resolution at oblique incidence angles of a flat panel imager for breast tomosynthesis. *Medical Physics.* **33,** 3159–3164.

Majewski, S., Kieper, D., Curran, E., et al. (2001). Optimization of dedicated scintimammography procedure using detector prototypes and compressible phantoms. *IEEE Transactions on Nuclear Science.* **3,** 822–829.

Malich, A., Boehm, T., Facius, M., Freesmeyer, M.G., Fleck, M., Anderson, R., and Kaiser, W.A. (2001a). Differentiation of mammographically suspicious lesions: evaluation of breast ultrasound, MRI mammography and electrical impedance scanning as adjunctive technologies in breast cancer detection. *Clinical Radiology.* **56,** 278–283.

Malich, A., Bohm, T., Facius, M., Freessmeyer, M., Fleck, M., Anderson, R., and Kaiser, W.A. (2001b). Additional value of electrical impedance scanning: experience of 240 histologically-proven breast lesions. *European Journal of Cancer.* **37,** 2324–2330.

Malich, A., Facius, M., Anderson, R., Bottcher, J., Sauner, D., Hansch, A., Marx, C., Petrovitch, A., Pfleiderer, S., and Kaiser, W. (2003). Influence of size and depth on accuracy of electrical impedance scanning. *European Radiology.* **13,** 2441–2446.

Malich, A. and Fuchsjager, M. (2003). Electrical impedance scanning in classifying suspicious breast lesions.[comment]. *Investigative Radiology.* **38,** 302–303.

Mankoff, D.A. and Eubank, W.B. (2006). Current and future use of positron emission tomography (PET) in breast cancer. [Review] [91 refs]. *Journal of Mammary Gland Biology & Neoplasia.* **11,** 125–136.

Manohar, S., Kharine, A., van Hespen, J.C.G., Steenbergen, W., and van Leeuwen, T.G. (2004). Photoacoustic mammography laboratory prototype: imaging of breast tissue phantoms. *Journal of Biomedical Optics.* **9,** 1172–1181.

McAdams, H.P., Samei, E., Dobbins, J., Tourassi, G.D., and Ravin, C.E. (2006). Recent advances in chest radiography. [Review] [130 refs]. *Radiology.* **241,** 663–683.

More, M.J., Goodale, P.J., Majewski, S., and Williams, M.B. (2006). Evaluation of gamma cameras for use in dedicated breast imaging. *IEEE Transactions on Nuclear Science., IEEE Transactions on* **53,** 2675–2679.

More, M.J., Heng, L., Goodale, P.J., Yibin, Z., Majewski, S., Popov, V., Welch, B., and Williams, M.B. (2007). Limited angle dual modality breast imaging limited angle dual modality breast imaging. *IEEE Transactions on Nuclear Science., IEEE Transactions on* **54,** 504–513.

Morimoto, T., Kimura, S., Konishi, Y., Komaki, K., Uyama, T., Monden, Y., Kinouchi, Y., and Iritani, T. (1993). A study of the electrical bio-impedance of tumors. *Journal of Investigative Surgery.* **6,** 25–32.

Nair, M.K., Grondahl, H.G., Webber, R.L., Nair, U.P., Wallace, J.A., Nair, M.K., Grondahl, H.G., Webber, R.L., Nair, U.P., and Wallace, J.A. (2003). Effect of iterative restoration on the detection of artificially induced vertical radicular fractures by tuned aperture computed tomography. *Oral Surgery, Oral Medicine, Oral Pathology, Oral Radiology & Endodontics.* **96,** 118–125.

Nan, Z., Thompson, C.J., Cayouette, F., Jolly, D., and Kecani, S. (2003). A prototype modular detector design for high resolution positron emission mammography imaging. *IEEE Transactions on Nuclear Science., IEEE Transactions on* **50,** 1624–1629.

Niklason, L.T., Christian, B.T., Niklason, L.E., et al. (1997). Digital tomosynthesis in breast imaging. *Radiology.* **205,** 399–406.

Ning, R., Tang, X., Conover, D., Yu, R., Ning, R., Tang, X., Conover, D., and Yu, R. (2003). Flat panel detector-based cone beam computed tomography with a circle-plus-two-arcs data acquisition orbit: preliminary phantom study. *Medical Physics.* **30,** 1694–1705.

Nioka, S. and Chance, B. (2005). NIR spectroscopic detection of breast cancer. *Technology in Cancer Research & Treatment.* **4,** 497–512.

Nioka, S., Wen, S., Zhang, J., Du, J., Intes, X., Zhao, Z., and Chance, B. (2005). Simulation study of breast tissue hemodynamics during pressure perturbation. *Advances in Experimental Medicine & Biology.* **566,** 17–22.

Nishikawa, R.M., Mawdsley, G.E., Fenster, A., and Yaffe, M.J. (1987). Scanned-projection digital mammography. *Medical Physics.* **14,** 717–727.

Nishikawa, R.M. and Yaffe, M.J. (1985). Signal-to-noise properties of mammographic film-screen systems. *Medical Physics.* **12,** 32–39.

Nunes, L., Schmidt, M., Orel, S., et al. (1997). Breast MR imaging: interpretation model. *Radiology.* **202,** 833–841.

Orel, S., Schnall, M., LiVolsi, V., and Troupin, R. (1994). Suspicious breast lesions: MR imaging with radiologic-pathologic correlation. *Radiology.* **190,** 485–493.

Palmedo, H., Biersack, H.J., Lastoria, S., Maublant, J., Prats, E., Stegner, H.E., Bourgeois, P., Hustinx, R., Hilson, A.J.W., and Bischof-Delaloye, A. (1998). Scintimammography with technetium-99m methoxyisobutylisonitrile: results of a prospective European multicentre trial. *European Journal of Nuclear Medicine.* **25,** 375–385.

Pani, R., De Vincentis, G., Scopinaro, F., Pellegrini, R., Soluri, A., Weinberg, I.N., Pergola, A., Scafe, A., and Trotta, G. (1998). Dedicated gamma camera for single photon emission mammography (SPEM). *IEEE Transactions on Nuclear Science.* **45,** 3127–3133.

Pani, R., Bennati, P., Cinti, M.N., et al. (2004). Imaging characteristics comparison of compact pixellated detectors for scintimammography. *Conference Record IEEE TNS/MIC.* **6,** 3748–3751.

Parmigiani, G., Berry, D.A., and Aguilar, O. (1998). Determining carrier probabilities for breast cancer-susceptibility genes BRCA1 and BRCA2. *American Journal of Human Genetics.* **62,** 145–158.

Perman, W., Heiberg, E., Grunz, J., et al. (1994). A fast 3D imaging technique for performing dynamic Gd-enhanced MRI of breast lesions. *Magnetic Resonance Imaging.* **12,** 545–551.

Pineda, A.R., Yoon, S., Paik, D.S., and Fahrig, R. (2006). Optimization of a tomosynthesis system for the detection of lung nodules. *Medical Physics.* **33,** 1372–1379.

Poplack, S.P., Tosteson, T.D., Kogel, C.A., and Nagy, H.M. (2007). Digital breast tomosynthesis: initial experience in 98 women with abnormal digital screening mammography.[see comment]. AJR *American Journal of Roentgenology.* **189,** 616–623.

Port, E.R., Park, A., Borgen, P.I., et al. (2007). Results of MRI screening for breast cancer in high-risk patients with LCIS and atypical hyperplasia. *Annals of Surgical Oncology.* **14,** 1051–1057.

Raylman, R.R., Majewski, S., Weisenberger, A.G., Popov, V., Wojcik, R., Kross, B., Schreiman, J.S., and Bishop, H.A. (2001). Positron emission mammography-guided breast biopsy. *Journal of Nuclear Medicine.* **42,** 960–966.

Raylman, R.R., Majewski, S., Wojcik, R., Weisenberger, A.G., Kross, B., Popov, V., and Bishop, H.A. (2000). The potential role of positron emission mammography for detection of breast cancer. A phantom study. *Medical Physics.* **27,** 1943–1954.

Reddy, D.H. and Mendelson, E.B. (2005). Incorporating new imaging models in breast cancer management. [Review] [66 refs]. Current *Treatment Options in Oncology.* **6,** 135–145.

Samani, A., Zubovits, J., and Plewes, D. (2007). Elastic moduli of normal and pathological human breast tissues: an inversion-technique-based investigation of 169 samples. *Physics in Medicine & Biology.* **52,** 1565–1576.

Santiago, J.F.Y., Gonen, M., Yeung, H., Macapinlac, H., and Larson, S. (2006). A retrospective analysis of the impact of 18F-FDG PET scans on clinical management of 133 breast cancer patients. *The Quarterly Journal of Nuclear Medicine & Molecular Imaging.* **50,** 61–67.

Sardanelli, F., Podo, F., Giuliano, D., et al. (2007a). Multicenter comparative multimodality surveillance of women at genetic-familial high risk for breast cancer (HIBCRIT Study): interim results. *Radiology.* **242,** 698–715.

Sardanelli, F., Podo, F. (2007b). Breast MR imaging in women at high-risk for breast cancer. Is something changing in early breast cancer detection? *European Radiology.* **17**(14), 873–887.

Saslow, D., Boetes, C.B., Burke, W., et al. (2007). American cancer society guidelines for breast screening with MRI as an adjunct to mammography. *CA Cancer Journal for Clinicians.* **57,** 75–89.

Schnall, M., Rosten, S., Englander, S., Orel, S., and Nunes, L. (2001). A combined architectural and kinetic interpretation model for breast MR images. *Academic Radiology.* **8,** 591–597.

Scopinaro, F., Schillaci, O., Ussof, W., et al. (1997). A three center study on the diagnostic accuracy of 99mTc-MIBI scintimammography. *Anticancer Research.* **17,** 1631–1634.

Scopinaro, F., Pani, R., De Vincentis, G., Soluri, A., Pellegrini, R., and Porfiri, L.M. (1999). High-resolution scintimammography improves the accuracy of technetium-99m methoxyisobutylisonitrile scintimammography: use of a new dedicated gamma camera. *European Journal of Nuclear Medicine.* **26,** 1279–1288.

Sechopoulos, I., Suryanarayanan, S., Vedantham, S., D'Orsi, C., Karellas, A., Sechopoulos, I., Vedantham, S., D'Orsi, C., and Karellas, A. (2007). Computation of the glandular radiation dose in digital tomosynthesis of the breast. *Medical Physics.* **34,** 221–232.

Shao, Y., Meadors, K., Silverman, R.W., Farrell, R., Cirignano, L., Grazioso, R., Shah, K.S., and Cherry, S.R. (2002). Dual APD array readout of LSO crystals: optimization of crystal surface treatment. *IEEE Transactions on Nuclear Science., IEEE Transactions on* **49,** 649–654.

Sinha, S.P., Goodsitt, M.M., Roubidoux, M.A., Booi, R.C., LeCarpentier, G.L., Lashbrook, C.R., Thomenius, K.E., Chalek, C.L., and Carson, P.L. (2007). Automated ultrasound scanning on a dual-modality breast imaging system: coverage and motion issues and solutions. *Journal of Ultrasound in Medicine.* **26,** 645–655.

Smith, M.F., Raylman, R.R., Majewski, S., and Weisenberger, A.G. (2004). Positron emission mammography with tomographic acquisition using dual planar detectors: initial evaluations. *Physics in Medicine & Biology.* **49,** 2437–2452.

Srinivasan, S., Pogue, B.W., Carpenter, C., Jiang, S., Wells, W.A., Poplack, S.P., Kaufman, P.A., and Paulsen, K.D. (2007). Developments in quantitative oxygen-saturation imaging of breast tissue in vivo using multispectral near-infrared tomography. [Review] [85 refs]. *Antioxidants & Redox Signaling.* **9,** 1143–1156.

Stack, J., Redmond, A., Codd, M., et al. (1990). Breast disease: tissue characterization with Gd-DTPA enhancement profiles. *Radiology.* **174,** 491–494.

Stavros, A.T., Thickman, D., Rapp, C.L., Dennis, M.A., Parker, S.H., and Sisney, G.A. (1995). Solid breast nodules: use of sonography to distinguish between benign and malignant lesions. [see comments]. *Radiology.* **196,** 123–134.

Stebel, L., Carrato, S., Cautero, G., et al. (2005). A modular prototype detector for scintimammography imaging. *Conference Record IEEE TNS/MIC.* **5,** 3027–3031.

Steinberg, B.D., Carlson, D.L., and Birnbaum, J.A. (2001). Sonographic discrimination between benign and malignant breast lesions with use of disparity processing. *Academic Radiology.* **8,** 705–712.

Stelling, C., Wang, P., and Lieber, A. (1985). Prototype coil for magnetic resonance imaging of the female breast. *Radiology.* **154,** 457–463.

Stojadinovic, A., Moskovitz, O., Gallimidi, Z., et al. (2006). Prospective study of electrical impedance scanning for identifying young women at risk for breast cancer. *Breast Cancer Research & Treatment.* **97,** 179–189.

Surry, K.J.M., Mills, G.R., Bevan, K., Downey, D.B., and Fenster, A. (2007). Stereotactic mammography imaging combined with 3D US imaging for image guided breast biopsy. *Medical Physics.* **34,** 4348–4358.

Suryanarayanan, S., Karellas, A., Vedantham, S., Glick, S.J., D'Orsi, C.J., Baker, S.P., and Webber, R.L., (2000). Comparison of tomosynthesis methods used with digital mammography. *Academic Radiology.* **7,** 1085–1097.

Tesic, M.M., Piccaro, M.F., Munier, B., Tesic, M.M., Piccaro, M.F., and Munier, B. (1999). Full field digital mammography scanner. *European Journal of Radiology.* **31,** 2–17.

Thomas, A., Fischer, T., Frey, H., et al. (2006). Real-time elastography—an advanced method of ultrasound: First results in 108 patients with breast lesions. *Ultrasound in Obstetrics & Gynecology.* **28,** 335–340.

Thompson, C.J., Murthy, K., Weinberg, I.N., and Mako, F. (1994). Feasibility study for positron emission mammography. *Medical Physics.* **21,** 529–538.

Thunberg, S., Adelow, L., Blom, O., et al. (2004). Dose reduction in mammography with photon counting imaging. *Proceedings SPIE.* **5368,** 457–465.

Tornai, M.P., Bowsher, J.E., Jaszczak, R.J., Pieper, B.C., Greer, K.L., Hardenbergh, P.H., and Coleman, R.E. (2003). Mammotomography with pinhole incomplete circular orbit SPECT.[see comment]. *Journal of Nuclear Medicine.* **44,** 583–593.

Van Vaals, J., Brummer, M., Dixon, W., Tuithof, H., Engels, H., Nelson, R.G.B., Chezmas, J., and den Boer, J. (1993). Keyhole method for accelerating imaging of contrast agent uptake. *Journal of Magnetic Resonance Imaging.* **3,** 671.

Wang, G.C., Huber, J.S., Moses, W.W., Qi, J., and Choong, W.S. (2006). Characterization of the LBNL PEM camera. *IEEE Transactions on Nuclear Science., IEEE Transactions on* **53,** 1129–1135.

Wang, X., Xu, Y., Xu, M., Yokoo, S., Fry, E.S., and Wang, L.V. (2002). Photoacoustic tomography of biological tissues with high cross-section resolution: reconstruction and experiment. *Medical Physics.* **29,** 2799–2805.

Warner, E., Plewes, D.B., Hill, K.A., et al. (2004). Surveillance of BRCA1 and BRCA2 mutation carriers with magnetic resonance imaging, ultrasound, mammography and clinical breast examination. *Journal of American Medical Association.* **292,** 1317–1325.

Webber, R.L., Horton, R.A., Tyndall, D.A., and Ludlow, J.B. (1997). Tuned-aperture computed tomography (TACT). Theory and application for three-dimensional dento-alveolar imaging. *Dento-Maxillo-Facial Radiology.* **26,** 53–62.

Webber, R.L., Webber, S.E., and Moore, J. (2002). Hand-held three-dimensional dental X-ray system: technical description and preliminary results. *Dento-Maxillo-Facial Radiology.* **31,** 240–248.

Weinberg, I.N., Beylin, D., Zavarzin, V., Yarnall, S., Stepanov, P.Y., Anashkin, E., Narayanan, D., Dolinsky, S., Lauckner, K., and Adler, L.P. (2005). Positron emission mammography: high-resolution biochemical breast imaging. *Technology in Cancer Research & Treatment.* **4,** 55–60.

Wu, T., Moore, R.H., Rafferty, E.A., and Kopans, D.B. (2004). A comparison of reconstruction algorithms for breast tomosynthesis. *Medical Physics.* **31,** 2636–2647.

Wu, T., Stewart, A., Stanton, M., et al. (2003). Tomographic mammography using a limited number of low-dose cone-beam projection images. *Medical Physics.* **30,** 365–380.

Yuan-Chuan, T., Heyu, W., and Janecek, M. (2006). Initial study of an asymmetric PET system dedicated to breast cancer imaging. *IEEE Transactions on Nuclear Science., IEEE Transactions on* **53,** 121–126.

Yutani, K., Shiba, E., Kusuoka, H., Tatsumi, M., Uehara, T., Taguchi, T., Takai, S.I., and Nishimura, T. (2000). Comparison of FDG-PET with MIBI-SPECT in the detection of breast cancer and axillary lymph node metastasis. *Journal of Computer Assisted Tomography.* **24,** 274–280.

Zhang, Y., Chan, H.P., Sahiner, B., et al. (2006). A comparative study of limited-angle cone-beam reconstruction methods for breast tomosynthesis. *Medical Physics.* **33,** 3781–3795.

Zhi, H., Ou, B., Luo, B.M., Feng, X., Wen, Y.L., and Yang, H.Y. (2007). Comparison of ultrasound elastography, mammography, and sonography in the diagnosis of solid breast lesions. *Journal of Ultrasound in Medicine.* **26,** 807–815.

Ziegler, C.M., Franetzki, M., Denig, T., Muhling, J., and Hassfeld, S. (2003). Digital tomosynthesis-experiences with a new imaging device for the dental field. *Clinical Oral Investigations.* **7,** 41–45.

P • A • R • T • 3

SURGERY

CHAPTER 13
SURGICAL SIMULATION TECHNOLOGIES

M. Cenk Cavusoglu
Case Western Reserve University, Cleveland, Ohio

Virtual environment-based surgical simulation is an emerging area of research on the application of virtual environment technologies to the training of surgery and other medical interventions.

Currently, surgeons are trained through apprenticeship. The basic techniques are taught with simple training equipment, but the rest of the training is either with books describing surgical procedures and techniques, or in the operating room by watching and participating in actual operations, and rarely in animal laboratories. There are inherent limitations associated with each of the established training methods. The limitation of reading about surgery is that it provides no practical experience. The limitation of conventional apprenticeship-based training in the operating room is the unpredictable availability of case material and the potential for serious injury to the patient as the student navigates the learning curve for the technique. This method of training also limits the diffusion of knowledge, since only a limited number of people can be trained by one experienced surgeon. The mandatory restriction of the work week for medical and surgical residents in the United States to 80 h will lead to a significant reduction in the total amount of teaching that can be done in the operating room. Of the existing training methods, the hands-on practical courses offer the best learning experience, but still fall short of the mark. The limitation of hands-on practical courses is the lack of standardization and the lack of realistic models of the various pathological conditions. The dry models (e.g., Styrofoam approximations of the anatomy) lack the realism provided by live tissue. The wet models (e.g., animal laboratories) are difficult to set up and fail to mimic true pathological conditions. Furthermore, animal models are complicated by ethical issues, problems of anesthesia, lack of reproducibility, and formidable cost. Although some basic dexterity training can be achieved, the forced feedback derived from tissues is quite variable, depending on the quality of the models. Cadavers are expensive and difficult to procure, transport, and preserve. Furthermore, the mechanical properties of the tissue, the visual appearance of anatomy, and the intraoperative bleeding that is encountered in live surgery cannot be provided by cadaveric specimen training.

Virtual environments present a complement to the contemporary apprenticeship-based training scheme of surgery and other medical interventions. With virtual environments, it is possible to create

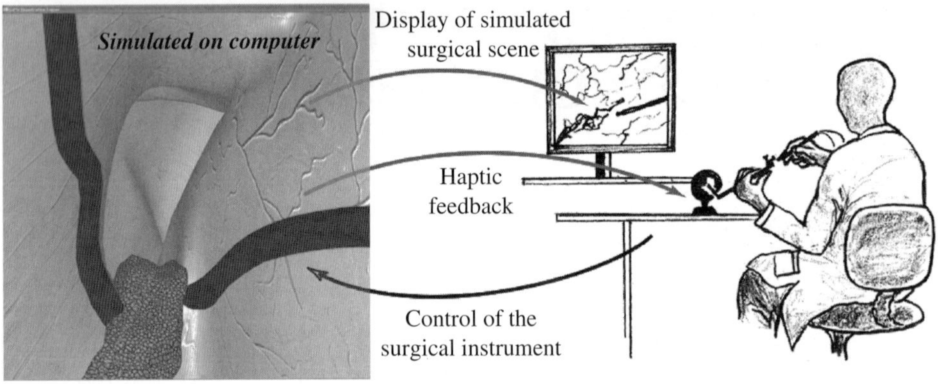

FIGURE 13.1 Surgical training simulator concept.

an interactive three-dimensional simulation milieu in which the surgeon, using haptic interfaces, can manipulate, cut, or suture dynamically and geometrically correct models of organs and tissues simulated on a computer (Fig. 13.1). Development of a virtual environment-based simulator for surgical training is analogous to the flight simulators that are currently used for pilot training. Virtual environments provide a setting in which there is no risk to patients and, therefore, less stress. They are interactive and three-dimensional in contrast to books, and they are relatively inexpensive compared to training in the operating room or animal labs. It also provides the trainees with the chance for multiple and repeatable trials. Virtual environments also give a unique advantage as it is possible to generate arbitrary anatomies and pathologies with which the surgeons can be trained for cases that they will encounter only rarely during their entire career, but nonetheless must be capable of doing. Virtual environment-based surgical simulation also permits standardization of training and accreditation in surgery.

13.1 VIRTUAL ENVIRONMENTS: A GENERAL PERSPECTIVE

Our sense of physical reality is a construction from the symbolic, geometric, and dynamic information directly presented to our senses. A large part of our sense of physical reality is a consequence of internal processing, including our prior experiences, rather than something that is developed only from the immediate sensory information we receive. The sense of reality can therefore be induced by presenting artificially synthesized sensory stimuli to realize the sensory and motor consequences of a real environment.[1] A virtual environment is a real or an imagined environment that is simulated on a computer and experienced by the user through artificially synthesized sensory stimuli. It is typically in the form of an interactive three-dimensional world created through computer graphics, audio, and haptics.

Milgram[2,3] described the taxonomy of real, virtual, and mixed environments as a continuum. Real and completely virtual environments form the ends of the continuum. In between these, there is a variety of forms of mixed reality, where real and virtual environments mixed at different levels. In an *immersive* virtual environment, the user is fully immersed in a completely computer-generated artificial, three-dimensional world, where the goal is to achieve the user feel "present" within this artificial world. In a *nonimmersive* virtual environment, the user remains as an observer working on the artificial world from outside. *Augmented reality* is a form of mixed reality where perception is predominantly from the real environments, while synthetic computer-generated data are overlaid to enhance the user experience. Most virtual environment-based medical simulations are in the form of nonimmersive virtual environments. This is mostly as a result of the nature of the surgical procedures being simulated, such as minimally invasive surgery. The limitations of the existing state-of-the-art user interface hardware, such as head-mounted displays and haptic interface devices, also limit the application of immersive virtual environments in surgical simulation. The most striking application of augmented reality in surgical simulation is to give the surgeon "x-ray vision," by projection of interior anatomical structures, such as the location of a tumor, obtained from preoperative medical images onto the surgical scene where these structures are not readily visible.

There are several terms that are used somewhat interchangeably, including *virtual reality*, *artificial reality*, *virtual worlds*, and *virtual environments*. Among these, the terms *virtual reality* and *virtual environments* are the most commonly used. *Virtual reality* is the term typically used by the popular press, while *virtual environments* is the term used by the scientific community. This is partly to emphasize the fact that a virtual environment does not necessarily try to replicate the reality, and also to distance the field from the hype that surrounds the term virtual reality in the popular press.[4]

13.2 DEVELOPMENTS IN SIMULATION-BASED MEDICAL EDUCATION

A variety of simulation approaches and tools have proliferated in the past 20 years. These include the sophisticated advanced cardiac life-support training systems, complex task trainers for endoscopic and catheter-based procedures, ultrasound simulators, and computer-controlled mannequin-based intervention simulators. Virtual environment-based devices are also under intense development, and several systems are commercially available.

The Harvey cardiology patient simulator (CPS), a life-size mannequin capable of simulating the bedside findings of a wide variety of cardiovascular conditions, may be the most widely used and most thoroughly studied and validated simulator-supported part-task skills trainer. Harvey is capable of replicating 27 physical conditions (2 normal conditions and 25 cardiovascular diseases), and is used for individual, small group, and large group instruction with or without the presence of a teacher. Harvey and its complementary computer-based curriculum (UMedic) have recently become key features of the curricula at every medical school in the United Kingdom.

Virtual environment-based surgical simulators for surgical training has been proposed in the early 1990s.[5] However, technological limitations, and lack of well-controlled clinical trials that demonstrate the effectiveness of such systems, limited the initial adoption of virtual environment-based surgical training simulators. By early 2000s, randomized double-blind studies demonstrating the efficacy of virtual environment-based surgical training simulators started to appear in the literature.[6] In 2004, the U.S. Food and Drug Administration's (FDA) approval of a new device (carotid artery stenting systems) included a requirement for training of physicians, which, as part of it, incorporates virtual environment-based simulators.[7] Currently, training on virtual environment-based simulators is not accepted as an alternative to actual procedural experience, but instead, considered as an integral part of a comprehensive curriculum designed to meet specific educational goals.

13.2.1 Applications of Virtual Environment-Based Surgical Simulators

Virtual environment-based training simulators have been developed for various surgical applications. Simulators can be grouped into general categories based on the nature of the surgical intervention[8]:

Needle and Catheter-Based Procedures. Needle and catheter-based procedures generally have simple user interfaces with very restricted interaction with biological tissue. As a result, the simulators constructed for these procedures require less sophisticated methods to generate sufficient visual realism and haptic feedback. Their simplicity makes them relatively inexpensive. They are typically used for teaching widely-performed, relatively straightforward procedures with well-defined algorithms. Simulations of spinal biopsy,[9] nerve blocks,[10] vascular access,[11] and interventional cardiology[12] are some successful examples of simulations of needle- and catheter-based procedures.

Minimally Invasive Surgery. Minimally invasive surgery is a revolutionary surgical technique, where the surgery is performed with instruments and viewing equipment inserted through small incisions (typically, less than 10 mm in diameter) rather than by making a large incision to expose and provide access to the operation site. Minimally invasive operations include laparoscopy (abdominal cavity), thoracoscopy (chest cavity), arthroscopy (joints), pelviscopy (pelvis), and angioscopy (blood vessels). The main advantage of this technique is the reduced trauma to healthy tissue, which is the leading cause of patients' postoperative pain and long hospital stay. The hospital stay and rest periods, and therefore the procedure costs, can be significantly reduced with minimally invasive surgery. However, minimally invasive procedures are more demanding on the surgeon, requiring more difficult surgical techniques.

The virtual environments-based training simulators in the literature are mostly for minimally invasive surgery applications. This is not a coincidence. In addition to the need for better training tools for minimally invasive surgery, the constraints which make minimally invasive surgery difficult are the same reasons that make building simulators for minimally invasive surgery more manageable with existing technology. It is significantly easier to imitate the user interface for minimally invasive surgery, limited and well-constrained haptic interaction, and limited amount and quality of feedback (visual and otherwise) available.

Examples of simulators for minimally invasive surgery include Refs. 13 to 16. Several commercial laparoscopic surgery training simulators are also available, including systems developed by Surgical Science,[17] Mentice,[18] Immersion Medical,[19] and Simbionix.[20]

Open Surgery. In open surgery, the surgeon has a direct visual view of the operation site, and directly interacts with the biological tissue for manipulation. Open surgery is significantly less structured compared to minimally invasive surgery. Furthermore, the surgeon has significantly more freedom of motion, and the amount and quality of tactile and visual feedback is higher. As a result, simulation of open surgery is remains challenging. Considerable advances in haptic devices and algorithms, deformable object modeling and simulation, user interface development, and real-time computer graphics are needed for realistic simulation of open surgery. The existing simulations, as a result, focus more on training simulators for individual skill rather than complete procedures. Examples of open surgical simulators include Refs. 21 to 23.

13.2.2 Components of Virtual Environment-Based Surgical Simulators

The construction of a virtual environment-based surgical simulation starts with development of three-dimensional geometric models of the structures in the surgical anatomy (Fig. 13.2). The geometric models are constructed from medical diagnostic images, and can be generic or patient specific. Typically, computerized tomography and magnetic resonance images are used for construction of anatomical models. Computerized tomography images typically have higher image resolution. Magnetic resonance images, on the other hand, have better contrast in soft tissues. Magnetic resonance imaging is also preferable as it does not involve ionizing radiation. The volumetric data of the medical diagnostic images are first segmented to identify individual anatomical entities, and then converted to geometric models for use in the subsequent parts of the development. Two types of geometric models are typically generated. Surface models are triangulated meshes that represent the boundaries of the anatomical entities. Volumetric geometric models are tetrahedral meshes that represent the geometry of the interior of the anatomical entities. Surface geometry is used in graphical rendering of the virtual environment, while volumetric geometry is used in simulation of the physical behavior of the anatomical entities.

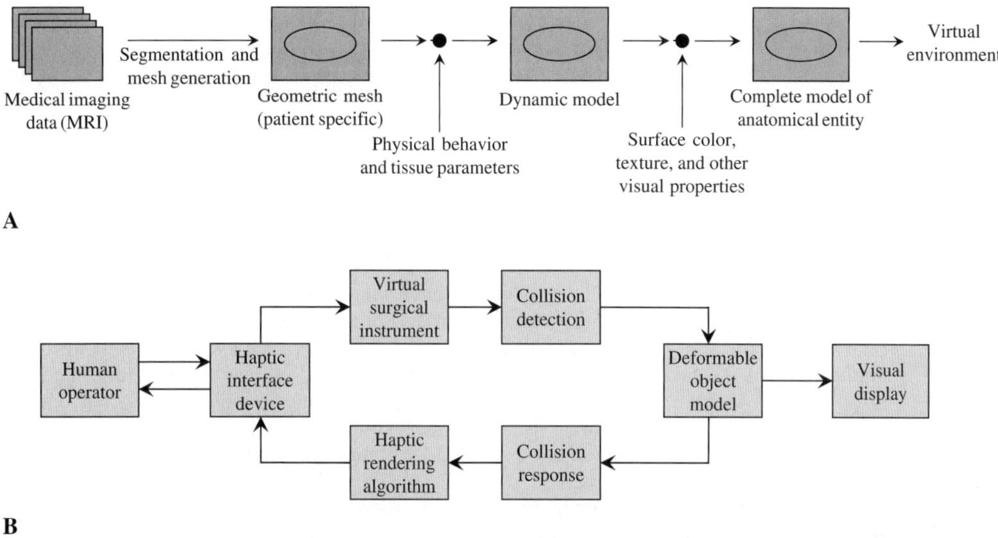

FIGURE 13.2 Development process (*a*) and components (*b*) of virtual environment-based surgical simulators.

Following the construction of the geometric models from medical diagnostic images, physical models corresponding to individual anatomical entities of interest are constructed. The physical models are used to simulate the physical deformations of the anatomy during surgical manipulation. The physical models also determine how the surface geometry models used in graphical rendering are modified as a result of the physical deformations. The resulting surface geometry models are then embedded with surface color, texture, and other visual properties, and rendered using computer graphics techniques in the virtual environment to create a realistic surgical scene.

During the simulation, the user interacts with the virtual environment, and the surgical anatomy simulated therein, using virtual instruments controlled through haptic interfaces. *Haptic interface* refers to a form of user interface that is based on the sense of touch and typically provides a form of force or tactile feedback to the user.

13.3 RESEARCH CHALLENGES IN SURGICAL SIMULATION TECHNOLOGY

The fundamental research problems in virtual environment-based medical training simulations can be grouped into three general categories. The first group of problems is related to the enabling technologies and the underlying scientific questions, which directly impact the realism of the virtual environment. These include modeling, characterization, and simulation of deformable organs, haptic interaction with deformable models simulated in virtual environments, realistic rendering of medical scenes, and development of distributed and networked virtual environments for complex and large-scale surgical simulations. The second group of problems is related to the pedagogical aspects of the training, namely to identify what to teach and how to teach, in terms of the basic motor skills (such as using surgical instruments, suturing, and knot tying), spatial skills (including navigation, exposure, and camera handling skills), tasks, and complete procedures. Finally, the third group of problems concerns verification of skill transfer from training simulator to real surgery. It is obviously important that the skills learned from the simulator are not skills in a new computer game, but rather, skills transferable to actual surgery. This subject has begun to receive significant attention in recent years.

Constructing realistic and efficient deformable models for soft tissue behavior is the main challenge in achieving realism in surgical training simulators. The deformable tissue models have to be interactive, efficient enough to be simulated in real time, visually and haptically realistic, and able to be cut and sutured. The state of the art for interactive deformable object simulation is not sufficiently advanced to build realistic real-time simulations on consumer level computer systems, and requires supercomputer level computational power and networked simulation technologies.

13.3.1 Patient-Specific Models in Surgical Simulation

A key requirement in development of virtual environment-based surgical simulators is the availability of visually and geometrically realistic models of the anatomy. It is essential to have a library of anatomical models with relevant pathologies to be able to develop an educational curriculum. For applications of surgical simulators beyond training, namely, surgical rehearsal and planning, it is also necessary to have the capability to construct patient-specific models of the anatomy. As discussed above, the geometric models used in surgical simulations are constructed from medical diagnostic images, such as magnetic resonance and computerized tomography images. The medical diagnostic images are first segmented to identify the image regions corresponding to the individual anatomical structures. The segmented images are then processed through mesh generation algorithms to create surface and volumetric geometric models needed for the visualization and physical modeling, respectively. Both medical image segmentation and mesh generation are very active areas of research. Level set methods are certainly the most popular techniques to capture the structures of interest during segmentation. The fast marching methods[24] and dynamic implicit surfaces[25] are two classes of level set algorithms that are widely used. These algorithms are relatively insensitive to noise, yield smooth surfaces, and have the topologies of the extracted surfaces robust to the choice of the threshold. There are also a number of commercial software packages available (e.g., Amira[26]), which provide manual or semiautomated segmentation and mesh generation tools. In spite of the availability of variety of tools for segmentation and mesh generation, these tasks remain to be labor intensive, requiring significant user interaction during initial segmentation, and post-processing for improving the quality of segmentation and generated meshes. Automation of image segmentation and mesh generation are key requirements for the use of patient-specific models in surgical simulators.

13.3.2 Deformable Object Modeling and Simulation

Most biological tissue is elastic. Therefore, a realistic simulation of surgical manipulation in a virtual environment requires modeling of physical deformations of soft tissue. There are two widely used types of physically based deformable object models used in the literature, namely, lumped element models (also known as mass-spring-damper models) and finite element models.

Lumped element models are meshes of mass, spring, and damper elements.[27–29] They are the most popular models for real-time surgical simulators, because they are natural extensions of other deformable models used in computer animation, conceptually simple, and easy to implement. A common problem with the lumped parameter models used in literature is the selection of component parameters, spring and damper constants, and nodal mass values. There is no physically based or systematic method in the literature to determine the element types or parameters from physical data or known constitutive behavior. The typical practice in the literature is somewhat ad hoc, the element types and connectivities are empirically assumed, usually based on the structure of the geometric model at hand, and the element parameters are either hand tuned to get a reasonable looking behavior or estimated by a parameter optimization method to fit the model response to an experimentally measured response.[30,31] There are several simulation libraries that are available for development of surgical simulations using lumped element models.[32]

Linear finite element models are used as a step to get closer using models with physically based parameters.[33–35] Linear finite element models are computationally attractive as superposition can be used, and it is possible to perform extensive off-line calculations to significantly reduce the real-time computational burden. However, linear models are based on the assumption of small deformation, which is not valid for large manipulations of the soft tissue during parts of surgery.

These models cannot handle rigid motions either. Linear models lose their computational advantage under topology changes, for example, as a result of cutting, as the off-line calculations cannot be used. Nonlinear finite element models are highly accurate models, which take into account nonlinear constitutive behaviors of the materials as well as large deformation effects. Nonlinear finite element models have been used extensively in biomechanics literature to model tissue deformations with off-line computations.[36] These models are computationally intensive, and therefore development of suitable algorithms for their real-time simulation is required.[15,37–41] Hybrid modeling approaches employing models of different types have also been proposed to address computational limitation while taking advantage of the strength of each of the modeling approaches. For example, Delingette[42] proposed to use lumped element models locally where there is topological change (such as cutting) and use a linear finite element model for the rest.

An important characteristic of the surgical manipulation is its topology changing nature. During surgical manipulation, the soft tissue are routinely cut, punctured, sutured, etc. Such manipulations bring significant modeling and computational challenges. These types of manipulations require models to include highly nonlinear and discontinuous deformable object behavior, such as, plasticity and fractures.[43] They also require online modification of the geometric models, and sometimes remeshing of the object.[44] The mesh modifications typically increase the number of elements used in the computation, increasing the computational complexity of the models. Furthermore, when geometric models of objects are modified, most precomputations performed become invalid, increasing the computational complexity even more.

The measurement of the tissue parameters for live tissue is a difficulty that is widely recognized in the literature. Not only the mechanical characteristics of tissue are highly nonlinear and time dependant, but also there is significant variability between different subjects.[45,46] However, it is important to realize that, for a training simulator, it is only necessary to provide qualities of the tissue behavior that the human operator can actually sense. Psychophysics studies on the haptic sensory-motor abilities of the human operator[47–49] reveal that humans are haptically more sensitive in detecting changes in mechanical impedances than they are in identifying the absolute values of these impedances. These results coupled with the inherent variability of the actual tissue properties suggest that it would be acceptable for a training simulator to use approximate tissue parameter values, such as those available in the literature.[50,51] However, it is important to include the nonlinear shape of the constitutive behavior of the tissue, as these characteristic nonlinearities yield the changes in the perceived tissue impedance during manipulation that the humans are good at detecting, and they usually relate to the damage occurring to the tissue that the trainees need to learn to identify. The time-dependent biphasic behavior of the tissue[52–54] and the strain rate effects, such as creep, are critical for accurate predictive modeling of surgical outcomes for surgical planning applications. However, such complex behaviors of tissue are not critical when teaching trainees the advanced endoscopic navigation and manipulation techniques, the steps of advanced endoscopic procedures, or strategies to avoid pitfalls. Therefore, including these types of tissue behaviors in a training simulator is not essential. Simulation of these tissue behaviors is also prohibitively computationally expensive for a real-time interactive simulation.

13.3.3 Collision Detection and Response

The simulation of tool-tissue and tissue-tissue interactions require the detection of contact locations. Collision detection is one of the most computationally intensive components of a surgical simulation. Furthermore, surgical simulations require collision detection to be performed at interactive speeds, at the update rates of the underlying physical models. Therefore, development of computationally efficient collision-detection algorithms is of great importance.

Collision-detection algorithms have been the focus of much research in the computer graphics literature (see Refs. 55 to 57 for review of general collision-detection algorithms). Most of these studies have focused on solving the collision-detection problem for rigid objects. Collision-detection algorithms for rigid bodies heavily rely on precomputed data structures, such as bounding volume hierarchies. However, these algorithms cannot be directly applied or do not necessarily result in efficient algorithm for deformable objects, since the data structures used to improve collision-detection efficiency need to be updated or reconstructed when the underlying object geometries change. Therefore, in surgical simulations, it is necessary to employ algorithms specialized in collision detection for deformable objects.[58–60]

In order to improve computational efficiency, most collision-detection algorithms use a two-stage approach. The first stage, which typically relies on forms of bounding volume hierarchies[60,61] or space partitioning[62,63], bounds the region of intersection. The second stage then determines the exact location of the collision, typically using ray-polygon[64,65] or polygon-polygon[66] intersection algorithms.

13.3.4 Haptic Interaction with Simulated Deformable Objects in Virtual Environments

The value of haptic interaction in surgical simulation applications has led to a great deal of research interest in the challenges involved in providing haptic force-feedback in virtual environment simulations with deformable surfaces.[67,68]

Ensuring stability of the haptic interaction is a fundamental concern in haptic systems. Stability of haptic systems, and the stability-performance trade-off has been subject to much research in the haptics literature[69,70]. The virtual coupling networks,[71] and time domain passivity observer algorithms[72] are effective algorithms to guarantee stability of haptic interaction with virtual environments.

The human sense of touch is remarkably sensitive, and can distinguish between changes in force into the range of hundreds of hertz. It is generally accepted that the update rate of the haptic interface must be 10 to 20 times higher than the highest frequency event that is to be simulated. Therefore, in order to render events in the 50 to 100 Hz range matching the capabilities of the PHANTOM or similar haptic interfaces, 1 kHz is widely considered the minimum update rate for realistic haptic feedback. On the other hand, the simulation of the deformable object models are typically linked to the graphical update rates of 10 to 60 Hz because of computational limitations. This 2 order of magnitudes difference between the physical model and haptic update rates is one of the major issues in haptic interaction with deformable objects. One common method of bridging this gulf is through multirate simulation. The core of the multirate simulation approaches is to divide the necessary computational tasks into those that must be performed at the servo-loop update rate of the haptic interface and those that can be performed at the same rate as the overall simulation. The algorithm is divided into two basic blocks, as shown in Fig. 13.3*a*. The "global" simulation incorporates the entire virtual environment and runs at the visual update rate in the order of magnitude of 10 Hz. A "local" simulation runs at the haptic device update rate and simulates the behavior of a subset of the global model (Fig. 13.3*b*). After each update of the global model, a low-order approximation model is generated and passed to a second simulation, running either in a separate process or thread in single-computer operation, or running on a second computer in networked operation. This second simulation uses the low-order approximation model to provide force output to the user and then sends the state of the haptic instrument back to the global model, which then recomputes a new low-order approximation for the next cycle.[73,74]

13.3.5 Realistic Graphical Rendering of Surgical Scenes

After the geometric model of the anatomy is constructed from medical diagnostic imaging data, it needs to be incorporated into the virtual surgical environment and displayed in a realistic manner. Therefore, the development of the virtual environment-based surgical simulators requires real-time realistic rendering of the surgical scene. The visual realism of the virtual environment is critical for a training simulator for several reasons. Teaching correct identification of critical structures and anatomical landmarks to a nonexpert requires a visual model which is as faithful to the reality as possible. Visual realism and availability of the visual cues used in depth perception in an endoscopic view, which is monoscopic, is also important to teach minimally invasive navigation skills to a

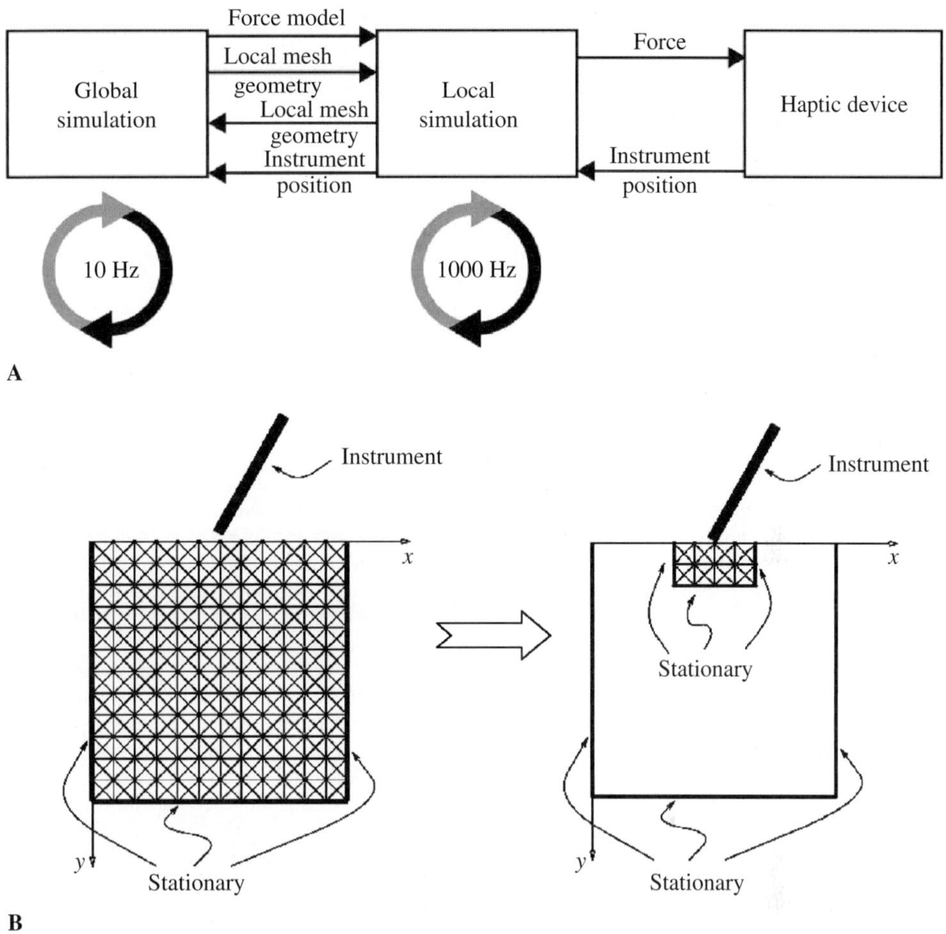

FIGURE 13.3 Multirate simulation for high-fidelity haptic interaction with virtual environments.

novice. The visual realism of the virtual environment is also important for the trainee to achieve a sense of immersion into the simulation, facilitating the trainee's engagement with the training task, which is essential for effective training.

The availability of powerful graphics capabilities at the new relatively low-cost consumer level graphics adapters facilitated the application of advanced rendering algorithms in interactive virtual environments, which was previously possible only with high-end graphics workstations. With the new programmable vertex and pixel shaders, it is possible to create realistic graphical a visually realistic reproduction of the surgical scene by applying advanced illumination models together with texture and bump mapping, extended to include the effects of glossiness and multilayered nature of the tissue, and superimposing capillaries and other visual details onto the gross geometry.[75]

13.3.6 Networked and Distributed Virtual Environments

In a surgical simulation, software modules numerically simulate the physics of a target environment. Highly accurate simulations for compelling virtual environments for training, especially, simulations involving models with geometric and material nonlinearities, topology changing manipulations, and large number of objects, may require computational power beyond what is available in single processor desktop computers or workstations. It is necessary to pursue the development of network-enabled virtual environments to perform distributed simulations on parallel (or cluster) computers. There are several studies in the literature which applied parallel high-performance computing techniques to surgical simulation. Szekely et al.[76] developed a custom-built hardware system to perform parallel computation of finite element models in real time. Wu et al.[37] developed a parallel implementation of the multigrid FEM algorithm on a cluster computer as a proof of concept to incorporate as part of an interactive surgical simulation. The implementation of Wu uses a readily accessible hardware platform; however, the implementation is rather customized. These studies demonstrate the feasibility of employing parallel computation to simulate larger-scale models in real-time interactive surgical simulation applications. More recently, Cai et al. developed network middleware for networked virtual environments, as part of the GiPSi/GiPSiNet surgical simulation framework.[77]

13.3.7 Open Architecture Software Frameworks for Surgical Simulation

The current state of the field of medical simulation is characterized by scattered research projects using a variety of models that are neither interoperable nor independently verifiable. Simulators are frequently built from scratch by individual research groups without input and validation from a larger community. The challenge of developing useful medical simulations is often too great for many individual research groups since expertise from large number of different fields is required. Therefore, model and algorithm sharing and collaborative development of surgical simulations with multiple research groups are very desirable.

The open source/open architecture software development model provides an attractive framework to address the needs of interfacing models from multiple research groups and the ability to critically examine and validate quantitative biological simulations. Open source models provide means for quality control, evaluation, and peer review, which are critical for basic scientific methodology. Furthermore, since subsequent users of the models and the software code have access to the original code, this also improves the reusability of the models and interconnectibility of the software modules. On the other hand, an open architecture simulation framework allows open source or proprietary third-party development of additional models, model data, and analysis and computation modules.

There are several technical issues that need to be addressed for the successful development of such a framework for model and algorithm sharing.

Modularity Through Encapsulation and Data Hiding. Maintaining the integrity of the data of the individual models in an open architecture simulation is an important requirement. Moreover, the application programmers interface (API) and the overall framework also need to be able to support hierarchical models and abstraction of the input-output behavior of individual layers or subsystems for the level of detail desired from the simulation model.

The object-oriented programming concepts of encapsulation and data hiding facilitate the modularity of the components while maintaining the data integrity. It also provides mechanisms to interface and embed the constructed models and other computational modules to a larger, more sophisticated model.

Abstraction. In the context of surgical simulation, model abstraction is an important consideration. Within a general modeling and simulation framework, different applications and different problems require different types or levels of abstraction for each of the processes and components in the model. Therefore, the simulation framework developed needs to be able to accommodate different types and levels of abstraction for each of the different subcomponents in the model hierarchy without artificially limiting the possibilities based on the requirements of a specific application or a modeling approach.

Heterogeneous Physical Mechanisms and Models of Computation. Another issue that arises with the varying types of abstractions is the requirement on the simulation engine to be able to handle heterogeneous physical mechanisms (e.g., solid mechanics, fluid mechanics, and bioelectricity) and models of computation (e.g., differential equations, finite state machines, and hybrid systems). The simulator and the application interfaces need to have support for hybrid models of computation, that is computation of continuous and discrete deterministic processes, and stochastic processes, which can be used to model basic biological functions.

Support for Parallel and Distributed Simulation. In a surgical simulation, software modules numerically simulate the physics of a target environment. Highly accurate simulations for surgical planning and compelling virtual environments for training typically require extensive computation available beyond basic desktop computers or single-processor workstations. It is therefore necessary for the simulation framework to support parallel and distributed simulations. Beyond just parallel processing, development of network-enabled virtual environments is desirable to extend the accessibility of surgical simulations and to allow computation to take place in existing computing facilities while supporting planning and training from a variety of locations. This would allow sharing of computational resources and ease the logistical requirements for deploying virtual environment-based simulators.

Validation. Validation of the models and the underlying empirical data is a basic requirement for reusability of the models.

Customization with Patient-Specific Models. In surgical planning and preoperational rehearsals, it is necessary to use patient-specific models during simulation. Therefore, the models in the simulation need to be customizable. This ties to the open architecture design of the simulation framework. The open architecture approach should allow loading and working with custom data sets generated by third parties.

There are several open source surgical simulation frameworks available, including, SPRING,[32] GiPSi,[78] and SOFA.[79]

13.4 CONCLUSION

Very significant technical and practical challenges need to be overcome for widespread adoption of virtual environment-based simulations in surgical training. Commercial success of this technology requires a successful business model which combines technological innovation with medical needs and practical realities of existing medical education system. An important requirement is the development of simulation systems together with an innovative education curriculum that will incorporate the system rather than focusing on development of individual stand-alone systems.

REFERENCES

1. Ellis, S. R., Origins and elements of virtual environments. *Virtual Environments and Advanced Interface Design.* 1995 [cited; 14–62].
2. Milgram, P. and F. Kishino, A taxonomy of mixed reality visual displays. *IEEE Transactions on Information Systems* E77–D, 1994. **12**:1321–29.
3. Milgram, P., H. Takemura, et al., Augmented reality: a class of displays on the reality-virtuality continuum. In *SPIE Proceedings: Telemanipulator and Telepresence Technologies*. 1994. Boston, MA.
4. Stuart, R., *The Design of Virtual Environments*. 1996: McGraw-Hill, New York.
5. Satava, R. M., Nintendo surgery. *Journal of the American Medical Association*, 1992. **267**(17):297–304.
6. Seymour, N. E., et al., Virtual reality training improves operating room performance: results of a randomized, double-blinded study. *Annals of Surgery*, 2002. **236**(4):458–63; discussion 463–64.
7. Gallagher, A. G. and C. U. Cates, Approval of virtual reality training for carotid stenting: what this means for procedural-based medicine. *Journal of American Medical Association*, 2004. **292**(24):3024–26.

8. Liu, A., et al., A survey of surgical simulation: applications, technology, and education. *Presence: Teleoperators and Virtual Environments*, 2003. **12**(6):599–614.
9. Cleary, K. R., C. E. Lathan, and C. Carignan, Simulator/planner for CT-directed needle biopsy of the spine. In *SPIE Conference 3262 on Surgical-Assist Systems*. 1998. San Jose, CA.
10. Blezek, D. J., et al., Simulation of Spinal Nerve Blocks for Training Anesthesiology Residents. In *SPIE Conference 3262 on Surgical-Assist Systems*. 1998. San Jose, CA.
11. Ursino, M., et al., CathSim: an intravascular catheterization simulator on a PC. *Studies in Health Technology and Informatics*, 1999. **62**:360–66.
12. Cotin, S., et al., ICTS, an interventional cardiology training system. *Studies in Health Technology and Informatics*, 2000. **70**:59–65.
13. Bro-Nielsen, M., et al., PreOp Endoscopic Simulator: A PC-Based Immersive Training System for Bronchoscopy. In *Medicine Meets Virtual Reality: 7*. 1999. Amsterdam: IOS Press.
14. Kuhnapfel, U., H. Cakmak, and H. Maass, Endoscopic surgery training using virtual reality and deformable tissue simulation. *Computers and Graphics*, 2000. **24**:671–82.
15. Szekely, G., et al., Virtual reality-based simulation of endoscopic surgery. *Presence: Teleoperators and Virtual Environments*, 2000. **9**(3):310–33.
16. Tendick, F., et al., A virtual environment testbed for training laparoscopic surgical skills. *Presence: Teleoperators and Virtual Environments*, 2000. **9**(3):236–55.
17. *The LapSim laparoscopic training tool*. 2008 [cited April 2008]; available from: http://www.surgical-science.com/.
18. *Mentice Medical Simulators*. 2008 [cited April 2008]; available from: http://www.mentice.com/.
19. *Medical and Surgical Simulators*. 2008 [cited April 2008]; available from: http://www.immersion.com/medical/.
20. *Medical Training Simulators and Clinical Devices for Minimally Invasive Surgery*. 2008 [cited April 2008]; available from: http://www.simbionix.com/.
21. Bro-Nielsen, M., et al., VR simulation of abdominal trauma surgery. *Studies in Health Technology and Informatics*, 1998. **50**:117–23.
22. O'Toole, R. V., et al., Measuring and developing suturing technique with a virtual reality surgical simulator. *Journal of American College of Surgeons*, 1999. **189**(1):114–27.
23. Webster, R. W., et al., A prototype haptic suturing simulator. *Studies in Health Technology and Informatics*, 2001. **81**:567–69.
24. Sethian, J. A., *Level Set Methods and Fast Marching Methods: Evolving Interfaces in Computational Geometry, Fluid Mechanics, Computer Vision, and Materials Science*. 2d ed. *Cambridge Monographs on Applied and Computational Mathematics*. 1999, Cambridge, UK; New York: Cambridge University Press. xx, 378.
25. Osher, S. and R. P. Fedkiw, *Level Set Methods and Dynamic Implicit Surfaces*. 2003, New York, NY: Springer. xii, 273.
26. *AMIRA: Visualize, Analyze, Present*. 2008 [cited April 2008]; available from: http://www.amiravis.com/.
27. Fung, Y. C., *Biomechanics: Mechanical Properties of Living Tissues*. 2d ed. 1993, New York, NY: Springer-Verlag. xviii, 568.
28. Metaxas, D. N., *Physics Based Deformable Models: Applications to Computer Vision, Graphics, and Medical Imaging*. Kluver Academic. 1997, Boston, MA.
29. Terzopoulos, D., et al., Elastically Deformable Models. In *Proceedings of SIGGRAPH 87: 14th Annual Conference on Computer Graphics*. 1987: ACM. Anaheim, CA.
30. d'Aulignac, D., M. C. Cavusoglu, and C. Laugier, Modeling the dynamics of the human thigh for a realistic echographic simulator with force feedback. In *Proceedings of the Second International Conference on Medical Image Computing and Computer-Assisted Intervention*. 1999. Cambridge, UK.
31. Joukhadar, A., F. Garat, and C. Laugier, Parameter identification for dynamic simulation. In *Proceedings of the IEEE International Conference on Robotics and Automation* (*ICRA'97*). 1997. Albuquerque, New Mexico.
32. Montgomery, K., et al., Spring: a general framework for collaborative, real-time surgical simulation. In *Medicine Meets Virtual Reality* (*MMVR 2002*). 2002. Amsterdam: IOS Press.
33. BroNielsen, M., Finite element modeling in surgery simulation. In *Proceedings of the IEEE/RSJ International Conference on Intelligent Robotics and Systems*. 1998. Victoria, Canada.
34. Cotin, S., H. Delingette, and N. Ayache, Real-time elastic deformations of soft tissues for surgery simulation. *IEEE Transactions on Visualization and Computer Graphics*, 1999. **5**(1):62–73.

35. James, D. L. and D. K. Pai, ARTDEFO: Accurate real time deformable objects. In *Proceedings of SIGGRAPH 99: 26th International Conference on Computer Graphics and Interactive Techniques*. 1999: ACM. Los Angeles, CA.
36. Nielsen, P. M., et al., Mathematical model of geometry and fibrous structure of the heart. *American Journal of Physiology,* 1991. **260**(4 Pt 2):H1365–78.
37. Wu, X., T. G. Goktekin, and F. Tendick, An interactive parallel multigrid FEM simulator. In *Proceedings of the International Symposium on Medical Simulation* (*ISMS 2004*). 2004: Springer-Verlag, Berlin, Heidelberg.
38. Wu, X. and F. Tendick, Multigrid integration for interactive deformable body simulation. In *Proceedings of the International Symposium on Medical Simulation* (*ISMS 2004*). 2004: Springer-Verlag, Berlin, Heidelberg.
39. Zhuang, Y. and J. Canny, Haptic interaction with global deformations. In *Proceedings of the IEEE International Conference on Robotics and Automation* (*ICRA 2000*). 2000. San Francisco, CA.
40. Cotin, S., H. Delingette, and N. Ayache, Real-time elastic deformations of soft tissues for surgery simulation. *IEEE Transactions on Visualization and Computer Graphics*, 1999. **5**(1):62–73.
41. Picinbono, G., H. Delingette, and N. Ayache, Nonlinear and anisotropic elastic soft tissue models for medical simulation. In *Proceedings of the IEEE International Conference on Robotics and Automation* (*ICRA 2001*). 2001. Seoul, Korea.
42. Delingette, H., S. Cotin, and N. Ayache, Efficient linear elastic models of soft tissues for realtime surgery simulation. In *Medicine Meets Virtual Reality: 7*. 1999. Amsterdam: IOS Press.
43. O'Brien, J. F. and J. K. Hodgins, Graphical modeling and animation of brittle fracture. In *Proceedings of the 26th Annual Conference on Computer Graphics and Interactive Techniques*. 1999: ACM Press/Addison-Wesley Publishing Co. Los Angeles, CA.
44. Mor, A. B. and T. Kanade, Modifying Soft Tissue Models: Progressive cutting with minimal new element creation. In *Proceedings of the Third International Conference on Medical Image Computing and Computer-Assisted Intervention*. 2000: Springer-Verlag. Pittsburgh, PA.
45. Brouwer, I., et al., Measuring in vivo animal soft tissue properties for haptic modeling in surgical simulation. *Studies in Health Technology and Informatics*, 2001. **81**:69–74.
46. Ottensmeyer, M. P., In vivo measurement of solid organ visco-elastic properties. *Studies in Health Technology and Informatics*, 2002. **85**:328–33.
47. Dhruv, N. and F. Tendick, Frequency dependence of compliance contrast detection. In *Proceedings of the Symposium on Haptic Interfaces for Virtual Environment and Teleoperator Systems, part of the ASME Int'l Mechanical Engineering Congress and Exposition* (*IMECE 2000*). 2000. Orlando, FL.
48. Jones, L. A. and I. W. Hunter, A perceptual analysis of stiffness. *Experimental Brain Research*, 1990. **79**(1):150–56.
49. Jones, L. A. and I. W. Hunter, A perceptual analysis of viscosity. *Experimental Brain Research*, 1993. **94**(2): 343–51.
50. Duck, F. A., *Physical Properties of Tissue*. 1990, London, UK: Academic Press.
51. Yamada, H., *Strength of Biological Materials*. 1970, Baltimore, MD: Williams & Wilkins.
52. Mendis, K. K., R. L. Stalnaker, and S. H. Advani, A constitutive relationship for large deformation finite element modeling of brain tissue. *Journal of Biomechanical Engineering*, 1995. **117**(3):279–85.
53. Miller, K., Constitutive model of brain tissue suitable for finite element analysis of surgical procedures. *Journal of Biomechanics*, 1999. **32**(5):531–37.
54. Miller, K., et al., Mechanical properties of brain tissue in-vivo: experiment and computer simulation. *Journal of Biomechanics*, 2000. **33**(11):1369–76.
55. Jiménez, P., F. Thomas, and C. Torras, 3D collision detection: a survey. *Computers and Graphics*, 2001. **25**(2):269–85.
56. Lin, M. C., et al., Collision detection: algorithms and applications. In *Algorithms for Robotic Motion and Manipulation*, J.-P. Laumond and M.H. Overmars, Editors. 1997, A K Peters, Ltd.
57. Lin, M. C. and D. Manocha, Collision and proximity queries. In *Handbook of Discrete and Computational Geometry*, J.E. Goodman and J. O'Rourke, Editors. 2004, CRC Press.
58. Teschner, M., et al., Collision detection for deformable objects. *Computer Graphics Forum*, 2005. **24**(1):61–81.
59. Larsson, T. and T. Akenine-Möller, Collision detection for continuously deforming bodies. In *Proceedings of Eurogrpahics 2001*. 2001. 325–33. Manchester, UK.
60. van den Bergen, G., Efficient collision detection of complex deformable models using AABB trees. *Journal of Graphics Tools*, 1997. **2**(4):1–13.

61. Klosowski, J. T., et al., Efficient collision detection using bounding volume hierarchies of k-DOPs. *IEEE Transactions on Visualization and Computer Graphics*, 1998. **4**(1):21–36.

62. van den Bergen, G., *Collision Detection in Interactive 3D Computer Animation*. 1999, Printed by University Press Facilities, Technische Universiteit Eindhoven, 1999: Eindhoven. viii, 181.

63. Fuchs, H., Z. M. Kedem, and B.F. Naylor, On visible surface generation by a priori tree structures. In *Proceedings of the 7th Annual Conference on Computer Graphics and Interactive Techniques*. 1980, ACM: Seattle, WA.

64. Möller, T. and B. Trumbore, Fast, minimum storage ray-triangle intersection. *Journal of Graphics Tools*, 1997. **2**(1):21–28.

65. Badouel, D., A. S. Glassner, An efficient ray-polygon intersection. In *Graphics Gems*. 1990, Academic Press Professional, Inc. 390–93.

66. Lin, M. C. and J. F. Canny, A fast algorithm for incremental distance calculation. In *Proceedings of the IEEE International Conference on Robotics and Automation,* 1991. Sacramento, CA.

67. Basdogan, C. and M. A. Srinivasan, Haptic rendering in virtual environments. In *Handbook of Virtual Environments: Design, Implementation, and Applications*, K.M. Stanney, Editor. 2002, Lawrence Erlbaum Associates.

68. Salisbury, K., F. Conti, and F. Barbagli, Haptic rendering: introductory concepts. *IEEE Computer Graphics and Applications*, 2004. **24**(2):24–32.

69. Colgate, J. E. and G. G. Schenkel, Passivity of a class of sampled-data systems: application to haptic interfaces. *Journal of Robotic Systems*, 1998. **14**(1):37–47.

70. Diolaiti, N., et al., Stability of haptic rendering: discretization, quantization, time delay, and Coulomb effects. *IEEE Transactions on Robotics and Automation*, 2006. **22**(2):256–68.

71. Adams, R. J. and B. Hannaford, Stable haptic interaction with virtual environments. *IEEE Transactions on Robotics and Automation*, 1999. **15**(3):465–74.

72. Hannaford, B. and J. H. Ryu, Time domain passivity control of haptic interfaces. In *IEEE Transactions on Robotics and Automation*. 2002. **18**(1):1–10.

73. Cavusoglu, M. C. and F. Tendick, Multirate simulation for high fidelity haptic interaction with deformable objects in virtual environments. In *Proceedings of the IEEE International Conference on Robotics and Automation* (*ICRA 2000*). 2000. San Francisco, CA.

74. Jacobs, P. and M. C. Cavusoglu, High fidelity haptic rendering of stick-slip frictional contact with deformable objects in virtual environments using multi-rate simulation. In *Proceedings of the IEEE International Conference on Robotics and Automation* (*ICRA 2007*). 2007. Rome, Italy.

75. Brown, N., et al., Virtual environment-based training simulator for endoscopic third ventriculostomy. In *Proceedings of Medicine Meets Virtual Reality XIV* (*MMVR 2006*). 2006. Long Beach, CA.

76. Szekely, G., et al., Modelling of soft tissue deformation for laparoscopic surgery simulation. *Medical Image Analysis*, 2000. **4**(1):57–66.

77. Cai, Q., V. Liberatore, and M. C. Cavusoglu, GiPSiNet, An open source/open architecture network middleware for surgical simulations. In *Proceedings of Medicine Meets Virtual Reality XIV* (*MMVR 2006*). 2006. Long Beach, CA.

78. Cavusoglu, M. C., T. Goktekin, and F. Tendick, GiPSi: a framework for open source/open architecture software development for organ level surgical simulation. In *IEEE Transactions on Information Technology in Biomedicine*, 2006. **10**(2):312–21.

79. Allard, J., et al., SOFA—an open source framework for medical simulation. *Studies in Health Technology and Informatics*, 2007. **125**:13–18.

CHAPTER 14
COMPUTER-INTEGRATED SURGERY AND MEDICAL ROBOTICS

Russell Taylor
Department of Computer Science Center for Computer-Integrated Surgical Systems and Technology, The Johns Hopkins University, Baltimore, Maryland, U.S.A.

Leo Joskowicz
School of Computer Science and Engineering Computer-Aided Surgery and Medical Image Processing Laboratory, The Hebrew University of Jerusalem, Israel

14.1 INTRODUCTION: COUPLING INFORMATION TO SURGICAL ACTION

The growing demand for complex and minimally invasive surgical interventions is driving the search for ways to use computer-based information technology as a link between the preoperative plan and the tools utilized by the surgeon. Computers, used in conjunction with advanced surgical assist devices, will fundamentally alter the way that procedures are carried out in twenty-first century operating rooms.

Computer-integrated surgery (CIS) systems make it possible to carry out surgical interventions that are more precise and less invasive than conventional procedures, while judiciously tracking and logging all relevant data. This data logging, coupled with appropriate tracking of patient outcomes, will make possible a totally new level of quantitative patient outcome assessment and treatment improvement analogous to “total quality management” in manufacturing.

The goals of CIS systems are to enhance the dexterity, visual feedback, and information integration of the surgeon. While medical equipment is currently available to assist the surgeons in specific tasks, it is the synergy between these capabilities that gives rise to a new paradigm. The goal is to complement and enhance surgeons’ skills and always leave them in control, never to replace them.

CIS systems are instances of an emerging paradigm of human-computer cooperation to accomplish delicate and difficult tasks. In some cases, the surgeon will supervise a CIS system that carries out a specific treatment step such as inserting a needle or machining bone. In other cases, the CIS system will provide information to assist the surgeon's manual execution of a task, for example, through the use of computer graphic overlays on the surgeon's field of view. In some cases, these modes will be combined.

From an engineering systems perspective, the objective can be defined in terms of two interrelated concepts:

- *Surgical CAD/CAM systems* transform preoperative images and other information into models of individual patients, assist clinicians in developing an optimized interventional plan, register this preoperative data to the patient in the operating room, and then use a variety of appropriate means, such as robots and image overlay displays, to assist in the accurate execution of the planned interventions
- *Surgical assistant systems* work interactively with surgeons to extend human capabilities in carrying out a variety of surgical tasks. They have many of the same components as surgical CAD/CAM systems, but the emphasis is on intraoperative decision support and skill enhancement, rather than careful preplanning and accurate execution.

Two other concepts related to CIS are *surgical total information management* (STIM) and *surgical total quality management* (STQM), which are analogous to total information management and total quality management in manufacturing enterprises.

Table 14.1 summarizes some of the factors that must be considered in assessing the value of CIS systems with respect to their potential application. Although the main focus of this chapter is the technology of such systems, an appreciation of these factors is very important both in the development of practical systems and in assessing the relative importance of possible research topics.

The CIS paradigm started to emerge from research laboratories in the mid-1980s, with the introduction of the first commercial navigation and robotic systems in the mid-1990s. Since then, a few hundreds of CIS systems have been installed in hospitals and are in routine clinical use, and a few tens of thousands of patients have been treated with CIS technology, with their number rapidly growing. The main clinical areas for which these systems have been developed are neurosurgery, orthopedics, radiation therapy, and laparoscopy. Preliminary evaluation and short-term clinical studies indicate improved planning and execution precision, which results in a reduction of complications and shorter hospital stays. However, some of these systems have in some cases a steep learning curve and longer intraoperative times than traditional procedures, indicating the need to carry out preoperative analysis and elaborate a surgical plan of action. This plan can range from simple tasks such as determining the access point of a biopsy needle, to complex gait simulations, implant stress analysis, or radiation dosage planning. Because the analysis and planning is specific to each surgical procedure and anatomy, preoperative planning and analysis software is usually customized to each clinical application. These systems can be viewed as medical CAD systems, which allow the user to manipulate and visualize medical images, models of anatomy, implants, and surgical tools, perform simulations, and elaborate plans. To give the reader an idea of the current scope of these systems, we will briefly describe two planning systems, one for orthopedics and one for radiation therapy.

In orthopedics, planning systems are generally used to select implants and find their optimal placement with respect to anatomy. For example, a planning system for spinal pedicle screw insertion shows the surgeon three orthogonal cross sections of the acquired CT image (the original *xy* slice and interpolated *xz* and *yz* slices) and a three-dimensional image of the vertebrae surfaces. The surgeon selects a screw type and its dimensions, and positions it with respect to the anatomy in the three cross-sectional views. A projection of the screw CAD model is superimposed on the images, and its position and orientation with respect to the viewing plane can be modified, with the result displayed in the other windows. Once a satisfactory placement has been obtained, the system stores it with the screw information for use in the operating room. Similar systems exist for total hip and total knee replacement, which, in addition, automatically generate in some cases machining plans

TABLE 14.1 Key Advantages of CIS Systems

Advantage	Important to whom	How quantify	Summary of key leverage
New treatment options	Clinical researchers Patients	Clinical and preclinical trials	Transcend human sensory-motor limits (e.g., in microsurgery). Enable less invasive procedures with real-time image feedback (e.g., fluoroscopic or MRI-guided liver or prostate therapy). Speed clinical research through greater consistency and data gathering.
Quality	Surgeons Patients	Clinician judgment; revision rates	Significantly improve the quality of surgical technique (e.g., in microvascular anastomosis), thus improving results and reducing the need for revision surgery.
Time and cost	Surgeons Hospitals Insurers	Hours, hospital charges	Speed or time for some interventions. Reduce costs from healing time and revision surgery. Provide effective intervention to treat patient condition.
Less invasive	Surgeons Patients	Qualitative judgment; recovery times	Provide crucial information and feedback needed to reduce the invasiveness of surgical procedures, thus reducing infection risk, recovery times, and costs (e.g., percutaneous spine surgery).
Safety	Surgeons Patients	Complication and revision surgery rates	Reduce surgical complications and errors, again lowering costs, improving outcomes and shortening hospital stays (e.g., robotic total hip replacement, steady-hand brain surgery).
Real-time feedback	Surgeons	Qualitative assessment Quantitative comparison of plan to observation Revision surgery rates	Integrate preoperative models and intraoperative images to give surgeon timely and accurate information about the patient and intervention (e.g., fluoroscopic x-rays without surgeon exposure, percutaneous therapy in conventional MRI scanners). Assure that the planned intervention has in fact been accomplished.
Accuracy or precision	Surgeons	Quantitative comparison of plan to actual	Significantly improve the accuracy of therapy dose pattern delivery and tissue manipulation tasks (e.g., solid organ therapy, microsurgery, robotic bone machining).
Documentation and follow-up	Surgeons Clinical researchers	Databases, anatomical atlases, images, and clinical observations	CIS systems inherently have the ability to log more varied and detailed information about each surgical case than is practical in conventional manual surgery. Over time, this ability, coupled with CIS systems' consistency, has the potential to significantly improve surgical practice and shorten research trials.

(cut files) for intraoperative surgical robots. Other systems also extract kinematic or fine-element models and perform gait and stress analysis that help surgeons estimate the effectiveness of the proposed solution.

Another example of a complex planning system is in the field of radiation therapy. The goal of radiation therapy is to kill tumor cells by exposing them to a radiation beam while affecting as little as possible the surrounding healthy cells. One way of achieving this is to expose the tumor cells to radiation beams from different directions so that the cumulative radiation effect on the tumor cells destroys them while preserving the surrounding healthy cells. The planning task consists of identifying the tumor and the critical areas where no radiation should be present from MRI images, and then selecting the number of beams, their radius, intensity, duration, and placement that maximizes the radiation to the tumor cells while minimizing the radiation to other cells, especially to improve them.

To make our discussion more concrete, we briefly present two examples of deployed CIS systems: ROBODOC® (Integrated Surgical Systems, Davis, California) an active medical robotics system, and the StealthStation® (Medtronic Surgical Navigation Technology, Boulder, Colorado), an intraoperative navigation system used in neurosurgery and orthopedics.

The ROBODOC system[1–7] is an active medical robot developed clinically by Integrated Surgical Systems from a prototype developed at the IBM T. J. Watson Research Center in the late 1980s (Fig. 14.1).

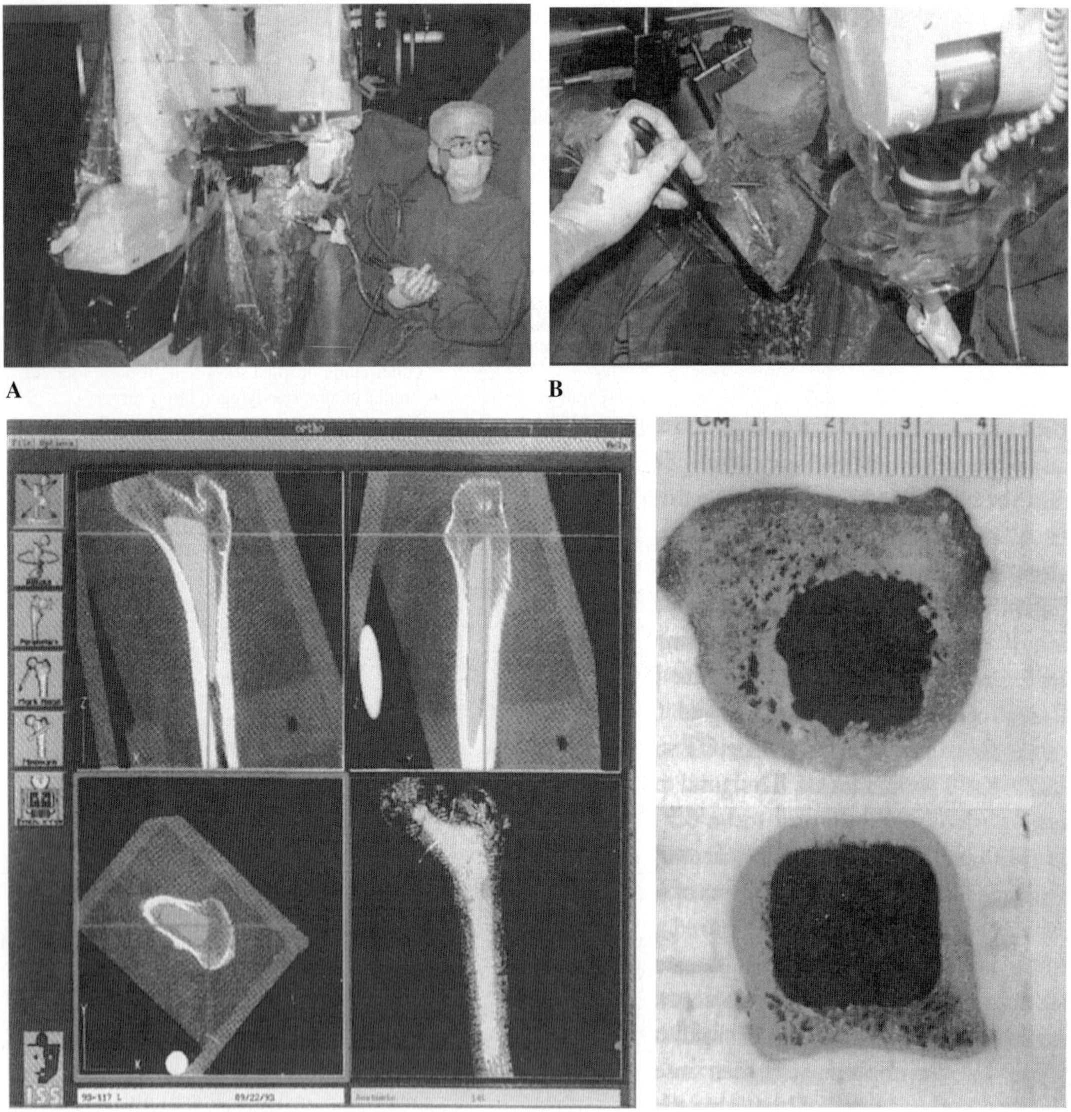

FIGURE 14.1 (*a*, *b*) ROBODOC system for orthopedic replacement surgery (photos by author). (*c*) Early version ROBODOC planning screen and (*d*) comparative cross sections showing conventionally broached (top) and robotically machined (bottom) cadaver femurs.[1,156,157]

ROBODOC is a computer-integrated system for cementless primary total hip replacement. In primary total hip replacement procedures, a damaged joint connecting the hip and the femur is replaced by a metallic implant inserted into a canal broached in the femur. ROBODOC allows surgeons to plan preoperatively the procedure by selecting and positioning an implant with respect to a computer tomography (CT) study and intraoperatively mill the corresponding canal in the femur with a high-speed tool controlled by a robotic arm. It consists of an interactive preoperative planning software, and an active robotic system for intraoperative execution. Preclinical testing showed an order-of-magnitude improvement in precision and repeatability in preparing the implant cavity. As of 2001, about 40 systems were in clinical use, having performed an estimated 8000 procedures, with very positive results documented in follow-up studies.

The StealthStation[8] is representative of current surgical navigation systems (Fig. 14.2). It allows surgeons to intraoperatively visualize the relative locations of surgical tools and anatomy in real time and perform surgical actions accordingly. The anatomical model used for navigation is constructed from preoperative CT or MRI data. The locations of instruments and rigid anatomy are obtained in real time by attaching to them frames with light-emitting diodes that are accurately tracked with a stereoscopic optical tracking camera. The preoperative model is registered to the intraoperative situation by touching with a tracked probe predefined landmarks or points on the anatomy surface and

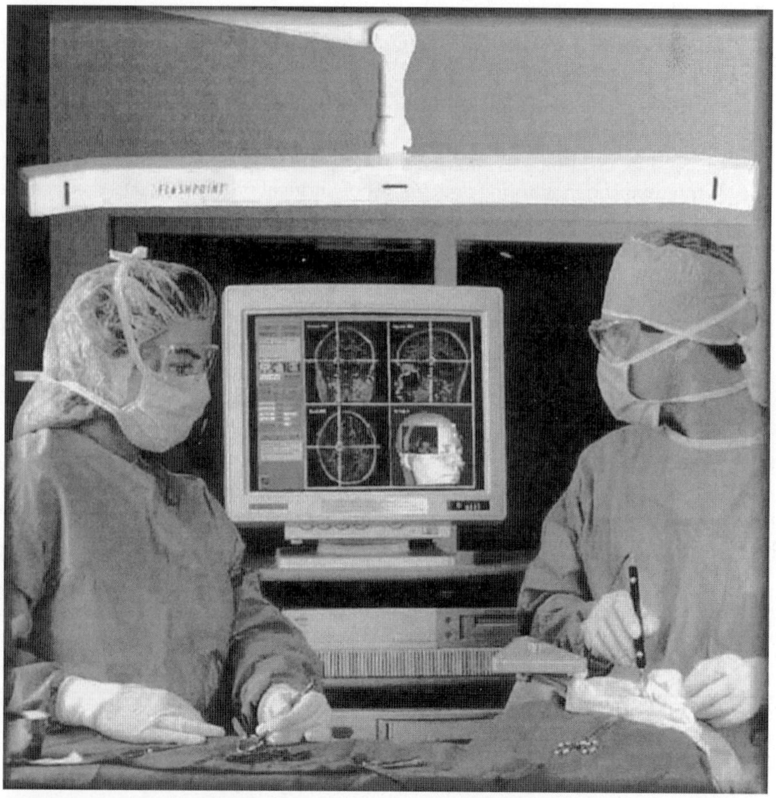

FIGURE 14.2 A CIS navigation system in action. The surgeon (left) is performing a brain tumor biopsy with the help of a navigation system. He is holding a pointer with light-emitting diodes whose position and orientation is precisely determined in real time by a stereo tracking camera (top). The computer display (center) shows the preoperative MRI and the current position of the pointer. The image shows three orthogonal cross sections and a three-dimensional reconstruction of the MRI data. The cross hair in each view shows the position of the pointer. The surgeon moves the pointer toward the desired position by watching the pointer location move on the screen.

matching them to their corresponding location on the model. Intraoperative navigation allows for less invasive surgery and more precise localization without the need of repeated intraoperative x-ray or ultrasound two-dimensional imaging. For example, to perform a biopsy of a tumor on the brain, the surgeon directs the instrumented drill on the patient's skull with the help of the images, and drills directly toward the tumor instead of making an incision on the skull and visually looking for the tumor.

The key technical enabling factors that led the development of CIS systems were the increasing availability of powerful imaging modalities, such as CT, MRI, NMT, and live video, powerful computers with graphics capabilities, novel algorithms for model construction and navigation, and integrative systems and protocol development. This article reviews the main technical issues of CIS systems. It is organized as follows: The next section presents an overview of CIS systems, their main elements architecture, and information flow. The following section describes the main enabling technologies of CIS systems: imaging devices, image processing, visualization and modeling, preoperative analysis and planning, registration, tracking and sensing, robotics, human-machine interfaces, and systems integration technology. Then, we describe in detail examples of CIS systems, including navigation systems, augmented reality navigation systems, and virtual reality systems. We conclude with perspectives and possible directions for future development.

14.2 AN OVERVIEW OF CIS SYSTEMS

Figure 14.3 shows a generic block diagram of a CIS system. At the core is a computer (or network of computers) running a variety of modeling and analysis processes, including image and sensor processing, creation and manipulation of patient-specific anatomical models, surgical planning, visualization, and monitoring and control of surgical processes. These processes receive information about the patient from medical imaging devices and may directly act on the patient through the use of specialized robots or other computer-controlled therapy devices. The processes also communicate with the surgeon through a variety of visualization modules, haptic devices, or other human-machine interfaces. The surgeon remains at all times in overall control of the procedure and, indeed, may do all of the actual manipulation of the patient using hand tools with information and decision support

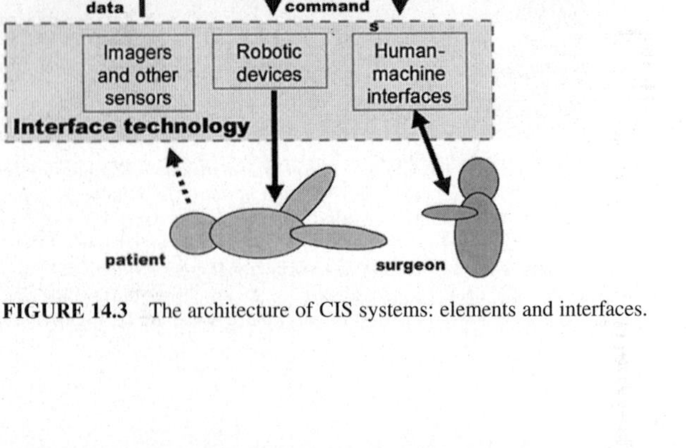

FIGURE 14.3 The architecture of CIS systems: elements and interfaces.

from the computer. The modeling and analysis processes within the computer will often rely upon databases of prior information, such as anatomical atlases, implant design data, or descriptions of common surgical tasks. The computer can also retain nearly all information developed during surgical planning and execution, and store it for postoperative analysis and comparison with long-term outcomes.

Essential elements of CIS systems are devices and techniques to provide the interfaces between the "virtual reality" of computer models and surgical plans to the "actual reality" of the operating room, patients, and surgeons. Broadly speaking, we identify three interrelated categories of interface technology: (1) imaging and sensory devices, (2) robotic devices and systems, and (3) human-machine interfaces. Research in these areas draws on a broad spectrum of core engineering research disciplines, such as materials science, mechanical engineering, control theory, and device physics. The fundamental challenge is to extend the sensory, motor, and human-adaptation abilities of computer-based systems in a demanding and constrained environment. Particular needs include compactness, precision, biocompatibility, imager compatibility, dexterity, sterility, and human factors.

Figure 14.4 illustrates the overall information flow of CIS systems from the surgical CAD/CAM paradigm perspective. The CIS systems combine preoperative and intraoperative modeling and planning with computer-assisted execution and assessment. The structure of the surgical assistant systems is similar, except that many more decisions are made intraoperatively, since preoperative models and plans may sometimes be relatively less important. Broadly speaking, surgery with a CIS system comprises three phases, all drawing upon a common technology base.

- *Preoperative phase*. A surgical plan is developed from a patient-specific model generated from preoperative images and a priori information about human anatomy contained in an anatomical atlas or database. Planning is highly application dependent since the surgical procedures are greatly different. In some cases, it may be simple interactive simulations or the selection of some key target positions, such as performing a tumor biopsy in neurosurgery. In other cases, such as in craneofacial surgery, planning can require sophisticated optimizations incorporating tissue characteristics, biomechanics, or other information contained in the atlas and adapted to the patient-specific model.
- *Intraoperative phase*. The images, patient-specific model, and plan information are brought into the operating room and registered to the patient, on the basis of information from a variety of sensors, such as a spatial tracking system and/or intraoperative imaging device. In some cases, the

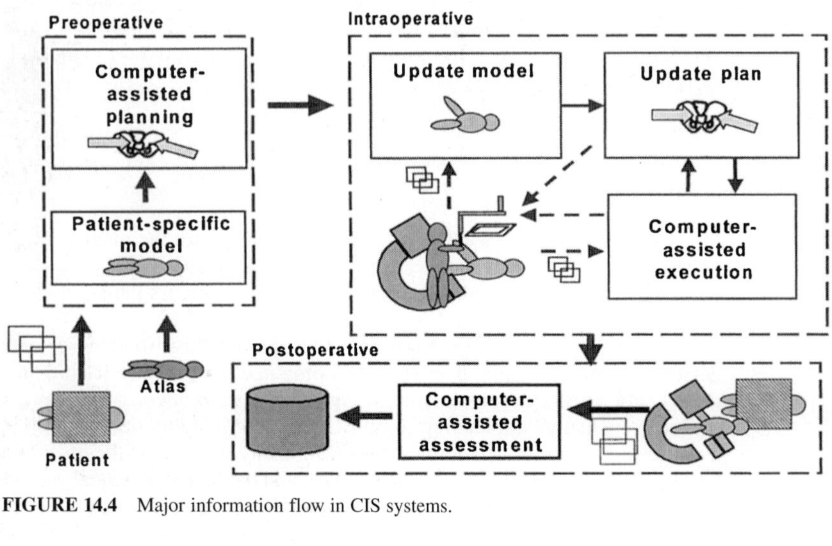

FIGURE 14.4 Major information flow in CIS systems.

model and plan may be further updated, based on the images. The computer then uses a variety of interface devices to assist the surgeon in executing the surgical plan. Depending on what is most appropriate for the application these interfaces may include active devices such as robots, "smart" hand tools, and information displays. As the surgery proceeds, additional images or other measurements may be taken to assess progress and provide feedback for controlling tools and therapy delivery. On the basis of this feedback, the patient model may be updated during the procedure. This updated model may be used to refine or update the surgical plan to ensure that the desired goals are met. Ideally, intraoperative imaging and other feedback can ensure that the technical goals of the surgical intervention have been achieved before the patient leaves the operating room. Further, the computer can identify and record a complete record of pertinent information about the procedure without significant additional cost or overhead.

- *Postoperative phase*. The preoperative and intraoperative information are combined with additional images and tests, both to verify the technical results of the procedure and to assess the longer-term clinical results for the patient. Further, the results of many procedures may be registered back to an anatomical atlas to facilitate statistical studies relating surgical technique to clinical outcomes.

Note that the above description is of an idealized CIS system: specific systems do not necessarily require all these capabilities, and some of them are beyond the current state of the art. However, we will use this generic description to organize the technical discussion in the following section.

From a surgeon's perspective, the key difference between advanced medical equipment and a CIS system is the information integration, both between phases and within each phase. This new capability requires in most cases modifications to existing surgical protocols, and in a few cases radically new protocols. It could also enable more surgeons to perform certain difficult procedures that require much coordination and knowledge available to only a few experienced specialists, or perform procedures that are currently not feasible.

14.3 THE TECHNOLOGY OF CIS SYSTEMS

This section describes the main technical elements of CIS systems. We begin with a brief summary of medical imaging devices, and then present methods for image processing, visualization, and modeling. We describe next preoperative planning and analysis, followed by registration of data from various sources. Then we discuss tracking and sensing, robotics, man-machine interfaces, and systems integration technology.

14.3.1 Medical Imaging

Medical images, both preoperative and intraoperative, are the main sources of information for CIS systems.

Since they are used in all CIS systems, we briefly discuss their technical characteristics and typical uses.

We distinguish between preoperative and intraoperative imaging devices. Preoperative imaging devices, such as film and digital x-rays, computed tomography (CT), magnetic resonance imaging (MRI), and nuclear magnetic tomography (NMT), in various forms, are used to obtain images for diagnosis and surgical planning. In most cases, the imaging devices are large and are located outside the surgical suite. Two-dimensional film x-ray images are the most common, with superb spatial resolution, gray-value range, and contrast, and negligible noise and geometric distortion. However, they are two-dimensional projections of spatial structures, and are not amenable to processing for further use unless scanned. CT and MRI images are used to visualize anatomical structures, with CT best suited for bony structures and MRI best suited for soft tissue. They consist of a series of two-dimensional parallel cross-sectional images with high spatial resolution, little geometric distortion and intensity bias, good signal-to-noise ratio, and a wide field of view. Typical data sets consist of 80 to 150 images of size 512 × 512 12-bit gray-level pixel images with pixel size of 0.4 × 0.4 mm at 1- to 2-mm intervals. They can be used to visualize anatomical structures, perform spatial measurements, and extract three-dimensional anatomical models. NMT images show functional anatomy, such as nerve activity, and are mostly used in the brain. They also consist of a series of two-dimensional parallel slices, although their quality is lower. They are usually viewed in conjunction with MRI images. The main drawback of preoperative images is that they are static and don't always reflect the position and orientation of anatomical structures which have moved between the time the images were taken and the surgery is performed.

Intraoperative imaging devices include fluoroscopic x-ray, ultrasound, and video image streams from endoscopes, laparoscopes, and surgical microscopes. Fluoroscopic x-ray is widely used in orthopedics to visualize and adjust the position of surgical instruments with respect to bones, or to locate kidney stones. The images are obtained from a mobile C-arm unit, which allows capturing two-dimensional projection images from different viewpoints while the patient lies on the table. The circular images are usually displayed on a video monitor. They have a narrow field of view (6 to 12 in, 400 pixels in diameter), limited spatial resolution and contrast, and present varying, position-dependent intensity and geometric distortions. They are mostly used for qualitative evaluation, and have cumulative radiation as a side effect. Ultrasound images (both static and as sequences) are used to obtain images of anatomy close to the skin. Unlike x-ray images, they have no ionizing radiation, but present significant imaging artifacts, such as speckling, noise, and spatial distortion. They also have a narrow field of view and have the resolution and image quality of the standard video monitor where they are displayed. Video image streams became commonplace with the introduction of minimally invasive surgery in the 1980s. They are used to support tumor biopsies, gall bladder removals, and colon explorations, among many others. They allow the surgeon to visualize in real time anatomy and surgical instruments inserted in a body cavity. The limitations of these imaging devices are that they have a narrow field of view (about 3 in), have no depth perception, uneven illumination, distortion due to the use of wide-angle lenses, and require direct line of sight. Surgeons must learn how to move and point the camera while respecting various point-of-entry and location constraints. The main advantage of intraoperative images is that they provide an up-to-date image of the surgical situation. However, the field of view and image quality are far inferior to preoperative images. More recent intraoperative imaging devices include surgical open MRI, surgical CT, and three-dimensional (3D) ultrasound, which overcome some of the limitations of the more common imaging devices.

The main limitation of current practice is that there is no quantitative correlation between high-quality preoperative images and intraoperative images. The surgeon must mentally establish the spatial correlation between the images and base decisions on this correlation.

14.3.2 Image Processing, Visualization, and Modeling

After image acquisition, the first task is usually visualization for diagnosis, evaluation, and planning. The visualization can take place on displays other than those of the devices where they were acquired, and can require various image-processing techniques for better evaluation. These include image balancing and enhancement, distortion and contrast correction, denoising, and spatial aggregation. For example, individual two-dimensional x-ray and ultrasound images can be processed using an array of standard image processing techniques to improve their clinical value. They can be visualized using zooming, cropping, and other imaging techniques. They can also be combined to create new, multimodal images.

Visualization of CT, MRI, and nuclear medicine images can greatly benefit from specialized visualization techniques, since they are series of two-dimensional cross sections. Instead of having the surgeon mentally correlate consecutive slices and create a mental three-dimensional view, it is desirable to directly reconstruct the three-dimensional information and show it as a new computed image. There are two families of visualization algorithms: volume visualization and surface visualization. We describe them briefly next.

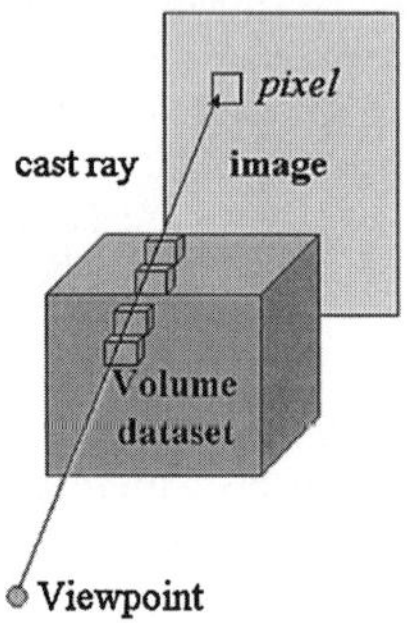

FIGURE 14.5 Volumetric rendering by ray casting. (*Adapted from Ref. 9.*)

Volume visualization algorithms[9] take as input slices and produce a three-dimensional image from any desired viewpoint. The most common method of generating the three-dimensional images is ray casting (Fig. 14.5). The data set is viewed as a volumetric data set, in which the space is divided into small volume units, called *voxels*. The voxels are rectangular blocks whose upper and lower faces are consecutive slice pixels in the vertical direction, and whose height is the slice interval distance. To each voxel is associated an intensity value, which is interpolated from the nearby pixel intensity values. To obtain the three-dimensional image, rays emanating from the viewpoint's location toward the image plane are cast on the volume. The pixel intensities in the new image are computed according to an attenuation function, which indicates how to compose the voxel intensity values that the ray traverses. Different choices of attenuation function produce various effects, such as opaque bodies, semitransparency, or anatomy isolation according to predefined intensity ranges. For example, if only bony surfaces are to be shown, only voxels whose intensity values are within the range of bone intensity are considered in the attenuation function. The advantage of this method is its simplicity, as no previous segmentation or surface extraction is necessary. However, it is computationally expensive, as hundreds of thousands of voxels need to be examined for each new image. Various hardware (Z buffering) and software techniques (precomputed views, ray arrays) have been developed to speed up the rendering process. Another disadvantage is that no model of the anatomy is created, restricting the types of analysis that can be performed on it. Volume visualization is best suited for complex anatomy with fine details, such as the brain gray matter.

Surface-based visualization algorithms rely on geometric surface models of the anatomy to be visualized. The inputs are usually objects described as triangular meshes extracted from the original data representing the surface of the anatomical structures of interest, such as the skull, femur, kidneys, and colon. The objects are then displayed as CAD models on viewers that can take advantage of standard graphics hardware. The main advantage of surface-based visualization is that it has to handle smaller data sets and is thus computationally much more efficient than volume visualization, allowing for near-real-time positioning and manipulation on standard computers. Another advantage is that CAD models of implants and surgical instruments can be readily incorporated into the image. However, surface-based visualization requires extracting the surface models, which can be difficult for complex anatomical structures with many fine details and complex geometry. Surface-based algorithms are best suited for anatomy with relatively large and clearly defined surfaces, such as bones and intestinal conduits.

Model construction algorithms are a prerequisite to surface-based visualization and for all tasks that require a geometric model of the anatomy: preoperative planning, contour-based registration, anatomical atlas construction, and matching. Their input is a series of slices, and a predefined intensity threshold interval that defines the image intensity ranges of the anatomy of interest. The output is one or more triangular meshes describing the geometry of the surfaces. Mesh extraction algorithms can be divided into two families: 2D contour extraction algorithms and 3D surface reconstruction algorithms. Contour extraction algorithms work by segmenting (manually or automatically) the contour of the anatomy of interest in each slice, and then connecting the resulting successive 2D contours to form a 3D surface. A point p_1 on the contour extracted in slice i is connected to the next point p_2 on the same contour at a predefined distance, and both are connected to the closest point p_3 in slice $i + 1$ to form a triangle $p_1p_2p_3$ which represents a surface element. By alternating between consecutive slices, a triangulated ribbon is created between the boundary contours. The drawback of this method is that ambiguities can arise as to how points should be selected to create triangles, resulting in topologically inconsistent surfaces (holes, self-intersections, etc.).

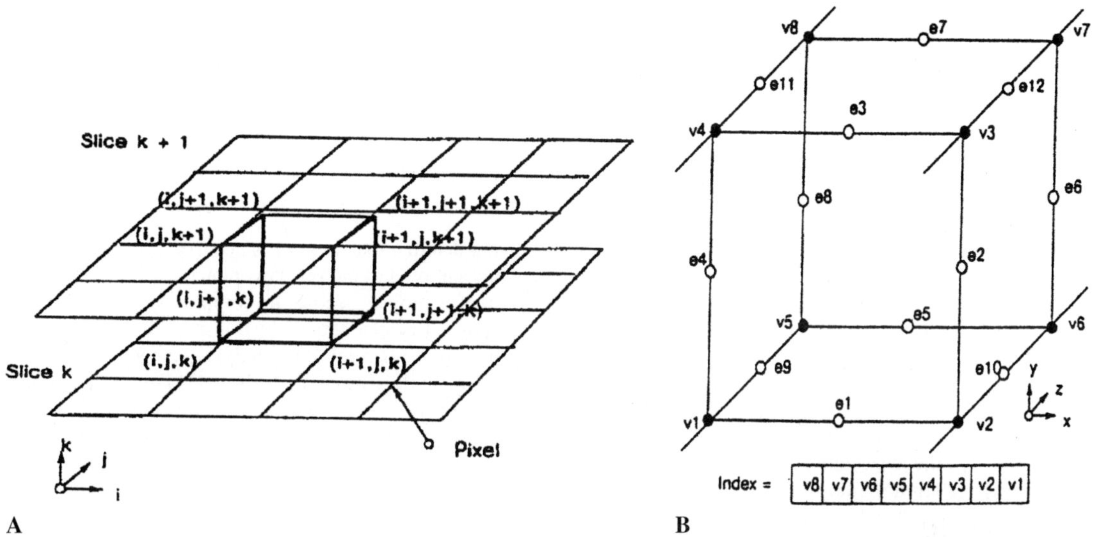

FIGURE 14.6 (*a*) Principle of the marching cubes algorithm: indexes for the marching cube and (*b*) coding scheme. (*Reproduced with permission from Ref. 10.*)

To alleviate this problem, surface reconstruction algorithms work directly on the volumetric data to identify the voxels, which are intersected by the object surface and determine its geometry. The most commonly used algorithm in this category is the so-called marching cubes algorithm.[10] The algorithm proceeds as follows: A moving cube whose vertices are the pixels of two subsequent slices is formed. The eight vertices of the cube have associated with them a binary number (0 or 1), which indicates if the corresponding pixel intensity value is above or below a prespecified threshold (Fig. 14.6). When all eight vertices have a value of 0 (1), the voxel is entirely outside (inside) the anatomical object of interest. Cubes with mixed values (one or more 0 and 1) are at the boundary of the object. Depending on which vertex values are zero or one, one or more triangular surfaces cutting the cube can be constructed. There are $2^8 = 256$ cases, which can be reduced by symmetry to 14 cases and stored in a lookup table for reference. The algorithm proceeds by moving the cube from the topmost, upper corner of the first two slices to the lowest, bottom corner of the last two slices in sequence. Depending on the vertex values, the table is accessed and the corresponding triangles are constructed. The advantage of this algorithm is its locality, and that the surfaces constructed are topologically consistent (ambiguities in surface construction can be resolved locally). Variants of this algorithm include a tetrahedron instead of a cube, for which there are only two cases with no ambiguities, but which produce 2 to 5 times more triangles. The resulting meshes are typically several tens to several hundreds of thousands of triangles, depending on the slice spacing on the original data set. Mesh simplification algorithms can then be applied to the resulting models to reduce their complexity with minimal loss of accuracy.

While surface models are the most commonly used in CIS systems, they are by no means the only types of models. Functional models, containing relevant information specific to an anatomical structure or procedure can also be extracted with custom techniques. For example, a kinematic model of the leg bones and joints is of interest when planning a total knee replacement. To construct this model, geometric entities such as the mechanical axis of the femur, the center of the femoral head, and other anatomical landmarks should be extracted. Each surgical application requires the construction of its model and the simulation associated with it.

Another type of model used in CIS is a digital atlas. Digital atlases are constructed from detailed imaging data of a person and are used for visualization, planning, and educational purposes. An example of this type of data is the Visible Human Project, which has detailed CT, MRI, and photographic data of a male and a female. The data are carefully segmented and labeled, and a database of organs is constructed from the data. The model can then be inspected, for example, using the VOXEL-MAN software,[11] or used to match to other patient data.

14.3.3 Preoperative Analysis and Planning

Once the diagnosis has been made and it has been decided that surgery is necessary, the next step is to carry preoperative analysis and elaborate a surgical plan of action. This plan can range from simple tasks such as determining the access point of a biopsy needle, to complex gait simulations, implant stress analysis, or radiation dosage planning. Because the analysis and planning is specific to each surgical procedure and anatomy, preoperative planning and analysis software is usually custom to each clinical application. These systems can be viewed as medical CAD systems, which allow the user to manipulate and visualize medical images, models of anatomy, implants, and surgical tools, perform simulations, and elaborate plans. To give the reader an idea of the current scope of these systems, we will briefly describe two planning systems, one for orthopedics and one for radiation therapy.

In orthopedics, planning systems are generally used to select implants and find their optimal placement with respect to anatomy. For example, a planning system for spinal pedicle screw insertion shows the surgeon three orthogonal cross sections of the acquired CT image (the original *xy* slice and interpolated *xz* and *yz* slices) and a three-dimensional image of the vertebrae surfaces. The surgeon selects a screw type and its dimensions, and positions it with respect to the anatomy in the three cross-sectional views. A projection of the screw CAD model is superimposed on the images, and its position and orientation with respect to the viewing plane can be modified, with the result displayed in the other windows. Once a satisfactory placement has been obtained, the system stores it with the screw information for use in the operating room. Similar systems exist for total hip and total knee replacement, which, in addition, automatically generate in some cases machining plans (cut files) for intraoperative surgical robots. Other systems also extract kinematic or finite-element models and perform gait and stress analysis that help surgeons estimate the effectiveness of the proposed solution.

Another example of a complex planning system is in the field of radiation therapy. The goal of radiation therapy is to kill tumor cells by exposing them to a radiation beam while affecting as little as possible the surrounding healthy cells. One way of achieving this is to expose the tumor cells to radiation beams from different directions so that the cumulative radiation effect on the tumor cells destroys them while preserving the surrounding healthy cells. The planning task consists of identifying the tumor and the critical areas where no radiation should be present from MRI images, and then selecting the number of beams, their radius, intensity, duration, and placement that maximizes the radiation to the tumor cells while minimizing the radiation to other cells, especially those in the critical areas. This problem is formulated as a geometric minimum-maximum constrained optimization problem, and solved with a combination of geometric and nonlinear optimization techniques. The planning system includes a data visualization and volume definition module, and outputs a series of location commands to the robotic arm carrying the radiation source, and the beam information at each location.

14.3.4 Registration

Multimodal registration is one of the key steps for information integration in CIS systems. The goal of the registration process is to allow the combination of data from several modalities, possibly taken at different times, so that they can be viewed and analyzed jointly. Registering two data sets consists of finding a transformation that aligns common features in two modalities, so that their spatial locations coincide. Registration is necessary for many tasks such as

- Combine information of the same patient taken with different modalities, such as CT and MRI or MRI and PET
- Combine information of the same patient before, during, and after surgery, such as preoperative CT and intraoperative x-ray fluoroscopy, preoperative MRI and intraoperative video from a microscope or an endoscope, or CT and x-rays from before and after surgery
- Create real-time virtual reality views of moving anatomy and surgical tools by matching preoperative models from CFT or MRI with intraoperative tracking data
- Perform a statistical study of patient data

Most CIS applications require more than one transformation to link two data sets, and thus have more than one registration problem. For example, in the ROBODOC system, the preoperative plan has to be registered to the intraoperative position of the bone so that the robot tip can machine the desired canal shape in the planed position. To obtain this transformation, we must compute the transformation from the bone coordinate system to the implanted fiducials, then from the fiducials to the robot tip, to the robot coordinate system, and then to the cut volume. The series of mathematical transformations that align one data set with another is called the *registration chain*.

The registration task is in fact not one but many different problems. There are great differences on technical approaches, depending on the type of data to be matched, the anatomy involved, and the clinical and technical requirements of the procedure. There is a vast body of literature on registration, which is comprehensively surveyed in Refs. 12 and 13 and can be classified according to the following characteristics:

- *Modalities*. Refer to the sources from which data are acquired, for example, x-ray, CT, MRI, PET, video, tracker. The combinations can be unimodal (same data source) or multimodal (different data sources), which can be two images, an image to a model, or an image to a patient (tracker data).
- *Dimensionality*. Refers to the spatial and temporal dimensions of the two data sets to be matched (two- or three-dimensional, static or time varying). The registration dimensionality can be static 2D/2D (x-ray images), 2D/3D (ultrasound to MRI), 3D/3D (PET to MRI) or time varying, such as digital subtraction angiography (DSA).
- *Registration basis*. Refers to the image features that will be used to establish the alignment. These can be extrinsic registration objects, such as a stereotactic frame or fiducial markers, or intrinsic, such as anatomical landmarks, anatomical contours, or pixel intensity values.
- *Nature and domain of mathematical transformation*. Refers to the type of mathematical transformation that is used to perform the alignment. The transformation can be rigid, affine, projective, or generally curved (deformable registration), and can be applied to parts of the image (local) or to the entire image (global).
- *Solution method*. Refers to how the transformation is computed. This can include direct solutions when an analytic solution or an appropriate approximation is found, or iterative solutions, where there is a search and numerical optimization methods are used.
- *Type of interaction*. Refers to the type of input that the user has to supply. The registration is interactive when it is performed entirely by the user, automatic when no user intervention is required, or semiautomatic when the user supplies an initial estimate, helps in the data segmentation, or steers the algorithm by accepting or rejecting possible solutions.
- *Subject*. Refers to the patient source from which the images are taken; it can be the same patient (intrasubject), two different patients (intersubject), or a patient and an atlas.
- *Anatomy*. Refers to the anatomy being imaged. This can be the head (brain, skull, teeth, nasal cavities), the thorax (heart, breast, ribs), the abdomen (kidney, liver, intestines), the pelvis and the perineum, or the limbs (femur, tibia, humerus, hand).

The main steps of registration algorithms are summarized in Table 14.2. Before attempting to match the datasets, each data set should be corrected for distortions so that the errors resulting from

TABLE 14.2 Basic Steps of a Registration Algorithm

Input: Two data sets to be matched, image acquisition parameters
  Process each data set separately to correct for geometric and intensity distortion and to reduce noise

While *there is dissimilarity* **and** *there is improvement* **do:**
  Extract features or regions of interest from both images
  Pair features from each data set
  Formulate a similarity measure based on pairing
  Find the transformation T that most reduces the dissimilarity
  Transform one of the data sets by T

Output: Transformation T

imaging artifacts do not affect the accuracy of the registration process. Next, what should be matched is identified in each image. This can be point landmarks, contours, surfaces, pixel values and their gradients, or regions of interest. The pairwise correspondence between these is established so that a measure of similarity between the data sets can be established. The more the features are apart, the larger the dissimilarity is. The similarity is usually formulated as a constrained minimization problem whose minimum is the transformation T that reduces the dissimilarity the most. If no closed form solution exists, the local minimum is found by numerical optimization. One of the data sets is moved by the transformation, and the process is repeated until the match is sufficiently good or no further improvement is possible.

Technically, registration techniques can be classified as rigid or deformable, and geometry or intensity based. Rigid registration computes a transformation of position and orientation between two data sets. It is applicable to rigid structures that change their position but not their shape, such as bones, implanted fiducials, and stereotactic frames, as an approximation to quasi-rigid structures, such as tumors or brain white matter. It is also used as the first step of deformable registration, which computes a general global or local curved map. Deformable registration is necessary for matching soft tissue organs (e.g., brain images before and after brain shift) for time-dependent comparisons (e.g., tumor growth evaluation), and for cross-patient and atlas comparisons. The main difficulties of deformable registration are that the problem is ill posed, since there are usually infinitely many transformations that match the data, and error measurements and comparisons are difficult. The geometric approach uses the spatial disparity (usually the distance) between geometric entities, such as points, contours, or surfaces. The intensity-based approach uses the pixel intensity values and the intensity gradient between pixels to maximize the image correlation.

Examples of common registration tasks are

- Rigid geometric registration between a surface model obtained from preoperative CT and intraoperative surface data on the same anatomy obtained by touching landmarks or collecting sample points with a tracker. This method is widely used in CIS orthopedic systems, such as pedicle screw fixation, total hip and knee replacement, and trauma.
- Deformable intensity-based registration between brain MRI data sets before and after brain shift.

14.3.5 Positional Tracking and Other Sensing

An important feature of many CIS systems is the ability to accurately determine in real time the location of selected anatomical structures, surgical instruments, and implants during surgery. This information is necessary for visualization, navigation, and guidance. The component that delivers this information to the CIS system is called a *tracker* or a *localizer*.

There are many technologies available for positional tracking, including encoded mechanical linkages, acoustic tracking, electromagnetic tracking, optical tracking using specialized devices, and optical tracking using conventional computer vision methods. Typically, these systems measure the motion relative to some base device of individual elements (which we will call *markers*) attached to the objects to be tracked. Several excellent surveys are available on this subject.[14,15] Each method has advantages and drawbacks. The main comparison parameters include setup requirements, work volume characteristics, number of objects that can be tracked simultaneously, the update frequency, the static and dynamic accuracy, the variability and repeatability of the readings, and cost.

Currently, the most commonly used position tracking approaches are based on specialized optical devices such as the Optotrak® and Polaris® systems (Northern Digital, Waterloo, Ontario) and Pixsys® and FlashPoint® systems (Image Guided Technologies, Boulder, Colorado). These devices use two or more optical cameras to identify light-emitting diodes or reflective markers in the camera image and compute their location by stereo triangulation. They can be quite accurate, providing 3D localization accuracies ranging from 0.1 to about 0.5 mm in typical applications. Their drawbacks include cost and the necessity of maintaining a clear line of sight between the sensors and the markers. Magnetic tracking systems such as the Polhemus® (Rockwell International, Milwaukee, Wisconsin), Flock-of-Birds® (Ascension Technology, Burlington, Vermont), and Aurora® (Northern Digital, Waterloo, Canada) systems are also widely used. These systems do not have line-of-sight constraints, but may be subject to field distortion from materials in the operating room.

Force sensors are commonly used in medical robotic systems to measure and monitor tool-to-tissue and tool-to-surgeon interaction forces.[16–21] Generally speaking, the technology used in these sensors is the same as that used in other applications, although specific issues of sterility and compactness often present unusual design strategies.

More broadly, a very wide variety of sensors may be used to determine any number of local tissue properties. Examples include electrical conductivity, optical coherence tomography, near-infrared sensing, and temperature sensing, to name a few.

14.3.6 Robotics

Medical robot systems have the same basic components as any other robot system: a controller, manipulators, end effectors, communications interfaces, etc. Many of the design challenges are familiar to anyone who has developed an industrial system. However, the unique demands of the surgical environment, together with the emphasis on cooperative execution of surgical tasks, rather than unattended automation, do create some unusual challenges. Table 14.3 compares the strengths and weaknesses of humans and robots in surgical applications.

Safety is paramount in any surgical robot, and must be given careful attention at all phases of system design. Each element of the hardware and software should be subjected to rigorous validation at all phases, ranging from design through implementation and manufacturing to actual deployment in

TABLE 14.3 Complementary Strengths of Human Surgeons and Robots

	Strengths	Limitations
Humans	Excellent judgment. Excellent hand-eye coordination. Excellent dexterity (at natural "human" scale). Able to integrate and act on multiple information sources. Easily trained. Versatile and able to improvise.	Prone to fatigue and inattention. Tremor limits fine motion. Limited manipulation ability and dexterity outside natural scale. Bulky end effectors (hands). Limited geometric accuracy. Hard to keep sterile. Affected by radiation, infection.
Robots	Excellent geometric accuracy. Untiring and stable. Immune to ionizing radiation. Can be designed to operate at many different scales of motion and payload. Able to integrate multiple sources of numerical and sensor data.	Poor judgment. Hard to adapt to new situations. Limited dexterity. Limited hand-eye coordination. Limited ability to integrate and interpret complex information.

the operating room. Redundant sensing and consistency checks are essential for all safety-critical functions. Reliability experience gained with a particular design or component adapted from industrial applications is useful but not sufficient or even always particularly relevant, since designs must often be adapted for operating room conditions. It is important to guard against both the effects of electrical, electronic, or mechanical component failure and the more insidious effects of a perfectly functioning robot system correctly executing an improper motion command caused by improper registration between the computer's model of the patient and the actual patient. Further excellent discussion may be found in Refs. 22 and 23 and in a number of papers on specific systems.

Sterility is also a crucial concern. Usually, covering most of the robot with a sterile bag or drape and then separately sterilizing the instruments or end effectors provides sterility. Autoclaving, which is the most universal and popular sterilization method, can unfortunately be very destructive for electromechanical components, force sensors, and other components. Other common methods include gas (slow, but usually kindest to equipment) and soaking.

Manipulator design is very important in medical robots. Several early systems (e.g., Ref. 24) used essentially unmodified industrial robots. Although this is perhaps marginally acceptable in a research system that will simply position a guide and then be turned off before any contact is made with a patient, any use of an unmodified robot capable of high speeds is inherently suspect. Great care needs to be taken to protect both the patient and operating room personnel from runaway conditions. It is generally better to make several crucial modifications to any industrial robot that will be used in surgery. These include

- Installation of redundant position sensing
- Changes in gear ratios to slow down maximum end-effector speed
- Thorough evaluation and possible redesign for electrical safety and sterility

Because the speed/work volume design points for industrial and surgical applications are very different, a more recent trend has emphasized design of custom manipulator kinematic structures for specific classes of applications.[25–30]

Many surgical applications (e.g., in laparoscopy or neuroendoscopy) require surgical instruments to pass through a narrow opening into the patient's body. This constraint has led a number of groups to consider two rather different approaches in designing robots for such applications. The first approach (e.g., Figs. 14.7*b*, 14.8, 14.9, and 14.10)[25,26,31,32] uses goniometers, chain drives, parallel

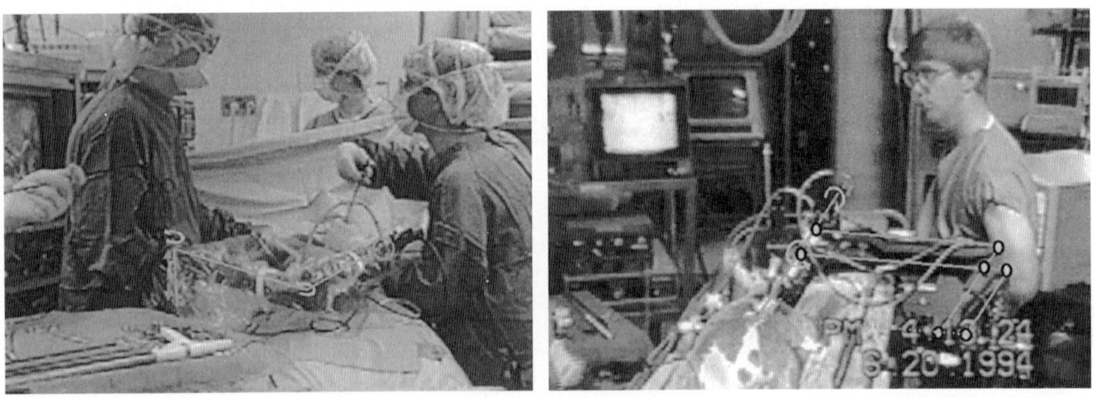

A **B**

FIGURE 14.7 Two robotic assistants for laparoscopic surgery. (*a*) The AESOP® system is a widely deployed commercial system for manipulating a laparoscopic camera. The robot combines active joints with a 2-degree-of-freedom wrist to achieve four controlled motions of the endoscope while preventing lateral forces from being exerted at the entry point into the patient's body. (*b*) The experimental IBM/JHU LARS system uses a five-bar linkage to decouple rotational and translational motions at the entry point. Both approaches have been used in a number of experimental and clinically deployed surgical robots. (*AESOP photo courtesy Computer Motion, Inc.*)

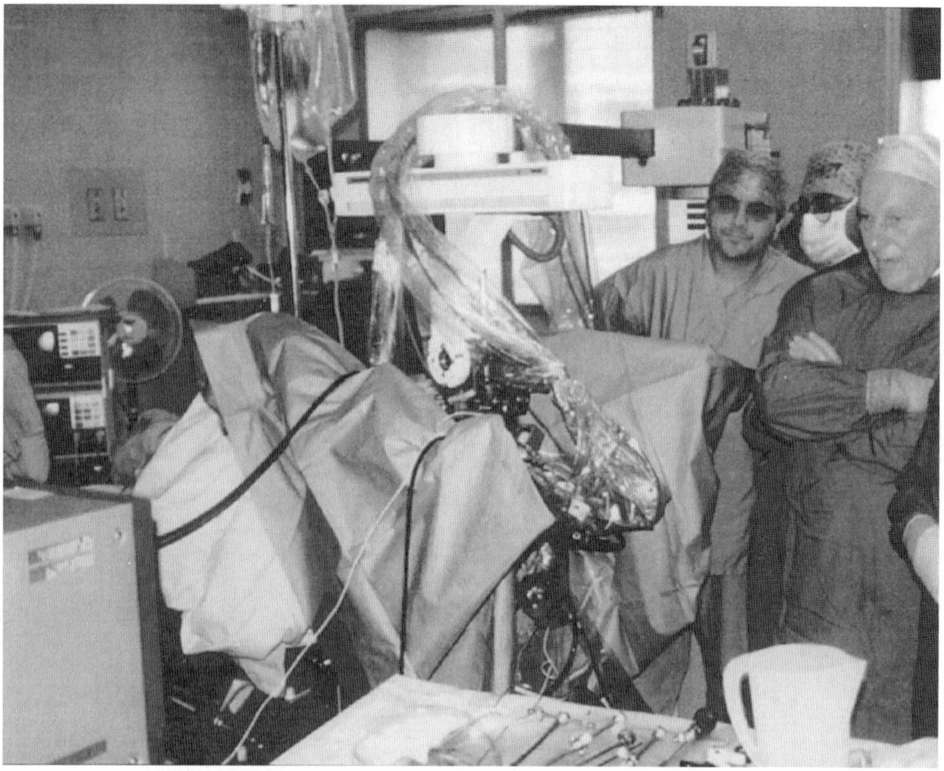

FIGURE 14.8 Robot system for transurethral prostate surgery.[25] This system uses goniometer arcs to provide conical motions about an apex point remote from the mechanism. (*Photo courtesy Brian Davies.*)

five-bar linkages, or other means to decouple instrument motions about an "isocenter" which is placed at the entry portal. The second approach (e.g., Fig. 14.7*a*)[33–35] relies on passive compliance to cause the surgical instrument to comply with the entry portal constraint. In this case, the robot's "wrist" typically has two unactuated, but encoded, rotary axes proximal to the surgical instrument holder. Both approaches have merit, and they can be combined fruitfully.[36] The first approach is usually more precise and provides a more stable platform for stereotactic procedures. The second approach has the advantages of being simple and of automatically accommodating patient motions. A fuller discussion of the trade-off can be found in Ref. 36.

Surgical manipulators are not always active devices. Often, the human surgeon provides some or all of the motive power, while the computer provides real-time navigational or other assistance.[25,27,32,37–39]

Because medical robots are often used together with imaging, materials are also an important concern in surgical manipulator design equipment.[27,40] Figure 14.9 shows one example of a simple 1-degree-of-freedom radiolucent mechanism that can be used to drive needles into soft tissue.[27] This device is designed for use with fluoroscopic x-rays or CT scanners, and it can be employed either with a simple support clamp or as the end effector of an active robot. Fiducial geometry can be added easily to the robot or end effectors to assist in registration of the robot to the images (Fig. 14.11).[41–45]

Development of robotic devices for use with magnetic resonance imaging (MRI) poses special challenges because of the strong magnetic fields and RF signals involved. Figures 14.12 and 14.13 show two typical systems.[40,46]

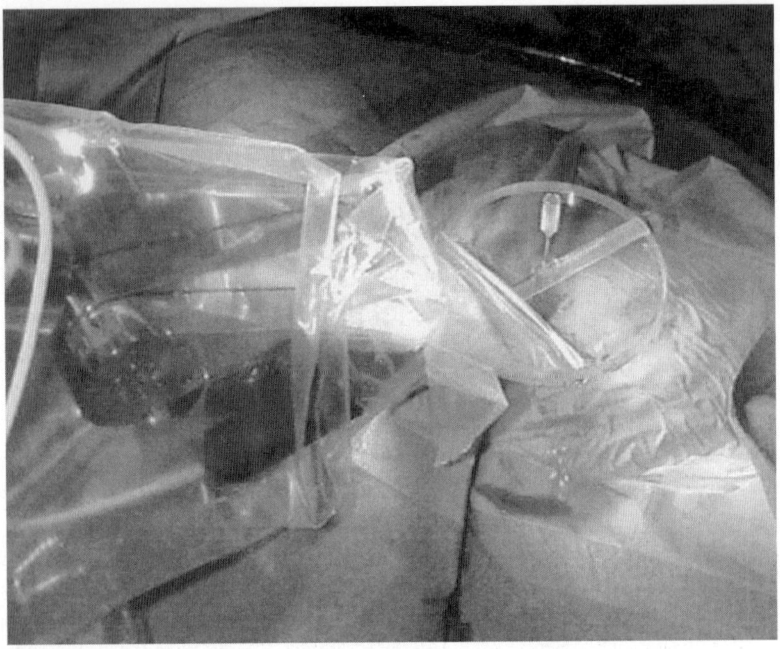

FIGURE 14.9 RCM robot with radiolucent PAKY needle driver used in percutaneous kidney stone removal.[127,158–162] *(Photo courtesy Dan Stoianovici.)*

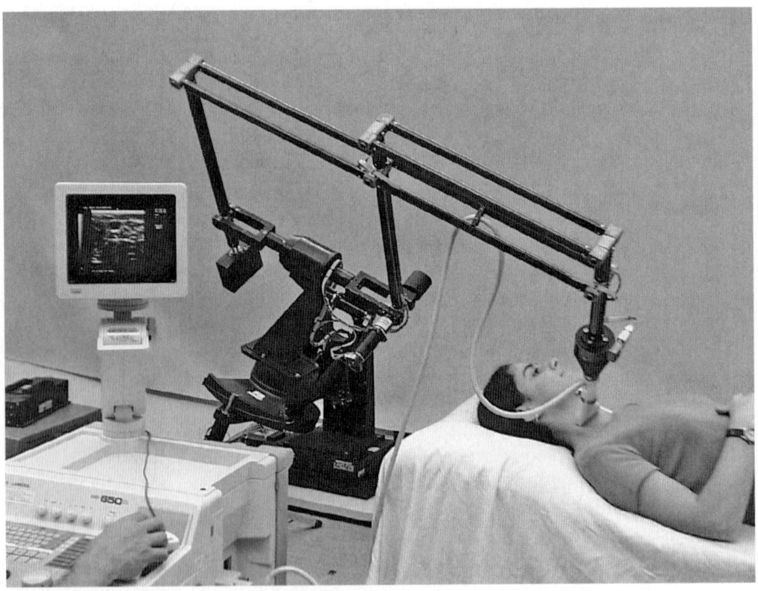

FIGURE 14.10 Robotic system for diagnostic ultrasound.[148] *(Photo courtesy S. Salcudean.)*

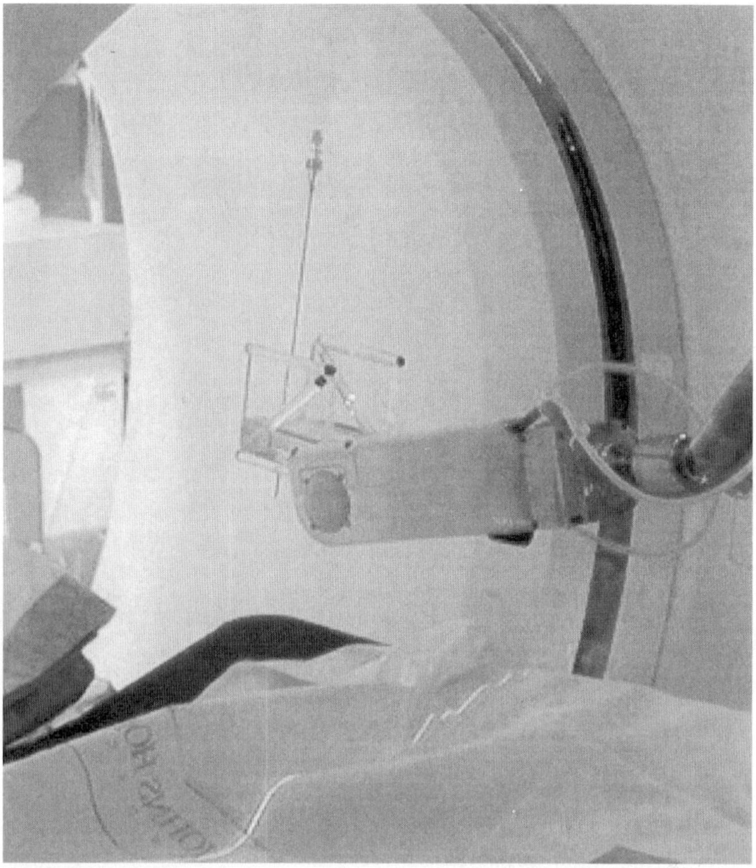

FIGURE 14.11 RCM robot with radiolucent CT-compatible needle driver.[42,44,45]

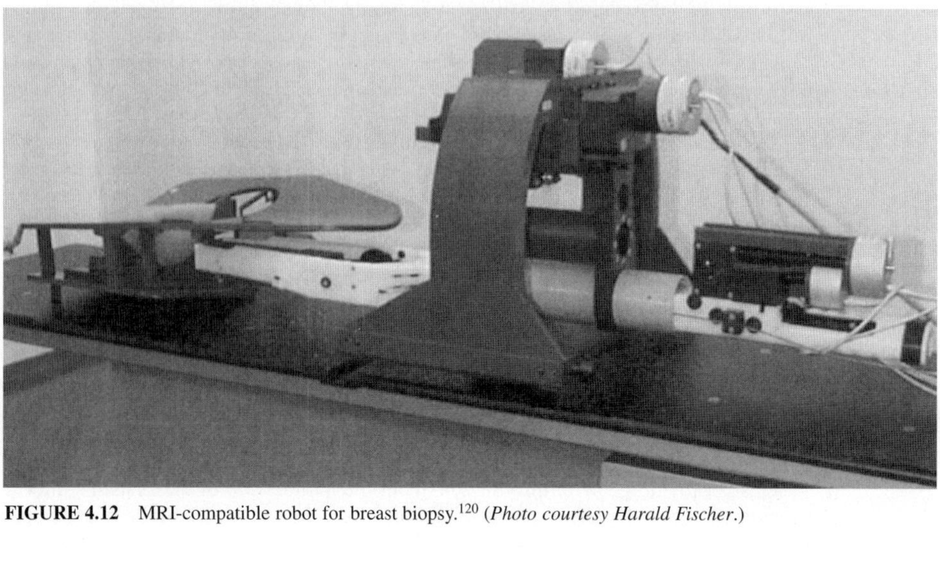

FIGURE 4.12 MRI-compatible robot for breast biopsy.[120] (*Photo courtesy Harald Fischer.*)

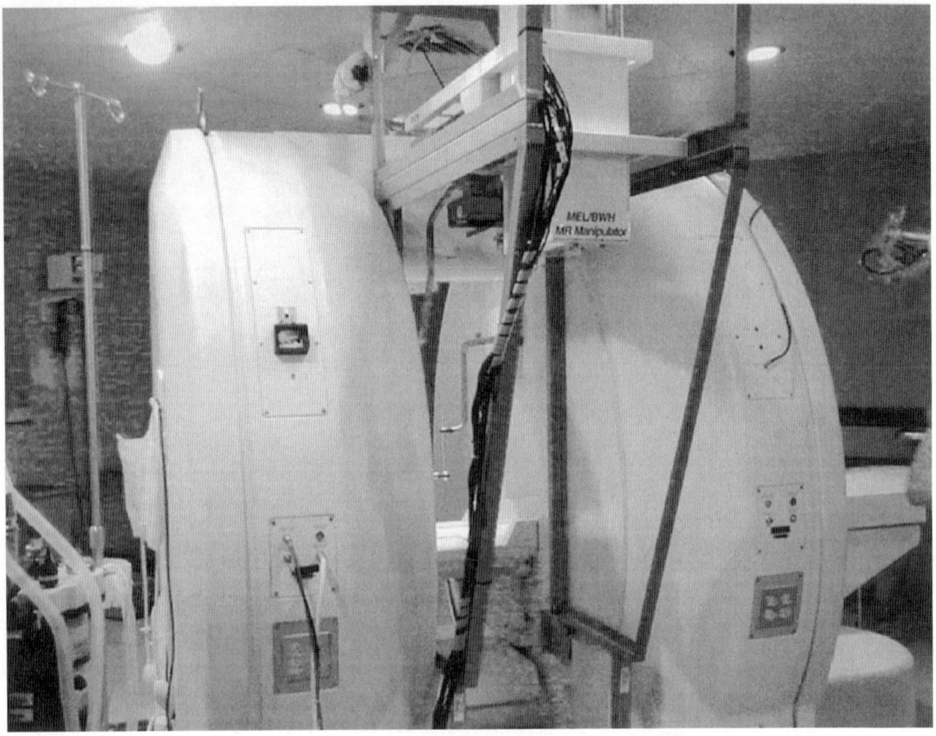

FIGURE 14.13 Robot system for use in open-magnet MRI system.[117]

14.3.7 Human-Machine Interfaces

Computer-based systems that work cooperatively with humans must communicate with them, both to provide information and to receive commands and guidance. As with surgical robots, surgical human-machine interfaces (HMIs) have much in common with those for other application domains, and they draw upon essentially the same technologies (speech, computer vision and graphics, haptics, etc.) that have found use elsewhere. In many cases, HMI subsystems that have been developed for other uses may be adapted with little change for surgical use. However, attention must be given to the unusual requirements of surgical applications.[47] Surgeons tend to have very high expectations about system responsiveness and transparency but have very low tolerance for interfaces that impede their work. On the other hand, they can also be quite willing to put up with great inconvenience if the system is really performing a useful function that truly extends their capabilities.

Surgeons overwhelmingly rely on vision as their dominant source of feedback during surgery. Indeed, the explosion in minimal access surgery over the past decade has very largely been the result of the availability of compact, high-resolution video cameras attached to endoscopic optics. In these cases, the surgeon's attention is naturally focused on a television monitor. In such cases, it is often possible for the computer to add computer graphics, text, and other information to the video stream.[48,49] Similarly, surgical navigation systems [8,9,45–52] provide computer graphic renderings and feedback based on tracked surgical instrument positions and preoperative images. The so-called virtual fluoroscopy systems[58–61] show predicted x-ray projections based on intraoperative fluoroscopic images and tracked instrument positions. One very important challenge in the design of such systems is providing useful information about the *imprecision* of the system's information, so that the surgeon does not make decisions based on a false determination of the relative position of a surgical instrument and target anatomy. One common approach is to display a circle or ellipse representing likely registration uncertainty, but significant advances are needed both in the modeling of such errors and in the human factors associated with their presentation.

One limitation of video overlay systems is the limited resolution of current-generation video cameras. This is especially important in microsurgical applications, where the structures being operated on are very small, or in applications requiring very good color discrimination. Consequently, there is also interest in so-called optical overlay methods in which graphic information is projected into the optical path of a microscope[62] or presented on a half-silvered mirror[63,64] so that it appears to be superimposed on the surgeon's field of view in appropriate alignment. The design considerations for these systems are generally similar to those for systems using video displays, but the registration problems tend to be even more demanding and the brightness of the display can also be a problem.

All of the common interfaces (mice, joysticks, touch screens, push buttons, foot switches, etc.) used for interactive computer applications are used to provide input for surgical systems as well. For preoperative planning applications, these devices are identical to those used elsewhere. For intraoperative use, sterility, electrical safety, and ergonomic considerations may require some design modifications. For example, the LARS robot[48] repackaged the pointing device from an IBM Thinkpad® computer into a three-button "mouse" clipped onto the surgeon's instruments. As another example, a tracked stereotactic wand has been used to provide a configurable "push button" interface in which functions are selected by tapping the tip of the pointer onto a sterilized template.[65]

Surgeons routinely use voice to communicate with operating room personnel. Further, their hands (and feet) are frequently rather busy. Accordingly, there has long been interest in using voice as a two-way command and control system for surgical applications.[35,48,66–68]

Force and haptic feedback is often important for surgical simulation[68,69] and telesurgery applications.[19,21,70–73] Again, the technical issues involved are similar to those for other virtual-reality and telerobotics applications, with the added requirement of maintaining sterility and electrical safety.

14.3.8 Systems

Computer-integrated surgery is highly systems oriented. Well-engineered systems are crucial both for use in the operating room and to provide context for the development of new capabilities. Safety, usability and maintainability, and interoperability are the most important considerations. We discuss them briefly next.

Safety is very important. Surgical system designs must be both safe, in the sense that system failures will not result in significant harm to the patient and the system will be perceived to be safe. Good system design typically will require careful analysis of potential failure sources and the likely consequences of failures. This analysis is application dependent, and it is important to remember that care must be taken to ensure that system component failures will not go undetected and that the system will remain under control at all times. Wherever possible, redundant hardware and software subsystems should be provided and cross-checked against each other. Rigorous software engineering practices must be maintained at all stages. Discussion of general safety issues for surgical robots may be found in Refs. 22 and 74–77. An excellent case study of what can happen when good practices are ignored may be found in Ref. 78, which discusses a series of accidents involving a radiation therapy machine.

Many discussions of safety in CIS systems tend to focus on the potential of active devices such as robots or radiation therapy machines to do great harm if they operate in an uncontrolled manner. This is a valid concern, but it should not be forgotten that such "runaway" situations are not usually the main safety challenge in CIS systems. For example, both robotic and navigation assistance systems rely on the accuracy of registration methods and the ability to detect and/or compensate for patient motion to ensure that the surgical instruments do not stray from the targeted anatomy. A human surgeon acting on incorrect information can place a screw into the spinal cord just as easily as a robot can. This means that analysis software and sensing must be analyzed just as carefully as motion control. Surgeons must be fully aware of the limitations as well as the capabilities of their systems and system design should include appropriate means for surgeons' "sanity checking" of surgical actions.

System usability and maintainability are also important design considerations. Clearly, the ergonomic design of the system from the surgeon's perspective is important.[79,80] However, the interfaces provided for the operating room staff that must set up the equipment, help operate it, and provide routine maintenance are also crucial both for safety and economic reasons. Similarly, CIS systems should include interfaces to help field engineers troubleshoot and service equipment. In this regard, the ability of computer-based systems to log data during use can be especially useful in post-failure analysis and in scheduling preventive maintenance, as well as in providing data for improvement in surgical outcomes and techniques. Although most systems make some use of such facilities, they are probably underused in present-day commercial systems.

System interoperability is currently a major challenge. Commonly accepted open standards permitting different equipment to work together in a variety of settings are badly needed. Several companies have proposed proprietary standards for use by alliances of vendors, and there has been some academic and government-supported work to provide tool kits, especially in software. However, these efforts are still very fragmented.

14.4 EXAMPLES OF CIS SYSTEMS

There are already a few dozen CIS systems available commercially or as prototypes in research laboratories worldwide. Although it is not practical to present an exhaustive survey, this section describes a few examples of integrated systems that use parts of the technology described above. For the purposes of this overview, we distinguish between four types of systems:

1. Information enhancement systems
2. Robotic systems for precise preoperative plan execution
3. Robotic systems for human augmentation
4. Other robotic systems

Note that many real systems could logically fit in several of these categories.

14.4.1 Information Enhancement Systems

The purpose of information enhancement systems is to provide the surgeon and surgical team with accurate, up-to-date, and useful data and images during the surgery so that they can best develop and update their plan of action and perform surgical actions. To achieve this goal, information enhancement systems usually combine information from different modalities, such as preoperative CT and MRI data, real-time tracking data of tools and anatomy, intraoperative images such as ultrasound and fluoroscopic x-ray images, video sequences from endoscopic cameras, and more. In some cases, such as virtual diagnostic endoscopy, a simulated environment replaces the actual procedure. Information enhancement systems are by far the most commonly used CIS systems. What distinguishes them from other CIS systems is that it is the surgeon who performs all surgical gestures without any physical assistance from mechanical devices.

We classify information enhancement systems into three categories:

1. Navigation systems
2. Augmented reality navigation systems
3. Virtual reality systems

We describe them briefly next.

Navigation Systems. The purpose of intraoperative navigation systems is to provide surgeons with up-to-date, real-time information about the location of surgical tools and selected anatomy during surgery. The goal is to improve the surgeon's hand/eye coordination and spatial perception, thereby improving the accuracy of the surgical gestures. They support less invasive procedures, can shorten surgery time, and can improve outcomes.

The basic elements of a navigation system are

1. A real-time tracking system to follow one or more moving objects (anatomy, surgical tools, or implants)
2. Tracking-enabled tools and reference frames
3. A display showing the intraoperative situation
4. A computer to integrate the information (Fig. 14.2)

Since the patient is usually not immobilized, a dynamic reference frame is attached to the anatomy to correct the relative position of the tools to the images.

What is displayed depends on the type of images that are available. The navigation systems can be based on

- Preoperative images, such as CT or MRI augmented with CAD models of tools and implants
- Intraoperative images, such as fluoroscopic x-ray, ultrasound, or open MR images augmented with projections of tool CAD models and implant axes
- Intraoperative video streams from an endoscopic camera or a surgical microscope, shown alongside or fused with preoperative CT or MRI images

Navigation systems based on preoperative CT or MRI images are typically used as follows: Shortly before surgery, a preoperative CT or MRI study of the anatomy of interest is acquired. In some cases, fiducial markers that will be used for registration are attached to the patient skin or implanted to the anatomy so that they appear in the images. The data are downloaded to a computer, and a model of the anatomy is created. When there are fiducials, they are identified and their precise relative spatial location is computed. The surgeon can visualize the data and elaborate the surgical plan. Before the surgery starts, the preoperative data, model, and plan are downloaded to the computer in the operating room. A dynamic reference frame is attached to the patient, and the intraoperative situation is registered with the preoperative data by either touching the fiducials with a tracked tool, or by acquiring a cloud of points on the surface of the anatomy. Once the registration has taken place, a display showing the preoperative images and model with the CAD models of the tools superimposed is created on the basis of the current tool and anatomy position obtained from the tracker (Fig. 14.14). Several commercial systems are currently available for a variety of procedures. Clinical studies report millimetric accuracy on tool and implant positioning. These types of systems have been applied extensively in orthopedics, (the spine,[58,81,82]) pelvis,[83,84] fractures,[85–89] hip,[56,90,91] and knee[57,92–94] neurosurgery, and craneofacial and maxillofacial surgery.

Navigation systems based on intraoperative images combine intraoperative images with position data from surgical tools and implants to create augmented intraoperative views. An example of such system is the FluoroNav system, which uses fluoroscopic x-ray images.[61] During surgery, a tracking device is attached to the fluoroscopic C arm, and one or more images are acquired with it. Projections of the tools are then superimposed on the original images and updated in real time as the tools move (Fig. 14.15). Since the camera and the tools are tracked simultaneously, there is no need for registration. The advantages of these systems are that they do not require a preoperative study and that no registration is necessary. However, the views remain two dimensional, requiring the surgeon to mentally recreate the spatial intraoperative situation. Recent clinical studies show that these systems are having excellent acceptance, since they are closest to current practice, and beginning to be used successfully.[95]

Other navigation systems combine video stream data obtained from endoscopic cameras or surgical microscopes, with data from preoperative studies, such as CT or MRI. The camera is tracked, so its position and orientation during surgery are known and can be shown, after registration,

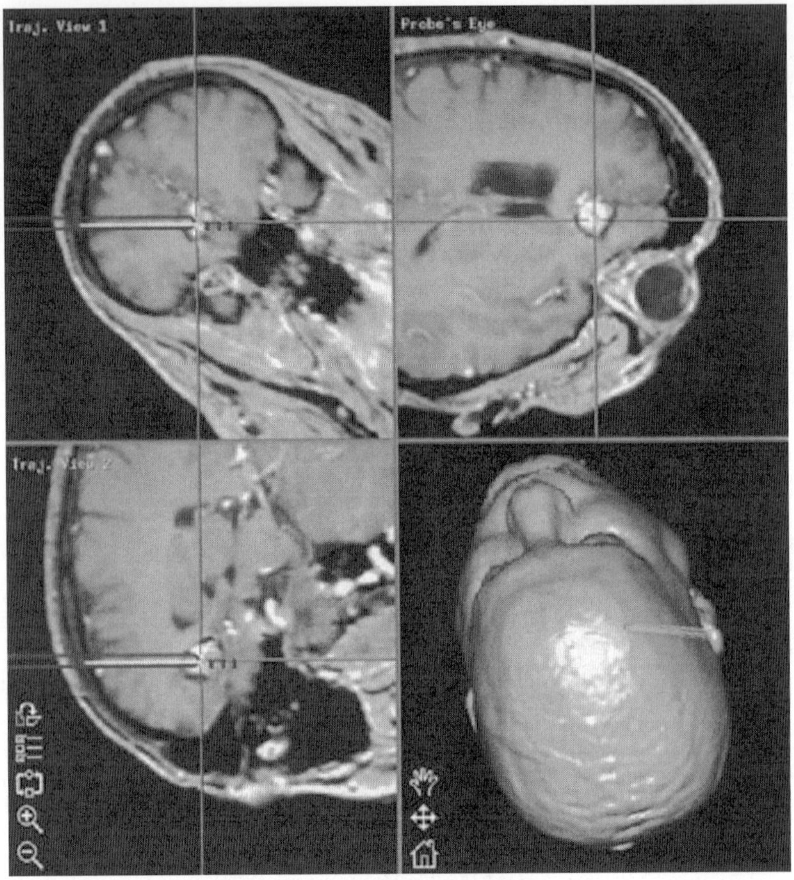

FIGURE 14.14 Typical screen display of a CIS navigation system in action. The top left, right, and bottom windows show orthogonal cross-sectional views of the MRI data set. The cross hair in each shows the position of the tool tip at the center of the tumor. The bottom right window shows the spatial view, with the tool shown in light gray. (*Photo courtesy of BrainLab.*)

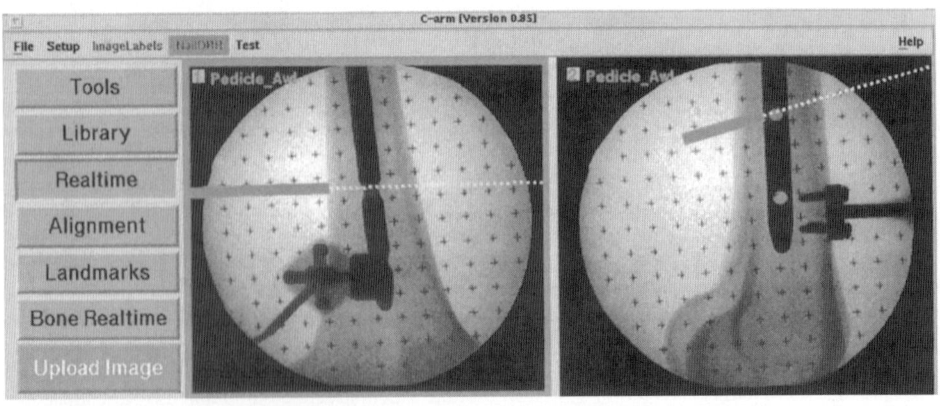

FIGURE 14.15 Screen display of a fluoroscopy-based navigation system during intramedullary nail distal locking. The windows show AP and lateral fluoroscopic x-ray images with the tool (solid line) and its extension (dotted line). The goal is to align the tool with the nail's hole axis.[59,61] (*Photo Courtesy of L. P. Nolte.*)

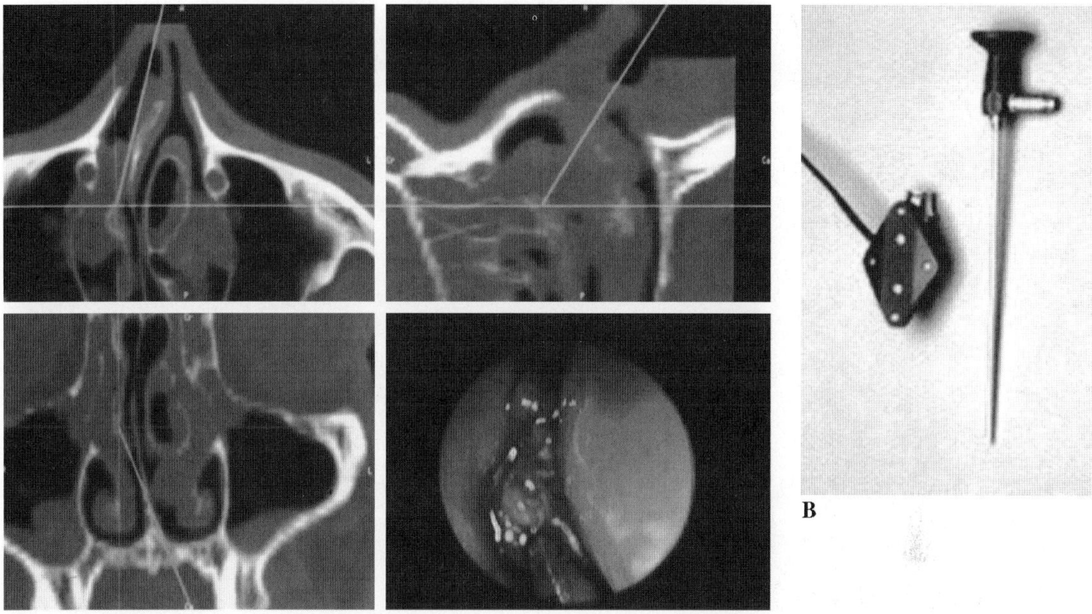

A

FIGURE 14.16 (*a*) Typical screen display of a CIS navigation system for endoscopic surgery. The left windows show orthogonal cross-sectional views of the CT data set and the endoscope image. The diagonal line (which is green in the original image) shows the position of the endoscope. (*b*) The endoscope and the tracking plate. (*Reproduced from Ref. 98.*)

together with the preoperative images. The video stream can be shown side by side with a preoperative study, as shown in Fig. 14.16, or selected information from it can be inserted in the video stream. The main advantage of these systems is that they allow surgeons to see beyond the surfaces shown in the video and to obtain spatial location information that overcomes the narrow field of view of the cameras.[96]

Augmented Reality Navigation Systems. One of the drawbacks of the navigation systems described above is that they require the surgeon to constantly shift attention from the patient to the computer display and back. Augmented reality navigation systems attempt to overcome this drawback by bringing the display right where the surgeon needs it. The data is viewed through glasses worn by the surgeon, projected directly on the patient, or displayed on a transparent screen standing between the surgeon and the patient. The surgeon's head is usually tracked, so that the data can be displayed from the correct viewpoint.

Two examples of this type of system are the augmented reality CIS system for neurosurgery[97] and the CMU image overlay system[63] for orthopedics. The augmented reality CIS system for neurosurgery projects colored segmented volumetric data of brain tumors and other neural structures directly on the patient's skull (Fig. 14.17). This allows the surgeon to directly see where to start the minimally invasive procedure. The HipNav navigation system was developed to assist orthopedic surgeons in positioning the acetabular cup in total hip replacement surgery. In this system, a transparent glass that serves as a projection screen is placed between the surgeon and the patient on the operating table. After registration, the hip and pelvis models extracted from the preoperative CT data are projected on the glass screen, thereby providing the surgeon with an x-ray-like view of what lies beneath.

Virtual Reality Diagnosis Systems. The third type of information-enhancing system is virtual reality diagnosis systems. These systems, typically used in diagnostic endoscopy and colonoscopy,

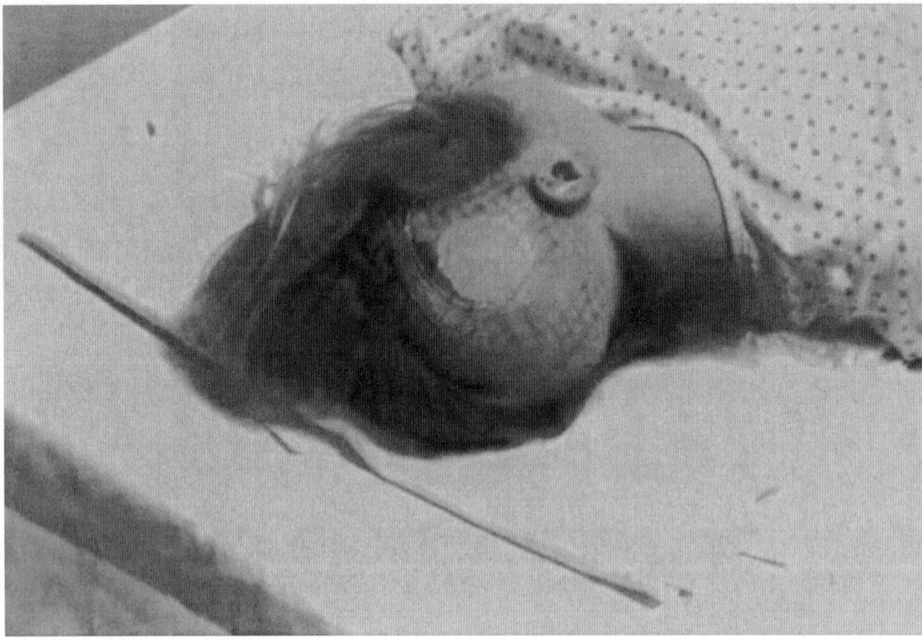

FIGURE 14.17 Augmented reality CIS system for brain tumor surgery. The tumor image (round area) and brain structure (below tumor image) are projected directly on the patient's skull. (*Photo courtesy of Ron Kikinis.*)

replace an actual exploration on the patient with a virtual exploration on MRI images. A three-dimensional reconstruction of the anatomical structures of interest, typically tubelike, is constructed from the data set, and a fly-through inspection path inside the structure is computed. The clinician is then presented with a virtual movie that simulates the actual endoscopic exploration (Fig. 14.18). On the basis of these images, the clinician can look for and identify certain pathologies, such as tumors, and then determine if an actual examination or surgery is necessary. Several algorithms have been developed for model construction, fast visualization, and computation of fly-through path.[98]

14.4.2 Robotic Systems for Precise Preoperative Plan Execution

One of the drawbacks of navigation systems is that they cannot guarantee that a planned surgical gesture, such as screw placement or needle insertion, will be executed precisely as planned. To ensure not only precise positioning but also precise execution, surgical robots have been developed. We describe next two examples of the most common types of active surgical robots: the ROBODOC system discussed earlier and the LARS robot for percutaneous therapy.

Robotic Orthopedic Surgery. Because bone is rigid and relatively easy to image in CT, and because geometric precision is often an important consideration in orthopedic surgical procedures, orthopedic surgery has been an important domain for the development of CIS systems. For example, the ROBODOC system has been in clinical use since 1992 and combines CT-based preoperative planning with robotic machining of bone. Both ROBODOC and a very similar subsequently introduced system called CASPAR®[99] have been applied to knee surgery[100–102] as well as hip surgery. Other robotic systems have been proposed or (in a few cases) applied for hip or knee surgery.[38,39,103–107]

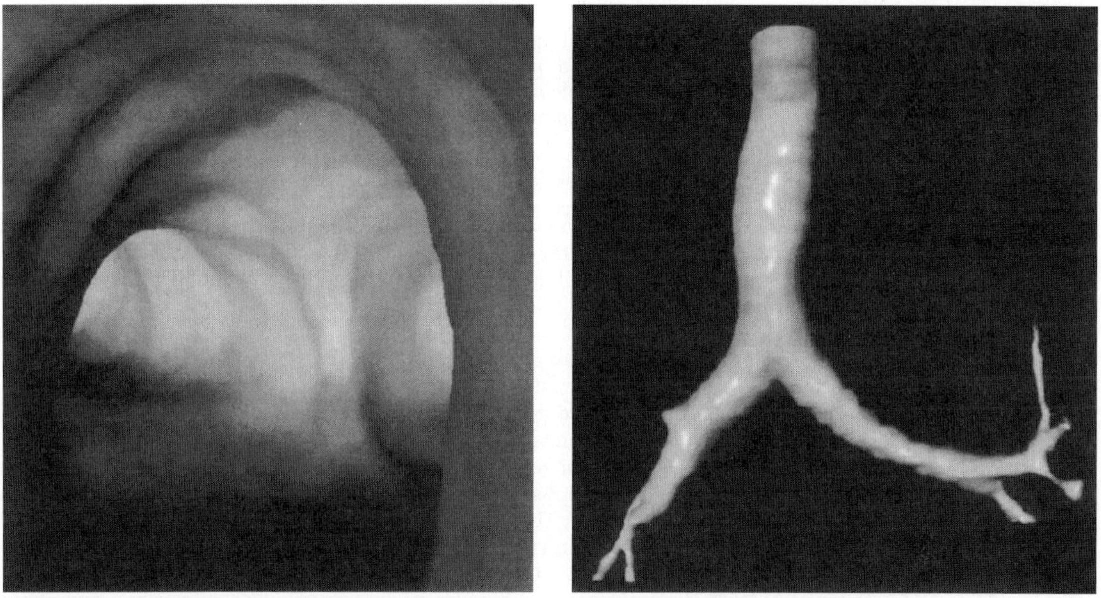

A B

FIGURE 14.18 Virtual endoscopy: (*a*) three-dimensional reconstruction of structure to be viewed and (*b*) view from the inside fly-through. (*Reproduced from Ref. 98.*)

These applications fit naturally within the context of surgical CAD/CAM systems. For example, Fig. 14.19 shows the information flow for the current ROBODOC implementation. The information flow in the CASPAR system is very similar. CT images of the patient's bones are read into a planning workstation and a simple segmentation method is used to produce an accurate surface model of key anatomical areas. After some key anatomical measurements are made from the images, the surgeon selects an implant design from a library and determines its desired placement in the patient by manipulating a CAD model of the implant with respect to selected mutually orthogonal cross sections through the CT data volume. The planning workstation computes a cutter trajectory relative to CT coordinates and all of the planning information is written to a magnetic tape along with the patient images and model.

In the operating room, robotic hip replacement surgery proceeds much as manual surgery until after the head of the femur (for the case of primary hip surgery) or failing implant (for revision

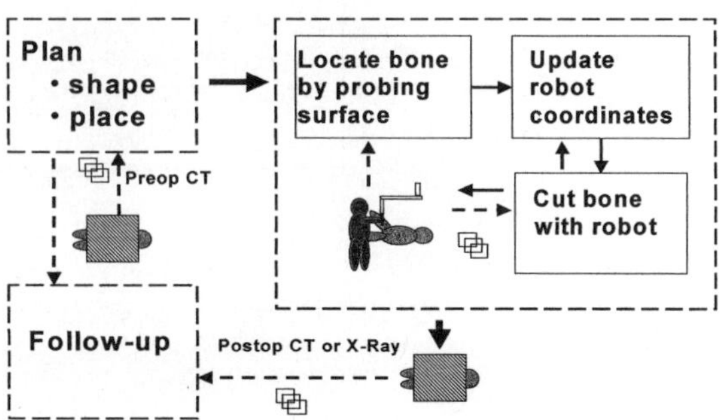

FIGURE 14.19 Information flow in a typical orthopedic robotic system (in this case, the ISS ROBODOC system).

surgery) is removed. Then the femur is fixed to the base of the robot and a redundant position sensor is attached to the bone to detect any slipping of the bone relative to the fixation device. Then a 3D digitizer is used to locate a number of points on the bone surface. These points are used to compute the coordinate transformation between the robot and CT images used for planning and (thus) to the patient's bone. The surgeon then hand-guides the robot to an approximate initial position using a force sensor mounted between the robot's tool holder and the surgical cutter. The robot then cuts the desired shape while monitoring cutting forces, bone motion, and other safety sensors. The surgeon also monitors progress and can interrupt the robot at any time. If the procedure is paused for any reason, there are a number of error recovery procedures available to permit the procedure to be resumed or restarted at one of several defined checkpoints. Once the desired shape has been cut, surgery proceeds manually in the normal manner. The procedural flow for robotic knee replacement surgery is quite similar.

Robotically Assisted Percutaneous Therapy. One of the first uses of robots in surgery was positioning of needle guides in stereotactic neurosurgery.[24,108,109] This is a natural application, since the skull provides a rigid frame of reference. However, the potential application of localized therapy is much broader. Percutaneous therapy fits naturally within the broader paradigm of surgical CAD/CAM systems. The basic process involves planning a patient-specific therapy pattern, delivering the therapy through a series of percutaneous access steps, assessing what was done, and using this feedback to control therapy at several time scales. The ultimate goal of current research is to develop systems that execute this process with robotic assistance under a variety of widely available and deployable image modalities, including ultrasound, x-ray fluoroscopy, and conventional MRI and CT scanners.

Current work at Johns Hopkins University is typical of this activity. Our approach has emphasized the use of "remote center-of-motion" (RCM) manipulators to position needle guides under real-time image feedback. One early experimental system,[110,111] shown in Fig. 14.20, was used to establish the feasibility of inserting radiation therapy seeds into the liver under biplane x-ray guidance. In this work, small pellets were implanted preoperatively and located in CT images used to plan the pattern

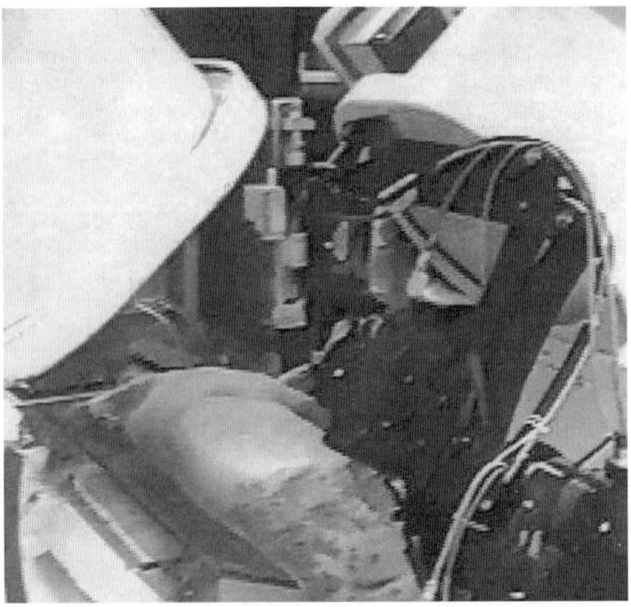

FIGURE 14.20 Early percutaneous therapy experiments at Johns Hopkins University using the LARS robot.[110,111]

of therapy seeds. The fiducial pellets were relocated in the biplane x-rays and used to register the preoperative plan to a modified LARS robot[112,113] used to implant the treatment seeds. Although this experiment and related work directed at placing needles into the kidney[114,115] established the basic feasibility of our approach, we concluded that significant improvements in the robot would be needed.

Subsequent work has focused on development of a modular family of very compact component subsystems and end effectors that could be configured for use in a variety of imaging and surgical environments. Figure 14.9 shows a novel RCM linkage with a radiolucent needle driver ("PAKY") developed by Stoianovici et al. that forms a key component in this next generation system. Figure 14.11 shows the RCM device with a novel end-effector developed by Susil and Masamune that permits the computer to determine the needle pose to be computed with respect to a CT or MRI scanner using a single image slice.[42,44,45] This arrangement can have significant advantages in reducing setup costs and time for in-scanner procedures and also eliminates many sources of geometric error. Figure 14.21 shows another variation of the RCM used as a high dexterity wrist in a system designed for manipulating ultrasound probes for diagnosis and ultrasound-guided biopsies.[116]

Related work at Brigham and Women's Hospital in Boston is illustrated in Fig. 14.13. This system[117] is designed to operate in an open-magnet MRI system and uses a common control architecture developed jointly by MIT, Brigham and Women's Hospital, and Johns Hopkins.[118,119] One early application will be MRI-guided prostate therapy. Figure 14.12 shows another MRI-compatible robot system, this one designed for breast biopsy.[120]

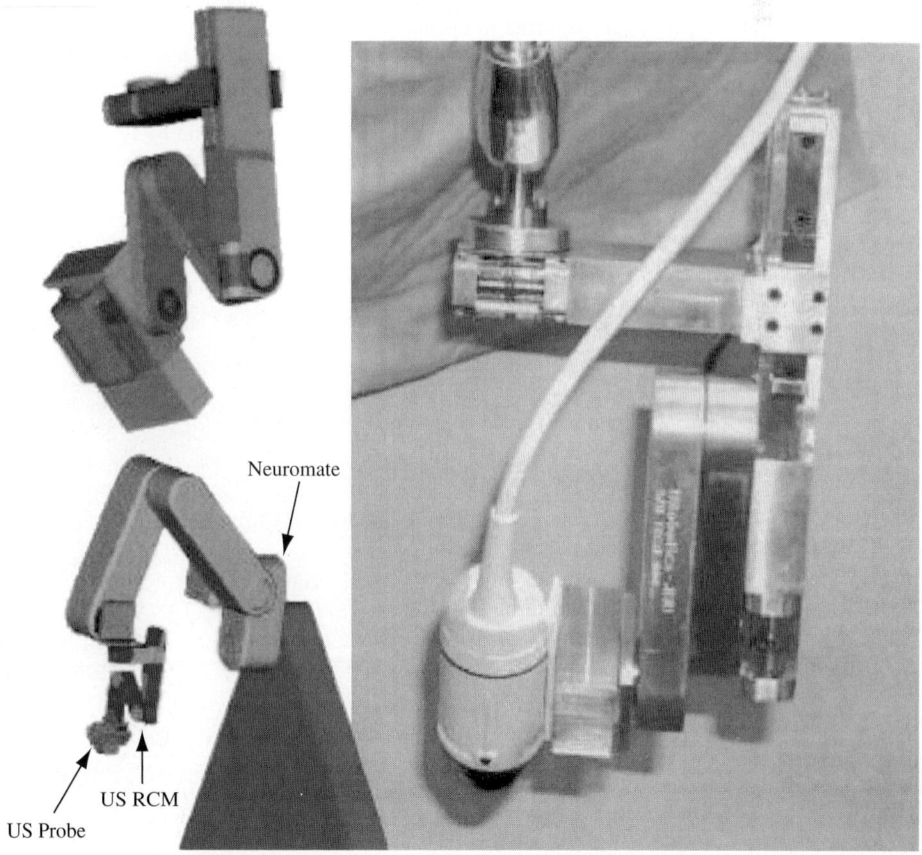

FIGURE 14.21 Dexterous RCM end effector for ultrasound and similar applications[116] mounted on an Integrated Surgical Systems Neuromate robot. (*Photo courtesy Randy Goldberg.*)

14.4.3 Robotic Systems for Human Augmentation

The emphasis in surgical assistant robots is the use of these systems cooperatively to enhance human performance or efficiency in surgery. Much of the past and current work on surgical augmentation[67,70,73,121–125] has focused on teleoperation. There is considerable interest in the use of master-slave manipulator systems to improve the ergonomic aspects of laparoscopic surgery. Figure 14.22 shows a typical example (the Da Vinci® system[122] marketed by Intuitive Surgical). In this case, three slave robots are used. One holds an endoscopic camera and two others manipulate surgical instruments. In the case of the Da Vinci, the surgical instruments have high dexterity wrists, as shown in Fig. 14.22*b* Other systems with varying degrees of complexity (e.g., the Zeus® system marketed by Computer Motion) are also in use, and this area of application may be expected to grow in the future.

Although the primary impact of teleoperated robots in surgical applications over the next years will probably be in applications in which the surgeon remains close to the patient, there has also been considerable interest in remote telesurgery.[70,126,127] In addition to the design issues associated with local telesurgery, these systems must cope with the effects of communication delays and possible interruptions on overall performance.

The manipulation limitations imposed by human hand tremor and limited ability to feel and control very small forces, together with the limitations of operating microscopes have led a number of groups to investigate robotic augmentation of microsurgery. Several systems have been developed for teleoperated microsurgery using a passive input device for operator control. Guerrouad and Vidal[128] describe a system designed for ocular vitrectomy in which a mechanical manipulator was constructed of curved tracks to maintain a fixed center of rotation. A similar micromanipulator[129] was used for acquiring physiological measurements in the eye using an electrode. While rigid mechanical constraints were suitable for the particular applications in which they were used, the design is not flexible enough for general-purpose microsurgery and the tracks take up a great deal of space around the head. An ophthalmic surgery manipulator built by Jensen et al.[130] was designed for retinal vascular microsurgery and was capable of positioning instruments at the surface of the retina with submicrometer precision. While a useful experimental device, this system did not have sufficient range of motion to be useful for general-purpose microsurgery. Also, the lack of force sensing prevented the investigation of force/haptic interfaces in the performance of microsurgical tasks.

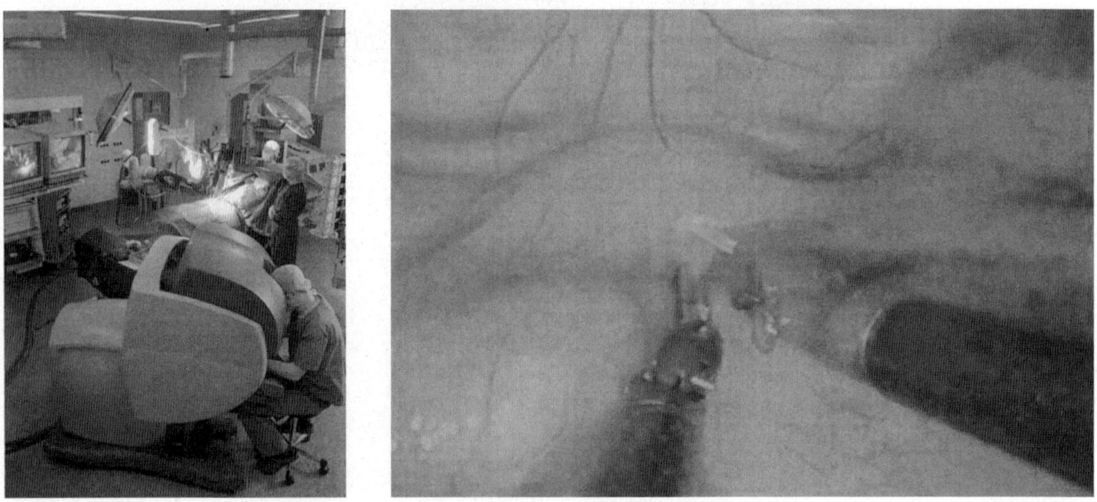

A B

FIGURE 14.22 Telesurgical augmentation system: In this "telepresence" system the surgeon sits at a control console [(*a*) foreground] and manipulates a pair of "master" robot arms while "slave" robots [(*a*) background and (*b*)] mimic his motions inside the patient's body.[122] (*Photos courtesy Intuitive Surgical Systems.*)

Many microsurgical robots[70,124,131–133] are based on force-reflecting master-slave configurations. This paradigm allows an operator to grasp the master manipulator and apply forces. Forces measured on the master are scaled and reproduced at the slave and, if unobstructed, will cause the slave to move accordingly. Likewise, forces encountered by the slave are scaled and reflected back to the master. This configuration allows position commands from the master to result in a reduced motion of the slave and for forces encountered by the slave to be amplified at the master.

While a force-reflecting master-slave microsurgical system provides the surgeon with increased precision and enhanced perception, there are some drawbacks to such a design. The primary disadvantage is the complexity and cost associated with the requirement of providing two mechanical systems, one for the master and one for the slave. Another problem with telesurgery in general is that the surgeon is not allowed to directly manipulate the instrument used for the microsurgical procedure. While physical separation is necessary for systems designed to perform remote surgery, it is not required during microsurgical procedures. In fact, surgeons are more likely to accept assistance devices if they are still allowed to directly manipulate the instruments.

The performance augmentation approach pursued by the CIS group at Johns Hopkins University, which has also been explored independently by Davies et al.,[37–39] and which has some resemblances to the work of Kazerooni,[134] emphasizes cooperative manipulation, in which the surgeon and robot both hold the surgical tool. The robot senses forces exerted on the tool by the surgeon and moves to comply. Our initial experiences with this mode in ROBODOC indicated that it was very popular with surgeons and offered means to augment human performance while maximizing the surgeon's natural hand-eye coordination within a surgical task. Subsequently, we incorporated this mode into the IBM/JHU LARS system.[26,36,49,135–139] Figure 14.23 shows one early experiment using LARS to evacuate simulated hematomas with a neuroendoscopic instrument.[54,140–142] We found that the surgeon took slightly longer (6 vs. 4 min) to perform the evacuation using the guiding, but evacuated much less surplus material (1.5 percent excess vs. 15 percent).

More recently, we have been exploring the extension of these ideas into microsurgery and other precise manipulation tasks. We have extended our model of cooperative control, which we call

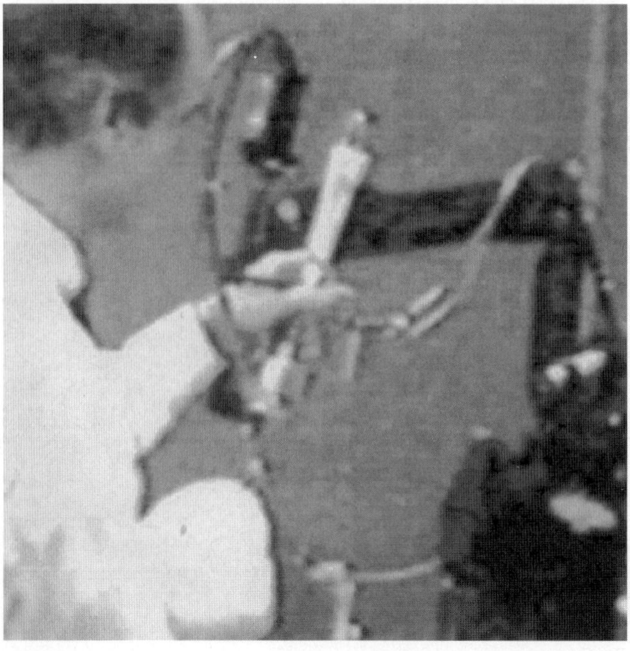

FIGURE 14.23 Cooperative guiding using LARS for a neuroendoscopy experiment.[54,140–142]

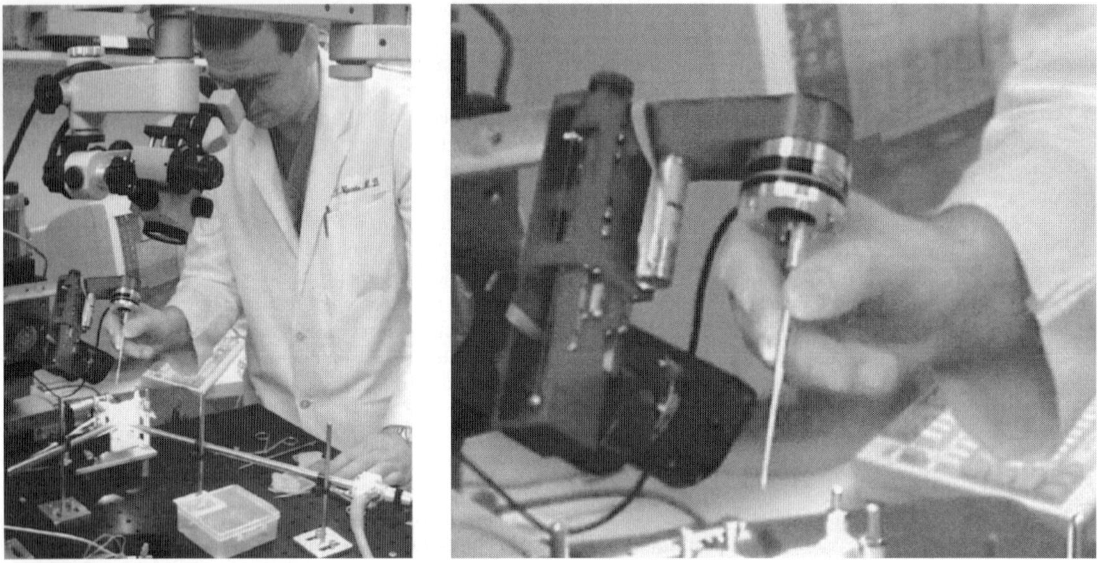

FIGURE 14.24 Microsurgical augmentation experiments with the Johns Hopkins steady-hand robot.[163] Shows the current generation of the robot being used to evaluate robotically assisted stapedotomy. The current generation comprises an RCM linkage,[164] a custom end-effector assembly,[21,165,166] and off-the-shelf components. (*Photo courtesy Dan Rothbaum.*)

"steady hand" guiding, to permit the compliance loop to be closed on the basis of a scaled combination of forces exerted by the surgeon and tissue interaction forces, as well as on other sensors such as visual processing. The result is a manipulation system with the precision and sensitivity of a machine, but with the manipulative transparency and immediacy of handheld tools for tasks characterized by compliant or semirigid contacts with the environment.[18] We have also begun to develop higher levels of control for this system, incorporating more complex behaviors with multiple sensing modalities,[72,143–146] using microsurgical tasks drawn from the fields of ophthalmology and otology. Figure 14.24 shows a typical experiment using our current robot to evaluate robot-assisted stapedotomies. Figure 14.25 shows a comparison of instrument tremor and drift with and without robotic assistance. We have also demonstrated 30:1 scaling of forces in compliant manipulation tasks.

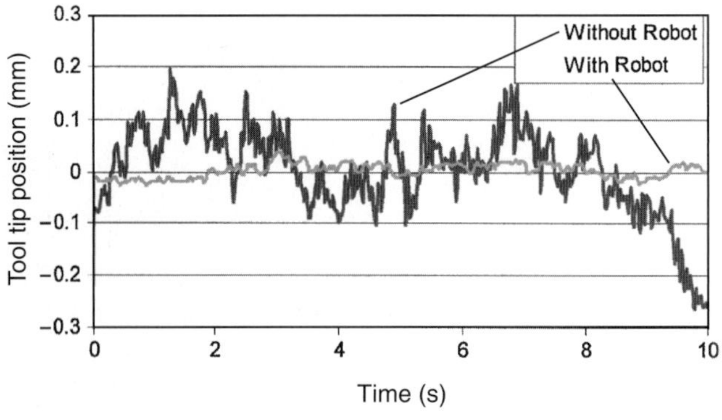

FIGURE 14.25 Comparative performance of human tremor and drift without a robot and with steady-hand manipulation augmentation.[167]

14.4.4 Other Robotic Assistants

The use of robotic systems to assist surgeons by performing routine tasks such as laparoscopic camera manipulation is becoming commonplace.[33,35,135,147] Some of the manipulator design issues associated with such systems were discussed in Sec. 14.3.6. For human-machine interfaces, these systems provide a joystick or foot pedal to permit the surgeon to control the motion of the endoscope. However, other interfaces include voice, tracking of surgeon head movements, computer vision tracking of surgical instruments, indication of desired gaze points by manipulating a cursor on the computer screen, etc. Figure 14.7*a* shows a typical installation of a voice-controlled commercial system (the AESOP™, developed by Computer Motion, Inc.).

More recently, there has been interest in robotic systems for manipulating ultrasound probes.[116,148–151] Figures 14.10 and 14.21 show typical current research efforts in development of such robotic systems. Most of this activity has targeted diagnostic procedures such as systematic examination of carotid arteries for occlusions. However, these systems have the potential to become as ubiquitous as the robotic endoscope holders discussed above. Our research group at Johns Hopkins University has begun to explore applications such as precise ultrasound-guided biopsies and other interventional procedures.

There has also been work in the use of flexible robotic devices for intralumenal applications such as colonoscopy and angioplasty.[152–155] Generally, these devices are snakelike, though there have been a few efforts[155] to develop autonomous crawlers.

14.5 PERSPECTIVES

Computer-integrated surgery is a new, rapidly evolving paradigm that will change the way surgery will be performed in the future. Technical advances in medical imaging, tracking, robotics, and integration are paving the way to a new generation of systems for minimally invasive surgery.

We believe that computer-integrated surgery (CIS) will have the same impact on health care in the coming decades that computer-integrated manufacturing has had on industrial production in the recent past. Achieving this vision will require both significant advances in basic engineering knowledge and the development of robust, flexible systems that make this knowledge usable in real clinical applications.

It is important to remember that the ultimate payoff for CIS systems will be in improved and more cost-effective health care. Quantifying these advantages in practice can be problematic, and sometimes the final answer may take years to be demonstrated. The consistency, enhanced data logging, and analysis made possible by CIS systems may help in this process. It will not be easy to figure out how to apply these capabilities. However, we believe that the CIS paradigm is here to stay.

14.6 BRIEF UPDATE FOR THE SECOND EDITION

In the past 5 years, since the appearance of the First Edition, significant developments have occurred in the field of computer-integrated surgery and medical robotics. An overview of these advancements is beyond the scope of this section. The list of references has been updated and revised (Refs. 168–225). We highlight a few important points, which in our opinion, are of relevance to the field. Further information may be found in published survey articles.[168–170]

14.6.1 Medical Imaging Devices

There has been a significant improvement in medical imaging devices, which now produce higher resolution images. There are more modalities, and their intraoperative use is more common. An example is 3D ultrasound and video from a variety of laparoscopic and endoscopic devices. In parallel, medical image processing is gaining momentum and has seen significant developments of methods for volumetric visualization, image segmentation, real-time image fusion as well as atlas, and statistical-based shape models of bone and organs.

14.6.2 Image Processing, Visualization, and Modeling

Medical image processing and visualization have greatly benefited from the increase in speed and performance of standard computing equipment. Specialized automatic and semiautomatic segmentation techniques for an ever-increasing number of image modalities and anatomical structures have been developed over the past 5 years.[171] The most commonly studied anatomical structures include the brain and its vasculature, the heart, the liver, the colon, and bones. Three-dimensional visualization is gaining acceptance in the clinical environment, especially for the visualization of complex anatomical structures and pathologies. A current trend is patient-specific modeling for preoperative planning and interventional procedures.

14.6.3 Preoperative Analysis, Planning, and Registration

Preoperative analysis and planning has remained very much procedure and equipment-specific. It is usually incorporated within the systems (Fig. 14.26*c*). Work on registration has emphasized multimodal and nonrigid registration, incorporating real-time laparoscopic video and ultrasound images.[171]

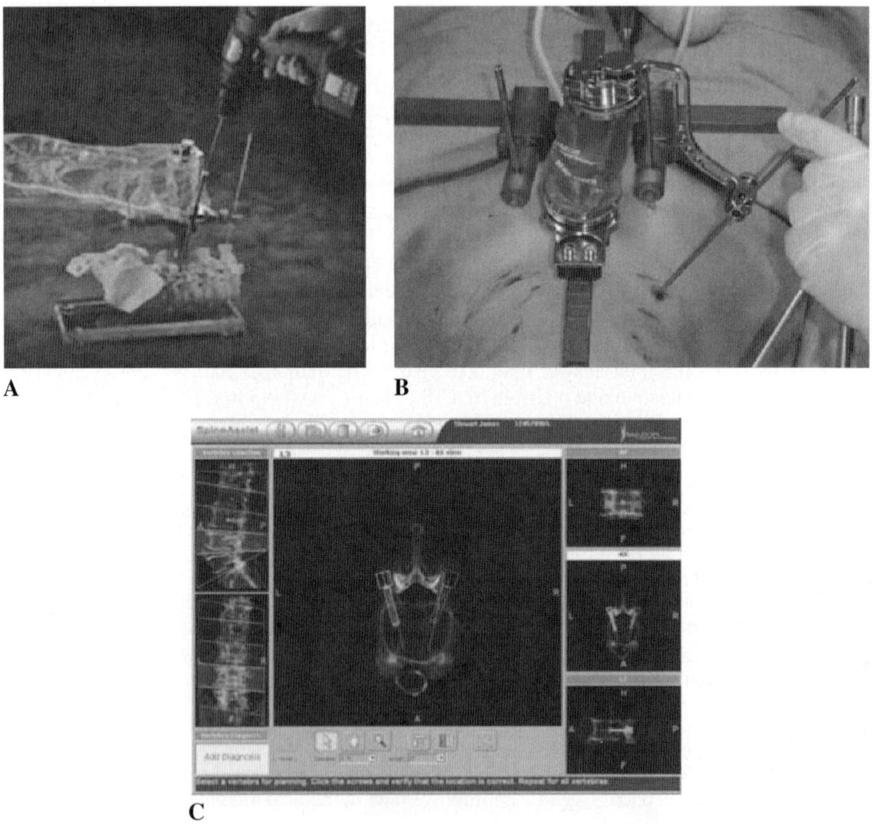

FIGURE 14.26 The SpineAssist System for pedicle screw insertion.[172] (*a*) In vitro demonstration showing the miniature robot clamped to the spinal process and guiding the pedicle screw hole drilling; (*b*) in vivo minimally invasive procedure; (*c*) screen dump showing preoperative pedicle screws planning on CT axial (center), sagittal, and coronal (center and bottom right) images (*Photos: Moshe Shoham*).

14.6.4 Positional Tracking and Other Sensing

A new generation of very compact electromagnetic positional trackers[173–175] that can be built into catheters, needles, and other instruments inserted into a patient's body has led to renewed interest in applications in which line-of-sight restrictions associated with optical tracking are important.[176–181] There has also been increased interest in developing "smart" surgical instruments that sense local tissue properties such as tissue ischemia.[182,183]

14.6.5 Robotics

Medical robotics has also seen new devices and applications. For recent comprehensive surveys in medical robotics, see Refs.168,169,184, and 185. Recent papers by the authors of this chapter[172,186–192] are typical of the breadth of work in this field. One common theme has been development of small robots that mount or rest on the patient's body, thus simplifying the problem of controlling relative motion between the robot and patient[172,186,187,193,194] (Fig. 14.27). Another theme has been the development of snake-like manipulators, providing high dexterity in limited space inside the patient's body,[188,195,198–202] or for semiautonomous mobility inside the patient.[193,203,204] Yet another noteworthy trend has been an increasing interest in MRI-compatible robots[205–209] (Fig. 14.28).

14.6.6 Systems

Navigation has become the standard of care in a growing variety of procedures, especially in neurosurgery[210] and orthopedics.[185,211] Other nonrobotic systems providing various forms of "augmented reality" support for the surgeon are also being developed[192,212–216] (Fig. 14.29).

Robotic systems for precise placement of needles into the patient's body under real-time image guidance[218] are continuing to develop rapidly, and systems are in various states of research and clinical deployment.

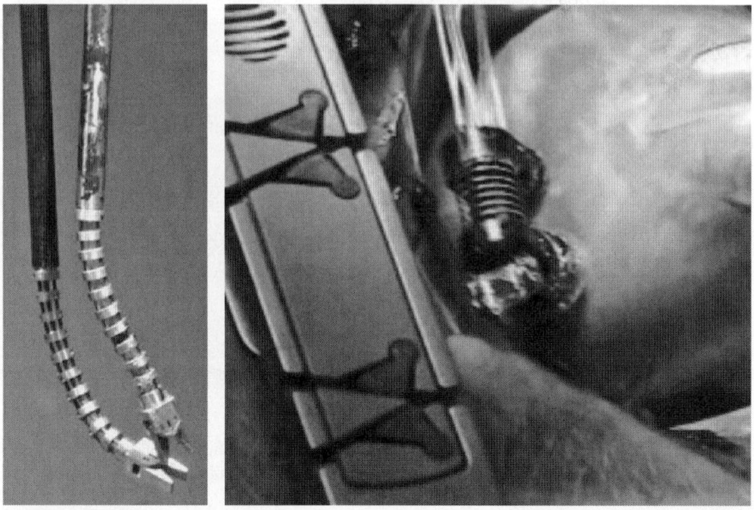

A B

FIGURE 14.27 Dexterity and mobility inside the patient's body. (*a*) 4.2-mm diameter snake-like robot designed for minimally invasive surgery of the throat and upper airway[195–197] (*Photo: N. Simaan*); (*b*) CMU HeartLander robot[193] (*Photo: C. Riviere*).

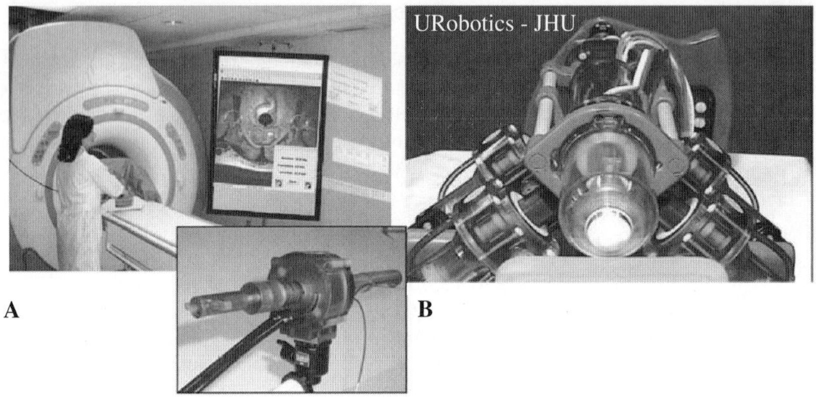

FIGURE 14.28 Robots for prostate needle placement under MRI guidance. (*a*) Clinically-applied robot for transrectal needle placement[209] (*Photo: G. Fichtinger*); (*b*) robot for percutaneous prostate brachytherapy[205] (*Photo: D. Stoianovici*).

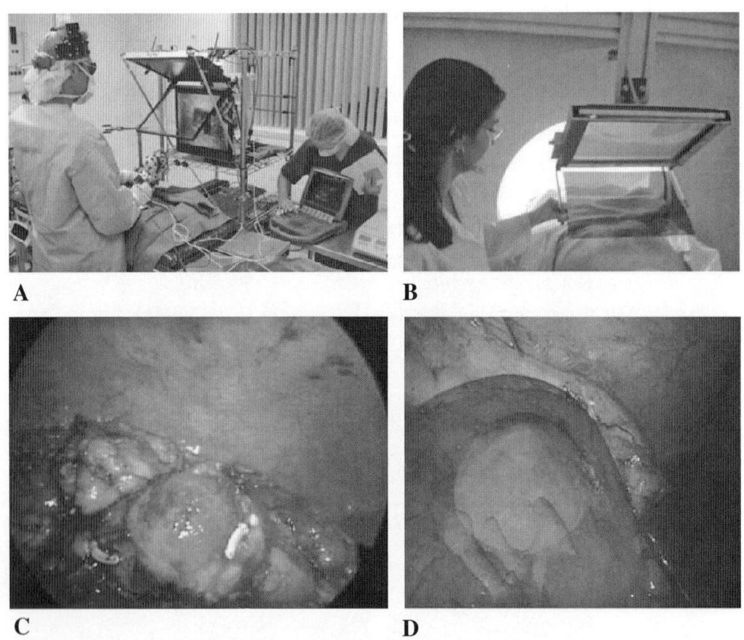

FIGURE 14.29 Augmented reality in surgical assistance. (*a*) UNC navigationally guided system for RF ablation of liver tumors[212] (*Photo: Henry Fuchs*); (*b*) JHU passively aligned system for in-scanner needle placement[217] (*Photo: JHU*); (*c*) clinically-applied video overlay of CT-based model in laparoscopic partial nephrectomy[214,215] (*Photo: Y. Sato*); (*d*) video overlay of CT-based model during laparoscopic partial nephrectomy using only stereo video for registration and tracking[216] (*Photo: JHU*).

Within the area of telesurgery, the commercially deployed Da Vinci Surgical System (Intuitive Surgical, Mountain View, California) has won widespread acceptance, with over 400 systems deployed for a variety of laparoscopic procedures, including heat surgery and prostatectomies.[219–221] Another recently deployed commercial telesurgical system (Artisen System, Hansen Medical, Palo Alto, California) is used for manipulating ablation catheters inside the heart.[222]

Finally, there are several ongoing efforts within the medical robotics and computer-assisted surgery community to develop common open-source software environments to facilitate research.[223–225]

ACKNOWLEDGMENTS

Any survey or critical summary must necessarily draw upon the work of many people. We would like especially to acknowledge the contributions of many colleagues over the past decade who have helped develop an evolving shared understanding of medical robotics and computer-integrated surgery. We are especially grateful to those individuals who generously provided photographs and other information about the specific systems that we have used as examples. In some cases, these colleagues have also worked with us in developing some of these systems.

We also gratefully acknowledge the many agencies and organizations that have contributed financial and other support to the development of much of the work that we have reported. The National Science Foundation supports the Engineering Research Center for Computer-Integrated Surgical Systems and Technology under cooperative agreement number EEC9731478. Further support has been provided by other NSF grants, the National Institutes of Health, the Whitaker Foundation, IBM Corporation, Integrated Surgical Systems, the Johns Hopkins University, and numerous other government, industry, and academic sources. We also acknowledge the partial support of the Israeli Ministry of Trade and Industry, through the IZMEL Consortium for Image-Guided Therapy.

REFERENCES

1. Taylor, R. H., et al., "An Image-directed Robotic System for Precise Orthopedic Surgery," *IEEE Transactions on Robotics and Automation,* 1994, **10**(3):261–275.
2. Mittelstadt, B. D., et al., "The Evolution of a Surgical Robot from Prototype to Human Clinical Trial," *Proc. Medical Robotics and Computer Assisted Surgery,* 1994, Pittsburgh.
3. Paul, H., et al., "Accuracy of Implant Interface Preparation: Hand-held Broach vs. Robot Machine Tool," *Proc. Orthopedic Research Society,* 1992, Washington, D.C.
4. Joskowicz, L., and R. H. Taylor, "Preoperative Insertability Analysis and Visualization of Custom Hip Implants," *1st International Symposium on Medical Robotics and Computer Assisted Surgery,* 1994, Pittsburgh.
5. Bauer, A., "Primary THR Using the ROBODOC System," *CAOS/USA,* 1999, Pittsburgh.
6. Joskowicz, L., et al., "Computer Integrated Revision Total Hip Replacement Surgery: Preliminary Report," *Second Annual International Symposium on Medical Robotics and Computer Assisted Surgery,* 1995, Baltimore.
7. Taylor, R. H., et al., "Computer-Integrated Revision Total Hip Replacement Surgery: Concept and Preliminary Results," *Medical Image Analysis,* 1999, **3**(3):301–319.
8. Smith, K. R., K. J. Frank, and R. D. Bucholz, "The Neurostation—a highly accurate minimally invasive solution to frameless stereotactic neurosurgery," *Comput. Med. Imaging Graph.,* 1994, **18**:247–256.
9. Levoy, M., "Efficient ray tracing of volume data," *ACM Transactions on Graphics,* 1990, **9**:245–261.
10. Lorensen, W. E., and H. E. Cline, "Marching Cubes: a high resolution 3D surface reconstruction algorithm," *Computer Graphics,* 1987, **21**:163–169.
11. Hohne, K. H., M. Bomans, and M. Reimer, "A 3D anatomical atlas based on a volume model," *IEEE Computer Graphics and Applications,* 1992, **2**(1):72–78.

12. Lavallee, S., "Registration for Computer-Integrated Surgery: Methodology, State of the Art," in *Computer-Integrated Surgery,* R. H. Taylor et al. (eds.), 1996, MIT Press, Cambridge, Mass., pp. 77–98.

13. Maintz, J. B., and M. A. Viergever, "A survey of medical image registration," *Medical Image Analysis,* 1998, **2**(1):1–37.

14. Reinhardt, H. F., "Neuronagivation: A ten years review," in *Computer-Integrated Surgery,* R. Taylor et al., (eds.), 1996, MIT Press, Cambridge, Mass., pp. 329–342.

15. Maciunas, R. J., *Interactive Image-Guided Neurosurgery,* American Association of Neurological Surgeons.

16. Taylor, R. H., et al. (eds.), "An Image-Directed Robotic System For Precise Orthopedic Surgery," *Computer-Integrated Surgery, Technology and Clinical Applications,* 1995, pp. 379–396.

17. Taylor, R. H., et al. (eds.), *Computer-Integrated Surgery, Technology and Clinical Applications,* 1995, MIT Press, Cambridge, Mass.

18. Taylor, R., et al., "A Steady-Hand Robotic System for Microsurgical Augmentation," *International Journal of Robotics Research,* 1999, **18**(12).

19. Howe, R. D., et al., "Remote Palpation Technology," *IEEE Engineering in Medicine and Biology,* 1995, pp. 318–323.

20. Glucksberg, M. R., and R. Dunn, "Direct measurement of retinal microvascular pressures in the live, anesthetized cat," *Microvascular Research,* 1993, **45**(2):158–165.

21. Berkelman, P. J., et al., "A Miniature Instrument Tip Force Sensor for Robot/Human Cooperative Microsurgical Manipulation with Enhanced Force Feedback." in *Medical Image Computing and Computer-Assisted Interventions,* 2000, Springer, Pittsburgh.

22. Taylor, R. H., "Safety," in *Computer-Integrated Surgery,* R. H. Taylor et al. (eds.), 1996, MIT Press, Cambridge, Mass., pp. 283–286.

23. Davies, B. L., "A discussion of safety issues for medical robots," in *Computer-Integrated Surgery,* R. H. Taylor et al. (eds.), 1996, MIT Press, Cambridge, Mass., pp. 287–298.

24. Kwoh, Y. S., J. Hou, E. A. Jonckheere, et al., "A robot with improved absolute positioning accuracy for CT guided stereotactic brain surgery," *IEEE Trans. Biomed. Eng.,* 1988, **35**(2):153–161.

25. Nathan, M. S., et al., "Devices for Automated Resection of the Prostate," in *Proc. 1st International Symposium on Medical Robotics and Computer Assisted Surgery,* 1994, Pittsburgh.

26. Eldridge, B., et al., "A Remote Center of Motion Robotic Arm for Computer Assisted Surgery," *Robotica,* 1996, **14**(1):103–109.

27. Stoianovici, D., et al., "An efficient needle injection technique and radiological guidance method for percutaneous procedures," in *First Joint Conference: CRVMed II & MRCAS III,* March 1997, Grenoble, France.

28. Erbse, S., et al., "Development of an automated surgical holding system based on ergonomic analysis," in *Proc. First Joint Conference of CVRMed and MRCAS,* 1997, Grenoble, France, Springer.

29. Grace, K. W., et al., "Six degrees of freedom micromanipulator for ophthalmic surgery," in *IEEE Int. Conf. Robotics and Automation,* 1993, Atlanta, IEEE.

30. Brandt, G., et al., "A compact robot for image-guided orthopedic surgery: concept and preliminary results," in *Proc. First Joint Conference of CVRMed and MRCAS,* 1997, Grenoble, France, Springer.

31. Neisius, B., P. Dautzenberg, and R. Trapp, "Robotic Manipulator for Endoscopic Handling of Surgical Effectors and Cameras," in *Proc. Medical Robotics and Computer Assisted Surgery,* 1994, Pittsburgh.

32. Taylor, R. H., et al., "A Model-Based Optimal Planning and Execution System with Active Sensing and Passive Manipulation for Augmentation of Human Precision in Computer-Integrated Surgery," in *Proc. 1991 Int. Symposium on Experimental Robotics,* 1991, Toulouse, France, Springer-Verlag.

33. Sackier, J. M., and Y. Wang, "Robotically Assisted Laparoscopic Surgery: from Concept to Development," in *Computer-Integrated Surgery,* R. Taylor et al. (eds.), 1996, MIT Press, Cambridge, Mass., pp. 577–580.

34. Wang, Y., "Robotically Enhanced Surgery," in *Medicine Meets Virtual Reality II,* 1994. San Diego.

35. Hurteau, R., et al., "Laparoscopic Surgery Assisted by a Robotic Cameraman: Concept and Experimental Results," in *IEEE Conference on Robotics and Automation,* 1994, San Diego.

36. Funda, J., et al., "Comparison of two manipulator designs for laparoscopic surgery," in *1994 SPIE Int. Symposium on Optical Tools for Manufacturing and Advanced Automation,* 1994, Boston.

37. Troccaz, J., M. Peshkin, and B. L. Davies, "The use of localizers, robots, and synergistic devices in CAS," in *Proc. First Joint Conference of CVRMed and MRCAS,* 1997, Grenoble, France, Springer.

38. Ho, S. C., R. D. Hibberd, and B. L. Davies, "Robot Assisted Knee Surgery," *IEEE EMBS Magazine, Sp. Issue on Robotics in Surgery,* April–May 1995, pp. 292–300.

39. Harris, S. J., et al., "Experiences with robotic systems for knee surgery," in *Proc. First Joint Conference of CVRMed and MRCAS,* 1997, Grenoble, France, Springer.

40. Masamune, K., et al., "A newly developed sereotactic robot with detachable driver for neurosurgery," in *Proc. 2nd Int. Symp. on Medical Robotics and Computer Assisted Surgery* (*MRCAS*), 1995, Baltimore, Center for Orthop. Res. Shadyside Hospital, Pittsburgh.

41. Taylor, R. H., et al., "Computer-Integrated Revision Total Hip Replacement Surgery: Concept and Preliminary Results," *Medical Image Analysis,* 1999, **3**(3):301–319.

42. Susil, R. C., J. H. Anderson, and R. H. Taylor, "A Single Image Registration Method for CT Guided Interventions," in *2nd Int. Symposium on Medical Image Computing and Computer-Assisted Interventions* (*MICCAI99*), 1999, Cambridge, England, Springer.

43. Yao, J., et al., "A C-arm fluoroscopy-guided progressive cut refinement strategy using a surgical robot," *Computer Aided Surgery,* 2000, **5**(6):373–390.

44. Masamune, K., et al., "Development of CT-PAKY frame system—CT image guided needle puncturing manipulator and a single slice registration for urological surgery," in *Proc. 8th annual meeting of JSCAS,* 1999, Kyoto.

45. Masamune, K., et al., "Guidance system for robotically assisted percutaneous procedures with computed tomography," *Journal of Computer Aided Surgery,* 2000. 2001, **6**(6):370–375.

46. Masutani, Y., et al., "Computer Aided Surgery (CAS) System for Stereotactic Neurosurgery," in *Proc. Computer Vision and Robotics in Medicine* (*CVRMED*), 1995. Nice, France, Springer.

47. "Human-Machine Interfaces," in *Computer-Integrated Surgery,* R. H. Taylor et al. (eds.), 1996, MIT Press, Cambridge, Mass, pp. 201–254.

48. Taylor, R. H., et al., "A Telerobotic Assistant for Laparoscopic Surgery," in *Computer-Integrated Surgery,* R. Taylor et al. (eds.), 1996, MIT Press, Cambridge, Mass., pp. 581–592.

49. Funda, J., et al., "Image Guided Command and Control of a Surgical Robot," in *Proc. Medicine Meets Virtual Reality II,* 1994, San Diego.

50. Adams, L., et al., "CAS—A Navigation Support for Surgery," in *3D Imaging in Medicine,* 1990, Springer-Verlag, Berlin, pp. 411–423.

51. Kosugi, Y., et al., "An Articulated Neurosurgical Navigation System Using MRI and CT Images," *IEEE Transactions on Biomedical Engineering,* February 1988, pp. 147–152.

52. Watanabe, E., T. Watanabe, and S. Manka, et al., "Three-dimensional digitizer (neuronavigator): New equipment for computed tomography-guided stereotaxic surgery," *Surg. Neurol.,* 1987, 27:543–547.

53. Cutting, C. B., F. L. Bookstein, and R. H. Taylor, "Applications of Simulation, Morphometrics and Robotics in Craniofacial Surgery," in *Computer-Integrated Surgery,* R. H. Taylor et al. (eds.), 1996, MIT Press, Cambridge, Mass., pp. 641–662.

54. Auer, L. M. "Virtual Endoscopy for Planning and Simulation of Minimally Invasive Neruosurgery," in *Proc. First Joint Conference of CVRMed and MRCAS,* 1997, Grenoble, France, Springer.

55. Bucholz, R. D., et al., "Intraoperative Localization Using a Three Dimensional Optical Digitizer," in *Proceedings Medical Robotics and Computer Assisted Surgery,* 1994, Shadyside Hospital, Pittsburgh.

56. DiGioia, A. M., et al., "HipNav: Pre-operative Planning and Intra-operative Navigational Guidance for Acetabular Implant Placement in Total Hip Replacement Surgery," *Computer Assisted Orthopedic Surgery,* 1996.

57. Picard, F., et al., "Computer-assisted navigation for knee arthroplasty: Intra-operative measurements of alignment and soft tissue balancing," in *First Annual Meeting of CAOS International,* 2001, Davos, Switzerland.

58. Nolte, L. P., et al., "Use of C-arm for Surgical Navigation in the Spine," in *CAOS/USA '98,* 1998, Pittsburgh.

59. Hofstetter, R., et al., "Principles of Precise Fluoroscopy Based Surgical Navigation," in *4th International Symposium on CAOS,* 1999, Davos, Switzerland.

60. Hofstetter, R., et al., "Fluoroscopy based surgical navigation-concept and clinical applications," in *Proceedings of Computer Assisted Radiology and Surgery,* CAR '97, 1997, Elsevier, Berlin.

61. Hofstetter, R., et al., "Fluoroscopy as an imaging means for computer-assisted surgical navigation," *Computer-Aided Surgery,* 1999, **4**(2):65–76.

62. N. Hata, W. M. Wells, M. Halle, S. Nakajima, P. Viola, R. Kikinis, and F. A. Jolesz, "Image guided microscopic surgery system using mutual information based registration," in *VBC,* 1996, Hamburg.

63. Blackwell, M., et al., "An Image Overlay System for Medical Data Visualization," *Medical Image Analysis,* 2000, **4**(1):67–72.

64. Masamune, T., et al., "Three dimensional slice image overlay system with accurate depth perception for surgery," in *Medical Image Computing and Computer-Assisted Intervention,* MICCAI 2000, 2000, Pittsburgh, Springer.

65. Nolte, L. P., H. Visarius, et al., *Computer Assisted Orthopedic Surgery,* 1996. Hofgrefe & Huber.

66. Uecker, D. R., et al., "A Speech-Directed Multi-Modal Man-Machine Interface for Robotically Enhanced Surgery," in *First Int. Symp. on Medical Robotics and Computer Assisted Surgery* (*MRCAS '94*), 1994, Shadyside Hospital, Pittsburgh.

67. Reichenspurner, H., et al., "Use of the voice controlled and computer-assisted surgical system zeus for endoscopic coronary artery surgery bypass grafting," *J. Thoracic and Cardiovascular Surgery,* 1999, **118**(1).

68. Confer, R. G., and R. C. Bainbridge, "Voice control in the microsurgical suite," in *Proc. of the Voice I/O Systems Applications Conference '84,* 1984, American Voice I/O Society, Arlington, Va.

69. d'Aulignac, D., R. Balaniuk, and C. Laugier, "A haptic interface for a virtual exam of the human thigh," in *IEEE Conf. on Robotics and Automation, 2000,* San Francisco.

70. Mitsuishi, M., et al., "A Telemicrosurgery System with Colocated View and Operation Points and Rotational-force-feedback-free Master Manipulator," in *Proc. 2nd Int. Symp. on Medical Robotics and Computer Assisted Surgery,* MRCAS '95, 1995, Baltimore, Center for Orthop. Res, Shadyside Hospital, Pittsburgh.

71. Howe, R. D., and M. R. Cutkosky, "Dynamic Tactile Sensing: Perception of Fine Surface Features with Stress Rate Sensing," *IEEE Trans. Robotics & Automation,* 1993, **9**(2):140–151.

72. Kumar, R., et al., "Preliminary Experiments in Cooperative Human/Robot Force Control for Robot Assisted Microsurgical Manipulation," in *IEEE Conference on Robotics and Automation,* 2000, San Francisco.

73. Green, P., "Telepresence Surgery," in *NSF Workshop on Computer Assisted Surgery,* 1993, Washington, D.C.

74. Taylor, R., et al., "Redundant Consistency Checking in a Precise Surgical Robot," *in 12th Annual Conference on Engineering in Medicine and Biology,* 1990, Philadelphia, IEEE Press.

75. Taylor, R., et al., "Taming the Bull: Safety in a Precise Surgical Robot," in *Intl. Conf. on Advanced Robotics* (*ICAR*), 1991, Pisa, Italy.

76. B. Davies, "A Discussion of Safety Issues for Medical Robots," in *Computer-Integrated Surgery,* R. Taylor, et al., (eds.), 1996, MIT Press, Cambridge, Mass., pp. 287–296.

77. Varley, P., "Techniques of development of safety-related software in surgical robots," *IEEE Trans. on Information Technology in Biomedicine,* 1999, **3**(4):261–267.

78. Levensen, N. G., and C. S. Turner, "An investigation of the Therac-25 accidents," *Computer,* 1993, **26**(7):18–41.

79. Rau, G., et al., "Aspects of Ergonomic System Design Applied to Medical Work Stations," in *Computer-Integrated Surgery,* R. H. Taylor et al. (eds.), 1996, MIT Press, Cambridge, Mass. pp. 203–222.

80. Sheridan, T., "Human Factors in Telesurgery," in *Computer-Integrated Surgery,* R. H. Taylor et al. (eds.), 1996, MIT Press, Cambridge, Mass., pp. 223–230.

81. Merloz, P., et al., "Computer-assisted versus manual spine surgery: Clinical report," in *Proc. First Joint Conference of CVRMed and MRCAS,* 1997, Grenoble, France, Springer.

82. Nolte, L. P., et al., "A Novel Approach to Computer Assisted Spine Surgery," in *First Int. Symp. on Medical Robotics and Computer Assisted Surgery* (*MRCAS 94*), 1994, Shadyside Hospital, Pittsburgh.

83. vanHellenMondt, G., M. deKleuver, and P. Pavlov, "Computer assisted pelvic osteotomies; clinical experience in 25 cases," in *First Annual Meeting of CAOS International,* 2001, Davos, Switzerland.

84. Arand, M., L. Kinzl, and F. Gebhard, "CT-based navigation in minimally invasive screw stabilization of the iliosacral joint," in *First Annual Meeting of CAOS International,* 2001, Davos, Switzerland.

85. Joskowicz, L., et al., "FRACAS: A System for Computer-Aided Image-Guided Long Bone Fracture Surgery," *Journal of Computer Assisted Surgery,* 1999.

86. Tockus, L., et al. "Computer-Aided Image-Guided Bone Fracture Surgery: Modeling, Visualization, and Preoperative Planning," in *MICCAI '98,* 1998, Cambridge, Mass.

87. Verheyden, A., et al., "Percutaneous stabilization of dorsal pelvic ring fractures—transiliosacral screw placement in the open MRI," in *First Annual Meeting of CAOS International,* 2001, Davos, Switzerland.

88. Grutzner, P., et al., "Computer-aided reduction and fixation of long bone fractures," in *First Annual Meetings of CAOS International,* 2001, Davos, Switzerland.

89. Suhm, N., et al., "Computer assisted distal locking of intramedullary implants: A controlled clinical study including 84 patients," in *First Annual Meeting of CAOS International,* 2001, Davos, Switzerland.

90. DiGioia, A. M., B. Jaramaz, and R. V. O'Toole, "An Integrated Approach to Medical Robotics and Computer Assisted Surgery in Orthopedics," in *Proc. 1st Int. Symposium on Medical Robotics and Computer Assisted Surgery,* 1994. Pittsburgh.

91. Digioia, A., et al., "Clinical Measurements of Acetabular Component Orientation Using Surgical Navigation Technologies," in *First Annual Meeting of CAOS International,* 2001, Davos, Switzerland.

92. Kunz, M., et al., "Development and verification of a non-CT based total knee arthroplasty system for the LCS prosthesis," in *First Annual Meeting of CAOS International,* 2001, Davos, Switzerland.

93. Stulberg, S. D., P. Loan, and V. Sarin, "Computer-Assisted Total Knee Replacement Surgery: An Analysis of an Initial Experience with the Orthopilot (TM) System," in *First Annual Meeting of CAOS International,* 2001, Davos, Switzerland.

94. Saragaglia, D., et al., "Computer-Assisted Total Knee Replacement Arthroplasty: comparison with a conventional procedure. Results of a 50 cases prospective randomized trial," in *First Annual Meeting of CAOS International,* 2001, Davos, Switzerland.

95. Wirth, S., et al., "C-arm based computed tomography: A comparative study," in *Proc. of the 15th Conf. on Computer-Aided Radiology and Surgery,* 2001, Elsevier, Berlin.

96. Shahidi, R., "Advances in video laparoscopic surgery using three-dimensional image enhanced endoscopy," *MDVista Journal,* 2000, May, pp. 56–65.

97. Grimson, W. E. L., et al., "An automatic registration method for frameless stereotaxy, image guided surgery and enhanced reality visualization," *IEEE Trans. on Medical Imaging,* 1996, **15**(2):129–140.

98. Ecke, U., et al., "Virtual Reality: preparation and execution of sinus surgery," *Computer-Aided Surgery,* 1998, **4**(2):45–50.

99. Peterman, J., et al., "Implementation of the CASPAR System in the reconstruction of the ACL," in *CAOS/USA,* 2000, Shadyside Hospital, Pittsburgh.

100. Wiesel, U., et al., "Total Knee Replacement Using the Robodoc System," in *Proc. First Annual Meeting of CAOS International,* 2001, Davos, Switzerland.

101. Tenbusch, M., et al., "First results using the Robodoc system for total knee replacement," in *First Annual Meeting of CAOS International,* 2001, Davos, Switzerland.

102. Mai, S., C. Lorke, and W. Siebert, "Motivation, Realization, and First Results of Robot Assisted Total Knee Arthroplasty," in *Proc. 1st Annual Meeting of CAOS International.* 2001, Davos, Switzerland.

103. Garbini, J. L., et al., "Robotic Instrumentation in Total Knee Arthroplasty," in *Proc. 33rd Annual Meeting, orthopedic Research Society,* 1987, San Francisco.

104. Fadda, M., et al., "Computer-Assisted Knee Arthroplasty at Rizzoli Institutes," in *Proc. 1st International Symposium on Medical Robotics and Computer Assisted Surgery,* 1994, Pittsburgh.

105. Kienzle, T. C., et al., "An integrated CAD-robotics system for total knee replacement surgery," in *Proc. IEEE Int. Conf. on Robotics and Automation,* 1993, Atlanta.

106. Leitner, F., et al., "Computer-assisted knee surgical total replacement," in *Proc. First Joint Conference of CVRMed and MRCAS,* 1997, Grenoble, France, Springer.

107. Marcacci, S., et al., "Computer-Assisted Knee Arthroplasty," in *Computer-Integrated Surgery,* R. H. Taylor et al. (eds.), 1996, MIT Press, Cambridge, Mass. pp. 417–423.

108. Cinquin, P., et al., "IGOR: Image Guided Operating Robot," *Innovation et Technonogie en Biologie et Medicine,* 1992, pp. 374–394.

109. Lavallee, S., et al., "Image-Guided Operating Robot: A Clinical Application in Stereotactic Neurosurgery," in *Computer-Integrated Surgery,* R. H. Taylor et al. (eds.), 1996, MIT Press, Cambridge, Mass., pp. 343–352.

110. Bzostek, A., et al., "A Testbed System for Robotically Assisted Percutaneous Pattern Therapy," in *Medical Image Computing and Computer-Assisted Surgery,* 1999. Springer, Cambridge, England.

111. Schreiner, S., et al., "A system for percutaneous delivery of treatment with a fluoroscopically-guided robot," in *Joint Conf. of Computer Vision, Virtual Reality, and Robotics in Medicine and Medical Robotics and Computer Surgery,* 1997. Grenoble, France.

112. Taylor, R., et al., "An Experimental System for Computer Assisted Endoscopic Surgery," in *IEEE Satellite Symposium on Neuroscience and Technoloy,* 1992, Lyons, IEEE Press.

113. Taylor, R. H., et al., "A Telerobotic Assistant for Laparoscopic Surgery," in *IEEE EMBS Magazine, Special Issue on Robotics in Surgery,* 1995, pp. 279–291.

114. Bzostek, A., et al., "An automated system for precise percutaneous access of the renal collecting system," in *Proc. First Joint Conference of CVRMed and MRCAS,* 1997, Grenoble, France, Springer.

115. Caddedu, J. A., et al., "A Robotic System for Percutaneous Renal Access," *Urology,* 1997.

116. Goldberg, R., A Robotic System for Ultrasound Image Acquisition, 1999, Johns Hopkins University, Baltimore.

117. Chinzei, K., et al., "MR Compatible Surgical Assist Robot: System Integration and Preliminary Feasibility Study," in *Proceedings of Third International Conference on Medical Robotics, Imaging and Computer Assisted Surgery,* 2000, Pittsburgh.

118. Bzostek, A., et al., "Distributed Modular Computer-Integrated Robotic Systems: Implementation Using Modular Software and Networked Systems," in *Medical Image Computing and Computer-Assisted Interventions,* 2000, Pittsburgh, Springer.

119. Schorr, O., et al., "Distributed Modular Computer-Integrated Robotic Systems: Architecture for Intelligent Object Distribution," in *Medical Image Computing and Computer-Assisted Interventions,* 2000, Pittsburgh, Springer.

120. Kaiser, W. A., et al., "Robotic system for biopsy and therapy of breast lesions in a high-field whole-body magnetic resonance tomography unit," *J. Investigative Radiology,* 2000, **35**(8):513–519.

121. Green, P., et al., "Mobile Telepresence Surgery," in *Proc. 2nd Int. Symp. on Medical Robotics and Computer Assisted Surgery,* MRCAS '95, 1995, Baltimore. Center for Orthop. Res., Shadyside Hospital, Pittsburgh.

122. Guthart, G. S., and J. K. Salisbury, "The Intuitive Telesurgery System: Overview and Application," in *Proc. of the IEEE International Conference on Robotics and Automation* (*ICRA2000*), 2000, San Francisco.

123. Charles, S., R. E. Williams, and B. Hamel, "Design of a Surgeon-Machine Interface for Teleoperated Microsurgery," *Proc. of the Annual Int'l Conf. of the IEEE Engineering in Medicine and Biology Society,* 1989, **11**:883–884.

124. Salcudean, S. E., S. Ku, and G. Bell. "Performance measurement in scaled teleoperation for microsurgery" in *First Joint Conference Computer Vision, Virtual Realtiy and Robotics in Medicine and Medical Robotics and Computer-Assisted Surgery,* 1997, Grenoble, France, Springer.

125. Ku, S., and S. E. Salcudean, "Dexterity enhancement in microsurgery using a motion-scaling system and microgripper," in *IEEE Int. Conf. on Systems, Man and Cybernetics,* 1995, Vancouver, B.C.

126. Satava, R., "Robotics, telepresence, and virtual reality: A critical analysis fo the future of surgery," *Minimally Invasive Therapy,* 1992, **1**:357–363.

127. Lee, B. R., J. T. Bishoff, S. Micali, L. L. Whitcomb, R. H. Taylor, and L. R. Kavoussi, "Robotic Telemanipulation for Percutaneous Renal Access," in *16th World Congress on Endourology,* 1998, New York.

128. Guerrouad, A., and P. Vidal, "S.M.O.S.: Stereotaxical Microtelemanipulator for Ocular Surgery," *Proc. of the Annual Int'l Conf. of the IEEE Engineering in Medicine and Biology Society,* 1989, **11**:879–880.

129. Pournaras, C. J., et al., "New ocular micromanipulator for measurements of retinal and vitreous physiologic parameters in the mammalian eye," *Exp. Eye Res.,* 1991, **52**:723–727.

130. Jensen, P. S., et al., "Toward robot assisted vascular microsurgery in the retina," *Graefes Arch. Clin. Exp. Ophthalmol.,* 1997, **235**(11):696–701.

131. Charles, S., "Dexterity enhancement for surgery," *Proc. First Int.'l Symp. Medical Robotics and Computer Assisted Surgery,* 1994, **2**:145–160.

132. Hunter, I. W., et al., "Ophthalmic microsurgical robot and associated virtual environment," *Computers in Biology and Medicine,* 1995, **25**(2):173–182.

133. Schenker, P. S., H. O. Das, and R. Timothy, "Development of a new high-dexterity manipulator for robot-assisted microsurgery," in *Proceedings of SPIE—The International Society for Optical Engineering: Telemanipulator and Telepresence Technologies,* 1995, Boston.

134. Kazerooni, H., and G. Jenhwa, "Human extenders," *Transaction of the ASME: Journal of Dynamic Systems, Measurement and Control,* 1993, **115**(2B):218–290, June.

135. Taylor, R. H., et al., "Telerobotic assistant for laparoscopic surgery," *IEEE Eng. Med. Biol.,* 1995, **14**(3):279–288.

136. Funda, J., et al., "Constrained Cartesian motion control for teleoperated surgical robots," *IEEE Transactions on Robotics and Automation,* 1996.

137. Funda, J., et al., "Control and evaluation of a 7-axis surgical robot for laparoscopy," in *Proc. 1995 IEEE Int. Conf. on Robotics and Automation,* 1995, Nagoya, Japan, IEEE Press.

138. Funda, J., et al., "An experimental user interface for an interactive surgical robot," in *1st International Symposium on Medical Robotics and Computer Assisted Surgery,* 1994, Pittsburgh.

139. Funda, J., et al., "Optimal Motion Control for Teleoperated Surgical Robots," in *1993 SPIE Intl. Symp. on Optical Tools for Manuf. & Adv. Autom.,* 1993, Boston.

140. Kumar, R., et al., "Performance of Robotic Augmentation in Microsurgery-Scale Motions," in *2nd Int. Symposium on Medical Image Computing and Computer-Assisted Surgery,* 1999, Cambridge, England, Springer.

141. Goradia, T. M., R. H. Taylor, and L. M. Auer, "Robot-assisted minimally invasive neurosurgical procedures: First experimental experience," in *Proc. First Joint Conference of CVRMed and MRCAS,* 1997, Grenoble, France, Springer.

142. Kumar, R., et al., "Robot-assisted microneurosurgical procedures, comparative dexterity experiments," in *Society for Minimally Invasive Therapy 9th Annual Meeting,* Abstract Book, vol 6, supplement 1, 1997, Tokyo.

143. Kumar, R., An Augmented Steady Hand System for Precise Micromanipulation, Ph.D. thesis, Computer Science, The Johns Hopkins University, Baltimore, 2001.

144. Kumar, R., and R. Taylor, "Task-Level Augmentation for Cooperative Fine Manipulation Tasks in Surgery," in *MICCAI 2001,* 2001.

145. Kumar, R., et al., "An Augmentation System for Fine Manipulation," in *Medical Image Computing and Computer-Assisted Interventions,* 2000, Pittsburgh, Springer.

146. Kumar, R., P. Jensen, and R. H. Taylor, "Experiments with a Steady Hand Robot in Constrained Compliant Motion and Path Following," in *8th IEEE International Workshop on Robot and Human Interaction* (*ROMAN*), 1999, Pisa, Italy.

147. Faraz, A., and S. Payandeh, "A robotic case study: Optimal design for laparoscopic positioning stands," *J. Robotics Research,* 1998, 17(9):986–995.

148. Abolmaesumi, P., et al., "A User Interface for Robot-Assisted Diagnostic Ultrasound," *IEEE Robotics and Automation Conference,* 2001, Seoul.

149. Goldberg, R., A Modular Robotic System for Ultrasound Image Acquisition, M.S. thesis, Mechanical Engineering, Johns Hopkins University, Baltimore, 2001.

150. Degoulange, E., et al., "HIPPOCRATE: an intrinsically safe robot for medical applicaions," in *IEE/RSH International Conference on Intelligent Robots and Systems,* 1998, Victoria, B.C.

151. Mitsuishi, M., et al., "Remote Ultrasound Diagnostic System," in *Proc. IEEE Conf. on Robotics and Automation,* 2001, Seoul.

152. Carrozza, M., et al., "The development of a microrobot system for colonoscopy," in *Proc. CVRMed and MRCAS—1205,* 1997, Grenoble, Springer Verlag.

153. Ikuta, K., M. Tsukamoto, and S. Hirose, "Shape Memory Alloy Servo Actuator System with Electric Resistance Feedback and Application for Active Endoscope," in *Computer-Integrated Surgery,* R. H. Taylor et al. (eds.), 1996, MIT Press, Cambridge, Mass, pp. 277–282.

154. Sturges, R., and S. Laowattana, "A voice-actuated, tendon-controlled device for endoscopy," in *Computer-Integrated Surgery,* R. H. Taylor, et al. (eds.), 1996, MIT Press, Cambridge, Mass.

155. Asari, V. K., S. Kumar, and I. M. Kassim, "A fully autonomous microrobotic endoscopy system," *Journal of Intelligent and Robotic Systems: Theory and Applications,* 2000, **28**(4):325–342.

156. Mittelstadt, B., et al., "Accuracy of Surgical Technique of Femoral Canal Preparation in Cementless Total Hip Replacement," in *Annual Meeting of American Acadamy of Orthopedic Surgeons,* 1990, New Orleans.

157. Mittelstadt, B., et al., "The Evolution of a Surgical Robot from Prototype to Human Clinical Use," in *Computer-Integrated Surgery,* R. H. Taylor et al., (eds.), 1996, MIT Press, Cambridge, Mass., pp. 397–407.

158. Bishoff, J. T., et al., "RCM-PAKY: Clinical application of a new robotics system for precise needle placement," *Journal of Endourology,* 1998, **12**:S82.

159. Cadeddu, J. A., et al., "A Robotic System for Percutaneous Renal Access Incorporating a Remote Center of Motion Design," *Journal of Endourology,* 1998, **12**:S237.

160. Stoianovici, D., J. A. Cadeddu, L. L. Whitcomb, R. H. Taylor, and L. R. Kavoussi, "A Robotic System for Precise Percutaneous Needle Insertion," *Thirteenth Annual Meeting of the Society for Urology and Engineering,* 1988, San Diego.

161. Stoianovici, D., et al., "Friction Transmission with Axial Loading and a Radiolucent Surgical Needle Drive," 1997, Johns Hopkins University (provisional patent application filed 17 February 1997).

162. Stoianovici, D., et al., "A Modular Surgical Robotic System for Image-Guided Percutaneous Procedures," in *Medical Image Computing and Computer-Assisted Interventions* (*MICCAI-98*), 1998, Cambridge, Mass., Springer.

163. Berkelmann, P. J., et al., "Performance Evaluation of a Cooperative Manipulation Microsurgical Assistant Robot Applied to Stapedotomy," in *Medical Image Computing and Computer-Assisted Interventions* (*MICCAI 2001*), 2001.

164. Stoianovici, D., et al., "A modular surgical robotic system for image guided percutaneous procedures," in *International Conference on Medical Image Computing and Computer-Assisted Intervention.* 1998, Cambridge, Mass.

165. Barnes, A., H. Su, and W. Tam, "An End-Effector for Minimally Invasive Robot Assisted Surgery," 1996, Johns Hopkins University, Dept. of Mechanical Engineering, Baltimore.

166. Barnes, A., A modular robotic system for precise minimally invasive surgery, M.S. thesis, Mechanical Engineering, The Johns Hopkins University, Baltimore, 1999.

167. Gomez-Blanco, M. A., C. N. Riviere, and P. K. Khosla, "Intraoperative instrument motion sensing for microsurgery," in *Proc. 20th Annu. Conf. IEEE Eng. Med. Biol. Soc.,* 1999, Atlanta.

168. Taylor, R. H. and P. Kazanzides, "Medical Robotics and Computer-Integrated Interventional Medicine," in *Biomedical Information Technology*, D. Feng, (ed.), Elsevier, 2007, pp. 393–416.

169. Taylor, R. H. "A Perspective on Medical Robotics," *IEEE Proceedings,* September 2006, **94**: 1652–1664.

170. Kazanzides, P. "Robots for Orthopaedic Joint Reconstruction," In: *Robotics in Surgery: History, Current and Future Applications*, R. A. Faust, (ed.), Nova Science Publishers, 2007, pp. 61–94.

171. *Proceedings of the 6-10th International Conference on Medical Image Computing and Computer Aided Intervention.* Lecture Notes in Computer Sciences, Springer-Verlag, 2003–2008.

172. Shoham, M. et al., "Robotic assisted spinal surgery—from concept to clinical practice," *Computer-Aided Surgery,* 2007, **12**:105–115.

173. The Aurora Electromagnetic Measurement System, Northern Digital, Inc., http://www.ndigital.com/medical/aurora.php, 2008.

174. Flock of Birds, Ascension Technology Corporation, http://www.ascension-tech.com/products/flockofbirds.php, 2008.

175. AXIEM™ Electromagnetic Tracking Technology, Medtronic Surgical Navigation, http://www.medtronicnavigation.com/procedures/navigation/tracking/axiem_electromagnetic_tracking.jsp, 2008.

176. Fischer, G. S. and R. H. Taylor, "Electromagnetic Tracker Measurement Error Simulation and Tool Design," In: *MICCAI*, Palm Springs, CA, 2005, pp. 73–80.

177. Wu, X. and R. H. Taylor, "A Framework for Calibration of Electromagnetic Surgical Navigation Systems," in *IROS*, Las Vegas, 2003, pp. 547–552.

178. Banovac, F. et al., "Precision Targeting of Liver Lesions Using a Novel Electromagnetic Navigation Device in Physiologic Phantom and Swine," *Medical Physics,* August 2005, **32**:2698–2705.

179. Poulin, F. and L. Amiot, "Electromagnetic Tracking in the OR: Accuracy and Sources of Intervention," in *Proceedings of CAOS USA 2001*, Pittsburgh, 2001, pp. 233–235.

180. Wilheim, D. H. Feussner, A. Schneider, and J. Harms, "Electromagnetically Navigated Laparoscopic Ultrasound," *Surgical Technology International,* 2003, **11**:50–54.

181. Wood, B. J. et al., "Navigation with Electromagnetic Tracking for Interventional Radiology Procedures: A Feasibility Study," *Journal of Vascular and Interventional Radiology,* April 2005, **16**:493–505.

182. Fischer, G., J. Zand, M. Talamini, M. Marohn, T. Akinbiyi, K. Kanev, J. Kuo, P. Kazandzides, and R. H. Taylor, "Intra-Operative Ischemia Sensing Surgical Instruments," in *International Conference on Complex Medical Engineering*, Takamatsu, Japan, 2005, p. Accepted.

183. Fischer, G. S., J. Zand, T. M., M. Marohn, T. Akinbiyi, K. Kanev, J. Kuo, P. Kazandzides, and R. H. Taylor "Intraoperative Ischemia Sensing Surgical Instruments," in *International Conference on Complex Medical Engineering*, Takamatsu, Japan, 2005.

184. Pott, P., H. Scharf, and M. Schwarz, "Today's State of the Art in Surgical Robotics," *Computer Aided Surgery,* March 2005, **10**:101–132.

185. Liebergall, M., L. Joskowicz, and M. R., "Computer-aided orthopaedic surgery," in: *Rockwood and Green's Fractures in Adults, 6th Edition*, R. Bucholz and J. Heckman, (eds.), Lippincott Williams and Wilkins, 2006, pp. 739–770.

186. Joskowicz, L., M. Freiman, R. Shamir, M. Shoham, E. Zehavi, and Y. Shoshan, "Image-Guided System with Miniature Robot for Precise Positioning and Targeting in Keyhole Neurosurgery," *Computer-Aided Surgery,* 2006, **11**:181–183.

187. Yaniv, Z. and L. Joskowicz, "Precise Robot-Assisted Guide Positioning for Distal Locking of Intramedullary Nails," *IEEE Transactions on Medical Imaging,* 2005, **24**:624–635.

188. Simaan, N., R. Taylor, A. Hillel, and P. Flint, "Minimally Invasive Surgery of the Upper Airways: Addressing the Challenges of Dexterity Enhancement in Confined Spaces," in *Surgical Robotics—History, Present and Future Applications,* R. Faust, (ed.), Nova Science Publishing, 2007, pp. 223–242.

189. Mitchell, B., J. Koo, I. Iordachita, P. Kazanzides, A. Kapoor, J. Handa, R. Taylor, and G. Hager, "Development and Application of a New Steady-Hand Manipulator for Retinal Surgery," in *International Conference on Robotics and Automation*, Rome, 2007, pp. 623–629.

190. Iordachita, I., A. Kapoor, B. Mitchell, P. Kazanzides, G. Hager, J. Handa, and R. Taylor, "Steady-Hand Manipulator for Retinal Surgery," in *MICCAI Workshop on Medical Robotics*, Copenhagen, 2006, pp. 66–73.

191. Fischer, G. S., A. Deguet, L. M. Fayad, S. J. Zinreich, R. H. Taylor, and G. Fichtinger, "Musculoskeletal Needle Placement with MRI Image Overlay Guidance," in *Annual Meeting of the International Society for Computer Assisted Surgery*, Montreal, Canada, 2006, pp. 158–160.

192. Fichtinger, G., A. Degeut, M. K., G. S. Fischer, E. Balogh, H. Matthieu, R. H. Taylor , S. J. Zinreich, and L. M. Fayad, "Image Overlay Guidance for Needle Insertions in CT Scanner," *IEEE Transactions on Biomedical Engineering,* 2005, **52**:1415–1424.

193. Patronik, N., M. Zenati, and C. Riviere, "Preliminary evaluation of a tethered robotic device for navigation on the beating heart," *Computer Aided Surgery,* 2005, **10**:225–232.

194. Wei, W., R. Goldman, N. Simaan, H. Fine, and S. Chang, "Design and Theoretical Evaluation of Micro-Surgical Manipulators for Orbital Manipulation and Intraocular Dexterity," in *IEEE International Conference on Robotics and Automation* (*ICRA'07*), Rome, 2007, pp. 3389–3395.

195. Simaan, N., R. Taylor, and P. Flint, "High Dexterity Snake-like Robotic Slaves for Minimally Invasive Telesurgery of the Throat," in *International Symposium on Medical Image Computing and Computer-Assisted Interventions*, 2004, pp. 17–24.

196. Wei, W., K. Xu, and N. Simaan, "A Compact Two-armed Slave Manipulator for Minimally Invasive Surgery of the Throat," in *BioRob'2006* (*The first IEEE/RAS-EMBS International Conference on Biomedical Robotics and Biomechatronics*), Pisa, Italy, 2006, pp. 287–292.

197. Kapoor, A., N. Simaan, and R. H. Taylor, "Telemanipulation of Snake-Like Robots for Minimally Invasive Surgery of the Upper Airway," in *MICCAI Medical Robotics Workshop*, Copenhagen, 2006, pp. 17–25.

198. Kapoor, A., N. Simaan, and R. H. Taylor, "Suturing in Confined Spaces: Constrained Motion Control of a Hybrid 8-DOF Robot," in *International Conference on Advanced Robotics*, Seattle, WA, 2005, pp. 452–459.

199. Degani, A., H. Choset, A. Wolf, and M. Zenati, "Highly Articulated Robotic Probe for Minimally Invasive Surgery," in *IEEE International Conference on Robotics & Automation*, Orlando, 2006, pp. 4167–4172.

200. Hongo, K., S. Kobayashi, Y. Kakizawa, J.-I. Koyama, T. Goto, H. Okudera, K. Kan, M. G. Fujie, H. Iseki, and K. Takakura, "NeuRobot: Telecontrolled Micromanipulator System for Minimally Invasive Microneurosurgery-Preliminary Results," *Neurosurgery,* October 2002, **51**:985–988.

201. Ikuta, K., K. Yamamoto, and K. Sasaki, "Development of Remote Microsurgery Robot and New Surgical Procedure for Deep and Narrow Space," in *IEEE Conference on Robotics and Automation*, Taiwan, 2003, pp. 1103–1108.

202. Webster, R. J., A. M. Okamura, and N. J. Cowan, "Toward Active Cannulas: Miniature Snake-Like Surgical Robots," in *EEE/RSJ International Conference on Intelligent Robots and Systems*, Beijing, 2006, pp. 2857–2863.

203. Stefanini, C., A. Menciassi, and P. Dario, "Modeling and Experiments on a Legged Microrobot Locomoting in a Tubular, Compliant and Slippery Environment," *International Journal of Robotics Research,* May-June 2006, **25**:551–560.

204. Dario, P., B. Hannaford, and A. Menciassi, "Smart Surgical Tools and Augmenting Devices," *IEEE Transactions on Robotics and Automation,* October 2003, **19**:782–792.

205. Stoianovici, D., A. Patriciu, Doru Petrisor, Dumitru Mazilu, M. Muntener, and L. Kavoussi, "MRI-Guided Robot for Prostate Interventions," in *Society for Minimally Invasive Therapy (SMIT) 18th Annual Converence*, Pebble Beach, 2006.

206. Krieger, A., R. C. Susil, C. Menard, J. A. Coleman, G. Fichtinger, E. Atalar, and L. L. Whitcomb, "Design of A Novel MRI Compatible Manipulator for Image Guided Prostate Intervention," *IEEE Transactions on Biomedical Engineering,* 2005, **52**:306–313.

207. Harada, K., K. Tsubouchi, M. G. Fujie, and T. Chiba, "Micro Manipulators for Intrauterine Fetal Surgery in an Open MRI," in *IEEE International Conference on Robotics and Automation (ICRA)*, Barcelona, Spain, 2005, pp. 504–509.

208. Louw, D. F., T. Fielding, P. B. McBeth, D. Gregoris, P. Newhook, and G. R. Sutherland, "Surgical Robotics: A Review and Neurosurgical Prototype Development," *Neurosurgery,* 2004, **54**:525–537.

209. Susil, R. C. et al., "Transrectal Prostate Biopsy and Fiducial Marker Placement in a Standard 1.5T MRI Scanner," *Journal of Urolology,* January 2006, **175**:113–120.

210. Joskowicz, L. "Advances in Image-Guided Targeting for Keyhole Neurosurgery: A Survey Paper," *Touch Briefings Reports, Future Directions in Surgery 2006,* vol. II, 2007.

211. DiGioia, A., B. Jaramaz, F. Picard, and L. P. Nolte, *Computer and Robotic Assisted Knee and Hip Surgery*: Oxford Press, 2004.

212. Fuchs, H., A. State, H. Yang, T. Peck, S. Lee, M. Rosenthal, A. Bulysheva, and C. Burke, "Optimizing a Head-Tracked Stereo Display System to Guide Hepatic Tumor Ablation," in *Medicine Meets Virtual Reality (MMVR)*, Long Beach, 2008, p. (to appear).

213. Stetten, G. D. and V. S. Chib, "Overlaying Ultrasonographic Images on Direct Vision," *Journal of Ultrasound in Medicine,* 2001, **20**:235–240.

214. Ukimura, O. and I. S. Gill, "Imaging-Assisted Endoscopic Surgery: Cleveland Clinic Experience," *Journal of Endourology,* April 2008, **22**:in press.

215. Ukimura, O. et al., "Augmented Reality Visualization During Laparoscopic Urologic Surgery: The Initial Clinical Experience," in *The 102nd American Urological Association (AUA 2007) Annual Meeting*, Anaheim, 2007, p. V1052.

216. Vagvolgyi, B., C. E. Reiley, G. D. Hager, R. Taylor, A. W. Levinson, and L.-M. Su, "Toward Direct Registration of Video to Computer Tomography for Intraoperative Surgical Planning During Laparoscopic Partial Nephrectomy," in *World Congress of Endourology*, Cancun, 2007, p. (Poster).

217. Fichtinger, G., A. Deguet, K. Masamune, G. Fischer, E. Balogh, H. Mathieu, R. H. Taylor, S. J. Zinreich, and L. M. Fayad, "Image Overlay Guidance for Needle Insertions in CT Scanner," *IEEE Transactions on Biomedical Engineering,* 2005, **52**:1415–1424.

218. Webster, R. J., J. S. Kim, N. J. Cowan, G. S. Chirikjian, and A. M. Okamura, "Nonholonomic Modeling of Needle Steering," *International Journal of Robotics Research,* 2006, **25**:509–525.

219. Guthart, G. S. and J. K. Salisbury, "The Intuitive Telesurgery System: Overview and Application," in *Proceedings of the IEEE International Conference on Robotics and Automation (ICRA2000)*, San Francisco, 2000, pp. 618–621.

220. Chitwood, W. R., Jr. and L. W. Nifong, "Minimally Invasive Videoscopic Mitral Valve Surgery: The Current Role of Surgical Robotics," *Journal of Cardiac Surgery,* Jan-Feb 2000, **15**:61–75.

221. Ahlering, T., D. Woo, L. Eichel, D. Lee, R. Edwards, and D. Skarecky, "Robot-Assisted versus Open Radical Prostatectomy: A Comparison of One Surgeon's Outcomes," *Urology,* 2004, **63**:819–822.

222. Kanagaratnam, P. M. Koa-Wing, D. Wallace, A. Goldenberg, N. Peters, and D. D.W., "Experience of Robotic Catheter Ablation in Humans Using a Novel Remotely Steerable Catheter Sheath," *Journal of Interventional Cardiac Electrophysiology,* Jan. 18, 2008, **18**:1383–1875X.

223. Kapoor, A. A. Deguet, and P. Kazanzides, "Software Components and Frameworks for Medical Robot Control," in *Proc. of IEEE International Conference on Robotics and Automation*, 2006, 3813–3818.

224. Open Source Software in the Development and Testing of an Image-Guided Robot System, Dspace handle, http://hdl.handle.net/1926/227.

225. Gary, K. L. Ibanez, S. Aylward, D. Gobbi, M. Blake, and K. Cleary, "IGSTK: An Open Source Software Toolkit for Image-Guided Surgery," *IEEE Computer,* April 2006, **39**:46–53.

P • A • R • T • 4

REHABILITATION ENGINEERING AND PROSTHETICS DESIGN

CHAPTER 15
TECHNOLOGY AND DISABILITIES

Albert M. Cook
University of Alberta Edmonton, Alberta, Canada

15.1 INTRODUCTION

This chapter is about the design of electronic assistive devices and the role that they play in the lives of people who have disabilities. It is also a chapter about the role that rehabilitation engineers play in the design and application of these devices and the unique design constraints placed on them in meeting the needs of people who have disabilities. Electronic assistive technologies have a relatively brief history that parallels the development of electronics in general. However, the key to successful application of electronic assistive devices for persons who have disabilities lies in the development of a thorough understanding of the needs which the person has, the context in which the technology will be used, and the skills which the person brings to the task.

15.1.1 The Context for Rehabilitation Engineering

Rehabilitation engineering can be described as the design, development, and application of engineering methods and devices to the amelioration of the problems faced by persons who have disabilities. Future developments in assistive technologies and the successful application of these technologies to meet the needs of people who have disabilities will be driven by the combination of rapid technological advances coupled with the requirement to meet the needs of persons with disabilities. We must design devices that are as accessible to people who have disabilities as possible. When this is not possible, then we must provide adaptations that ensure accessibility in a timely manner. If we do not meet these objectives, then individuals with disabilities may be left behind as technological advances occur.

15.1.2 A Working Definition of Assistive Technologies

One widely used definition of *assistive technologies* is that provided in PL (Public Law) 100-407, the Technical Assistance to the States Act in the United States. The definition of an assistive technology device is

> Any item, piece of equipment or product system whether acquired commercially off the shelf, modified, or customized that is used to increase or improve functional capabilities of individuals with disabilities.

This definition has also been incorporated into other legislation in the United States and is used as a working definition in other countries as well (Cook and Polgar, 2008). Note that the definition includes commercial, modified, and customized devices. This allows us to include products made for the general population in our working definition of assistive technologies. This definition also emphasizes functional capabilities of individuals who have disabilities. The inclusion of customized devices emphasizes the role of the rehabilitation engineer in designing or modifying devices that meet the unique needs of an individual person who has a disability.

15.2 CONTROL INTERFACES FOR ELECTRONIC ASSISTIVE TECHNOLOGIES

There are three elements that make up the user interface for assistive technologies: the control interface, the selection set, and the selection method (Cook and Polgar, 2008). The *control interface* is the boundary between the user and an electronic or mechanical assistive technology device. This is what allows the individual to operate, or control, the device. For electronic assistive technology systems, control interfaces include joysticks for powered wheelchairs, keyboards and mouse input for computers, and communication devices and single switches used to control household devices such as lights or radios. Alternative control interfaces to these are also used, and they are described in later sections of this chapter.

The *selection set* is a presentation of the items from which the user makes choices. The elements in the selection set correspond to the elements of a specific assistive technology device output. Selection sets may have written letters, words and sentences, symbols used to represent ideas, computer icons, or line drawings/pictures. They may be presented in visual (e.g., letters on keys), tactile (e.g., Braille), or auditory (e.g., voice synthesis) form. We can define two *selection methods* through which the user makes selections using the control interface: *direct selection* and *indirect selection* (Cook and Polgar, 2008). For any particular application the three elements of the human/technology interface will be chosen based on the best match to the consumer's skills (motor, sensory, linguistic, and cognitive) (Cook and Polgar, 2008).

The fastest and easiest selection method to understand and use is *direct selection*. In this method, each possible choice in the selection set is available at all times and the user merely chooses the one that she wants. *Indirect selection* methods were developed to provide access for individuals who lacked the motor skills to use direct selection. Indirect selection methods are scanning, directed scanning, and coded access. Each of the indirect selection methods involves one or more intermediate steps between the user's action and the entry of the choice into the device. One of the most commonly used methods is *scanning*. Although there are a variety of implementations of scanning, they all rely on the basic principle of presenting the selection set choices to the user sequentially and having the user indicate when his choice is presented. The indication may be by a single movement of any body part. Since scanning is inherently slow, there have been a number of approaches that increase the rate of selection (Cook and Polgar, 2008). These involve selecting groups of characters first to narrow the choices, then selecting the desired item from the selected group.

In a hybrid approach, called *directed scanning*, the user first activates the control interface to select the direction (vertically or horizontally) in which the selection set is scanned by the device. The user then sends a signal (either by waiting or hitting an additional switch) to the *processor* to make the selection when the desired choice is reached. Joysticks or other arrays of switches (2–8 switches, including diagonal directions) are the control interfaces that are typically used with directed scanning.

Coded access requires the individual to use a unique sequence of movements to select a code corresponding to each item in the selection set. These movements constitute a set of intermediate steps that are required to make the selection using either a single switch or an array of switches as the control interface. One example of coded access used in electronic assistive devices is Morse code, in which the selection set is the alphabet. An intermediate step [e.g., holding longer (dash) or shorter (dot)] is necessary in order to make a selection. Two-switch Morse code is also used, in which one switch sends dots and the other sends dashes. As long as either switch is held down, the dots or dashes are sent. A major goal in the development of Morse code was its efficiency, and this can be very useful when speed of entry is the goal. Codes are usually memorized, and this means that the selection set need not be visually displayed. This allows use by individuals who have visual limitations. Coded access also requires limited physical skill but significant cognitive skill, especially memory and sequencing.

15.2.1 Methods of Activation Used for Control Interfaces

Control interfaces may be characterized by the way in which the consumer activates them (Cook and Polgar, 2008). Three types of action by the user can result in activation of the control interface: movement, respiration, and phonation. These are shown in Table 15.1. Movements can be detected in three basic ways. First, a force may be generated by a body movement and detected by the control interface. These mechanical control interfaces (e.g., switches, keyboard keys, joysticks, mouses, and trackballs) represent the largest category. Many mechanically activated switches are available for control of assistive devices. Most often movement of the hand, head, arm, leg, or foot activates these switches. Hand, foot, or head movement (e.g., chin) is generally used to activate multiple switch arrays, including some joysticks. These vary in the amount of force required, the sensory feedback provided, and the degree to which they can be mounted to a wheelchair, table, or other surface for easy access.

Electromagnetic control interfaces can also be used to detect movement at a distance through either light (visible or IR) or radiofrequency (RF) energy. These interfaces include head-mounted light sources or detectors and transmitters used with environmental control systems for remote control.

The third type of movement detection is electrical. These control interfaces sense bioelectric signals. Switches of this type require no force, and a common example of this type of interface is

TABLE 15.1 Methods of Activation for Control Interfaces

Signal sent, user action (what the body does)	Signal detected	Examples
1. Movement (eye, head, tongue, arms, legs)	a. Mechanical control interface: activation by the application of a force	a. Joystick, keyboard, tread switch
	b. Electromagnetic control interface: activation by the receipt of electromagnetic energy such as light or radio waves	b. Light pointer, light detector, remote radio transmitter
	c. Electrical control interface: activation by the detection of electrical signals from the surface of the body	c. EMG, EOG, capacitive or contact switch
	d. Proximity control interface: activation by a movement close to the detector, but without contact	d. Heat-sensitive switches
2. Respiration (inhalation/expiration)	a. Pneumatic control interface: activation by the detection of respiratory airflow or pressure	a. Puff and sip
3. Phonation	a. Sound or speech control interface: activation by the detection of articulated sounds or speech	a. Sound switch, whistle switch, automatic speech recognition

Source: From Cook AM and Hussey SM: *Assistive Technologies: Principles, and Practice,* (2d ed.), St. Louis, 2002, Mosby Yearbook Publishers, with permission.

capacitive switches used on some elevator buttons. Bioelectrical switches detect muscle electrical activity (EMGs) or eye movement (EOG) by attaching electrodes to the skin.

Another type of body-generated signal is respiration that is detected by measuring either airflow or air pressure using what is called a sip-and-puff switch activated by blowing air into the switch or sucking air out of it. Arrays of single puff-and-sip switches are often used for multiple functions. The most common use has been two puff-and-sip switches mounted side by side for wheelchair control. Puffing on both cause forward motion, sipping on both leads to reverse, and puffing on only one results in a turn in that direction.

15.2.2 Control Interfaces for Direct Selection

The most common control interface for direct selection is the keyboard. However, there are many different types of keyboards and each requires unique user skills. Some consumers have limited range of movement, but good fine motor control. In this case, a contracted keyboard (closely spaced keys over a small range) can be more effective than the standard keyboard. Other individuals have difficulty accessing small targets, but they have good range of movement. In this case, an expanded keyboard, in which the size of each key can be up to several inches, may allow direct selection. Different keyboard layouts can also be used (e.g., for left-hand- or right-hand-only typing). It is also possible to make the keys in different sizes and different shapes on the same keyboard. Touch screens allow a user to choose from the selection set by pointing directly to the item on the screen. Because the item chosen is the one that is pointed at, this method can be easier for some users to understand.

Automatic speech recognition (ASR), in which the individual uses sounds, letters, or words as a selection method, is another alternative to keyboard input. In most systems the speech recognition is *speaker-dependent*, and the user trains the system to recognize his voice by producing several samples of the same element (Comerford et al., 1997). ASR system use is increasing in the mainstream commercial market on the Internet, for dictation, for cell phone use, for personal digital assistants (PDAs), and for most other computer activities. Microsoft Vista* includes ASR as part of the built-in package of accessories. Persons with disabilities will be the beneficiaries of this expanded usage of ASR systems. These systems all use continuous ASR techniques in which the user can speak in almost normal patterns with sight pauses between words.

Speaker-independent systems recognize speech patterns of different individuals without training (Gallant, 1989). These systems are developed using samples of speech from hundreds of people and information provided by phonologists on the various pronunciations of words (Baker, 1981). The total recognition vocabulary is generally small. Discrete ASR systems are used in assistive technology applications for wheelchair control and electronic aids to daily living for appliance control. These systems require the user to pause between words and result in very abnormal speech patterns. They are only used in limited applications requiring a few commands to be recognized.

Often the microphones supplied with ASR systems are not adequate when the user has limited breath support, special positioning requirements, or low-volume speech (Anson, 1997). Many individuals who have disabilities may not be able to independently don and doff headset microphones that are normally supplied with commercial ASR systems. In these cases, desk-mounted types are often used. Current ASR systems utilize commonly available sound cards rather than separate hardware installed in the computer (Anson, 1999).

15.2.3 Control Interfaces for Indirect Access

Indirect methods of selection use a single switch or an array of switches. Cook and Polgar (2008) describe a variety of interfaces that are used for indirect selection.

---

*Microsoft, Seattle, Wash.

15.3 COMPUTER ACCESS BY PERSONS WITH DISABILITIES

Computer use by persons who have disabilities has opened up new opportunities for education, employment, and recreation. The computer offers (1) flexibility (multiple options with the same hardware), (2) adaptability (e.g., as user's skills change over time), (3) customization to a specific user and need (e.g., settings of scanning rate for indirect selection), and (4) specific applications and/or upgrades that can be based on software rather than hardware (e.g., specific user profile for Internet browsing in Braille) (Cook and Polgar, 2008). Computer use is often difficult for individuals who have motor and/or sensory impairments. Successful computer use requires sensory and perceptual abilities for processing computer outputs, motor control for generating input to the computer, and cognitive skills (e.g., problem solving, decision making, memory, language) for understanding the computer functions. When a person with one or more disabilities has difficulty carrying out these functions, engineers are called upon to adapt the computer to make it accessible.

15.3.1 Adapted Computer Inputs

The most common user computer input is provided via either the keyboard or mouse. We can provide adapted computer input in many ways, depending on the needs of the consumer. Keyboard alternatives have been discussed earlier in this chapter. There are also software adaptations for the most common problems experienced by people with disabilities when using a standard keyboard. These are shown in Table 15.2. These software adaptations are included in Accessibility Options in

TABLE 15.2 Minimal Adaptations to the Standard Keyboard and Mouse*

Need addressed	Software approach
Modifier key cannot be used at same time as another key	StickyKeys†
User cannot release key before it starts to repeat	FilterKeys†
User accidentally hits wrong keys	SlowKeys†, BounceKeys†, FilterKeys†
User cannot manipulate mouse	MouseKeys†
User wants to use augmentative communication device as input	SerialKeys† in Windows XP or an alternative (like AAC Keys)
User cannot access keyboard	On-screen keyboard (Windows XP and Vista), built-in ASR (Window Vista)

*Easy Access (part of Universal Access) in Macintosh operating system, Apple Computer, Cupertino, Calif.; Accessibility Options in Windows XP, Ease of Access in Windows Vista, Microsoft Corp., Seattle, Wash.

†Software modifications developed at the Trace Center, University of Wisconsin, Madison, Wis. These are included as before-market modifications to the Macintosh operating system or Windows in some personal computers and are available as after-market versions in others. The function of each program is as follows:

StickyKeys: User can press modifier key, then press second key without holding both down simultaneously.

SlowKeys: A delay can be added before the character selected by hitting a key that is entered into the computer; this means that the user can release an incorrect key before it is entered.

BounceKeys: Prevents double characters from being entered if the user bounces on the key when pressing and releasing.

FilterKeys: The combination of SlowKeys, BounceKeys, and RepeatKeys in Microsoft Windows.

MouseKeys: Substitutes arrow keys for mouse movements.

SerialKeys: Allows any serial input to replace mouse and keyboard, this function has largely been replaced by USB standard devices.

Source: From Cook AM and Polgar JM: *Cook and Hussey's Assistive Technologies: Principles and Practice,* (3d ed.), St. Louis, 2007, Mosby Yearbook Publishers, with permission.

Windows XP*, Easy Access in Windows Vista™, and Universal Access in Macintosh† operating systems. They are accessed and adjusted for an individual user through the control panel. Universal Access for the Macintosh includes Easy Access and Zoom. Easy access features are shown in Table 15.2. Zoom is described later in this chapter.

For persons who have cognitive difficulties we can increase access by using *concept keyboards*. These keyboards replace the letters and numbers of the keyboard with pictures, symbols, or words that represent the concepts required by the software. For example, a program designed to teach monetary concepts might use a concept keyboard in which each key is a coin, rather than a number or letter. The user can push on the coin and have that amount entered into the program. Such keyboards have been used in point-of-sale applications to allow individuals who have intellectual disabilities to work as cashiers. The Intellikeys keyboard‡ is often used as a concept keyboard.

Alternatives to the use of a mouse for computer input that are often used by persons with disabilities include trackballs, a head-controlled mouse, a continuous joystick, eye pointing, and the use of the arrow keys on the numeric keypad (called MouseKeys; see Table 15.2).§ Head control for mouse emulation employs an infrared system, which detects a reflected beam to measure head position relative to a fixed reference point for the cursor (the center of the screen). As the user moves her head away from this point in any direction, the cursor is moved on the screen. Commercial systems¶ use a wireless approach in which a reflective dot is placed on the user's forehead and serves as the reflective target. This allows the user to move around more freely. These head-controlled systems are intended for individuals who have limited arm and hand control and who can accurately control head movement. For example, persons with high-level spinal cord injuries who cannot use any limb movement often find these head pointers to be rapid and easy to use. On the other hand, individuals who have random head movement (e.g., due to cerebral palsy) or who do not have trunk alignment with the vertical axis of the video screen because of poor sitting posture often have significantly more trouble using this type of input device.

In some severe physical disabilities, the user may only be able to move his eyes. In this case, we can use a system that detects the user's eye movements to control mouse pointing. Two basic approaches are used in the design of eye-controlled systems. One of these uses an infrared video camera mounted below the computer monitor. An infrared beam is aimed at the eye and reflected back into the camera. As the user directs his eye gaze at different points of the computer monitor screen, signal-processing software is used to analyze the camera images and determine where and for how long the person is looking on the screen. The user makes a selection by looking at it for a specified period of time, which can be adjusted according to the user's needs. The EyeGaze System, Quick Glance, ERICA**, and Tobii†† are examples of this type. The design principles and approach to the ERICA system are described by Lankford (2000). The second approach uses a head-mounted viewer attached to one side of the frame of a standard pair of glasses in front of the eye. Eye movements are tracked and converted into keyboard input by a separate control unit. One example of this type of system is VisionKey.§§ An eye-controlled system is beneficial for individuals who have little or no movement in their limbs and may also have limited speech; for example, someone who has had a brain stem stroke, has amyotrophic lateral sclerosis (ALS), or high-level quadriplegia.

In each of these alternative pointing devices, input to the pointing device moves a pointer on the screen. One approach uses an onscreen keyboard that displays all of the keys on a standard keyboard. Once the pointer is moved to the desired item, the user can make a selection by either pausing for a preset time (called *acceptance time selection*) or pressing a switch (called *manual selection*). There is an on-screen keyboard utility in Windows™ with basic functionality. Two modes of entry are

*Microsoft, Seattle, Wash.
†Apple Computers, Cupertino, Calif.
‡Intellitools, Richmond, Calif., www.intellitools.com.
§Included with Windows and Macintosh operating systems.
¶HeadMouse, Origin Instruments, http://www.orin.com/; Tracker, Madentec Limited, http://www.madentec.com.
**Eye Response Technologies, Charlottesville, Va. www.eyeresponse.com.
††TobiiTechnology, San Francisco, Calif., www.tobii.com.
§§H.K. EyeCan Ltd., Ottawa, Canada, www.eyecan.ca.

available when an on-screen key is highlighted by mouse cursor movement: clicking and dwelling. In the latter the user keeps the mouse pointer on an on-screen key for an adjustable, preset time and the key is entered. The on-screen feature also allows entry by scanning, using a hot key or switch-input device. Several keyboard configurations are included, and an auditory click may be activated to indicate entry of a character.

The *graphical user interface* (GUI) is used as the selection set for mouse entry. There are limitations to the use of the GUI for people with disabilities. The first of these is that the GUI requires significant eye-hand coordination. Pointing devices rely on a significant amount of coordination between the body site (hand, foot, or head for most individuals with disabilities), executing the movement of the screen pointer and the eyes following the pointer on the screen and locating the targets. Second, it relies on a visual image of the screen for operation. If either of these is not present (e.g., muscle weakness or limited vision), then the GUI is difficult to use, and it must be adapted or an alternative found.

The sensory feedback provided by the particular type of pointing device can vary widely. For individuals who have some vision, a major form of feedback is vision, that is, following the cursor on the screen. Devices controlled by the hand (e.g., mouse, trackball, joystick) also provide rich tactile and proprioceptive feedback. Head- and eye-controlled pointing devices provide much less sensory feedback, and other means, such as an LED that lights when the signal is being received are included to aid the user. The type of sensory feedback affects the user's performance, and the more feedback available, the more likely the use will be successful.

15.3.2 Adapted Computer Outputs

User output from the computer is typically provided by either a video display terminal (VDT), a printer, or speech or sounds. Use of any of these requires an intact sensory system. Alternatives that can be provided may substitute auditory (e.g., speech) or tactile (e.g., Braille) for the VDT output or visual cues for sounds or speech. In the case of low vision, the standard size, contrast, and spacing of the displayed information is inadequate. For individuals who are blind, alternative computer outputs based on either auditory (hearing) or tactile (feeling) modes are used. Persons who are deaf or hard of hearing may also experience difficulties in recognizing auditory computer outputs. Adaptations that facilitate some of these functions are included in *Accessibility Options** in Windows. These include ShowSounds, which displays captions for speech and sounds, and SoundSentry, which generates a visual warning when the system generates a sound.

Alternatives to Visual Input for Individuals Who Have Low Vision. Individuals who have low vision require alternatives to the standard computer screen. Commercial screen magnifiers are used to compensate for several of these problems. The most common adaptation is screen-magnifying software that enlarges a portion of the screen. The unmagnified screen is called the *physical screen.* Screen magnifiers have three basic modes of operation. These are lens magnification, part-screen magnification, and full-screen magnification (Blenkhorn et at., 2002). At any one time the user has access to only the portion of the physical screen that appears in this magnified viewing window. Lens magnification is analogous to holding a handheld magnifying lens over a part of the screen. The screen magnification program takes one section of the physical screen and enlarges it. This means that the magnification window must move to show the portion of the physical screen in which the changes are occurring. Part-screen magnification displays a magnified portion of the screen referred to as the *focus* of the screen in a separate window usually at the top or bottom of the screen (Blenkhorn et al., 2002). Typical foci are the location of the mouse pointer, the location of the text-entry cursor, a highlighted item (e.g., an item in a pull-down menu), or a currently active dialog box. Screen readers automatically track the focus and enlarge the relevant portion of the screen.

Adaptations that allow persons with low vision to access the computer screen are available in several commercial forms. Lazzaro (1999) describes several potential methods of achieving computer access

*Microsoft, Seattle, Wash.

for people who have low vision. Some commonly used operating systems have built-in adaptations. The Macintosh operating system includes a screen magnification program called *Zoom.** This program allows for magnification from 2 to 20 times and has fast and easy text-handling and graphics capabilities. More information is available on the Apple accessibility Web site http://www.apple.com/accessibility. *Magnifier* is a minimal function screen magnification program included in Windows.† Magnifier displays an enlarged portion of the screen (in Windows XP, from 2 to 9 times magnification; in Windows Vista, from 2 to 16 times) and uses a part-screen approach and has three focus options: mouse cursor, keyboard entry location, and text editing. Accessibility Options for Windows XP, Ease of Access for Windows Vista, and Universal Access for Macintosh contain other adaptations such as color contrast, cursor size, and icon size.

Software programs that are purchased separately rather than being built-in offer wider ranges of magnification and have more features than built-in screen magnifiers. Hardware and software combinations have other features such as multiple enlarged windows, smoother scrolling, and a wider range of magnification. Cook and Polgar (2008) and Lazzaro (1999) describe commercial approaches to screen magnification utilities. Most of these approaches also allow adjustment of background and foreground colors to address difficulties with contrast.

Alternatives to Visual Input for Individuals Who Are Blind. For individuals who are blind, computer outputs must be provided in either auditory or tactile form or both. Auditory output is typically provided through systems that use voice synthesis, and tactile output is in Braille. These adaptations are generally referred to as *screen readers*. In its accessibility options, Windows™ includes a basic function screen reader utility, *Narrator*, and a program called *Toggle Keys* that generates a sound when CAPS LOCK, NUM LOCK, or SCROLL LOCK key is pressed.

Macros in screen reader programs are useful in moving between windows or locating key areas (e.g., a dialog box or a window requiring input from the user). Screen readers are ideally suited for applications that consist of text only.

GUI design uses an approach that creates many options for the portrayal of graphic information to video display control. Since each character or other graphical figure is created as a combination of dots, letters may be of any size or shape or color, and many different graphical symbols can be created. This is very useful to sighted computer users because they can rely on the use of "visual metaphors" (Boyd et al., 1990) to control a program. *Visual metaphors* use familiar objects to represent computer actions. For example, a trash can may be used for files that are to be deleted, and a file cabinet may represent a disk drive. The graphical labels used to portray these functions are referred to as *icons*. Screen location is important in using a GUI, and this information is not easily conveyed via alternative means such as screen readers. Visual information is spatially organized and auditory information (including speech) is temporal (time based). It is difficult to convey screen location of a pointer by speech alone. An exception to this is screen locations that never change (e.g., the edges of the screen such as "right border," "top of screen"). Another major problem is that mouse pointer location on the screen is relative, and the only information available is the direction of the movement and how far the mouse has moved. One approach to this problem is the Microsoft Screen Access Model.‡ This is a set of technologies designed to facilitate the development of screen readers and other accessibility utilities for Windows™ that provide alternative ways to store and access information about the contents of the computer screen. The Screen Access Model also includes software driver interfaces that provide a standard mechanism for accessibility utilities to send information to speech devices or refreshable Braille displays. GUI access also requires capability for locating open windows, monitoring them for changes, and outputting information to the user if changes occur. Screen reader programs also provide assistance in this "navigation" function by using keyboard commands such as movement to a particular point in the text, finding the mouse cursor position, providing a spoken description of an on-screen graphic or special function key, or accessing help information. Screen readers also monitor the screen and take action when a particular block

*Macintosh Operating System, Apple Computer, Cupertino, Calif., www.apple.com/accessibility.

†www.microsoft.com/enable/default.aspx.

‡www.microsoft.com/enable/products/microsoft.

of text or a menu appears (Lazzaro, 1999). This feature allows the user to automatically have pop-up window and dialog boxes read to her. Screen readers can typically be set to speak by line, sentence, or paragraph.

For Windows-based computers, the majority of commercial products include both a voice synthesizer and a software-based screen reader to provide access. Many of these bundled software programs also work with computer soundboards to generate high-quality synthetic speech. Tactile (Braille) display of screen information is the other major alternative for screen readers. This requires the use of a translator program to convert from text characters to Braille cell dot patterns. Computer output systems utilize either a refreshable Braille display consisting of raised pins or hard copy via Braille printers. Refreshable Braille displays consists of 20, 40, or 80 separate cells. Rather than the standard six-cell Braille used for print materials, a unique eight-dot cell format is available in which the seventh and eighth dots are used for indicating the location of the cursor and to provide single-cell presentation of higher-level ASCII characters. The latter feature is necessary since the normal 6-cell Braille display can only generate 64 permutations and full ASCII has 132 characters. Braille embossers produce hard copy (printed) output. Cook and Polgar (2008) describe a number of commercial approaches to screen readers with speech and Braille output as well as embossers for hard copy.

15.4 AUGMENTATIVE AND ALTERNATIVE COMMUNICATION

The term *augmentative and alternative communication* (AAC) is used to describe any communication that supplements speech. When someone is unable to speak and/or write so that all current and potential communication partners can understand them, then an AAC system is required. Communication requiring only the person's own body, such as pointing and other gestures, pantomime, facial expressions, eye-gaze and manual signing, or finger spelling is called *unaided communication. Aided AAC* may be either electronic or nonelectronic and includes a pen or pencil, a letter or picture communication board, a computer, a cell phone, and an electronic speech generating device (SGD).

Humans communicate in many ways, including speaking and writing, for example face to face, on the phone, and across the Internet. Writing includes drawing, plotting, graphing, and mathematics. Light (1988) describes four purposes of communicative interaction: (1) expression of needs and wants, (2) information transfer, (3) social closeness, and (4) social etiquette. Expression of needs and wants allows people to make requests for objects or actions. Information transfer allows expression of ideas, discussion, and meaningful dialogue. Social closeness connects individuals to each other, and social etiquette establishes cultural formalities in communication. For example, students will speak differently to their peers than to their teachers.

15.4.1 Needs Served by Augmentative Communication

In considering communication needs, we address three perspectives: individuals with developmental disorders; individuals with acquired conditions, and individuals with degenerative conditions. The focus of AAC interventions may vary across these groups. AAC interventions for children with developmental disabilities require integration into the child's daily experiences and interactions that take into account what we know about child development (Light and Drager, 2002). Adults with acquired disabilities such as traumatic brain injury (TBI), aphasia, and other static conditions may require the use of AAC interventions as part of the rehabilitation process (Beukelman and Ball, 2002). Persons who are recovering from injury or disease often experience changing levels of motor, sensory, and/or cognitive/linguistic capability that can benefit from the use of aided AAC.

15.4.2 Characteristics of Augmentative Communication Systems

Since speech allows communication at a rapid rate, between 150 and 175 words per minute (Miller, 1981), an individual using an AAC system must be as rapid as possible. In all AAC systems, some form of letter or symbol selection is required, and in many cases persons who are unable to speak use a keyboard to type their messages that are then spoken by an AAC device. If the person has limited motor skills, this can result in significantly lower rates of communication than for speech (as low as a few words per minute). Cook and Polgar (2008) describe other relationships between AAC characteristics and effective conversational skills.

AAC systems may be thought of as having three major components: (1) user interface, (2) processor, and (3) output. The user interface has been described earlier in this chapter. It includes the user control interface, selection method and selection set, and an optional user display to provide feedback for self-correction. AAC devices often use special symbols in the selection set. These include miniatures of objects, color or black-and-white pictures, line drawings, pictographic symbols, text characters, and multiple meaning icons* (Beukelman and Mirenda, 2005). For AAC systems, the processor has several specific functions: (1) selection technique, (2) rate enhancement and vocabulary expansion, (3) vocabulary storage, and (4) output control. The output is conversational and/or graphic communication. Communication takes place in many different settings.

In order to maximize the production of output, AAC devices use techniques to increase the rate of entry by the user. Any approach that results in the number of characters generated being greater than the number of selections that the individual makes will increase rate. Rate enhancement techniques can be grouped into two broad categories: (1) encoding techniques and (2) prediction techniques. There are several types of codes that are currently used in AAC devices. Numeric codes can be related to words or complete phrases or sentences. When the user enters one or more numbers, the device outputs the complete stored vocabulary item. Abbreviation expansion is a technique in which a shortened form of a word or phrase (the abbreviation) stands for the entire word or phrase (the expansion). When an abbreviation is entered, it is automatically expanded by the device into the desired word or phrase. Vanderheiden and Kelso (1987) discuss the major features of abbreviation expansion systems and the strategies for developing stored vocabulary using this approach. An alternative approach that is based on coding of words, sentences, and phrases on the basis of their meaning is called *semantic encoding* (Baker, 1982). In this approach, pictorial representations, called icons, are used in place of numerical or letter codes. For example, using a picture of an apple for "food," and a sun rising for "morning," then selecting "apple" "sunrise" as a code for "What's for breakfast" is easier to remember than an arbitrary numeric or letter code for the same phrase. The apple can also represent the color red, eating, fruit, etc.

It is also possible to realize significant increases in rate by using word prediction or word completion techniques with any selection method (Swiffin et al., 1987). Devices that use these techniques typically have a list on the screen that displays the most likely words based on the letters that have previously been entered. The user selects the desired word, if it is listed, by entering a number listed next to the word. If the desired word is not displayed, the user continues to enter letters, and the listed words change to correspond to the entered letters. In adaptive word completion, the ranking of the presented list is changed based on the user's frequency of use. Placing the word lists on the screen at the point in the document where the typed letters appear enables the user to keep his gaze fixed on one location while typing, and it also requires significantly fewer switch activations in scanning. One application of this approach, called Smart Lists,™† can be used with either keyboard or scanning entry. Smart Keys™‡ is similar to the Minspeak icon prediction. After each entry only the keys which contain a prediction based on that entry are left on the on-screen keyboard, making scanning significantly faster.

A selection set for AAC consists of a maximum of 128 selections on most devices, and many have far fewer available at any one time. However, even a child has a vocabulary of thousands of words. Thus, it is necessary to have methods to allow easy access to vocabulary items that are not displayed. The rate enhancement techniques are one way to do that, but they all require memory and cognitive skills such as sequencing. One approach is to present the selection sets on a dynamic display

*Minsymbols, Prentke Romich Co., Wooster, Ohio.
†Applied Human Factors, Helotes, Tex., www.ahf-net.com.
‡Applied Human Factors, Helotes, Tex., www.ahf-net.com.

accessed through a touch screen. The displayed information is changed based on previous entries. For example, a general selection set might consist of categories such as work, home, food, clothing, greetings, or similar classifications. If one of these is chosen, either by touching the display surface directly or using scanning, then a new selection set is displayed. For example, a variety of food-related items and activities (eat, drink, ice cream, pasta, etc.) would follow the choice of "foods" from the general selection set. Thus, the user does not have to remember what is on each level. Cook and Polgar (2008) describe typical approaches used in AAC system design.

15.5 AIDS FOR MANIPULATION

Many individuals who have limited function of their arms and hands experience difficulty in manipulating objects, controlling appliances (e.g., television, telephone), reading a book, or feeding oneself or self-care. Assistive technologies that aid manipulation may be simple mechanical aids (e.g., reachers, enlarged handle eating utensils), special-purpose electromechanical devices (e.g., page turners or feeders), or more general-purpose devices [e.g., *electronic aids to daily living* (*EADLs*) and robotics]. In this section we will discuss only EADLs. The others are described in Cook and Polgar (2008).

Many objects that need to be manipulated are electrically powered devices such as appliances (e.g., television, room lights, fans, and kitchen appliances such as blenders or food processors), which use standard house wiring (110 V ac in North America). *EADLs* are designed to allow people with limited upper extremity function to control these appliances. A typical EADL for turning appliances on and off is shown in Fig. 15.1. The user control interface may be a keypad as shown or a single switch with an indirect selection method. The appliances are plugged into modules that are controlled by the EADL. The most common type of on/off module is the X-10.* Three types of wireless transmission are used in EADL design. The most common is *infrared* (IR) transmission like that used in most TV remote units. A second method, also sometimes used for TV control, is *ultrasound* transmission. The third method, often used in garage door openers, is *radiofrequency* (RF) transmission. IR and ultrasound require line-of-sight transmission. RF transmission does not have this requirement. ZigBee is one form of wireless technology that is ideally suited for low data rate applications such as EADLs since it provides all the advantages of RF transmission and has low power consumption (meaning longer battery life) and long range of operation (range enough to control the whole home from anywhere inside it, not just the immediate room) (Bessell et al., 2006).

The system of Fig. 15.1 may be modified to include remote control over TV or VCR functions such as volume control, channel selection, play, fast forward, and reverse. In this case the level (for volume) or number (for channel) is under the control of the human user. Often these functions are incorporated into EADLs by modifying standard TV or VCR remote controls. This may be done by merely adding a single switch to the remote control or by more elaborate adaptations that allow indirect selection. Sometimes universal remote controls that can "learn" the signal for a particular TV or VCR are used. This allows several appliances to be controlled from the same EADL. Cook and Polgar (2008) describe several commercial approaches to this type of EADL.

Persons with physical disabilities of the upper extremities often have difficulty in carrying out the tasks associated with telephone use. These include lifting the handset, dialling, holding the handset while talking, and replacing the handset in its cradle. There are several options for accomplishing these tasks. Nonelectronic methods such as mouth sticks or head pointers can be used to press a button to open a line on a speakerphone, dial, and hang up. EADLs perform these same telephone tasks electronically. For persons who require single switch access to the system, the control interface is connected to a control unit that also interfaces with a display and with standard telephone electronics. A typical approach is for the device to present numbers sequentially on the display, and

*X-10 Powerhouse System, Northvale, N.J.

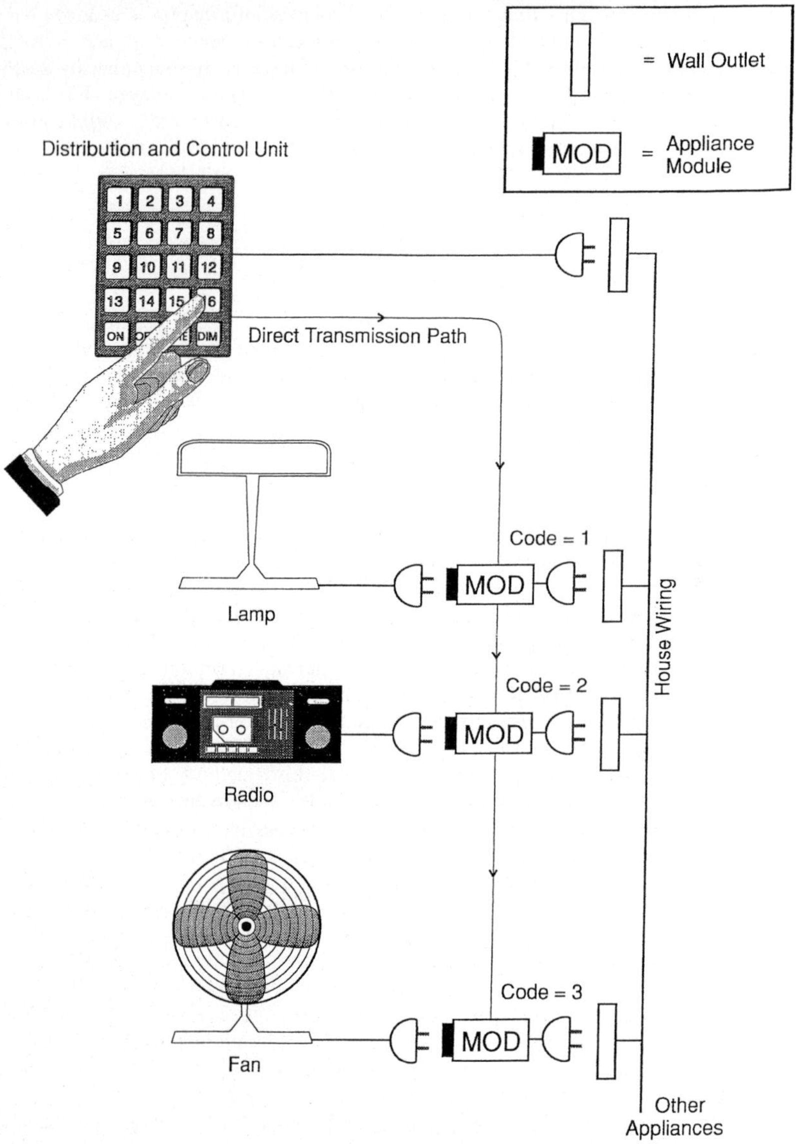

FIGURE 15.1 A direct-selection ECU. Each appliance has a numeric code, and the keypad is used to select the appropriate module. Control functions such as "on," "off," and "dim" are also activated by pressing the proper key on the keypad. This figure also illustrates the use of house wiring for distribution of the control signals to the appliance modules. (From Cook AM and Hussey SM: *Assistive Technologies: Principles and Practice,* (2d ed.), St. Louis, 2002, Mosby Yearbook Publishers, with permission.)

the user to press a switch when the desired number to be dialled is on the display. By repeating this process, any phone number can be entered and then sent through the standard telephone electronics for automatic dialling. Since many persons with disabilities respond slowly, all practical systems use stored numbers and automatic dialling. Another unique feature is the inclusion of a Help or Emergency phone number that can be dialled quickly. Most systems have a capacity of 50 to 100 stored numbers. Some telephones are IR-controlled, and they can be included with EADLs that learn device codes.

15.6 FUTURE TRENDS

The editors of *PC Magazine* identified 10 trends that are likely to have a profound impact on assistive technology design and application over the first 10 years of the twenty-first century (Miller et al., 1999). One prediction is that computers will have more human attributes such as reacting to spoken words (using ASR) or hand-written instructions. In general, the emphasis is on making the user interface more "friendly." Telephone access to the Internet via ASR is already available. ASR will continue to improve, but a major challenge will continue to exist for people who have unintelligible (dysarthric) speech. Current ASR systems do not provide good results for this population, and this is clearly an area in which assistive technologies must be developed to allow persons with speech disabilities to access the new user interfaces. Similar problems could occur for individuals who have poor fine motor control if user interfaces require recognition of handwriting.

Changes in the nature of networks are occurring that have the potential to benefit those who have disabilities. Existing networks are expanding into home, work, and community environments, providing the capability for unique and powerful connections. For example, automobile networks will be connected to toll booths and automated fuel pumps, reducing the need for physical manipulation and facilitating payment. They will also make assisted driving possible, with a potential benefit to persons with disabilities. Wireless networks provide connectivity as a function of local resources, not existing hard-wired communications providers. This offers the opportunity for people with disabilities to use their assistive technologies to connect to the network.

Creating an accessible environment for ICT is referred to as *universal design* (Emiliani, 2006). The goal of universal design is to have an easily adaptable environment based on embedded intelligence. The overall goal is to have access to information involving communities of users with a wide range of motor, sensory, and cognitive skills. To ensure that this connectivity is possible, rehabilitation engineers must also design assistive technologies that keep pace with constant changes in the design of network configurations where universal design is not feasible.

A major part of universal design is to increase the "embedded intelligence" of the Internet. People with disabilities will be able to download many applications from the Internet. A user will be able to store their customized programs on the network and download them as needed from any remote location. Applications such as hand- or fingerprint recognition built into a door knob will recognize the owner and avoid the necessity of manipulating a key. Because of the need for very small keyboards and more and more functions, embedded automatic speech recognition is being developed for PDAs (Kumagai, 2004). This feature could be very useful to individuals who have limited hand function or for those who cannot see the keyboard to make entries. Embedded information networks allow trainable hearing aids to adjust to changing noise levels in the environment automatically. For people who are blind, downloading a talking book program into a cell phone can provide access to digital libraries. Outputs in speech or enlarged visual displays can be added as needed by the user. A blind person could obtain a verbal description of a scene by using a built-in camera and network access and linking to online volunteers who provide descriptions of images. These applications will depend on the increasing application of universal design in information technology products such as ATMs, cell phones, vending machines, and other systems that are encountered on a daily basis.

In the future, appliances from watches to dishwashers will have embedded intelligence, making it possible to network them within a home and to control them remotely. For example, a meal can be started from work by turning on the stove remotely. One of the keys to these applications is the use of hardware and software that allows digitally controlled appliances to "self organize" into a community without a server to manage the network. This type of interconnectivity and remote control are ideal for individuals who use EADLs or who can't see appliance controls.

15.7 SUMMARY

Electronic assistive devices provide expanded opportunities for people who have disabilities. Those discussed in this chapter include access to computers for input and output functions, Internet access, EADLs for manipulation, and communication devices (AAC). As advances are made in electronics, computing, and network applications, there is a constant challenge to ensure that these systems remain accessible to persons who have disabilities. Rapidly changing communication technologies may result in the need to redesign accessible interfaces. Developments that broaden the scope, applicability, and usability of the user interface will be driven, at least in part, by the needs of people who have disabilities. Engineers who focus their efforts on rehabilitation applications can have a significant influence on these developments and on the lives of people who have disabilities.

REFERENCES

Anson D: Speech recognition technology. *OT Practice*, 59–62, January/February, 1999.

Anson DK: *Alternative Computer Access: A Guide to Selection*, Philadelphia, 1997, F. A. Davis Company.

Baker B: Minspeak, *Byte*, **7**:186–202, 1982.

Baker JM: How to achieve recognition: a tutorial/status report on automatic speech recognition, *Speech Technology*, 30–31,36–43, Fall 1981.

Bessell T, Randell M, Knowles G, and Hobbs D: Connecting People with the Environment—A New Accessible Wireless Remote Control, *Proceedings of the 2004 ARATA Conference*, retrieved from http://www.e-bility.com/arataconf06/papers/environmental_control/ec_hobbs_paper.doc, Nov. 17, 2006.

Beukelman DR and Mirenda P: *Augmentative and Alternative Communication, Management of Severe Communication Disorders in Children and Adults,* (3d ed.), Baltimore, 2005, Paul H. Brooks.

Blenkhorn P, Gareth D, and Baude A: Full-screen magnification for Windows using DirectX overlays, *IEEE Transactions on Neural Systems and Rehabilitation Engineering,* **10**:225–231, 2002.

Beukelman DR and Ball LJ: Improving AAC use for persons with acquired neurogenic disorders: understanding human and engineering factors, *Assistive Technology,* **14**:33–44, 2002.

Boyd LH, Boyd WL, and Vanderheiden, GC: The graphical user interface: crisis, danger, and opportunity, *Journal of Visual Impairment and Blindness,* **84**(10):496–502, 1990.

Comerford R, Makhoul J, and Schwartz R: The voice of the computer is heard in the land (and it listens too), *IEEE Spectrum,* **34**(12):39–47, 1997.

Cook AM and Polgar JM: *Cook and Hussey's Assistive Technologies: Principles and Practice,* (3d ed.), St. Louis, 2008, Mosby Yearbook Publishers.

Emiliani PL: Assistive technology (AT) versus mainstream technology (MST): the research perspective. *Technology and Disability,* **18**:19–29, 2006.

Gallant JA: Speech-recognition products, *Emergency Department News,* 112–122, Jan. 19, 1989.

Lazzaro JL: Helping the web help the disabled, *IEEE Spectrum,* **36**(3):54–59, 1999.

Lankford C: Effective eye-gaze input into Windows™, *Eye Tracking Research and Applications Symposium,* Palm Beach Gardens, 23–27, 2000.

Kumagai J: Talk to the machine, *IEEE Spectrum,* **39**(9):60–64, 2004.

Light J: Interaction involving individuals using augmentative and alternative communication systems: state of the art and future directions, *Augmentative and Alternative Communication,* **4**(2):66–82, 1988.

Light JC and Drager KDR: Improving the design of augmentative and alternative technologies for young children, *Assistive Technology,* **14**:17–32, 2002.

Miller MJ, Kirchner J, Derfler FJ, Grottesman BZ, Stam C, Metz C, Oxer J, Rupley S, Willmott D, and Hirsch N: Future technology, *PC Magazine,* **18**(12):100–148, 1999.

Swiffin AL, et al.: Adaptive and predictive techniques in a communication prosthesis, *Augmentative and Alternative Communication,* **3**(4):181–191, 1987.

Vanderheiden GC and Kelso DP: Comparative analysis of fixed-vocabulary communication acceleration techniques, *Augmentative and Alternative Communication,* **3**:196–206, 1987.

CHAPTER 16
APPLIED UNIVERSAL DESIGN

Ronald S. Adrezin
United States Coast Guard Academy, New London, Connecticut

16.1 MOTIVATION

Engineers are expert problem solvers. They love challenges and regularly handle the stress and excitement of balancing cost with safety and reliability. However, many wonderful devices on the market were not designed by engineers. So what makes engineers so valuable? They can apply their skills across industries. An engineer can safely strip every ounce out of a weight-critical design. And when a problem is properly defined, an engineer can solve it in a cost-effective manner.

Designing a product that is accessible to persons with disabilities will increase your market share and produce a better product for all. If this accessibility is designed into the product, there is a negligible effect on the price. This is the heart of what we call *universal design*. By applying one's creativity, countless products can be manufactured that do not neglect people below the fifth or above the ninety-fifth percentiles. These individuals may be found among your family, friends, neighbors, and colleagues. Do not exclude them!

It is my sincere hope that this chapter will assist you in designing for persons with disabilities. The consumers of these products have been divided into three broad categories. The first includes custom devices designed for a sole user. Here, the design team knows the needs, desires, and anthropometrics of the final user, who is generally part of the team. A second category covers devices to be marketed to persons with a common disability. Examples include hearing aids, wheelchairs, and environmental control units. Their design may include the ability to be customized by the end user. The last category describes products to be used by the general population. These mass-produced devices include television remote controls, appliances, toys, and computers. Whether for a sole user, a group of persons with a common disability, or a mass-produced product where universal design principles are applied, I have attempted to provide engineers with a practical starting point. This chapter stresses new designs of devices for persons with disabilities. It is not focused on the selection or customization of existing assistive devices.

Engineers sometimes forget the importance of form while focusing on function. Persons with disabilities are often subjected to stares and the stigmas attached to the use of many assistive devices. In the design process, therefore, you must consider the aesthetics of the device. There is often an assumption that everyone loves technology as much as engineers. For instance, there was a time when many counselors would push a person with a spinal chord injury into the field of computer programming. Yes, the interface to the computer was available but not necessarily the person's interest. Can everyone in the general population become a programmer? So why should everyone with a disability?

It is our role to utilize technology to expand the options available. As a result of the Americans with Disabilities Act,* companies must make reasonable accommodations to allow those with disabilities to succeed in the workplace.

It is my hope that readers will consider lending their talents to this challenging but satisfying field. I also encourage you to fully incorporate universal design into all your products.

16.2 DESIGN METHODOLOGY

This section has been developed to supplement the many fine design textbooks available. The order of the subsections from problem definition to embodiment design is similar to the organization of many of these texts. The conceptual generation stage includes techniques such as brainstorming and functional decomposition. This section will simply present functional decomposition as an example. Embodiment design, where the design concept begins its physical form, combines product architecture, configuration, and parametric design.[1] Here, the focus is on human factors and universal design. Evaluation methods and detail design are not included, but your concepts should satisfy universal design principles in the evaluation stage.

16.2.1 Problem Definition

This subsection addresses special issues in the problem definition stage of the design process. It then demonstrates how techniques such as quality function deployment can be applied to this field.

16.2.2 Avoid an Ill-Defined Problem

A properly defined engineering problem is essential to a successful design. You must understand the desires and needs of the device's user, as well as those who will interact with, prescribe, service, or pay for this device. (Read Sec. 16.2.5 for more details.) Many articles and texts treat this topic, and it is there that I refer you.[1–3,7] As you study this chapter, pay careful attention to the person's age, prognosis, and the many social-psychological issues as the problem is defined. If the user is a child, his or her size will change, as will his or her physical and cognitive abilities. A person with a disease may have his or her condition improve or worsen. The prognosis is the best indication of what might happen. Finally, if the device has any negative connotations associated with it, it might not be used in public or at all.

16.2.3 Striving to Increase Independence

Assistive devices for persons with disabilities are not designed to "fix" the person but rather to improve the person's surroundings.[4] Devices that can improve and enhance a person's independence are of great value. A device that helps a person bathe his or her elderly parent is useful. Imagine a product that allows this parent to bathe himself or herself; now that is wonderful! Whether applying universal design principles to develop a product to satisfy an aging population, an adult to succeed in the workplace, a teen to attend school, or a child to participate in social activities with both able-bodied and disabled friends, an engineer has the ability to increase a person's independence and improve the quality of his or her life. In addition, for often a negligible differential in per-unit cost when designed into the product, a company will increase its market share by tapping into this large population.

*The Americans with Disabilities Act was signed into law in 1990 and went into effect in January 1992. *Reasonable accommodations* refer to efforts that may include, among other adjustments, making the workplace structurally accessible to disabled individuals, restructuring jobs to make best use of an individual's skills, modifying work hours, reassigning an employee with a disability to an equivalent position as soon as one becomes vacant, acquiring or modifying equipment or devices, appropriately adjusting or modifying examinations, training materials, or policies, and providing qualified readers for the blind or interpreters for the deaf.

16.2.4 Reality Check

Commitment to a design refers to the point at which you have invested too many resources to make substantial revisions. At this point, your options may be to continue with your current design or scrap it entirely. Best practice suggests that you keep your design on paper (or computer) as long as possible before investing funds on the product's manufacture.[7] As part of good design practice, before you are committed to a design, do a reality check. This is where you ensure that the features that you have selected to satisfy your customers are appropriate. Simply selecting to meet the requirements calculated to be of greatest importance as a result of a focus group may lead to a design that no one wants. For example, you might miss the features that are commonplace and therefore expected. This may result from a focus group's failure to list important features because they assume that all products will have them. Examples include a remote control for a television, the automatic shutoff of a coffee pot, the ability to fold a manual wheelchair, and the light weight of a walker. When designing products for a broad population, the statistics from the quality function deployment, if improperly interpreted, may lead to the production of a two-door minivan with seven sporty bucket seats that cannot accommodate infant seats. However, when applied correctly, techniques such as quality function deployment will aid the design team in fully understanding the customers' needs and wants. It is one of many important tools that will lead to a successful, safe, and cost-effective design.

16.2.5 Quality Function Deployment

Brief Overview. Quality function deployment (QFD) is a powerful and widely used method to define your customers, determine their needs, benchmark the competition, and define engineering parameters and targets that, when met, will lead to a successful product. The QFD diagram, referred to as the *house of quality* because of its shape (Fig. 16.1), provides an important view of the customers' needs. Understanding your customers and the environment in which you must compete is crucial to your problem definition.

There are variations to the house of quality.[1,3,5,7] Some people try to quantify the relative importance of each requirement[1]; others are more qualitative. There may be multiple QFDs corresponding to elements of the design process. Figure 16.1 shows a house of quality with each "room" numbered. Figure 16.2 illustrates an example of the following hypothetical product: A manufacturer of toaster ovens would like its next generation of products to satisfy universal design requirements. Figure 16.3

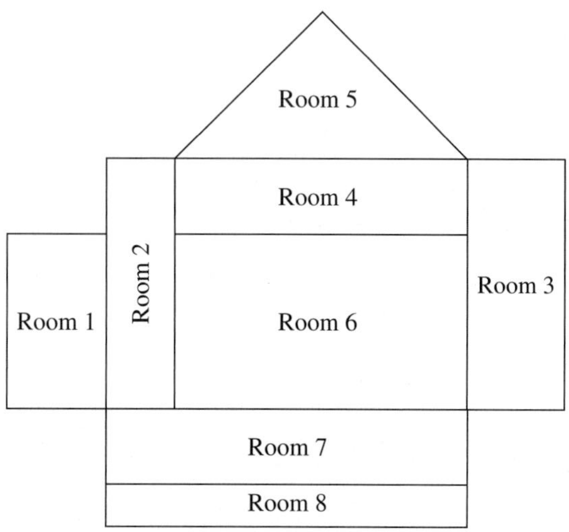

FIGURE 16.1 House of quality.

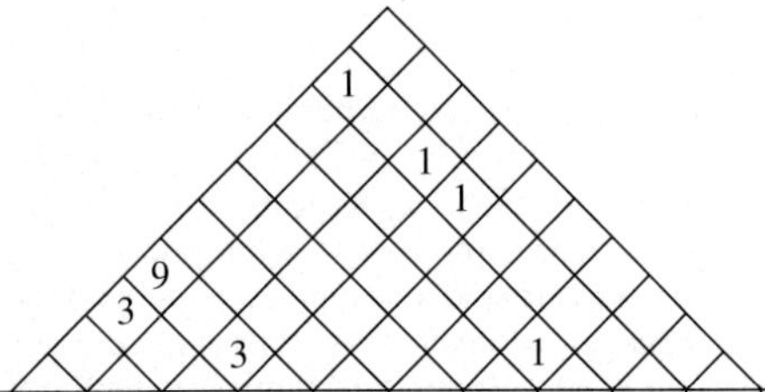

	User with low vision	User with arthritis	User with no disabilities	Hold temperature within X degrees [°C]	Force to open door [N]	% of food burned	Evenness [1–5 scale]	% of focus groups finding design appealing	% of input/output devices compatible with	Size of smallest font [point]	Size of smallest input device [cm^2]	Maximum exterior case temperature [°C]	Sales price [$]	Competitor A	Competitor B	Competitor C	No product
Cooks well	5	5	5	9		9	9							4	4	4	1
Easy to open	2	5	4		9									3	3	3	
Cannot burn food	5	4	4			9	3							1	1	1	
Looks nice	3	4	3					9		1	1	1		3	2	4	
Compatible with I/O	4	5	1						9					1	1	1	
Easy to read settings	5	3	3					3	3	9				2	2	3	
Easy to adj. settings	2	5	3						3		9			3	4	2	
Low price	2	3	5	3			3		3				9	4	5	4	5
Case not too hot	3	5	3			1						9		1	1	1	5
Easy to clean	5	5	5		1	3								3	4	4	5
Can hear when done	4	3	3											2	1	1	

	Hold temperature within X degrees [°C]	Force to open door [N]	% of food burned	Evenness [1–5 scale]	% of focus groups finding design appealing	% of input/output devices compatible with	Size of smallest font [point]	Size of smallest input device [cm^2]	Maximum exterior case temperature [°C]	Sales price [$]
Competitor A	5	0.1	NA	3	40	0	6	3	200	30
Competitor B	4	0.2	NA	2	25	0	6	2	210	15
Competitor C	4	0.2	NA	4	60	0	8	3	190	65
No product										0
Target	4	0.1	0	4	80	100	18	9	30	60

FIGURE 16.2 Partial QFD, toaster oven example.

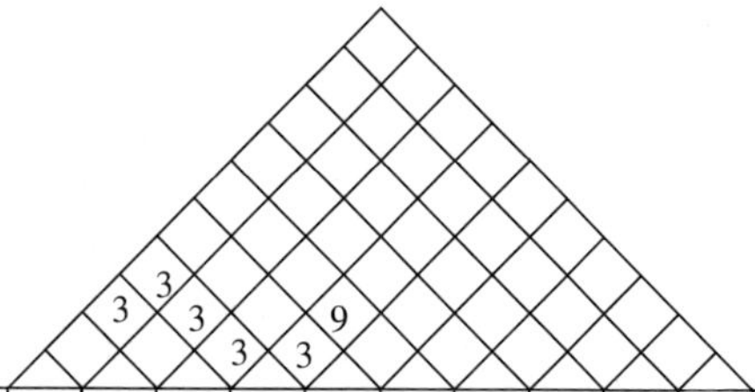

	Infant and parent	Nurse	Insurer	Max. heart rate [beats per minute]	Max. respiration rate [breaths per minute]	Pulse oximetry [%]	# of apnea events missed	Time between apnea event and alarm [seconds]	% of false positives	Log memory capacity [days]	Weight [kg]	% of caregivers who can troubleshoot correctly	Alarm volume [dB]	Home apnea monitor	Video monitor	Adult present with infant	No product or adult present
Detects apnea	5	5	5	9	9	9	9	3	9			3		4	2	4	
Notifies caregiver	5	5	5					9	3	1			9	5	3	5	
Portable	3	3									9			2	1	5	
Easy to use	4	4							9		3	9		3	4	4	5
Simple to clean	3	3		1	1	1					1			4	5		
Safe	5	5	5	9	9	9	9	9	9	9		9	3	5	5	5	
Easy to troubleshoot	3	5		1	1	1		1		9		9		4	4		
Logs events	2	5		1	1	1	1			9				4	5	4	
Use in auto/stroller/crib	4	3		3	3	3		3	3		9		9			4	
Setup quickly	3	5		3	3	3					3	9		2	2	5	5
Few false positives	5	5		3	3	3	1	1	9			1		3	1	4	
Home apnea monitor				250	120	100	0	20	50	30	2.5	60	70				
Video monitor				0	0	0	10			1	2	80					
Adult present with infant				0	0	0	0										
No product				0	0	0											
Target				250	120	100	0	10	5	60	2	90	70				

FIGURE 16.3 Partial QFD, device to detect apnea in an infant at home.[9]

TABLE 16.1 Additional Customer Requirements for a System to Detect Apnea

Captures all events	Panic button	Easy installation
No false positives	Electrical safety	Comprehensive instructions
Doesn't irritate the skin	Patient comfort	Per patient basis adjustability
Can't harm the baby	Visible vital signs	User-friendly interface
Doesn't impact handling the baby	No bigger than a band-aid	Plug-and-play capabilities
Washable	Will not burn patient	Aesthetically pleasing
Easy to take on/off	Rechargeable	Wireless
Waterproof	Reusable construction	Portable
Not attached to the baby at all	Replaceable battery	Labeled connections
Easy to operate	Long battery life	Reads EKG signal
Disconnect alarm	Easily sterilized	Reads respiratory rate
Animal/kid proof	Disposable parts	Reads heart rate
Low battery indicator	Updatable software	Type of data storage
Indication options (alarm/flash/etc.)	Updatable circuitry	Adjustable time of stimulation
Dispatch service	Crush resistant	Fast response time
Tracks events in detail	Will not tangle	Cost
Doesn't wake the baby	Will not overheat	Replacement availability
Ability to transfer data	Strong connections	Not small enough to swallow
Short set-up time	Easily adjustable settings	

demonstrates elements of a QFD for a system to detect when a baby stops breathing. Table 16.1 shows examples of additional customer requirements for this QFD. Figure 16.4 is a rendering of a pod that may be transported by ground vehicle or helicopter to an emergency. A fire protection version must be accessible to all, including those in wheelchairs, for protection from wild fires. Figure 16.5 is a partial QFD for this pod.[8] In this brief overview of QFD, select issues will be highlighted in each room. Follow both Figs. 16.1 and 16.2 in the house tour below. A completed QFD would rarely fit on a single page as in these three examples.

Room 1: Customer requirements. These are generated by focus groups, surveys, interviews, etc. The requirements include expecters, spokens, unspokens, and exciters.[1] *Expecters* are standard features that one would expect in a product. *Spokens* are features that the customer will tell you are desired. *Unspokens* are important features that the customer has forgotten, was unwilling to mention, or did not realize at the time. These first three categories must be addressed for consumer satisfaction. The last category, *exciters*, are typically unique features of your product that will boost sales. Since technology advances quickly and competition is stiff, today's exciters will become next quarter's spokens and next year's expecters. This is evidenced in both the computer and consumer electronics industry. Some requirements are directed toward function and others toward form. Requirements also may include price, serviceability, etc.

Room 2: Identification of the customers and their ranking of the customer requirements. When identifying your customers, consider internal customers as well. Are you developing a product that your manufacturing personnel can produce? Does your sales force need a claim of cheapest, fastest, or lightest? List salespersons, assemblers, etc., as customers in the house of quality. Figure 16.1 primarily illustrates external customers that an engineer new to this field may be unfamiliar with. Multiple house-of-quality diagrams may need to be generated to handle all the customers on manageable-sized diagrams. In addition to the primary customer, the device user, other customers include all who must interact with it. For example, will a family member or health professional need to customize or maintain this device? How about the insurance agency or organization that may be paying for it? Have their requirements been addressed? Typically, each class of customer ranks the importance of each requirement. One common ranking scheme is to have the customer list all requirements in the order of importance beginning with one. Although this forces the customer to distinguish between requirements, it does not show the relative weight of each. A second approach is to mark each requirement that is extremely important with a 5, very important with a 4, and continue down to 1 for minimally important. (Blank can be reserved for not important at all.)

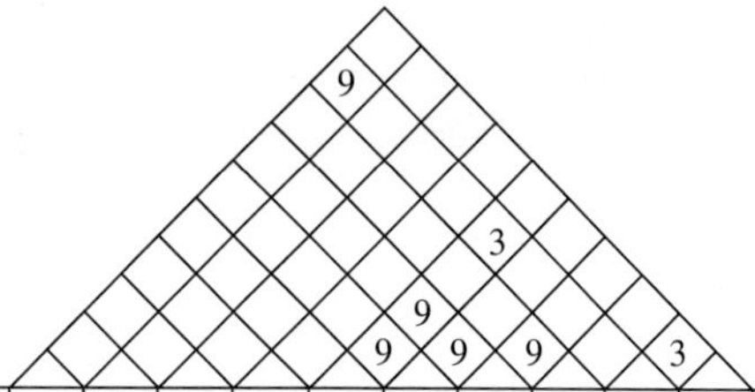

	Person seeking shelter	Emergency personnel - ground	Emergency personnel - air	Maximum occupancy	% Who could self access from wheelchair	Deployment time [minutes]	# of deployments before major repairs	Weight [kg]	Center of gravity [x, y, z in cm]	Mass moment of inertia [3 × 3 matrix in N-m]^2	Interior dimensions [cm]	Hours of safe air [hours/person]	Max. external temp. vs. duration [°C versus hrs]	Fire tents	Home	Automobile	No product
Shelter many people	5	5	5	9	9	3		9	3	9	9	1		1			
Ample clean air	5	5	5					9		1	1	9		3	3	3	
Wheelchair access	5	5			9	1					1						
Safe internal temp.	5	5	5					9				1	9	1			
Quickly deployed	5	5	5			9		1	1	1				3			
Quickly retrieved	5	5	5	9		3		9	1	1				5			
Reusable	2	5	5				9					9	3				
Safe to lift by helicopter			5			1		9	9	9	3			5			
Can be pulled by unmanned vehicle	3	5		9		1		9	9	9	3			3			
Minimize weight	1	2	5	9				9	9	9	9	9	3	5			
Moderate price	2	3	3	9	3	3	3	9	1	1	1	3	9	5			
Fire tents				1		1	1	5				0.1					
Home				20													
Automobile				4													
No product																	
Target				12	100	3	5	675				8					

FIGURE 16.4 Partial QFD, rescue pod that may be used as a fire shelter.

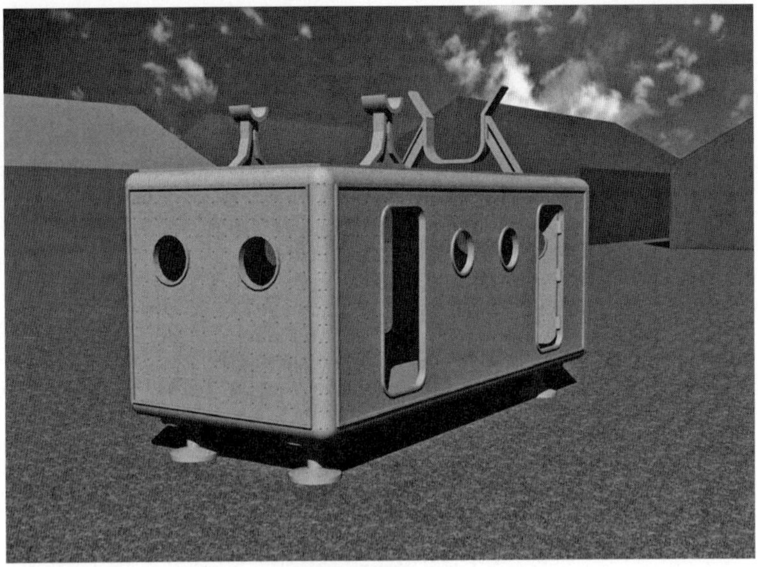

FIGURE 16.5 Rendering of a pod concept.[8]

Room 3: Identification and customer evaluation of the competition or environmental scan. The competition must be identified. Once again, look internal as well. Will this new product compete with your existing product? If so, list it here. An important competitor to list when developing any assistive technology product is "no product at all." For example, how many of you have had a grandparent who could clearly benefit by a hearing aid but refused it, stating, "I have heard all that I need to hear already!"? In this room, the customers assess how satisfied they are with the competition for each requirement. A scale from 1 to 5 may be used, with 5 representing completely satisfied and 1 not satisfied at all. Although the competitor "no product at all" may score a 1 on its ability to amplify in this hearing aid example, it would score straight 5s on great comfort, good looks, low cost, and serviceability.

Room 4: Engineering parameters. How do we ensure that the entire design team is visualizing the same magnitude when the members hear customer requirements such as low cost or very powerful? If customers indicate that they want a powerful automobile, one engineer may be envisioning 200 hp, and another, 400. Clearly, each would lead to very different design concepts in the conceptual design phase. Furthermore, what is a low-cost automobile, $6000, $16,000, or $26,000? The engineering parameters would include the sales price and the vehicle's horsepower. Engineering parameters (also called *engineering characteristics*) are measures that allow us to quantify the customer requirements. If property selected and our room 8 target is met, we will have increased confidence in the future success of our product.

Room 5: Correlation matrix. Is there a strong interdependence between our engineering parameters? In the room 4 automotive example, is there a relationship between the horsepower of the vehicle and its cost? The following scale is often used: 9 (strong relationship), 3 (moderate), and 1 (weak), and the space is left blank if there is no relationship at all. This room will result in an increased awareness of trade-offs at the beginning of the design process.

Room 6: Relationship matrix. Applying the scale from room 5, consider the following questions: Have I developed engineering parameters that will clearly show if I have satisfied each customer requirement? In other words, do I have enough 3s and 9s in each row? Are my engineering parameters repetitive, with unnecessary measures of a requirement? Restated, do I have too many 3s and 9s in each row? Each engineering parameter may have a substantial cost associated with it. It may require significant testing or analysis.

Room 7: Benchmarking. For each competitor listed in room 3, apply the engineering parameters to their products. In the automotive example in room 4, what is the horsepower and sales price of each of your competitors? Some benchmarking (measuring your product against the competition) may only require reading published specifications; others might require expensive testing.

Room 8: Target. You have made it to the last room in the house of quality. Now we understand who the customers are and what they want. We have sized up our competition, in both our customers' eyes and our own tests. Engineering parameters have been developed to allow us to measure success throughout the design process. With this understanding, it is now time to select the product's targets. We will develop our target for each engineering parameter. This is often selected with the help of experts: marketing people who understand what price the market will bear; senior engineers who can assess technical feasibility in the selection of weight, power, and speed requirements; and strategic planners who can ensure that the product is consistent with the company's mission.

One model for selecting an appropriate target is illustrated in Fig. 16.6. It is a graph of price versus differentiation. *Differentiation* refers to the uniqueness of the product or service. Most successful businesses operate in one of the four corners. For example, a successful business in the low-price/low-differentiation corner (3) is Wal-Mart. Products found here include many remote controls and walkers. The high-price/low-differentiation corner (4) would include many sneaker manufactures whose products are similar, but they distinguish themselves through extensive advertising. The Ferrari is in the high-price/high-differentiation corner (2) with its impressive power, design, and sticker price. Many custom assistive devices would fit here. They are designed specifically for the consumer, but this may result in a high price. The final corner (1), low price/high differentiation includes consumer electronics manufactures that can add exciters to their products quickly and cheaply. When a business that is successful in operating in a particular corner adds a product line that pulls it toward the center (danger zone), that business often has problems as it begins to lose its market identity, and thus eventual profitability. Does this shift follow the corporation's strategic plan? This model is used to define a company's targeted strategic market segment based on its competitive advantages and manufacturing strategies.[6]

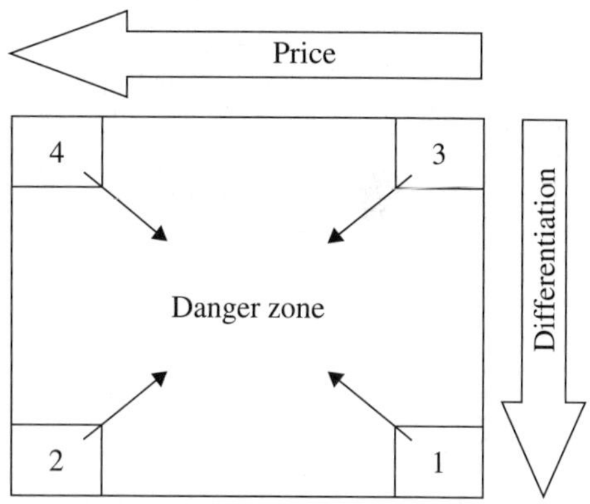

FIGURE 16.6 Target strategy.

16.2.6 The Team

The balance of the team and their involvement will primarily depend on whether the product is targeted for one specific person (denoted here as *sole user*), a class of persons with specific types of disabilities, or a general consumer product applying universal design principles to maximize its customer base. The members of the team include those drawn from the QFD customers list, as shown in Table 16.2. The specific backgrounds of the engineering team are left for other sources to detail.[1,3] This section will focus on the consumer and medical team.

Sole User. The most critical member of the design team is the user of the product. Methods, such as quality function deployment, stress understanding the customers' requirements, so why not involve the user of this custom device in the process? Just as a product that is high-tech but almost works is of little value to the customer, a device that works flawlessly but is too large and visually unappealing (function without form) may also be put aside. An example, most would agree that a device that improves its wearer's vision by 25 percent is significant, but if it were built into a helmet, most would not trade in their eyeglasses. Section 16.3.4 provides further details.

TABLE 16.2 Potential Customers to Satisfy with Your Design

Category*	Member	Description
A,C	Client/user/patient	Person who will use the product.
B,C	Client's family	They have valuable insight. They also may interact with the device.
B	Home health aide	Assists client with activities of daily living (ADL).
C	Insurance company (public or private)	May fund the purchase of an assistive device.
C	Vocational rehabilitation	May fund the purchase of an assistive device.
D	Assembler	
D	Repairperson	
D	Engineering technologist	Often the assistive technology provider that installs or adapts a device for client.
E	Audiologist	Concerned with alternative and augmented communication (AAC) devices; *www.asha.org*
E	Speech pathologist	Concerned with alternative and augmented communication (AAC) devices; *www.asha.org*
E	Physical therapist	Works with mobility aids; *www.apta.org*
E	Occupational therapist	Works with devices that assist in the activities of daily living (bathing, toileting, cooking, etc.). Concerned with devices necessary to perform at an occupation; *www.aota.org*
E	Recreational therapist	Concerned with devices that allow a client to enjoy avocations, dine out, and play sports.
E	Physician	In addition to traditional medical duties, prescribes devices. Coordinates the care of the client. A physiatrist specializes in rehabilitation/physical medicine.
E	Nurse	Cares for the client. Interacts with the devices.
E	Certified orthotist/prosthetist	Fits and produces orthotic/prosthetic device.
F	Salesperson	May need certain claims (e.g., fastest, lightest, least expensive) to sell the device. May be a therapist, etc.

*Category classification: A, primary user of the device; B, may interact with the device while in use; C, pays for the device; D, maintains, builds, or modifies the device; E, medical personnel who may train the user or prescribe the device; F, other.

Other team members include the user's family. They are particularly important when the user is a child or a cognitively impaired adult. If the device is an alternative or augmentative communication aid, a speech pathologist is needed. The speech pathologist would perform the evaluation of the user and often would provide training with the device. Similarly, a physical therapist might be involved when the device is a walking aid such as a walker, cane, or crutch. Activities of daily living (bathing, cooking, toileting, etc.), vehicle modifications, specialized seating to minimize the formation of pressure sores, and workplace accommodations are examples of situations where an occupational therapist may be critical to the team. Nurses and physicians are just two more professions that might be required to design an appropriate device. Note that the team leader is often not an engineer but a clinician (a medically trained person such as a physician or therapist).

Multiple Users. The issues discussed earlier still apply in the design of mass-produced products, but the single user on the team may be replaced by focus groups, surveys, etc. Examples of other methods for gathering required information can be found in both marketing and design texts.[7]

16.2.7 Necessary Research

Engineers are experts at gathering and interpreting technical information. The medical world, however, introduces an entirely foreign vocabulary. Those trained as biomedical engineers have begun to learn medicine as a second language, but for the rest, it is just one more challenge. Traditionally, it is the biomedical engineer's job to speak the language of the clinician, not the clinician's responsibility to learn our engineering jargon. The medical team members will lead you through the medical issues briefly described below. For example, they will determine the user's diagnosis and prognosis. Together you will determine the product's efficacy and safety. Hybrid areas such as ergonomics are concerned with the interaction of a person and his or her surroundings. An ergonomist (typically with a clinical background) will be aware of the proper positioning of a person while performing a specified task. An engineer, however, is of great value in the measurement of specific forces on the body, as well as the estimation of joint forces that may be created by the use of products under development. Both anthropomorphic and traditional analysis software is useful in these activities.

Pathology → Impairment → Disability → Handicap. *Pathology* is the underlying cause of the disability. In this context, it refers to diseases and traumatic events such as amputations and spinal chord injuries. *Impairment*, the effect of the pathology on the body, describes the loss of specific functions. For example, the individual cannot move his or her right leg. *Disability* often refers to one or more impairments that interfere with specific activities. Examples include an inability to walk or feed oneself. *Handicap* generally implies the loss of one or more of life's major functions.

EXAMPLE *A dancer, Tom, suffers a traumatic head injury as the result of a drunk driver. He can walk but becomes dizzy when making any quick movements while standing. Pathology: traumatic head injury; Impairment: cannot move quickly while standing; Disability: cannot dance; handicap: ??? Tom might consider himself handicapped due to his inability to dance, since that was a major life function for him. But what if he performs in a wheelchair? He might decide that he has overcome his handicap. A second person with a balance disorder might not consider it a handicap at all if he or she had no interest in dancing to begin with.*

Handicap is a term left to the person with disabilities to apply. A great percentage of those who society views as having handicaps would not describe themselves that way.[10] Despite this definition, the term *handicap* has specific legal meanings that are often not politically correct.

Diagnosis versus Prognosis. In the preceding section, the diagnosis by the clinician would tell us the pathology. But the engineer generally focuses on the impairment and disability, so how does the pathology affect our design? The answer is the *prognosis*. Will the user be regaining function? Is the level of impairment increasing with time? What is the projected timetable? Is the person medically stable? Are there important secondary and tertiary effects of the pathology?

EXAMPLE *Amy has been diagnosed with amyotrophic lateral sclerosis (ALS), also known as Lou Gehrig's disease. The design team is assembled to create a device or modify the environment to allow her to continue to teach college physics. At the time the design team is assembled, Amy has begun to lose function in her legs and uses a self-propelled wheelchair. The team developed some initial concepts. These included building a ramp and a platform in front of the chalkboard so that she may write as she had before. A second idea is to reposition an overhead projector so that she may comfortably write on transparencies while seated in her wheelchair. The second concept was chosen due to cost and safety concerns. Shortly after it was adapted, Amy lost control of her arms. If the team had considered the prognosis, it would have realized the path of the progression of ALS. Eventually, Amy will only be able to communicate through her eyes. Locked-in syndrome, where she understands everything as always but cannot easily communicate, is one of the final stages. An appropriate device might be a computer and projector to display her notes for her class. As the disease progresses, the input device can be repeatedly replaced. Ultimately, Amy may require a blink switch or eye-tracking device.*

Sources. Engineers are familiar with such databases for articles as the Engineering Index[11] and sources for manufacturers, including the *Thomas Register*.[12] Medical articles can be searched online with the database Medline.[13] The medical members of the team can aid in this search. What about existing medical devices? The *Medical Device Register*[14] lists medical device manufacturers by product and location. The National Institute on Disability and Rehabilitation Research supports the

TABLE 16.3 Sources on the Web

Description	URL
ABLEDATA: Links to manufacturers of assistive technology	*www.abledata.com*
American Foundation for the Blind: Reviews products for persons who are blind or have low vision. Produces fact sheets on many topics.	*www.afb.org*
Canadian Institutes of Health Research: Begun in June 2000, it is a federal agency that supports medical research.	*www.cihr.ca*
Canadian Standards Association (CSA): Works with standards and the certification and testing of products.	*www.csa.ca*
Eastem Paralyzed Veterans Association (EPVA): Provides materials on the Americans with Disabilities Act, workplace accommodation, and more.	*www.unitedspinal.org*
FDA: Checks the codes and standards that affect durable medical equipment and other medical devices.	*www.fda.gov*
Health Canada: The federal department responsible for helping the people of Canada maintain and improve their health.	*www.hc-sc.gc.ca*
Medical Device Register: Directory of medical products manufacturers.	*www.mdrweb.com*
Medline: Online database of medical and biomedical engineering articles; searches and abstracts are free, but there is a fee for ordering the full article.	*www.ncbi.nlm.nih.gov/PubMed/ gateway.nlm.nih.gov.gw.cmd*
National Institute on Disability and Rehabilitation Research, U.S. Department of Education: Supports research in assistive technology.	*www.ed.gov/about/offices/list/ osers/nidrr/index.html*
National Institutes of Health (NIH): A first stop to leam about many disorders including clinical trials.	*www.nih.gov*
Patent site: Conduct free patent searches and view recent patents online.	*www.uspto.gov*
Rehabilitation Engineering and Assistive Technology Society of North America (RESNA): Professional society with a strong focus on assistive technology; members are engineers and clinicians; sponsors a licensing exam for assistive technology providers.	*www.resna.org*
Sites for designing accessible software and Web sites.	*www.w3.org/TR/WAI-AUTOOLS* *www.microsoft.com/enable/* *www.access-board.gov*
Thomas Register: Directory of manufacturers.	*www.thomasnet.com*
Whitaker Foundation: Supports biomedical engineering education and research.	*www.whitaker.org*

database ABLEDATA,[15] which lists assistive technology. Table 16.3 lists a few traditional engineering Web sites but focuses on assistive technology sites.

16.2.8 Conceptual Design

After completion of techniques such as QFD, we have a strong understanding of the customers' product requirements. The problem is defined in a written problem statement or product design specification, and the design team is finally ready to brainstorm its initial concepts. It is important to consider all options for each of the product's functions. What are my options for turning my device on? Should it use a lever, button, sensor, or timer? What about voice activation? How should information be displayed? Does it require a gauge, light-emitting diode (LED), buzzer, or synthetic speech?

Functional Decomposition. Functional decomposition is a method of exploring many design options for each product function. Figure 16.7 shows the overall system diagram for the toaster oven example. Inside the box is the overall function of the product. At the top of the box, there are the objects with which the toaster oven will interface. It must accept pans and trays and sit on a countertop or be installed below an upper cabinet.

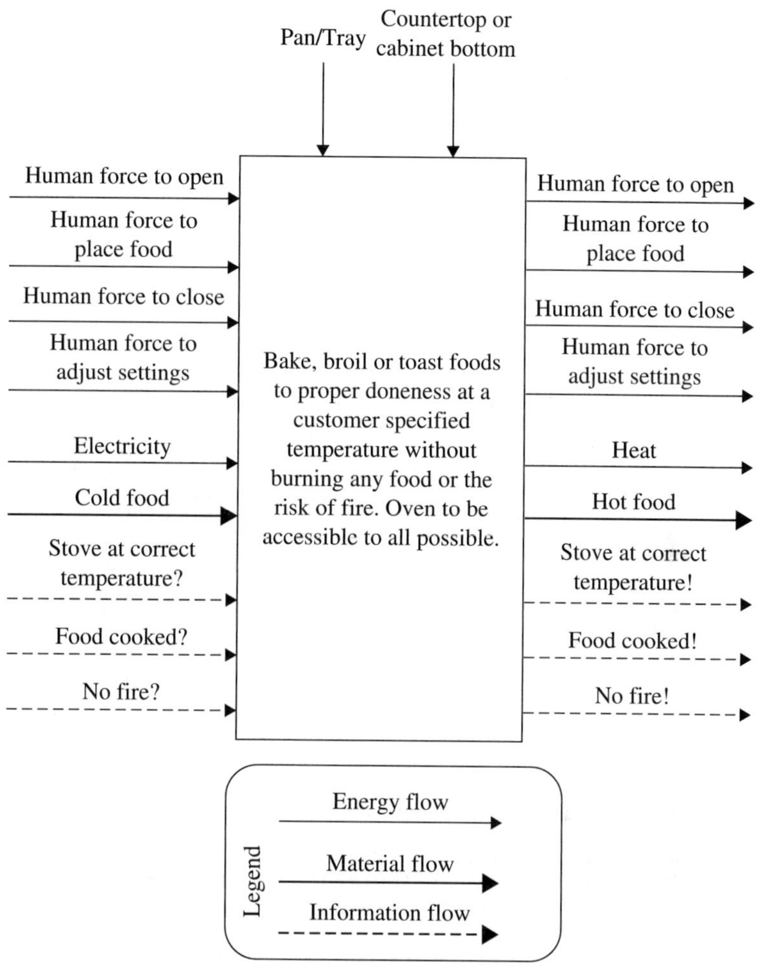

FIGURE 16.7 Overall system diagram, toaster oven example.

The legend shows lines with arrowheads for energy, material, and information flow. Anything that does not remain in the toaster oven must be shown to leave. For example, food is considered a material flow. It enters cold and then leaves hot. The design team can then brainstorm ways to go from cold to hot. An example of information flow is "No fire?" and "No fire!" The question mark designates that we need an answer. The exclamation point tells us that we have an answer. Once again, the team will brainstorm, this time searching for methods of preventing fires due to grease, etc.

The overall system diagram is reduced to subfunction diagrams. Figure 16.8 shows four of the subfunctions. These shall be further subdivided as necessary. These diagrams allow us to separate each function of the product for individual and thorough consideration. Subfunction 3, for example, notifies the cook when the oven is preheated. How will this be accomplished? Tone, light, speech synthesizer, flag, or LED display? Table 16.4 is designed to heighten awareness of sample input and output devices used by persons with disabilities. Ideally, the product should suit all cooks, including those with disabilities. At times, appropriate jacks need to be designed into the product so that specialized input-output (I/O) devices can be used. For example, a person with a hearing impairment

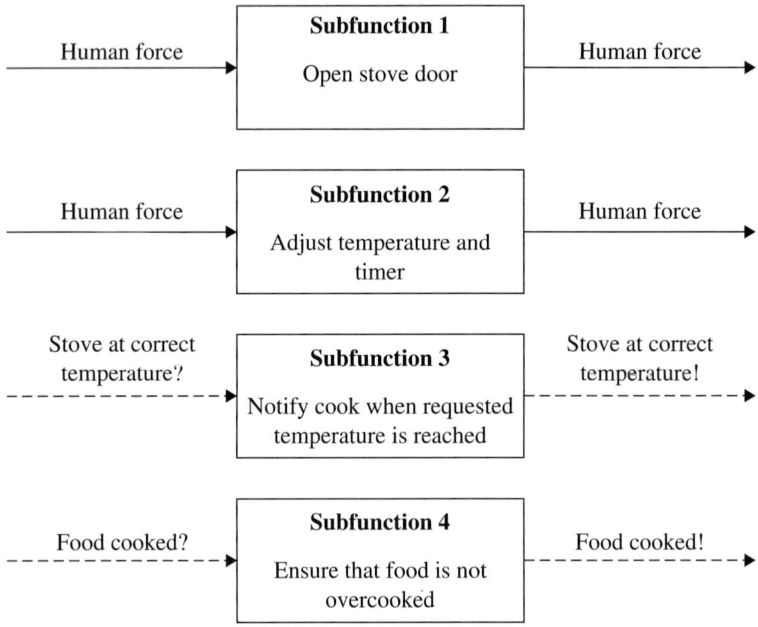

FIGURE 16.8 Subfunctions, toaster oven example.

would simply connect his or her own amplified bell. Of course, try to build such features into your product. Requiring an interface would lead to its own subfunctions, such as "Connect external devices." Brainstorming might result in concepts that include quick connectors, Bluetooth, and infrared sensors (control the appliance from your wheelchair or recliner).

While brainstorming subfunction 2, questions that may arise include: Do I need any human force at all, or can it be voice-activated? Is it better to turn a knob, push a slider, or use an electronic keypad? Can it be controlled by remote? Why not have all controls and feedback designed into a remote unit?

The resources in Table 16.3, especially ABLEDATA,[15] will help you customize and update Table 16.4 as technology changes. During the evaluation phase, remember to consider universal design principles in the assessment of all concepts.

16.2.9 Embodiment Design

Once again, I refer you to your design texts for a review of embodiment design. Since this is the time when the product takes shape, I introduce the topics of human factors and universal design. Because of the equal importance of both form and function, the design team should include an industrial designer from the initial design stages. In addition, consultants with expertise in the area of accessibility for persons with various disabilities must also be included. It is far less expensive and more effective to apply universal design principles in the earliest stages. In addition, both the industrial designer and the consultants will be invaluable in the development of the QFD.

Human Factors. Human factors or ergonomics are critical in any design with which a person will interface. Are the controls, warning lights, etc., laid out in a logical way? Does the color red mean hot and blue cold? Brake on the left and accelerator on the right? Rewind before the fast-forward button? Is it simple to operate? We also desire to minimize the energy that must be expended. Are

TABLE 16.4 Sample Input/Output Devices

Name	Description
Amplification/magnification	Sound may need to be amplified or a display magnified.
Braille display	Multiple-character display in which pins extend to represent Braille characters and are continuously refreshed by the computer.
EEG switch	Receiver worn on the forehead can detect EEG signals to activate a switch.
Electromyographic (EMG) switch	A surface electrode detects a muscle contraction and triggers this switch; it can use small, controlled muscle movements.
Environmental control unit (ECU)	A "black box" that accepts most input devices (e.g., sip and puff and touch switches) and may be connected to multiple devices (e.g., telephones, bed controls, lamps, and appliances); it has the ability to scan through different options, such as "call home," "turn lamp on," and "increase the volume of the television," with a minimum of one switch.
Eye/eyebrow switch and eye trackers	Detect blinks, eyebrow motion, or the wrinkling of the forehead; eye trackers are more sophisticated systems that can detect the coordinates of the eye to replace a computer mouse, etc.
Flashers	A smoke detector, door bell, or a baby's cry can alert a person who is deaf with a flashing light.
Functional electrical stimulation (FES)	Electrodes inserted into muscles to activate (stimulate) selected muscles for those with paralysis.
Optical pointer	Laser that can be mounted on a user to allow for precise pointing.
Proximity and temperature sensors	Technologies include ultrasound and can detect the presence of a person through his or her motion or body temperature.
Remote I/O devices	These include remote keyboards that allow you to roll up in a wheelchair near your personal computer without having to physically connect or carry a laptop; television, lamp, and appliance remotes can be purchased at local electronics stores; these include Bluetooth, infrared and FM-based systems.
Scanning device	Using as little as a single input device, the device switches between multiple output options.
Sip-and-puff switch	Ultrasensitive pneumatic switch actuated by slight mouth pressure.
Skin surface stimulation/subdermal stimulation[10]	Electrodes are placed on the surface of the skin or implanted to provide sensory feedback.
Speech output	These include computer-generated speech synthesizers and systems that replay human speech.
Tactile	Includes textured surfaces, scales, thermometers, and watch faces that can be felt (raised and Braille lettering).
Touch pads	Adhesive-backed flexible plastic pad; it is activated by touch and can be washed.
Touch switch	Single switch activated by very light pressure.
Vibrators	Includes smaller vibrators used in pagers and larger units that may be placed underneath a mattress to wake a person who is deaf.
Voice- and sound-activated systems	From systems that respond to a clap to word processors that can type what you speak, the sophistication and price cover a broad spectrum.

the controls positioned appropriately? Is there a concern for repetitive-motion injuries? A person might have limited neuromuscular control or may be wearing gloves while operating the device outdoors. The person may have low vision or be in a dimly lit room. Is the user color-blind?

When designing for a specific person, certain anthropometric measurements (mass, lengths, radii of gyrations, etc., of the human body) can easily be made. These include height, weight, and reach. What if you are creating a product for the mass market? One approach is to use anthropometric tables. You can estimate, for example, the height of the fifth, fiftieth, and ninety-fifth percentiles of American women. However, who do you design for? If you design for even the ninety-fifth percentile, you are still excluding the tallest 5 percent. What if you are attempting to estimate the mass of someone's leg to be used in a gait analysis (how someone walks)? The tables are based on cadaveric studies with a sample of generally fewer than a dozen. Did any of the cadavers fit the build of your target consumer?[16]

Disability categories include vision, hearing, speech, limb loss, neuromuscular impairment, other, and multiple impairments.[10] Categories may easily be subdivided. For example, vision may be divided into low vision and blind. Each may lead to different solutions. Similarly, is a person hard of hearing or profoundly deaf? The following is a list of suggestions or questions to consider in your design. It is a starting point, not a comprehensive list. Some are geared more to the design of a device for a sole user and others to a mass market:

1. What are a child's personality traits, intelligence, developmental and functional levels, physical size, and growth factors? Do we understand their physical, financial, and social environment?[18]
2. What is the diagnosis and prognosis?
3. Is the product compatible with the user's existing I/O devices? If computer-based, can it be operated without a pointing device such as trackball or mouse? Will it interface with a voice dictation system? What about speech output? Can keystroke commands be entered sequentially? For example, pressing the Control, Alternate, and Delete buttons simultaneously is impossible for many people.[17,18]
4. Is documentation in Braille, electronic format, large print, or on audiotape, etc.?[17,19]
5. How can print be made more readable for someone with low vision? Use an 18-point font (but no less than 16 points) in standard roman or sans serif. Avoid decorative fonts, italics, and all capital letters. Bold type increases the thickness of the letters and is preferable. Avoid the use of color fonts for headings. However, if used, consider dark blues and greens. Maximize contrast. Some people prefer white or light-yellow letters on a black background over the reverse. Avoid glossy paper due to the glare. Use a line spacing of 1.5 rather than single space. Spacing between letters should be wide. Since low-vision devices such as closed-circuit televisions and magnifiers often require a flat surface to read, use a margin of 1.5 in (but no less than 1 in).[19]
6. How can one design a product to be easier to use by someone with low vision? Maximize contrast between components. For example, use a dark switch on a light device or a light handle on a dark door. Avoid glares.[20]
7. How can my software application be improved to help those with visual impairments? Use standard user-interface elements compatible with screen readers. Is the application compatible with screen-magnification and speech-synthesis software? Do not require a pointing device and allow the user to modify the interface. For example, can the user select the font style, color, and size? What about the background color? Do not place time limits on input activities or messages. Do not rely on color alone to convey information. For example, a green-filled circle that becomes red when done may not be seen.[18]
8. Have I considered the ergonomics of the design? Is the device easy to grip? What does it weigh? How must the user be positioned to operate the device? Will its use lead to back or neck pain? Are repetitive-motion injuries a concern? There is commercial software available to determine forces at the back and extremities for various anatomic positions and loading cases. Parameters such as the user's height may be specified.

Universal Design. Over the years, industry has moved away from telling consumers that they know what is best for them to seeking their input early on in the design process. Designing quality into the product has also become the norm. There is a great need for universal design to become the industry standard as well. Universal design results in a more usable product for all consumers, improves sales by increasing the customer base, and is good for society as a whole. There will likely be great resistance and some problems in the transition phase as industry learns these new requirements. Ultimately, it will be profitable, as corporations have seen with total quality management.

Universal Design Principles. Universal design, as in all other design requirements, depends on sufficient and correct background information. Many codes and standards actually meet only minimum requirements. For example, the standard recommended pitch for a wheelchair ramp requires significant upper body strength. A less steep incline is actually preferred. Simply observing the letter of the law does not necessarily lead to a satisfactory design. Check with the experts.

An accommodation that benefits one type of disability may cause new concerns for others. A curb cut, for example, is an absolute necessity for persons in wheelchairs but will make it difficult for a person who is blind to use a cane to detect where the sidewalk ends and the roadway begins. As a result, the ramp portion of the curb cut is often textured to provide tactile feedback. Elimination of the need to step up onto a sidewalk has also benefited countless persons pushing baby carriages or hand trucks.

Increasing the size and contrast of the letters on a remote control will not only aid users with low vision but also will aid the general population in low light. Choose color combinations that can be seen by those with color blindness.[21] Also, larger switches arranged in an expected, logical order will make for a better product. Those with limited mobility, including the millions with arthritis, will be able to operate such a remote with ease.

Devices that increase a person's independence are essential. But do not forget to apply universal design to fun products too! Work, school, and activities of daily living are not enough. Persons with disabilities do not lose their desire to participate in leisure activities.

In addition to the universal design principles that follow, Table 16.5 shows a set of principles developed by the Center for Universal Design at North Carolina State University.

1. Maximum inclusion will increase your market share and result in a better product for all consumers.
2. Provide appropriate interfaces (jacks, plugs, etc.) to allow a user to connect his or her own specialized I/O devices.
3. Designing for inclusion has a significant positive societal impact.

16.3 SPECIAL TOPICS

16.3.1 Stochastic Processes

The human body is subjected to many environmental forces that may be treated as stochastic (random) processes. For example, how would you estimate the forces on an individual during an automobile crash? How about the stress on a hip as a person transverses a rocky terrain? A second area of interest focuses on the treatment of uncertainties in the measurement of anthropometric data or human performance. Refer to Sec. 16.2.9 ("Human Factors") for more details. A clinician estimates the mass of a man's arm as 0.4 kg from anthropometric tables, but how do we quantify the effects that might occur due to an error in the estimate? One method to quantify the effect of stochastic processes is the Monte Carlo simulation.[22–25]

The Monte Carlo simulation allows an engineer to methodically study the effect of a parameter on the results. The parameter's range is identified, and then a random sample is selected from within this range. Imagine using a roulette wheel in Monte Carlo to select these values. In practice, programs such as MS Excel and MathWorks Matlab or random-number tables are used to select the values. The Monte Carlo simulation will be demonstrated by example.

EXAMPLE *A medical device manufacture is developing a hearing aid that will reduce the chances of injury to its user during a car accident. The manufacturer would like to know the forces on an individual's head during an accident. An automobile manufacturer has software to simulate the forces on the head for any size driver during a simulated car accident. What height should the manufacturer choose? Can we just estimate the worst case? Is the shortest driver less safe because of his or her proximity to the steering column and air bag? Would a very tall driver experience added forces if he or she is too tall for the headrest? Would an average size driver be more likely to strike the top of the steering wheel?*

What heights do we analyze? How many do we choose? Have we selected appropriately?

TABLE 16.5 Universal Design Principles

1. *Equitable use.* The design is useful and marketable to people with diverse abilities.

   Guidelines:

   a. Provide the same means of use for all users: identical whenever possible; equivalent when not.
   b. Avoid segregating or stigmatizing any users.
   c. Provisions for privacy, security, and safety should be equally available to all users.
   d. Make the design appealing to all users.

2. *Flexibility in use.* The design accommodates a wide range of individual preferences and abilities.

   Guidelines:

   a. Provide choice in methods of use.
   b. Accommodate right- or left-handed access and use.
   c. Facilitate the user's accuracy and precision.
   d. Provide adaptability to the user's pace.

3. *Simple and intuitive use.* Use of the design is easy to understand, regardless of the user's experience, knowledge, language skills, or current concentration level.

   Guidelines:

   a. Eliminate unnecessary complexity.
   b. Be consistent with user expectations and intuition.
   c. Accommodate a wide range of literacy and language skills.
   d. Arrange information consistent with its importance.
   e. Provide effective prompting and feedback during and after task completion.

4. *Perceptible information.* The design communicates necessary information effectively to the user, regardless of ambient conditions or the user's sensory abilities.

   Guidelines:

   a. Use different modes (pictorial, verbal, tactile) for redundant presentation of essential information.
   b. Provide adequate contrast between essential information and its surroundings.
   c. Maximize "legibility" of essential information.
   d. Differentiate elements in ways that can be described (i.e., make it easy to give instructions or directions).
   e. Provide compatibility with a variety of techniques or devices used by people with sensory limitations.

5. *Tolerance for error.* The design minimizes hazards and the adverse consequences of accidental or unintended actions.

   Guidelines:

   a. Arrange elements to minimize hazards and errors: most used elements, most accessible; hazardous elements eliminated, isolated, or shielded.
   b. Provide warnings of hazards and errors.
   c. Provide fail-safe features.
   d. Discourage unconscious action in tasks that require vigilance.

6. *Low physical effort.* The design can be used efficiently and comfortably and with a minimum of fatigue.

   Guidelines:

   a. Allow user to maintain a neutral body position.
   b. Use reasonable operating forces.
   c. Minimize repetitive actions.
   d. Minimize sustained physical effort.

7. *Size and space for approach and use.* Appropriate size and space are provided for approach, reach, manipulation, and use, regardless of user's body size, posture, or mobility.

   Guidelines:

   a. Provide a clear line of sight to important elements for any seated or standing user.
   b. Make reach to all components comfortable for any seated or standing user.
   c. Accommodate variations in hand and grip size.
   d. Provide adequate space for the use of assistive devices or personal assistance.

Note: The principles of universal design address only universally usable design, whereas the practice of design involves more than consideration for usability. Designers must also incorporate other considerations, such as economic, engineering, cultural, gender, and environmental concerns, in their design processes. These principles offer designers guidance to better integrate features that meet the needs of as many users as possible.

Source: Reprinted with permission of North Carolina State University, The Center for Universal Design, 1997.

For simplification of this example, let us assume that the peak force on the head during a crash is a function of height only and follows the following hypothetical equation:

$$
\begin{aligned}
F &= 2h^4 + 7 && \text{when } h < 60 \text{ in} \\
&= 2h^3 + 6h && \text{when } 60 \le h < 72 \text{ in} \\
&= 2h^5 && \text{when } 72 \le h \text{ in}
\end{aligned}
$$

where F is the peak force on the head and h is the subject's height when standing.

Steps

1. *Determine the range of heights.*
2. *Select initial sample size n.*
3. *Using a random-number generator that can produce a uniform random distribution, select n values of h.*
4. *Calculate a total of n peak forces by calculating the force for each height.*
5. *Apply all relevant statistical measures to these peak forces. They might include mean, standard deviation, correlation coefficients, etc.*
6. *Repeat steps 2 to 5 with a larger sample size.*
7. *Compare the statistical measures from each sample size. Repeat steps 2 to 5 with an ever-increasing sample size until the results of these statistical measures converge. Use these results in your design.*

Suppose that h is in the range from 58 to 77 in and n is initially selected to be 10. A random-number generator has generated the sample heights using the random number seed 123 shown in Table 16.6.

Figure 16.9 shows the mean, standard deviation, and maximum for the peak force for n = 10 above, where n = 15 and the random seed is arbitrarily chosen as 7,638, n = 20 with seed 418, n = 50 with seed 6,185, n = 100 with seed 331, and n = 200 with seeds 43 and 3,339. Note the range of values at n = 200 when two different seeds were selected. The engineer would then decide if he or she is satisfied with the results. Remember, in an actual computer simulation, the CPU time may be significant, and a sample of even n = 10 may be expensive.

TABLE 16.6 Random Heights

Height, in
58.25513474
69.04791406
71.38007752
65.59837642
76.76573992
59.89321574
75.82985931
76.9483932
63.6593524
74.27295755

16.3.2 Weight Is Critical

Many products that a person with disabilities may use are carried, worn, or are mounted on a wheelchair. The heavier the product, the more energy that a person must exert to carry it. When a device is mounted on a self-propelled wheelchair, the user must also expend additional energy to account for this weight. On an electric wheelchair, the added load will shorten the interval between recharges and reduce available power. The reduction of weight as a critical factor is one that is shared with the aerospace industry. Additional engineering efforts to reduce the product's weight will yield significant benefits to the consumer.

EXAMPLE *Lisa, a 15-year-old high school student, wears an ankle-foot orthosis (AFO). This AFO, worn around her calf and under her foot, supports her ankle. To the casual observer, the AFO seems light. Through Lisa's daily activities, the extra weight is noticed. Fig. 16.10 shows her AFO. An engineer may initially check that the peak stresses do not exceed their limit. But as an aerospace engineer would ask, why do we allow all these areas of low stress? If the material is thinned or removed from the low-stress regions, the AFO will not fail, and its weight will be reduced. Figure 16.11 shows a*

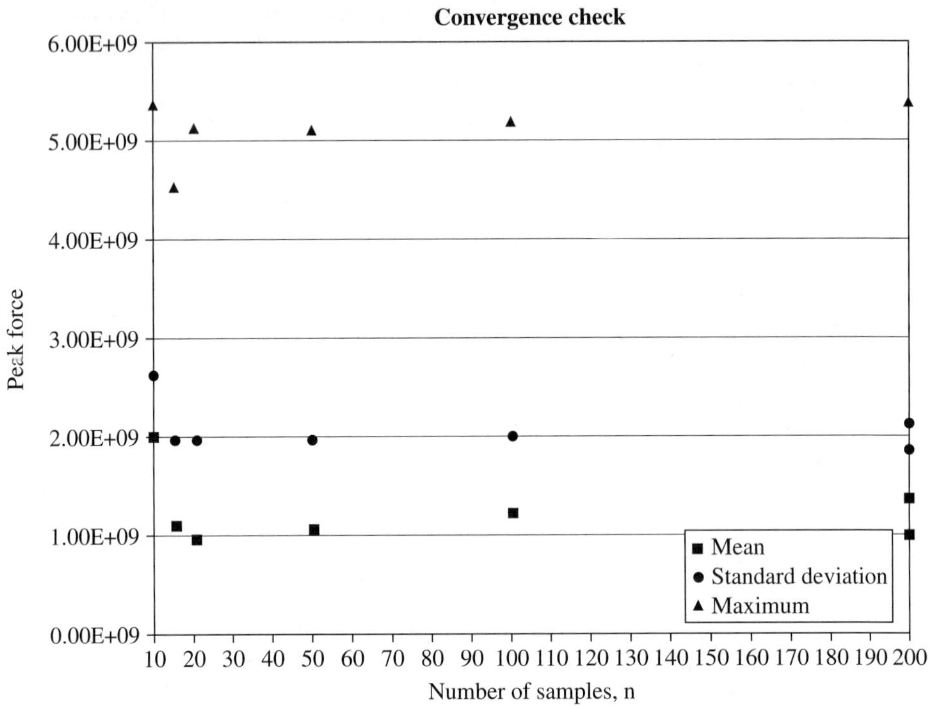

FIGURE 16.9 Monte Carlo simulation sample results.

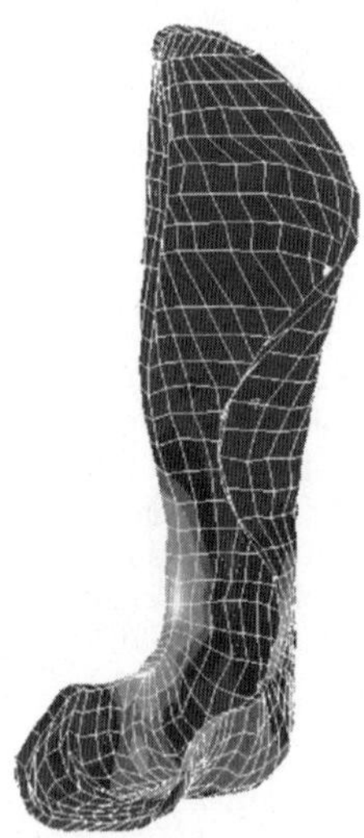

FIGURE 16.10 FEM of a standard ankle-foot orthotic. *(Reprinted with permission of Khamis Abu-Hasaballah and the University of Hartford.)*

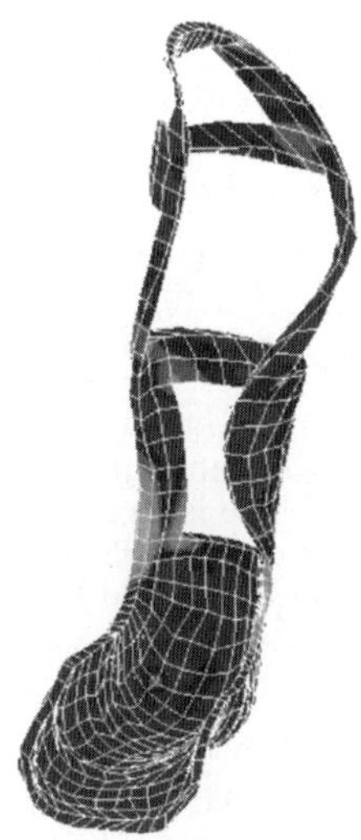

FIGURE 16.11 FEM of an ankle-foot orthotic after weight reduction. *(Reprinted with permission of Khamis Abu-Hasaballah and the University of Hartford.)*

finite-element model of the AFO after non-load-bearing material is reduced. An added benefit is the reduction of perspiration experienced due to wearing an AFO in the summer. Technology transfer from other industries would certainly benefit Lisa.

16.3.3 Design for Failure

Engineers are constantly considering failure modes in their designs. When designing a device for persons with disabilities, great care must continue. What will happen to its user if a failure occurs? Could the person become injured? Trapped until someone happens by? Who would repair this device? Can it be completed onsite? Would it require special training or tools? From the instant the device fails, how long will it take before the user has the repaired or replaced device in use? If this product is important to users, how could they do without it? If it is not that important, they probably would not have purchased the unit in the first place. If this is a custom design for a sole user who you know personally, it is even easier to picture the possible impact of a failure.

16.3.4 Social-Psychological Perspective

A team of talented engineers is asked to design a device that will automatically open doors for a teenage girl who has no use of her arms. The team, after 3 months, produces a device that can open standard doors, sliding doors, light doors, heavy doors, and even bifold doors with ease. It is lightweight and works off a single AA battery that lasts for a year. The team proudly delivers the invention to the client, but she refuses to wear it. You see, the device is built into a helmet with a robotic arm jutting out. Most teens will not leave their homes if they are wearing the "wrong" clothes. Why would a teen with a physical disability be any different? Many people, young or old, will not use the appropriate assistive technology because of the stigma attached. They might avoid using a wheelchair that is too ungainly, even if they are in a wheelchair already. Many of us have friends and family members who would benefit from a hearing aid but refuse one because of what they fear people might say. Others may be concerned that it would make them feel old.

These are complex issues that must be considered in the design of a product. The following are questions to consider: Will my client use the device as intended if it is designed and fabricated? What if the device could be hidden? Can it be made aesthetically pleasing? What if through universal design the product was desired by the general population, thereby eliminating the stigma?[10]

16.4 DESIGN FOR UNDERDEVELOPED REGIONS

People around the world all deserve effective available medical care. In underdeveloped regions of the world, medical care does not meet the standards that we expect in wealthier nations. Even when medical staff is available, medical equipment is often not present, in disrepair or of insufficient quantities. Groups, including Engineers Without Borders[27] provide critical engineering skills to impoverished villages by providing clean water and many important services. Specialty organizations such as Engineering World Health[28] focus on supplying and maintaining critical medical equipment.

There are often political, transportation, and distribution issues working in these regions. In the United States, labor tends to be expensive compared to the parts required in a consumer or medical device. Designing for underdeveloped regions often requires a paradigm shift. Parts may be prohibitively expensive for a local economy preventing a donated medical device from being repaired. Labor is often inexpensive and abundant. This shift has a major impact on the engineering design.

Whether a consumer product or a medical device, reliable power is not always present. For example, is their reliable continuous power at home or daily power suitable for charging a system a few hours each day? If not, is there a central location such as a school or clinic with available power? How are sudden power interruptions handled by the system?

As an alternative to shipping completed products to underdeveloped regions, can the device be designed for construction and repair with local resources? Can it be designed with yesterday's technology to reduce the cost and then ship the parts for local assembly? For example, if a system can use computer hardware 2- to 4-years old, there may be sources willing to donate their older systems. Whatever the design, let us not forget those in poorer nations.

16.5 WHAT'S NEXT?

Toward the final stages of the embodiment design phase, there are often two or three "most promising" designs that the team may still be considering. There are still many factors to consider. These include technical feasibility, safety, cost, and many manufacturing issues. Is the device at risk for failure due to fatigue or corrosion? Are all applicable codes and standards satisfied? Must the product be registered with the Food and Drug Administration (FDA) or other regulatory agency? Will it require clinical trials? Once the final design is selected, it is time for the detail design phase.

The detail design phase will include the preparation of detail drawings and product specifications. A bill of materials must be prepared along with a detailed cost estimate. A final design review is conducted before releasing all drawings to be manufactured.

REFERENCES

1. Dieter, G. E., *Engineering Design: A Materials and Processing Approach,* 3d ed., McGraw-Hill, New York, 2000.
2. Lumsdaine, E., Lumsdaine, M., and Shelnu, H. J., *Creative Problem Solving and Engineering Design*, McGraw-Hill, 1999.
3. Shetty, D., *Design for product success,* Society of Manufacturing Engineers, Dearborn, Mich., 2002.
4. *www.resna.org.*
5. Ulrich, K. T., and Eppinger, S. D., *Product Design and Development,* 2d ed., McGraw-Hill, New York, 2000.
6. Birch, John, *Strategic Management Process,* The Birch Group, New Britain, Conn., 1997.
7. Ullman, D. G., *The Mechanical Design Process,* 2d ed., McGraw-Hill, New York, 1997.
8. Ford, E. J., Adrezin, R. S., Filburn, T., Norwood, P. M., Wei, F. -J., Gallagher, F., Lang, S. A., Feasibility of Helicopter Transported Pods to Support Homeland Security, *AHS 63rd Annual Forum*, Virginia Beach, VA, May 2007.
9. Hill, J. M., Adrezin, R. S., Eisenfeld, L., Wireless Central Apnea Response System for Neonatal Intensive Care, *Proceedings of Biomed 3rd Frontiers in Biomedical Devices Conference*, Irvine June, 2008.
10. Smith, R. V., and Leslie, J. H., Jr., *Rehabilitation Engineering,* CRC Press, Boca Raton, Fla., 1990.
11. *Engineering Index, www.ei.org.*
12. *Thomas Register, www.thomasregister.com.*
13. *Medline, www.ncbi.nlm.nih.gov/PubMed/.*
14. *Medical Device Register,* Medical Economics Co., Montvale, N.J., 2000.
15. ABLEDATA, Silver Spring, Md., *www.abledata.com.*
16. Chaffin, D. B., Andersson, G. B. J., and Martin, B. J., *Occupational Biomechanics,* 3d ed., Wiley, New York, 1999.
17. Missouri Assistive Technology Project, Basic Questions to Ask When Purchasing Technology, Missouri Technology Center for Special Education, Kansas City, Mo., September 1996.
18. National Technology Access Program, *Creating Applications Accessible to People Who Are Visually Impaired,* American Foundation for the Blind, New York, June 1998.
19. Orr, A. L., *Tips for Making Print More Readable,* American Foundation for the Blind, New York, June 1999.

20. AFB Aging Program, *A Checklist for Environmental Safety and Access,* American Foundation for the Blind, New York, August 1998.

21. Guyton, A. C., *Textbook of Medical Physiology,* 7th ed., Saunders, Philadelphia, Pa. 1986.

22. Adrezin, R., and Benaroya, H., Monte Carlo simulation of a partially submerged compliant structure, *ASME IMECE,* November 1998, pp. 191–198.

23. Benaroya, H., *Mechanical Vibration: Analysis, Uncertainties, and Control,* Prentice-Hall, Upper Saddle River, N.J., 1998.

24. Adrezin, R., and Benaroya, H., Nonlinear stochastic dynamics of tension leg platforms, *Journal of Sound and Vibration,* **220**(1):27–65 (1999).

25. Adrezin, R., and Benaroya, H., Dynamic modelling of tension leg platforms, in *Stochastically Excited Nonlinear Ocean Structures,* World Scientific, Singapore, 1998.

26. Nowak, M. D., Abu-Hasaballah, K. S., and Cooper, P. S., Design enhancement of a solid ankle-foot orthosis: Real-time contact pressures evaluation, *J. Rehabil. Res. Dev.,* **37**(3):273–281 (2000).

27. Engineers Without Borders USA, http://www.ewb-usa.org/.

28. Engineering World Health, http://www.ewh.org/.

CHAPTER 17
HOME MODIFICATION DESIGN

Blair A. Rowley
Wright State University, Dayton, Ohio

There are many areas of the home both inside and out that may require modification to accommodate individuals with disabilities. This chapter discusses two major indoor areas, the kitchen and the bathroom. The considerations that follow should be used as starting points in meeting the unique needs of each person who has a disability.

17.1 GENERAL CONSIDERATIONS

17.1.1 Electrical

The main electrical consideration is safety. The electrical service in the kitchen and bathroom must incorporate ground-fault monitors as required by local codes. Additional consideration involves the accessibility of switches and outlets. Lighting is also a factor in meeting the needs of the visually impaired.

17.1.2 Lighting

Lighting should be nonglare, and areas of lighting should be nonreflective, using low-sheen laminates. Natural lighting, if available, is preferred. Other lighting sources involve incandescent tungsten, halogen, or fluorescent lighting. The following are considered when using these.

Incandescent Tungsten. This is a harsh light that creates a sharper edge to objects, allowing them to be easily differentiated. The yellow and red characteristics of this light give it a better definition to objects.

Halogen. This is similar to tungsten, except the color characteristics are more constant over the color spectrum. It is also a brighter light and adds dimension if other lighting is used. It is an excellent light to highlight ceilings and walls and to reduce glare without using a diffuser.

Fluorescent. There are choices in selecting fluorescent bulbs with different color lighting. A full-spectrum fluorescent light allows the eyes to see items in a natural state; it is a soft light that may blend objects into the background, making them harder to see. Those that give off blue and green colors may be harder on some eyes yet advantageous for people with color impairments.

17.1.3 Switches

Switches and other type of electrical controls for the disabled are designed for ease of operation and should be placed in an accessible location, where they cannot be accidentally turned on by being bumped into. Depending on the type of disability the user has, these controls can vary greatly and most likely will have to be tailored to each individual's need.

17.1.4 Main Light

The location of all wall switches should not exceed 48 in above the floor. A dimmer switch with a lever handle can control the proper amount of lighting for the main kitchen light fixture and should be placed by the main door on a wall. Additional simple on/off switches can be located by other entrances.

17.1.5 Sink and Range Fluorescent Lights

The best switch locations are a few inches below the overhang of the kitchen counter, roughly at 28 to 30 in of height. Placing these switches at the back wall extends the reach of a seated individual too far, especially over a hot range, so this is *not* a good solution.

17.1.6 Electric Disposal

The disposal switch should be placed where a disabled individual cannot turn it on accidentally by bumping it with his or her wheelchair. The switch should also be located so that no one can operate it and be in contact with the sink at the same time.

17.1.7 Electric Fan

A control knob with a three-speed clicking-type lever handle is a good choice. This variable control can accommodate people with a multitude of disabilities.

17.2 THE KITCHEN

17.2.1 Kitchen Layout

When designing a kitchen for use by persons with mobility impairments, especially those who use wheelchairs, careful layout of the kitchen is crucial to maintaining accessibility. People who are mobility impaired may

- Have walking and standing limitations that require them to sit while working
- Use a mobility aid such as crutches, canes, or walkers
- Use a wheelchair

One of the key issues to consider when designing for persons with mobility impairments is adequate space to maneuver a mobility aid such as a wheelchair or walker.

17.2.2 Maneuvering Space

Space to maneuver close to cabinets, appliances, and work areas must be provided. Each feature must have at least 30 by 48 in of clear floor space arranged for either parallel or perpendicular approach by wheelchair. Clear floor space may extend under the counters and into knee-space areas up to 19 in.

17.2.3 Knee Space

Adequate knee space under counter surfaces is important for people who need to sit while performing kitchen tasks. The space should allow them to pull up under the counter for work areas, sinks, and cook tops. Knee room should be provided beside appliances such as ranges, ovens, and dishwashers. Knee spaces should be at least 30 in wide, 27 in high, and 19 in deep. A width of at least 36 in is preferred because this provides additional turning space, which is especially important in small kitchens.

17.2.4 Turnaround Space

A space large enough for a person to turn around 180 degrees should be provided in the kitchen. If the kitchen is very small, the space can be provided immediately adjacent to the kitchen.

Pivoting Turn. Sufficient space for a complete pivoting turn can be provided with a 5-ft clear diameter floor area. This allows a full turning radius of 360 degrees. The best location for the turning space is away from appliance areas and between walls or cabinets only.

T-Turn. A T-shaped turning space allows a three-point turn to be accomplished. By making one of the necessary kitchen knee spaces 3 ft wide or wider, one leg of the T can be accomplished within the knee space. This arrangement can solve maneuvering problems in very small kitchens.

17.2.5 Laying It All Out

Efficient kitchens are usually designed around a work triangle. This triangle is formed by the location of the refrigerator, sink, and range. The arrangement of the surrounding work center depends on the available space. In general, an L-shaped kitchen provides the best access.

17.2.6 U-Shaped Work Center

Advantages to using a U-shaped work center include

- Plenty of room to maneuver a wheelchair
- Room for two cooks
- Reduced traffic flow problems
- Reduced risk of bumping into appliances

17.2.7 L-Shaped Work Center

Advantages to using an L-shape work center are

- Traffic flow does not interfere with work triangle
- Plenty of room for storage next to each workstation
- Room for two people or a wheelchair

17.2.8 Island and Peninsula Work Centers

A work center with this layout shortens the work triangle, an advantage for people with low vision or those who use walkers or crutches. Open appliance doors may, however, block aisle space needed for a wheelchair.

17.2.9 Corridor and Pullman Work Centers

A corridor work center places appliances across an aisle. A Pullman design has all appliances on one wall. Like island work center designs, these designs shorten the work triangle. The distances between appliances can make working in a kitchen with this type of design tiring for people with mobility impairments. Table 17.1 summarizes the preceding information.

TABLE 17.1 Recommended Work Triangle Dimensions

Appliance/fixture	Standard, ft	Wheelchair, ft	Walker/crutches, ft
Total distance connecting refrigerator, range, and sink	12–22	14–24	10–20
Refrigerator to sink	4–7	6–9	2–5
Sink to range	4–6	6–8	2–4
Range to refrigerator	4–9	6–11	2–7

Source: Whirlpool Home Appliances.

Table 17.2 provides some comfort zones for kitchen dimensions. These are ranges for some kitchen dimensions to maintain usability.

TABLE 17.2 Comfort Zones

Comfort zones	Standing/walking unassisted, ft	Walking with assistance,* ft	Sitting, ft
Minimum aisle space	3	4	4.5
Maximum aisle space between counters	6	6	6.5
Minimum space between workstations			
One cook	4	5	5.5
Two or more cooks	4.5	5.5	6

*Leaning on another person or using a cane, crutches, or walker.
Source: Whirlpool Home Appliances.

17.2.10 Design Notes

- The spaces recommended in Tables 17.1 and 17.2 generally are adequate for most people who use standard-sized manual or electric wheelchairs.
- More space than the minimum is recommended when designing a kitchen for use by more than one person.
- People who use electric scooters for mobility will require more space to maneuver because most scooters are much less maneuverable than a power wheelchair.
- Always consider the specific needs of the person for whom the kitchen is being designed before implementing a standard design.
- Be sure to use nonskid floor coverings.

- Design eating areas with room for round tables for families with deaf members. This provides individuals with a clear view of each other to facilitate communication.
- Keep the pathway for bringing groceries into the house as short and straight as possible.
- Keep the work triangle small for persons with visual impairments.

17.2.11 Refrigerator/Freezer

A refrigerator/freezer in a side-by-side configuration with good door storage spaces, a built-in icemaker, and a cold-water dispenser is recommended.

Dimensions. *Height.* Forty-eight inches is the maximum height a wheelchair-assisted individual should be expected to reach into a refrigerator/freezer.

Width. Between 32 and 48 in; standard to extrawide dimensions are recommended. Due to a lower reach height, a wider refrigerator/freezer will allow more accessible storage space.

Depth. Standard dimensions are best used along with rollout drawers.

Adaptive Features. *Location.* The best alternative is to position the refrigerator/freezer away from any corners in the kitchen so that doors open 180 degrees. This allows plenty of space to open the doors and for wheelchair accessibility to the interior of the refrigerator/freezer.

Loop Handles. Due to the tight seal and weight of refrigerator/freezer doors, a significant force and space are required to open and close them. Loop handles should be the same dimensions as handrails, $1^1/_4$ to $1^1/_2$ in in diameter for the handgrip, and they should be mounted $1^1/_2$ in away from the refrigerator door. Sometimes a short leather or nylon loop can be used, e.g., a short dog leash. These are excellent features to ease access for those with degraded motor coordination and for visually impaired individuals.

Powered Doors. A self-opening and closing feature is a good idea for individuals with loss of strength and motor coordination. This can best be accomplished using a custom-designed system with electrical servomotors and a touch-sensitive switch.

Rollout Basket Shelves. Due to standard depth of a refrigerator, the reach must be accommodated for wheelchair-assisted individuals. Simple plastic-covered wire baskets with wheels on a rail allow access to the rear of the refrigerator. A lock-in mechanism should be designed into the shelf at its maximum extension, which should be set at two-thirds its depth.

Side-by-Side Layout of Refrigerator/Freezer. The best configuration is for the two units to sit side by side with their doors opening from the middle. This makes it easier to move items between the two units.

Water Dispenser. Built into refrigerator at 32 in above the ground, this is the average counter top height for wheelchair-assisted individual.

Icemaker. This eliminates the nuisance of filling up and emptying ice trays for mobility-impaired individuals. Location of icemaker dispenser should be next to the water dispenser.

17.2.12 Dishwasher

The assistive kitchen dishwasher is designed for wheelchair-assisted people with varying disabilities but also accommodates people with visual impairments. Since it is impossible to come up with one universal design for all disabilities, adaptations are presented.

Dimensions

- Standard height to fit under the countertop or countertop height for a roll-around unit
- Standard width of a conventional dishwasher
- Standard depth of a conventional dishwasher

Adaptive Features. *Location.* The dishwasher should be located so that it is accessible from either side. It should be raised off the floor 6 to 8 in to ease access.

Controls. Controls for the dishwasher should be designed to require little force to operate and not require gripping, twisting, or fine finger dexterity.

Lever Handle or Blade Control Knob. These are excellent controls for setting different types of wash cycles, and their position can be labeled to assist those with visual disabilities.

Electronic Touch-Pad Controls. These are the best controls for those with degraded finger/hand mobility and strength.

Rolling Table. This item is essential for loading and unloading the dishwasher. It should be countertop height with handles for ease of mobility.

Alternative Design. If space is a concern, compact dishwashers are available on the market that fit on top of a countertop with the following dimensions: 19.5 in high by 21.5 in wide by 22.5 in deep. These have the standard drop-down doors with rollout baskets.

Drop-Down Front Door. Most standard dishwashers are equipped with drop-down doors. As an added feature, grip handles are nice for both inside and outside the dishwasher for ease of opening and closing the door.

Roll-Out Basket. Most standard dishwashers are also equipped with this feature, so this should not be an additional need unless absent.

17.2.13 Microwave

Controls. The choice of controls depends on the disability that is being accommodated. It is important to note that many companies offer optional Braille controls for those who are visually impaired.

Dial Controls

Advantage

- More accessible for the visually impaired (vs. electric touch controls)

Disadvantages

- Require grasping and twisting motions
- Difficult for persons with limited motor capabilities to operate

Electrical Touch Controls

Advantages

- Single-touch operation
- Requires little force for operation
- Requires no gripping or twisting
- Does not require fine finger dexterity
- Some manufacturers offer plastic overlay panels with raised tactile openings or labeling to aid the visually impaired

Disadvantage

- May not be accessible to those with visual impairments

Redundant Cueing/Feedback to the User. Controls should provide redundant cueing or feedback to the user in order to be accessible to persons with visual and hearing impairments.

Examples of Redundant Cueing/Feedback

- Click stops. These provide distinct audible sound and tactile cues.
- High-contrast labeling.
- Raised markers.

Knee Space. Knee space needs to be available to wheelchair users to allow them access to the microwave. Make sure that the microwave is placed on a countertop that provides adequate knee space.

Minimum Requirements

- *Height*: 27 in
- *Depth*: 19 in
- *Width*: 30 in

Recommended Dimensions

- *Height*: 29 in or greater to allow for wheelchair armrests
- *Width*: 36 in

Reach Ranges. Make sure that the microwave is situated so that its location complies with reach range requirements.

Reach Range for Persons Seated in Wheelchair

- *Down*: 12 to 15 in above the floor
- *Out* (over the counter): 44 in above the floor (maximum)
- *Up*: 48 in above the floor (maximum)

Side Reach for Persons Seated in a Wheelchair

- *Lateral*: 12 in (maximum)
- *Down*: 9 in above the floor (minimum)
- *Up*: 54 in above the floor (maximum)

Reach for Standing Person, Mobility Impaired

- *Up*: 72 in above the floor
- *Down*: 24 in above the floor

Clear Space. A minimum of 10 in of clear space must be available immediately adjacent to the microwave to allow for transfer of foods in and out of the microwave.

17.2.14 Oven

A wall oven is the recommended type of oven to be used when accommodating persons with disabilities. This type of oven can be installed at the most appropriate height for the user, and the controls can be placed within reach of a standing or sitting user. Wall ovens come in several widths (24, 27, and 30 in). There are three types of doors that can be used: drop-front, side-hinged, and swinging doors.

Height. Lowered wall ovens are usually installed 30 to 40 in above the floor. When installing the wall oven, it is important to make sure that its height is appropriate for the user.

Knee Space. Knee space must be available to wheelchair users to allow them to access the oven. For a drop-front door, knee space must be provided on either side of the oven. For a side-hinged or swinging door, knee space must be provided directly under the oven or on the side closest to the door handle.

Minimum Requirements and Recommended Dimensions. The same as for microwaves.

Reach Ranges. The same as for microwaves.

Controls. The type of control chosen should be based on the individual's disability. The following control types can be used for the oven, and the advantages and disadvantages are provided for each type.

Lever Type. Advantages include

- They do not require grasping for operation.
- Their shape provides a natural pointer that indicates the control's position.

Blade Knobs. Control with a large straight blade across the center; use the blade to turn the knob. Advantages include

- Blade shape is asymmetrical. It extends on one side, which forms a pointer that helps indicate the control's position.
- The shape acts as a lever. Turning is accomplished with reduced effort.

The disadvantage is that it requires grasping for operation.

Electrical Touch Controls. Advantages include

- Single-touch operation.
- Requires little force for operation.
- Requires no gripping or twisting.
- Does not require fine finger dexterity.
- Some manufacturers offer plastic overlay panels with raised tactile openings or labeling to aid the visually impaired.

The disadvantage is that they may not be accessible to those with visual impairments.

Redundant Cueing/Feedback to the User. Controls should provide redundant cueing or feedback to the user in order to be accessible to persons with visual and hearing impairments.

Examples of Redundant Cueing/Feedback

- Click stops. These provide distinct audible sounds and tactile cues.
- High-contrast labeling.
- Raised markers.

Transfer of Foods. The most used oven rack should be placed so that it is at the same height as the adjacent counter space. This facilitates easy sliding of hot pans from the oven to the counter.

Drop-Front Door. Pullout shelf next to the oven, just below the countertop and at the same height as the oven rack.

Side-Hinged Door. Shelf below the oven, 10 in wide, extends the full width of the oven (minimum).

1. Permanent shelf, that is, the front edge of the counter.
2. Pull-out shelf, located directly under the countertop.

Safety. It is recommended that only electrical ovens be used because (1) there are no products of combustion such as carbon monoxide when using electrical ovens and (2) individuals with an impaired sense of smell will not be able to detect a gas leak.

17.2.15 Range

It is recommended that a cooktop be used because it can be installed at the most appropriate height for the user, its side or front controls are easily reached by most individuals, and counter installation can allow open space below the cooktop for easy access.

Height. It is recommended that the cooktop be installed at a height of 30 to 32 in above the floor. However, to ensure adequate clear space adjacent to the cooktop, make sure that the cooktop is installed at the same height as the adjacent countertop.

Knee Space. Knee space needs to be available for wheelchair users to allow them to access the cooktop. Ideally, space should be available under the cooktop to allow easiest access.

Minimum Requirements and Recommended Dimensions. The same as for microwaves.

Reach Ranges. The same as for microwaves.

Clear Space. Adequate clear space beside burners is required. The recommended minimum amount of clear space is 12 in.

Controls. Controls should never be located at the rear of the unit. Controls should be located on or near the front of the cooking unit. This ensures that there is no need to reach over or around any burners. Also, controls located near or at the front are more accessible for persons with visual impairments. There are several different types of controls that can be used with the cooktop. The choice of control type should be based on the individual's disability. These control types, along with their advantages and disadvantages, are provided below.

Lever Type. Advantages include

- They do not require grasping for operation.
- Their shape provides a natural pointer that indicates the control's position.

Blade Knobs. Control with a large straight blade across the center; use the blade to turn the knob. Advantages include

- Blade shape is asymmetrical. It extends on one side and forms a pointer that helps indicate the control's position.
- The shape acts as a lever. Turning is accomplished with reduced effort.

The disadvantage is that they require grasping for operation.

Electrical Touch Controls. Advantages include

- Single-touch operation.
- Requires little force for operation.
- Requires no gripping or twisting.
- Does not require fine finger dexterity.
- Some manufacturers offer plastic overlay panels with raised tactile openings or labeling to aid the visually impaired.

The disadvantage is that they may not be accessible to those with visual impairments.

Redundant Cueing/Feedback to the User. Controls should provide redundant cueing or feedback to the user in order to be accessible to persons with visual and hearing impairments.

Examples of Redundant Cueing/Feedback.

- Click stops. Provide distinct audible sounds and tactile cues.
- High-contrast labeling.
- Raised markers.

Range Hood. Range hoods come in a variety of widths (30, 36, and 48 in). Controls for the range hood may be located on the lower front panel of the hood to decrease the reach-range requirements for operation. However, it is recommended that these controls be located on the cooktop panel or in nearby base cabinets just below the countertop.

To adapt existing controls located on the range hood itself, a conventional toggle switch can be installed at a lower position as an auxiliary control. The hood controls should be set and left on so that the toggle switch can be used for on/off operation.

Safety. Install the cooking unit near to the sink so that the spray hose can reach some of the burners in case of nongrease-based fires. Cooking units that have flush burners should be specified such that pots and pans can be slid from the cooking surface to the counter without having to be lifted. The counter surface next to the stove should be able to withstand hot items. The burners, cooktop, and counters should be at a smooth common level, with no more than a $^1/_8$-in raised edge, flush is preferred. Burners should be staggered so that the user does not have to reach over a hot burner to get to a rear burner. Placing an angled mirror over the cooktop allows people in wheelchairs to see the contents of pots. It is recommended that only electrical cooktops be used because (1) there are no products of combustion such as carbon monoxide when using electrical cooktops and (2) individuals with an impaired sense of smell will not be able to detect a gas leak.

17.2.16 Kitchen Sink

The adapted kitchen sink is designed for wheelchair-seated people with varying disabilities but also accommodates visually impaired people. Since it is impossible to come up with a universal design for all disabilities, some alternative suggestions are provided.

Design Concept. The adaptive sink design features two bowls with an electric waste disposal in the left sink bowl. Drains are positioned at the center of the left bowl and at the rear inner corner of the right bowl so as to position the plumbing away from the individual's knees in a wheelchair. Since the right basin has its drain positioned at the corner, the bottom of the sink should be sloped toward the drain hole. Lever handles are mounted halfway between the two sink bowls with 300-degree range of motion for maximum flexibility. Another faucet with a flexible rubber hose is provided with a 7-ft reach. A removable sloping protection panel is mounted in front of the plumbing pipe under the sink to protect the knees of a wheelchair-assisted individual.

Dimensions. The recommended countertop height is 27 to 34 in from the finished floor to the underside of the countertop. The upper limit was chosen for the sink height due to the bowl depth being 6.5 in. This allows ample knee space for a wheelchair-assisted individual.

The shallow basin (6.5 in) allows the 27-in minimum knee height from the finished floor to the bottom of the sink necessary for a wheelchair-assisted individual. The total sink dimension (bowl only is 20 in wide by 20 in deep). The maximum depth reach for a wheelchair-assisted person is 44 in, so there is plenty of margin to reach beyond the back of the sink. The width of the right-hand sink plus the counter is 40 in. The wheelchair is generally 26 in wide, so this distance is 14 in wider than the necessary space needed to accommodate a wheelchair-assisted individual's knees under the sink and the counter (40 in).

Adaptive Features

- *Height and reach*: Must be accessible by someone in a wheelchair with limited mobility.
- *Knee space*: Must allow wheelchair to fit under sink to provide maximum access.
- *Bowl depth*: Must be designed for accessible reach.
- *Faucet and drain position*: Must be designed for accessible reach and not hinder knee position under sink.

- *Faucet and hose attachment*: Designed to reach countertops.
- *Single-lever faucet*: Adapted to blind individuals or persons with degraded hand coordination.
- *Protective panel*: Plumbing drain pipe is shielded from knees of individual in a wheelchair.

Other adaptive features considered but not used in the preceding adaptive kitchen sink design include

- Hot water dispensers to prevent individuals from having to carry pots of water to and from a range
- Adjustable-height basin that lowers and raises electrically with a touch of a button
- Pedal-operated faucets
- Motion sensors that, when tripped, activate hot or cold water at a preset rate and temperature for a finite amount of time and shut off automatically

Electric Disposal. A disposer can be installed in any sink that has a full-size drain opening. For an assistive kitchen design, switch location, safety, and disposal location are the main design objectives. The on and off switch should be placed in an accessible area, possibly under the front lip of the countertop. Care should be taken not to position the switch where a wheelchair can accidentally bump the switch while the person is washing the dishes. It should also be located so that a person cannot contact the sink and switch at the same time. The electrical connection should be away from the water line and should be protected with a conduit pipe to eliminate any shock hazard. The disposal should be located away from any wheelchair-accessible area.

17.2.17 Counters

Standard kitchen counters are 36 in high. This is adequate for disabled and nondisabled standing people but too high for people who are seated. Counter heights of 30, 32, and 34 in are more comfortable for a seated person to use for food preparation. This disparity will obviously make the design of a kitchen for use by standing and seated people difficult.

For work such as mixing or beating, a 27-in height is desirable.

NOTE: The usual height for a wheelchair armrest is 29 in. Adequate knee space requires at least 24 in.

Accessible Solutions and Adaptations. *Uniform-Height Counters.* A uniform lowered height is not a recommended solution for a number of reasons:

- This is inconvenient for standing users.
- Appliances such as dishwashers, trash compactors, and ranges are designed for 36-in counter heights.
- Lowered counters may make resale of the house difficult without restoring counters to the standard height.

Dual-Height Counters. A dual-height kitchen includes lowered counter segments to provide work areas for seated people. Each lowered segment must have clear knee space below. Clear vertical space of 30 in at the front of the counter will provide enough clearance for most wheelchairs.

Electrically Adjustable Height. Motor-driven adjustable height counter segments that allow their height to be adjusted at the press of a switch provide a uniquely flexible, highly accessible solution.

Manually Adjustable Segments. A design of this type allows counter height to be adjusted with minimal work. An adaptable design approach such as this is ideal for a rental unit where tenants may change relatively frequently. This can be accomplished in a couple of ways:

Wall-mounted brackets. Counters may be mounted with heavy-duty commercial shelf brackets and standards. Shelving of this type is seen in many retail store shelving units.

Movable wood support. A wooden support strip can be attached to the sides of base cabinets and the countertop to allow for some adjustability.

Breadboards, Chopping Blocks, and Pullout Work Surfaces. Provide a variety of work heights for different jobs. These accessories work best when at a height of 27 in and at least 30 in wide by 24 in deep.

17.2.18 Simple Modifications

The following suggestions are modifications that can be readily and inexpensively made to existing kitchens to make them more accessible.

Carts. A rolling, drop-leaf cart can provide an accessible work surface:

- The leaf can be raised to provide additional workspace.
- The cart can be rolled to the refrigerator or stove to transport food.

A Sturdy Work Table. Providing a heavy-duty kitchen table, which can take the abuse of food preparation work and is located as close as possible to the sink and appliances, is a workable and low-cost solution.

Design Notes

- Use solid surface material for countertops (easy cleaning).
- Round corners on all countertops, especially for visually impaired persons.
- Use contrasting colors on counter edges to increase visibility for those with visual impairments.
- Install drawer organizers.
- Ensure that a fire extinguisher is in easy reach of oven and range and is usable by persons with impaired mobility and dexterity.
- A mirror suspended above the cooking area allows vision into pots for a seated person.
- Include pullout shelving or readily accessible counter space near ovens and microwave to allow for sliding transfer of hot items.
- Be creative when designing a multilevel kitchen. Incorporate desks, eating bars, and tables.

Cabinets and Storage. Storage space is a particularly troublesome issue for people with limited mobility. For many, a significant portion of conventional kitchen storage space is out of reach. In addition, available base cabinet space is reduced when making a kitchen accessible to people who use wheelchairs. By selecting more efficient and accessible storage options, much of this space can be recovered.

Table 17.3 provides some information on shelving height for people with various mobility limitations.

Accessible Storage Solutions. *Full-Extension Drawers.* A deep drawer that extends the full depth of the base cabinet and is mounted on full-extension slides is very useful. These drawers are similar to those found in an office file cabinet (Table 17.4).

TABLE 17.3 Comfort Zones

Comfort zones	Standing/walking unassisted, in	Walking with assistance,* in	Sitting, in
Maximum upper cabinet reach			
Over a counter	68	63	60
Without a counter	77	68	48
Maximum vision for items on a high shelf	61	61	48
Maximum height of storage for daily use	74	65	45

*Leaning on another person or using a cane, crutches, or walker.
Source: Whirlpool Home Appliances.

TABLE 17.4 Recommended Drawer Heights

Purpose	Height, in
Silver, small tools	3–4
Spices	3–4
Linens	3–4
Saucepans	6–7
Canned foods	6–7
Canisters	11–12
Large packaged foods	11–12
Shallow utensils, stored vertically	12–13

Carts. Rolling carts that fit into knee space under countertops can provide additional storage. In addition, they

- Can be easily rolled out to provide knee space
- Can provide additional workspace
- Can provide a safe way to transport food and utensils

Countertop Storage Unit. The space between countertop and upper cabinets can provide easily reachable open storage.

Overhead Cabinet Doors. Traditional swinging wall cabinet doors can be a hazard for blind people. Hardware that allows the cabinet doors to swing up and stay open can reduce this problem.

Concealed Knee Space. Retractable doors can be used to conceal knee space. Special hardware allows the door to be pushed back under the counter after opening.

Pantry. A pantry can provide easily accessible storage space. Height-adjustable shelving can tailor the space to individual needs. Shallow shelves keep items within easy reach. The pantry can be a reach-in unit with storage shelving on the doors or even a walk-in design.

Other Accessible Storage Options. Additional options for accessible storage include

- Storage bins
- Pull-out storage
- Revolving shelves
- Swing-out shelves

Add Storage Bins. The addition of pullout storage bins to shelves and cabinets can help make existing storage space accessible.

Lower Existing Cabinets. Existing overhead cabinets can be lowered as far as the top surface of existing counters if necessary. This provides accessible storage at minimal cost. Cabinets may be lowered to 12 to 15 in above the counters, while keeping the counter surface usable.

Add a Freestanding Storage Cabinet. If floor space is available, a freestanding storage cabinet can provide accessible storage space.

Design Notes. All drawers, doors, and hardware should be selected to provide easy access for people with limited dexterity. Recommended features include the following:

- Sliding or folding doors for cabinets provide for the least interference.
- Magnetic catches should be used on the doors.
- Large loop handles also should be used on doors and drawers.
- Toe space on base cabinets should be at least 9 in high and 6 in deep to allow wheelchair users to maneuver closer to the counters.

17.3 THE BATHROOM

Accessible bathrooms should be designed to accommodate the maximum amount of maneuvering possible for physically challenged persons, their wheelchairs, and the possibility of a second person assisting.

17.3.1 Commode

Location

- Ample space around the commode is necessary for side or front approach by wheelchair or walker user.
- The commode is best located in a corner where a wall is behind and beside the commode to easily install grab bars.
- Clearance of 18 in is needed between center line of commode and side wall for adequate shoulder space.

Seat Height

- An accessible toilet seat height varies from user to user.
- Adjusting the seat height aids people who have difficulty rising.
- A commode seat should be at a height of 15 to 19 in above the floor.
- A good rule of thumb is an 18-in height, which is the same as most wheelchair seats.

If a shower commode wheelchair is used, the chair and commode opening must line up. In general, this requires the commode opening to be 20 in from back wall. Adequate space is needed on both sides of the commode so that there is no obstruction.

Safety Bars

- Mounted onto commode to provide user with grab bars.
- Good for person who has limited range of motion and cannot reach grab bars on walls.

Toilet Paper Dispenser

- Dispenser should be below any grab bars located around the commode area.
- Dispenser should be within easy reach of the person.

17.3.2 Door

Clear Opening

- Doors should have a clear opening of between 32 and 36 in.
- The clear opening is measured from the face of the door in a 90-degree open position to the stop on the opposite jamb; the door itself has to be wider than the clear opening in order to comply.

Level Surface

- The clear opening should lead to a level surface for a minimum of 5 ft in the direction that the door swings.
- A 60- by 60-in clear space is best and complies with all approaches.
- There are exact requirements for given approaches; please see Americans with Disabilities Act Accessibility Guidelines (ADAAG Sec. 4.13 and Fig. 25) for exact requirements.

Threshold

- The threshold maximum height is $^1/_2$ in.
- There must not be any sharp inclines or abrupt changes.
- A beveled threshold is recommended.

Force to Open Door

- The pressure required to open doors with door closures should be limited to 3 to 6 ft · lb.
- There should be a 3-s minimum closing time to a point 3 in from the latch.
- An automatic door opener may be used in different situations.

17.3.3 Electrical Controls (Wall Switches and Thermostat for Paraplegic Users)

Safety

- Ground fault circuit indicator (GFCI)–protected electrical receptacles, approved by *National Electrical Code*
- Plastic plug inserts for childproofing electrical receptacles whenever toddlers and young children are present in the environment
- Shatterproof light fixtures
- Use of ground wire with wiring and proper installation

Lighting

- Natural
    - Window at natural height

- Glass blocks that admit light but obscure vision; to install
  1. Reinforced wood framed floor
  2. Bracing at side wall
  3. Provide for trim at top, curbs at floor level, and wall anchors
  4. Set glass blocks with mortar
  5. Caulk around glass wall
- Artificial
  - Above sink with light beams (recommend two minimum) directed toward bowl and away from user's vision field
  - Above and on both sides of grooming mirror/area

In the bathing area, there should be lights above the shower stall or directed into stall above or around the door or curtain.

Electrical Power Outlets

- AC with ground fault interrupters near or within sink reach area for various electrical grooming appliances
- Locate 15 in minimum above floor and $^1/_8$ in minimum from any corners
- When installed above sink, recommend $^1/_5$ in above sink top
- Wall switch located at entry 48 in above floor and 3in in from door molding

Infrared or Sunlamp

- Flush mounting in the ceiling
- 115 V ac, 250 to 300 W
- Beam downward just outside shower stall exit
- Function: for warmth and drying comfort

Fan Connection

- 115 V ac, 100 W
- Locate in ceiling, middle of bathroom
- Install concentric with ventilation porting

17.3.4 Flooring

Nonslip Surface. A nonslip surface should be used to prevent slipping and rolling resistance to wheelchairs.

Color and Patterns

- Providing high contrasts allow for visual acuity.
- Patterns and edgings can guide people with low vision.
- Floors should be relatively light in color, with 30 to 50 percent reflectance.
- Examples of color schemes: cool colors (blues and greens), pastel colors, subdued color with intense color accents, or intense colors.

Fire Code. All flooring and materials must meet *National Fire Code*, Class I.

Clear Floor Space for Commode Area

- Ample floor space in front of and beside the toilet fixture is necessary for users to approach the seat and make a safe transfer.
- If the commode can be approached from the front and side and a sink is installed next to it, the floor space must be at least 4 ft by 5 ft, 6 in:
  - The 4-ft dimension extends into room from side wall next to commode fixture.
  - The 5-ft, 6-in measurement is measured from the wall behind toilet to wall in front of toilet.
- If possible, always design the layout of an accessible bathroom to allow both a front and side transfer to the commode.

Clear Floor Space for Shower and Sink Area

- Clear floor space under the lavatory must be a minimum area of 30 in wide by 48 in long that extends a maximum of 19 in under the lavatory.
- Minimum clear floor space for a roll-in shower is 3 ft by 3 ft.

Clear Floor Space for Entire Bathroom

- Adequate floor space is necessary for a person to maneuver a wheelchair or walker around the bathroom without any obstruction.
- At least a 60-in turning radius is recommended.

Clear Floor Space for Door Area

- Clear, unobstructed floor space is necessary at the door area to allow the door to open and close easily.
- Clear floor space includes the area on the hinge side of the door extending the width of the door and the area past the latch side of the door.
- A wider floor space is needed on the pull side of the door to provide space to open the door.
- Less area is needed on the push side of the door.
- Space must be available on the pull side of the door to operate the door latch, pull the door open, and remain out of the way of the swinging door.
- An outward-swinging door is preferable to provide more accessibility.

17.3.5 Grab Bars

Resistance Force. Grab bars need to be capable of resisting at least 250 lb of force. However, very large persons may require more strength in the grab bar.

Diameter of Bars. The bars should have a diameter in the range of $1^1/_4$ to $1^1/_2$ in.

Clear Space. The space between the grab bar and the walls should be at least $1^1/_2$ in.

Locations of Applicability

- *Roll-in showers.* In 36- by 36-in stalls, bars should be located on the side wall and the wall opposite the seat. In 30- by 60-in stalls, bars should be located on both side walls and the rear wall.
- *Tubs.* Bars should be located on the rear wall, side wall, and side wall opposite controls.
- *Toilet stalls.* Bars should be located on side wall and the wall flush against the commode.

17.3.6 Sink

Type of Sinks

- Wall-mounted and countertop lavatories are accessible.
- Countertop sinks are more accessible due to large surface area to place toiletries.
- Countertop space can be adjusted according the consumer's needs.
- A self-supporting sink can have an optional, removable vanity cabinet underneath.

Dimensions

- Depth of the sink (front to back) for persons using a wheelchair to be able to pull underneath sink.
- Accessible sinks should have dimensions of about 20 in wide by 18 to 27 in deep.
- Sink must have at least 29 in of clearance from the floor to the bottom of apron at front of sink.
- Adequate knee space under sink provides clearance for turns as well as space for close approach to sink by wheelchair users.
- Sink bowl should not be any deeper than $6^1/_2$ in.

Mirror. Mirror must be mounted no higher than 40 in off floor. Examples of accessible mirrors include

- Tilted mirror angled toward floor to accommodate user
- Full-length mirror

Faucet Systems

- Faucets should operate without gripping or twisting of handles.
- For persons who can operate faucet with closed fist, handle should not require more than 5 lb of force.

Accessible faucet handle designs include

- Faucet setup with timer for water to run for period of time and then shut off automatically
- Faucet that is electronically controlled to eliminate the need to turn handles:
  - Senses the presence of the user's hands
  - Automatically turns water on and off
  - Temperature and flow rate of water are preset
  - Particularly useful for people with severe hand limitations
- Faucets with single or double loop or lever handle designs

Plumbing

- Piping underneath sink must not interfere with clear floor space and knee space for wheelchair users and must be insulated to prevent heat injury to legs.
- Wheelchair user needs a clear floor space in front of sink area of approximately 30 by 48 in and knee height to bottom of sink of 22 in.

Reinforcement of Walls. Bathroom walls around sink area may need to be reinforced for proper support of wall-mounted sink.

17.3.7 Storage

Knee Space Underneath Shelves. For a frontal approach to items on shelves, the bottom shelves can be eliminated. This design limits the total shelving space available to user, though.

Depth of Shelves. This should be no greater than 18 in from the front of the closet to the back of the closet. This may vary, depending on the size and limitations of person.

Closet Doors. Several options exist:

- Door swings back 180 degrees so that wheelchair users can make a close parallel approach to reach items from the side.
- Eliminate the door, especially if the bathroom is not very large.

Height Range of Shelves

- An adequate reach range for a wheelchair user to make a side reach is 9 to 54 in above the floor.
- A good height range for storage is 15 in to 48 in above the floor.

Storage Location and Size

- Placed in an area of bathroom that is easily accessed by disabled user.
- Must not obstruct any of the bathroom appliances.
- Amount of storage necessary varies from individual to individual.
- Users may want room for medical supplies and equipment.
- Others may need only a small amount of storage space.

Pull-Out Drawers or Shelves

- Full-extension drawers can be installed in bathrooms up to 60 in off the floor.
- Higher drawers should be shallow for easy access.
- Lower drawers can be deeper.
- For a built-in storage drawer system, use full-extension drawer slides. These slides allow drawers to be pulled out of the cabinet for easy viewing and reaching to contents. These drawers should not be placed more than 42 in above the floor for wheelchair users.

Handles

- Handles on storage closets and drawers should be accessible.
- Standard round doorknobs should be avoided for users with weak grasp.
- Handles should consist of a single lever or open-loop handle.

ACKNOWLEDGMENTS

I acknowledge the contributions of my graduate students in helping assemble this information. Information was gathered from practical field experience, the literature, and interviews with users and rehabilitation engineers.

REFERENCES

Frechette, Leon A., *Accessible Housing,* McGraw-Hill, New York, N.Y., 1996.

Germer, Jerry, *Bathrooms: Design-Remodel-Build,* Creative Homeowners Press, Upper Saddle River, N.J., 1995.

Kearne, Deborah S., *The ADA in Practice,* R. S. Means Company, Kingston, Mass., 1995.

Kira, Alexander, *The Bathroom Criteria for Design,* Bantam Books, New York, N.Y., 1967.

Loversidge, Robert D. Jr., and Laura V. Shinn, *Access for All: An Illustrated Handbook of Barrier Free Design for Ohio,* Schooley Caldwell Associates and the Ohio Governor's Council on People with Disabilities, Cleveland, Ohio, 1994.

Mace, Ronald L., *The Accessible Housing Design File,* Barrier Free Environments, Inc., Van Nostrand Reinhold, New York, N.Y., 1991.

Mean ADA Compliance Pricing Guide, R. S. Means Company, and Adaptive Environments Center, Kingston, Mass., 1994.

Wing, Charlie, *The Visual Handbook of Building and Remodeling,* Rodale Press, Emmaus, Pa., 1990.

Wylde, Margaret, et al., *Building for a Lifetime: The Design and Construction of Fully Accessible Homes,* Taunton Press, Newtown, Conn., 1994.

CHAPTER 18
INTELLIGENT ASSISTIVE TECHNOLOGY

Julie S. Weber (corresponding contributor)
University of Michigan, Ann Arbor, Michigan

Martha Pollack
University of Michigan, Ann Arbor, Michigan

Brett Clippingdale
University of Michigan, Ann Arbor, Michigan

Mark Hodges
University of Michigan, Ann Arbor, Michigan

18.1 INTRODUCTION

Over the past decade, there has been a surge of interest in the development of assistive technologies (AT): technologies that provide support to people with various types of disabilities. A notable feature of this research activity has been its reliance on advanced information and communication technologies (ICT), including probabilistic inference mechanisms and machine-learning algorithms developed in the artificial intelligence research field; low-cost, reliable sensors of many kinds; and ubiquitous wireless networks. Several book-length surveys of the AT field have been written: for example, Cook and Hussey[1,2] give a comprehensive description of work in AT, but not limited to approaches that rely on high-tech solutions; a National Research Council report[3] is also quite broad, but focuses on AT for older adults; and Bardram et al.[4] discuss the use of advanced computing in healthcare applications, including, but not limited to, AT.

We will describe current and emerging AT systems, with an emphasis on the underlying technology that makes those systems feasible. For additional information about AT for cognition, refer to Ref.[5] In the interest of space, we focus here on AT specifically for the domain of cognitive impairments. This class of technology is particularly important in light of the unprecedented demographic changes currently underway. It is predicated that by 2050, 20 percent of the U.S. population will be over the age of 65, and nearly 8 percent will be older than 80; and similar rates are expected internationally.[6] Aging is, of course, a significant risk factor for illnesses that cause cognitive decline—as just one example, as many as 20 percent of those between 85 and 89 years, and nearly a third of those over the age of 90 have Alzheimer's disease.[7] Of course, the AT systems that we describe can also be useful for younger people with cognitive impairments, for example, those who have had a traumatic brain injury or who have a developmental delay.

People with cognitive impairments exhibit an immense variety of configurations of capabilities and disabilities, and hence one of the key challenges for designers of AT for cognitive impairment is to ensure that the technology can be readily customized to the needs of individual users, where preferably this customization is automated. That said, there are certain fundamental types of support that AT for cognition can provide, and we focus here on three:

- Memory aids that facilitate the effective performance of daily activities
- Navigational aids that enhance orientation
- Evaluation systems that perform naturalistic assessment of functional performance

Within each class of systems, an important capability is that of recognizing the activities performed by the user. We thus begin by summarizing approaches to activity recognition, and then turn to each of the three classes of systems listed above.

18.2 ACTIVITY RECOGNITION

To make informed decisions and suggestions, effective intelligent assistance often requires an understanding of which tasks or activities have been performed. For example, a prompting system for overseeing an individual's self-administration of medication should not provide a cue to take the medication if an individual has already been observed to have taken it. The same system is even more helpful if it can issue a warning when it observes the person beginning to administer medicine before it is time to do so, or if that particular dose of the medication has already been taken. As another example, a system that provides cues to guide a severely impaired individual through the process of hand-washing must recognize the attempt at washing hands, understand the steps being performed, and identify any errors that may have been made (for instance, using a towel before wetting the hands). To provide a type of navigational support that will be discussed later in this chapter—guiding someone to his/her destination—it is necessary for a guidance system to recognize the destination as well as the activities that may be performed there. For instance, at dinnertime, an individual may require guidance to the dining room, with a stop in the bathroom for hand-washing along the way. Finally, to assess an individual's performance on a set of functional activities, an evaluative system should have the ability to recognize the activities that are being performed in combination with a quality metric to determine performance levels. This is illustrated in the example just above, in which an individual begins to use a towel without wet hands, a clear indicator of poor performance. A great deal of research on AT for cognition has therefore emphasized the problem of activity recognition.

18.2.1 Formal Definition of Activity Recognition

We can define the activity recognition problem as follows: provided a set of observations, determine the task or activity that a person is performing. We must then identify the set of possible activities to be recognized, the source of the observations, and the algorithms used to map from observations to activities. When the observations are certain—that is, there is no noise within the data collected—the problem reduces to that of plan recognition, a well-studied problem in artificial intelligence.[8] However, in general in AT applications, the observations are obtained from sensor readings, with which there is generally a significant amount of associated noise. In that case, we typically extend the problem, to infer not a specific activity, but rather a probability distribution over possible activities.

18.2.2 Choosing Activities to Recognize

When designing an activity recognition system, a key decision that must be made is which activities the system should be able to recognize. Different systems take different approaches to activity recognition. Some attempt to differentiate between individuals' motion patterns, or modes of physical movement, which includes activities like running, walking, or jumping. Other systems approach activity recognition on the level of interaction with objects, differentiating amongst tasks such as preparing a meal, eating a meal, and watching television. Yet another class of activity recognition systems attempt to differentiate among destinations to which an individual is traveling, as a particular location may be associated with a particular set of activities (e.g., dinner is usually served in the dining room).

18.2.3 Sensors

Next we must consider *how* to observe an individual to determine the task or activity that he or she is performing at a given time. There are two broad classes of sensors that can be used to make these observations: simple, or information-poor, sensors and information-rich sensors. A simple sensor is associated with a single-valued piece of data; an example is a contact switch that returns a binary value, indicating whether or not contact has been made with the sensor at the time of a query. An information-rich sensor, such as a video camera, provides more complex data for potential analysis, the most general forms being audio and visual information, which can each be subdivided and analyzed in a number of different ways to retrieve many different types and amounts of useful information. While a single information-rich sensor collects much more data than a single simple sensor, information-rich sensor data are often more difficult for a system to process; conversely, data acquired by a simple sensor may provide very little information despite being easier to analyze.

An inherent advantage to video cameras and microphones, the most commonly used rich sensors, is their ability to perform passive observation, requiring no action on behalf of the individuals being observed. In addition, by definition they provide a great deal of information. One of the most notable disadvantages, however, is that individuals commonly express privacy concerns about the invasive nature of this type of sensor, that is, the fact that they feel they are being "watched."[9]

Rather than use a small number of information-rich sensors, an alternative is to use a large number of information-poor sensors. This is primarily done in one of two ways: by placing these sensors throughout an individual's home environment, or by placing sensors on a wearable platform to be worn by the individual being observed. With sensors placed throughout an environment, a system can identify the objects with which an individual is interacting. Examples of sensors used for this purpose include contact switches, motion detectors, sensors to measure electric current or water flow, and radio frequency identification (RFID) systems. RFID systems consist of several tags and one or more readers that can detect tags within a certain range. By placing an RFID reader on a bracelet worn by the individual being observed, a system can detect the tagged objects that are in close proximity (approximately 10 cm for the Intel iBracelet[10]) to a user's hand and, therefore, those objects with which the individual might be interacting. The objects with which a person interacts tend to correspond to his or her actions, and this is the basis of activity detection with this approach.

The other commonly employed method for utilizing information-poor sensors is to place them on a wearable platform. This approach is frequently used to observe an individual's movement; however, it can also be used to gather observations about the individual's environment. Typically, sensors in such systems include accelerometers in all three dimensions, placed in one or more locations around the body to observe motion. Other wearable sensing platforms make use of ambient temperature readings, barometric readings, and measurements of galvanic skin response or skin temperature.

Unfortunately, there are a number of limitations associated with different types of sensors. Certain classes of sensors are fairly unreliable, and data can be noisy. Of course, sensor networks, composed of multiple sensors communicating amongst one another, are more susceptible to sensor failure, because the likelihood of a single sensor failing increases with the number of sensors in the network. And certain types of sensors have other limitations; for example, motion sensors will detect *any* motion in their environment, that is, there is no way for them to exclusively detect human (let alone a single human's) movement.

18.2.4 Algorithms for Activity Recognition

Once a system has access to an individual's task data, it can identify patterns in that data that allow it to infer the activity that is most likely being performed at a given time using a classifier algorithm, which classifies the activity as one of a set of possibilities. For instance, if an individual is in the kitchen, he/she may be performing any one of the following activities, potentially among others: preparing a meal, setting the table, clearing the table, or cleaning the room.

Before a system can perform classification, it must generate a model of the sensor signals it might observe and their correlation to members of the set of potential activities. This process of generating the model typically relies on labeled data: sets of examples of sensor readings that have been manually labeled with the type of activity that produced each example. In other words, the system needs to have access to a set of examples of sensor data that it knows were, say, observed during meal preparation; another set of examples it knows were collected during dish-washing; and so on.

There are many different types of classifiers and many ways in which a model can be generated on receipt of labeled training data. Broadly, and for the purposes of this discussion of activity recognition, there are two types of classifiers: deterministic and probabilistic. Deterministic classifiers generate a model that will determine, for any new set of data, the activity that is most likely being performed. A probabilistic classifier, on the other hand, will generate a probability distribution over the possible activities being performed at any given time. This section highlights a single type of deterministic classifier, a decision tree, and three probabilistic classifiers—Bayes nets, hidden Markov models, and dynamic Bayesian networks—with a focus on how each model is used once generated. The subsequent section describes a set of techniques for generating each type of classification model from acquired sensor data.

Deterministic Classifiers. Deterministic classifiers take as input a set of sensor readings and as output predict the class or category of the data provided. A widely used form of deterministic classifier is a decision tree, which is a model that encodes a set of "decision criteria" used as a means for classifying a set of sensor-based observations. Given input data, a decision tree algorithm will traverse the tree, beginning at the root, and check the decision criterion encoded at each branch-point against the data provided as input. Upon reaching a leaf of the tree, a class value is predicted for the given input data. When performing activity recognition, input data would come from sensor observations, and the predicted class value would be the system's best guess as to which activity was being performed, given the associated set of sensor readings.

Suppose that we would like to distinguish between two activities being performed by Mrs. Jones, an older adult who lives alone. These activities are *setting* the table and *clearing* the table. Let us assume for simplicity of exposition that there is a contact or light sensor inside the cupboard (sensor C) and one inside the dishwasher (sensor D), and no other sensors, that these sensors are robust to noise, and that at the time of observation, an individual is always performing one of our two activities: either setting or clearing the table.* Further, suppose that using labeled training data, a classification system has learned the decision tree displayed in Fig. 18.1.

There are two decision criteria inside of the decision tree in Fig. 18.1. First, at the root, the system asks whether its user has been observed to have interacted with the dishwasher, that is, whether the dishwasher sensor was observed to have fired. If so, its prediction is that the user was clearing the table; and if not, it consults another decision criterion. This second criterion relates to whether the sensor in the cupboard was observed to be active, and if so, the system predicts that the user was setting the table; otherwise, if the cupboard sensor was inactive (in addition to the dishwasher sensor), then the system predicts that the user was performing the activity of clearing the table.

*A caveat about this example, which will act as a basis for further discussion of AI techniques for assisted cognition throughout this chapter, is that it is highly simplified and solely used for illustration of the techniques that will be presented; there is a much broader set of activities that are useful to recognize within the domain of AT, including medication administration, hydration, exercise, and many others.

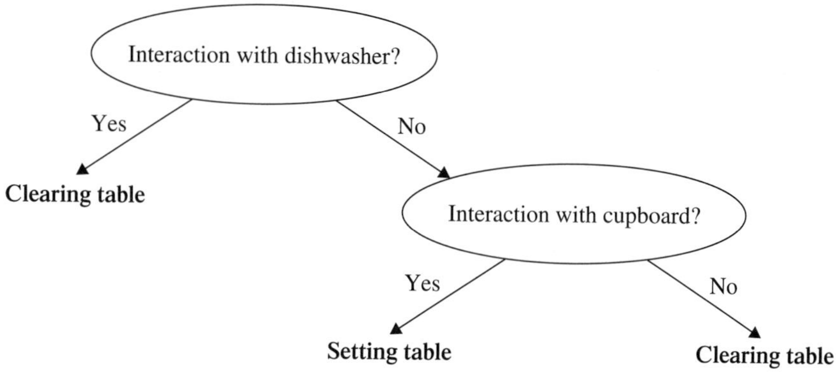

FIGURE 18.1 A decision tree using rules based on sensor data.

Probabilistic Classifiers. The decision tree approach is deterministic: it assumes that there is always a single, well-defined function mapping from sensor data to activities. But of course there are many alternative means for performing certain activities, which is a fact that can complicate the mapping. For instance, an individual may decide to set the table using clean dishes taken directly from the dishwasher, or clear the table and return an unused glass directly to the cupboard. In some situations we could handle this with more complex and detailed rules, but in general, it is preferable to use alternative methods that explicitly reason about probabilistic connections between sensor data and activities.

Probabilistic classifiers model probability distributions over all possible sensor observations and use inference techniques to determine the most likely state of the world at any given time, based on these observations. The most frequently used methods for performing probabilistic inference are Bayesian classifiers,[11] hidden Markov models (HMMs),[12] and dynamic Bayes nets (DBNs).[13] Collectively, these are known as *graphical models*, because they allow modeling with an explicit graphical representation of probabilistic dependencies. We discuss each model in turn.

Bayesian Classifiers. Bayesian inference is a very well-studied approach to reasoning about probabilities. Within the AI literature, most Bayesian inference is underpinned with the use of Bayesian networks (BN), which provide a compact way of encoding probabilistic relations between random variables. Figure 18.2 provides an illustration of a BN for our running example. The nodes

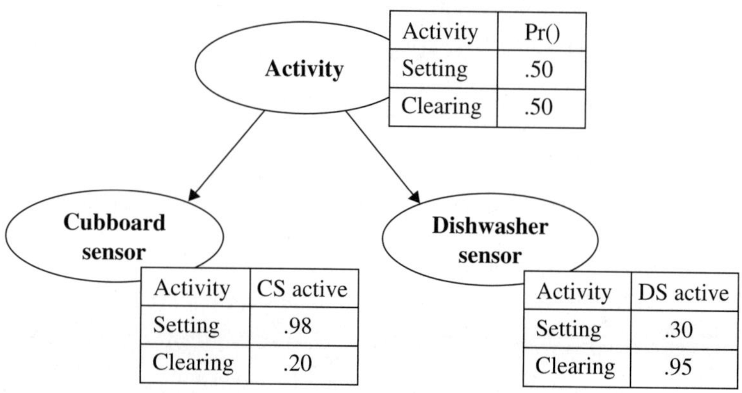

FIGURE 18.2 A Bayesian network to distinguish between setting and clearing the table, with associated probabilities in their conditional probability tables.

represent features of the world, such as the activity being performed or the firing of a sensor, while the arcs represent causal influences between those features. The third component of BNs are conditional probability tables (CPT), which provide the probabilities of a given node taking particular value, conditioned on the value of its parent nodes in the graph. Thus, for example, in Fig. 18.2, the "cupboard sensor" node has a CPT that indicates that the probability of that sensor firing is .98 if the activity being performed is setting the table, and .20 if the activity is clearing the table.

As mentioned above, the primary advantage of BNs is that they allow one to exploit conditional independencies, and thus, in general, to encode a smaller set of probability values than would be needed to specify the full joint probability distribution for a given problem. For instance, in our simple example, there are three nodes each representing a binary random variable, and consequently, the full joint would require eight values. However, we have assumed that in this domain, the firing of the cupboard sensor and that of the dishwasher sensor are independent conditioned on the activity; that is, letting C, D, and A represent each of the random variables:

$$P(C|A,D) = P(C|A) \qquad \text{and} \qquad P(D|A,C) = P(D|A)$$

As a result, we need to only specify four values in the CPTs: those encoding $P(C|A = set)$, $P(C|A = clear)$, $P(D|A = set)$ and $P(D|A = clear)$. Here we have a 50 percent reduction in the number of values required; in practice, the reduction will depend on the degree of independence amongst the domain variables.

As is well known, Bayesian inference allows one to reason both from causes to effects, as well as from effects to causes; the latter is typically achieved using Bayes' rule:

$$P(X|Y) = \frac{P(Y|X)P(X)}{P(Y)}$$

For instance, suppose that in our example, we know that both the dishwasher sensor and the cupboard sensor have fired, that is, C = true and D = true. Our goal in activity recognition is to determine a probability distribution over the possible values for A, that is, we are interested in $P(A|C = true, D = true)$. By Bayes rule we know:

$$P(A|C = true, D = true) = \frac{P(C = true, D = true|A) \cdot P(A)}{P(C = true, D = true)}$$

We show how to calculate this for $A = clear$. Because C and D are conditionally independent given A, we can easily compute the first factor in the numerator:

$$P(C = true, D = true|A = clear) = P(C = true|A = clear) \cdot P(D = true|A = clear)$$
$$= .2(.95) = .19$$

The second factor in the numerator is the prior probability that $A = clear$; let us assume that this is equal to .5.

Finally, we can compute the denominator using marginalization, we know:

$$\begin{aligned}
&P(C = true, D = true) \\
&\quad = P(C = true, D = true|A = clear)P(A = clear) + P(C = true, D = true|A = set)P(A = set) \\
&\quad = P(C = true|A = clear)P(D = true|A = clear)P(A = clear) \\
&\qquad + P(C = true|A = set)P(D = true|A = set)P(A = set) \\
&\quad = (.2)(.95)(.5) + (.98)(.3)(.5) = .24
\end{aligned}$$

Plugging these values back into Bayes rule, we obtain

$$P(A = clear|C = true, D = true) = \frac{.19(.5)}{.24} = .40$$

In other words, if both sensors fire, there is a 40 percent probability that the table is being cleared.

A number of algorithms have been developed for efficiently performing Bayes inference on BNs. One of the best known is the junction tree algorithm,[14] which creates a cycle-free, moralized maximum spanning tree (a junction tree), and uses a message-passing scheme to propagate evidence throughout the graph and determine the probabilities of each node. Unfortunately, exact inference is often infeasible due to the size of BNs and particularly when they are polytrees, that is, contain more than a single (undirected) path between nodes. As a result, a number of approximation algorithms have been developed. Most of these algorithms are based on some form of randomized sampling, and examples include likelihood weighting[15] and Markov chain Monte Carlo (MCMC).[16]

MCMC approximation initializes the observed nodes with arbitrary values, then samples the likelihood of each hidden node's values, given the evidence variables that affect it—those in its *Markov blanket* of parents, children, and children's parents. This is done repeatedly in a random walk over the nodes in the graph, and the actual probabilities are determined by normalizing the frequency of each value for each hidden node. Using our example, if, given an evidence variable configuration where both cupboard and dishwasher sensors are "true," the random walk finds 12 instances in which activity is clearing the table, and 18 states where it is setting the table, then the approximate value of (A = *clear*) would be 12/(18 + 12), or 40 percent.

In our running example, we assumed that all sensor observations are independent. When this assumption is true, it is associated with a special case of a Bayes net, called a *naïve* Bayesian classifier, for which

$$P(Cause, Effect_1, Effect_2, \ldots, Effect_n) = P(Cause)\sum_i P(Effect_i|Cause)$$

This classifier is called *naïve* because its simplicity may reflect naivety about actual conditional independence of each of the effects, given the cause. However, in real-world use, even when the effects are not independent, this classifier is often quite accurate.

Hidden Markov Models. One limitation of Bayesian classifiers is that they do not consider temporal effects with respect to a set of tasks or activities. For example, they do not exploit the fact that one would typically set the table before eating a meal. A well-known formalism that accounts for temporal effects is the hidden Markov model, or HMM.[12] HMMs are based on the Markov assumption, which states that the present is a sufficient statistic to predict the future, in other words, for any timepoint t, the state X_t is a function of the state transition distribution from the state X_{t-1} and any observation of evidence variables O_t.

A typical HMM is displayed in Fig. 18.3. Similar to BNs, each transition arc is assigned a probability value. The HMM in Fig. 18.3 is particularly simple; in general, the sequence of states need not be linear. If there is more than one variable representing a given state, then these variables are combined into a *mega-variable* to maintain the single-state-per-time-slice invariant of HMMs.

Several algorithms are available for reasoning with HMMs. For example, the forward-backward algorithm[17] efficiently calculates the likelihood of a sequence of underlying states, given the probability distributions over state transitions and observations, and the Viterbi algorithm[18] determines the most likely sequence of prior events that would lead to a particular state.

Although HMMs can be very efficient, as was the case for BNs, reasoning with them may become intractable as the size of the model grows. Due to the HMM restriction of a single state variable, every member of a state mega-variable X_t is dependent on every evidence variable E_t (comprising observed state), and thus, the worst case computational complexity of this model is exponential: $|X|^{|E|}$.

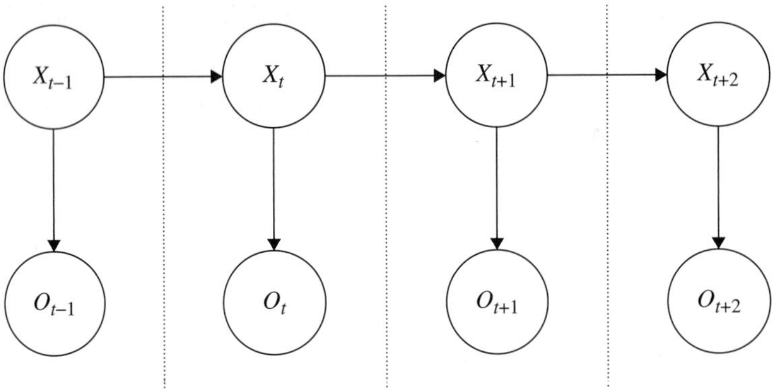

FIGURE 18.3 A hidden Markov model (HMM), modeling the actual, hidden state (X) based on observed state (O) at each time interval.

Dynamic Bayesian Networks. One way to reduce computational complexity, while still modeling the temporal dependencies that are so important in activity recognition, is to use a dynamic Bayesian network, or DBN.[13] A DBN can be seen as a hybrid of a Bayes net and an HMM. Similar to a Bayes net, a DBN allows factorization of states and observations: there is no need for mega-variables, because individual features are each represented. For example, the DBN in Fig. 18.4 splits the observations into two: triggering of the dishwasher sensor and triggering of the cupboard sensor. Although in this simplistic example there is only a single state variable (A) representing the activity performed, in general, DBNs, like Bayes nets, may represent multiple features of state.

At the same time, a DBN is similar to an HMM in that it explicitly encodes state and observation values at each time point, along with transition probabilities. Thus, for instance, in Fig. 18.4, there are nodes representing the values of C (a triggering of the cupboard sensor) at each of times $t - 1$, t, and $t + 1$.

Like a static Bayesian network, a DBN exploits conditional independence to achieve a compact representation. For example, suppose we wish to model a network with 15 Boolean state and observation variables in each time slice, and in which each variable depends on four parent variables from the previous time slice. An HMM's probability matrix for this problem would include all 2^{15} states,

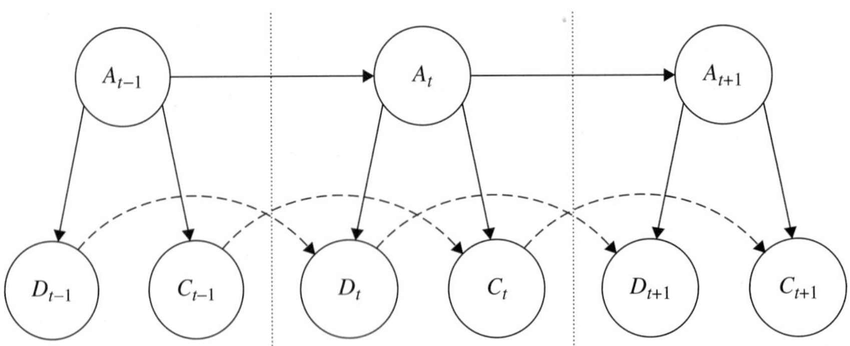

FIGURE 18.4 A dynamic Bayesian network (DBN), modeling nodes for user activity (A), dishwasher sensor (D), and cupboard sensor (S) at each time interval.

and thus would need to represent $2^{2\times15}$ (more than 1 billion) transitions; a DBN, by comparison, would have only 15×2^4 (or 240) transitions to model.

With this representation, it is possible to perform exact inference by *unrolling* the desired number of time slices into a single Bayesian network and using, for example, the junction tree algorithm discussed earlier in this section. However, DBNs can still grow very large; although their representations are typically much more compact than those for HMMs (depending on conditional dependencies), approximate inference methods (such as the Markov chain Monte Carlo technique introduced earlier) are often required.

18.2.5 Learning Classifiers

There is a rich literature on learning both deterministic and probabilistic classifiers, which we only touch on here. For more information, please see Ref. 19.

Learning a Decision Tree. Several supervised learning algorithms, such as ID3[20] and C4.5,[21] learn decision trees recursively: at each node in the decision tree, a rule or criterion is used to determine how that node will categorize the data, and the process is then repeated for each of the subnodes that are created, using only the data sets that are assigned to the subnode. Heuristics based on information-theoretic principles are used to select the best criterion at each branching point of a tree. More specifically, an algorithm will select a criterion that results in the greatest amount of *information gain* at each node, maximally reducing the overall entropy of the as-yet unclassified data associated with a given node.

One potential difficulty in decision-tree learning is *overfitting* the data; generating a model that is too specific to the training data and does not generalize to new data instances. A decision tree that chooses new decision criteria to exhaustion, that is, until every instance has been classified into a homogeneous category such that the entropy is zero at every leaf node, is likely to overfit the data that was used to train it, especially in the case of noisy data. To avoid overfitting in decision trees, a technique called *pruning* can be employed. A pruning algorithm removes those nodes from a decision tree that are least useful in classifying training instances. For example, a pruning algorithm may consider every new tree in which a single, internal node (and its associated subtree) has been removed and replaced with the class label associated with the largest number of data instances. The tree with highest accuracy when classifying elements of the training set becomes the new tree, with (perhaps many) less nodes.

Learning Probabilistic Classifiers. There are also numerous techniques for using supervised learning for probabilistic classifiers. A particularly powerful approach is the Baum-Welch algorithm,[22] which performs iterative learning of HMMs by beginning with a single estimation of an HMM and iteratively modifying it to better fit the training data. It is an expectation-maximization (EM) algorithm, in which learning occurs in two iterated steps: expectation, in this case determining the likelihood that the HMM observed the training data, and maximization, adjusting the parameters of the HMM so that this likelihood will be increased. EM algorithms have been shown to be very powerful in practice.

18.3 ACTIVITY GUIDANCE AND MEMORY SUPPORT

Now that we have seen what is involved in automatically recognizing activities, we can turn to the question of what AT systems do, given the ability to recognize activities. An important capability involves guidance by intelligent cueing. In order to provide appropriate cues, an activity guidance system must combine information obtained from an activity recognition engine, regarding which activities are likely being performed, with knowledge about the activities that a user *should* be performing, as well as *how* those activities should be performed.

TABLE 18.1 Mrs. Jones' Daily Plan

Activity	Earliest start time	Latest start time	Duration
Breakfast	7:00 am	9:00 am	30–60 min
Lunch	11:30 am	1:30 pm	30–60 min
Dinner	5:00 pm	8:00 pm	30–60 min
Medication	12:00 pm	2:00 pm	5 min
Exercise	12:00 pm	9:00 pm	15–20 min

18.3.1 Planning by Rewriting

One approach to providing cueing support is to remove the activities that have been performed from the set of those that are required to be performed within an individual's daily plan, generating a simple cueing (or reminder) plan that initially includes a reminder for each remaining activity, and then using a technique called *iterative plan-repair* to refine that reminder plan.

For example, consider the daily plan displayed in Table 18.1, which we imagine belongs to Mrs. Jones. If an activity recognition system has inferred that Mrs. Jones has already eaten breakfast, say because she has just cleared the table, then an initial reminder plan for the remainder of Mrs. Jones' day might look like the one displayed in Fig. 18.5. This diagrams each of the scheduled reminders as well as their dependencies; a reminder for dinner is dependent on the lunch activity having been successfully completed. Furthermore, the goal is met only when all reminders have been issued and activities completed.

The system has scheduled a naïve reminder for the earliest possible start time of each activity. As a result, the reminder plan requires two reminders be issued at once—at noon, which is likely to be during Mrs. Jones' lunch. To create an improved plan for issuing reminders to Mrs. Jones (so as to increase satisfaction and the likelihood of compliance, and to minimize the amount of overreliance), a plan repair algorithm such as the *planning-by-rewriting* paradigm[23] can be adopted. This technique allows the user or a care provider to provide a set of rules that may be added to those used as a basis for improving a reminder plan. In other words, an initial set of generic rewrite rules can be provided, and they can be supplemented by specialized rules pertaining to a given individual.

Suppose the optimization rules for Mrs. Jones's reminder plan are those displayed in Table 18.2. These *rewrite* rules are applied using a local search technique,[24] in which a set of new reminder plans is generated by incorporating these three rules, one at a time. The search process then selects from amongst these new reminder plans, choosing the plan that receives the highest score from a prespecified quality metric as the next plan to be refined. This process continues until either time runs out (essentially indicating, in this domain, that a reminder must be issued immediately) or no higher quality plan can be generated.

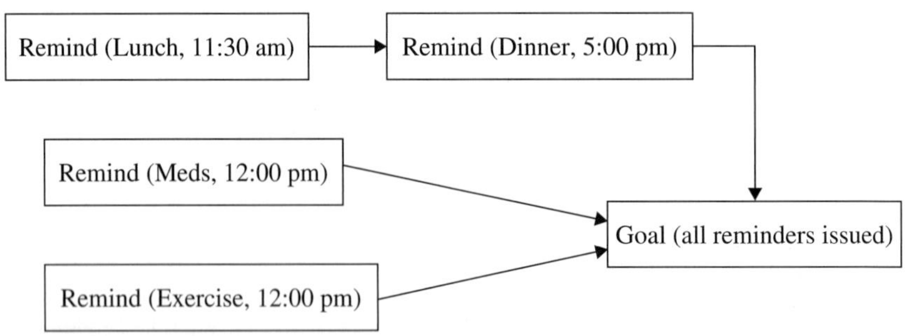

FIGURE 18.5 An initial reminder schedule for the remainder of Mrs. Jones' daily plan.

TABLE 18.2 Rewrite Rules for Mrs. Jones' Reminder Plan

Rule 1	Rule 2	Rule 3
Space out reminders as much as possible	Remind at the latest possible start time	Merge reminders issued at the same time

The Autominder system,[25] a cognitive orthotic designed to assist people with memory impairment in going about their activities of daily living, uses the planning-by-rewriting paradigm in its development of a reminder plan for each user. In Autominder, the quality metric established for assessing the relative quality of a given reminder plan is based on the following set of factors: (1) number of reminders: the smaller the number of reminders that must be issued, the less likely that a user will become overreliant on the system; (2) timing of reminders: reminders issued later in the interval of possibility will also decrease user reliance; (3) spacing between reminders: reminder plans are more efficient, and likely more effective, if reminders are spaced out throughout the day and between activities of similar types than if they are clustered in one part of the day. Other potential quality metrics for intelligent cueing using planning-by-rewriting may specify the priority of certain reminders over others, or place a loose cap on the number of reminders issued for a given category of activity.

18.3.2 Reinforcement Learning

An alternate approach to intelligent cueing for daily activities relies on techniques adopted from the AI subfield called *reinforcement learning*.[26] Such an approach extends the capabilities of the iterative refinement-based planning system described above in that neither rewrite rules nor a quality metric need to be manually defined; instead the effectiveness of alternative reminding strategies are learned by observing the individual's performance over time. Where ordinary rules are fixed and nonadaptive, reinforcement learning can produce a user model that is adapted to a given individual's behavior, and automatically adjusted if that behavior changes over time.

In general, a reinforcement learning system begins with an initial *policy* that determines which actions it will take (i.e., cues that it will issue) in which system states, or settings. After each action, a *payoff* will be computed, indicating the learning system's performance with respect to that action, in that setting. This payoff will spawn the generation of an updated policy (that incorporates actions with the highest expected payoff in each setting), and the state-action-payoff process repeats as the policy is continually updated.

The Autominder system, mentioned above, was expanded with a reinforcement learning mechanism for generating reminders.[27] The payoff function implemented by this reminding mechanism was designed to penalize the system for every reminder that is issued (to discourage user reliance) and reinforce behavior that leads to high user success or compliance. The objective function, then, equated to maximizing the expected summed payoff for a given day. Testing of the reinforcement learning component of the Autominder system was performed only in simulation; however, it was a promising initial step toward development of a system that adapts to its users and their changing needs.

18.3.3 (Partially Observable) Markov Decision Processes

Another approach to activity support models the entire interaction with a user as a set of states and observations, where prompting decisions (or *actions* in the state space) are made by considering the present state of an individual and the intended future results of taking a particular action. As an example, consider the situation in which it has just been observed that Mrs. Jones has finished setting the table. Then, if it is known that Mrs. Jones is often forgetful of what to do next (e.g., prepare dinner), and that in the past reminders have served useful in this context, a reminder could be issued, with the likely desired effect that Mrs. Jones will respond and begin to prepare her meal.

A Markov decision process, or MDP,[28] is a model similar to a Bayesian network in which states and actions may be represented graphically. The primary distinction is that in an MDP, *values* are associated with each state of the world, and *rewards* are then associated with the performance of any action, depending on the value of the state that results from taking the action in the current state. Because the outcome of an action may be uncertain, the reward is actually a weighted sum of the values in the possible outcome states. *Partially observable* Markov decision processes, or POMDPs,[29] are an extension of MDPs, in which it is assumed that states are unknown. That is, in a POMDP, not only can one represent the fact that the outcome of a given action is uncertain, but one can also encode situations in which there is not even certainty about what state was reached after the action was taken. States are thus replaced with observations, in a manner that recalls HMMs. POMDPs are widely used in the literature for plan-based reasoning in uncertain environments.

Given either an MDP or a POMDP, one needs to compute a *policy,* which is, a function from states (in the case of an MDP) or observations (for a POMDP) to actions. Ideally, one would like an optimal policy, i.e., one that guarantees maximal reward relative to an aggregation function, where a typical aggregation function discounts future rewards so that in the limit, no further reward is received. Several well-known algorithms, including value-iteration and policy-iteration, can be used to calculate optimal policies for MDPs. In general, computation of an optimal policy for POMDPs has high complexity, and so approximation techniques to compute near-optimal policies are used instead.[30]

Figure 18.6 displays a sample graphical representation of a component of a POMDP, called a *policy tree*, which encodes a policy for our simple example. Each node in the tree represents an action that can be taken by the assistance system (where actions are either to "do nothing" or issue a prompt to eat a meal), and arcs represent observations (restricted only to the cupboard sensor for the example, as described in Fig. 18.6).

We assume that the system begins in a state in which the user is equally likely to be setting the table or not setting the table [$P(set) = 0.5$]. Although not shown here, we assume that there is a positive reward for issuing an appropriate prompt (e.g., to eat the meal, as the table has just been set) and a negative reward for issuing an errant prompt (e.g., to eat the meal when the person has instead cleared the table). Intuitively, if the cupboard sensor is observed to fire, then the observation probabilities indicate that it is even more likely that the user is setting the table, and this has led to a policy in which a prompt is issued in response. Otherwise, if the cupboard sensor is not observed, then it is much less likely that the user is setting the table, and here the policy reflects this by including its "do nothing" action.

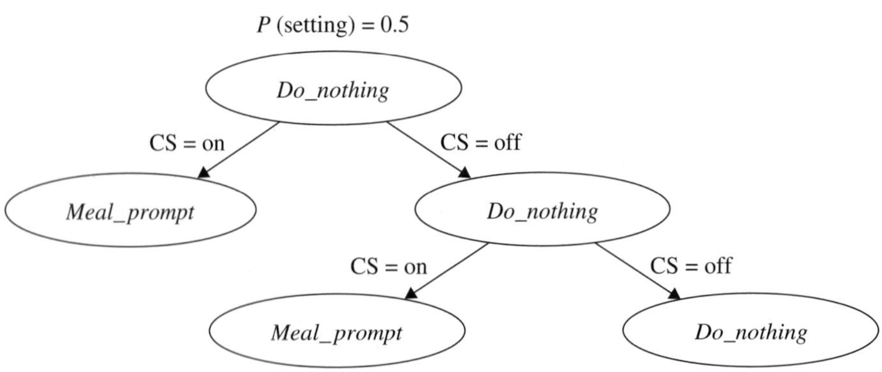

FIGURE 18.6 A simplistic version of a POMDP policy tree.

The COACH system[31] provides an example of POMDP modeling for activity cueing. As an initial step toward general toileting support for individuals with dementia,* this system monitors the activity of hand-washing, providing appropriate prompts as necessary to promote successful completion of the entire task. The COACH system is configured to accept video input, from which it tracks towel and hand movements using a Bayesian estimation technique called *particle filtering*. This process requires the system to recognize congruously moving color patterns as the main source of information extracted from the video sensor. In turn, the color-tracking information is provided to a belief monitor, which attempts to determine the individual's state, comprising attitude and planstep information, where attitude relates to the individual's current level of dementia and planstep refers to the step of the hand-washing activity currently being performed. Then, given an estimate of the individual's current state, the POMDP uses its policy to determine the most appropriate action to be taken by the system. In general, actions in COACH are prompts specific to the individual's progress and carried out by a synthesized voice that suggests the next step required to move forward in the hand-washing activity. The system may also determine that a human caregiver's assistance is required and alert the caregiver accordingly. When tested with individuals experiencing mild-to-severe dementia, the COACH system yielded promising results, suggesting that such a system may be a useful tool for both mitigating the burden on human caregivers and promoting independence of older adults with dementia.

18.4 NAVIGATION

We now turn to another type of support for individuals with cognitive impairment, that of assisting an individual in navigating his or her environment. We consider two problems inherent in providing navigational assistance: acquiring or developing a map of the environment and localizing (or pinpointing) an individual within that environment. In addition, we briefly discuss the process of recognizing an individual's destination, as this permits path planning as well as replanning when the user of a navigational support system deviates from a given path.

Though the overarching goals of navigational support systems are fairly universal, these systems can be categorized into interior and exterior navigational aids. Interior navigational aids provide support for someone in the home or other indoor environment, whereas exterior navigation refers to guidance outdoors. In an interior environment, navigational support may come from a *smart robot* that guides an individual from location to location.[32] Outdoors, navigational aids such as global positioning systems, or GPS, which are familiar navigational supports, can assist their users in moving from one place to the next.

18.4.1 Mapping and Localization

Typically, in exterior navigational support, the problem of mapping an unknown environment is trivial, because maps, both paper-based and computerized, are very easily accessible, and thus new maps need not be generated. Furthermore, localization is itself trivial in an outdoor environment, where GPS devices can provide accurate information.

However, this is often not true for indoor environments: instead, maps may not exist, and GPS may not work; even if it does, the error associated with the GPS signals (between 5 and 15 m[33]) may be too imprecise. Thus, both map-generation and localization must occur. One way to perform map generation is to make use of a mobile robot, having it randomly walk (or roll) around the environment, collecting data using whatever types of sensors it has on board, typically including sonar and laser range-finders.

*Caregivers have indicated a strong desire for support with toileting assistance among other tasks that also currently require human assistance.

The resulting description of the sensed environment, which will include features such as doors, walls, rooms, and corridors, can then be manually labeled with place-names (e.g., indicating which room is the dining room, which is the bedroom) Once a map has been created, the process of localization consists of performing pattern-matching between current sensor readings and those recorded in the map; techniques for this process of environment-mapping make use of the types of probabilistic inference described above in the discussion of activity recognition. Recent advances in automated navigation have focused on simultaneous localization and mapping or simultaneous localization and mapping, SLAM.[34]

18.4.2 Destination Prediction

If an AT system can recognize a user's destination, it can then assist him or her in getting there. Destination prediction may be important both indoors and outdoors. The problem is to infer where a person wants to get to, given information about their current route as well as other commonsense information (such as time of day or day of week). Another relevant piece of information may be the sequence of a user's destinations: for example, in an exterior environment, it may be useful to know that the person has walked to the bus-stop and is now traveling north on a bus. (The rate of change in the current location can be used to infer mode of transportation.)

One way to model a sequence of destinations is to use a Markov chain. In an n-order Markov chain, the $(n + 1)^{st}$ state is determined by the prior n states in the model. This type of model has been used in destination prediction with time-lapse GPS data that is clustered into meaningful locations.[35] A similar technique is used in a separate initiative to infer an individual's destination and mode of transportation.[36] However, rather than the second-order Markov model used in Ref. 35, this system utilizes a more efficient hierarchical DBN, which can learn an individual's transportation routine and detect potential user errors by recognizing deviations from its calculated norms.

The Opportunity Knocks system[37] is a complete navigational support system for people with cognitive impairment intending to travel within their communities (e.g., people with developmental delays who ride buses to work). This system makes use of a hierarchical DBN with three levels. The bottom level reasons about a user's current actual location and mode of transportation. The middle level reasons about the user's destination. And the top level computes the probability of *novelty*, which is the term the system designers used to describe a person doing something unexpected. The system is implemented on a cell phone with GPS, and when the novelty probability exceeds some threshold, the user is alerted to a problem, and real-time path planning is invoked to create a plan that gets the user back on track toward his or her inferred goal. Although only preliminary tests were conducted, the overall approach of this system seems highly promising.

18.5 ASSESSMENT

Most of this chapter has focused on assisting an individual with a cognitive impairment to successfully complete a task or daily routine. Another important focus within the domain of cognitive assistive technology is the *assessment* of a cognitive impairment: determining whether an individual has a cognitive impairment and, if so, its associated level of severity.

Assessment is of particular importance due to the inherent difficulty in recognizing cognitive impairments during routine doctor's visits. Cases of dementia or probable dementia, for example, often go undiagnosed by primary-care physicians.[38] Additionally, because cognitive ability can vary from day to day, and caregivers cannot typically observe patients on a daily basis, they are often forced to rely on questioning, requiring them to "play detective" to determine whether a patient has dementia.[39] Perhaps surprisingly, traumatic brain injury, or TBI, can also be difficult to recognize. While it will of course be obvious that a patient has had an accident that could potentially cause a TBI, the physical damage to the brain cannot always be detected with imaging tests. Moreover, patients with TBI do not always recognize the changes in their behavior, as documented in a recent study of service members returning from the Iraq War.[40]

18.5.1 Assessment via Mobility

Based on scientific findings indicating that slowed mobility may be a predictor of future cognitive decline in older adults,[41] one technique for assessing the onset of dementia is to observe an individual's mobility. One way to do this is to measure walking speed using passive infrared motion sensors placed along a corridor within an individual's residence.[42] Not all homes have an ideal hallway—one that is both long enough to measure speed of mobility and devoid of closets or other adjoining rooms that may divert a walker's course. Thus, an alternate approach is to measure the time required for an individual to move from one room or space to another. In this approach, motion detectors or RFID systems are used to determine whether an individual is in each room of interest.[43] The time it takes to move between two rooms, then, is measured as the time between when activity is no longer observed in one room and is once again observed in the next.

Because sensors cannot perfectly determine an individual's location within a living environment, probabilistic inference may need to be used to estimate the individual's location. For example, an HMM can be configured such that the location of the individual is the hidden variable and the sensors triggered are the observations. Once an estimate is made regarding an individual's location, the time required to transition from one area to another can be computed. In practice, a variation of the HMM, called a *hidden semi-Markov model* (HSMM), has been employed for this task: it discards the unrealistic assumption made in HMMs that "dwell" time—the time spent in one location—will be geometrically distributed. This geometric distribution assumption would mean that the probability of spending a given length of time in one location would decrease exponentially with the length of time. An HSMM allows an arbitrary distribution to be utilized instead.[44,45]

The problem of mobility assessment becomes more complicated when more than one person—or even a pet—is in the home. This problem can be alleviated by placing contact switches on external doors to detect each instance of someone entering or exiting the living space.[42] Alternatively, individuals can wear RFID tags, for which readers can be placed near the main corridor or in particular rooms of interest to help identify the individual being observed.[46] Or, if one is using the hallway monitoring approach, one can configure an HMM for each individual that models his or her walking speed. When motion is detected and measured in the corridor, each individual's HMM can be compared to determine which individual was most likely to have been in the corridor.[43]

18.5.2 Assessment via Task Performance

Another approach to assessment of cognitive status involves observing an individual performing a task or set of tasks. Computerized games may be one good choice of task for assessing the onset of dementia in older adults: between the years 2000 and 2004, the proportion of adults aged 65 years and over who actively use the Internet increased from 15 to 22 percent, and the proportion is expected to continue to grow. Moreover, more than one-third of those adults who browse the Internet also play online computerized games.[47] In addition, games are generally an enjoyable activity for the individual being assessed. Performance on mentally challenging games presents what is thought to be a natural avenue for measuring cognitive abilities, and because the games are being played on a computer, it is easy to collect a variety of measurements about game play.

One study monitored older adults as they played the FreeCell solitaire game.[48] Rather than simply using an individual's winning percentage, a very limited measurement of cognitive impairment, this study computed the ratio between the number of steps required by the individual to win a game and the number of steps required by an automated solver to win the same game. Using this measure, it was possible to distinguish people with cognitive impairment from those without, at least within a small pilot study.[48] Other studies have developed new games, with associated metrics that aim at evaluating verbal fluency, memory, and the ability to attend to multiple activities.[49] For example, to measure verbal fluency, one can use a word jumble in which individuals are provided seven letters of a scrambled word and are asked to create as many words as possible using only those seven letters. Another game is a computerized matching game that measures working memory and adjusts the difficulty of the game by adjusting the cognitive difficulty of the matches (different representations of the same class of object, for example, digital and analog clock faces) and the number of cards to be matched. The suite of games developed in Ref. 49 not only allows different abilities to be tested but also provides individuals a chance to either choose games that are more interesting to them, or avoid playing games that they dislike.

REFERENCES

1. Cook, Albert M., and Susan Hussey. *Assistive Technologies: Principles and Practice*, 2d ed. Mosby, 2001.
2. Cook, Albert M., and Janice Miller Polgar. *Cook and Hussey's Assistive Technologies: Principles and Practice*, 3d ed. Mosby, 2007.
3. Pew, R., and S. V. Hemel, eds. *Technology for Adaptive Aging.* Washington, DC: National Academies Press, 2004.
4. Pervasive Computing, In *Healthcare* (Hardcover) by Bardram, Jakob E. Mihailidis, A., Wan, D., eds., CRC Press, 2006.
5. LoPresti, E. F., A. Mihailidis, and N. Kirsch. Assistive Technology for Cognitive Rehabilitation: State of the Art. *Neuropsychological Rehabilitation,* **14**(1/2):5–39, 2004.
6. 15: United States Census Bureau: International database. http://www.census.gov/ipc/www/idb/. July 2007.
7. Dementia.com: About dementia. http://www.dementia.com/bgdisplay.jhtml?itemname=dementia_about. March 2008.
8. Kautz, H. *A Formal Theory of Plan Recognition.* PhD Thesis, University of Rochester, 1987.
9. Beaudin, Jennifer S., Stephen S. Intille, and E. Morris Margaret. To Track or Not To Track: User Reactions to Concepts in Longitudinal Health Monitoring. *Journal of Medical Internet Research,* **8**(4), 2006.
10. Fishkin, Kenneth P., Matthai Philipose, and Adam Rea. Hands-on RFID: Wireless Wearables for Detecting Use of Objects. In *Proceedings of the International Semantic Web Conference 2005*, pp. 38–43, 2005.
11. Wright, S. Correlation and Causation. *Journal of Agricultural Research,* **20**:557–585, 1921.
12. Rabiner, Lawrence R. A Tutorial on Hidden Markov Models and Selected Applications in Speech Recognition, *Proceedings of the IEEE,* **77**(2), 257–286, February 1989.
13. Dean, T., and Keiji Kanazawa. A Model for Reasoning About Persistence and Causation. *Computational Intelligence Journal*, **5**(3):142–150, 1989.
14. Lauritzen, Steffen L., and David J. Spiegelhalter. Local Computations with Probabilities on Graphical Structures and their Application to Expert Systems. *Journal of the Royal Statistical Society*, Series B **50**:157–224. Blackwell Publishing, 1988.
15. Fung, R., and K. Chang. Weighing and Integrating Evidence for Stochastic Simulation in Bayesian Networks. In *Uncertainty in Artificial Intelligence,* 5, pp. 209–219, New York, N.Y., 1989. Elsevier Science Publishing Company, Inc.
16. Metropolis, N., and S. Ulam, The Monte Carlo Method. *Journal of the American Statistical Association*, **44**(247):335–341, 1949.
17. Forney, G. D. The Forward-Backward Algorithm. In *Proceedings of the 34th Allerton Conference on Communications, Control and Computing*, pp. 432–446, 1996.
18. Forney Jr., G. D. The Viterbi Algorithm, *Proceedings of IEEE Transactions*, **61**:268–278, March 1973.
19. James, M. *Classification Algorithms*, New York, N.Y. Wiley-Interscience, 1985.
20. Quinlan, J. R. Induction of Decision Trees. In *Journal of Machine Learning*. Springer, 1986.
21. Quinlan, J. R. *C4.5: Programs for Machine Learning*. Morgan Kaufmann Publishers, 1993.
22. Baum, L. E., T. Petrie, G. Soules, and N. Weiss, A Maximization Technique Occurring in the Statistical Analysis of Probabilistic Functions of Markov Chains. *The Annals of Mathematical Statistics,* **41**(1):164–171, 1970.

23. Ambite, Jose Luis, and Craig A. Knoblock. Planning by Rewriting: Efficiently Generating High-Quality Plans. In *Proceedings of the Fourteenth National Conference on Artificial Intelligence*, Providence, RI, 1997.

24. McCarthy, C. E., and M. Pollack. A Plan-Based Personalized Cognitive Orthotic. *AIPS,* 2002.

25. Pollack, M. E., Brown, L., Colbry, D., McCarthy, C. E., Orosz, C., Peintner, B., Ramakrishnan, S., and Tsamardinos, I. Autominder: An Intelligent Cognitive Orthotic System for People with Memory Impairment. *Robotics and Autonomous Systems,* **44**(3–4):273–282, 2003.

26. Sutton, R. S., and A. G. Barto. *Reinforcement Learning: An Introduction.* MIT Press, Cambridge, Mass., 1998.

27. Rudary, M., Singh, S. B., and Pollack, M. E. Adaptive Cognitive Orthotics: Combining Reinforcement Learning and Constraint-Based Temporal Reasoning. In *Proceedings of the Twenty-First International Conference on Machine Learning*, pp. 719–726. New York: Association for Computing Machinery, 2004.

28. Puterman, M. L. Markov Decision Processes: Discrete Stochastic Dynamic Programming, John Wiley & Sons, Inc., New York, N.Y., 1994.

29. Cassandra, A. R., L. P. Kaelbling, and M. L. Littman. Acting Optimally in Partially Observable Stochastic Domains. In *Proceedings of the AAAI*, pp. 1023–1028, 1994.

30. Cassandra, A. R. *Exact and Approximate Algorithms for Partially Observable Markov Decision Processes.* PhD thesis, Brown University, 1998.

31. Hoey, J., A. von Bertoldi, P. Poupart, and A. Mihailidis, Assisting Persons with Dementia During Handwashing Using a Partially Observable Markov Decision Process, In *ICVS '07*, 2007.

32. Pineau, J., M. Montemerlo, M. Pollack, N. Roy, and S. Thrun. *Towards Robotic Assistants in Nursing Homes: Challenges and Results*'. Special issue on Socially Interactive Robots, Robotics and Autonomous Systems, **42**(3–4):271–281, 2003.

33. Wing, Michael G., Eklund, Aaron, and Kellogg, Loren D. Consumer-Grade Global Positioning System (GPS) Accuracy and Reliability. *Journal of Forestry*, 103(4): June 2005, 169–173(5), Society of American Foresters, 2005.

34. Leonard, J. J., and H. F. Durrant-Whyte. Simultaneous Map Building and Localization for an Autonomous Mobile Robot. In *Proceedings for IEEE International Workshop on Intelligent Robots and Systems*, pp. 1442–1447, Osaka, Japan, 1991.

35. Ashbrook, D., Starner, T. Learning Significant Locations and Predicting User Movement with GPS. In *International Symposium on Wearable Computing*, Seattle, Wash., 2002.

36. Patterson, D. J., Liao, L., Fox, D., Kautz, H. Inferring High-Level Behavior from Low-Level Sensors. In Dey, A., A. Schmidt, and J. F. McCarthy, eds., *Proceedings of UBICOMP 2003,* vol. LNCS 2864., Springer-Verlag, pp. 73–89, 2003.

37. Patterson, D. J., Liao, L., Gajos, K., Collier, M., Livic, N., Olson, K., Wang, S., Fox, D., and Kautz, H. Opportunity Knocks: A System to Provide Cognitive Assistance with Transportation Services. In *UbiComp 2004: Ubiquitous Computing*, vol. 3205 of Lecture Notes in Computer Science, pp. 433–450, Berlin, Heidelberg, Springer, 2004.

38. Holsinger, T., Deveau, J., Boustani, M., John W. Williams, J. Does This Patient Have Dementia? *JAMA*, **297**(June 2007):2391–2404, 2007.

39. Wilson, D., Consolvo, S., Fishkin, K., Philipose, M. In-Home Assessment of the Activities of Daily Living of the Elderly. *Extended Abstracts of CHI 2005: Workshops—HCI Challenges in Health Assessment,* April 2005.

40. Zoroya, G. Scientists: Brain Injuries from War Worse Than Thought. *USA Today,* September 2007.

41. Pavel, M., Adami, A., Morris, M., Lundell, J., Hayes, T. L., Jimison, H., Kaye, J. A. Mobility Assessment Using Event-Related Responses. *1st Transdisciplinary Conference on Distributed Diagnosis and Home Healthcare,* pp. 71–74, 2006.

42. Hayes, T. L., M. Pavel, and J. A. Kaye. An Unobtrusive In-home Monitoring System for Detection of Key Motor Changes Preceding Cognitive Decline. *Proceedings of the 26th Annual International Conference of the IEEE EMBS,* San Francisco, Calif., 2004.

43. Pavel, M., Hayes, T., Tsay, I., Erdogmus, D., Paul, A., Larimer, N., Jimison, H., Nutt, J. Continuous Assessment of Gait Velocity in Parkinson's Disease from Unobtrusive Measurements. *Proceedings of the 3rd International IEEE EMBS Conference on Neural Engineering*, pp. 700–703, 2007.

44. Misha, Pavel, Tamara L. Hayes, Andre Adami, Holly Jimison, and Jeffrey Kaye. Unobtrusive Assessment of Mobility. *Proceedings of the 28th IEEE EMBS Annual International Conference,* New York City, N.Y., Aug. 30–Sep. 3, 2006.

45. Levinson, S. Continuously Variable Duration Hidden Markov Models for Automatic Speech Recognition, *Computer, Speech, and Language*, **1**(1):29–45, 1986.

46. Hayes, T. L., M. Pavel, N. Larimer, I. A. Tsay, J. Nutt, and A. G. Adami. Distributed Healthcare: Simultaneous Assessment of Multiple Individuals Pervasive Computing, *IEEE,* **6**(1):36–43, January–March 2007.

47. Pew Internet Project. *Older Americans and the Internet.* Pew Internet and American Life Project, www.pewinternet.org,. March 2004.

48. Jimison, H. B., Pavel, M., McKanna, J., Pavel, J. Unobtrusive Monitoring of Computer Interactions to Detect Cognitive Status in Elders. *IEEE Transactions on Information Technology in Biomedicine,* **8**(3):248–252, 2004.

49. Jimison, Holly B, M. Pavel, K. Wild, P. Bissell, J. McKanna, D. Blaker, and D. Williams. A Neural Informatics Approach to Cognitive Assessment and Monitoring. *Proceedings of the 3rd International IEEE EMBS Conference on Neural Engineering*, pp. 696–699, 2007.

CHAPTER 19
REHABILITATORS

David J. Reinkensmeyer
University of California, Irvine, California

19.1 INTRODUCTION

Millions of people in the United States currently require rehabilitation therapy due to neurologic injury and disease. In the case of stroke alone, there are approximately 600,000 new survivors each year and over 2 million survivors with chronic movement deficits.[1] Recent evidence suggests that intensive therapy improves movement recovery.[2–9] However, such therapy is expensive because it relies on individualized interaction with rehabilitation therapists. The type and quality of therapy also vary greatly between clinics and therapists. Little technology is available to assist patients in practicing therapy on their own. Therapy techniques that require expert feedback or that incorporate manual manipulation of the patient's limbs are often inaccessible once formal therapy is discontinued.

To address these needs, mechatronic and robotic devices are being developed to automate movement therapy after neurologic injury. This chapter discusses the rationale for these rehabilitators, reviews practical design considerations, and discusses their future development.

19.2 RATIONALE FOR REHABILITATORS

19.2.1 Target Populations and Therapies

Stroke survivors are a key target population for rehabilitators. Stroke is a leading cause of severe disability in the United States, with roughly 1 of 100 Americans having experienced a stroke.[1] The incidence of stroke doubles with each decade after age 55. Consequently, as baby boomers age, there will likely be an increase in the number of people experiencing strokes and requiring rehabilitation therapy.

Stroke causes an array of motor impairments.[10] Hemiparesis, or weakness on one side of the body, arises due to destruction of the neural systems and outflow pathways responsible for controlling muscles.[11,12] The degree of hemiparesis varies from complete paralysis to mild weakness, depending on the severity of damage and the location of the lesion. Stroke also impairs interjoint coordination, making it difficult to contract muscle groups independently[13–17] and to steer the arm along smooth, coordinated paths.[18,19] In many patients, muscle tone, or the resistance felt when movement is imposed on a passive limb, is increased due to changes in stretch reflex sensitivity (i.e., spasticity) and a loss of soft tissue suppleness (i.e., contracture).[20–22] When combined, these impairments decrease the ability to use the upper and lower extremities for activities of daily living, such as dressing and walking.

Stroke-induced motor impairments are amenable to rehabilitative treatment. Recent evidence from both animal and human research suggests that improved recovery is possible for both the upper and lower extremities with intensive movement practice. In studies of the upper extremity, repetitive-movement practice improved movement ability of the hand and arm after stroke.[5,23,24] This improved movement ability arose at least in part from cortical reorganization. It has been hypothesized that intensive movement practice facilitates "rewiring" of the brain, with undamaged cortical areas assuming control functions previously allocated to damaged ones.[23,25]

A large number of therapeutic techniques besides simple repetitive-movement practice have been developed, many of them requiring manual intervention or detailed feedback from therapists.[10] While none of these techniques has been identified as superior, a number have been shown to produce better recovery when more therapy is given.[2,3,6,7]

Other neurological conditions relevant to rehabilitators are traumatic brain injury (TBI) and spinal cord injury (SCI). About 500,000 people in the United States receive hospital treatment for TBI yearly, and about 20 percent of TBI survivors have long-term impairment.[26] When damage extends to motor regions of the brain, motor impairments similar to those seen in stroke often arise. SCI affects 10,000 new people per year in the United States, and over 200,000 SCI patients are alive today.[26] Displacement of the spinal column crushes the spinal cord, paralyzing muscles that are innervated by nerves below the lesion level. Locomotion is commonly affected since leg muscles are innervated by lower spinal nerves.

Rehabilitative therapy has been shown effective in improving walking ability after both, brain and spinal cord injuries. Of special promise here is a technique referred to as *step training with body weight support*.[27,28] In this technique, the patient is suspended over a treadmill, bearing only a fraction of his or her full weight, while therapists provide manual assistance to one or both legs and the torso to assist in locomotion. In one clinical trial, significantly more SCI subjects who received such step training achieved independent overground walking when compared with a group that received conventional physical therapy.[29] Those who could walk before receiving locomotor training were able to walk further and at greater speeds after training. Rhythmical flexor and extensor electromyographic (EMG) activity can be elicited during stepping with manual assistance even in human subjects who have a clinically complete thoracic SCI.[30] Thus even high-level, complete spinal cord injury patients can generate locomotor muscle activity with step training, suggesting that a core of circuitry responsible for locomotion pattern generation resides in the spinal cord. This circuitry apparently "listens" to proprioceptive and cutaneous input from the legs and adapts based on its ongoing sensory experience.

19.2.2 Rehabilitator Designs

A number of devices for providing therapy to the arm and legs after brain and spinal cord injury have been developed. This section introduces three illustrative designs for arm rehabilitators and two for locomotion rehabilitators. The next section reviews clinical results with these devices. For descriptions of other upper extremity rehabilitators, the reader is referred to Refs. 31 to 35, and for other lower extremity, locomotor, and postural rehabilitators, the reader is referred to Refs. 36 to 38. Rehabilitators also have been developed for rodents to facilitate research in animal models of neurologic injury.[39,40]

The *MIT-MANUS* device (*manus*, from the Latin for "hand") was the first rehabilitator to undergo intensive clinical testing.[4,41] This device is a planar, two-revolute-joint, backdrivable robotic device that attaches to the patient's hand and forearm through a brace (Fig. 19.1). The device can assist or resist in horizontal movement of the arm across a tabletop. It can also accurately measure planar movement of the hand, providing feedback to the patient via a computer screen.

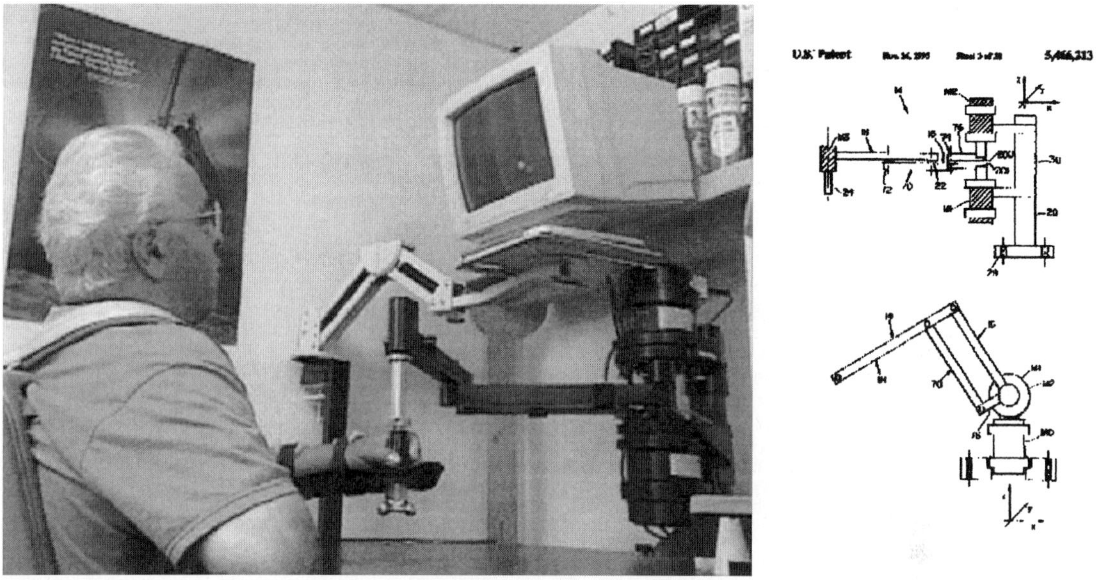

A B

FIGURE 19.1 MIT-MANUS. (*a*) The patient attaches to the robot through a splint. The patient can move the robot or the robot can move the patient in the horizontal plane. The patient receives feedback of the hand trajectory on the computer screeen. (*From H. I. Krebs, B. T. Volpe, M. L. Aisen, and N. Hogan, Increasing productivity and quality of care: Robot-aided neurorehabilitation, Journal of Rehabilitation Research and Development* **37**:*639–652, 2000. Used with permission.*) (*b*) Details of the mechanism design. MIT-MANUS uses a five bar-linkage design with the elbow and shoulder motors mechanically grounded at the base and their axes colinear. (*From N. Hogan, H. I. Krebs, J. Charnarong, and A. Sharon, Interactive robot therapist, 1995, U.S. Patent No. 5466213.*)

The *MIME* (*Mirror Image Movement Enhancer*) arm rehabilitator incorporates a PUMA 560 industrial robot arm to manipulate the patient's arm[42] (Fig. 19.2) This device can move the patient's arm in three-dimensional space. For hemiparetic patients, the motion of the patient's unimpaired arm can be tracked with a mechanical digitizing stylus, and that motion can be used to control the trajectory of the impaired arm.

The *ARM Guide* (*Assisted Rehabilitation and Measurement Guide*) rehabilitator is a singly actuated, 3-degrees-of-freedom device for assisting in reaching movements[43] (Fig. 19.3). The device consists of a linear guide that can be oriented at different yaw and pitch angles. The patient reaches along the linear guide. Like MIT-MANUS and MIME, the device can assist or resist in movement and can measure hand movement.

The *Mechanized Gait Trainer* (*MGT*) is a singly actuated mechanism that drives the feet through a gaitlike trajectory[44] (Fig. 19.4). The device consists of two foot plates connected to a doubled crank and rocker system. An induction motor drives the cranks via a planetary gear system. The rear ends of the foot plates follow an ellipsoid-like movement. Different gears can be incorporated to vary stride length and timing. The planetary gear system also moves the patient harness in a locomotion-like trajectory through two cranks attached to suspension ropes. The torque generated by the motor is sensed and displayed online to provide a biofeedback signal to the patient.

The *Lokomat* is a motorized exoskeleton worn by the patients during treadmill walking[45] (Fig. 19.5). This device has four rotary joints that accommodate hip and knee flexion/extension for each leg. The joints are driven by precision ball screws connected to dc motors. Parameters such as the hip width, thigh length, and shank length can be manually adjusted to fit individual patients. The weight of the exoskeleton is supported by a parallelogram mechanism that moves in the vertical direction and is counterbalanced by a gas spring. The hip and knee motors can be programmed to drive the legs along gaitlike trajectories.

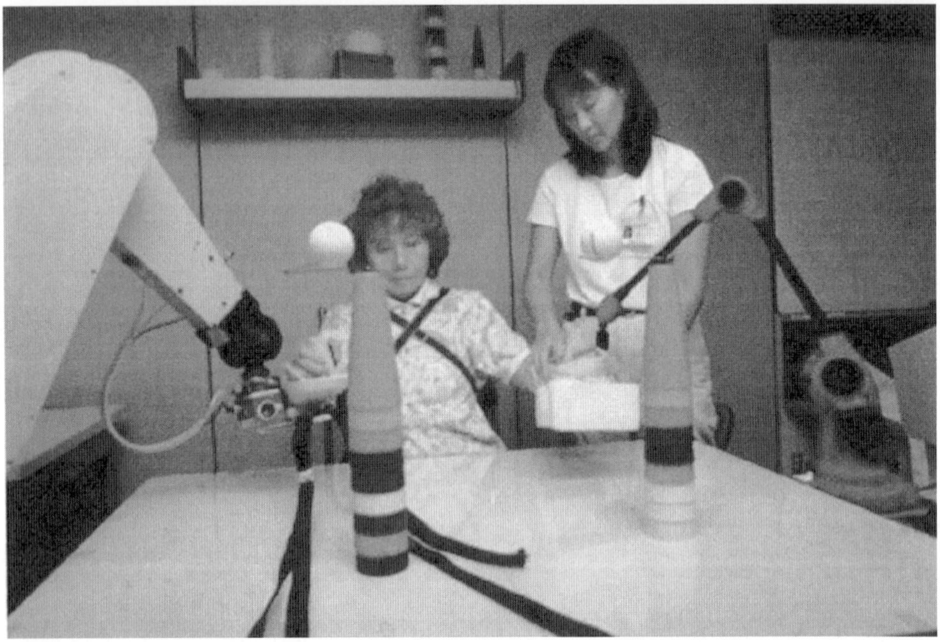

FIGURE 19.2 MIME rehabilitator being used in bimanual mode. When the patient moves her unimpaired arm (left arm), a mechanical digitizing stylus senses the movement. The PUMA 560 robot arm then moves the patient's impaired arm (right arm) along a mirror-symmetrical trajectory. (*From C. G. Burgar, P. S. Lum, P. C. Shor, and H. F. M. Van der Loos, Development of robots for rehabiltitation therapy: The Palo Alto VA/Stanford experience, Journal of Rehabilitation Research and Development* ***37****:663–673, 2000. Used with permission.*)

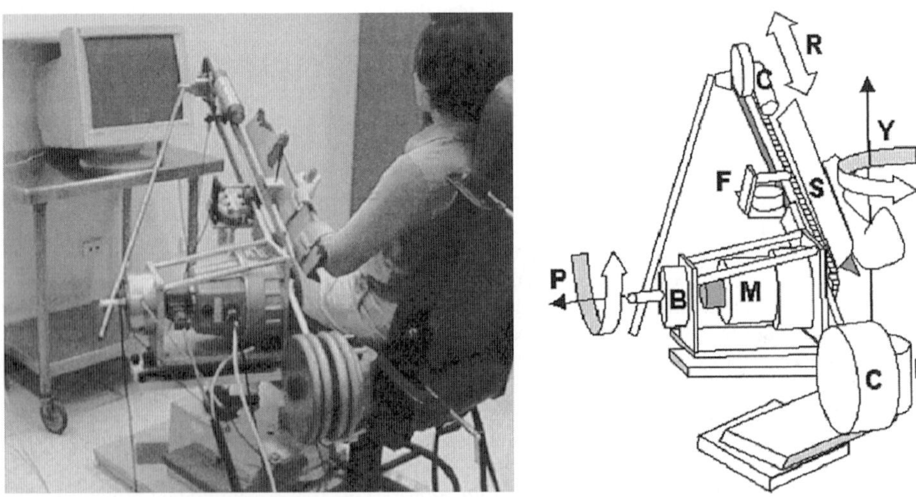

FIGURE 19.3 The ARM Guide. The patient's arm is attached to a hand splint (*S*) that is attached to an orientable linear track. A dc servo motor (*M*) can assist in movement of the subject's arm in the reaching direction (*R*) along the linear track. Optical encoders record position in the reach (*R*), pitch (*P*), and yaw (*Y*) axes. A six-axis force sensor (*F*) records the forces and torques at the interface between the device and the subject. The device is statically counterbalanced with two counterbalance weights (*C*).

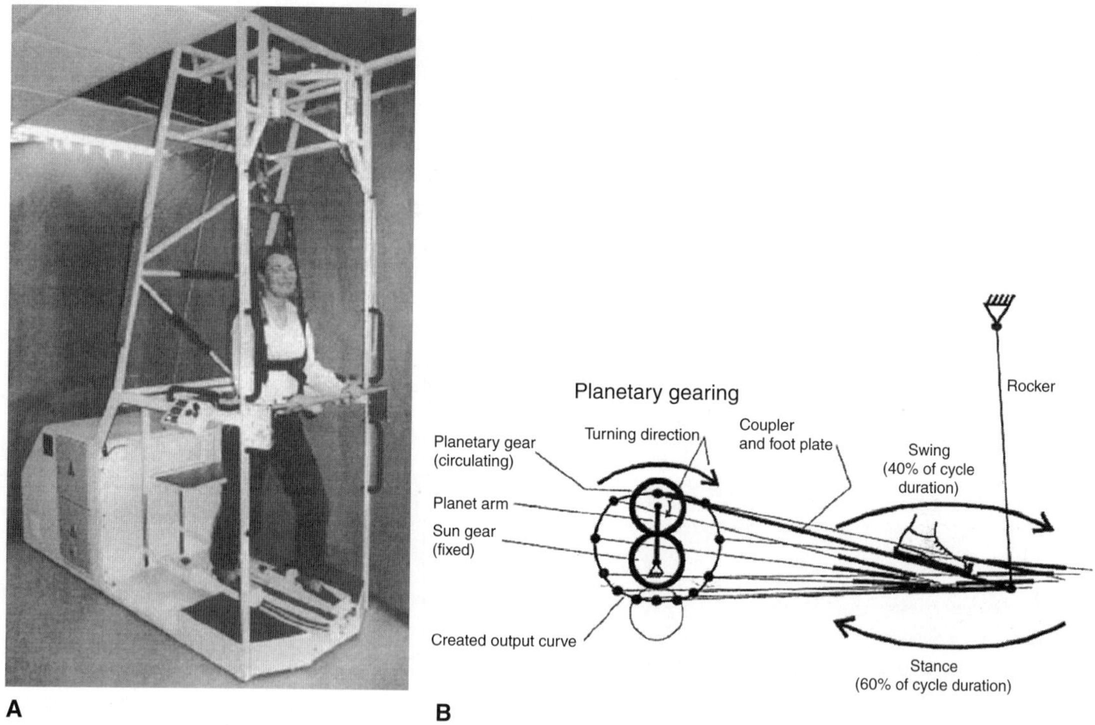

FIGURE 19.4 The Mechanized Gait Trainer (MGT). (*a*) The patient is supported by an overhead harness as the device drives the feet and torso in a steplike pattern. (*b*) A modified crank and rocker system that includes a planetary gear system simulates the stance and swing phases of gait. (*From: S. Hesse and D. Uhlenbrock, A mechanized gait trainer for restoration of gait, Journal of Rehabilitation Research and Development* ***37****:701–708, 2000. Used with permission.*)

19.2.3 Can Therapy Be Automated?

Recent research using these devices suggests that rehabilitator-based therapy can enhance movement recovery following neurologic injury. In the first clinical trial of robot-aided neurorehabilitation, MIT-MANUS was used to assist acute stroke patients in sliding their arms across a tabletop.[4,41,46] The subjects performed a daily series of movement tasks such as moving to targets and tracing figures. The robot helped complete the movement using an impedance-type controller. It was found that patients who received robot-assisted therapy recovered more than those receiving a sham treatment did, according to a coarse clinical rating scale of arm movement ability. A subsequent study indicated that these relative improvements were maintained in the robot group at a 3-year follow-up.[47]

A therapy study of the MIME device has produced similar results with chronic stroke patients.[42] In this study, the robot was position controlled so as to drive the subject's arm through a desired trajectory, as specified either by the trajectory of the contralateral (unimpaired) arm in real time (bimanual mode) or as measured previously (unimanual mode). Chronic stroke subjects exercised 3 h/week, performing reaching exercises and tracing shapes. At the end of 2 months, the robot exercise group exhibited enhanced movement ability, as measured by clinical scales similar to those used in the MIT-MANUS study, as well as in terms of measurements of active range of motion and strength. Encouragingly, the improvements in movement ability were comparable with those of a control group that received a matched amount of traditional tabletop occupational therapy exercise.

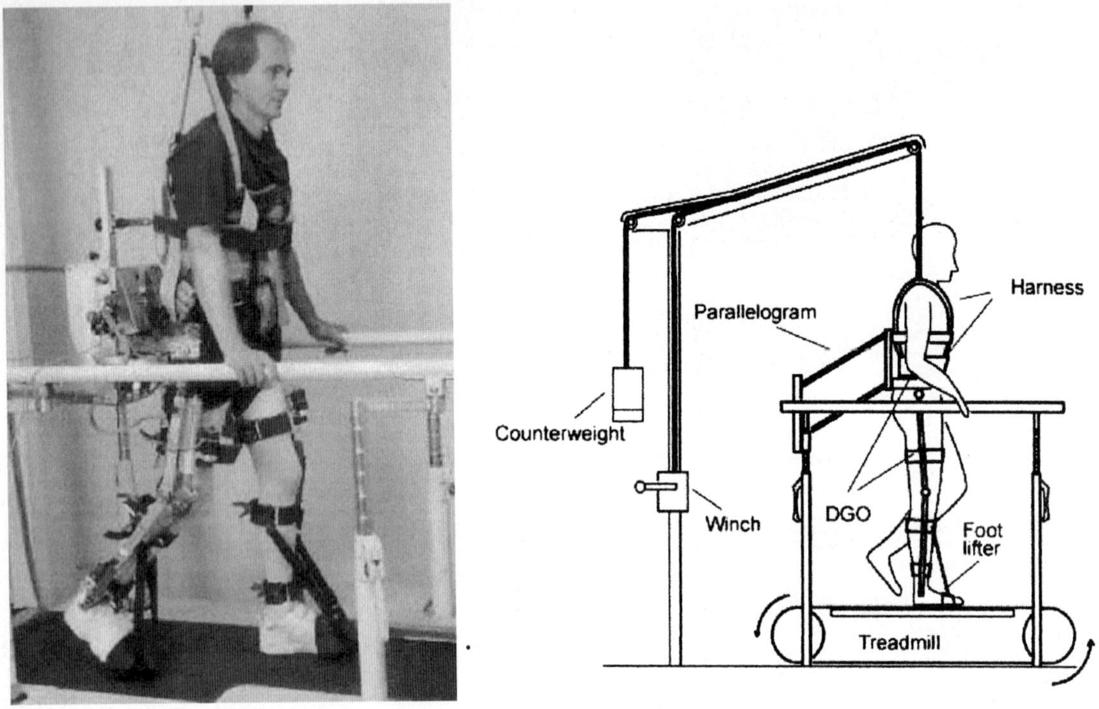

A B

FIGURE 19.5 The Lokomat. (*a*) A motorized orthosis is attached around the upper and lower segment of each leg and drives hip and knee movement in the sagittal plane as the patient walks on a treadmill. (*b*) The patient is suspended from a counterbalanced harness. A parallelogram mechanism with a gas spring supports the weight of the driven gait orthosis (DGO). (*From G. Colombo, M. Joerg, R. Schreier, and V. Dietz, Treadmill training of paraplegic patients with a robotic orthosis, Journal of Rehabilitation Research and Development 37:693–700, 2000. Used with permission.*)

A clinical trial is also being performed with the ARM Guide.[48] In this trial, one group of chronic stroke patients is receiving mechanically assisted reaching exercise with the ARM Guide. A second group is receiving a matched amount of unassisted, repetitive reaching exercise. All subjects are evaluated using a set of clinical and biomechanical measures of arm movement. The seven subjects who have received therapy with the ARM Guide at the time of writing have shown significant improvement in the measures. However, the amount of improvement in seven unassisted exercise subjects has been comparable. Thus these results also support the concept that rehabilitator-assisted manipulation of the arm following stroke is beneficial but highlight the need to clarify which aspects of that therapy are essential. For example, it may be that the repetitive movement attempts by the patient, rather than the mechanical assistance provided by the rehabilitator, are the primary stimuli to recovery.

Clinical trials with locomotion rehabilitators are just beginning. The MGT has been used to train two patients who were 2 months poststroke.[44] The patients received 4 weeks of gait training with the device, consisting of five 20-min sessions per week. The patients improved markedly in their overground walking ability. Therapeutic results have not been reported for the Lokomat, although several spinal cord injured patients have tested the device.[45] The device was able to produce gaitlike patterns in the patients, reducing the labor burden on the therapists who were assisting in the step training.

19.3 DESIGN OF REHABILITATORS

This section reviews practical design considerations for rehabilitators using design features of the MIT-MANUS, MIME, and ARM Guide arm rehabilitators and the MGT and Lokomat locomotion rehabilitators for reference.

19.3.1 Connecting the Patient to the Machine

The design of the interface between the patient's limbs and the rehabilitator is a key consideration if the device is to be used comfortably, safely, and with a minimal level of supervision. In the case of therapy for the arm, many stroke patients do not have hand grasp ability and thus cannot grip a handle. During manual therapy with a human therapist, the therapist can compensate for the patient's loss of hand grasp by using his or her own hands to grip the patient's arm. Although replicating the gentle grip of a therapist is difficult, simple approaches can provide safe attachment for many patients.

One of these simple approaches is to make use of existing hand splinting technology. A wide variety of splints are available from rehabilitation therapy supply houses such as Sammons-Preston. These splints are made of thin sheets of thermoplastics that can be heated in a water bath or with a heat gun and then formed into the desired shape. Common configurations for hand splints are ball-, cone-, and U-shaped. Padded hook-and-loop straps can be glued to the splints and secured around the forearm and back of the hand. The MIT-MANUS and MIME devices make use of cone-type splints, whereas the ARM Guide uses a custom-designed grip in which the forearm lies in a padded aluminum trough and the hand wraps around a cylinder that can be slid into the palm and locked.

Many patients also have decreased range of motion of the arm, constraining the set of postures into which they can self-attach their arms to a machine. Commonly affected degrees of freedom are forearm supination and shoulder external rotation. It is thus important to avoid having the patient maneuver his or her hand through a complex attachment geometry. The MIT-MANUS, the MIME, and the ARM Guide allow attachment of the hand in a pronated posture directly in front of the torso.

With respect to therapy for locomotion, therapists typically grasp the patient's leg with both hands. A common technique is to grasp the lower shank with one hand below the knee and with the other hand above the ankle. The therapist may alter contact force during specific phases of the gait cycle in order to stimulate (or avoid stimulation) of tendons and cutaneous reflexes. A gentle touch is essential to avoid skin damage, since decreased skin health and sensation are common after spinal cord injury.

The existing locomotion rehabilitator designs rely on simple attachment schemes. The MGT attaches to the patient's foot via a foot plate, whereas the Lokomat attaches to the thighs and shanks through padded straps. Skin irritation has been reported with the Lokomat if the exoskeleton is not properly adjusted.[45] For both devices, modified parachute or rock-climbing-type harnesses provide an attachment to the torso that allows partial body weight support through an overhead cable.

Cutaneous reflexes are an important consideration in the design of attachment interfaces for locomotion rehabilitators. Cutaneous input significantly modulates muscle activity during stepping, and cutaneous reflexes are often hyperactive following neurologic injury. By virtue of their mechanical contact with the limb, rehabilitators alter cutaneous input to the limb. In SCI rodents, attaching small robotic devices to the paws disrupts stepping, presumably by stimulating cutaneous reflexes.[40] Further research is needed to determine whether attaching rehabilitators to the lower extremities in humans excites cutaneous reflexes and to identify attachment points for which that excitation is minimized or utilized.

19.3.2 Mechanism Design

The design of a kinematic linkage for a rehabilitator is constrained by many factors, including the desired movements to be performed, cost, and safety. Current rehabilitator designs reflect a compromise between these factors.

The MIT-MANUS device relies on a SCARA-like* or five-bar mechanism to achieve two-dimensional movement of the patient's hand in the horizontal plane (see Fig. 19.1). An advantage of this mechanism is that it allows both motors to be affixed at the robot base (or grounded). Thus, instead of placing the elbow motor at the elbow joint (and requiring the shoulder motor to move the mass of the elbow motor), the five-bar linkage allows the elbow motor to be affixed across from the shoulder motor and the linkage to remain lightweight. A variation on this design allows both motors to remain stationary and on the same side of the linkage, which is useful if the device's base is to be placed next to the patient's shoulder.[49] A mechanism that allows the actuators to remain grounded while providing 2-degree-of-freedom end-effector movement on the surface of a sphere, or even 3-degree-of-freedom spatial motion, also has been conceived.[50]

The MIME device uses an elbow manipulator kinematic configuration with a spherical shoulder, hinge elbow, and spherical wrist, allowing arbitrary positioning and orientation of the end effector with highly geared dc motors (see Fig. 19.2). The device is powerful enough to move a patient's arm throughout the workspace against gravity.

The ARM Guide incorporates a linear bearing that can be pointed in different yaw and pitch directions by rotating it about two revolute axes (see Fig. 19.3). Magnetic particle brakes can lock the bearing in a desired orientation. Movement along the linear bearing can then be assisted or resisted via a motor with a cable chain drive. Thus movement across a large workspace can be achieved using only one actuator. This design can be viewed as analogous to a five-bar mechanism, with the revolute elbow joint replaced with a prismatic joint and the shoulder joint actuated only with a brake.

The MIT-MANUS and MIME devices and the ARM Guide all attach to the patient's hand at their end effectors. Attaching at multiple positions on the upper extremity is also possible and may allow improved control over joint loading.[51] Exoskeleton designs that parallel the degrees of freedom of the upper extremity have been proposed.[52]

With respect to locomotion rehabilitators, the Lokomat device uses an exoskeleton approach to interface with the leg (see Fig. 19.5). This device has rotary degrees of freedom at the hip, knee, and ankle and allows for vertical torso movement via a four-bar linkage. The four-bar linkage also counterbalances the weight of the leg exoskeletons through a gas spring. The MGT device incorporates a single-degree-of-freedom crank and rocker linkage to drive the foot along a fixed steplike trajectory (see Fig. 19.4). Another crank connected to the foot crank also drives the torso periodically in the sagittal plane in a gaitlike pattern.

19.3.3 Backdrivability

An important issue in rehabilitator design is backdrivability, defined as low intrinsic endpoint mechanical impedance[53] or simply as the ability to move a device by pushing on its linkages. Good backdrivability has several advantages for rehabilitator design. It allows the patient to move relatively freely when the actuators are not powered. Thus a backdrivable device can record movements of the patient in order to quantify recovery progress. The MIT-MANUS device has been used in this way to assess the smoothness of reaching movements following stroke, providing insight into possible fundamental subunits of movement.[54] The ARM Guide has also been used in this way to assess the role of abnormal limb tone during reaching movements.[20] Backdrivable machines can also be made to fade to nothing by reducing the amount of assistance they provide as patient recovery improves. Additionally, a backdrivable device can be controlled in such a way that it deviates for the

*Selectively compliant, articulated robot arm.

desired path when the patient exerts uncoordinated forces, providing direct and natural kinematic feedback of movement control errors. In contrast, a nonbackdrivable device must rely on force sensing and visual, tactile, or auditory feedback of the sensed force to provide feedback of movement error. A possible safety advantage is that a properly controlled backdrivable machine can "get out of the way" of the patient if the patient rapidly changes his or her pattern of force development.[54]

Backdrivability with substantial actuator power is difficult to achieve. Modern robotic devices commonly incorporate dc electric motors because of their low cost, ease of operation, and good controllability. However, dc electric motors generate maximum power at high speeds and thus must be geared down to produce high torque at lower speeds. Devices that rely on highly geared motors are in turn difficult to backdrive because of the frictional resistance of the gear train and because the frictional resistance of the motors is amplified by the gear ratio. The PUMA robot used in the MIME device is an example of a geared device that is strong but difficult to backdrive. The Lokomat is another example of a device that is difficult to backdrive because of its use of ball-screw drives.

Backdrivable robots can be made using several approaches. Directly driving the robot linkages using large, nongeared electric motors, such as those offered by PMI, Inc., is a common technique and is used by the MIT-MANUS device. The ARM Guide achieves backdrivability using a cable-chain drive attached to its actuated degree of freedom. A clever design for backdrivability that should be mentioned is the 3-degree-of-freedom PHANToM haptic input device manufactured by Sensable Technologies, Inc. This device uses small, coreless dc brushed motors (such as those available from Micromo, Inc., and Maxon, Inc.) with cable and capstan drives in which the motor rolls around the cable to produce excellent backdrivability.

Some backdrivability can be endowed to a nonbackdrivable device by sensing the contact force between the device and the environment and moving the actuators to control that force. However, this approach is intrinsically limited by delays in sensors, processors, and actuators.[55,56] Adding a spring in series with a stiff, position-controlled device and controlling the length of the spring provides instantaneous compliant behavior, enhancing backdrivability and allowing good force control across a wide range of forces.[57]

A related concept to backdrivability is *Z-width*, defined as the range of mechanical impedances that a robotic device can achieve while maintaining stable contact with a human.[58] Counterintuitively, intentionally incorporating a passive, mechanical viscosity into a device can allow higher stiffnesses to be achieved, thus expanding Z-width.[58] When low impedance is desired, the passive viscosity can be actively canceled with the robot actuators.

Minimizing the inertia of the linkages is also important for maintaining good backdrivability and maximizing the Z-width of a machine. Carbon fiber and thin-wall aluminum tubing are common choices for strong, lightweight linkages.

Achieving backdrivability often increases cost and complexity. In direct-drive configurations, larger, more expensive motors are needed to produce high torques. Cabling systems such as those used by the PHANToM robot may add complexity. Designing a machine that can actively drive a limb against gravity over a large workspace while maintaining good backdrivability is a key design challenge. Present designs either sacrifice backdrivability for power, as in the case of the MIME and Lokomat devices, or use passive structural support to support the weight of the arm and maintain backdrivability, as in the case of the MIT-MANUS device, the ARM Guide, and the MGT device.

19.3.4 Controller Design

Early research with simple bimanual rehabilitators indicated that simple proportional position feedback control laws can be used to assist in impaired movements.[33,59] In this scheme, the controller specified an actuator force proportional to the error between a reference trajectory and the actual movement trajectory. The reference trajectory was chosen as the normative or "desired" trajectory for the limb. Thus the more the limb deviated from the desired trajectory, the more force was provided by the rehabilitator to drive the limb toward the desired trajectory. The firmness of the assistance was determined by the gain of the position controller.

In the first clinical trial of a rehabilitator, the MIT-MANUS device used a version of this scheme in which the stiffness and damping of the controller were designed to be isotropic and soft using impedance-control techniques.[46] The ARM Guide has also used a version of position control to deliver therapy.[60] In this approach, a smooth desired trajectory is initialized when the patient initiates a movement from a starting position outside a position threshold window. The gains of the position controller are set to be low at first, producing soft assistance, and then are gradually increased, producing increasingly firmer assistance.

Therapy has also been provided using stiff position control with the MIME device.[42] For this device, a desired movement trajectory is initialized when the patient generates a threshold contact force against the machine. MIME then servos the arm along the desired movement trajectory with a high-gain position controller. In bimanual therapy mode, the sensed movement of the contralateral arm determines the desired trajectory of the rehabilitator (see Fig. 19.2).

Counterbalancing has also been proposed as an assistive technique for therapy.[60] In this approach, the rehabilitator compensates for the gravitational forces resisting movement of the arm. In the case of counterpoise control, the tone of the arm can also be measured and actively counteracted. The patient then uses any residual force-generating ability to move. Such control is an enhanced version of two common clinical devices—the mobile arm support and the overhead sling—both of which act to relieve gravity. A clever arm orthosis that counterbalances its own weight plus the weight of the user's arm using springs instead of inertia-increasing counterweights is described in Ref. 61. The benefits of these passive counterbalancing approaches are that they allow patients to reach under their own control and that they are relatively inexpensive. However, some patients may exhibit position-dependent weakness that limits their effectiveness.[60]

With respect to locomotion rehabilitation, the MGT and Lokomat devices have also initially used proportional position-control algorithms to drive the legs along step trajectories. It has been proposed that the nonbackdrivable Lokomat device can be made more responsive to patient movement using the above-mentioned technique of sensing contact forces between the legs and device and moving the device to control those forces.[45] Some work has been done to quantify the magnitude and pattern of forces actually applied by therapists during locomotion training.[62] In addition, dynamic motion optimization has been used as a tool for identifying possible torso movement trajectories for facilitating leg movement during locomotion training.[63]

19.3.5 Safety

Safety is of paramount importance when attaching a robotic device to a human. A sensible approach is to use redundant precautions. At the hardware level, actuator size can be limited. A breakaway connector that separates at a prescribed force/torque level can be used to attach the device to the patient's limb. Sensors can be built into contact locations with the patient such that if contact is lost, power is cut to the device, thus reducing the risk of the device swinging freely and colliding with the patient. The rehabilitator's linkage can be designed so that its workspace matches that of the limb as closely as possible, reducing the chance of moving the limb into harmful postures. Mechanical hard stops can also be used to limit motion, and limit switches at those stops can cut power to the actuators when triggered. Software can also set limits on actuator force, position, and velocity, allowing added flexibility in specifying the form of the limiting relationship. A watchdog timer can be used to continually check that the rehabilitator controller is running on time and has not malfunctioned. Handheld or foot-activated cutoff switches can also be incorporated such that the patient can voluntarily cut power to the device.

Care can also be taken in the design of the control algorithm for the device. As mentioned earlier, a backdrivable device may enhance safety since the device can "get out of the way" of the patient if the patient exerts an uncontrolled force, provided the device is controlled with a suitably soft impedance controller. To date, however, the nonbackdrivable MIME device has been operated safely and has not increased joint pain or decreased joint range of motion in over 10 chronic stroke patients.[64] In addition, Food and Drug Administration (FDA)–approved active dynamometers such as the Biodex machine are nonbackdrivable.

19.3.6 Assessment Procedures

A useful feature of rehabilitators is their ability to measure and assess movement ability and recovery. A variety of assessment procedures have been developed for arm rehabilitators. Range, accuracy, and speed of motion are common measures of movement ability. Smoothness of movement, quantifiable using jerk or the number of movement subunits, has been proposed as a measure of recovery.[46] The amount of assistance needed to steer a limb along a trajectory can also be used to quantify patient progress, and off-axis force generation during steered movement can be used to quantify abnormal coordination.[13,17,33] Imposing movement on the arm with the device, either when the arm is relaxed or during voluntary movement, and measuring the resulting resisting force provides a means to quantify abnormal tone.[20] Similar assessment procedures, along with established gait-analysis techniques, can be applied during locomotion rehabilitation.

19.3.7 Networking

As therapy becomes increasingly automated and accessible from home, development of efficient information-transfer software for communication between patients and medical professionals is needed. The feasibility of rehabilitator-based teletherapy for the arm and hand after stroke was recently demonstrated.[65] In this scheme, a library of status tests, therapy games, and progress charts written in the Java programming language were housed on a Web site. This library was used with a low-cost, force-feedback joystick capable of assisting or resisting in movement. The system was used to direct a therapy program, mechanically assist in movement, and track improvements in movement ability.

19.4 THE FUTURE OF REHABILITATORS

Many fundamental questions concerning the nature of rehabilitation and neural recovery remain unanswered. Without answers to these questions, it is impossible to optimize rehabilitator designs. This section briefly summarizes three key unanswered questions and then brashly attempts to predict what future rehabilitators will be like despite these uncertainties. For more discussion along these lines, see Ref. 66.

19.4.1 Three Things a Rehabilitator Designer Would Like to Know

One question that a rehabilitator designer would like answered is, "What types of movements should be practiced?" Specifically, in the case of arm rehabilitation, should individual joint movements be practiced, or should functional multijoint movements be practiced? Are large excursions needed, or will smaller movements suffice? Is three-dimensional motion better than planar motion? Is bimanual therapy better than unimanual therapy? Is some combination of these approaches better than any one approach? For locomotion rehabilitation, the general type of movement to be practiced is clearer—that is, stepping—but what stepping trajectory should be practiced? Should a normative trajectory be practiced? Should variability be incorporated into the practiced trajectory? What torso movements should be practiced? The answers to these questions clearly impact rehabilitator design in terms of size, strength, kinematics, and controller parameters.

A second major unanswered question is, "How should the device mechanically interact with the patient?" Should it assist movement, resist movement, tune itself to the level of the patient, or simply "go along for the ride," measuring the patient's movement. As noted earlier, preliminary clinical results with the ARM Guide suggest that unassisted movement exercise may be as effective as mechanically assisted exercise in promoting movement recovery.[48] Other therapy techniques besides assisting in movement have been developed, many of which could be automated.[10] Rehabilitators with strong actuators, precise sensors, and smart processors offer the possibility of applying novel therapeutic manipulations unachievable by therapists, such as state-dependent force fields that are sculpted to take advantage of implicit learning capability[67] or dynamically optimized torso-shifting strategies for assisting in locomotion.[63] The optimal therapy technique will likely depend on the lesion characteristics, stage of recovery, and impairment profile for both arm and leg rehabilitators, further complicating the problem of designing optimal devices and protocols.

A third major unanswered question is, "What should the rehabilitator quantify?" As mentioned earlier, range, speed, tone, straightness, coordination, and smoothness of movement are all affected after neurologic injury, but it is unclear how each of these relates to recovery progress. Which measure or combination of measures is the most sensitive and reliable assessor of ongoing recovery? Which measures are best at motivating and directing patient effort?

Answering these questions will be difficult because it will require many carefully crafted, controlled clinical trials. However, the answers are essential to improving rehabilitator designs in a rational manner.

19.4.2 What Will Rehabilitators Look Like in the Future?

Despite these uncertainties, it is interesting to try to predict what rehabilitators will look like in the future. A best guess is that future devices will be wearable so that the patient can use them to assist in activities throughout the day. These worn devices will address multiple motor systems, including hand movement, arm movement, posture, and locomotion. If simply assisting in movement is found to be a reasonable therapeutic strategy, future devices will likely seek to infer the motor intent of the patient. Then, if the patient imagines or wills a movement (e.g., the patient simply thinks "reach" or "walk"), the device will complete the movement appropriately, even if the patient is severely impaired. As the patient regains movement ability, the devices will then adapt to the level of the patient. Future rehabilitators will also be embedded with smart sensors and networked so that both the patient and the patient's health providers receive continuous information about the patient's status.

19.4.3 What Technology Is Needed to Improve Rehabilitators?

What design problems must be overcome to move toward this future? First, actuators and energy sources must be developed that are lightweight yet powerful enough to allow wearable devices. Novel actuators and energy sources, such as fuel-cell-powered piezo-hydraulic actuators and monopropellant-powered pneumatic actuators, are being developed for wearable exoskeletons targeted at military applications (see http://www.darpa.mil/DSO/thrust/md/Exoskeletons/briefings.html). An attractive possibility from an energetic perspective is to use the patient's muscles themselves as the actuators via electrical stimulation of nerves. Millimeter-sized muscle stimulators are being developed that can be implanted near the motor points of individual muscles and controlled via wireless communication from outside the body.[68] Such functional neuromuscular stimulation could provide the supplemental force needed to complete movements and has already shown promise as a therapeutic technique after stroke.[69] Another possibility is to directly stimulate neural networks in the central nervous system with implantable microelectrode arrays.[70] It is currently possible to drive simple limb movements in frogs,[71] rats,[72] and cats[73] via spinal microstimulation.

Second, better algorithms are needed to infer the intent of the patient for each movement. Inferring motor intent from downstream measures of the patient's residual muscle activation (such as force, movement, and EMG) will likely only go so far. Tapping into upstream signals in the cerebral cortex using implantable microelectrode arrays or electroencephalogram techniques may allow greater control, especially for severely impaired patients. Brain-computer interfaces for completely paralyzed patients have been developed that allow typing at slow rates using thought alone.[74] Better brain-computer interfaces will be possible with implanted microelectrode arrays.[75] It was recently demonstrated that hand trajectories during reaching can be inferred in real time from neural signals recorded from microelectrode arrays implanted in monkey motor cortex.[76] Rehabilitator control algorithms that receive information directly from the cortex will also need to be adaptive so that direct cortical control is reduced as biological motor pathways are restored. It is interesting to note that current brain-computer interfaces require substantial patient practice to achieve control. An analogy can thus be made with rehabilitators in that both technologies allow a patient to learn to make new movements by altering neural pathways. Melding the technologies may be synergistic.

Third, sensors and software need to be developed to interpret and monitor daily activity of patients. Micromachined inertial sensors[77] and vision chips,[78] which are rapidly improving in quality and cost, will likely play a role in generating the raw signals for assessing movement. Processing algorithms are needed to log functional activity throughout the day by categorizing movements (e.g., drinking, opening a door, combing hair) based on sensor readings. Algorithms are also needed to interpret the quality of each movement (e.g., smoothness, speed, range) to provide a continuous measure of movement recovery.

19.4.4 Rehabilitators and Neuroregeneration Approaches

This chapter has focused on the design of mechatronic/robotic devices for stimulating nervous system recovery. Clearly, however, the development of new cells and connections to replace dead and diseased ones holds great promise for restoring normal movement. Rehabilitators will likely play key roles in the development of cell- and molecule-based neuroregeneration techniques. For example, rehabilitators may act synergistically with neuroregeneration techniques by maintaining the suppleness and mobility of the arms and legs and by preconditioning residual neural movement control circuitry through repetitive sensory-motor training. Thus, as new connections develop, they will find relatively intact motor systems to control. Also, the repetitive sensorimotor stimulation provided by rehabilitators may provide directional guidance to regenerating fibers so that they make appropriate functional connections. Rehabilitators will also provide a means to more precisely quantify the functional effects of neuroregeneration techniques, thus providing a more rational basis for evaluating and optimizing them.

19.5 CONCLUSION

Rehabilitator design is an evolving art and science. As reviewed earlier, progress has been made in designing patient-machine interfaces, mechanical linkages, control algorithms, safety mechanisms, assessment procedures, and networking software. Even with the current uncertainties in optimal therapeutic parameters, existing rehabilitators have been successful in enhancing movement recovery. As scientific advances are made in understanding neurorecovery mechanisms and technological advances are made in sensors, actuators, and computational algorithms, rehabilitators will continue to improve, making rehabilitation therapy increasingly accessible and effective.

REFERENCES

1. G. E. Gresham, P. W. Duncan, and W. B. Stason (1995), *Post-Stroke Rehabilitation,* AHCPR Publication No. 95-0662, U.S. Department of Health and Human Services, Agency for Health Care Policy and Research, Rockville, Md.
2. D. S. Smith, E. Goldenberg, A. Ashburn, G. Kinsella, K. Sheikh, P. J. Brennan, T. W. Meade, D. W. Zutshi, J. D. Perry, and J. S. Reeback (1981), Remedial therapy after stroke: A randomised controlled trial, *British Medical Journal* **282**:517–520.
3. R. S. Stevens, N. R. Ambler, and M. D. Warren (1984), A randomized controlled trial of a stroke rehabilitation ward, *Age and Aging* **13**:65–75.
4. M. L. Aisen, H. I. Krebs, N. Hogan, F. McDowell, and B. Volpe (1997), The effect of robot-assisted therapy and rehabilitative training on motor recovery following stroke, *Archives of Neurology* **54**:443–446.

5. C. Butefisch, H. Hummelsheim, P. Denzler, and K. Mauritz (1995), Repetitive training of isolated movement improves the outcome of motor rehabilitation of the centrally paretic hand, *Journal of the Neurological Sciences* **130**:59–68.

6. A. Sunderland, D. J. Tinson, E. L. Bradley, D. Fletcher, R. Langton Hewer, and D. T. Wade (1992), Enhanced physical therapy improves recovery of arm function after stroke: A randomized controlled trial, *Journal of Neurology, Neurosurgery, and Psychiatry* **55**:530–535.

7. M. Dam, P. Tonin, S. Casson, M. Ermani, G. Pizzolato, V. Iaia, and L. Battistin (1993), The effects of long-term rehabilitation therapy on poststroke hemiplegic patients, *Stroke* **24**:1186–1191.

8. E. Taub, N. Miller, T. Novack, E. Cook, W. Fleming, C. Nepomuceno, J. Connell, and J. Crago (1993), Technique to improve chronic motor deficit after stroke, *Archives of Physical Medicine and Rehabilitation* **74**:347–354.

9. S. Wolf, D. Lecraw, L. Barton, and B. Jann (1989), Forced use of hemiplegic upper extremities to reverse the effect of learned nonuse among chronic stroke and head-injured patients, *Experimental Neurology* **104**:125–132.

10. D. J. Reinkensmeyer, J. P. A. Dewald, and W. Z. Rymer (1996), Robotic devices for physical rehabilitation of stroke patients: Fundamental requirements, target therapeutic techniques, and preliminary designs, *Technology and Disability* **5**:205–215.

11. R. W. Bohannon (1997), Measurement and nature of muscle strength in patients with stroke, *Journal of Neurologic Rehabilitation* **11**:115–125.

12. S. C. Gandevia (1993), Strength changes in hemiparesis: Measurements and mechanisms, in A. F. Thilmann, D. J. Burke, and W. Z. Rhymer, (eds.), *Spasticity: Mechanisms and Management,* 111–122, Springer-Verlag, Berlin.

13. D. J. Reinkensmeyer, J. P. A. Dewald, and W. Z. Rymer (1999), Guidance based quantification of arm impairment following brain injury: A pilot study, *IEEE Transactions on Rehabilitation Engineering* **7**:1–11.

14. J. P. Dewald and R. F. Beer (2001), Abnormal joint torque patterns in the paretic upper limb of subjects with hemiparesis, *Muscle and Nerve* **24**:273–283.

15. R. F. Beer, J. D. Given, and J. P. Dewald (1999), Task-dependent weakness at the elbow in patients with hemiparesis, *Archives of Physical Medicine and Rehabilitation* **80**:766–772.

16. J. P. A. Dewald, P. S. Pope, J. D. Given, T. S. Buchanan, and W. Z. Rymer (1995), Abnormal muscle coactivation patterns during isometric torque generation at the elbow and shoulder in hemiparetic subjects, *Brain* **118**:495–510.

17. P.S. Lum, C. G. Burgar, D. Kenney, and H. F. M. Van der Loos (1999), Quantification of force abnormalities during passive and active-assisted upper-limb reaching movements in post-stroke hemiparesis, *IEEE Transactions on Biomedical Engineering* **46**:652–662.

18. M. F. Levin (1996), Interjoint coordination during pointing movements is disrupted in spastic hemiparesis, *Brain* **119**:281–293.

19. R. F. Beer, J. P. Dewald, and W. Z. Rymer (2000), Deficits in the coordination of multijoint arm movements in patients with hemiparesis: Evidence for disturbed control of limb dynamics, *Experimental Brain Research* **131**:305–319.

20. D. J. Reinkensmeyer, B. D. Schmit, and W. Z. Rymer (1999), Assessment of active and passive restraint during guided reaching after chronic brain injury, *Annals of Biomedical Engineering* **27**:805–814.

21. K. L. Harburn and P. J. Potter (1993), Spasticity and contractures, in *Physical Medicine and Rehabilitation: State of the Art Reviews*, **7**:113–132.

22. N. J. O'Dwyer, L. Ada, and P. D. Neilson (1996), Spasticity and muscle contracture following stroke, *Brain* **119**:1737–1749.

23. R. J. Nudo, B. M. Wise, F. SiFuentes, and G. W. Milliken (1996), Neural substrates for the effects of rehabilitative training on motor recovery after ischemic infarct, *Science* **272**:1791–1794.

24. E. Taub, G. Uswatte, and R. Pidikiti (1999), Constraint-induced movement therapy: A new family of techniques with broad application to physical rehabilitation—A clinical review, *Journal of Rehabilitation Research and Development* **36**:237–251.

25. J. Liepert, H. Bauder, H. R. Wolfgang, W. H. Miltner, E. Taub, and C. Weiller (2000), Treatment-induced cortical reorganization after stroke in humans, *Stroke* **31**:1210–1216.

26. B. H. Dobkin (1996), *Neurologic Rehabilitation*, F. A. Davis, Philadelphia, Pa.

27. I. Wickelgren (1998), Teaching the spinal cord to walk, *Science* **279**:319–321.
28. H. Barbeau, K. Norman, J. Fung, M. Visintin, and M. Ladouceur (2000), Does neurorehabilitation play a role in the recovery of walking in neurological populations? *Annals of the New York Academy of Sciences* **860**:377–392.
29. A. Wernig, A. Nanassy, and S. Muller (1999), Laufband (treadmill) therapy in incomplete paraplegia and tetraplegia, *Journal of Neurotrauma* **16**:719–726.
30. S. J. Harkema, S. L. Hurley, U. K. Patel, P. S. Requejo, B. H. Dobkin, and V. R. Edgerton (1997), Human lumbosacral spinal cord interprets loading during stepping, *Journal of Neurophysiology* **77**:797–811.
31. F. Amirabdollahian, R. Loureiro, B. Driessen, and W. Harwin (2001), Error correction movement for machine assisted stroke rehabilitation, in M. Mokhtari (ed.), *Integration of Assistive Technology in the Information Age*, vol. **9**, 60–65, IOS Press, Amsterdam.
32. G. Arz and A. Toth (2001), REHAROB: A project and a system for motion diagnosis and robotized physiotherapy delivery, in M. Mokhtari (ed.), *Integration of Assistive Technology in the Information Age*, vol. **9**, 93–100, IOS Press, Amsterdam.
33. P. S. Lum, S. L. Lehman, and D. J. Reinkensmeyer (1995), The bimanual lifting rehabilitator: A device for rehabilitating bimanual control in stroke patients, *IEEE Transactions on Rehabilitation Engineering* **3**:166–174.
34. J. A. Cozens (1999), Robotic assistance of an active upper limb exercise in neurologically impaired patients, *IEEE Transactions on Rehabilitation Engineering* **7**:254–256.
35. R. Rao, S. K. Agrawal, and J. P. Scholz (2000), A robot test-bed for assistance and assessment in physical therapy, *Advanced Robotics* **14**:565–578.
36. S. Okada, T. Sakaki, R. Hirata, Y. Okajima, S. Uchida, and Y. Tomita (2000), TEM: A therapeutic exercise machine for the lower extremities of spastic patients, *Advanced Robotics* **14**:597–606.
37. N. A. Siddiqi, T. Ide, M. Y. Chen, and N. Akamatsu (1994), A computer-aided walking rehabilitation robot, *American Journal of Physical Medicine and Rehabilitation* **73**:212–216.
38. Z. Matjacic, I. Johannesen, and T. Sinkjaer (2000), A multi-purpose rehabilitation frame: A novel apparatus for balance training during standing of neurologically impaired individuals, *Journal of Rehabilitation Research and Development* **37**:681–691.
39. D. J. Reinkensmeyer, W. K. Timoszyk, R. D. de Leon, R. Joynes, E. Kwak, K. Minakata, and V. R. Edgerton (2000), A robotic stepper for retraining locomotion in spinal-injured rodents, in *2000 International Conference on Robotics and Automation*, 2889–2894. San Francisco, Calif.
40. W. K. Timoszyk, R. D. de Leon, N. London, R. Joynes, K. Minakata, V. R. Edgerton, and D. J. Reinkensmeyer (2002), Robot-assisted locomotion training after spinal cord injury: Comparison of rodent stepping in virtual and physical treadmill environments, *Robotica* (to appear).
41. B. Volpe, H. Krebs, N. Hogan, L. Edelstein OTR, C. Diels, and M. Aisen (2000), A novel approach to stroke rehabilitation: Robot-aided sensorimotor stimulation, *Neurology* **54**:1938–1944.
42. C. G. Burgar, P. S. Lum, P. C. Shor, and H. F. M. Van der Loos (2000), Development of robots for rehabilitation therapy: The Palo Alto VA/Stanford experience, *Journal of Rehabilitation Research and Development* **37**:663–673.
43. D. J. Reinkensmeyer, L. E. Kahn, M. Averbuch, A. N. McKenna-Cole, B. D. Schmit, and W. Z. Rymer (2000), Understanding and treating arm movement impairment after chronic brain injury: Progress with the ARM Guide, *Journal of Rehabilitation Research and Development* **37**:653–662.
44. S. Hesse and D. Uhlenbrock (2000), A mechanized gait trainer for restoration of gait, *Journal of Rehabilitation Research and Development* **37**:701–708.
45. G. Colombo, M. Joerg, R. Schreier, and V. Dietz (2000), Treadmill training of paraplegic patients with a robotic orthosis, *Journal of Rehabilitation Research and Development* **37**:693–700.
46. H. I. Krebs, N. Hogan, M. L. Aisen, and B. T. Volpe (1998), Robot-aided neurorehabilitation, *IEEE Transactions on Rehabilitation Engineering* **6**:75–87.
47. B. Volpe, H. Krebs, N. Hogan, L. Edelstein, C. Diels, and M. Aisen (1999), Robot training enhanced motor outcome in patients with stroke maintained over 3 years, *Neurology* **53**:1874–1876.
48. L. E. Kahn, M. Averbuch, W. Z. Rymer, and D. J. Reinkensmeyer, Comparison of robot-assisted reaching to free reaching in promoting recovery from chronic stroke, in M. Mokhtari (ed.), *Integration of Assistive Technology in the Information Age*, 39–44, IOS Press, Amsterdam.

49. H. Kazerooni and H. Ming-Guo (1994), The dynamics and control of a haptic interface device, *IEEE Transactions on Robotics and Automation* **10**:453–464.

50. B. D. Adelstein (1998), *Three degree of freedom parallel mechanical linkage*, U.S. Patent No. 5816105, 1998.

51. D. Khalili and M. Zomlefer (1988), An intelligent robotic system for rehabilitation of joints and estimation of body segment parameters, *IEEE Transactions on Biomedical Engineering* **35**:138–146.

52. S. H. Scott (1999), *Kinesiological instrument for limb movements*, U.S. Patent No. 6155993, 1999.

53. H. I. Krebs, B. T. Volpe, M. L. Aisen, and N. Hogan (2000), Increasing productivity and quality of care: Robot-aided neuro-rehabilitation, *Journal of Rehabilitation Research and Development* **37**:639–652.

54. H. I. Krebs, M. L. Aisen, B. T. Volpe, and N. Hogan (1999), Quantization of continuous arm movements in humans with brain injury, *Proceedings of the National Academy of Science USA* **96**:4645–4649.

55. D. A. Lawrence (1989), Actuator limitations on achievable manipulator impedance, in *Proceedings 1989 IEEE International Conference on Robotics and Automation*, 560–565.

56. D. A. Lawrence (1988), Impedance control stability properties in common implementations, in *Proceedings of the 1988 IEEE International Conference on Robotics and Automation*, vol. **2**, 1185–1190.

57. D. W. Robinson, J. E. Pratt, D. J. Paluska, and G. A. Pratt (1999), Series elastic actuator development for a biomimetic walking robot, in *Proceedings of the 1999 IEEE/ASME International Conference on Advanced Intelligent Mechatronics*, 561–568.

58. J. E. Colgate and J. M. Brown (1999), Factors affecting the Z-Width of a haptic display, *Proceedings 1994 IEEE International Conference on Robotics and Automation*, vol. **4**, 3205–3210.

59. P. S. Lum, D. J. Reinkensmeyer, and S. L. Lehman (1993), Robotic assist devices for bimanual physical therapy: Preliminary experiments, *IEEE Transactions on Rehabilitation Engineering* **1**:185–191.

60. D. J. Reinkensmeyer, C. D. Takahashi, W. K. Timoszyk, A. N. Reinkensmeyer, and L. E. Kahn (2000), Design of robot assistance for arm movement therapy following stroke, *Advanced Robotics* **14**:625–638.

61. T. Rahman, W. Sample, R. Seliktar, M. Alexander, and M. Scavina (2000), A body-powered functional upper limb orthosis, *Journal of Rehabilitation Research and Development* **37**:675–680.

62. A. Bejczy (1999), Towards development of robotic aid for rehabilitation of locomotion-impaired subjects, presented at *the First Workshop on Robot Motion and Control* (RoMoCo'99), 9–16, Kiekrz, Poland.

63. C. E. Wang, J. E. Bobrow, and D. J. Reinkensmeyer (2001), Swinging from the hip: Use of dynamic motion optimization in the design of robotic gait rehabilitation, *Proceedings of the 2001 IEEE International Conference on Robotics and Automation*, 1433–1438, Seoul, Korea.

64. P. C. Shor, P. S. Lum, C. G. Burgar, H. F. M. Van der Loos, M. Majmundar, and R. Yap (2001), The effect of robot-aided therapy on upper extremity joint passive range of motion and pain, in M. Mokhtari (ed.), *Integration of Assistive Technology in the Information Age: Proceedings of the 7th International Conference on Rehabilitation Robotics, Institut National des Télécommunication*, 79–83, IOS Press, Amsterdam.

65. D. Reinkensmeyer, C. Pang, J. Nessler, and C. Painter (2001), Java therapy: Web-based robotic rehabilitation, in M. Mokhtari (ed.), *Integration of Assistive Technology in the Information Age*, vol. **9**, 66–71, IOS Press, Amsterdam.

66. D. J. Reinkensmeyer, N. Hogan, H. I. Krebs, S. L. Lehman, and P. S. Lum (2000), Rehabilitators, robots, and guides: New tools for neurological rehabilitation, J. Winters and P. Crago (eds.), in *Biomechanics and Neural Control of Posture and Movement*, 516–533, Springer-Verlag, Berlin.

67. J. L. Patton and F. A. Mussa-Ivaldi (2001), Robot teaching by exploiting the nervous system's adaptive mechanisms, in M. Mokhtari (ed.), *Integration of Assistive Technology in the Information Age: Proceedings of the 7th International Conference on Rehabilitation Robotics, Institut National des Télécommunication*, 3–7, IOS Press, Amsterdam.

68. G. E. Loeb, R. A. Peck, W. H. Moore, and K. Hood (2001), BION system for distributed neural prosthetic interfaces, *Medical Engineering and Physics* **23**:9–18.

69. M. Glanz, S. Klawansky, W. Stason, C. Berkey, and T. C. Chalmers (1996), Functional electrostimulation in poststroke rehabilitation: A meta-analysis of the randomized controlled trials, *Archives of Physical Medicine and Rehabilitation* **77**:549–553.

70. H. Barbeau, D. A. McCrea, M. J. O'Donovan, S. Rossignol, W. M. Grill, and M. A. Lemay (1999), Tapping into spinal circuits to restore motor function, *Brain Research Reviews* **30**:27–51.

71. E. Bizzi, S. F. Giszter, E. Loeb, F. A. Mussa-Ivaldi, and P. Saltiel (1995), Modular organization of motor behavior in the frog's spinal cord, *Trends in Neurosciences* **18**:442–446.

72. M. C. Tresch and E. Bizzi (1999), Responses to spinal microstimulation in the chronically spinalized rat and their relationship to spinal systems activated by low threshold cutaneous stimulation, *Experimental Brain Research* **129**:401–416.

73. V. K. Mushahwar, D. F. Collins, and A. Prochazka (2000), Spinal cord microstimulation generates functional limb movements in chronically implanted cats, *Experimental Neurology* **163**(2):422–429.

74. J. R. Wolpaw, N. Birbaumer, W. J. Heetderks, D. J. McFarland, P. H. Peckham, G. Schalk, E. Donchin, L. A. Quatrano, C. J. Robinson, and T. M. Vaughan (2000), Brain-computer interface technology: A review of the first international meeting, *IEEE Transactions on Rehabilitation Engineering* **8**:164–173.

75. M. A. Nicolelis (2001), Actions from thoughts, *Nature* **409**:403–407.

76. J. Wessberg, C. R. Stambaugh, J. D. Kralik, P. D. Beck, M. Laubach, J. K. Chapin, J. Kim, S. J. Biggs, M. A. Srinivasan, and M. A. Nicolelis (2000), Real-time prediction of hand trajectory by ensembles of cortical neurons in primates, *Nature* **408**:361–365.

77. N. Yzadi, F. Ayazi, and K. Najafi (1998), Micromachined inertial sensors, *Proceedings of the IEEE* **86**:1640–1659.

78. GVPP, Generic Visual Perception Processor Web Site.

CHAPTER 20
THE DESIGN OF ARTIFICIAL ARMS AND HANDS FOR PROSTHETIC APPLICATIONS

Richard F. Weir
Rehabilitation Institute of Chicago, Chicago, Illinois

Jonathon W. Sensinger
Mahidol University, Nakhon Pathom, Thailand

20.1 INTRODUCTION

The design of fully functioning artificial arms and hands replacement with physiological speeds-of-response and strength (or better) and that can be controlled almost without thought is the goal of upper-extremity prosthetics research. Unfortunately, current prosthetic components and interface techniques are still a long way from realizing this goal. The current state-of-the-art prosthesis can be considered to be a tool rather than a limb replacement.

The prosthesis as a tool makes no pretense of trying to replace the lost limb physiologically but is there as an aid to help provide some of the functions that were lost. The prosthesis as a tool is an interchangeable device that is worn and used as needed, and then ignored. Much effort in the field of upper-extremity prosthesis research is directed toward the creation of prostheses as true limb replacements; however, in current practice we are mostly limited to prostheses as tools.

The major causes of the limitation of prostheses as tools and not limb replacements are practical ones due to the severe weight, power, and size constraints of hand/arm systems as well as the difficulty in finding a sufficient number of appropriate control sources to control the requisite number of degrees of freedom. Of these, it is the lack of independent control sources that imposes the most severe impediment to the development of today's prosthetic hand/arm systems. As a result, upper-limb prosthetics research is somewhat dominated by considerations of control. Still, the importance of better actuators and better multifunctional mechanisms must not be ignored. Control is useless if effective hand and arm mechanisms are not available.

The problems associated with the design of artificial hand and arm replacements are far more challenging than those associated with the design of robotic arms or terminal devices. In fact, robotics and prosthetics design has much less in common than one might expect. Robotics concepts have had little impact on commercial prosthetics because of the severe physical constraints required for a prosthetic device to be successful. Although some size, weight, and power constraints must be placed on robots and manipulators, robotic actuators can often be as large and as heavy as required to achieve a specific result. Power is usually not an issue since it can be obtained from the power mains. Prosthetic arm and hand design can be viewed as a subset of the greater field of robot and manipulator arm and end-effector design.

Robot arms look impressive. However, announcements by robot arm designers who, when searching for an application for their new mechanical arms, claim their new robot will be a boon to the field of prosthetics, should be treated with skepticism. The issue has never been about an inability to build mechanical arms and hands. The MIT/Utah dexterous hand (Jacobsen et al., 1984) is an example of a mechanical hand that mimics the function of a hand. This hand was designed for use in research studying robot dexterity. This device could never be used in prosthetics because the actuators and computer system required to control this hand occupy the space of two small filing cabinets, and power is supplied externally from electrical mains. The real issue in upper-limb prosthetics, of which most robot arm designers seem to be unaware, is "How does one interface this arm to the person?" and "How is the arm to be controlled?"

Eugene F. Murphy, Ph.D. (1955), a former Chief of the Research and Development Division, Prosthetic and Sensory Aids Service, Veterans Administration (Hays, 2001), probably articulates best the awe and frustration associated with the task of trying to replicate the function of the natural hand by mechanical means, when he wrote in "Engineering—Hope of the Handless":

> The human hand, with its elaborate control system in the brain, is doubtless the most widely versatile machine that has ever existed anywhere. Its notorious deficiency lies in its persistent inability to create a similar machine as versatile as itself. This circumstance accounts for the fact that, while there has been from earliest times a great need for hand replacements, all attempts to produce successful hand substitutes have thus far ended in only a rather crude imitation of a very few of the many attributes of the living counterpart. For want of complete knowledge of the natural hand-brain complex, and of the ingenuity requisite even to the most modest simulation of the normal hand, artificial hands have always resembled the natural model in a superficial way only. Voltaire is said to have remarked that Newton, with all his science, did not know how his own hand functioned.

The design of artificial arms and hands is a multidisciplinary endeavor. A designer needs an understanding of the mechanics of mechanisms such as gears, levers, points of mechanical advantage, and electromechanical design such as switches, dc motors, and electronics. In addition to these skills, the prosthesis designer must also have knowledge of musculoskeletal anatomy, and muscular- as well as neurophysiology.

It is the goal of this chapter to serve as a resource for designers of artificial limbs who come to the problem with different areas of expertise. As such, I am compelled to refer the reader to the *Atlas of Amputations and Limb Deficiencies* (Smith et al., 2004). This text is a comprehensive guide to the surgical, prosthetic, and rehabilitation techniques employed in current clinical practice. From a historical perspective *Human Limbs and Their Substitutes* (Klopsteg and Wilson, 1954) is invaluable and contains much biomechanical data on amputees that is still valid. If one is unaware of the history, one is doomed to repeat it. Consequently, both these texts are referenced throughout this chapter. Also, following the philosophy of "Why reinvent the wheel?" wherever possible examples are provided of commercially available devices that use the mechanisms, algorithms, or control approaches mentioned in the text.

It is hoped that the reader will find the information in this chapter to be practical and useful and an aid in eliminating much of the start-up time usually associated with familiarizing oneself with a new topic. Ultimately it is hoped that the information imparted will aid and facilitate in the design of better artificial arm and hand replacements for people with upper-limb amputations and deficiencies.

20.2 THE NATURE OF THE PROBLEM

There are over 30 muscles acting on the forearm and hand. The human hand has 27 major bones, and at least 18 joint articulations with 27 or more degrees of freedom (DOF). The arm contributes another 7 degrees of freedom. The primary role of the arm is to position the hand in space. The primary role of the hand is to enable a person to interact with the environment. Control of a person's arm is directed at controlling the position of the arm's hand. Even though people control their arms with great facility, this is a highly complex and demanding task.

A backhoe is essentially a mechanical arm that is under the control of an operator. To control this mechanical arm the operator uses both arms, both feet, both eyes, and all of his or her concentration (Fig. 20.1). The driver uses both arms to pull levers, both feet to press pedals to operate the arm, and both eyes to monitor the task being performed by the digger. All this to control a single mechanical arm. Now consider a person with bilateral (both arms) high-level upper-extremity (e.g., above the elbow) amputations and one begins to have some appreciation of the task such a limbless person faces in controlling a prosthetic arm or arms.

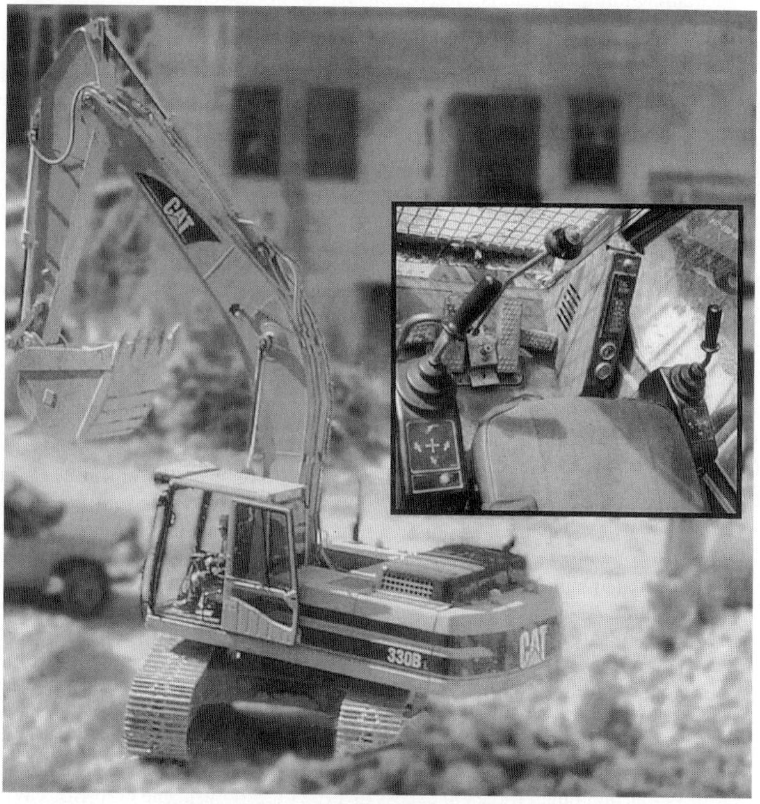

FIGURE 20.1 A digger, or backhoe, is essentially a large mechanical arm. To control this arm, an operator needs to use both hands (to operate the joysticks, see inset), both feet (to operate multiple pedals), both eyes, and almost all of their concentration (to watch what they are doing). These are the requirements for a "whole" individual to control just one artificial arm. Consider now the control problems experienced by a person who has lost both arms at the shoulder. These individuals do not have hands to help in the control of their artificial arms, their feet are needed for walking, and the mental burden placed on the person to control their prosthetic arms cannot be so great that controlling their prostheses takes more effort than it is worth. (*Many thanks to Mr. John Marbes of American Demolition for taking me on to the job site and allowing me to take these pictures.*)

As for performance, the anatomical hand is capable of speeds in excess of 40 rad/s (2290 degrees/s) and grasps involving all fingers of the hand can exert up to about 400 N (90 ft · lb) of force. Average physiological speeds for everyday pick-and-place tasks have been found to be in the range of 3 to 4 rad/s (172 to 200 degrees/s), while most activities of daily living (ADLs) require prehension forces in the range 0 to 67 N (0 to 15 ft · lb) [these forces are dependent on the coefficient of friction between the gripping surface and the object held (Heckathorne, 1992)].

For the wrist and forearm, normal ranges of motion (ROM) (Fig. 20.2, top) are 85 to 90 degrees of pronation, 85 to 90 degrees of supination; 15 degrees of radial deviation, 30 to 45 degrees of ulnar deviation; and 80 to 90 degrees of wrist flexion and 70 to 90 degrees of wrist extension (Magee, 1987). It has been found that for ADLs, 100 degrees of forearm rotation, 80 degrees of wrist flexion-extension, and 60 degrees of radial-ulnar deviation is sufficient (Heckathorne, 1992). The forearm can achieve maximum rotational velocities in excess of 14 rad/s (800 degrees/s) for pronations (inward rotations) and 20 rad/s (1150 degrees/s) for supinations (outward rotations).

For the elbow, normal range of motion (Fig. 20.2, bottom left) is 140 to 150 degrees of flexion and 10 to 15 degrees of hyperextension. Peak anatomic elbow speeds of 261 degrees/s (4.5 rad/s) have been found (Doubler, 1982) for 90-degree movements, and the average male can generate an elbow torque of 138 N · m (102 ft · ft · lb) in flexion with the elbow at 90 degrees. In extension the average male can generate 75 percent of the maximum flexion torque.

For the upper arm, normal ranges of motion (Fig. 20.2, center) are 90 degrees of medial (inward, toward the midline) humeral rotation and 40 degrees of lateral (outward, away from the midline) humeral rotation; 180 degrees of flexion (forward, rotation of the arm about the shoulder) and 45 degrees of extension (backward rotation of the upper arm about the shoulder); and 180 degrees of elevation (abduction, outward rotation about the shoulder) and 20 degrees of depression (adduction, inward rotation of the upper arm about the shoulder).

For the shoulder, the normal ranges of motion (Fig. 20.2, bottom center and right) are 40 degrees of elevation and 10 degrees of depression, 15 degrees of extension (scapular adduction) and 20 degrees of flexion (scapular abduction). The primary power source for body-powered prostheses uses a combination of glenohumeral flexion (forward rotation of upper arm about the shoulder) and biscapular abduction (shrugging of the shoulders). This motion can result in excursions of up to 10 cm (4 in) with a force of 178 to 266 N (40 to 60 ft · lb). Knowledge of the normal ranges of motions for the arm and hand is important, particularly when designing body-powered systems. For more in-depth information, Sarrafian (1992) provides extensive anatomical range-of-motion data relating individual muscle contributions to different arm motions.

Another property of the physiologic arm is that it has "give," that is, it is compliant or spring-like. This compliance is not a fixed quantity but can be varied, depending on the task requirements: a stiff arm for bracing oneself against an expected blow or a relaxed arm for playing the piano. This inherent compliance of the human arm also provides protection for the joints and musculoskeletal system. Because the musculoskeletal system is compliant, it can withstand external shock loads far better than can a stiff-jointed equivalent.

Interaction with the real world is something current robotics and prosthetics actuators (dc electric motors with gear trains) do not do well. When a stiff robot arm comes into contact with a hard surface, a phenomenon, known as *contact instability*, can arise unless the robot satisfies certain passivity requirements (Colgate and Hogan, 1989).

The performance of current artificial mechanisms come nowhere close to meeting the maximum speed and force of which the anatomic arm and hand are capable, although hand mechanisms are available (NU-VA Synergetic Prehensor, Hosmer-Dorrance, CA) that can attain speeds in excess of 3 rad/s and pinch forces in excess of 110 N (25 ft · lb). The Otto Bock Wrist Rotator is the only commercially available electric wrist rotator. It is slow (1 rad/s) and produces minimal torque. Motion Control is set to release a much faster and stronger wrist rotator which is integrated into the hand, and Otto Bock is working on a faster and stronger wrist rotator as well. All other prosthetic wrist components are body-powered and, when used, are used for positioning purposes.

Current electric-powered prosthetic elbows can attain up to 18 N · m (13 ft · ft · lb) of "live-lift" (lift by the elbows' own motor mechanism) and speeds of up to 4 rad/s (Dynamic Arm, Otto Bock). Body-powered elbows are limited by the speed and strength of the user and the efficiency of the linkage used to connect the user and the component. Humeral rotation for elbow components, with

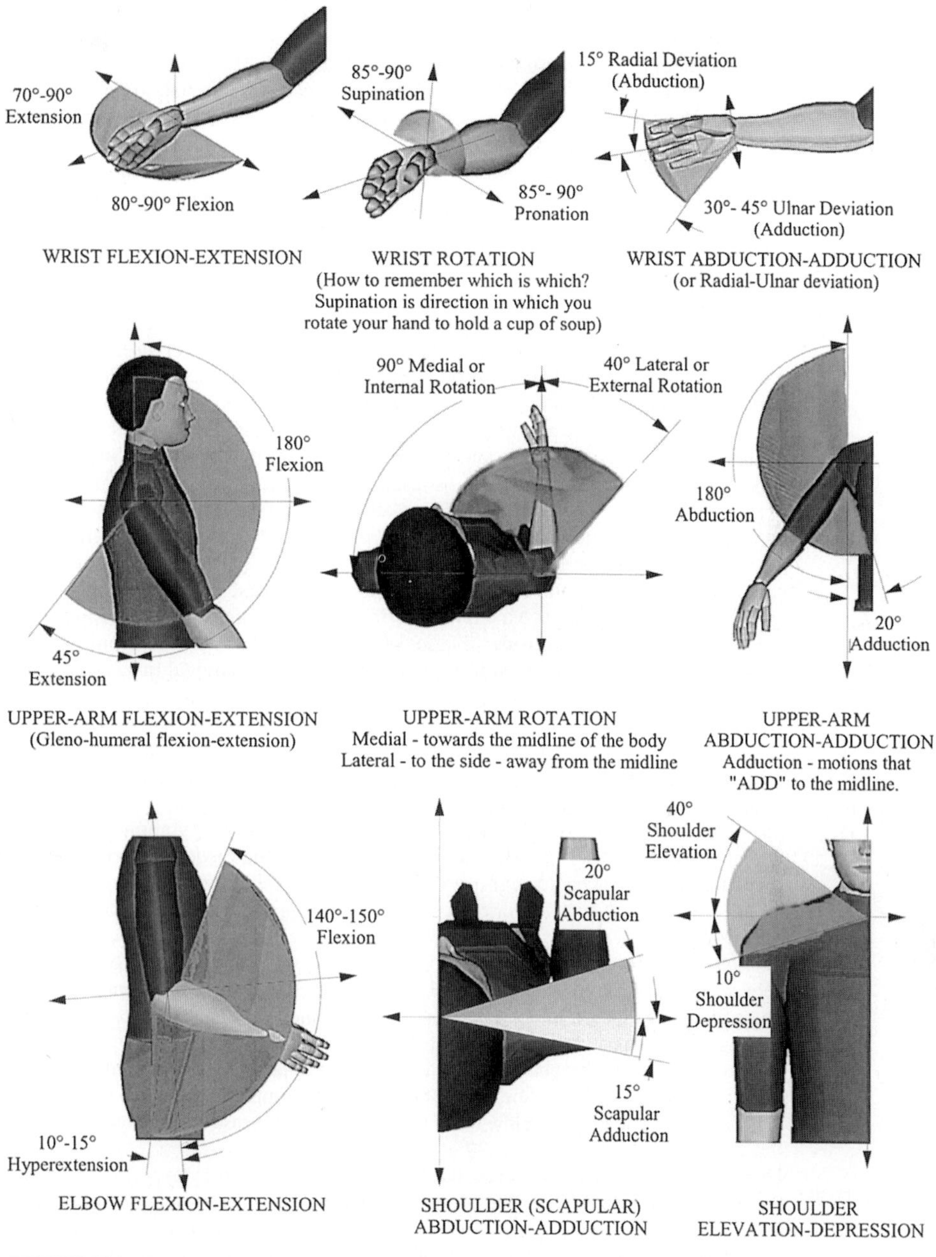

FIGURE 20.2 Ranges-of-motion for the wrist (top), upper-arm (center), elbow (bottom-left), and shoulder (bottom-center and right). Normal ranges-of-motion are for the wrist and forearm –85° to –90° of pronation, 85° to 90° of supination; 15° of radial deviation, 30° to 45° of ulnar deviation; and 80° to 90° of wrist flexion and 70° to 90° of wrist extension. For the elbow: 140° to 150° of flexion and 10° to 15° of hyperextension. For the upper arm: 90° of medial humeral rotation and 40° of lateral humeral rotation; 180° of flexion and 45° of extension; and 180° of adduction and 20° of adduction. For the shoulder: 40° of elevation and 10° of depression, 15° of scapular adduction and 20° of flexion. (*Many thanks to Ms. Pinata Hungspreugs for her help in making this image.*)

the exception of the RIMJET body-powered humeral rotator (RIMJET, FL), is achieved with manually positioned friction joints or turntables. The only shoulder joints available are also passive, manually positioned units that use friction or a lock to hold their position.

Thus it is apparent that, although the user-prosthesis interface is a major impediment to the advancement of prosthetic technology, there is much room for improvement in the prosthetic components themselves. The limitations of current systems are not due to a lack of innovative design but rather due to the very severe nature of the physical constraints that are placed on the designer and the inability of current technology to match the power density of natural muscle.

20.2.1 Socket User Interface

The socket user interface is potentially the most important component of a prosthetic system, yet it is often overlooked by engineers. The comfort of the socket or user interface will often define whether a prosthesis will be worn by a user. The inside of a socket is a hot and sweaty environment that can be uncomfortable to wear for long periods at a time. Thus it does not matter how sophisticated the limb is that is mounted on the socket if the socket itself is not comfortable. The perception of this interface also has a substantial impact on the acceptable weight of a prosthesis: a poor interface requires a prosthesis that weighs less than the anatomical counterpart to maintain a perception of equal weight. Likewise, almost all socket user interfaces are compliant, and this compliance has an effect on the position and force accuracy of the distal components that may mitigate the effect of design and control paradigms (Sensinger and Weir, 2007). The socket user interface affects sensor contact and migration, and has an effect for better or worse in the thermal dissipation—often a critical factor in users who have a reduced surface area through which to dissipate heat. For all of these reasons it is critical to consider the socket user interface when designing prosthetic components. Available options are described in order of complexity or surgical invasiveness.

Harness. In addition to providing a control source through body-powered movement, the harnesses may be used to suspend the prosthesis (Fryer and Michael, 2004). This support method transfers the weight of the prosthesis to the superior aspect of the shoulder and clavicle.

Supracondylar Support. Subjects with a below elbow amputation who cannot capture pronation/supination of their residual limb may suspend their socket from the humeral epicondyles (Brenner, 2004). Such a design prevents pronation/supination of the forearm, and as such is contraindicated for subjects who are capable of capturing this important movement.

Suction. If subjects do not have substantial scarring, it is often possible to achieve an intimate fit between the socket and the residual limb, in turn allowing for suction (Brenner, 2004; Daly, 2004). Some liners may also be used to achieve suction. These liners are then attached to the socket through a pin-locking device or lanyard. Suction distributes the weight over a larger surface area, providing a more comfortable weight distribution than a harness or supracondylar support. Weight is still transferred through the skin and soft tissue, rather than directly through bone, and as such is not as comfortable as the anatomical counterpart. Slow leaks over time may decrease the reliability of suction sockets.

Vacuum. Small vacuum pumps have recently been added to experimental upper-limb prosthetic sockets to avoid the effects that slow leaks have over time on suction sockets. Vacuum serves the added purpose of creating a stronger interface such that subjects may confidently hang from their limb without the socket falling off. The added weight of the pump is justified by the lesser perception of this weight due to a better interface. This claim is doubtful, however, because loads are still transferred through the skin and soft tissue.

Dynamic Sockets. Dynamic sockets change the intimacy and strength of the fit, depending on the loads sensed in the socket. If loads are minimal, then the socket is loose, allowing for a more relaxed fit. If loads increase, however, the socket automatically tightens on the user, providing a stronger and more intimate fit at the potential cost of reduced comfort. The concept of a dynamic socket is an interesting proposal, but the added complexity and weight are likely to prevent it from clinical realization.

Marquart Angulation Osteotomy. The previously mentioned methods have dealt almost exclusively with suspension in the presence of gravity. Suspension in the presence of rotational torques, however, is also important. Although many sockets have wings around the shoulder to prevent the prosthesis from slipping around the cylindrical residual limb, the rotational movement of the humerus is not captured, and as such there is no way to capture humeral rotation—an important movement for many tasks of daily living. In order to solve this problem a humeral angulation osteotomy can be performed to create a boney element for suspension and rotational control of a transhumeral prosthesis. This option is only available if there is sufficient bone length available to perform the procedure. The angulation osteotomy, in addition to providing rotational control, also provides as a limited suspension mechanism against gravity (Owens and Ouellette, 2004).

Subfascial Implant Supported Attachment (SISA). A technique similar to angulation osteotomy for subjects who do not have a sufficiently long humerus has recently been proposed through a surgical implant. Termed *subfascial implant supported attachment* (SISA), these implants may be a clinically viable method of suspension and humeral control once future refinements of the condyle geometry are achieved (Witsø et al., 2007).

Osseointegration. In Sweden, pioneering work in the area of direct skeletal attachment has been performed by Brånemark and his team (Brånemark, 1997; Brånemark et al., 2001). Called *osseointegration,* these surgeons and orthopedic engineers have created interfaces for direct skeletal attachment systems for upper and lower limb amputations. With osseointegration, a prosthesis is attached directly to the skeleton by way of a titanium abutment that protrudes through the skin from the cut end of the bone. Brånemark's techniques appear to have greatly diminished the infection problem that persisted in previous efforts (Hall and Rostoker, 1980). Should direct skeletal attachment prove itself viable, it could revolutionize the prosthetic fitting of amputees.

20.2.2 Mechatronics

Form versus Function. The role of form, or cosmesis, in prosthetics cannot be overstated. Often a prosthesis designer will sacrifice cosmetic appeal to achieve increased prehensile function. However, the relative importance of appearance versus function is highly dependent on the individual amputee. Some amputees may be solely concerned with visual presentation and reject a conventional body-powered, cable-operated prosthesis, which is deemed to be very functional, because of the unsightly appearance of the control harness or of a hook-shaped terminal device. Others might find the function provided by these devices sufficient to outweigh their poor appearance.

It is common for an amputee to have two prostheses, a functional one for work and an interchangeable cosmetic one for social occasions, that is, different tools for different jobs. Choice of prosthesis is ultimately based on many psychological, cultural, and practical factors. Other factors affecting the issue are age, sex, occupation, degree of physical activity, the amputee's attitude toward training, the type of amputation involved, and whether it is unilateral or bilateral limb loss. (Beasley and de Bese, 1990; Pillet and Mackin, 1992).

Cosmesis is the term used in prosthetics to describe how a particular device looks. A device is considered to be cosmetic in appearance if it is aesthetically pleasing and looks like the limb it seeks to replace in both its lines and color. However, a device might be statically "correct" in appearance but it can look "wrong" or lifeless when it is in motion. In this instance, the device has good *static cosmesis* and poor *dynamic cosmesis.*

People see what they expect to see, so if a person with an artificial limb replacement looks and moves in an expected manner, the fact of the artificial limb will often go unnoticed by casual observers. Oftentimes a hand replacement can have only a vague resemblance to the natural hand but because it is moved in a natural-looking manner, it can pass undetected unless closely scrutinized. Here the device has poor *static cosmesis* and good *dynamic cosmesis.*

Dynamic cosmesis is frequently the more important of the two forms of cosmesis but it is frequently overlooked. Dynamic cosmesis can be enhanced by preserving as much of the amputee's residual motion as possible. For example, a partial hand prosthesis should not interfere with residual wrist motion because the wrist is used extensively in the positioning of the hand in space. Finally, a device

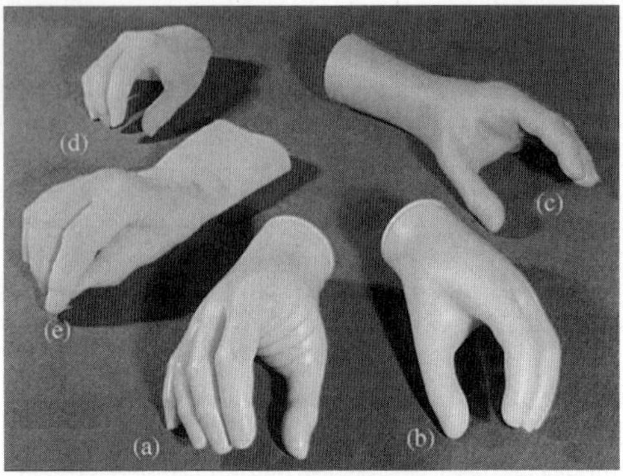

FIGURE 20.3 Photograph of various mechanism liners (*a*, *b*) and their associated cosmetic glove covers (*c, d, e*). Hand liner (*b*) is an older version of liner (*a*). Liner (*a*) has "grooves" or serrations added (in the thumb finger web space) in an attempt to reduce the elastic forces the liner imposes on the hand mechanism when it is trying to open or close the hand. Cosmetic glove (*c*) is made from polyvinyl chloride (PVC) while gloves (*d* and *e*) are made from silicone rubber. Silicone cosmetic gloves can be made with much more lifelike detail but tend not to be as sturdy as their PVC counterparts.

can be considered to be *functionally cosmetic* if at a glance it is not immediately recognizable as an artificial hand regardless of whether it is in motion or not or whether it is hand-like when stationary.

Cosmetic gloves, made of polyvinyl chloride (PVC) or silicone, are frequently employed to cover artificial hand mechanisms to give them good static cosmesis (Fig. 20.3). These coverings serve to increase the passive adaptability of a prosthetic hand to the shape of a grasped object and to increase the coefficient of friction of the hand. The price paid for this increased cosmesis and grasping function is a restricted range of motion and hindered performance (speed/force output) of the hand. This is because the hand motors must overcome the elastic forces inherent in the glove. The ideal glove should enhance the cosmesis of the prosthesis without interfering with its performance.

Limb replacements should be anthropomorphic in general shape, outline, and size. This does not mean an artificial hand or arm should look exactly like its human counterpart. However, there should be a joint that operates like an elbow joint where one would expect to see an elbow joint and the various limb segments should be of a size consistent with a normal human being, that is, any replacement should have similar kinematics and kinetics. With regard to the issue of hand size, artificial hands are usually smaller than their physiological counterparts. This is because artificial hands are perceived to be larger than they really are, probably due to their rigid structure and largely static appearance.

Final weight of a prosthesis is critical to the success of any prosthetic fitting. Contrary to what one might think, one cannot make an artificial limb replacement the same weight as the limb it replaces. The weight of an adult male arm is about 10 kg (20 lb). The weight of any total arm replacement should not exceed 3 kg or a little over 6 lb. Artificial arms need to be as light as possible or else they will end up gathering dust in a closet.

The lack of an intimate connection between the amputee and limb replacement means that the prosthesis is perceived as an external load and therefore as something that must be carried. To be effective, artificial arms should be worn by their users for periods in excess of 8 to 12 a day. To gain some insight into how this might feel, consider carrying a 6-lb laptop computer slung from your shoulder for a day.

Prehension or Grasp. Hand function is generally limited to those modes of prehension that are used the most often. Numerous studies of how the hands grasp objects have been performed [(Schlesinger et al., 1919; Keller et al., 1947; Napier, 1956; Kamakura et al., 1980) to name but a few]. Broadly speaking, hand tasks can be subdivided into nonprehensile functions and prehensile functions. Nonprehensile functions of the hand are those functions where grasping is not required; for example, pushing an object, holding an object between the body and forearm, flicking, brushing, percussive motions such as playing the piano, and so on. Prehensile hand functions are those cases where an object is grasped and held partly or wholly within the hand. The 6 grasping patterns adapted by Keller et al. (1947) from Schlesinger et al.'s (1919) 12 patterns are the most widely accepted in the field of prosthetics (Fig. 20.4) and have endured the test of time. These patterns are

1. Tip prehension
2. Palmar prehension
3. Lateral prehension
4. Hook prehension
5. Spherical prehension
6. Cylindrical prehension

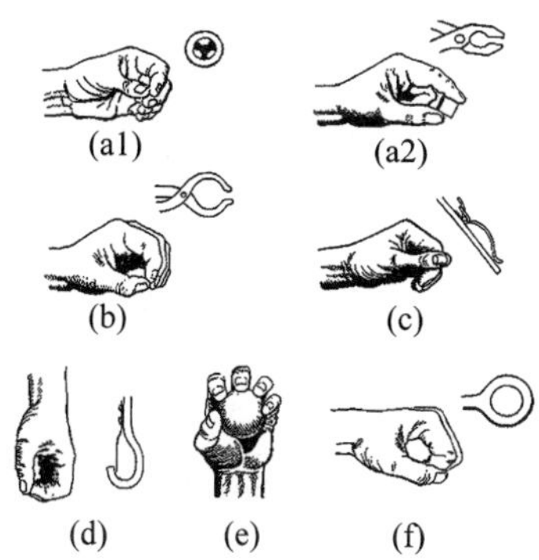

FIGURE 20.4 Schematic of the prehension patterns of the hand as defined by Keller et al. (1947): (*a*1) palmar prehension (three jaw chuck), (*a*2) palmar prehension (two finger), (*b*) tip prehension, (*c*) lateral prehension, (*d*) hook prehension, (*e*) spherical prehension, (*f*) cylindrical prehension. In a hand-like prosthesis, it takes two to four independently controlled degrees of freedom to implement these prehension patterns. In a non-hand-like device, a single degree-of-freedom device such as a split hook can be used.

Napier (1956) described tip prehension, palmar prehension, and lateral prehension as precision grips and spherical and cylindrical prehension as power grasp, while hook prehension falls outside of both these categories. Precision grips primarily involve the thumb working in opposition with the index and middle fingers. Tip prehension, or fingernail pinch, is used mainly to grasp small objects. In lateral prehension, the thumb holds an object against the side of the index finger as is the case when using a key. In palmar prehension (sometimes referred to as tridigital pinch or three-jaw chuck), the thumb opposes either a single finger or two or more fingers.

Power grasps use all the fingers of the hand to provide an encompassing grasp that firmly stabilizes the object being held. Hook prehension is achieved by flexing the fingers into a hook; the thumb is either alongside the index finger or opposes the index and middle fingers to lock the object held. Carrying a briefcase is a good illustration of this kind of prehension. Keller et al. found that palmar prehension or tridigital pinch was the most frequently used prehensile pattern for static grasping, while lateral prehension is used most often for dynamic grasping.

The finding by Keller et al. (1947) that palmar prehension was the most frequently used pattern and the reduction of most prosthetic terminal devices to a single DOF has meant that most prosthetic terminal devices incorporate palmar prehension as the dominant grasp pattern. The persistence of this pattern combined with a wide width of opening in prosthetic hand designs and its general acceptance over the years tend to support this compromise (Heckathorne, 1992).

A study done at the University of California, Los Angeles (UCLA), (Taylor, 1954) on human prehension force indicated that adult males could produce maximum mean forces of 95.6 N (21.5 ft · lb) of palmar prehension, 103 N (23.2 ft · lb) for lateral prehension, and 400 N (90 ft · lb) for cylindrical grasp. In the light of another, unpublished, UCLA study that showed forces up to 68 N (15 ft · lb) were needed for carrying out activities of daily living, Peizer et al. (1969) proposed that 68 N (15 ft · lb) be a minimum standard for the maximum prehension force for electric prehensors (Heckathorne, 1992).

Dominant and Nondominant Hands. The issue of hand dominance, whether one is right or left handed, must also be considered. People use their dominant hand differently from their nondominant hand. The role of the nondominant hand is to hold things while the dominant hand is working, or waiting to work, on them. A unilateral amputee will always use their prosthesis in a nondominant role, even if the prosthesis is a replacement for what was once the amputee's dominant hand. The unilateral amputee will also tend to pick things up with his/her dominant hand and then place them into the nondominant hand. Consequently, van Lunteren et al. (1983) suggested that there is a difference in the type of grasps that ought to be incorporated in devices for unilateral as opposed to bilateral amputees. However, Toth (1991; Heckathorne et al., 1995) showed that the findings of Keller et al. (1947) held regardless of whether the dominant or nondominant hand was used.

The Rancho Los Amigos Easy-Feed Hand (Lansberger et al., 1998) is an example of a new body-powered hand design that is based on this observation that prosthetic hands for persons with unilateral amputations tend to be used to hold objects placed into them with the sound hand. The Easy-Feed hand is a body-powered children's prosthesis that is easy to push objects into but difficult to pull things out of, making it good for grasping or hanging onto objects. This hand is being commercialized as the Live Touch hand from TRS, Boulder, Colorado.

Hand Width of Opening. Most manipulations of the hand are precision manipulations of the palmar prehension kind where the thumb directly opposes the index finger and/or the middle finger. In this mode, most of the hand's actions are performed with a hand opening of about 5 cm (2 in) (Keller et al., 1947). When designing for dominant hand function, palmar prehension is the desirable pattern with emphasis not so much on wide opening. For nondominant hand function where the hand is used essentially as a portable vice with objects being placed into it, a wide opening becomes more important. From a design perspective, allowing the hand mechanism to open 10 cm (3.5 to 4 in), instead of 5 cm (2 in) enables the mechanism to perform the cylindrical prehension power grasp with minimal extra design effort. In general, an artificial hand should be able to open at least 10 cm (3.5 to 4 in), or enough to grasp a beverage can or a Mason jar, which are common household items.

Passive Adaptation During Grasping. The grip of the hand is improved by the ability of the hand to passively adapt to the shape of an object grasped. A grasped object depresses, or indents, the skin and underlying soft tissues of the hand, at first meeting little reaction. Consequently, the soft tissue adapts easily to the shape of the object grasped. However, the mechanical properties of the soft tissue are nonlinear, and the conforming tissue becomes more rigid as pressure is increased. The rise in tissue stiffness after conformation to shape enables objects to be grasped securely. This feature of the human hand would seem to be useful for robotic and prosthetic systems. In prosthetics, the passive adaptability, afforded by the soft tissue of the hand, is mimicked, to some extent, by lining the prosthesis mechanism with a soft plastic and covering it with a cosmetic glove. In robotics, it is common to use a compliant coating on an end effector to stabilize a robot arm during contact with hard surfaces.

Non-Hand-Like Prehensors. The reduction of most prosthetic terminal devices to a single degree of freedom (DOF) was a compromise to make the best use of the available control sources. A standard transhumeral (above-elbow) body-powered prosthesis has two control cables (two active DOF). The terminal device invariably takes the form of a split hook. A split hook is used when maximum function is desired (Fig. 20.5). Although a split hook is a single DOF device, depending on which part of the hook is used, a split hook can reproduce tip, palmar, lateral, cylindrical, or hook prehension, making it a very simple and versatile device. This is another contributing factor to the success of body-powered prostheses over externally powered prostheses.

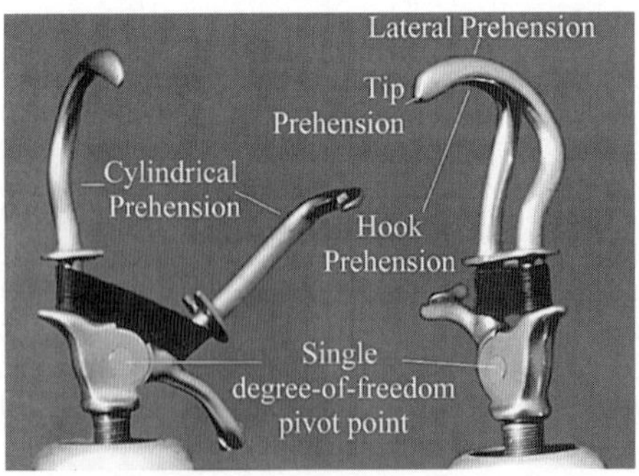

FIGURE 20.5 A split hook with the prehension surfaces pointed out of the page. Here a single degreee-of-freedom device can recreate four of the prehension patterns of Keller et al. (1947): tip prehension; lateral prehension; cylindrical prehension; and hook prehension. This is one of the reasons why the hook, though often thought unsightly, has been so successful in the field of prosthetics.

The use of split hooks highlights the trade-off made between form and function. The hook bears little resemblance to the natural hand but is widely used because of the function it affords if only one DOF is available for terminal device control. Split hooks are available in many variations on a basic theme from Hosmer-Dorrance Corp. and Otto Bock Healthcare.

Fryer and Michael (1992) provide a thorough review of the various types of hooks currently available.

In an effort to capitalize on the function of the split hook, the Hosmer-Dorrance NU-VA Synergetic Prehensor uses a split hook in an externally powered configuration. Other commercially available, externally powered, non-hand-like prehensors include the Otto Bock Greifer and the RSLSteeper Powered Gripper. The NU-VA Synergetic Prehensor, the Otto Bock Greifer, and the Steeper Powered Gripper incorporate many of the previously mentioned prehension patterns (Fig. 20.6).

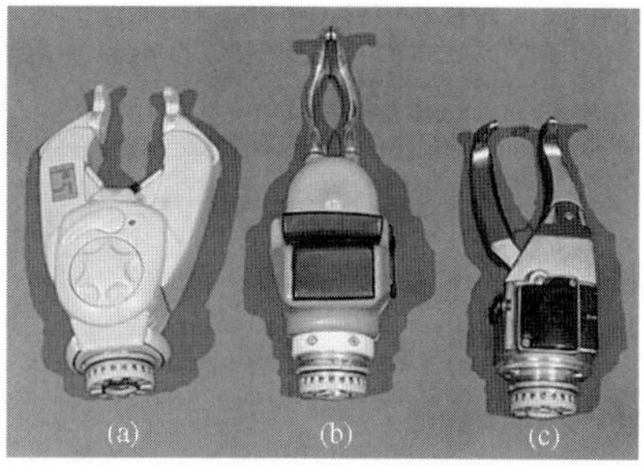

FIGURE 20.6 Examples of powered non-hand-like prehensnion devices. (*a*) Otto Bock Greifer (Otto Bock Orthopedic Industry Inc., Duderstadt, Germany), (*b*) NU-VA Synergetic Prehensor (Hosmer-Dorrance Corp., Campbell, California), (*c*) RSLSteeper Powered Gripper (RSLSteeper, Ltd., England). Both the NU-VA Synergetic Prehensor and the RSLSteeper Powered Gripper use the principle of synergetic prehension to maximize performance, while the Greifer uses Otto Bock's automatic transmission. The NU-VA Synergetic Prehensor sought to capitalize on the success of the split hook by basically creating a powered version of it. All the mechanisms are shown here with an Otto Bock quick-wrist disconnect, a de facto standard type of wrist interface for powered components. The NU-VA Synergetic Prehensor and the Otto Bock Griefer are capable of high pinch forces, high speeds, and large widths-of-opening, making them very functional at the expnese of cosmesis.

Hand-Like Prehensors. The de facto standard for externally powered hand-like prosthesis is the single DOF Otto Bock Sensor Hand Speed (Fig. 20.7). When used in a prosthetic fitting, a plastic hand form liner is pulled over the mechanism and a PVC or silicone rubber cosmetic glove is then pulled over the liner. This gives the hand good overall *static* cosmesis at the expense of reduced overall mechanism performance. RSLSteeper Ltd. (Roehampton, England) and Centri (Sweden) also manufacture single

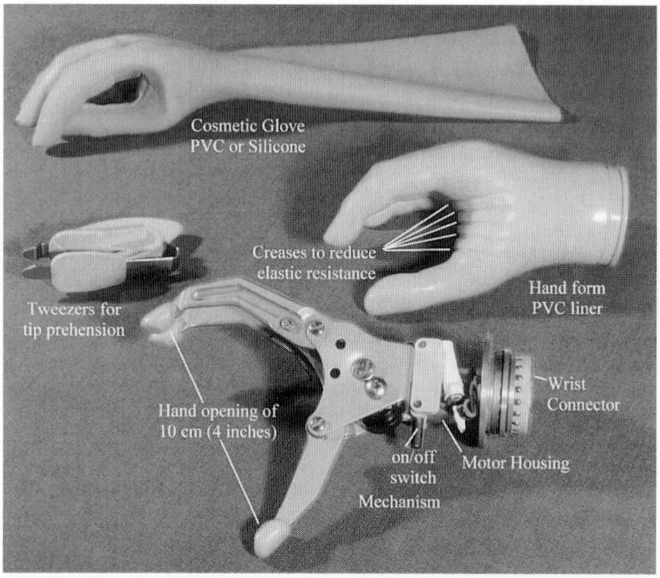

FIGURE 20.7 Otto Bock System Electric Hand (Otto Bock Orthopedic Industry Inc., Duderstadt, Germany). The hand consists of a mechanism over which a liner is placed. A cosmetic glove is then pulled over the liner (Note: Otto Bock does not provide siliocne gloves). Liner creases have been placed in the finger thumb web space in an effort to reduce its elastic resistance. Also shown is a pair of tweezers that are provided with each hand to make tip prehension possible. Prosthetic hands have very poor tip prehension without the aid of some sort of extra tool such as these tweezers.

DOF devices for the adult. Single DOF child-size hands are also available from Systemteknik, Variety Village, Otto Bock Orthopaedic Inc., and RSLSteeper Ltd., among others. Michael (1986) provides a nice overview of the commercially available externally powered hand mechanisms of the day while Heckathorne (1992) provides in-depth descriptions and technical specifications of all the externally powered components available at the time of writing.

Touch Bionics has recently introduced the i-Limb Hand, in which each finger has a separate motor. This prosthetic hand is able to easily conform around objects, since each finger continues to flex until it meets resistance. The position of the thumb may be manually adjusted, providing palmer prehension or lateral prehension. Whether this hand will prove robust enough remains to be seen.

The liner and cosmetic glove act as springs to oppose the opening of the hand by the mechanism, thus degrading the overall performance of the hand. De Visser and Herder (2000) advocated the use of compensatory mechanisms to reduce the effect of the liner and glove on the mechanisms' performance. Palmar prehension, in these hand-like prehensors, is achieved by single joint fingers that are fixed in slight flexion at a position approximating the interphalangeal joint. The resulting finger shape also creates a concave inner prehension surface that can be used to provide cylindrical prehension (Heckathorne, 1992).

All these mechanisms are typically used in a prosthesis that has no wrist flexion or extension. This can be a problem when trying to pick up small objects from a surface. The fixed wrist combined with poor line of sight of the object to be grasped can lead to nonphysiological movements, resulting in poor *dynamic* cosmesis.

Planes of Motion of the Thumb. The physiological thumb has two axes of rotation, the metacarpophalangeal (MP) joint and the carpometacarpal (CP) joint, giving it many degrees of freedom. Blair and Kramer (1981) claim that the thumb accounts for up to 40 percent of the function of the hand. In general, prosthetic hands have a single axis of rotation for the thumb. This axis of rotation should be chosen to be at a point between the two natural pivot points to optimize the device's overall function and cosmesis.

Operating under the assumption that a practical prosthetic hand can have only one axis of rotation for the thumb, Lozac'h et al. (1992) and Vinet et al. (1995) performed a series of experiments to find if there was a preferred working plane for a single DOF active thumb. From these experiments he determined that the preferred working plane of the thumb lay between 45 and 55 degrees (Fig. 20.8). These findings conform to those reported by Taylor (1954) who, from a statistical analysis on natural unrestricted prehension, concluded that "In palmar prehension, the thumb approaches the fingers in a plane inclined approximately 45 degrees to the palmar plane."

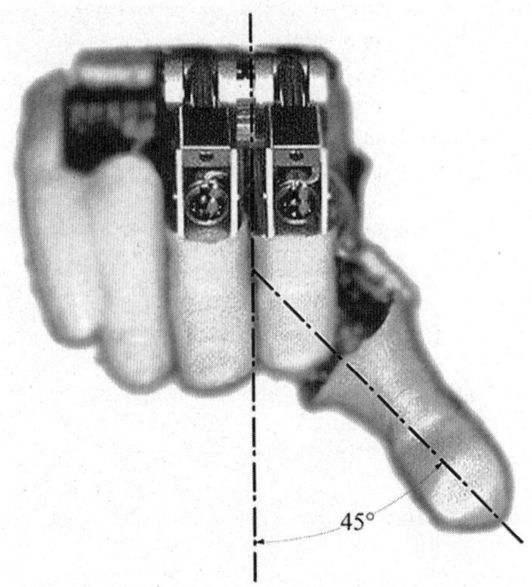

FIGURE 20.8 Preferred operating plane of the thumb in an artificial hand. The physiological thumb has two axes of rotation, the metacarpophalangeal (MP) joint and the carpometacarpal (CP) joint. A practical prosthetic hand can have only one axis of rotation for the thumb. Lozac'h (1984; Vinet et al., 1995) determined that the preferred working plane of the thumb lay between 45 and 55 degrees.

This finding was implemented in a single DOF, multifunctional hand design (Lozac'h et al., 1992; Vinet et al., 1995). Because the hand had articulated fingers that could move independently of each other, it was capable of forming an adaptive grip with which to grasp objects. An adaptive grip meant it required much lower forces than conventional prosthetic hands to hold objects. Lozac'h et al. (1992) also found that the hand reduced the number of arm and body compensatory movements during both the approach and utilization phases of prehension. As well as greatly improving the object visibility, the prehension cosmesis (dynamic cosmesis), and the grip stability, particularly for large objects. Unfortunately they also found that they had to further improve the design and the long-term reliability.

The finding that the preferred working plane of the thumb lay between 45 and 55 degrees is not reflected in many other prosthetic or orthotic devices. Kenworthy (1974) designed a hand in which the thumb moved at 90 degrees to the fingers, that is, the hand used a side pinch type of grip (lateral prehension). This hand was developed for use with the CO_2-powered arms (Simpson, 1972) of the Orthopaedic Bio-Engineering Unit (OBEU) of Princess Margaret Rose Orthopaedic Hospital, Edinburgh, Scotland.

The motivation for placing the thumb at this angle came from trying to improve the visibility of the object to be grasped during the final stages of the grasping process and to improve flat surface operation. It was an attempt to overcome the poor dynamic cosmesis that results from the use of a traditional "pincer" grip prostheses (such as the Otto Bock Electrohand) with a rigid wrist.

Traditional pincer grip prostheses are easy to use when picking up tall objects (greater than 25 mm above the surface), but the only way that low objects (less than or equal to 25 mm) can be grasped is by approaching the object from above. This requires the amputee to maintain an unsightly line-of-attack (poor dynamic cosmesis) in order to see the object being grasped and to permit flat surface operation. This unusual motion in turn draws attention to the user.

Kenworthy's hand had the fingers fixed with only the thumb being able to move. Although flat surface operation is important, it is perhaps not the most important feature of prosthesis design. This hand was designed primarily for use in bilateral arm systems in which one hand was a conventional pincer-type hand and the other was of Kenworthy's design. The 90 degrees of the Kenworthy hand was chosen so that at least one hand of a bilateral arm system could have flat surface operation.

Another hand, developed by Davies et al. (1977) also at the OBEU, was a monofunctional body-powered device in which the thumb moved about an axis inclined at an angle of 60 degrees to the middle and index fingers. This hand, called the OBEU hand, was a compromise between the more traditional pincer type of hand and the Kenworthy hand. The motivation for this hand was to retain the pincer-type function while improving the overall visibility of the object to be grasped. Additionally, flat surface operation could be achieved by allowing the fingers and thumb to "sweep" the surface. In this design, both the thumb and fingers moved simultaneously. The 60 degrees for the OBEU hand was chosen because it allowed the loci of the tips of the thumb and index and middle finger to move approximately in a horizontal plane when the wrist axis is at about 25 degrees to the horizontal so that they can sweep the surface. Thus, both these designs were an attempt to improve the dynamic cosmesis of the prosthesis while using single DOF hand-like mechanisms.

Multifunctional Mechanisms. There have been many attempts to design fully functional arms and hands but it was not until after the Second World War and in particular during the 1960s and 1970s that much time, effort, and money was invested in the development of externally powered multifunctional hand-arm systems (Jacobsen et al., 1982). Much of the impetus for the research of the 1960s was as a result of the thalidomide drug that was prescribed to a large number of pregnant women in Europe, Canada, and Australia. The drug acted on the fetus in such a way as to inhibit the development of the limbs, causing the child to be born with one or more fetal size limbs that never developed further.

Worldwide, many new government initiatives were established to help in the development of externally powered, multifunctional, complete arm systems for these children. Prime among these being the Edinburgh Arm (Simpson, 1969), the Boston Arm (Mann, 1968; Mann and Reimers, 1970), the Philadelphia Arm (Taylor and Wirta, 1969; Taylor and Finley, 1971), the Waseda Hand (Kato, 1969), the Belgrade hand (Razic, 1972; Stojiljkovic and Saletic, 1974), the Sven Hand (Herberts et al., 1978), and the Utah Arm (Jacobsen et al., 1982).

Although many ideas were tried and tested during this period, only a few devices ever made it from the laboratory into everyday clinical practice. The Edinburgh Arm, which was pneumatically powered, saw some clinical usage. It was mechanically complex and as a result prone to failure. Although this arm is not available today, it is important because it was an implementation of Simpson's ideas on extended physiological proprioception (EPP). The Boston Arm, developed at MIT, was the first myoelectrically controlled elbow. This elbow was extensively redesigned (Williams, 1989) to become commercially available today as the Boston Digital Arm (Liberating Technology, MA). The Utah Arm is commercially available through Motion Control Inc. (Sears et al., 1989).

The Sven Hand was extensively used in research, particularly in regard to multifunction control using pattern recognition of myoelectric signals (Lawrence and Kadefors, 1971). Henry Lymark, the director of the Handikappinstitutet of Stockholm, Sweden, later created a simplified version of the Sven Hand, called the ES Hand. This hand possessed an adaptive grip and a passive two-position thumb. It was powered by a single motor with differential drives to the fingers. Lymark visited our laboratory (NUPRL) in 1987 and demonstrated this hand. Unfortunately, he died soon after his visit and the ES Hand essentially died with him.

The Philadelphia Arm of Taylor and Wirta (1969) and Taylor and Finley (1971) also found use as a research tool for multifunction control using weighted filters for the pattern recognition problem, but was never used clinically. The Belgrade hand was never used clinically to any great extent but has influenced the robotics field in the form of the Belgrade/USC robotic hand (Beattie et al., 1994).

The U.S. Defense Agency Research Projects Agency (DARPA) has recently funded two projects to create self-contained, modular, multifunctional prostheses. These prostheses are tasked to have the same anthropomorphic constraints of the fiftieth percentile female, yet to be as strong as the average soldier along with numerous other design requirements. Over 50 institutions have collaborated on two independent projects, which have looked at each component of prosthesis design, from socket user interface to mechatronics to control to sensor design to energy supply. Through the support of commercial companies like Otto Bock and Liberating Technologies Inc., existing electromechanical technologies have been refined, providing complex multifunctional hands that use existing motor technologies optimized at every level. Advances have also been made in more exotic technologies such as hydraulic actuation (Fite et al., 2008). Perhaps one of the more interesting designs of the DARPA project has been in the use of cobots (Faulring et al., 2006), which tap a central disk that continuously rotates to independently provide energy to each degree of freedom. Each drive mechanism has a small continuously variable transmission, and the design is theoretically elegant in that the high inertial forces of the fingers as they flutter back and forth in rapid movement are mitigated by the constantly rotating drum through which energy is tapped.

In practice, size constraints, technology limitations, and complexity of the associated local control have put the performance of this interesting technology on par with more conventional motor-gear systems. The cobot system also takes up most of the forearm, so at least in the near future it appears as if conventional systems will be used. The Intrinsic hand (Weir et al., 2007a; 2007b) designed by the author's group and Otto Bock, Vienna, was based on the observation that to fit persons with transradial amputations—the most prevalent level for upper-limb amputation—all the actuators used to drive the hand must reside in the hand. The Intrinsic hand had 15 motors in the hand and 3 in the wrist and in theory has the same performance capability as both the hydrogen peroxide arm and the cobot arm in terms of speed, torque, and power consumption. To build this intrinsically actuated hand, we had to develop custom brushless dc electric motors that were capable of providing high torque at physiological hand speeds. These motors are small enough to be fitted into the volume available for a 50 percent female finger, yet capable of providing sufficient torque and speed for a 50 percent male hand. These motors were coupled with high-torque capacity Wolfrom transmissions to form the drivetrains for each of the DOFs to be driven in the hand.

Each finger has three articulations with two motors. The distal and medial phalanges are driven by one motor and coupled by a differential drive mechanism. The proximal phalange has its own motor. In the palm, the index, ring, and little fingers have ab/adduction motors. The thumb has four DOF, each with its own motor. The wrist does flexion-extension, radial-ulnar deviation, and wrist rotation. It is the intrinsic hand architecture that has been chosen for the final phase of the DARPA project.

In reality, although the DARPA projects have achieved amazing degrees of dexterity and come closer to anthropomorphically sized, self-contained, weight-appropriate prostheses, the amount of complexity required to achieve these results has likely prevented them from clinical viability; with so many parts it is inevitable that some will quickly fail when users subject them to tasks never considered by the designers.

Most of the early artificial arms for the high-level amputee were designed as complete arm systems. But as these systems failed to provide the expected function, there was a move away from designing complete arm prostheses to the design of specific or modular components, such as externally or body-powered elbow joints, powered or passive wrist rotators, passive humeral rotators, and whole ranges of different hooks, hands, and prehensors. The current trend is to use a "mix and match" approach to optimize the function available. This modular approach has the advantage of providing great flexibility and practicality for system design. However, it will probably never be able to attain the high functional goals that may be possible from a more integrated standpoint—though the DARPA project may yet prove us wrong.

In the end, most multifunctional prosthesis designs are doomed by practicality. Most mechanisms fail because of poor durability, lack of performance, and complicated control. No device will be clinically successful if it breaks down frequently or if the socket is uncomfortable. A multifunctional design is by its nature more complex than a single degree-of-freedom counterpart. From a maintenance standpoint, this means the device will have more components that are likely to fail. Articulated joints on fingers are more likely to fail than monocoque, or solid finger, designs.

Prosthesis users are not gentle with their devices; they expect them to work in all sorts of situations never dreamed of by their designers. This was one of the reasons why the Sven Hand was simplified to the ES hand so that it might find some clinical application. However, in the end, a compromise must be made if increased function is to be achieved. Some of the robustness and simplicity of a single degree-of-freedom device must be traded to achieve the performance possible with a multi-degree-of-freedom (MDOF) hand.

Another practical consideration is performance. The hand must be able to generate enough torque and speed, and have a sufficient width of opening to be useful to the user. Many devices have been designed in the laboratory that have insufficient performance once a cosmetic glove is added. A cosmetic glove is standard for prosthetic hands and unless a mechanism is specifically designed not to require a glove, the effect of the glove on performance must be taken into consideration.

The ES hand was designed to work in its own cover. The Belgrade Hand needed an additional cover. Current commercially available single DOF hands today are capable of forces of about 30 ft · lb (133.5 N) and speeds in excess of 3 rad/s. The pinch force of a multifunctional hand does not have to be as high because the adaptive nature of the grip enables objects to be encompassed within the hand. Given the severe design constraints that exist in terms of size, weight, and power, achieving these performance criteria is challenging.

The Case for a Reduced Degree-of-Freedom Multifunctional Hand. A compromise to the dilemma of practicality and robustness versus the increased function possible with a MDOF hand is to limit the device to the minimum number of degrees of freedom necessary to replicate the grasp patterns of Keller et al. (1947). This idea of limiting the function of the hand to a number of DOFs sufficient to recreate the grasp patterns of Keller et al. turns up in many unrelated fields when compromise must be made between function and some other variable.

Professional scuba diver gloves trade function for warmth in order to extend dive times (Fig. 20.9). A mitten is warmest while a glove with individual fingers is the most functional. Professional scuba diver gloves are a compromise, having the thumb and index fingers free and the middle, ring, and little

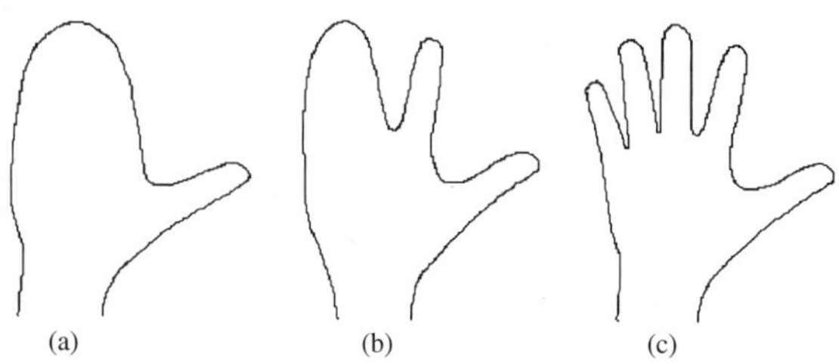

FIGURE 20.9 Sketches of the three types of gloves used by scuba divers: (*a*) a mitten is warmest, but has the poorest function; (*b*) compromise glove provides warmth and allows diver to achieve the prehension patterns of Keller et al. (1974); (*c*) standard glove with individual fingers provides the least warmth but the most function.

fingers together. This configuration affords the diver the basic prehension patterns of the hand while at the same time keeping the bulk of the hand warm.

In the area of remote manipulation, three DOF have been used by the SARCOS system (Jacobsen et al., 1990). The SARCOS system (Jacobsen et al., 1990) uses a three-DOF hand for the slave manipulator terminal device and limits the hand of the operator to the same three DOF when controlling the master arm. Constraining the operator's hand to the same DOF as the slave and vice versa enables the operator to extend his or her proprioception into the remotely controlled terminal device. Forces experienced by the slave are reflected back to the master and experienced by the operator. In this mechanism, clever choice of the DOFs to be controlled have resulted in a device that can reproduce Keller et al.'s prehension patterns with only three DOF. The thumb has two DOF for thumb flexion and extension and thumb abduction and adduction, while the three fingers (middle, ring, and little) have three DOF for finger flexion and extension. The index finger was kept rigid, providing a stable platform against which to operate.

For space suit gloves, the Direct-Link Prehensor (1991a; 1991b) limits the motions of the operator's hand to three DOF. Space suit gloves are bulky and stiff due to the suit's pressurization. This stiffness results in limited external dexterity and excessive hand fatigue. Also, as in the case with diver's gloves, tactile sensation and manual dexterity are lost because the hand is gloved. The Direct-Link Prehensor is a two-finger device, with the thumb mounted at 45 degrees to the fingers per the work of Lozac'h (Lozac'h, 1984).

In the area of surgery, Beasley (1983) described a surgical procedure to provide a functional four-DOF hand for persons with C5-C6 quadriplegia. This procedure is a three-stage reconstruction, which makes possible precision prehension with careful positioning of the stabilized thumb to oppose the actively flexed index and middle fingers. The result is a functional hand that retains some of its sense of touch.

In the field of functional electrical stimulation (FES), surgical techniques similar to those of Beasley (1983) have been combined with implantable four-channel FES electrodes to enable patients with flail arms to reproduce the palmar and lateral grasp patterns of Keller et al. (Triolo et al., 1996).

In three of these instances, the exceptions being the surgical intervention and FES, tactile sensation was compromised either by gloves or the remote nature of the terminal device (SARCOS). Vision, proprioceptive feedback from the joints, and diffuse skin pressure were the main sources of feedback. In the case of the surgery and FES, vision and sensation (feedback) were intact but muscular function (control) was impaired. In all instances, restricting hand function to three of four DOF necessary to recreate Keller et al.'s prehension patterns optimized hand function versus the number of available control sources and increased overall function.

Assuming sufficient control sites can be found, then a prosthetic hand capable of implementing the Keller's grasp patterns should also optimize function versus the available number of control sites. At first glance it would appear that such an artificial hand-like prehensor would require three or four DOF to adequately reproduce all six prehension patterns—at least one, more usually two, for the thumb, one for the index finger and one for the remaining three fingers.

However, if the fingers are of a single joint monocoque design and the middle, ring, and little (MRL) fingers are lumped together to move as a unit while the index finger can move on its own and if the thumb is limited to a single DOF and is oriented such that it operates along its preferred plane, 45 degrees (Lozac'h, 1984; Vinet et al., 1995), then a three-DOF mechanism results. But if one considers the role of the thumb during grasping, then it can be seen that the resulting prehension pattern is a function of the timing of thumb closure (assuming a fully open position to start with). A "close" signal to both thumb and all fingers together would result in tridigital or palmar prehension. Delaying closure of the thumb, a fraction would result in tip prehension because the MRL finger unit will not mate with the thumb and will pass on to close on themselves. (It is assumed that current sensing or limit switches are used to switch off stalled motors.) Delaying thumb closure more would result in lateral prehension because neither the index finger nor MRL fingers will mate with the thumb. The thumb will then close down on the side of the index finger. Power grasps result from the monocoque shape of the fingers and a wide width of opening. With such a system, a single "open" signal drives all motors (thumb and finger motors) back to the same start position. Two "close" signals, one for both the index and the MRL finger drives and a second for the thumb would be required. This implies a $1^1/_2$-DOF system. If a wiffle tree structure is used to drive the fingers, then a single motor could be used to drive all the fingers. It should be noted that prehension (grasping) should not be confused with manipulation. For dexterous manipulation, many more degrees of freedom of control are required. The work of Santello et al. (1998; 2002) and Santello and Soechting, 1998) shows that much of hand grasping can be represented by two or three principal components, providing further evidence that grasping/prehension is a low-dimensional task. To achieve full dexterous manipulation, however, requires at least nine independently controlled DOFs (Mason and Salisbury, 1985) as well as good finger tip sensation (Cutkosky, 1989)

Power Sources. As is the case for all portable devices, power is scarce. Choice of power source defines a prosthesis in that it determines the choice of actuator. If the power source is to be the amputee, that is body-power, then the actuator is the amputee's own musculature, and the prosthesis should not require excessive effort to use. Mechanical mechanisms need to be efficient and frictional losses need to be minimized to avoid tiring the user over the course of the day. If the artificial limb is externally powered (i.e., uses a power source other than the body, usually electric storage), the limb should be able to run for a day from the same power source without needing to be replaced or recharged. In addition, it is desirable for the power source to be contained within the prosthesis.

Electrochemical batteries are the main source of energy for modern, externally powered prosthetic arms, although pneumatic gas cylinders have been used in the past. There are a number of other technologies that could replace batteries as portable sources of electricity in the future. These include electromechanical flywheel systems that store energy in a rotating disc and miniature Wrenkel-type internal combustion engines; however, the most promising technology is that of ethanol- or methanol-based fuel cells. These devices are already moving into production for interim cell phone products. All are heavy and occupy space. If electricity is the power source, then for the foreseeable future dc electric motors will be the actuators. The problem of portable prosthesis power is analogous to the power issues in the laptop computer and cellular phone industry where a major contributor to the weight and space of these portable devices is the battery.

Unpowered or Passive Prostheses. There is a class of terminal devices that do not offer prehensile function. Devices in this class, usually hands, are regarded as passive or passively functional prostheses. They have no moving parts and require no cables or batteries for operation. They are typically lightweight and reliable. Generic (standard) passive hand prostheses may consist of a cosmetic outer glove over a soft plastic hand with wire reinforcements in the fingers. Traditionally, cosmetic gloves have been made of PVC, although silicone is becoming the material of choice (Fig. 20.3). Individualized hands, when expertly done, have a preferable appearance to generic hand replacements. Highly realistic hands, fingers, and finger parts can be custom sculpted and painted to an individual's size and skin coloring. Such prostheses confer to persons what Beasley has called the highly important function of "social presentation" (Beasley and de Bese, 1990).

Passive work prostheses may be a simple post to provide opposition, or they may incorporate specialized features to aid in certain occupations. A custom-designed system that serves only one function may aid the wearer more than one that is supposed to be multifunctional. In such cases, the prosthetic device is worn on those occasions when it is needed. These devices range from tool adapters to sports mitts.

In the past, a prosthetic fitting was deemed to have been unsuccessful if the patient did not wear an actively controlled prosthesis for prehensile function. In a recent study, Fraser (1998) showed that amputees used their prostheses most frequently for nonprehensile tasks, such as stabilizing, pushing, or pulling an object. In addition, Fraser (1998) showed that those amputees with passive or cosmetic prostheses used their devices for nonprehensile tasks on average just as frequently as those amputees with active prostheses. These results show that just because a prosthetic device is passive, or cosmetic, does not imply it is not functional.

Body-Powered Power Sources. In a body-powered device the amputee's body operates the prosthesis with its own muscular power, usually via a cable link called a *Bowden cable* (Fig. 20.10). A Bowden cable consists of two parts, an outer housing and an inner tension cable. The housing is fixed

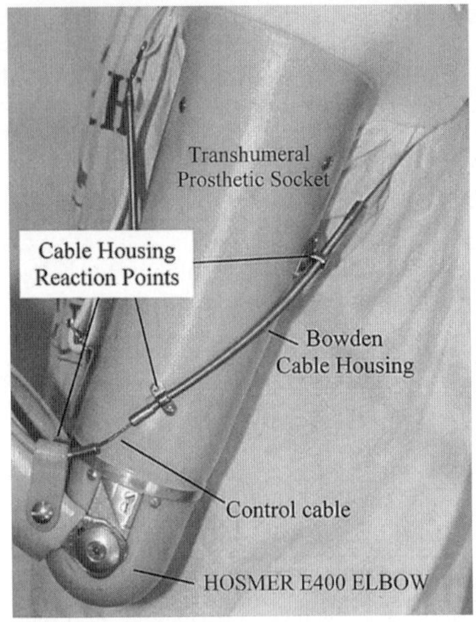

FIGURE 20.10 Photograph of how a Bowden cable is set up for use as the control cable of a transhumeral (above-the-elbow) body-powered prosthesis. The housing acts as a guide or channel for the control cable, which transmits forces developed by a harnessed body part, in this case the contralateral shoulder, to the prosthesis. Retainers on the housing fasten it to the prosthesis, which serve as reaction points in the transmission of force by the cable. (*Photograph courtesy of Mr. C. Heckathorne of the Northwestern University Prothetics Research Laboratory, Chicago, IL.*)

at both ends and serves as a flexible bridge between two points, maintaining a constant length regardless of any motion. The cable is free to slide within the housing.

The Raleigh Bicycle Co., UK, first introduced Bowden cables as bicycle brake actuators in the later part of the nineteenth century. They were then adopted by the fledgling aircraft industry of the early twentieth century for the control of aircraft flight surfaces. At the end of World War II, many former aircraft designers, in particular engineers at Northrop-Grumman, California, were set to the task of designing better prostheses for returning U.S. veterans. One of their more important contributions was the use of Bowden cables to operate upper-limb prostheses.

The typical prosthetic-control system consists of a Bowden cable with appropriate terminal fittings. The terminal fittings are used to attach one end of the cable to a harnessed body control point and the other end to the prosthetic component to be controlled. The housing through which the cable slides acts as a guide or channel for the transmission of force by the cable. Retainers on the housing fasten it to the prosthesis, which serve as reaction points in the transmission of force by the cable.

The basic configuration of Bowden cables has changed little over the intervening years and is still in use today. In fact, if prehensile function is the primary goal of the prosthetic fitting, the device of choice for most amputees is a body-powered, Bowden cable-operated prosthesis with a split hook-shaped terminal device. This is in spite of all the technological advances in electronics, computers, and dc motor technology that have occurred since the end of World War II.

Low technology does not imply wrong or bad technology. Ease of maintenance, ease of repair in the event of failures in the field (one can use a piece of string to get one if the control cable should break), and the intuitive understanding of pulling on one end of the cable to effect motion at the other

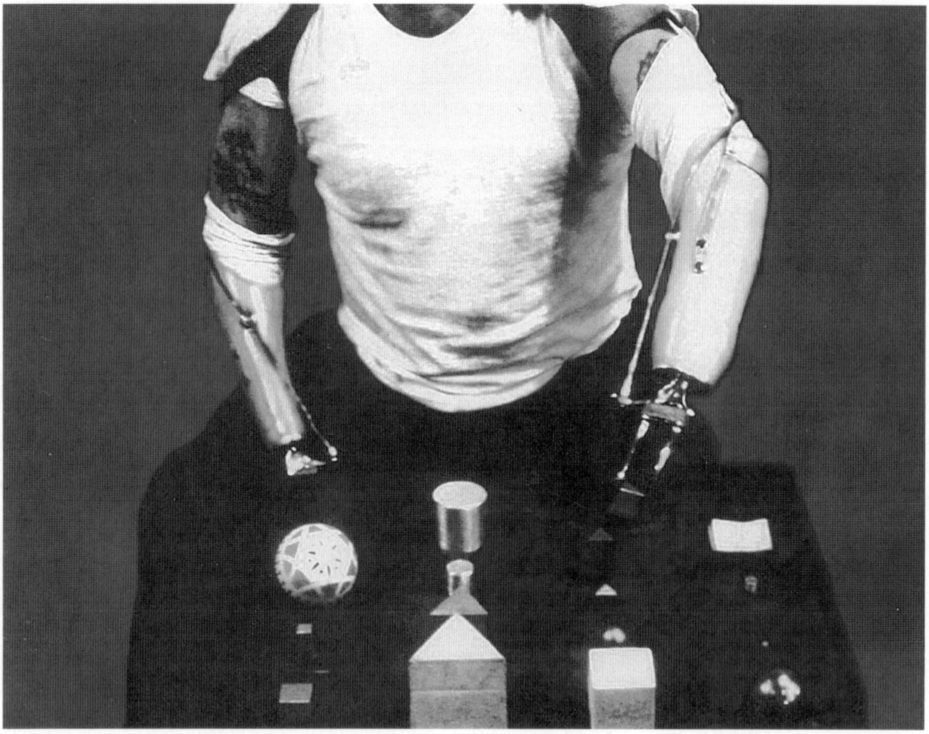

FIGURE 20.11 Photograph of a person with bilateral transradial (below-the-elbow) amputations using body-powered prostheses to perform standard object manipulation tasks during an occupational therapy session. Tasks of this nature usually take the form of pick and place trials. These trials require the subject to move objects of various sizes and shapes as quickly as possible between two different locations. This teaches the subject how to coordinate the prosthesis control while moving the terminal device. In another set of trials, the subject moves objects of various sizes and shapes as quickly as possible from one hand to the other, for the purpose of teaching bimanual dexterity. Such tasks are used for training and evaluation purposes.

are probably major reasons for the success of Bowden cables in prosthetics. These benefits are in addition to the ability of users to sense prosthesis state by the "pull" or "feel" of the control cable and harness on their skin.

For transradial (below-elbow) prostheses, only one Bowden cable is needed to open and close the terminal device (Fig. 20.11). In transhumeral (above-elbow) prostheses two Bowden cables are needed, one to lock and unlock the elbow and another to flex and extend the elbow when the elbow is unlocked or to open and close the terminal device when the elbow is locked (Fig. 20.12). Both the transradial and transhumeral prostheses use a harness worn about the shoulders to which the cables are attached.

A combination of glenohumeral flexion and shoulder abduction is the primary body-control motion used to affect terminal device opening and closing or elbow flexion and extension. Typically a total excursion of 10 cm (4 in) and upward of 222 N (50 ft · lb) of force is possible using these motions. Elbow lock control is affected by a complex shoulder motion, which involves downward rotation of the scapula combined with simultaneous abduction and slight extension of the shoulder joint. Figure 20.13 shows the basic harnessing of these cables for each case. There are many different variations on these basic harnessing schemes, depending on specific needs of the amputee. These variations and their application are described in Fryer (1992). Fryer and Michael (1992) provide an excellent overview of available body-powered components.

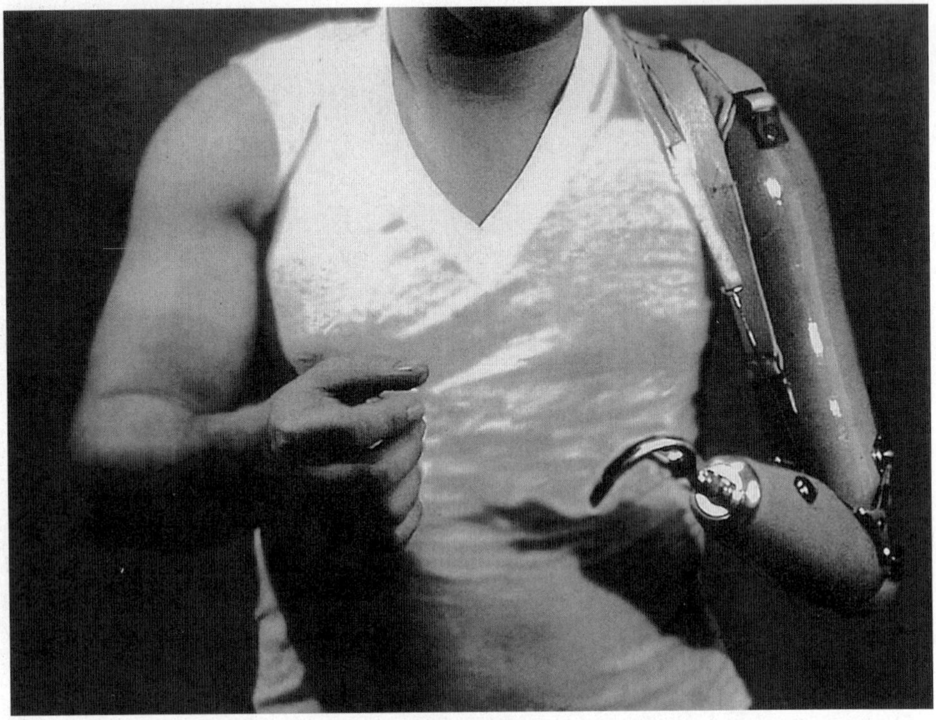

FIGURE 20.12 Photograph of a person with a unilateral transhumeral (above-the-elbow) amputation using a body-powered prosthesis. This picture clearly shows the elbow lock control cable (strap and cable on the anterior of the humeral section of the prosthesis). In a transhumeral prosthesis, this cable is needed to switch control from the elbow to the terminal device. When the elbow is locked the terminal device is under the control of the control cable; when the elbow is unlocked then the elbow is under the control of the control cable.

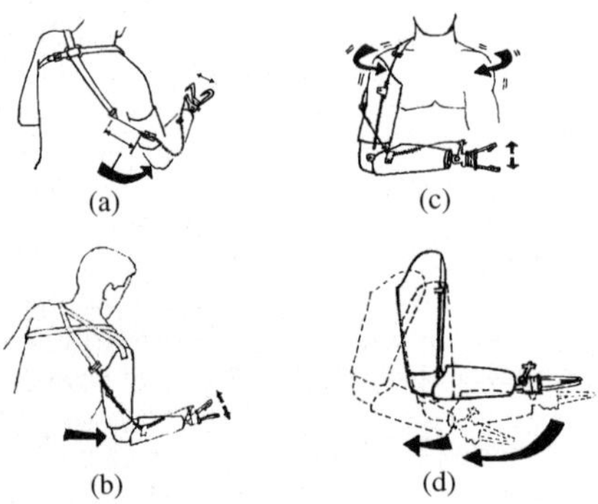

FIGURE 20.13 Schematics showing the harnessing and control motions used in both transradial and transhumeral body-powered prostheses. (*a*) Glenohumeral flexion—forward motion of the upper-arm about the shoulder. Ths schematic shows the harnessing for a transradial prosthesis. (*b*) Glenohumeral flexion for a person harnessed for a transhumeral prosthesis. (*c*) Biscapular abduction (rounding of the shoulders) used by person with either transradial or transhumeral amputations. A combination of glenohumeral flexion and biscapular abduction is the most common mode of body-powered prosthesis control. (*d*) Shoulder depression followed by glenohumeral extension is the contorl motion used by persons with transhumeral amputations to actuate the elbow lock.

TABLE 20.1 Force and Excursions for Different Body-Powered Control Sites for Average-Strength Male Amputees

	Force available		Excursion available	
Control source	N	ft · lb	mm	in
Arm flexion	280	63	53	2.10
Shoulder flexion	271	61	57	2.25
Arm extension	247	56	58	2.30

Source: Taylor, 1954.

Typical forces and excursions for different body-powered control sources for an average amputee can be found in Table 20.1. As can be seen, the average amputee has fairly high magnitude sources of force and excursion. By varying the locations of the reaction points of the Bowden cable or through the use of a pulley mechanism known as a force, or excursion, amplifier force can be interchanged with excursion or vice versa; however, the total power (force times excursion) remains constant.

In prosthetics, Bowden cables come in two sizes: standard and heavy duty. The basic configuration is a standard multistranded steel cable in a standard housing. A heavy-duty user will use Spectra® cable in a heavy-duty housing. Spectra®, a registered trademark of Allied-Signal, Inc., is composed of ultra high molecular weight polyethylene fibers. Its primary use outside of prosthetics is as deep sea fishing line because it does not stretch. In addition, Spectra® is very lightweight, quiet, strong, and has a low coefficient of friction, making it an ideal alternative for numerous prosthetic applications, especially children. Unfortunately, tying Spectra® cable to components is substantially more difficult than swaging standard cable, and Spectra® may develop creep over time.

Friction is the primary cause of transmission losses in a Bowden cable. If friction is an issue, then a heavy duty housing with a Teflon Liner and a standard cable can be used. In Europe, it is common to use a perlon cable in a standard housing for light to medium users. Although Spectra®, like perlon, can be used with standard cable housings, lower friction can be achieved by using Spectra® or perlon with a heavy duty housing with a Teflon insert. This solution provides a plastic—plastic interface, which reduces friction and wear, and increases lifetime.

TIP: Bowden housings are essentially tightly wound steel spirals (tightly wound spring) and as such can be screwed into an appropriately sized hole. For standard housing, use a $^1/_8$-in drill and a No. 8-32 tap (note that this is a nonstandard drill and tap combination).

Voluntary Opening versus Voluntary Closing Devices. Body-powered hands can be either voluntary opening or voluntary closing. Voluntary opening devices require a closing force, exerted usually by rubber bands, to be overcome before it will open (default to close position). The maximum pinch force in a voluntary opening device is limited to the closing force exerted by the rubber bands. Typically, a standard prosthesis rubber band results in 2 ft · lb of prehension force and a good user will have anywhere from three to eight rubber bands, depending on strength and personal preference.

Voluntary closing devices require an opening force to be overcome before the terminal device will close (default to open position). Pinch force in a voluntary closing terminal device is directly proportional to the force applied to the device.

The voluntary closing principle is the closest to natural hand prehension (Fletcher, 1954). However, tension must be maintained in the control cable to hold a constant gripping force or position, just as must be applied by the human hand to maintain grasp. The natural neuromuscular mechanism has the ability to maintain grasp over long periods of time without undue strain. Automatic or manual prehension locking mechanisms have been used for this function in voluntary closing devices. A voluntary opening device does not have this problem so long as the object held can withstand the maximum closing force.

Few voluntary closing body-powered devices are currently in use due to the fact that the default position of the hand is the open position and this causes the fingers to get caught in pockets, and so on. In addition, the automatic lock mechanism used to aid in the prehension process tends to fail.

TABLE 20.2 Force and Excursions Needed to Actuate a Number of Standard Body-Powered Prosthetic Components

	Force needed		Excursion needed	
Component/operation	N	ft · lb	mm	in
Elbow flexion (no load on hook)	40	9	51	2
Prehension, APRL* voluntary closing hook	40–155	9–35	38	1.5
Prehension, Sierra two-load† voluntary opening hook	44.4, 89	10, 20	38	1.5
Elbow lock actuation	9–18	2–4	15	0.6

*The Army Prosthetics Research Laboratory (APRL).

†The Sierra two-load hook, formerly the northrop two-load hook, was a voluntary opening hook with two closing force settings. A manually controlled switch on the side of the hook moved the hook between force settings.

Source: Taylor, 1954.

The Therapeutic Recreation Systems (TRS) (Boulder, CO) range of terminal devices and the Army Prosthetic Research Laboratory (APRL) hook, which was used predominantly by muscle tunnel cineplasty amputees, are examples of successful voluntary closing devices that are available. The APRL hook has automatic locking while the TRS devices do not.

Operating requirements (force and displacement) for a number of standard body-powered prosthetic components are given in Table 20.2. Neither the Army Prosthetics Research Laboratory (APRL) hook nor the Sierra two-load hook are used much today. It is most common to find a voluntary opening split hook on current body-powered systems.

Electric Power Sources (Batteries). Battery technology, specifically rechargeable battery technology, is vital to portable electronic equipment and is driven by the billions of dollars spent by the laptop, computer, and cellular phone industries. The field of prosthetics and orthotics (P&O) sits on the sidelines and picks up anything that looks like it could be of use. In an electrically powered prosthesis, the main current draw comes from the dc motor(s) used to actuate the device. In a dc motor, the output torque is directly proportional to the amount of current drawn. Motor use in prostheses is not continuous but is intermittent. Consequently, it is important not only to know how much current a battery can provide, but also how fast the battery can provide it.

The maximum amount of current drawn by a dc motor is the "stall" current. This is the current drawn by the motor when it is fully "on" but unable to move, such as occurs when a hand has grasped an object and the fingers can close no further. This is also the point of maximum torque output of the motor and is known as the *stall torque*. Running a dc motor in stall for extended periods of time will damage the motor. However, the stall current is the upper limit on the amount of current required by a dc motor–driven mechanism. As such the stall current determines the size of the MOSFET's (field effect transistor) and/or H-bridges used to deliver current to the motor.

Batteries are a chemical means of producing electricity, in which the choice of electrode materials is dictated by their relative location in the electrochemical series. Compounds that are at the extremes of the series are desirable. Many battery chemistries exist. Batteries are usually packages of a number of "cells" stacked in series to achieve a desired voltage. The voltage of the individual battery cells is dependent on the chemistry of the cell. The nonrechargeable off-the-shelf batteries that one buys in the store are referred to as *alkaline batteries*. In P&O, we are most interested in rechargeable batteries with solid chemistries, that is, nonliquid batteries.

Weight, capacity, and power-density are the primary selection considerations in externally powered prosthetic design applications. The most popular types of rechargeable batteries in use in prosthetics today are nickel-cadmium (NiCd), nickel-metal-hydride (NiMH), lithium-ion (Li-ion), and lithium polymer (Li-poly). Lithium (Li-ion and Li-poly) is fast becoming the chemistry of choice because of its high capacity-to-size (weight) ratio and low self-discharge characteristics.

The amount of time it takes to discharge a battery depends on the battery capacity, C, expressed in milliamp hours (mAh) (more is better) and the amount of current drawn by the load. Battery charge and discharge currents are normalized with respect to battery capacity and are expressed in terms of "C-rate." C-rate = C/1 hour, for example, a 150-mAh battery has a C-rate of 150 mA. The current corresponding to 1C is 150 mA, and for 0.1C, 15 mA. For a given cell type, the behavior of cells with varying capacity is similar at the same c-rate. More in-depth information about batteries can be found in the *Handbook of Batteries* (Linden, 1995). Recent advances at a nanoscale level have allowed lithium-ion batteries to rapidly discharge large amounts of current (A123 Systems, Watertown, Massachusetts). Although these batteries are not denser than conventional lithium-ion batteries, they are more suitable for short bursts of large current.

These are the important measures of performance in the cell phone and laptop industries because once the device is switched "on," the load current remains fairly constant. The *discharge rate* is an important measure for prosthetics applications because it is a measure of the rate at which current can be delivered to the load. It is the maximum allowable load or discharge current, expressed in units of C-rate. The higher the discharge rate, the faster a battery can meet the demand for current.

The *self-discharge rate* is the rate at which a battery discharges with no-load. Li-ion are a factor of two better than NiCd or NiMH. The number of charge and discharge cycles is the average number of time a battery can be discharged and then recharged and is a measure of the service life. For prosthetics applications, a battery ought to provide at least a day of use before needing to be recharged; thus, the average life expectancy for a rechargeable battery in prosthetics use should be about 3 years. Table 20.3 tabulates these quantities for the chemistries of interest.

The problem of *memory* that one hears about in association with NiCd batteries is relatively rare. It can occur during cyclic discharging to a definite fixed level and subsequent recharging. Upon discharging the cell potential drops several tenths of a volt below normal and remains there for the rest of the discharge. The total ampere-hour capacity of the cell is not significantly affected. Memory usually disappears if the cell is almost fully discharged (*deep discharged*) and then recharged a couple of times. In practice memory is often not a problem because NiCd battery packs are rarely discharged to the same level before recharging. Environmental concerns exist regarding the proper disposal of NiCd batteries because of the hazardous metal content. NiMH and Li-ion do not contain significant amounts of pollutants, but nevertheless, some caution should be used in their disposal. Discharge profiles for these three popular types of batteries are shown in Fig. 20.14.

Slow charging (charging time greater than 12 h) is straightforward for all battery chemistries and can be accomplished using a current source. Charge termination is not critical, but a timer is sometimes used to end slow charging of NiMH batteries. Li-ion slow-chargers should have a voltage limit to terminate charging of Li-ion batteries. *Trickle charging* is the charging current a cell can accept continually without affecting service life. A safe trickle charge for NiMH batteries is typically 0.03C. Fast charging (charge time less than 3 h) is more involved. Fast-charging circuits must be tailored

TABLE 20.3 Figures-of-Merit Used to Characterize the Common Rechargeable Battery Chemistries in Use Today

	Nickel-cadmium (NiCd)	Nickel-metal-hydride (NiMH)	Lithium-ion (Li-ion)	Lithium-metal (LiM)*
Cell voltage (V)	1.2	1.25	3.6	3.0
Energy density [watthour/liter (Wh/L)]	45	55	100	140
Energy density [watthour/kilogram (Wh/kg)]	150	180	225	300
Cost [$/watthour ($/Wh)]	0.75–1.5	1.5–3.0	2.5–3.5	1.4–3.0
Self-discharge rate (%/month)	25	20–25	8	1–2
Discharge rate	>10C	<3C	<2C	<2C
Charge/discharge cycles	1000	800	1000	1000
Temperature range (°C)	−10–+50	−10–+50	−10–+50	−30–+55
Memory effect	Yes	No	No	No
Environmental concerns	Yes	No	No	No

*Lithium-metal chemistry is a new chemistry that is not yet widely available.
The values shown here are based on an AA size cell.
Source: Kester and Buxton, 1998, p. 5.3.

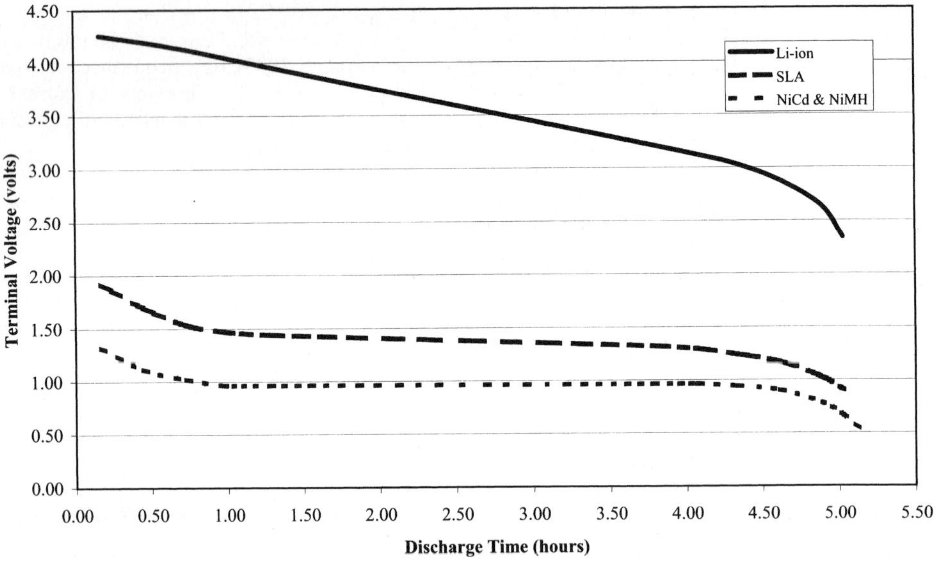

FIGURE 20.14 Discharge profiles of different kinds of batteries. A discharge current of 0.2C was used in each case. NiCd and NiMH batteries have a relatively flat profile while Li-ion batteries have a nearly linear discharge profile. This feature is useful when designing "fuel gauges" for Li-ion batteries. (*Generated using data supplied in: Kester and Buxton 1998.*)

to the battery chemistry and provide both reliable charging and charge termination. Overcharging can damage the battery by causing overheating and catastrophic outgassing of the electrolyte. The gas released from any outgassing may be dangerous and corrosive. In some instances, overcharging may cause the battery to explode (Kester and Buxton, 1998).

Standard operating voltages used in prosthetics are 4.8, 6, 9, and 12 V, depending on the manufacturer and component to be driven. All Otto Bock System 2000 children's hands (Fig. 20.15) (Otto Bock Orthopedic Industry Inc., Duderstadt, Germany) run off 4.8 V and will not run at higher voltages. Otto Bock adult hands (Fig. 20.7), Steeper hands (Fig. 20.6*c*) (RSLSteeper, Rochester, UK), VASI hands and elbows [Variety Ability System Inc. (VASI), Toronto, Canada], and Hosmer NYU elbow (Hosmer-Dorrance Corp., Campbell, California) are specified to run off 6 V but can sometimes be run at higher voltages to boost performance. The Hosmer NU-VA Synergetic Prehensor (Fig. 20.6*b*) and Motion Control ProControl system (Motion Control, Inc., Salt lake City, Utah) use 9 V. All three powered elbows, including the Motion Control Utah Arm, LTI Digital Arm [Liberating Technology, Inc. (LTI), Holliston, Massachusetts], and Otto Bock Dynamic Arm, run off 12 V, while Motion Control's electric hand is specified to run on any voltage between 6 and 18 V. The Touch Bionics i-Limb Hand runs off 7.2 V. In general, electric hands use 6 V while electric elbows use 12 V. Elbows need the extra voltage so that they can have a useful live-lift capacity. Typical currents are 2 to 3 A for hand mechanisms and 9 to 12 A for some of the brushless dc motors used in elbow prostheses.

The preponderance of 6 V for electric hands is due to the dominance and history of Otto Bock in the field of prosthetics. Otto Bock was one of the first companies to produce an electric hand with its associated electronics and power source in the early 1970s. Their standard battery is the 757B8 five-cell NiCd battery pack, where each cell has a voltage of 1.2 V. This is a custom-designed battery pack and battery holder. The battery holder is designed to be laminated into the prosthetic socket so that batteries can be easily interchanged should one discharge completely during use. Even if the battery chemistry has changed, this battery holder's form has been around for many years. The disadvantage of a custom form is that if the battery dies in the field and the user does not have any spares, then they are stuck without a working component. Liberating Technology Inc. and Motion Control elbows use custom battery packs, while the Hosmer-Dorrance elbows use packs made up of off-the-shelf AA rechargeable batteries (Fig. 20.16).

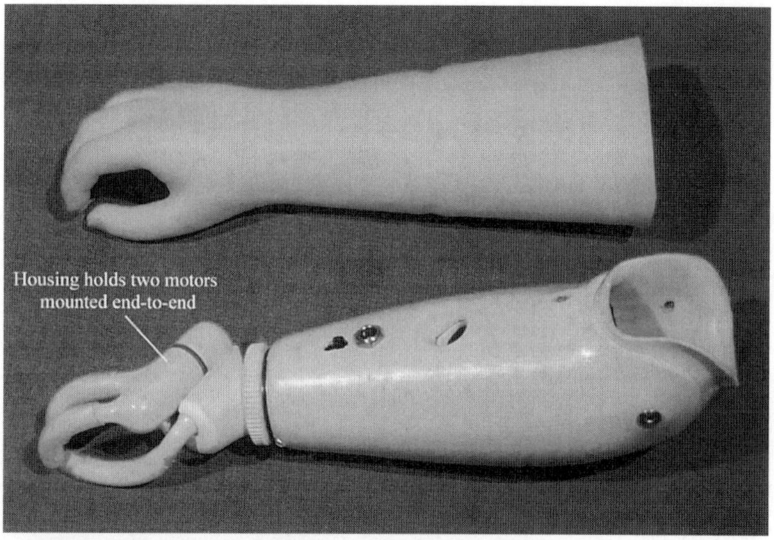

FIGURE 20.15 Otto Bock System 2000 children's Hand (Otto Bock Orthopedic Industry Inc., Duderstadt, Germany). This mechanism uses two gear motors attached end-to-end that operate using the principle of synergetic prehension. Notice this hand does not use a liner. The cosmetic glove is pulled directly over the mechanism. This is because for a child's hand the forces are not as high as for an adult mechanism and the tips will not punch through the glove at the lower grip force.

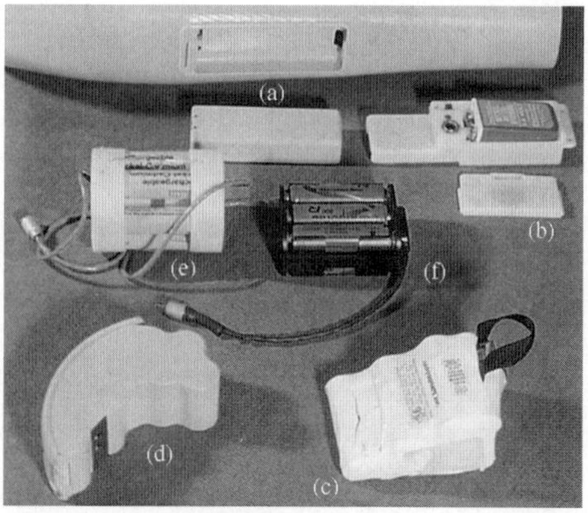

FIGURE 20.16 Battery packs is prosthetics come in all different shapes and sizes. (*a*) Standard Otto Bock (Otto Bock Orthopedic Industry Inc., Duderstadt, Germany) NiCd battery pack and holder. (*b*) The Hosmer-Dorrance (Hosmer-Dorrance Corp., Campbell, California) battery holder for a standard 9-V transistor battery (NiCd or NiMH). (*c*) Liberating Technology (Liberating Technology Inc., Holliston, Massachusetts) NiCD battery pack for the Boston Elbow II. (*d*) Motion Control's (Motion Control, Salt Lake City, Utah) custom battery pack for the Utah Arm, and (*e*) and (*f*) Hosmer-Dorrance (Hosmer-Dorrance Corp., Campbell, California) NiCd battery packs for their NY-Hosmer Elbow. Battery packs (*c*), (*e*), and (*f*) consist of multiple AA rechargeable batteries packaged together to create a battery of the desired output voltage and capacity.

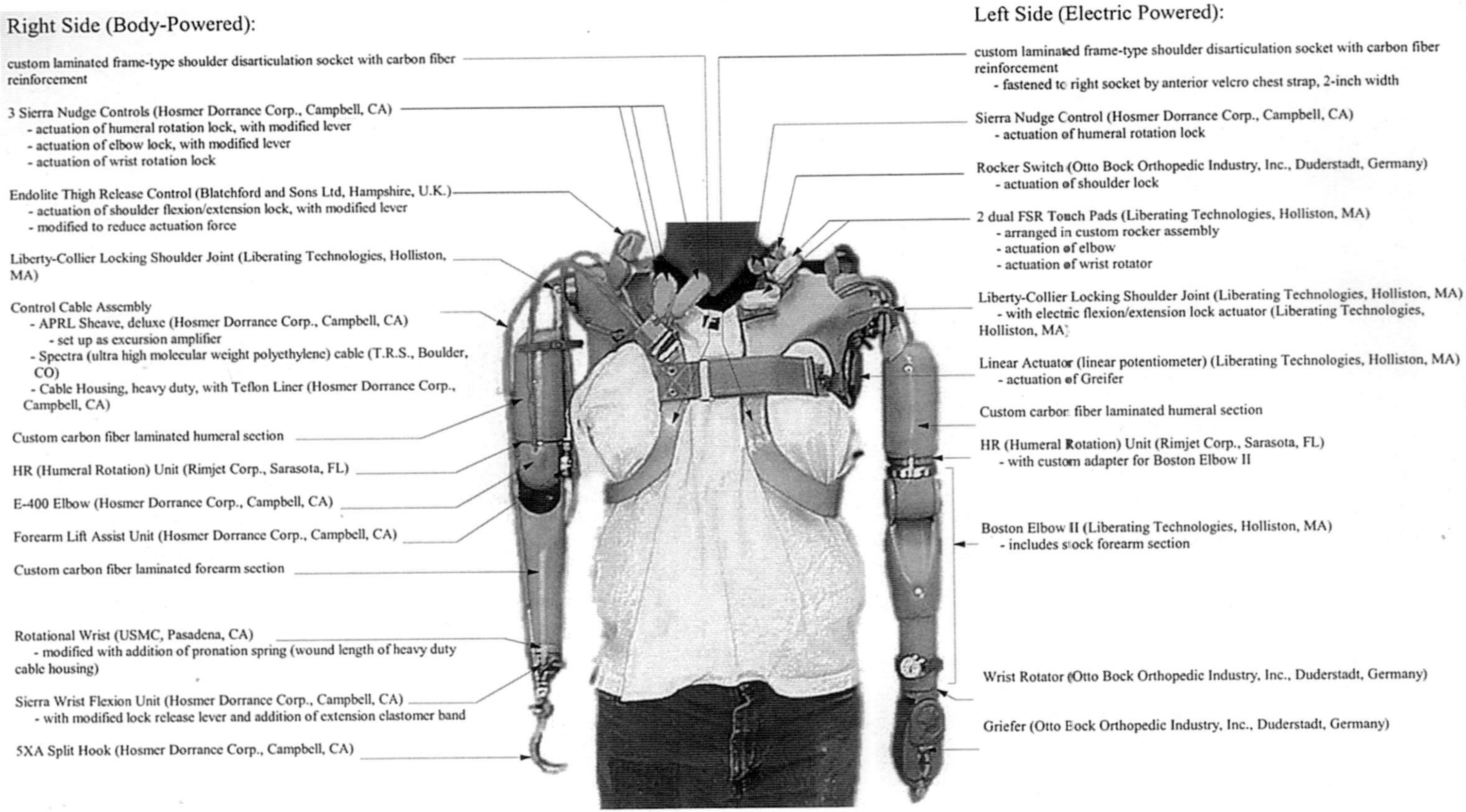

FIGURE 20.17 This photograph shows a person with bilateral shoulder disarticulations who has been fitted bilaterally using hybrid prostheses. The right side is fitted with a body-powered, single-control cable, four function system. This is a sequential control system in which the control cable controls elbow flexion-extension, wrist rotation, wrist flexion, or terminal device opening and closing, depending on which components are locked or unlocked by the chin-actuated mechanical switches. Chin-actuated levers lock and unlock a shoulder flexion-extension unit, a humeral rotator, an elbow, and a wrist rotator. A lever on the wrist locks and unlocks a wrist flexion unit. The terminal device is a voluntary-opening split hook. Shoulder flexion-extension and humeral rotation are under gravity control once they are unlocked. The left side, or electric-powered side, still uses mechanical chin-actuated levers to lock and unlock a shoulder flexion-extension joint and a humeral rotator, otherwise the remaining components are externally powered. The arm has an electric-powered elbow and wrist rotator that are controlled by chin movement against two rocker switches. Pulling on a liner potentiometer actuates the powered prehensor. Output speed, or force, of the prehensor is proportional to how much the transducer is pulled. For this system the body-powered side is used as the dominant arm, with the electric-powered side assisting in a nondominant role. The prostheses are used for activities of daily living. This fitting highlights a number of important issues that are discussed further in the text.

Our laboratory's preference is to use rechargeable batteries in a 9-V transistor battery form. This enables the prosthesis to be recharged overnight, while a standard 9-V transistor battery form allows commercially available off-the-shelf 9-V alkaline batteries to be easily purchased and used should the rechargeable battery run out of charge unexpectedly. Motion Control sells an Otto Bock battery case that has been modified to accommodate a standard 9-V transistor battery.

Hybrid Systems. When body-powered and externally powered systems are linked together, they are called *hybrid systems*. Hybrid systems are used most frequently with persons who have high-level amputations, that is, amputations above the elbow, or who have bilateral arm amputations. Such systems can provide the user with the high gripping and/or high lifting capacities of powered systems and the fine control of body-powered system. For example, providing a person with bilateral limb loss at the shoulder level with a body-powered limb on one side and with an electric-powered limb on the other side decouples the limbs (Fig. 20.17). The body motions used to operate the body-powered side do not influence the state of the powered limb and vice versa.

dc Electric Motors. By far the most common actuator for electric-powered prostheses is the dc electric motor with some form of transmission (Fig. 20.18). Although there is much research into other electrically powered actuator technologies, such as shape memory alloys and electro-active polymers, none is to the point where it can compete against the dc electric motor. A review of the available and developing actuator technologies with their associated advantages and disadvantages as well as their power and force densities can be found in Hannaford and Winters (1990) and Hollerbach et al. (1991). In both these reviews, biological muscle is used as the benchmark for comparison of these technologies.

For electric-powered prosthetic hand mechanisms, a coreless, brushless dc motor with a fitted gear head transmission is the actuator of choice. For elbows, coreless or brushless dc motors and a transmission are used. Brushless dc motors are becoming more common now that both the motor and its electronics are small enough to be accommodated in prosthetic components. Although brushless motors require much more complicated control electronics, their use is justified because they have substantially higher performance than their brushed counterparts. In addition, recent advances in surface-mounted integrated circuit (IC) technology greatly facilitate the design of controllers for these motors. A broad range of driver and controller ICs are available in surface-mount forms from companies like Texas Instruments, International Rectifier, Allegro, Motorola, ST Electronics, Vishay-Siliconix, Zetex, and others, and application notes explaining the use of these

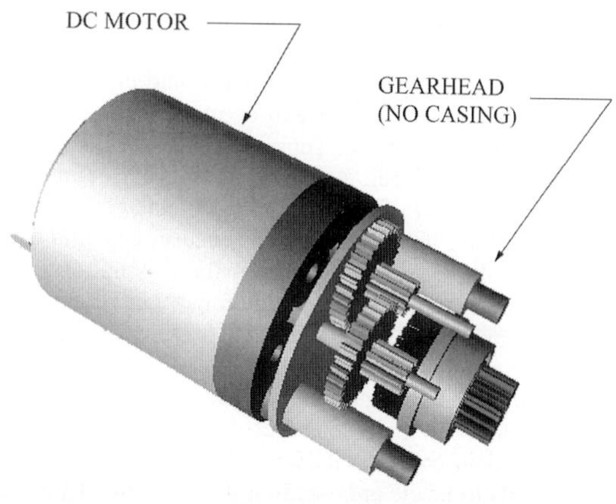

FIGURE 20.18 Drawing of a dc motor and gear head. The high output speed of small dc motors must be converted into a usable torque in order to build functional components. This transformation of speed into torque is performed by a gear train (shown in the figure without its casing).

chips are readily available on company web pages. Unfortunately, the connection between these chips and the motors is rarely straightforward, unless the same company manufactures both components. Both the chip and the motor have 2 sets of 3 wires, resulting in 36 possible permutations. Of these, six combinations may work, but only one may work smoothly. Until motor companies and chip manufacturers standardize the process, testing each permutation is likely to be the fastest way to obtaining the proper connection.

Sizing a dc Motor for Maximum Performance. In general, because there is no actuator technology that can match muscle tissue's speed and force capabilities for a given weight and volume, one chooses the largest motor-gear-head combination that will fit within the physical constraints of the mechanism being designed. When one discusses maximizing performance, one is talking about maximizing output speed and output torque to attain physiological speeds and torques.

The key issue to keep in mind when choosing a motor is that one trades output speed for output torque and vice versa (Fig. 20.19). Output power ($P = F \times V$) is constant. Choice of gear ratio depends on the no-load speed and stall torque of the motor selected, as well as the desired output speed and torque of the mechanism. One must also allow for the overall efficiency of the gear head and the maximum allowable intermittent output torque for a given gear head. The Micro Mo catalog provides worked examples on how to choose the correct motor and gear head for a particular output speed and force requirement (Faulhaber Micro Mo Application Notes). The maximum allowable intermittent output torque is a function of the tooth strength (this is a material property) of the gears and as such is an upper limit on the torque a particular gear can handle. So although a particular gear ratio might suggest that the output torque is attainable, the gears in the drivetrain might not be physically able to handle the loads placed on them. A further constraint is to ensure that the motor-gear-head maximum axial load will not be exceeded. This is usually not an issue when using spur gears on the output but if a worm gear, or lead screw, or some other rotation-to-linear conversion mechanism is used, then this parameter must be taken into consideration and thrust bearing used to protect the gear head, if necessary. A good reference is the *Handbook of Small Electric Motors* (Yeadon and Yeadon, 2001).

Manufacturers will often offer motors with different magnet materials. To maximize the performance (force-speed output) of a particular size of motor, choose the "rare earth" version. Also, when specifying the nominal drive voltage of the motor, consider deliberately overvoltaging the motor to boost overall performance at the cost of decreased efficiency. This can be done because prosthesis use is intermittent in nature. A nominal 6-V motor can be run at 9-V, yielding a 50 percent increase in output speed and torque. Care must be taken, however, because the stall current will also increase. Prolonged exposure to increased stall current can damage the motor unless the rise in current, as the motor stalls, is detected and the supply voltage cut off, or the current limited. Many motor manufactures are willing to optimize the windings of the motor for a given application. This easy procedure often results in improved performance and efficiency of the motor for a given application.

Current flowing in the motor can be monitored using a number of different ICs or power FETs available from any number of suppliers. These devices include current shunt ICs (Maxim, Texas Instruments, Zetex, Micrel, Allegro), sense FETs (Fairchild Semiconductor), HEX sense power FETs (International Rectifier), and fault-protected switches (fancy MOSFETs) (Micrel) to name but a few. Current shunt ICs are common because they find use in dc-to-dc converters; consequently, a large number of different manufacturers make them in many different forms and flavors (Fig. 20.20).

Although the output power of a motor might remain constant, how that power is used, that is, whether all the power is used to generate high force at low speed or high speed at low force, is up to the designer. Since there is no one motor small enough to be placed in an artificial hand that can meet both the speed and force requirements (even with overvoltaging), other techniques must be employed to increase hand mechanism speed of opening and closing and grip force. Two techniques are currently employed in commercially available prosthetic prehensors to increase the performance of prosthetic hands to levels approaching those of the physiological hand.

The first technique is to use a single large motor and an automatic transmission. In this case the motor opens and closes the hand in a high-speed, low-force gear ratio. When the hand closes against an object, the rise in force (as detected by an internal spring) automatically triggers the transmission to switch into a high-force, low-speed mode that allows the hand mechanism to build up prehension/pinch

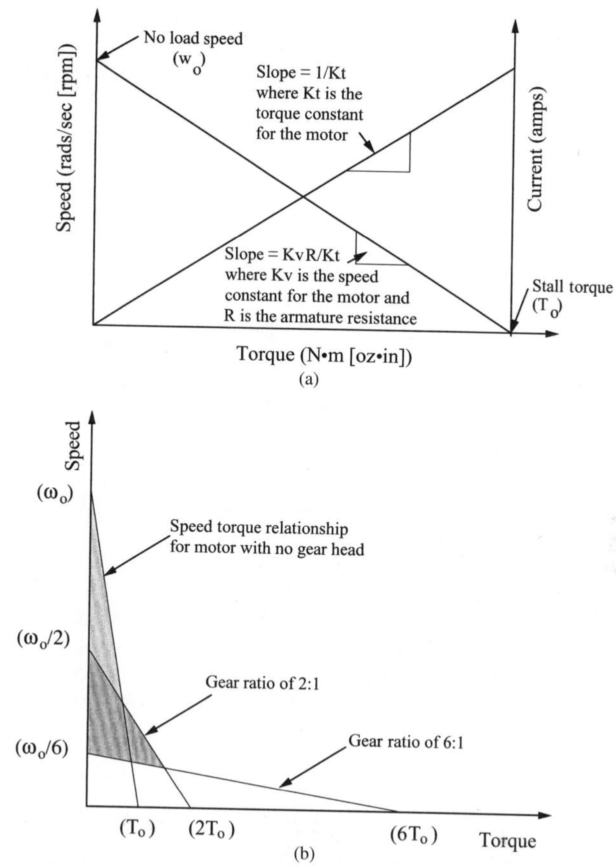

FIGURE 20.19 (*a*) Typical speed-torque and current-torque relationships for a dc motor. The key issue is that stall torque times no-load speed is constant (stall torque × no-load speed = const.) regardless of the ratio of the gear train driven by the motor. The main points of interest on this curve are no-load speed (outpur speed of the motor when running without load), the stall torque (torque generaed by the motor when fully "ON" but unable to move), and the area under the curve which is the total power available to the motor. Typical units are included in brackets—imperial equivalents are in the square brackets (careful use of the correct conversion factors is required when working with imperial units). (*b*) Adding a gear head to the motor output changes the no-load speed and stall torque of the drivetrain, but the area under the new speed-torque relationships remains the same as for the motor without the gear head (assuming a lossless gear head, that is, 100 percent efficient). One trades no-load speed for stall torque and vice versa but the total available power remains the same.

force. The main disadvantage of these mechanisms is associated with tightly grasped objects. In this instance, during opening, a perceptible amount of time appears to elapse before the hand visibly opens. This is because time must be allowed for the force built up during the grasping cycle to drop below the force threshold where the hand automatically switches from high force, low speed to low force, high speed. So although the hand is opening, the gear ratio is such that little motion occurs until the transmission switches into the high-speed mode. To user, this time spent "unwinding the hand" appears as if nothing is happening in response to the open command. A further disadvantage of automatic

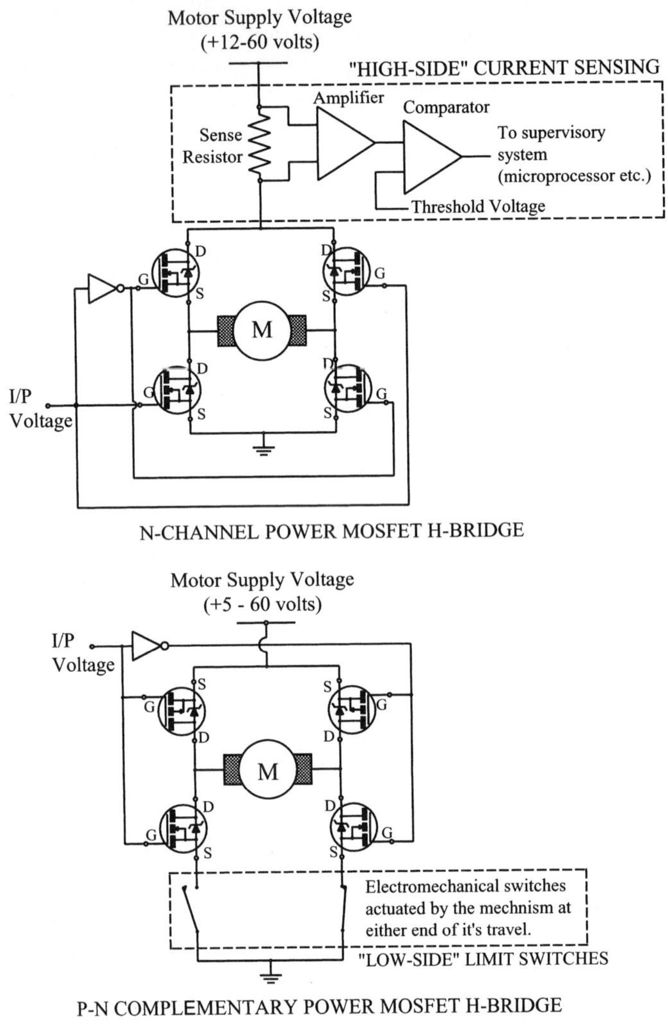

FIGURE 20.20 Diagram shows a full *n*-channel and *pn* (complementary)-channel H-bridges with their associated control. It is important to notice that for the *n*-channel H-bridge, *diagonally* opposite *n*-FETs are controlled as a pair; while for the *pn* H-bridge, FETs on the *same side* of the bridge are controlled as a pair. Also notice how the *p*-FET is wired as compared with the *n*-FET in terms of their drain and source connections. The use of the inverter symbol is to highlight that both sides of the bridge are never on at the same time, and in fact, break-before-make switching ought to be used to prevent current transients during the switching process. An implementation of high-side current monitoring is shown on the *n*-channel H-bridge while an implementation of limit switch protection of the motor is shown on the *pn* complementary H-bridge. (See text for further discussion.)

transmissions is that they are mechanically complex and are often beyond the means of the individual to design in a form compact enough for use in hand prostheses. The Otto Bock range of system electric hands for adults has used and refined its automatic transmission for many years, to the point where their design is a marvel of compactness and robustness (Fig. 20.7). The Motion Control hand, which owes much of its mechanical design to the Otto Bock hands, also uses an automatic transmission.

A variation of this design is the continuously variable transmission (CVT) which optimizes the power or efficiency of the gear for a given speed/torque. A CVT may be thought of a two-stage transmission, but with the capability to have an intermediate ratio as well. The Otto Bock Dynamic arm uses a CVT. CVTs do not suffer as much as two-stage transmissions from an unwinding delay.

Synergetic Prehension. The second technique is to use multiple smaller motors, configured for what Childress (1973) called *synergetic prehension.* In synergetic prehension, one motor is geared for high speed at low force and another is geared for high force at low speed. A simple synergetic prehensor consists of two motors, which open and close a split hook (Fig. 20.21*a*). One motor gives one tine of the hook high speed and excursion but little force (fast-side), the other motor gives the other tine of the hook high force but little speed and excursion (force-side). In this way the motors work in synergetic prehension to boost overall performance (Fig. 20.21*b*).

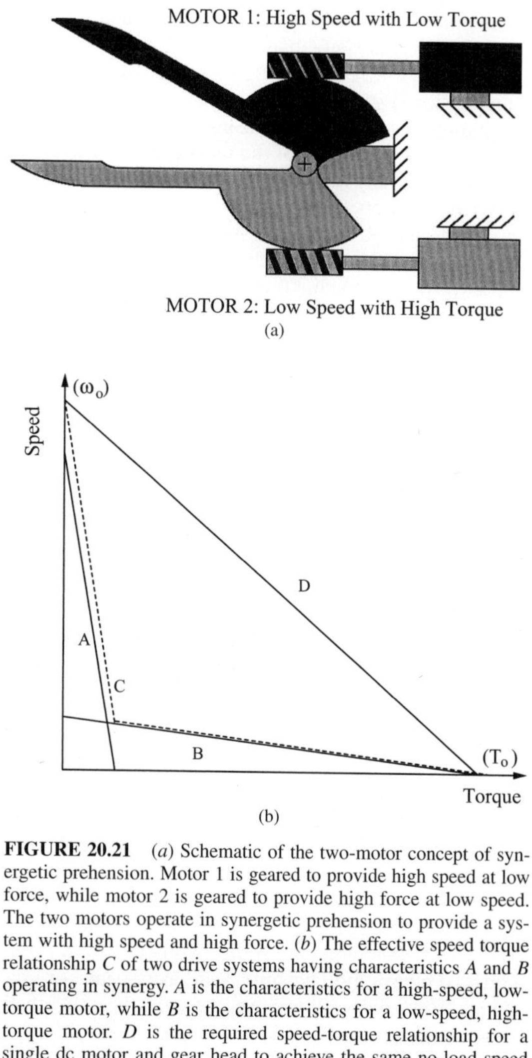

FIGURE 20.21 (*a*) Schematic of the two-motor concept of synergetic prehension. Motor 1 is geared to provide high speed at low force, while motor 2 is geared to provide high force at low speed. The two motors operate in synergetic prehension to provide a system with high speed and high force. (*b*) The effective speed torque relationship *C* of two drive systems having characteristics *A* and *B* operating in synergy. *A* is the characteristics for a high-speed, low-torque motor, while *B* is the characteristics for a low-speed, high-torque motor. *D* is the required speed-torque relationship for a single dc motor and gear head to achieve the same no-load speed and stall torque as the synergetic system.

The principle of *synergetic prehension* stems from Childress' (1973) observation that the act of grasping an object usually requires little real work. When an object is grasped, a force is exerted with very little excursion, while excursion of the grasping fingers usually occurs in space and requires very little force. In both cases, the work involved is minimal. The exception is grasping a compliant object where both force and excursion are required (e.g., squeezing a lemon). This condition, however, is not the usual case in prosthetics. Synergetic prehension can be readily implemented using multiple motors that operate together or in "synergy." Each synergetic motor pair controls a single DOF and has its own synergetic motor controller. The combination of the synergetic controller and synergetic motor pair allows it to be treated like a single motor. Placing a voltage across the input lines of the synergetic controller will drive the motors in the synergetic motor pair. The polarity of this voltage determines the direction the motors in the pair will rotate. Drive signals in the form of either pulse-width-modulated (PWM) signals for proportional speed and force control or on/off signals for switch or single speed control can be used.

The Hosmer-Dorrance NU-VA Synergetic Prehensor was developed using this theory and achieved angular velocities in excess of 3 rad/s and prehension forces greater than 20 ft · lb (89 N) using a small 9-V transistor battery (Fig. 20.6*b*). The Otto Bock System 2000 children's hands (Fig. 20.15) and the RSLSteeper Powered Gripper (RSLSteeper, UK) also use the principle of synergetic prehension (Fig. 20.6*c*). The main disadvantage associated with synergetic systems is the use of multiple motors. More motors means more parts that can fail in addition to, which the motor and its gear head tend to be, some of the most expensive components in a hand mechanism.

Not all commercially available hands use automatic transmissions or multiple motors operating in synergy. VASI's [Variety Ability System Inc. (VASI), Canada] range of children's hands, Centri AB's (Sweden) hands, and RSLSteeper's Adult Electric Hands (RSLSteeper, UK) are all examples of single motor designs with a fixed gear ratio. Typical performance for these devices is correspondingly lower [35 N (8 ft · lb) pinch, 10 cm/s (4 in/s) speed] than typical performance for those prehensors that utilize synergy or automatic transmissions [80 N (18 ft · lb) pinch, 11 cm/s (4.3 in/s) speed].

All hands need some form of "back-lock" mechanism to prevent the fingers from being forced open or "back-driven" once power is removed. This is so a hand mechanism will hold its position, or applied force, once the control signal is removed. Although this is nonphysiological, that is, muscles must keep contracting to maintain a position or an applied force, this preserves power. Synergetic mechanisms need a back-lock mechanism to prevent the "force-side" from back driving the "speed-side" in addition to maintaining applied force in the absence of power.

The RSLSteeper Electric Hands use a worm gear for this purpose. A worm gear is inherently nonbackdrivable. The VASI hands, the NU-VA Synergetic prehensor, and the LTI Digital Arm all use variations on a roller clutch (back-lock) first used in ViennaTone hands of the 1950s (Fig. 20.22). Locking occurs when a cam inside the mechanism wedges a roller(s) between itself and the outside cylindrical surface in response to an external torque. Driving the input shaft from the motor-side, causes the cam move away from the roller(s), allowing the roller(s) to move away from the outside surface, thus freeing up the mechanism. These roller clutches can resist external torques in either direction or only one direction, depending on the number and position of the roller(s) and shape of the cam. The location of these roller clutches involves a compromise. Placing them closer to the motor reduces the amount of backlash they introduce, but also substantially increases the inertia of the system, resulting in less responsive movements. The issue is magnified because a given gear ratio of N amplifies the inertia of the roller-clutch by N^2. As such, roller clutches should be placed as far away from the motor as possible while maintaining an acceptable limit of backlash and being capable of resisting the maximum force expected on the device. *Machinery's Handbook* (Oberg et al., 2000) is a good reference on different types of mechanisms and all issues pertaining to the design and machining of mechanical components, including material properties, tooling, machining, manufacturing, gearing, threading, fasteners, and the likes.

Back-locks are also found in some prosthetic elbows [Boston Digital Arm, (LTI MA), Otto Bock body-powered elbow and Dynamic Arm] as a means of holding elbow position in the absence of a drive signal. This ability allows users to park their prosthetic arm at any desired position and then remove (decouple) themselves from the arm's control.

The Otto Bock body-powered elbow mechanism and electric Dynamic Arm use a spring-like clamp that locks down onto a shaft when twisted in one direction but opens to release a shaft when

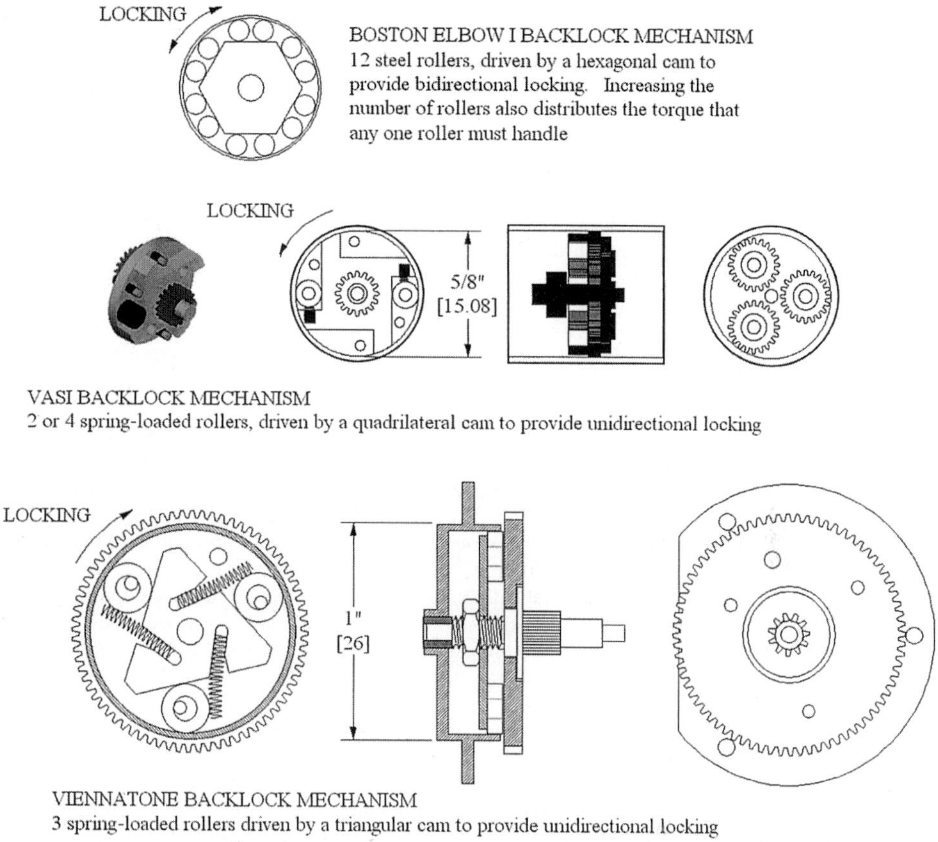

FIGURE 20.22 Back-lock mechanisms or roller clutches/brakes. The drawing shows three variations on a back-lock (roller clutch/brake) mechanism first used in the Viennatone Hands of the 1960s. Back locks find extensive use in prosthetic components because the components must often hold their position in the absence of power even in the presence of externally applied forces. Locking occurs when a cam inside the mechanism wedges a roller(s) between itself and the outside cylindrical surface in response to an external torque. Depending on the component, this ability to resist external loads can be in one or both directions. In synergetic mechanisms, the back lock prevents the high-speed, low-force side from being back driven, or forced open, by the high-force, low-speed side. The Boston Elbow I (Liberating Technology Inc., Holliston, Massachusetts) has a hexagon-shaped roller cam to provide bidirectional locking. VASI hands (Variety Ability Systems Inc., Toronto, Canada) has a quadrilateral cam that provides unidirectional locking, and the NU-VA Synergetic prehensor (Hosmer-Dorrance Corp. Campbell, California) uses a triangular cam to provide unidirectional locking. The NU-VA Synergetic prehensor back lock is very similar to the original Vienna tone design.

twisted in the other. This is a unidirectional mechanism whose main advantage is simplicity. A similar mechanism can be found in some children's bicycles where the child backpedals to brake the bike. A disadvantage of this type of mechanism is that over time the lock can slip because of wear and tear of the spring lock on the elbow shaft.

Electric Power Distribution. The torque output of a dc electric motor is linearly related to the amount of current the motor can handle. The limiting factor is usually heat. Current flow in the windings of the motor generates heat. If the heat in a motor can be dissipated fast enough, then the motor is able to handle more current. The same issue applies to the electronic components used to switch the direction of currents used to control the motor. In order to drive the motor, an H-bridge, generally made up of four power MOSFETs, is usually employed to direct current to the motor under the direction of a controller. As a rule, the higher the current, the larger the MOSFETs in the H-bridge must be to handle the current and to dissipate the heat generated.

The important issues from a prosthetics standpoint for the selection and/or design of bridge circuits are that they should be as small as possible and consume as little power as possible. In general, one wants as much of the battery's power as possible to be directed to drive the mechanism motors, rather than expending it running the prosthesis/bridge controller. *An empirical rule of thumb based on experience in our laboratory is that no more than 5 percet of the available power should be used to power the controller circuitry.*

MOSFET H-bridges come in two basic configurations: *n*-channel half-bridge and *p*- and *n*-channel (complementary half-bridge) (Fig. 20.23). Simplicity of the MOSFETs gate drive is the main advantage of the *p*- and *n*-complementary half-bridge. When an *n*-channel MOSFET is used for the high-side (or "upper") switch, the gate drive signal requires level shifting, resulting in increased complexity and cost. However, most power IC processes are optimized for *n*-channel devices. Also *n*-channel power MOSFETs (*n*-FETs) are more efficient than *p*-channel power MOSFETs (*p*-FETs) in terms of die size for a given current and voltage. For a given breakdown voltage, rating a *p*-FET can be 2.5 to 4 times the area of a comparable *n*-channel device.

The H-bridge and/or MOSFETs are some of the larger components required in the electronics used to control a prosthetic mechanism (Fig. 20.20). Surface-mount technology is employed in prosthetics control electronics packages to reduce overall circuit size. Surface-mount IC bridges and bridge drivers are available but there is a problem. In prosthetics, the supply voltage is usually 6 to 12-V. In the field of industrial motor control, the standard operating voltage, for which all the commercially available high-current IC bridges and controllers are designed, is anywhere from 12 to 60 V. This means one must either build one's own bridge using four discrete MOSFETs and some sort of MOSFET driver. Although this appears straightforward, H-bridge design can be something of a black art, particularly if two *n*-channel half-bridges are used, and the resulting bridge can take time to get working properly and can occupy a large amount of printed circuit board (PCB) space. An alternative (Vishay-Siliconix, 1992) is to use standard motor control components and use a charge pump to boost the supply voltage to a voltage sufficient to drive both upper and lower MOSFET gates directly. The use a charge pump resolves the issue of how to drive the gate of the high side (upper) *n*-FET above the half-bridge supply to fully turn the device "on."

Another possibility would be to use a number of low current (1 A max), surface-mount, single-chip H-bridges (e.g., Vishay-Siliconix Si9986, or Zetex) and wire them in parallel. These chips use complimentary *p*- and *n*-channel half-bridges in a standard eight-pin SOIC surface-mount package and as such can be run on supply voltages ranging from 4 to 13 V and have a smaller footprint than the standard TO-220 surface-mount package used for some power MOSFETs. Also using single-chip bridges, rather than building your own, enables a prosthetics designer to benefit from the protection features incorporated into these chips. One such protection feature ensures that both sides of the bridge are never turned on together. Turning on both sides of the bridge at the same time will create a short and burnout the bridge FETs very quickly. Another common cause of FET failure is not turning the FET "on" "hard" enough (i.e., not turning the FET all the way on or off). If multiple motors are to be used in a hand mechanism, these chips are a nice solution since a multiple motor configuration will generally use smaller motors that individually do not draw very high currents. A very good introduction to, and general reference on, electronics and electronics design is the *Art of Electronics* by Horowitz and Hill (1995).

Pneumatic Power. Historically, the other major source of external power in prosthetics was pneumatic power. The major attraction of pneumatic systems for prosthetics applications is their inherent compliance, which tends to give these systems a very natural look and feel. Pneumatic actuators were employed in a number of hand and arm designs in the 1970s. Cool and van Hooreweder (1971) developed a pneumatically powered hand prosthesis with adaptive internally powered fingers. This hand could achieve good grasping with low forces because it was able to adapt to the shape of the object grasped. The Edinburgh Arm was a pneumatically powered arm, which saw limited clinical usage (Simpson, 1972). Unfortunately, this arm was mechanically complex and prone to failure. Kenworthy (1974) also designed a CO_2-powered hand for use with the Edinburgh Arm. Otto Bock

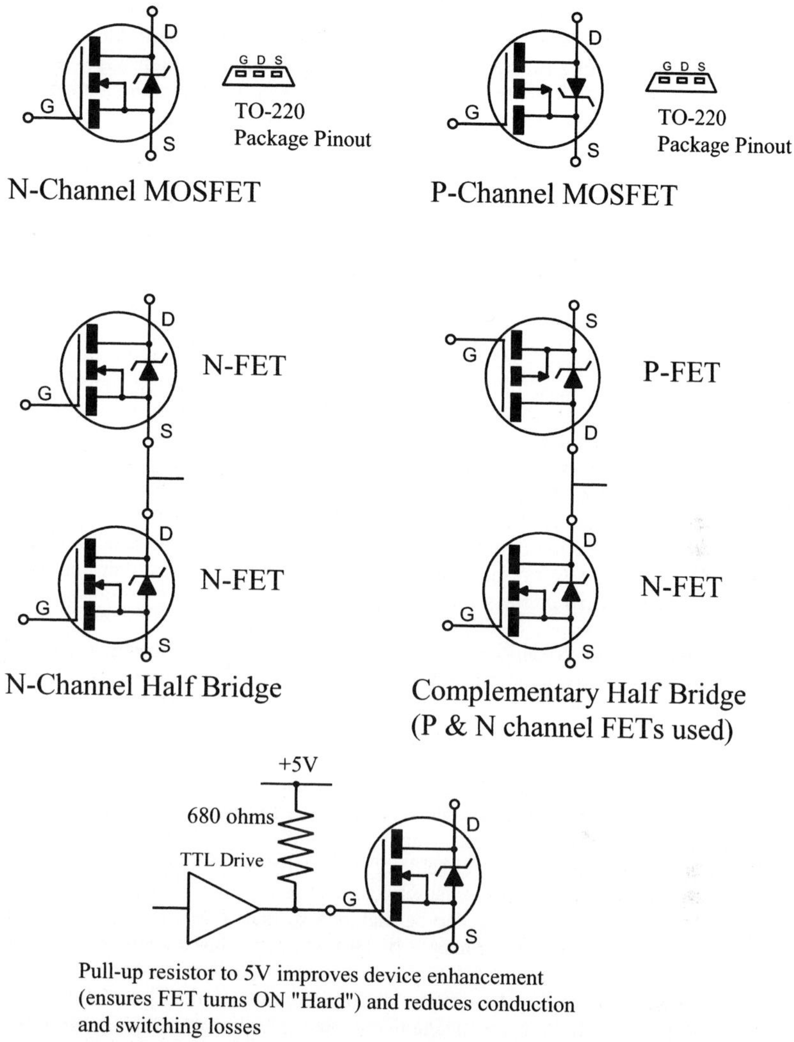

FIGURE 20.23 There are two types of power MOSFETs: *n* (top left) and *p* (top right). When used to drive a motor, or a speaker, these MOSFETs are usually configured as either an *n*-channel half-bridge (bottom left) or a complementary (*pn*) half-bridge (lower right). One talks about half-bridges because when driving multiphase motors a half-bridge is needed to drive each phase. Brushless motors need three half-bridges while dc motors need two. Oftentimes a logic circuit with logic circuit voltage levels (5 V) is used to drive the bridge FETs. To ensure that the FET turns on fully, it is common to use a pull-up resistor, as shown in the bottom diagram, to improve FET performance. Also shown are the associated pinouts for a standard TO-220 package. Note: FETs do not normally have logic-level gate drive signals, and consequently, this must be specified when ordering them.

Healthcare (Duderstadt, Germany) also sold a number of CO_2-powered systems up until the mid-1970s. A disadvantage associated with pneumatics is that a cylinder of gas [carbon dioxide (CO_2)] has to be secreted somewhere on the user and a ready supply of these cylinders must be available. Because the user has to have tubes running from the gas supply to his/her hand, self-containment of the whole prosthesis becomes an issue.

Currently, there are no pneumatically powered prostheses available. However, the BioRobotics Lab in Seattle, Washington, is experimenting with pneumatic McKibben muscle actuators to mimic the musculature of the natural arm. These actuators, which were first conceived of in the 1950s, consist of an inflatable elastic tube covered by a flexible braided mesh. When pressurized, the elastic tube inside expands but is constrained by the mesh. The flexible mesh shortens or contracts like a muscle due to the expanding tube. It has been found that McKibben muscles can exhibit passive behavior very similar to biological muscle since both have series and parallel elasticity (Klute et al., 1999). From a robotics perspective, McKibben muscles can have a high force-to-weight ratio. However, this ratio ignores the weight of the compressed air source and associated tubing, which is an issue for a self-contained prosthetic device. In addition, McKibben muscles have a shorter range-of-motion than human muscle and so far have not proven themselves to be reliable, long-term mechanisms.

Hydraulic Power. Although pneumatic systems found some measure of success in prosthetics, hydraulic systems did not. Hydraulic systems tend to be messy, with hydraulic units leaking hydraulic fluid. In addition, a fluid reservoir and fluid are also required, adding to the total weight of the mechanism. Microhydraulic systems have recently been revisited as part of the Defense Agency Research Projects Agency (DARPA) Revolutionizing Prosthetics initiative (Fite et al., 2008). Hydraulic systems have 3 times the power density of electromechanical motors (Hollerbach et al., 1991), and as such one would expect them to excel in the area of prosthetics. Unfortunately, effects of miniaturization on their transmission viscosity have prevented high performance in miniaturized applications. As a result, their performance has yet to rival conventional electromechanical motors when designed on the scale of a prosthetic hand.

Others (EAP, Nitinol, and Others). Other actuator, technologies such as nitinol, artificial muscles (electroactive polymers), and piezoelectric motors have lower power densities than electromechanical motors. Due to these problems along with other problems (low efficiency, high thermal dissipation, and so on), they have not yet seen commercial implementation in prostheses.

Safety. Safety considerations are an integral part of any design that has a person in the loop. Limit switches, or a suitable substitute (current sensing) should be used to shut off the motor at the limits of a component's range-of-motion (Fig. 20.20). These limit switches should be backed up by mechanical stops capable of physically stopping the component's drive should the electrical limit switches fail. This way, while the drive may burn out, the user remains safe. Manual overrides for mechanisms should also be included so that if a prehensor fails while it is gripping an object, the user can still open it manually. Motion control has a manual override built into the on-off switch of its new hand. Otto Bock has a breakaway mechanism that consists of a friction brake. In the Bock mechanism, there are multiple interdigitated plates that are preloaded by way of a set screw. The problem with the Bock mechanism is that it will protect the drivetrain from high external loads by slipping at a preset friction but it must be screwed tight enough that it cannot be manually unloaded.

As prostheses become faster and stronger, their inertia is increasingly a problem, since their work sphere includes the user's head. Severe injury or even death may result from a collision with a fast prosthetic elbow, unless adequate compliance is included or other means to ensure safety in the event of a collision (Zinn et al., 2004).

20.3 CONTROL

Although the physical design constraints of weight, volume, and power are severe, they are not so severe that multifunctional arms and hands cannot be built that would be of acceptable weight and size. The real problem is, as we have alluded to before, the issue of how to interface a multifunctional arm or hand to an amputee in a meaningful way. It is for this reason that upper-limb prosthetics is often dominated by consideration of control. That is, how can the prosthesis be controlled in such a fashion that it will be an aid, rather than a burden to the user?

Childress (1992) presented the following attributes of prosthesis control as desirable. Although some of these attributes may be difficult, if not impossible to achieve in practice, they are still seen as desirable goals:

1. **Low mental loading or subconscious control:** The prosthesis should be able to be used without undue mental involvement. The prosthesis should serve the user; the user should not be the servant of the prosthesis.
2. **User friendly or simple to learn to use:** Any device should be intuitive and natural. An amputee should be able to learn to use the prosthesis quickly and easily.
3. **Independence in multifunctional control:** Control of any function or degree of freedom should be able to be executed without interfering with the other control functions of a multifunctional prosthesis.
4. **Simultaneous, coordinated control of multiple functions (parallel control):** The ability to coordinate multiple functions simultaneously in effective and meaningful ways without violating the first and third attributes.
5. **Direct access and instantaneous response (speed of response):** All functions, if possible, should be directly accessible to the user and these functions should respond immediately to input commands.
6. **No sacrifice of human functional ability:** The prosthesis should be used to supplement, not subtract, from available function. The control system should not encumber any natural movement that an amputee can apply to useful proposes.
7. **Natural appearance:** Movements that appear mechanical in nature, attract unwanted attention in social situations, and may not be pleasing to the eye.

As one might imagine, the level of amputation has very important consequences for the control of a prosthetic device. The level of amputation determines the number of control sites available versus the number of control sites that are needed. This is an inverse relationship. That is, the higher the level of amputation, the fewer the available control sources but the greater the amount of function that must be replaced. A control source is the means used by the amputee to control a specific function, or degree of freedom, of the prosthesis, for example, opening and closing of an artificial hand. The fewer the number of independent control sources, the greater the number of compromises that must be made in order to achieve a clinically practical device.

Practical inputs typically come from muscular activity, (a) directly, (b) indirectly through joints, and (c) indirectly from by-products of muscular contraction (myoelectricity, myoacoustics, muscle bulge, and mechanical/electrical impedance). Although signals can be obtained from brainwaves, voice, feet, eyes, and other places, these sources of control have not been shown to be practical for artificial limb control (Childress, 1992).

The primary sources of control for body-powered devices are biomechanical in nature. Movement, or force, from a body joint or multiple joints is used to change position, or develop a force/pressure, which can be transduced by a harness and Bowden cable and/or mechanical switches. Typically, inputs such as chin and head force/movement, glenohumeral flexion/extension abduction/adduction, biscapular and scapular abduction, shoulder elevation and depression, chest expansion, or elbow or wrist movements are used. But direct force/motion from muscle(s) has also been used by way of surgical procedures such as muscle tunnel cineplasty (Sauerbruch, 1916) and the Krukenberg cineplasty (Krukenberg, 1917).

For externally powered devices, electromechanical switches and myoelectric control are the main sources of control. The usual input to most externally powered prosthetic components is the plus-minus drive wires of the dc motor used to drive the component. So long as the motor receives a voltage of either polarity across these wires, it will run in one direction or the other. The motor cares little how this voltage is developed. This voltage can be an on/off-type voltage in which the motor is fully "on" or fully "off" (switch control). Or it can take the form of a variable dc level voltage in which case motor speed is proportional to the dc voltage level (proportional control). Or it can be a stream of pulses in which the motor drive voltage level is proportional to the amount of "on" time of the pulses [pulse width modulation (PWM)]. PWM too is a type of proportional control. In all instances, a control source is needed to transduce some body motion or biological artifact into a voltage to drive the motor. Although biomechanical inputs are used most extensively in the control of body-powered prosthetic components, the same inputs can be used, through the use of appropriate electromechanical switches, or force transducers, to control externally powered components. Figure 20.17 shows a high-level bilateral hybrid fitting that highlights many of these issues.

Proportional Control

In proportional control, the amount/intensity of a controlled output variable is proportional to the amount of the input signal. For example, the output speed of a dc motor is proportional to the amount of voltage applied to its terminals. This is why dc motors are said to be speed controlled. This is also the reason why most of today's commercially available prosthetic components are speed controlled. Output speed is proportional to the amount of input signal. Proportional control is used where a graded response to a graded input is sought.

Position control is similar to speed control, except that in this case the position of the prosthetic joint is proportional to the input amount/intensity. The input amount/intensity might be the position of another physiological joint or a force level. If the position of another joint is used as the input, then the system is known as a *position-actuated, position servomechanism.* If the amount of force applied by some body part is the input, then the system is a force-actuated, position servomechanism. An example is the power steering of a car. Here, the position of the steering wheel is related directly (proportional) to the position of the front wheels. Such a system is an example of a position follower (the position of the wheels follows the position of the steering wheel) or a position servomechanism.

If a further constraint is added whereby the input and output are physically (mechanically) linked such that change in position of the output cannot occur without a change in position of the input and vice versa, then, as is the case in the power steering example, the system becomes an "unbeatable" position servomechanism or a system that has inherent extended physiological proprioception (EPP) (an EPP system)(Simpson, 1974). Unbeatable servomechanisms are a subset of position servomechanisms as a whole.

With position control, the amputee's ability to perceive and control prosthesis position is directly determined by his or her ability to perceive and control the input signal. A major disadvantage of position control is that, unlike velocity control, it must maintain an input signal to hold an output level other than zero. This means that power must be continuously supplied to the component to maintain a commanded position other than zero. This is one of the reasons why speed, or velocity, control is the dominant mode of control in externally powered prosthetics today in spite of the fact that it has been shown that position control for positioning of the terminal device in space is superior to velocity control (Doubler and Childress, 1984a; 1984b). Equally well it has been observed that velocity control may be better suited to the control of prehension (McKenzie, 1970; Carlson and Primmer, 1978), but this observation may be due to the poor performance of the prosthetic hand mechanisms of the day and consequently the manner in which amputees tended to use them.

Although proportional control for externally powered prostheses has been around since the 1970s, it is only comparatively recently that proportional controllers have become more widely accepted. This is because of the poor speed and speed-of-response of most of today's systems. If a mechanism is slow, a user will tend to drive it using either a full "open" signal or full "close" signal regardless of the type of controller, that is, slow devices will be used in essentially a switch or "bang-bang" mode. It is the bandwidth of the mechanism and controller together which determines speed-of-response. If the mechanism is fast but the controller introduces delays due to processing, then the speed-of-response of the overall system will be limited by the controller. However, it is only recently that any prosthetic components have had sufficiently high mechanical bandwidth that users could perceive, or have a use for, a proportional-type control. The Hosmer-Dorrance NU-VA Synergetic Prehensor, Otto Bock System Electric hands, the Motion Control Hand, the Touch Bionics i-Limb,

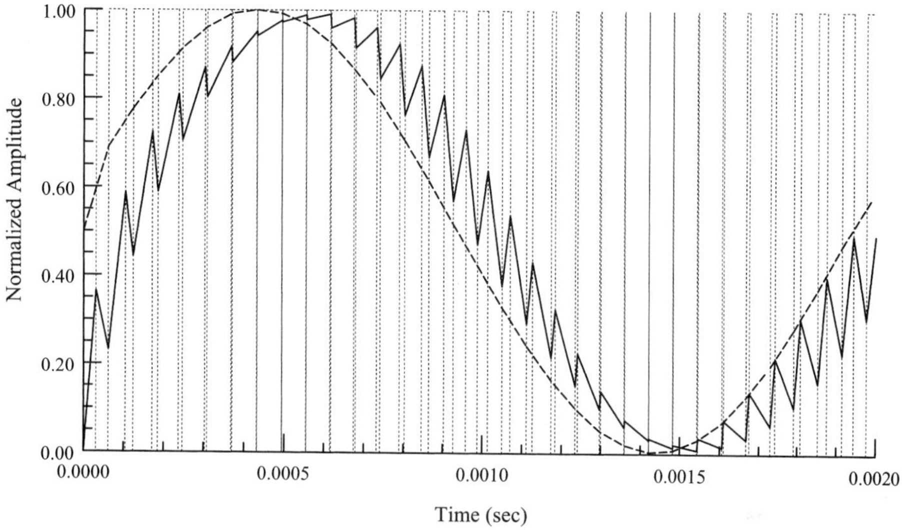

FIGURE 20.24 Plot showing a sine wave, a pulse width modulation (PWM) representation of the sine wave (jagged waveform), and the reconstructed sine wave following filtering of theh PWM stream by a simple RC filter. Notice that in the PWM stream the time between pulses (base period) remains constant; however, the duration, or the on time (duty cycle) of the pulse changes in proportion to the input sine wave amplitude. The restored sine wave signal has been phase-shifted by the filtering process and it has a lot of high-frequency components superimposed on the original signal, but an analysis of the power spectra of original sine wave and the reconstructed sine wave reveals the high-frequency components to be low magnitude by comparison to the main signal. The high-frequency components could be further reduced by using a higher-order filter, or a higher PWM frequency (1/base period) or both. The benefits of using pulse modulation for motor control are that smaller transistors can be used, possibly without heat sinking, because they are operated either in saturation or off and current pulses are more efficient at overcoming stiction in the motor, which improves overall motor efficiency.

the Utah Elbow, the Boston Digital Arm, and the Otto Bock Dynamic Arm all benefit from the use of proportional controllers. For some users, these devices need a proportional controller so that they can be controlled in a meaningful way because they are too fast to run in a switch control mode.

In this day and age of digital circuits and microprocessor-based controllers, pulse width modulation (PWM) is the preferred method of supplying a graded (proportional) control signal to a component. A PWM stream only requires a single digital output line and a counter on the microprocessor to be implemented while a conventional analog signal (linear dc voltage level) requires a full digital-to-analog (D/A) converter (Fig. 20.24). PWM techniques are used extensively in switched mode power supply design and audio amplifiers (Israelsohn, 2001), and as such there is a vast amount of resources available to the designer to choose from.

As implemented on most microprocessors, a period register is loaded with a base period (1/PWM frequency; PWM frequency is usually in the range of 30 kHz for switched mode power supplies, but can be as low as 300 Hz in some motor control applications), which is some fraction of the microprocessor's clock frequency (D'Souza and Mirta, 1997). A duty-cycle register is loaded with a percentage of the base period that corresponds to the desired proportional output voltage level as a percentage of the maximum possible output voltage. At the beginning of each period, the output at the PWM port is high and the microprocessor counts down until the duty cycle register is zero at which time the PWM port goes low. The microprocessor continues to count down until the base period register is zero at which time a new value for the duty cycle is loaded and the process repeats itself (Palmer, 1997).

A variation on PWM is pulse position modulation (PPM), also known as *pulse period modulation* or *pulse frequency modulation* (PFM). In this case, the duty-cycle pulse remains on for a fixed time while the base period is varied. The frequency of the pulses (how close together the pulses are) determines the voltage level. The neuromuscular system is an example of a pulse-position modulation system. A muscle is made up of many discrete motor units. A motor unit has an all or nothing response to a nerve impulse; in much the same way as a nerve impulse is a nonlinear (thresholded) all or nothing event. The level of sustained force output of a motor unit is dictated by the frequency of incidence of the nerve impulses, with the motor units' dynamics [mechanical properties—inertial and damping properties (acts as a mechanical filter)] holding the force output smooth between incoming impulses. The motor unit is pulse frequency modulated by the nervous system.

Finally, it is possible to have a combination of the two where one has variable duty-cycle pulses and variable periods. In all cases, the output PWM stream is a series of pulses in which the dc voltage level is proportional to the ratio of the amount of on time with respect to the amount of off time for the pulses in the stream.

To recover the analog voltage level from a pulse stream requires the use of a low-pass filter (Palacherla, 1997). When used to drive a motor (via an H-bridge), the inductance and inertia of the armature in the motor form a mechanical filter that provides the filtering necessary to smooth the pulses into a continuous signal. The use of a simple RC circuit can be used to smooth the pulse stream if the pulse stream is not being fed directly into a dc motor. If using a simple RC circuit, the cutoff frequency should be about two decades below the PWM frequency if a smooth output signal is sought. An RC filter is a first-order filter that has an attenuation of 20 dB/decade. Higher-order filters could of course be used with cutoff frequencies closer to the PWM frequency. For motors, a smooth signal is not vital.

Control Sources

Body-Powered Control. Body-powered control has been described above as a suitable energy source to power prostheses. It is also a good control source. Although friction in the cable limits the fidelity of force transmission or sensation, the coupling of a proximal joint to the distal prosthesis provides a good proprioceptive link, which in turn decreases the cognitive burden on the user. Body-powered control may be used without visual feedback, and with a moderate degree of certainty regarding the position and exerted force of the terminal device. The largest impediment to body-powered control is that there are a very limited number of joints which may be coupled to the artificial limb without impeding other functions. As a result, conventionally body-powered control may only be used to control single DOF at a time, precluding the use of multifunctional prostheses. Ironically, it is the area of multifunctional prostheses, where the high mental load of coordinating multiple DOFs is significant, where the proprioceptive feedback of body-powered control would otherwise excel. Body-powered control may be used to control a single DOF, and as such may be part of a hybrid multifunctional prosthesis.

FSRs and Potentiometers. Force-sensitive-resistors (FSRs) and potentiometers are clinically viable sensors at the shoulder disarticulation level, where some residual motion of the shoulder complex may be independently captured while the socket remains fixed to the rest of the body. Potentiometers have been demonstrated to provide higher fidelity control than FSRs, and both have been demonstrated to have higher fidelity than myoelectric sensors (Vodovnik and Rebersek, 1974). As a result, FSRs and potentiometers offer a viable addition to the ensemble of appropriate sensors for multifunctional prostheses, and should be considered as the primary control source for shoulder disarticulation subjects only controlling a single DOF. Over FSRs, two-DOF potentiometers are to be preferred due to their higher force fidelity and the fact that potentiometers may simply track the shoulder movement of subjects, rather than requiring hunting to find FSRs.

Myoelectric Control. Myoelectric control derives its name from the Latin word for muscle (*myo*) and the resulting by-product of electricity that muscle contraction creates. It is commonly called *electromyographic (EMG) control*, although strictly speaking *electromyography* refers to the recording of myoelectric signals, rather than to the actual signals themselves. When a muscle contracts, an electric potential is produced as a by-product of that contraction. If surface electrodes are placed on

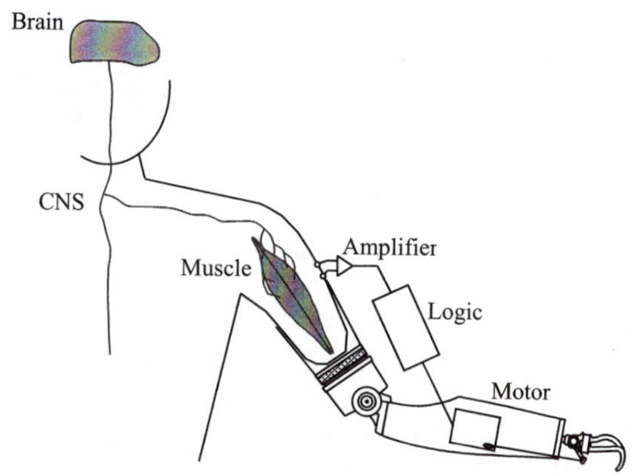

FIGURE 20.25 Muscle as a biological neural amplifier. The muscle in effect acts as a biological amplifier for the neural signal. The myoelectric signal caused by the neural signal activation of the muscle can then be detected at the skin surface and further amplified electronically for use in logic circuitry.

the skin near a muscle, they can detect this signal (Fig. 20.25). The signal can then be electronically amplified, processed, and used to control a prosthesis. Although the intensity of the EMG increases as muscle tension increases, the relationship is a complex nonlinear process that is dependent on many variables, including the position and configuration of the electrodes (Heckathorne, 1978; Heckathorne and Childress, 1981). Although the EMG is nonlinear, it is broadly monotonic, and the human operator perceives this response as more or less linear.

The first externally powered prosthesis was a pneumatic hand patented in Germany in 1915. Drawings of this hand and possibly the first electric hand were published in 1919 in *Ersatzglieder und Arbeitshilfen* (Borchardt et al., 1919). The first myoelectric prosthesis was developed during the early 1940s by Reinhold Reiter. He published his work in 1948 (Reiter, 1948) but it was not widely known, and myoelectric control had to wait to be rediscovered during the 1950s. Reiter's prosthesis consisted of a modified Hüfner hand that contained a control electromagnet controlled by a vacuum tube amplifier. The prosthesis was not portable but was instead intended for use at a workstation, although Reiter did hope that one day it might be portable. The Russian hand was the first semi-practical myoelectric hand to be used clinically. This hand also had the distinction of being the first-to-use transistors (germanium) to process the myoelectric control signal (Childress, 1985). In this country, following the Second World War the Committee on Artificial Limbs contracted with IBM to develop several electric-powered limbs. These were impressive engineering feats in their day but never found use outside the laboratory (Klopsteg and Wilson, 1954).

Myoelectric control has received considerable attention since it first appeared during the 1940s, and there is an extensive body of literature on myoelectric characteristics and properties (Basmajian and De Luca, 1985; Parker and Scott, 1985). It was considered to be the cutting edge of technology of the day and was advanced as a natural approach for the control of prostheses since it made it possible for amputees to use the same mental processes to control prosthesis function as had previously been used in controlling their physiological limb (Mann, 1968; Hogan, 1976).

Usually, the EMG is amplified and processed (bandlimited, rectified, and thresholded) to provide a dc signal that is related to the force of muscular contraction; this is then used to control the prosthesis (Scott, 1984) (Fig. 20.26). EMG processing in a typical prosthetic myoelectric control system involves two pairs of differential "dry" metal electrodes and a reference electrode (Fig. 20.27). Although the electrodes are referred to as dry, the environment inside a prosthetic socket causes the amputee's residual limb to sweat, which creates a conductive interface between the skin and the electrodes (Fig. 20.28). As a result, performance typically improves 5 min or so after donning the

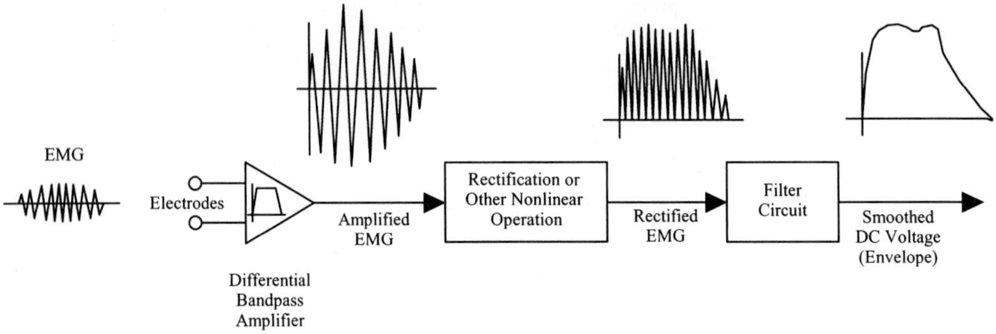

FIGURE 20.26 Schematic showing conventional myoelectric signal processing. A conventional myoelectric processing stream consists of differentially amplifying and bandlimiting the EMG signal. The amplified signal is then changed into a dc signal by rectification, by full wave rectification, squaring, root mean squaring (RMS), or some other appropriate nonlinear processing. The rectified signal is then filtered to obtain the envelope of the EMG signal. This voltage level can then be fed to the motor as a dc voltage level. All these processing steps introduce time delays into the overall control loop. The major delay is introduced by the time constant of smoothing (envelope) filter circuit. These delays can in turn reduce the bandwidth of the entire motor controller system.

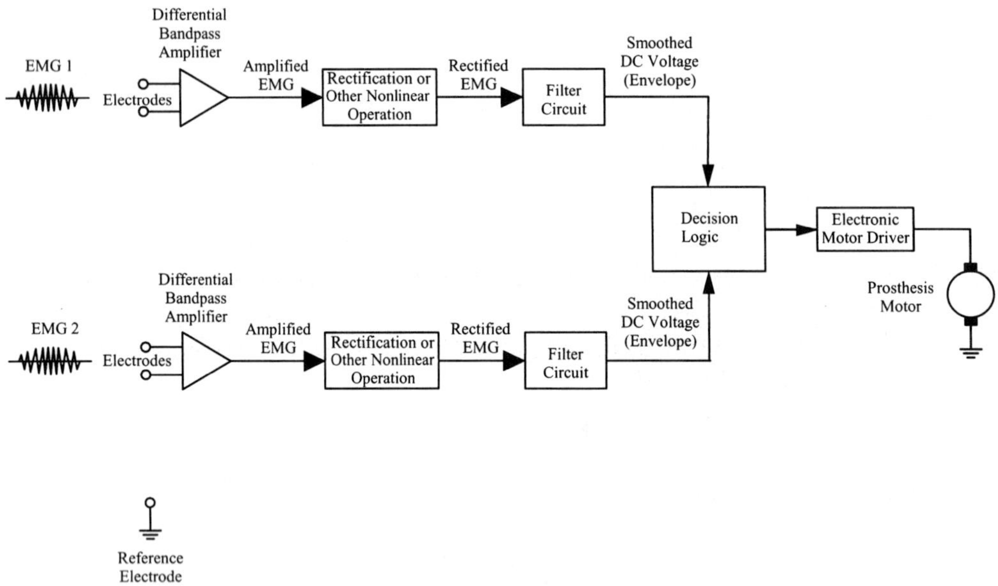

FIGURE 20.27 Schematic of the typical myoelectric processing scheme used in standard commercially available two-site myoelectrically controlled systems. (See also Figs. 20.28 and 20.29). The major difference here from Fig. 20.26 is that there must be some way to decide which of the two incoming signals to use to drive the motor. Usually a drive signal proportional to the magnitude of the difference between the two incoming signals is sent to the motor.

prosthesis. Traditionally, myoelectric control uses electrodes placed on the skin near each of a protagonist/antagonist pair of muscles to control a single DOF. For below-elbow fittings, this usually means electrodes on those muscle groups responsible for flexion and extension of the wrist and fingers (Fig. 20.29). Thinking about flexing or extending the "phantom" fingers controls closing or opening, respectively, of some terminal device.

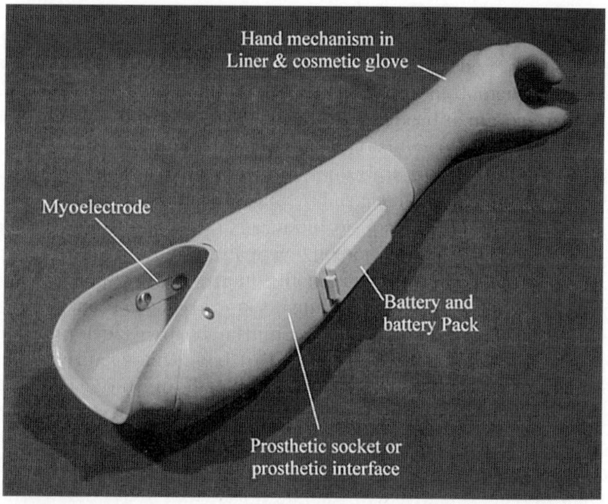

FIGURE 20.28 A standard transradial myoelectric prosthetic interface (socket). The battery pack, wrist unit, and myoelectrodes are all fitted into a custom-made laminated prosthetic socket and forearm. The socket is fabricated after a mold made from the amputee's residual limb.

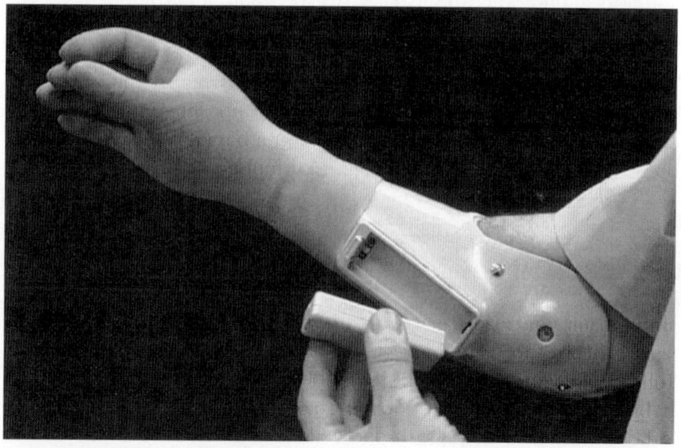

FIGURE 20.29 A person with a transradial amputation wearing a typical myoelectric prosthesis. The user is demonstrating how the battery pack is propped in and out. The battery pack housing is usually located on the medial surface of the prosthesis for appearance reasons and ease of access.

EMG signal amplitude is approximately 100 μV for a moderately contracted forearm muscle. This signal must be amplified to a signal with an amplitude in the range of 1 to 10 V before it can used. This implies that a gain of upward of 10,000 is needed. The bandwidth for the surface EMG signals is 10 to 300 Hz with most of the signals' energy in and around 100 Hz (Childress, 1992). Differential amplifiers are used to amplify the EMG because the small EMG signal is often superimposed on large common-mode signals that, at these gain levels, would saturate an amplifier in a single-mode configuration. A differential amplifier can remove the large common-mode signals, leaving only the potential difference (EMG signal) between the electrodes to be amplified. This has the effect of most effectively amplifying the EMG signal frequencies around 100 Hz. Because the large gain requirement would drive most op-amps to instability, these differential amplifiers are seldom single op-amps, but instead use multiple stages to meet the gain requirements.

Once the EMG signal has been amplified and bandlimited, it is then changed into a dc signal by rectification or squaring. This dc potential is then commonly smoothed with a low-pass filter to remove the pulses and extract the envelope of the signal. For on/off, or switch, control, the smoothed dc voltage, is then compared in a logic circuit with a threshold voltage. If the signal is greater than the threshold voltage, then power is supplied to the prosthesis motor, otherwise the power remains off. For proportional control, the smoothed voltage is fed to the motor.

When used for proportional control, the EMG signal is usually treated as an amplitude-modulated signal, where the mean amplitude of the cutaneous signal is the desired output from the myoelectric processor. However, in order to have accurate estimates of muscle force from EMG signals, a processing system with high signal-to-noise ratio (SNR) as well as short rise time (fast response) is required (Meek et al., 1990). Unfortunately, there is a fundamental filtering paradox whereby it is possible to have either fast response or high SNR, but not both (Jacobsen et al., 1984). To overcome this perceived problem, Meek et al. (1990) proposed using an adaptive filter in which the time constant of the low-pass filter used in the final stage of EMG processing (acquire signal envelope) was varied, depending on the rate of change of the EMG signal. Their assumption was that an amputee, when moving quickly, will tolerate noise (low SNR) but will not tolerate delays in control. When holding the prosthesis steady or performing slow, dexterous tasks such as treading a needle, the amputee will tolerate slow response as long as there is low noise (high SNR).

Designers need to be aware of this filtering paradox should they be involved in the design of high-bandwidth, myoelectrically controlled systems. It is also questionable whether the user needs an accurate measure of muscle force versus EMG signal amplitude. So long as the control signal is broadly monotonic, the user learns to equate a particular level of contraction with a particular control signal output.

Finally, all these processing steps take time! Any delay in the response of the output to a change in the input of greater than 250 μs is perceptible to the human operator as a "sluggish" response. Any delay at all decreases functional performance, and a delay greater than 100 μs creates clinically significant reduction in performance (Farrell and Weir, 2007).

Childress Pulse Width Modulation. Myopulse modulation (Childress, 1972) offers a means of processing myoelectric signals that maximizes the speed-of-response of an externally powered component (Fig. 20.30). This technique eliminates the delays that are introduced by analog or digital filtering methods, provides proportional control, and keeps the component count to a minimum, thus keeping size and power consumption down.

Because percent myoelectric signal "on" time (EMG signal level above an arbitrary threshold) is monotonically related to muscle output force level, a proportional signal can be achieved very simply. This controller simply converts a differentially amplified myoelectric signal directly into a pulse stream through the use of a pair of comparators. This pulse stream is then fed directly to the motor H-bridge without further processing. This controller is able to present a pulse stream to the drive motor in advance of the operator being able to detect motion by the innervated muscle, making it ideally suited for prosthetic mechanisms that require a quick speed-of-response. This controller is now commercially available through Hosmer-Dorrance Corp.

Another alternative method of myoelectric signal smoothing, called *autogenic backlash*, (Bottomley, 1965) produced a more or less consistent dc output from a fluctuating myoelectric signal while not sacrificing time response.

Comments on Myoelectrodes. The electrode spacing has two contrary effects. A differential amplifier subtracts out those elements of the measured signal that are common to the two inputs of the amplifier and leaves only the difference (Fig. 20.31). For prosthetic myoelectric control applications, each input to the amplifier is some form of button electrode that sits on the skin surface. It is important that this pair of button electrodes be oriented along the long axis of the muscle from which the EMG is being measured. This is because the EMG travels along the muscle's length, creating a difference in potential between the electrodes, that forms the input to the differential amplifier. The greater the distance between the electrodes, the larger the potential difference is.

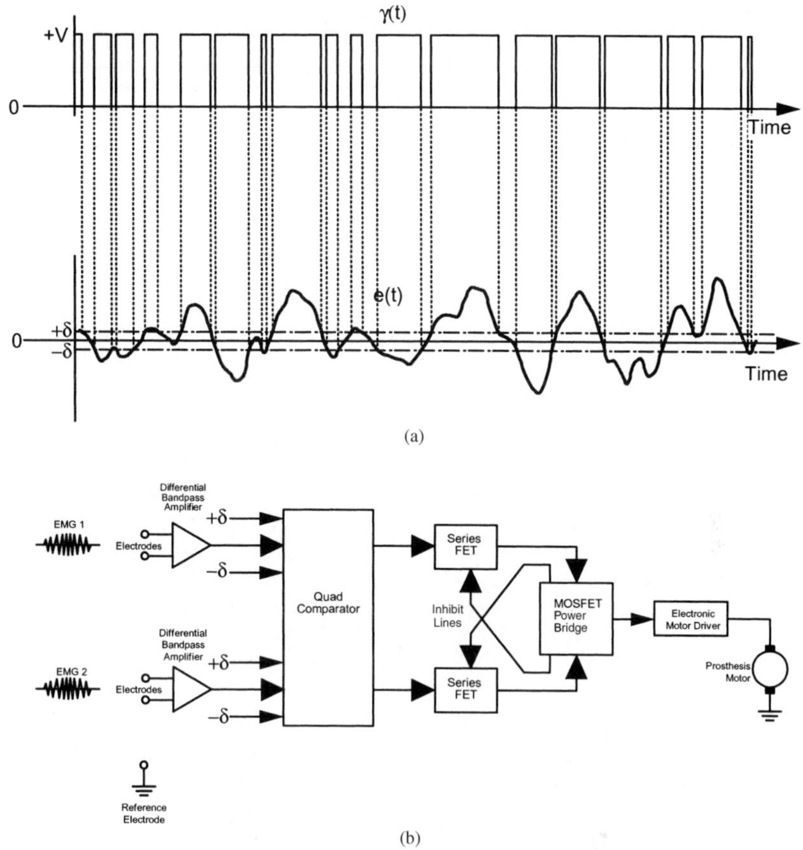

FIGURE 20.30 Myopulse modulation (Childress, 1973)—the voltage level seen at the motor is proportional to the ratio of on time of the pulses to off time. The mean of this ratio is in turn proportional to the intensity of muscle contraction and as such is a very simple means of providing proportional myoelectric control. The top trace [$\gamma(t)$] shows the switching response of a comparator in response to a time-varying EMG signal [$e(t)$] and is given by the expression:

$$\gamma(t) = \frac{V}{2}[1 + \mathrm{sgn}(|e(t)| - \delta)]$$

where $|e(t)|$ is the absolute magnitude of the amplified myoelectric signal, δ is the threshold, and V is the power supply voltage. The thresholds for switching are $+\delta$ and $-\delta$. One method of choosing these thresholds is to set them at levels corresponding to ±3 standard deviations of the quiescent (resting) signal amplitude. The lower schematic shows the key components needed to implement this kind of control. The advantages of this EMG processing approach are (1) the simple electronic implementation, (2) no electrical time constant delay (processing delay)—implies faster response, (3) control signal already in pulse modulation form, and (4) wide dynamic range of muscle output.

The unwanted large common-mode noise signals, on the other hand, are equally present at both electrodes regardless of the orientation of the electrodes. However, these common-mode noise signals are more likely to be the same at both electrodes if the electrodes are located physically close together. However, the potential difference of the actual EMG between the electrodes will be reduced. Thus one trades better common-mode rejection (CMRR) for reduced gain. Commercially available myoelectrodes from Otto Bock consist of a pair of bar electrodes spaced about 20 mm

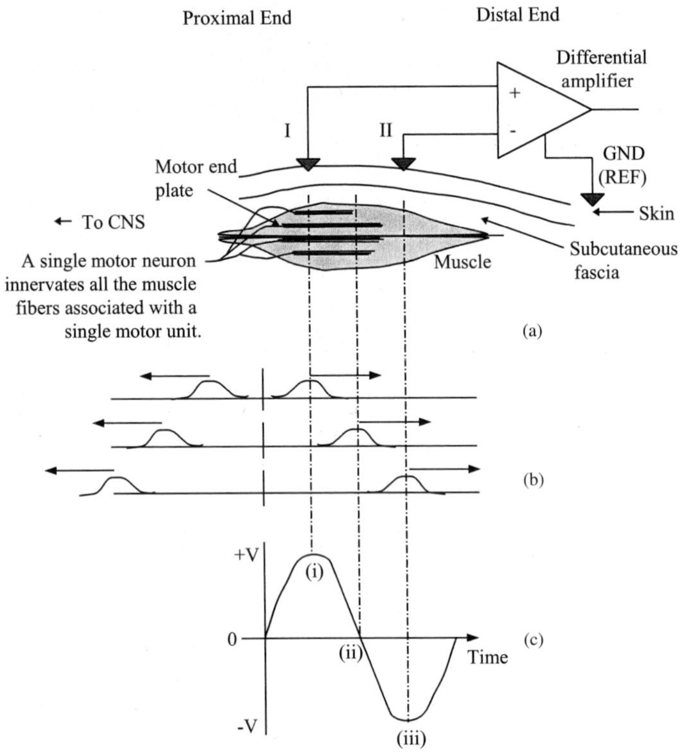

FIGURE 20.31 Schematic of how differential electrodes function. Dry button electrodes I and II are placed over a muscle belly on the skin surface in the line of the long axis of the muscle. These electrodes form the positive (I) and negative (II) inputs of a differential amplifier electrode pair. (*a*) In skeletal muscle, the individual muscle fibers are generally oriented along the long axis of the muscle. A single axon from the central nervous system innervates a single motor unit usuallly (for skeletal muscle) at the end of the muscle closest to the spinal chord (i.e., the proximal end). The points where the nerve fibers attach to the individual muscle fibers of a motor unit are called "motor end plates." When a nerve sends a signal to an individual muscle fiber to contract, the electric signal travels in both directions away from the motor end plate. For this reason the electrodes of the differential amplifier should be oriented along the long axis of the muscle's fibers. (*b*) Depolarization wave that travels in both directions away from the motor end plate along individual muscle fibers when activated by a motor nerve fiber. (*c*) Typical signal seen at the output of the differential amplifier for a single muscle fiber. At (i) the depolarization wave is directly under the positive input (I) with nothing under the negative input (II) to the differential amplifier and consequently registers as a positive going wave at the differential amplifier output; at (ii) the depolarization wave registers equally at the positive (I) and negative (II) inputs and is therefore cancelled out, giving a zero at the output of the differential amplifier; at (iii) the depolarization wave is now directly under the negative input (II) with noting under the positive input (I) so this registers at the differential amplifier output as a negative going wave. In reality, there are thousands of fibers all at different stages in their firing process, which results in the quasi-random signal seen at the skin surface.

apart, with a circular reference electrode located between them. The location of Otto Bock's reference electrode presents problems. A better configuration, from a CMRR standpoint, is the Hosmer-Dorrance electrode pair which consists of button electrodes 11 mm ($^7/_{16}$ in) in diameter spaced about 28 mm ($1^1/_8$ in) apart, with a separate reference electrode that is located as far away from any electrodes as possible within the confines of the prosthesis (Fig. 20.32).

A physically separate and remote reference electrode is desirable because the reference is not electrically isolated from the inputs to the differential amplifier. The reference electrode is in contact with the person and consequently is electrically coupled to both inputs of the amplifier by the electrical impedance of the body. This impedance is a function of distance that is, the further away the

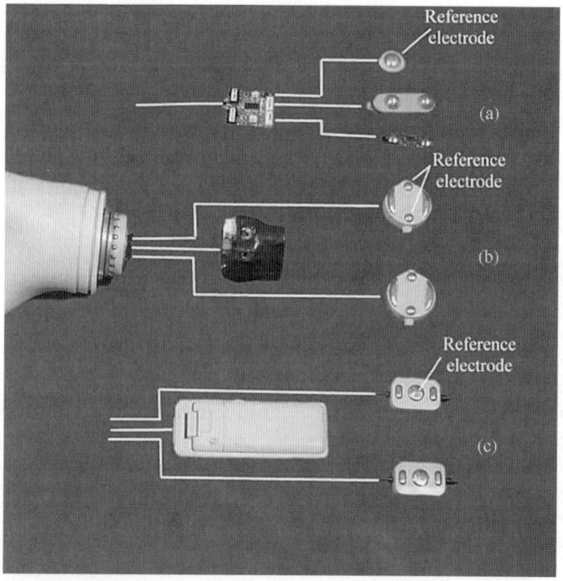

FIGURE 20.32 Photograph of different electrode configurations. (*a*) Hosmer-Dorrance Myopulse modulation electrodes and controller; note physically separate reference electrode to improve the common mode rejection ratio (CMRR). (*b* and *c*) Otto Bock electrodes with integrated reference electrodes.

reference is, the greater the attenuation. The reference electrode forms a "floating" ground signal rather than a "true" ground. Furthermore, the noise signal that can be introduced by the reference electrode is not necessarily a common-mode signal that will be removed by the differential amplification process.

The size of these electrodes could be greatly reduced, given the availability today of many low-offset, ultra-fast single supply op-amps for the cellular phone industry. The ultra-low offset voltage of these op-amps allows for higher gains to be used. This in turn would facilitate the design of smaller electrode pairs with higher common-mode rejection ratios. Such a reduction in size is necessary if multifunctional myoelectric control of prostheses is to become a reality.

Insulated Sensors. Surface myoelectric sensors have three inherent problems:

- Maintaining consistent contact in the same location
- Providing consistent signal properties in the presence of environmental fluctuations (perspiration and skin dryness)
- Integration with socket interface technologies such as silicon suspension sleeves

Two solutions have been proposed to these problems. Capacitive myoelectric sensors provide a noninvasive solution to the latter two problems. Implantable myoelectric sensors (IMES) provide a minimally invasive solution to all three problems. Both are described below.

Capacitive myoelectric sensors, also known as *insulated electrodes*, have been investigated since at least the early 1970s (David and Portnoy, 1972), but have only recently become clinically viable due to new semiconductor ceramic materials and signal-processing chips (Kajitani and Higuchi, 2007). These capacitive sensors are not influenced by the impedance of the interface, and as a result, their signals are not influenced by perspiration or dry skin. As a result, they do not require the settling in period associated with conventional myoelectric sensors. In addition, capacitive myoelectric sensors do not require direct contact with the skin, and, as such, may easily be used in conjunction with cloth socks or silicon liners without significant signal degradation. This latter distinction poses a significant clinical advantage: current attempts to integrate myoelectric sensors with silicon liners involve attaching the electrodes through the liners. The resulting tangle of wires that must be rolled onto the residual limb with the liner is not clinically viable. Capacitive sensors, by contrast, may be placed in the outer socket, allowing the user to easily roll on the silicon liner without having to deal with any wires. Capacitive myoelectric sensors still suffer from the practical problem of maintaining consistent contact in the same location, and they require a ground electrode to contact the skin. As multifunctional prostheses require multiple electrodes; however, their advantages are substantial enough that they are likely to be produced by several prosthesis companies.

IMES. *Implantable myoelectric sensors* (IMES) are small electrodes, the size of a grain of rice, that may be injected using a large needle (Weir et al., 2003). Their hermeneutically sealed packaging is based off the FDA-approved BION, which is used to stimulate muscle (Loeb et al., 2001; Salter et al., 2004; Popovic et al., 2007). IMES only record muscle signals, transmitting data and receiving power through induction. Inductive transfer does not require wires to pass through the skin, resulting in a clinically viable interface that is not prone to infection. Because the inductive coil is laminated into the socket, the entire interface is transparent to the user. Because these sensors are small, it is easy to simultaneously record from multiple muscles to control multifunctional prostheses. Because they are located within the muscle, they are not affected by environmental conditions such as dry skin or perspiration levels. Perhaps most importantly, because they are connected to the muscle, they do not migrate over time, and they never lose contact with the muscle. As a result, they provide a consistent signal even when torque is applied to the prosthesis, which may twist the socket such that contact is lost between the socket and the skin. The fact that the sensors may be implanted through a large needle makes the surgical procedure minimally invasive. All of these advantages make IMES a promising advancement in the field of myoelectric control. High cost due to the hermeneutically sealed package is likely to be the largest inhibitor to their acceptance. IMES are currently being tested in monkeys, and are awaiting FDA approval for implantation in humans.

Myoacoustic Control. Myoacoustic signals are auditory sounds created as a by-product of muscle contraction. A myoacoustic control system is very similar in structure to a myoelectric control system, but the elimination of unwanted acoustic noise appears to be a bigger problem than the elimination of unwanted electrical noise in myoelectric systems (Barry and Cole, 1990). It has not gained widespread use.

Muscle Bulge or Tendon Movement. Tendon or residual muscle movement can be used to actuate pneumatic sensors. These sensors, when interposed between a prosthetic socket and superficial tendons and/or muscle, can be used for prosthesis control. The Vaduz hand, which was developed by a German team headed by Dr. Edmund Wilms in Vaduz, Liechtenstein, following World War II, used muscle bulge to increase pneumatic pressure to operate a switch-controlled voluntary-closing position-servo hand (Childress and Weir, 2004). This hand was a forerunner of the pneumatic Otto Bock Hands of the 1970s and the electrically powered Otto Bock hands of today.

Simpson (1966) also used muscle bulge to provide a control signal for the proportional control of an Otto Bock gas-operated hand. The force applied by the muscle's bulge was proportional to the width-of-opening of the hand. This device was an example of a force-actuated, position servomechanism, and because the bulging muscle had to achieve a significant pressure to ensure sufficient force for control valve operation, a subconscious feedback path existed through the skin's own pressure sensors. This device was a precursor for Simpson's concept of extended physiological proprioception (EPP) (Simpson, 1974).

In 1999, the Rutgers multifunctional hand (Abboudi et al., 1999) received considerable media attention because they developed a multifunctional controller that allowed amputees to play the piano in a laboratory setting. This controller used multiple pneumatic sensors that were actuated by the movement of the superficial extrinsic tendons associated with individual finger flexors (Curcie et al., 2001). For this hand to be clinically viable, the developers need to resolve some of the issues that led to the failure of the previous attempts at using pressure transducers.

The problem with using pressure sensors in any practical prosthetic device is the system cannot differentiate between actual control signals from a tendon and external pressures and impacts from objects in the environment. A prosthesis wearer interacting with the real world will exert forces and moments on the socket, which may actuate the pressure sensors and issue commands to the drive system of the prosthesis. There is also the issue of socket fit; if the wearer gains weight the socket will get tighter, thereby actuating the sensors.

A more promising alternative to measuring pressure is measuring the movement of muscles or tendons, since this method is more impervious to external variables, yet captures the individual movement of the muscles. It is very difficult, however, to capture this movement. Zheng et al. (2005) have attempted to measure muscle movement using sonomyography. Although the technique has provided impressive results, the technology seems incapable at this time of being shrunk to a size that is compatible with prostheses. Miniature muscle tunnel cineplasties (Beasley, 1966; Marquardt, 1987; Childress and Weir, 2004), in which the tendons of muscles are connected to external cables, offer a more accurate measurement of tendon excursion. Due to the invasive nature of this method, however, it has not seen much clinical interest in the United States.

The concept of direct muscle attachment is not new. It had its origins in Italy at the turn of the twentieth century and was brought into clinical practice in Germany by Sauerbruch around 1915 (Sauerbruch, 1916). Sauerbruch's technique, called *muscle tunnel cineplasty*, fashions a skin-lined tunnel through the muscle (released at its insertion) and enables the muscle's power to be brought outside the body. Weir (1995; Weir et al., 2001) has shown the efficacy of tunnel cineplasty control when compared to the control of a conventional above-elbow, body-powered prosthesis. A similar but alternative surgical procedure, called *tendon exteriorization cineplasty* (Beasley, 1966), uses tendon transfers combined with skin flaps to bring a tendon loop outside the body.

The subconscious control possible with an EPP controller operating in conjunction with the proprioception of a surgically created muscle tunnel cineplasty presents the intriguing possibility of making independent multifunctional control of a prosthetic hand or arm a reality. Suitable control muscles and EPP controllers, in conjunction with powered fingers of an artificial hand, would be a step toward achieving the goal of meaningful, independent multifinger control of hand prostheses. In a prototype fitting (Fig. 20.33), a below-elbow amputee with tendon exteriorization cineplasties was fitted with an externally powered hand that utilized the subject's exteriorized tendons as control inputs to an EPP controller (Weir et al., 2001). Movement of the flexor tendon caused the hand to close. Movement of the extensor tendon caused the hand to open. This was the first clinical fitting of a powered-hand prosthesis, controlled directly by antagonist muscles (via exteriorized tendons) in a somewhat physiological manner.

The use of muscle/tendon cineplasty procedures would require changes in the way amputation surgery is performed at the time of initial amputation. Preservation of muscle tone and length are of paramount importance if future surgery is to be successful at creating muscle cineplasty interfaces. Muscle tone can be preserved by ensuring that residual muscles retain the ability to develop tension when voluntarily contracted. This requires that either myoplasty and/or myodesis be performed at the time of initial amputation. In myoplasty, agonist-antagonist residual muscle pairs are tied off

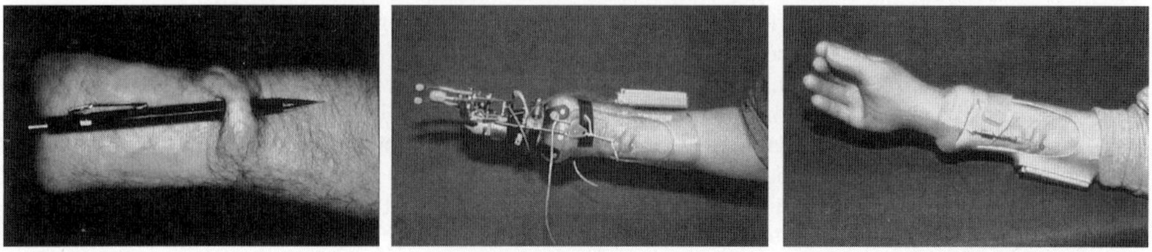

(a) (b) (c)

FIGURE 20.33 Prototype fitting of a person with a transcarpal amputation with tendon exteriorization cineplasties. The subject was fitted with an externally powered hand that utilized the subject's exteriorized tendons as control inputs to an EPP controller. (*a*) Photograph of a tendon exteriorization cineplasty—a pen is shown passing through the skin-lined tendon loop; (*b*) prototype version of the proof-of-concept EPP-controlled prosthesis; (*c*) Finished proof-of-concept prosthesis. Contraction of the flexor tendon caused the hand to close. Contraction of the extensor tendon caused the hand to open.

against each other. In myodesis, the residual muscle is stitched to the bone. In both cases, the residual musculature retains the ability to easily develop tension, thus preventing atrophy during the interval between initial amputation and the revisions necessary to create muscle/tendon cineplasty control interface. Myoplasty would generally be used on the superficial muscles while myodesis could be used on the deep muscles.

Neuroelectric Control. Neuroelectric control or the control of a prosthetic device by way of nerve impulses would appear to be a natural control approach. Although there is, and has been, research concerning prosthesis connections with nerves and neurons (Edell, 1986; Kovacs et al., 1989; Andrews et al., 2001), the practicality of human-machine interconnections of this kind are still problematic. Edell (1986) attempted to use nerve cuffs to generate motor control signals in experimental systems. Kovacs et al. (1989) explored the use of integrated circuit electrode arrays into which the nerve fiber was encouraged to grow. However, nervous tissue was sensitive to mechanical stresses, and this form of control required the use of implanted systems.

Andrews et al. (2001) reported on their progress in developing a multipoint microelectrode peripheral nerve implant. They use a 100 × 100 grid array of silicon microelectrodes that they insert into a peripheral nerve bundle using a pulse of air. This group is still working with animal models but claims to be able to identify individual neuron action potentials and also claims good long-term results so far. Concerns about how permanently electrode arrays are fixated have yet to be addressed.

A variation on the use of peripheral neural interfaces is the use of electroencephalogram signals (EEGs). These are electric signals that are detected on the surface of the skull and are emitted as a by-product of the natural functioning of the brain. Reger et al. (2000) demonstrated a hybrid neurorobotic system based on two-way communication between the brain of a lamprey and a small mobile robot. The lamprey brain was an in vitro preparation that was used to send and receive motor control and sensory signals. IEEE Spectrum (2001a) reported on research at Duke University, where researchers had implanted an electrode array into the cerebellum of a monkey and through the use of appropriate pattern recognition software had it control a remote manipulator at MIT over 1000 km away via the Internet. One of the main practical goals cited for this research is to put paralyzed people in control of artificial limbs. Although both these projects are long away from an amputee using their thoughts to control a prosthesis, it does show the shape of things to come.

Multifunctional Control. For prosthetic arms to be more than just position controllers for portable vices, multifunctional mechanisms that have the ability to have multiple degrees of freedom controlled simultaneously (in parallel) in a subconscious manner need to be developed. Commercially available multifunctional controllers are sequential in nature and take the form of two-site, three-state multifunctional controllers. Motion Control, Inc., in their ProControl hand-wrist controller, uses rapid cocontraction of the forearm extensors and flexors to switch control between hand opening and closing to wrist rotation. Otto Bock, GmbH, adopted Motion Control's control strategy in their wrist-hand controller. Motion Control, Inc., in their elbow controller, use dwell time (parking) to switch from elbow flexion and extension to hand opening and closure and cocontraction of biceps and triceps to switch control from the hand back to elbow.

Humans do not consciously control every joint of their arm for a given movement. Rather, they consciously choose a pattern and then their mind subconsciously controls each joint to generate that pattern. It is thus probable that subjects with an amputation can more intuitively generate a pattern for a given grasp or movement than that they can independently and simultaneously control multiple degrees of freedom. To implement grasp pattern control by way of myoelectric signals, a specific grasp pattern of the hand is tied to a specific pattern of EMG signals that the controller identifies. As an example, the user fires the muscles associated with palmar prehension or lateral prehension. The controller detects the resulting EMG signals generated by the residual musculature and through the appropriate use of pattern recognition and signal processing techniques extracts key features from these signals. These key features in turn enable the controller to recognize the grasp pattern associated with that EMG pattern, enabling the controller to actuate the appropriate motors to generate the desired hand grasp pattern.

In the Philadelphia Arm (Taylor and Finley, 1971) and Sven hand (Lawrence and Kadefors, 1971), multiple myoelectric signals were used as control inputs, which were processed using adaptive weighted filters. The weights on the filters were adjusted to tailor the filters to a specific individual. In the Philadelphia Arm, the choice of location for the myoelectrodes was based on muscle synergies associated with arm movements instead of phantom limb sensations used in the Sven hand. One of the findings with the Sven hand was that control using myoelectric signals from an intact limb was superior to control using a residual limb and phantom limb sensation. They theorized that this was due to the presence of an intact proprioception system.

At present, there is ongoing research into the multifunctional myoelectric control of artificial hand replacements using complex time, frequency, and time-frequency identification techniques to identify features in the EMG signals that describe a particular grasp pattern. A wide range of feature sets, including time-domain (Graupe and Cline, 1975; Graupe et al., 1982; Basmajian and De Luca, 1985; Kelly et al., 1990; Hudgins et al., 1993; Farry et al., 1996; Park and Lee, 1998; Han et al., 2000; Micera et al., 2000) and frequency domain (Englehart et al., 2001), combined with a wide range of classifiers, including fuzzy logic (Park and Lee, 1998; Chan et al., 2000; Han et al., 2000; Kiguchi et al., 2004; Ajiboye and Weir, 2005), neural networks (Graupe et al., 1982; Hudgins et al., 1993; Gallant et al., 1998; Bu and Fukuda, 2003; Fukuda et al., 2003; Huang et al., 2005; MacIsaac et al., 2006), and Bayesian statistics (Farina et al., 2004; Huang et al., 2005; Chu et al., 2006) have yielded high accuracy on able-bodied subjects. Several studies have produced high accuracy on subjects with an amputation (Gallant et al., 1998; Fukuda et al., 2003; Ajiboye and Weir, 2005; Huang et al., 2005; Chu et al., 2006; Hargrove et al., 2007). Currently, it is the features of Hudgins et al. (1993) that find the most widespread use. Several companies are working on the commercialization of microprocessors capable of pattern recognition. Clinically, robust algorithms will also have to be developed before these devices become a commercial reality.

Targeted Reinnervation. Kuiken et al. (2004; 2007b) has developed an intuitive, physiologically appropriate control source for multifunctional prostheses termed *targeted reinnervation*. Targeted muscle reinnervation (TMR) uses the residual nerves from an amputated limb and transfers them onto alternative muscle groups that are not biomechanically functional since they are no longer attached to the missing arm. The reinnervated muscles serve as biological amplifiers of the amputated nerve motor commands (Hoffer and Loeb, 1980; Kuiken, 2003). TMR thus provides physiologically appropriate EMG control signals that are related to previous functions of the lost arm. For example, transferring the median nerve to a segment of pectoralis muscle provides a "hand close" EMG. The patient thinks about closing his or her hand and the median nerve reinnervated segment of the pectoralis muscle contracts. The EMG from this reinnervated muscle segment is then used to provide a control input to close the motorized hand. By transferring multiple nerves, TMR EMG signals allow intuitive, simultaneous control of multiple joints in an advanced prosthesis. This procedure has been performed on over a dozen subjects. All tested subjects have shown a 2.5- to 7-fold increase in speed of task performance (Kuiken et al., 2004; Kuiken et al., 2007c; Miller et al., 2008). The procedure is now being provided outside of a research setting as a clinical service.

Similarly, targeted sensory reinnervation (TSR) may also be used to provide the amputee a sense of touch in the missing limb (Kuiken et al., 2007a). With this technique, a segment of skin near or overlying the TMR site is denervated and the regenerating afferent nerve fibers from the residual hand nerves are enabled to reinnervate this area of skin. As a result, when this skin is touched, the amputee feels as if their hand is being touched. Subjects have near-normal light touch thresholds—a stimulus of only a few grams force is perceived as being in the missing hand. They have normal hot and cold perception. They also feel sharp/dull and vibration (Kuiken et al., 2007a; Kuiken et al., 2007c).

Physiologically Appropriate Feedback. Physiologically correct feedback, beyond that provided by vision, is essential if low mental loading or coordinated subconscious control of multifunctional prostheses is to be achieved (Fig. 20.34). When prosthetic arm technology moved to externally powered systems, the control modalities shifted, with the exception of Simpson (1974) and a few others, from the position-based cable control of the body-powered systems almost exclusively to open-loop velocity control techniques (such as myoelectric and switch control). That is, prosthetic technology

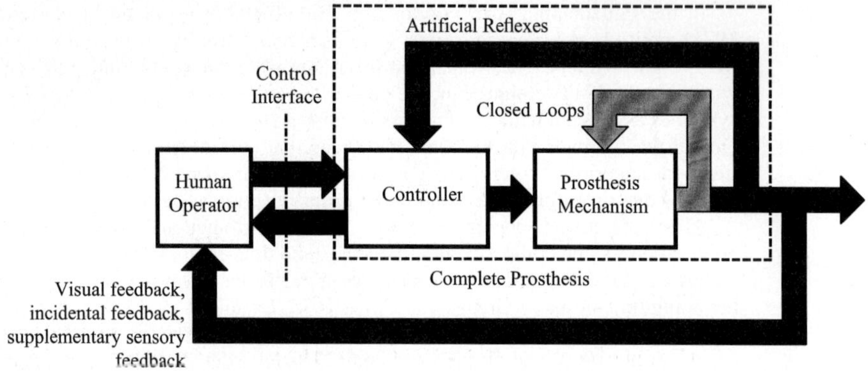

FIGURE 20.34 Feedback in human prosthetic systems. Most powered upper-limb prostheses are currently controlled primarily through *visual feedback* with some assistance from what has been called *incidental feedback*—whine, prosthesis vibration, socket forces, and so on, being examples of incidental feedback; that is, the motor feedback is incidental rather than by design. Attempts have been made to provide *supplementary sensory feedback (SSF)* through the use of vibrations of the skin, electrical stimulation of the skin, by auditory and visual signals, and by other means. However, because these methods are supplementary to the normal sensory feedback paths of the body, they fail to present the feedback information in physiologically useful manner and consequently have not seen much success. *Control interface feedback* means that the operator receives information concerning the state of the prosthesis through the same channel through which the prosthesis is controlled. Information concerning prosthetic joint position, velocity, and the forces acting on it is available to the operator through the proprioceptors of the controlling joint. Because feedback through the control interface is usually in forms that are easily interpreted by the user, it can be interpreted at a subconscious level, reducing the mental burden placed on the user. *Artificial reflexes* are closed loops within the controller/prosthesis mechanism itself that seek to remove the operator from the control loop, and as a result to also remove the mental burden placed on the user. Such systems use onboard intelligence to automatically respond to some external sensor input. To be effective, a user must have confidence in the artificial reflex or else they will not relinquish control to the reflex loop.

shifted away from cable inputs, which provide sensory and proprioceptive feedback, to techniques that provide little feedback to the operator beyond visual feedback.

Simplicity was probably the primary reason why prosthetics shifted to open-loop velocity control. The actuator of choice, the electric dc motor, is an inherently rate-controlled device (i.e., its output speed is directly proportional to the input voltage), and it can be readily controlled with on-off switches. This resulted in the primary use of open-loop, velocity-controlled, externally powered prostheses. In addition, a velocity-controlled system does not draw power to maintain a particular position.

Unfortunately, the user must integrate velocity in order to control position when using velocity control. Constant visual monitoring, due to the essentially open loop nature of myoelectric control, is therefore required for effective operation. For the control of multiple degrees of freedom, this places excessive mental load on the user, greatly diminishing any benefits a prosthesis of this complexity might offer. Visual and auditory feedback are slower, less automated, and less programmed than normal proprioceptive feedback, and therefore place a greater mental burden on the operator (Soede, 1982).

In contrast, Simpson (1974) advocated augmented cable control. He coined the phrase *extended physiological proprioception* (EPP) to indicate that the body's own natural physiological sensors are used to relate the state of the prosthetic arm to the operator. EPP can be thought of as the extension of one's proprioceptive feedback into an intimately-linked inanimate object. Consider a tennis player hitting a ball with a tennis racquet. The player does not need to visually monitor the head of the racquet to know where it will strike the ball. Through experience, the tennis player knows how heavy and how long the tennis racquet is. He or she knows where in space the head of the racquet is located based on proprioceptive cues from his/her wrist and hand; that is, how it feels in his/her hand. The tennis player has effectively extended his/her hand, wrist, and arm's proprioception into the tennis racquet.

The use of locking mechanisms to switch control from one component to the next in a sequential control cable system provides a similar type of control. The prosthesis, when locked, becomes a rigid extension of the user. The user can use this rigid extension to interact with the real world by pulling and pushing on objects. Because the prosthesis is rigid the user "feels" the forces exerted on the prosthesis and has a sense of feedback about what the prosthesis is doing. The user has extended their proprioception into the prosthesis, in a fashion similar to how the tennis racket becomes an extension of the player. When the device is unlocked, it can be easily positioned with minimal effort (Fig. 20.17). The locked/unlocked state of the prosthesis can be thought of as a form of impedance control—two-state impedance control. The prosthesis is either in a state of high impedance—rigid or locked, or in a state of low impedance—free or unlocked.

This same principle can be used to provide proprioceptive feedback to a powered prosthetic joint. Consider again parking a car that has power-steering. The driver feels, through the steering wheel, the interaction between the front wheels and the parking surface, curb, and so on. However, the user does not provide the power to turn the wheels; this comes from the engine. The driver is linked to the front wheels through the steering wheel and has extended his or her proprioception to the front wheels. Essentially, EPP control for externally powered prosthetic components can be thought of as power-steering for prosthetic joints.

An ideal EPP system is an *unbeatable position servomechanism.* It is the mechanical linkage between input and output that converts a simple position servomechanism or velocity controller into an *unbeatable* position servomechanism. The mechanical linkage closes the loop and provides the path for the force feedback. The mechanical linkage constrains both the input and output to follow each other. In theory, the input cannot get ahead of (or beat) the output and vice versa. In practice, a small error must exist for the controller to operate. This error can be made very small with an appropriate controller gain. Doubler and Childress (1984a; 1984b) quantifiably demonstrated the potential effectiveness of applying EPP to the control of upper-limb prostheses.

However, after being formalized and implemented by Simpson, control of powered limbs through EPP systems has been slow to gain acceptance. This is probably due to the harnessing that is required for these systems and if harnessing is required, why not just use a body-powered system. Until a high-bandwidth, externally powered, multifunctional prosthesis that needs parallel control of a number of degrees of freedom is developed, EPP control is unlikely to be rediscovered. Such a prosthesis might be a Boston Digital Arm with a powered humeral rotator. In that case, shoulder elevation and depression would control elbow flexion, while shoulder abduction and adduction would control humeral rotation.

Artificial Reflexes. An alternative approach to the problem of the lack of physiologically appropriate feedback associated with today's prosthetic components is to automate more of the control functions of a given system. These *artificial reflexes* strive to reduce both the mental burden placed on the user and the number of control sources required. Artificial reflexes seek to remove the operator from the control loop and use onboard intelligence to automatically respond to some external sensor input, and as such they can be thought of as being similar to an *artificial reflex loop.* By putting more intelligence into the device through the use of embedded microprocessors, and so on, more and more of the decision-making process can be automated—requiring less attention on the part of the operator. Artificial reflexes are essentially closed loops within the mechanism/prosthesis itself. This trend of putting more onboard intelligence into prosthetic components is a trend that will only increase in importance in the future.

Otto Bock has a hand that has a microprocessor-controlled slip detector (Otto Bock Sensor Hand). The thumb has a sensor that detects slippage of an object grasped by the prehensor and automatically increases prehension force until it detects that the slippage has stopped. Anecdotal evidence suggests that users of the Otto Bock Sensor Hand feel more confident that an object they grasp using only visual cues will be grasped properly because the slip detector prevents the object from falling.

Kyberd and Chappell (1994) use a system they call *hierarchical artificial reflexes* to automate the control process. In their multifunctional hand, they take the operator out of the loop and use onboard processing and sensors in the hand to tell the hand what grasp pattern to adopt. The operator only provides a conventional single DOF open or close EMG signal. The idea is that by allowing the processor to take control, it reduces the mental loading on the operator. A major factor in the success or failure of these devices is confidence in the mechanism on the part of the user, allowing them to relinquish control to the artificial reflex.

20.4 CONCLUSION

To put the current state of prosthesis control in the context of the evolution of control in airplanes, automobiles, and remote-manipulators, it can be seen that all these fields used similar control methodologies in their early days. However, prosthetics later diverged from the others with the advent of electric power and myoelectric control. In each field, flight surfaces, front wheels, remote manipulators, or prosthetic joints were controlled directly by linking the operator to the device. In early aircraft, control cables connected the joystick to the wing, tail flaps, and rudder. In early automobiles, a rack-and-pinion mechanism connected the driver directly to the front wheels. In early master/slave manipulators, master and slave were physically connected by cables. In early prostheses, a control cable connected the user to the artificial joint.

In each of these cases, the operator provides both power and control signals and transfers them to the machine via a mechanical linkage that physically interconnects the operator and the machine output. Feedback from the machine is transferred back to the operator via the same mechanical linkage, that is, feedback is returned to the user via the control interface (Fig. 20.34). The pilot could "feel" what was happening to the aircraft flight surfaces through the joystick. The amputee had a sense of prosthesis state through the control cable.

As aircraft got larger and faster, hydraulic power assist was added to the cable controls. As automobiles advanced, power steering was developed. The control input (the operator at a joystick or steering wheel) remained the same but instead of the operator providing both the power and control signals, power was now provided by hydraulic systems, which augmented the cable systems of aircraft and the steering of cars. The key is that the same type of feedback through the control linkage was maintained. Position, velocity, and force information were still fed back with these "boosted" systems. A similar pattern of development occurred with remote manipulators (i.e., human-powered cable systems were followed by electric-motor–boosted cable systems).

However, it was at this point, the advent of externally powered devices, that prosthetics diverged from the others and moved almost exclusively to open-loop velocity control techniques with its associated loss of feedback information. It is this of lack of subconscious sensory feedback to the user that has inhibited the use of many externally powered multifunctional prosthetic designs.

Meanwhile, in the area of remote manipulation electrohydraulic, or electromechanical, bilateral master/slave systems were developed for the nuclear power industry to reduce the mental burden placed on the operator by providing force reflection. Aircraft controls for large planes and some high-performance military aircraft, building on work from the field of teleoperation or remote manipulation, have done away with the direct physical interconnection of the pilot and flight surfaces and now use fly-by-wire systems.

Fly-by-wire systems owe much of their development to Goertz (1951), who built the first bilateral force reflecting master-slave remote manipulators, and Mosher (1967) at General Electric Corp., who built force-reflecting manipulators with power augmentation. In these systems, the pilot/operator is connected to the flight surfaces through electrical wire connections and use bilateral master/slave techniques with force feedback or force reflection to provide the operator with the appropriate feedback or feel. Automobiles are also beginning to go to steer-by-wire and brake-by-wire systems (2001b).

For the top-of-the-line fighter planes, a stage beyond fly-by-wire has been reached. These planes are so inherently unstable that a human operator is incapable of controlling them unaided; so now *boosted control* has been added to *boosted power*. Artificial-reflex–based systems are the logical conclusion of this trend to move more and more of the control from the operator to automated systems. In the end, the operator is just along for the ride. To some extent, operatorless systems are being explored in a new generation of military aircraft. These aircraft are essentially robot planes that are piloted from the ground. For these aircraft, performance is no longer limited by what the pilot can withstand.

As for arm prosthetics, the future of what can be achieved depends to a large extent on the interactions of physicians, surgeons, prosthetists, and engineers. If meaningful multifunctional control of prostheses is to be achieved, then physicians and surgeons need to perform innovative procedures that can be coupled with the novel components and controllers that you, the designer, have created.

REFERENCES

(1991a) Direct-Link Prehensor. In: *NASA Tech Briefs*, p. 78.

(1991b) Direct-Link Prehensor. In: Technical Support Package, *NASA Tech Briefs*. Moffett Field, Calif.: NASA Ames Research Center.

(2001a) A Mind-Internet-Machine Interaction, News Analysis, IEEE Spectrum. In: *IEEE Spectrum*, p. 33.

(2001b) By-Wire Technology Creates New Car Concept, Tech UpGrade. In: *DesignFax*, pp. 26–27: Adams Business Media.

Abboudi RL, Glass CA, Newby NA, Flint JA, Craelius W (1999) A biomimetic controller for a multifinger prosthesis. *IEEE Transactions on Rehabilitation Engineering* **7**:121–129.

Ajiboye AB, Weir RF (2005) A heuristic fuzzy logic approach to EMG pattern recognition for multifunctional prosthesis control. *IEEE Transactions on Neural Systems and Rehabilitation Engineering* **13**:280–291.

Andrews B, Warwick K, Jamous A, Gasson M, Harwin W, Kyberd P (2001) Development of an implanted neural control interface for artificial limbs. In: *Proceedings of the 10th World Congress of the International Society for Prosthetics and Orthotics (ISPO)*, p. TO8.6. Glasgow, Scotland.

Barry DT, Cole NM (1990) Muscle sounds are emitted at the resonant frequencies of skeletal muscle. *IEEE Transactions on Biomedical Engineering* **37**:525–531.

Basmajian J, De Luca C (1985) *Muscles Alive: Their Functions Revealed by Electromyography*, 5th ed. Baltimore, Md: Williams and Wilkins.

Beasley RW (1966) The Tendon Exteriorization Cineplasty. A Preliminary Report. In: *Inter-Clinic Information Bulletin* (ICIB), Committee on Prosthetics Research and Development, pp. 6–8. New York, N. Y.

Beasley RW (1983) Surgical treatment of hands for C5–C6 tetraplegia. *Orthopedic Clinics of North America* **14**:893–904.

Beasley RW, de Bese GM (1990) *Prosthesis for the Hand. Surgery of the Musculoskeletal System*, 2d ed. New York, N.Y.: Churchill Livingstone, Inc.

Beattie D, Iberall T, Sukhatme GS, Bekey GA (1994) EMG Control for a Robot Hand Used as a Prosthesis. In: *Proceedings of the Fourth International Conference on Rehabilitation Robotics (ICORR)* (Bacon DC, Rahmin T, Harwin WS, eds.), pp. 67–72. Wilmington, Del.

Blair SJ, Kramer S (1981) Partial-hand Amputation. In: *Atlas of Limb Prosthetics: Surgical and Prosthetic Principles*, pp. 159–173. St. Louis, Mo.: American Academy of Orthopaedic Surgeons (AAOS).

Borchardt M, Hartmann K, Leymann H, Radike R, Schlesinger G, Schwiening H (1919) *Ersatzglieder und Arbeitshilfen*. Berlin, Germany: Julius Springer.

Bottomley AH (1965) Myo-electric control of powered prostheses. *Journal of Bone & Joint Surgery—British,* Vol. **47**:411–415.

Brånemark P-I (1997) Osseointegration: Biotechnological Perspective and Clinical Modality. In: *Skeletal Reconstruction and Joint Replacement* (Branemark P-I, Rydevik BL, Skalak R, eds.), pp. 1–24. Chicago, Ill.: Quintessance Publishing Co. Inc.

Brånemark R, Brånemark PI, Rydevik B, Myers RR (2001) Osseointegration in skeletal reconstruction and rehabilitation: a review. *Journal of Rehabilitation Research & Development* **38**:175–181.

Brenner CD (2004) Wrist Disarticulation and Transradial Amputation: Prosthetic Management. In: *Atlas of Amputations and Limb Deficiencies*, 3d ed. (Smith DG, Michael JW, Bowker JH, eds.), pp. 223–230. Rosemont, Ill.: American Academy of Orthopaedic Surgeons.

Bu N, Fukuda O (2003) EMG-based motion discrimination using a novel recurrent neural network. *Journal of Intelligent Information Systems* **21**:113–126.

Carlson LE, Primmer KR (1978) Extended Physiological Proprioception for Electric Prostheses. In: Advances in External Control of Human Extremities, *Proceedings of the 6th International Symposium on External Control of Human Extremities*. Dubrovnik, Yugoslavia.

Chan FHY, Yang YS, Lam FK, Zhang YT, Parker PA (2000) Fuzzy EMG classification for prosthesis control. *IEEE Transactions on Rehabilitation Engineering* **8**:305–311.

Childress D (1972) An Approach to Powered Grasp. In: *Fourth International Symposium on External Control of Human Extremities: Advances in External Control on Human Extremities*, pp. 159–167. Dubrovnik, Yugoslavia: Yugoslav Committee for Electronics and Automation (ETAN).

Childress D (1985) Historical aspects of powered limb prosthetics. *Clinical Prosthetics and Orthotics* **9**:2–13.

Childress D (1992) Control of Limb Prostheses. In: *Atlas of Limb Prosthetics, Surgical Prosthetic, and Rehabilitation Principles*, 2d ed. (Bowker J, Michael J, eds.), pp. 175–199. St. Louis, MO.: Mosby-Year Book, Inc.

Childress DS (1973) An Approach to Powered Grasp. In: *Fourth International Symposium on External Control of Human Extremities*. Dubrovnik, Yugoslavia.

Childress DS, Weir RF (2004) Control of Limb Prostheses. In: *Atlas of Amputations and Limb Deficiencies-Surgical, Prosthetic and Rehabilitation Principles* 3d ed. (Smith DG, Michael JW, Bowker JH, eds.). Rosemont: American Acedemy of Orthopaedic Surgeons.

Chu JU, Moon I, Mun MS (2006) A real-time EMG pattern recognition system based on linear-nonlinear feature projection for a multifunction myoelectric hand. *IEEE Transactions on Biomedical Engineering* **53**:2232–2239.

Colgate E, Hogan N (1989) An Analysis of Contact Instability in Terms of Passive Physical Equivalents. In: *IEEE International Conference on Robotics and Automation*, pp. 404-409.

Cool JC, van Hooreweder GJ (1971) Hand prosthesis with adaptive internally powered fingers. *Medical & Biological Engineering* **9**:33–36.

Curcie DJ, Flint JA, Craelius W (2001) Biomimetic finger control by filtering of distributed forelimb pressures. *IEEE Transactions on Rehabilitation Engineering* **9**:69–75.

Cutkosky MR (1989) On grasp choice, grasp models and the design of hands for manufacturing tasks, *IEEE Transactions on Robotics and Automation*, **5**(3).

D'Souza S, Mirta S (1997) *Frequency and Resolution Options for PWM Outputs*. MicroChip Application Note AN539. In: MicroChip Technology Inc., Chandler, Ariz.

Daly W (2004) Elbow Disarticulation and Transhumeral Amputation: Prosthetic Management. In: *Atlas of Amputations and Limb Deficiencies*, 3d ed. (Smith DG, Michael JW, Bowker JH, eds.), pp. 234–249. Rosemont, Ill.: American Academy of Orthopaedic Surgeons.

David RM, Portnoy WM (1972) Insulated electrocardiogram electrodes. *Medical and Biological Engineering and Computing* **10**:742–751.

Davies EW, Douglas WB, Small AD (1977) A cosmetic functional hand incorporating a silicone rubber cosmetic glove. *Prosthetics & Orthotics International* **1**:89–93.

de Visser H, Herder JL (2000) Force-directed design of a voluntary closing hand prosthesis. *Journal of Rehabilitation Research and Development* **37**:261–271.

Doubler JA (1982) *An Analysis of Extended Physiological Proprioception as a Control Technique for Upper-Extremity Prostheses*. Evanston, Ill.: Northwestern University.

Doubler JA, Childress DS (1984a) An analysis of extended physiological proprioception as a prosthesis-control technique. *Journal of Rehabilitation Research & Development* **21**:5–18.

Doubler JA, Childress DS (1984b) Design and evaluation of a prosthesis control system based on the concept of extended physiological proprioception. *Journal of Rehabilitation Research & Development* **21**:19–31.

Edell DJ (1986) A peripheral nerve information transducer for amputees: long-term multichannel recordings from rabbit peripheral nerves. *IEEE Transactions on Biomedical Engineering* **33**:203–214.

Englehart K, Hudgins B, Parker PA (2001) A wavelet-based continuous classification scheme for multifunction myoelectric control. *IEEE Transactions on Biomedical Engineering* **48**:302–311.

Farina D, Fevotte C, Doncarli C, Merletti R (2004) Blind separation of linear instantaneous mixtures of nonstationary surface myoelectric signals. *IEEE Transactions on Biomedical Engineering* **51**:1555–1567.

Farrell TR, Weir RF (2007) The optimal controller delay for myoelectric prostheses. *IEEE Transactions on Neural Systems and Rehabilitation Engineering* **15**:111–118.

Farry KA, Walker ID, Baraniuk RG (1996) Myoelectric teleoperation of a complex robotic hand. *IEEE Transactions on Robotic Automation* **12**:775–788.

Faulhaber Micro Mo Application Notes, http://www.micromo.com/03application_notes.asp. In: MicroMo Electronics, Inc., 14881 Evergreen Avenue, Clearwater, Fla. 33762–3008.

Faulring EL, Colgate JE, Peshkin MA (2006) The cobotic hand controller: design, control and performance of a novel haptic display. *International Journal of Robotics Research* **25**:1099–1119.

Fite KB, Withrow TJ, Shen XR, Wait KW, Mitchell JE, Goldfarb M (2008) A gas-actuated anthropomorphic prosthesis for transhumeral amputees. *IEEE Transactions on Robotics* **24**:159–169.

Fletcher MJ (1954) New Developments in Hands and Hook. In: *Human Limbs and Their Substitutes* (Klopsteg PE, Wilson PD, eds.), pp. 359–408. New York, N. Y.: McGraw-Hill.

Fraser CM (1998) An evaluation of the use made of cosmetic and functional prostheses by unilateral upper limb amputees. *Prosthetics & Orthotics International* **22**:216–223.

Fryer CM (1992) Harnessing and Controls for Body-Powered Devices. In: *Atlas of Limb Prosthetics—Surgical, Prosthetic, and Rehabilitation Principles,* 2d ed. (Bowker J, Michael JW, eds.), pp. 133–151. St. Louis, Mo.: Mosby-Year Book, Inc.

Fryer CM, Michael JW (1992) Body Powered Components. In: *Atlas of Limb Prosthetics—Surgical, Prosthetic, and Rehabilitation Principles*, 2d ed. (Bowker J, Michael JW, eds.), pp. 107–132. St. Louis, Mo.: Mosby-Year Book, Inc.

Fryer CM, Michael JW (2004) Harnessing and Controls for Body-Powered Devices. In: *Atlas of Amputations and Limb Deficiencies*, 3d ed. (Smith DG, Michael JW, Bowker JH, eds.), pp. 131–143. Rosemont, Ill.: American Academy of Orthopaedic Surgeons.

Fukuda O, Tsuji T, Kaneko M, Otsuka A (2003) A human-assisting manipulator teleoperated by EMG signals and arm motions. *IEEE Transactions on Robotics and Automation* **19**:210–222.

Gallant PJ, Morin EL, Peppard LE (1998) Feature-based classification of myoelectric signals using artificial neural networks. *Medical & Biological Engineering & Computing* **36**:485–489.

Goertz RC (1951) Philosophy, Development of Manipulators. In: *Teleoperated Robotics in Hostile Environments.* (Martin HL, Kuban DP, eds.), pp. 257–262. Dearborn, Mich.: Society of Manufacturing Engineers.

Graupe D, Cline WK (1975) Functional separation of EMG signals via ARMA identification methods for prosthesis control purposes. *IEEE Transactions on Systems, Man, and Cybernetics* **2**:252–258.

Graupe D, Salahi J, Kohn KH (1982) Multifunctional prosthesis and orthosis control via microcomputer identification of temporal pattern differences in single-site myoelectric signals. *Journal of Biomedical Engineering* **4**:17–22.

Hall CW, Rostoker W (1980) Permanently attached artificial limbs. *Bulletin of Prosthetics Research* **10**:98–100.

Han JS, Song WK, Kim JS, WC B, Lee H, Bien Z (2000) New EMG Pattern Recognition Based on Soft Computing Techniques and its Application to Control a Rehabilitation Robotic Arm. In: *International Conference on Soft Computing*, pp. 1–4. Fukuoka, Japan.

Hannaford B, Winters J (1990) Actuator Properties and Movement Control: Biological and Technological Models. In: *Multiple Muscle Systems: Biomechanics and Movement Organization* (Winters, Woo, eds.), pp. 101–120: Springer-Verlag.

Hargrove L, Englehart K, Hudgins B (2007) A comparison of surface and intramuscular myoelectric signal classification. *IEEE Transactions on Biomedical Engineering* **54**:847–853.

Hays M (2001) Eugene F. Murphy, PhD, and early VA research in prosthetics and sensory aids. *Journal of Rehabilitation Research & Development* **38**:vii–viii.

Heckathorne CW (1978) *A Study of the Cineplastic Human Biceps: Relationship of the Surface Electromyogram to Force, Length, Velocity and Contraction Rate.* Master of Science Thesis, Department of Biomedical Engineering, Northwestern University, Evanston, Ill.

Heckathorne CW (1992) Components for Adult Externally Powered Systems. In: *Atlas of Limb Prosthetics, Surgical, Prosthetic, and Rehabilitation Principles*, 2d ed., pp. 151–175. St. Louis, Mo.: Mosby-Year Book, Inc.

Heckathorne CW, Childress DS (1981) Relationships of the surface electromyogram to the force, length, velocity, and contraction rate of the cineplastic human biceps. *American Journal of Physical Medicine* **60**:1–19.

Heckathorne CW, Toth PJ, Childress D (1995) Role of the Non-Dominant Hand in Manipulative Tasks. In: *Proceedings of the Eighth World Congress of the International Society for Prosthetics and Orthotics (ISPO)*, p. 146. Melbourne, Australia.

Herberts P, Petersén I (1970) Possibilities for control of powered devices by myoelectric signals. *Scandinavian Journal of Rehabilitation Medicine* (2):164–170.

Herberts P, Almstrom C, Caine K (1978) Clinical application study of multifunctional prosthetic hands. *Journal of Bone & Joint Surgery—British* **60-B**:552–560.

Hoffer JA, Loeb GE (1980) Implantable electrical and mechanical interfaces with nerve and muscle. *Annals of Biomedical Engineering* **8**:351–360.

Hogan N (1976) *Myoelectric Prosthesis Control: Optimal Estimation Applied to EMG and Cybernetic Considerations for Its Use in a Man-Machine Interface*. Boston, Mass.: Massachusetts Institute of Technology.

Hollerbach JM, Hunter IW, Ballantyne J (1991) A Comparative Analysis of Actuator Technologies for Robotics. In: *Robotics Review 2*, pp. 299–342. Cambridge, Mass.: MIT Press.

Horowitz P, Hill W (1995) *The Art of Electronics*, 2d ed. New York, N. Y.: Cambridge University Press.

Huang YH, Englehart KB, Hudgins B, Chan ADC (2005) A Gaussian mixture model based classification scheme for myoelectric control of powered upper limb prostheses. *IEEE Transactions on Biomedical Engineering* **52**:1801–1811.

Hudgins B, Parker P, Scott RN (1993) A new strategy for multifunction myoelectric control. *IEEE Transactions on Biomedical Engineering* **40**:82–94.

Israelsohn J (2001) Listening to Class D. In: *Electronics Design News (EDN)*, pp. 61–72.

Jacobsen SC, Meek SG, Fullmer RR (1984) An Adaptive Myoelectric Filter. In: *IEEE EMBS Conference*, pp. 15–17. Los Angeles, Calif.

Jacobsen SC, Knutti DF, Johnson RT, Sears HH (1982) Development of the Utah artificial arm. *IEEE Transactions on Biomedical Engineering* **29**:249–269.

Jacobsen SC, Smith FM, Iverson EK, Backman DK (1990) High Performance, High Dexterity, Force Reflective Teleoperator. In: *Proceedings of the 38th Conference on Remote Systems Technology*, pp. 180–185.

Kajitani I, Higuchi T (2007) A Myoelectric Sensor with Insulating Electrodes. In: *12th World Congress of the International Society of Prosthetics and Orthotics*, p. 292. Vancouver, Canada.

Kamakura N, Matsuo M, Ishii H, Mitsuboshi F, Miura Y (1980) Patterns of static prehension in normal hands. *American Journal of Occupational Therapy* **34**:437–445.

Kato I (1969) Multifunctional Myoelectric Hand Prosthesis with Pressure Sensory Feedback System—Wasada Hand—4P. In: Advances in External Control of Human Extremities, *Proceedings of the Third International Symposium on External Control of Human Extremities*, pp. 155–170. Dubrovnik, Yugoslavia.

Keller A, Taylor C, Zahn V (1947) Studies to Determine the Functional Requirements for Hand and Arms Prostheses. In: *Final Report to the National Academy of Science*. Los Angeles, Calif.: University of California at Los Angeles.

Kelly MF, Parker PA, Scott RN (1990) Myoelectric signal analysis using neural networks. *IEEE Engineering in Medicine and Biology* **9**:61–64.

Kenworthy G (1974) An artificial hand incorporating function and cosmesis. *Bio-Medical Engineering* **9**:559–562.

Kester W, Buxton J (1998) Battery Chargers. In: *Practical Design Techniques for Power and Thermal Management* (Kester W, ed), pp. 5.1–5.25. Norwood, Mass.: Analog Devices.

Kiguchi K, Tanaka T, Fukuda T (2004) Neuro-fuzzy control of a robotic exoskeleton with EMG signals. *IEEE Transactions on Fuzzy Systems* **12**:481–490.

Klopsteg PE, Wilson PD (1954) *Human Limbs and Their Substitutes*. New York, N. Y.: McGraw-Hill.

Klute GK, Czerniecki JM, Hannaford B (1999) McKibbon Artificial Muscles: Pneumatic Actuators with Biomechanical Intelligence. In: *IEEE/ASME Conference on Advanced Intelligent Mechatronics*. Atlanta, Ga.

Kovacs GT, Storment CW, Hentz VR, Rosen JM (1989) Fabrication Techniques for Directly Implantable Microelectronic Neural Devices. In: *Proceedings of RESNA 12th Conference*, pp. 292–293. New Orleans, La.

Krukenberg H (1917) *Über Plastische Umwertung von Armamputationsstümpfen*. Stuttgart, Germany: Verlag.

Kuiken TA (2003) Consideration of nerve-muscle grafts to improve the control of artificial arms. *Journal of Technology and Disability* **15**:105–111.

Kuiken TA, Dumanian GA, Lipschutz RD, Miller LA, Stubblefield KA (2004) The use of targeted muscle reinnervation for improved myoelectric prosthesis control in a bilateral shoulder disarticulation amputee. *Prosthetics and Orthotics International* **28**:245–253.

Kuiken TA, Marasco PD, Lock BA, RN H, Dewald JPA (2007a) Redirection of cutaneous sensation from the hand to the chest skin of human amputees with targeted reinnervation. *Proceedings of the National Academy of Sciences of the United States of America* **104**:20061–20066.

Kuiken TA, Miller LA, Lipschutz RD, Lock BA, Stubblefield K, Marasco PD, Zhou P, Dumanian GA (2007b) Targeted reinnervation for enhanced prosthetic arm function in a woman with a proximal amputation: a case study. *Lancet* **369**:371–380.

Kuiken TA, Miller LA, Lipschutz RD, Lock B, Stubblefield KA, Marasco P, Zhou P, Dumanian GA (2007c) Targeted reinnervation for enhanced prosthetic arm function in woman with a proximal amputation. *Lancet* **369**:371–380.

Kyberd PJ, Chappell PH (1994) The Southampton hand: an intelligent myoelectric prosthesis. *Journal of Rehabilitation Research & Development* **31**:326–334.

Lansberger S, Shaperman J, Lin A, Vargas V, Fite R, Setoguchi Y, McNeal D (1998) A Small Problem: Body-Powered Toddler Hand Design. In: *Proceedings of the 9th World Congress of the International Society for Prosthetics and Orthotics (ISPO)*, p. 222. Amsterdam, the Netherlands.

Lawrence P, Kadefors R (1971) Classification of myoelectric patterns for the control of a prosthesis. In: *Control of Upper Extremity Prostheses and Orthoses* (Herberts P KR, Magnusson RI, and Petersén I, eds.), pp. 190–200. Göteborg, Sweden: Charles C. Thomas.

Linden D (1995) *Handbook of Batteries*, 2d ed. New York, N. Y.: McGraw-Hill.

Loeb GE, Peck RA, Moore WH, Hood K (2001) BION (TM) system for distributed neural prosthetic interfaces. *Medical Engineering & Physics* **23**:9–18.

Lozac'h Y (1984) The Preferred Working Plane for an Active Thumb. In: *Proceedings of the 2nd International Conference on Rehabilitation Engineering (RESNA 84)*. Ottowa, Canada.

Lozac'h Y, Madon S, Hubbard S, Bush G (1992) On the Evaluation of a Multifunctional Prosthesis. In: *Proceedings of the 7th World Congress of the International Society for Prosthetics and Orthotics (ISPO)*, p. 185. Chicago, Ill.

MacIsaac DT, Parker PA, Englehart KB, Rogers DR (2006) Fatigue estimation with a multivariable myoelectric mapping function. *IEEE Transactions on Biomedical Engineering* **53**:694–700.

Magee DJ (1987) *Orthopedic Physical Assessment*. Philedelphia, Pa.: Saunders.

Mann RW (1968) Efferent and Afferent Control of an electromyographic Proportional Rate, Force Sensing Artificial Elbow with Cutaneous Display of Joint Angle. In: *Proceedings of the Symposium on the Basic Problems of Prehension, Movement, and Control of Artificial Limbs*, pp. 65–92. London, England.

Mann RW, Reimers SD (1970) Kinesthetic sensing for the EMG controlled "Boston Arm." *IEEE Transactions on Man-Machine Systems MMS* **11**:110–115.

Marquardt E (1987) Come-back of the pectoral cineplasty. *Journal of Association of Children's Prosthetic-Orthotic Clinics* **22**:32.

Mason M, Salisbury J (1985) *Robot Hands and the Mechanics of Manipulation*. Cambridge, Mass.: MIT Press.

McKenzie DS (1970) Functional Replacement of the Upper-Extremity Today. In: *Prosthetic and Orthotic Practice* (Murdoch G, ed), pp. 363–376. London, England: Edward Arnold, Ltd.

Meek SG, Wood JE, Jacobsen SC (1990) Model-Based, Multi-Muscle EMG Control of Upper-Extremity Prostheses. In: *Multiple Muscle Systems: Biomechanics and Movement Organization* (Winters JM, Woo SL-Y, eds.), pp. 360–376: Springer-Verlag.

Micera S, Sabatini A, Dario P (2000) On automatic identification of upper limb movements using small-sized training sets of EMG signal. *Medical Engineering & Physics* **22**:527–533.

Michael JW (1986) Upper-limb powered components and controls: current concepts. *Clinical Prosthetics and Orthotics* **10**:66–77.

Miller LA, Stubblefield KA, Lipschutz RD, Lock BA, Kuiken TA (2008) Improved myoelectric prosthesis control using targeted reinnervation surgery: a case series. *IEEE Transactions on Neural Systems and Rehabilitation Engineering* **16**:46–50.

Mosher RC (1967) *Handyman to Hardiman.* SAE Paper 67008.

Murphy EF (1955) Engineering; hope of the handless. *Artificial Limbs* **2**:1–3.

Napier JR (1956) The prehensile movements of the human hand. *Journal of Bone and Joint Surgery-British* **38**:902–913.

Oberg E, Jones FD, Horton HL, Ryffell HH (2000) *Machinery's Handbook*, 26th ed. New York, N. Y.: Industrial Press.

Owens P, Ouellette EA (2004) Wrist Disarticulation and Transradial Amputation: Surgical Management. In: *Atlas of Amputations and Limb Deficiencies*, 3d ed. (Smith DG, Michael JW, Bowker JH, eds.), pp. 219–222. Rosemont, Ill.: American Academy of Orthopaedic Surgeons.

Palacherla A (1997) *Using PWM to Generate Analog Output.* MicroChip Application Note AN538. In: MicroChip Technology Inc., Chandler, Ariz.

Palmer M (1997) *Using the PWM.* MicroChip Application Note AN564. In: MicroChip Technology Inc., Chandler, Ariz.

Park SH, Lee SP (1998) EMG pattern recognition based on artificial intelligence techniques. *IEEE Transactions on Rehabilitation Engineering* **6**:400–405.

Parker PA, Scott RN (1985) Myoelectric control of prosthesis. *CRC Critical Reviews in Biomedical Engineering* **13**:283–310.

Peizer E, Wright DW, Mason C, Pirello T Jr (1969) Guidelines for standards for externally powered hands. *Bulletin of Prosthetics Research* **10**:118–155.

Pillet J, Mackin EJ (1992) Aesthetic Restoration. In: *Atlas of Limb Prosthetics-Surgical, Prosthetic, and Rehabilitation Principles*, 2d ed. (Bowker J, Michael JW, eds.), pp. 227–239. St. Louis, Mo.: Mosby-Year Book, Inc.

Popovic D, Baker LL, Loeb GE (2007) Recruitment and comfort of BION implanted electrical stimulation: Implications for FES applications. *IEEE Transactions on Neural Systems and Rehabilitation Engineering* **15**:577–586.

Razic D (1972) Kinematics Design of a Multifunctional Hand Prosthesis. In: Advances in External Control of Human Extremities, *Proceedings of the Fourth International Symposium on External Control of Human Extremities* (Gavrilovic MM, Wilson ABJ, eds.), pp. 177–183. Dubrovnik, Yugoslavia.

Reger BD, Fleming KM, Sanguineti V, Alford S, Mussa-Ivaldi FA (2000) Connecting brains to robots: an artificial body for studying the computational properties of neural tissues. *Artificial Life* **6**:307–324.

Reiter R (1948) *Eine Neue Electrokunsthand.* Grenzgebiete der Medizin:133.

Salter ACD, Bagg SD, Creasy JL, Romano C, Romano D, Richmond FJR, Loeb GE (2004) First clinical experience with BION implants for therapeutic electrical stimulation. *Neuromodulation* **7**:38–47.

Santello M, Soechting JF (1998) Gradual molding of the hand to object contours. *Journal of Neurophysiology* **79**:1307–1320.

Santello M, Flanders M, Soechting JF (1998) Postural hand synergies for tool use. *Journal of Neuroscience* **18**:10105–10115.

Santello M, Flanders M, Soechting JF (2002) Patterns of hand motion during grasping and the influence of sensory guidance. *Journal of Neuroscience* **22**:1426–1435.

Sarrafian SK (1992) Kinesiology and Functional Characteristics of the Upper-Limb. In: *Atlas of Limb Prosthetics, Surgical, Prosthetic, and Rehabilitation Principles*, 2d ed., pp. 83–105. St. Louis, Mo.: Mosby-Year Book, Inc.

Sauerbruch F (1916) *Die Willkürlich Bewegbare Künstliche Hand.* Eine Anleitung für Chirurgen und Techniker. Berlin, Germany: Julius Springer-Verlag.

Schlesinger G, DuBois RR, Radike R, Volk S (1919) Der mechanische Aufbau der künstlichen Glieder. I.: Der Eratzrarm. In: *Ersatzglieder und Arbeitshilfen für Kriegsbeschädigte und Unfallverletzte* (Borchardt M, Hartmann K, Leymann H, Radike R, Schlesinger G, eds.) Berlin, Germany: Julius Springer-Verlag.

Scott RN (1984) An Introduction to Myoelectric Prostheses. In: *UNB Monographs on Myoelectric Prostheses.* New Brunswick, Canada: University of New Brunswick Bio-Engineering Institute.

Sears HH, Andrew JT, Jacobsen SC (1989) Experience with the Utah Arm, Hand, and Terminal Device. In: *Comprehensive Management of the Upper-Limb Amputee* (Atkins DJ, Meier RH, eds.), pp. 194–210. New York, N. Y.: Springer-Verlag.

Sensinger JW, Weir RF (2007) Modeling and measurement of rotational stiffness in trans-humeral pseudarthrosis. *IEEE Transactions on Neural Systems and Rehabilitation Engineering* TNSRE-2007–00063, accepted for publication.

Simpson DC (1966) Powered hand controlled by "muscle bulge." *Journal of Scientific Instruments* **43**:521–522.

Simpson DC (1969) An externally powered prosthesis for the complete arm. *Bio-Medical Engineering* **4**:106–110 passim.

Simpson DC (1972) The Control and Supply of a Multi-Movement Externally-Powered Upper-Limb Prosthesis. In: *Proceedings of the Fourth International Symposium on External Control of Human Extremities* (Gavrilovic MM, Wilson ABJ, eds.), pp. 247–254. Dubrovnik, Yugoslavia.

Simpson DC (1974) The Choice of Control System for the Multimovement Prosthesis: Extended Physiological Proprioception (e.p.p). In: *The Control of Upper-Extremity Prostheses and Orthoses* (Herberts P, Kadefors R, Magnusson R, Petersen I, eds.), pp. 146–150. Springfield, Ill.: Charles Thomas.

Smith DG, Michael JW, Bowker JH (2004) *Atlas of Amputations and Limb Decifiencies*, 3d ed. Rosemont, Ill.: American Academy of Orthopaedic Surgeons.

Soede M (1982) *Mental Control Load and Acceptance of Arm Prostheses*. Automedica, pp. 193–191.

Stojiljkovic ZV, Saletic DZ (1974) Tactile Pattern Recognition by Belgrade Hand Prosthesis. In: Advances in External Control of Human Extremities. In: *Proceedings of the Fifth International Symposium on External Control of Human Extremities*. Dubrovnik, Yugoslavia.

Taylor CL (1954) The Biomechanics of the Normal and of the Amputated Upper Extremity. In: *Human Limbs and Their Substitutes* (Klopsteg PE, Wilson PD, eds.) New York, N. Y.: McGraw-Hill.

Taylor D, Wirta R (1969) Development of a Myoelectrically Controlled Prosthetic Arm. In: Advances in External Control on Human Extremities. In: *Proceedings of the Third International Symposium on External Control of Human Extremities*. Dubrovnik, Yugoslavia.

Taylor D, Finley F (1971) Multiple-Axis Prosthesis Control by Muscle Synergies. In: *Control of Upper Extremity Prostheses and Orthoses* (Herberts P KR, Magnusson RI, Petersén I, eds.), pp. 181–189. Göteborg, Sweden: Charles C Thomas.

Toth PJ (1991) Hand Function Differentiation. In: *Biomedical Engineering*. Evanston, Ill.: Northwestern University.

Triolo R, Nathan R, Handa Y, Keith M, Betz RR, Carroll S, Kantor C (1996) Challenges to clinical deployment of upper limb neuroprostheses. *Journal of Rehabilitation Research & Development* **33**:111–122.

van Lunteren A, van Lunteren-Gerritsen GH, Stassen HG, Zuithoff MJ (1983) A field evaluation of arm prostheses for unilateral amputees. *Prosthetics & Orthotics International* **7**:141–151.

Vinet R, Lozac'h Y, Beaudry N, Drouin G (1995) Design methodology for a multifunctional hand prosthesis. *Journal of Rehabilitation Research & Development* **32**:316–324.

Vishay-Siliconix (1992) *Low Voltage Motor Drive Designs Using N-Channel Dual MOSFETs in Surface Mount Packages*. Application Note AN802. In: Vishay Intertechnology Inc., Malvern, Pa.

Vodovnik L, Rebersek S (1974) Information-content of myo-control signals for orthotic and prosthetic systems. *Archives of Physical Medicine and Rehabilitation* **55**:52–56.

Weir R, et al. (2007a) The Intrinsic Hand: An 18 Degree-of-Freedom Artificial Hand Replacement. In: *Proceedings of the 12th International Conference of the International Society for Prosthetics and Orthotics (ISPO)*, p. 273. Vancouver, Canada.

Weir R, et al. (2007b) New Multifunctional Prosthetic Arm and Hand Systems. In: *Proceedings of the 29th Annual International Conference of the IEEE Engineering in Medicine Society (EMBS)*, pp. 4359–4360. Lyons, France.

Weir REF, Troyk PR, DeMichele G, Kuiken TA (2003) Implantable Myoelectric Sensors (IMES) for Upper-Extremity Prosthesis Control. Preliminary work. In: *Proceedings of the 25th Silver Anniversary International Conference of the IEEE Engineering in Medicine and Biology Society (EMBS)*. Cancun, Mexico.

Weir RF (1995) Direct Muscle Attachment as a Control Input for a Position Servo Prosthesis Controller. In: *Biomedical Engineering*. Evanston, Ill.: Northwestern University.

Weir RF, Heckathorne CW, Childress DS (2001) Cineplasty as a control input for externally powered prosthetic components. *Journal of Rehabilitation Research & Development* **38**:357–363.

Williams TW (1989) Use of the Boston Elbow for High-Level Amputees. In: *Comprehensive Management of the Upper-Limb Amputee* (Atkins DJ, Meier RH, eds.), pp. 211–220. New York, N. Y.: Springer-Verlag.

Witsø E, Kristensen T, Sivertsen S, Havik S, Leif P, Funderud A, Magne T, Aursand HP, Benum P, Aamodt A (2007) Improved Comfort and Function of Arm Prosthesis After Implantation of a Humerus-T-Prosthesis in Transhumeral Amputees: The Subfascial Implant Supported Attachment (SISA) Project. In: *12th World Congress of the International Society for Prosthetics and Orthotics*. Vancouver, B.C.

Yeadon WH, Yeadon AW (2001) *Handbook of Small Electric Motors*. New York, N. Y.: McGraw-Hill.

Zheng Y, Chan MMF, Shi J, Chen X, Huang QH (2005) Sonomyography: monitoring morphological changes of forearm muscles in actions with the feasibility for the control of powered prosthesis. *Medical Engineering & Physics*.

Zinn M, Khatib O, Roth B, Salisbury JK (2004) Playing it safe. *IEEE Robotics and Automation Magazine* **11**:12–21.

CHAPTER 21
DESIGN OF ARTIFICIAL LIMBS FOR LOWER EXTREMITY AMPUTEES

M. Barbara Silver-Thorn
Marquette University, Milwaukee, Wisconsin

21.1 OVERVIEW

Artificial limbs for lower extremity amputees are designed and fabricated by prosthetists. These limbs include custom interfaces between the residual limb and prosthesis (prosthetic socket) and commercial components specifically selected for the individual. Biomedical engineers have been involved in the design of some of these commercial components and in the quantitative evaluation of these prostheses and the performance (e.g., walking and running) of the amputee with his or her prosthesis. Biomedical engineers have also been involved in the development of computer-aided design (CAD) and computer-aided manufacture (CAM) of these limbs. Future opportunities for biomedical engineers include continued development and incorporation of strong, lightweight materials in lower extremity prosthetic limbs, high-technology prosthetic components that improve lower extremity amputee performance, and prosthetic sockets and interface materials that minimize risk of dermatological breakdown of residual limb tissues. Additional opportunities involve the enhancement of CAD-CAM systems and technology, assessment of lower extremity prosthetic fit, evaluation of lower extremity amputee function, and development of sensors and technology to more reliably produce comfortable sockets and optimally align prostheses.

21.2 HISTORY OF LIMB PROSTHETICS

The earliest limb amputations generally resulted in death due to blood loss or infection. The amputation was a "guillotine" operation such that all tissues were divided at the same level in one stroke of the blade. Bleeding vessels were immediately cauterized with heated irons or boiling oil. The first recorded successful amputation dates back to 484 B.C., when Hegesistratus reportedly escaped from prison by cutting off one of his feet. (He built himself a wooden foot to compensate for the limb loss.)

The use of anesthesia (ether—Long, 1842; chloroform—Flourens, 1847) and antiseptics (Lister, 1860) significantly improved amputation surgery. Other medical advances contributing to the reduced morbidity of amputation included the use of ligatures or sutures (originally described by Hypocrites, reintroduced by Pare in 1529) to cauterize blood vessels and the tourniquet (von Gersdorff, 1517; Morel, 1674; Faby, 1853).

In addition to resourceful amputees, early prosthetists were blacksmiths, armor makers, and other skilled artisans. Artificial limbs in Europe, and later in America, used metal, wood, and leather. Notable lower extremity prostheses include the first transtibial prosthesis with an unlocked knee, a thigh corset and external hinges introduced in 1696 by Verduyn, a Dutch surgeon and the first transfemoral prosthesis with an articulating ankle and knee, the Anglesey leg (Fig. 21.1), introduced by Potts in 1816. This latter leg was introduced in the United States in 1839. The first artificial limb shop in the United States was opened by Hanger in Richmond, Virginia, during the Civil War. Hanger is also credited with replacing the plantar /dorsiflexion cords in the Anglesey leg with bumpers. In 1863, Parmalee introduced a transfemoral prosthesis with a suction socket, polycentric knee, and multiarticulated foot (Fig. 21.2). Other historical prosthetic developments include the introduction of the Canadian hip disarticulation prosthesis in the United States (McLaurin, 1954), the solid-ankle, cushioned-heel (SACH) foot (1956), and the patellar-tendon-bearing (PTB) prosthesis (University of California at Berkley, 1958). The first hydraulic knee, the Hydra-Cadence leg, was introduced by Stewart-Vickers in 1960.

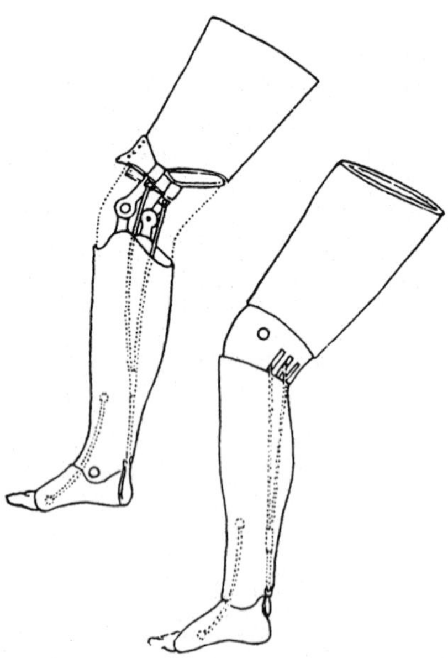

FIGURE 21.1 The Anglesey leg with articulated knee, ankle, and toes. (*Adapted from Ref. 5, Fig. 1.4.*)

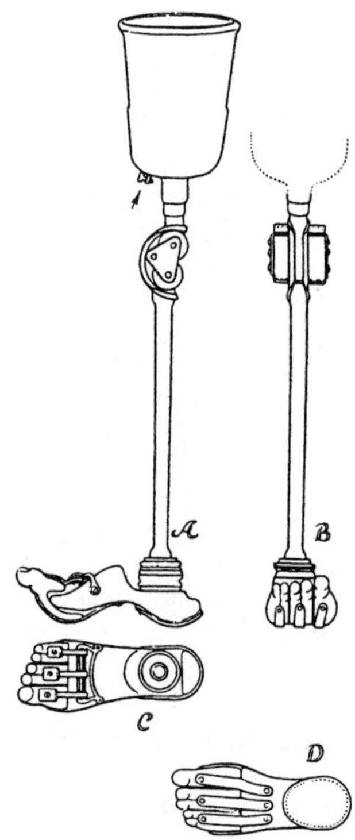

FIGURE 21.2 The Parmalee leg for transfemoral amputees incorporating a suction socket. (*Adapted from Ref. 5, Fig. 1.5.*)

As alluded to earlier, war resulted in many amputees and motivated investment in prosthetic development and training. In 1870 (after the Civil War), Congress passed a law providing artificial limbs to all persons honorably discharged from the U.S. military or navy who had lost a limb in service. This law also entitled these individuals to a new prosthesis every 5 years. In 1945 (after World War II), in response to veterans' demands for more functional prostheses, the National Academy of Sciences (NAS) initiated a study to develop design criteria to improve function for artificial limbs. This Committee on Artificial Limbs (CAL) contracted with universities, industry, and healthcare providers in this initiative. The Veterans Administration established prosthetic laboratories in New York, the University of California at Berkley (lower extremity), and the University of California at Los Angeles (upper extremity) in 1947. In 1949, the American Orthotics and Prosthetics Association developed educational criteria and examinations to certify prosthetists and orthotists. From 1947 to 1976, NAS sponsorship and support from the Veterans Administration, CAL, the Committee on Prosthetics Research and Development (CPRD), and the Committee on Prosthetic-Orthotic Education (CPOE) influenced the development of prosthetics and orthotics. (A detailed history of lower extremity amputation and prosthetics is summarized in Chap. 2 of Sanders' text.[1])

21.3 AMPUTATION SURGERY

Amputation is defined as the removal, usually by surgery, of a limb, part, or organ.[2] Its purpose is to remove dead or diseased tissue, to relieve pain, to obtain healing, and/or to rehabilitate the individual. If the amputation level is properly selected and the surgery is performed well, amputation should be considered not as a salvage procedure but as a rescue procedure that is the first step in rehabilitation.

Causes of amputation include trauma (loss of arterial supply, avulsion, and thermal injury), disease, and congenital deformity.[3] Disease categories leading to amputation include vascular or circulatory disease (e.g., arteriosclerosis, diabetes mellitus, Buerger's disease), cancer, and infection.[4] Since the United States does not have national healthcare, accurate records regarding the incidence and level of amputation are unavailable. However, random polls by the U.S. Public Health Service indicate that there are approximately 1.53 amputees per 1000 population, not including patients in institutions.[4] A 1991 U.S. National Health Survey indicates that the total number of amputees in the United States is 1.5 million, with 75 percent of these amputations (lower and upper extremity) attributed to disease, 23 percent to trauma, and 3 percent to birth defects. Most *lower* extremity amputations are performed secondary to peripheral vascular disease (Fig. 21.3), with primary incidence among the 61- to 70-year age group.[5] Lower extremity amputation is often preceded by attempts at limb salvage through revascularization procedures. Although the data are dated (pre-1975), such data indicate that 10 percent of lower extremity amputees lose their other leg within 1 year, 20 percent within 2 years, and 33 percent within 5 years.[1]

The level of amputation is selected based on the potential for healing and future function. Vascular surgeons, who may or may not have special training in prosthetic rehabilitation, perform most amputations. Orthopedic surgeons, who complete a course in prosthetics as part of their residency, perform amputations necessitated by trauma, malignancy, and other nonvascular causes.[5] Factors influencing the level of vascular amputation include the local blood supply, the nutritional state of the patient, and the probability of successful fitting. Level selection for traumatic amputations or major tumors is based on the nature of the injury and the viability of the remnant tissues.

In the management of acute and chronic ischemia, the vascular status and potential need for amputation are evaluated, followed by assessment of the level of amputation.[6] The primary determinant in assessing the level of vascular amputation is the adequacy of skin blood flow. Assessment measures include segmental blood pressure using Doppler flowmetry, transcutaneous oxygen tension, quantitative skin fluorescence, isotope clearance, and/or laser Doppler and maintenance of normal skin temperature. (Moore,[6] Chaps. 4 through 9, reviews relevant methodological details and

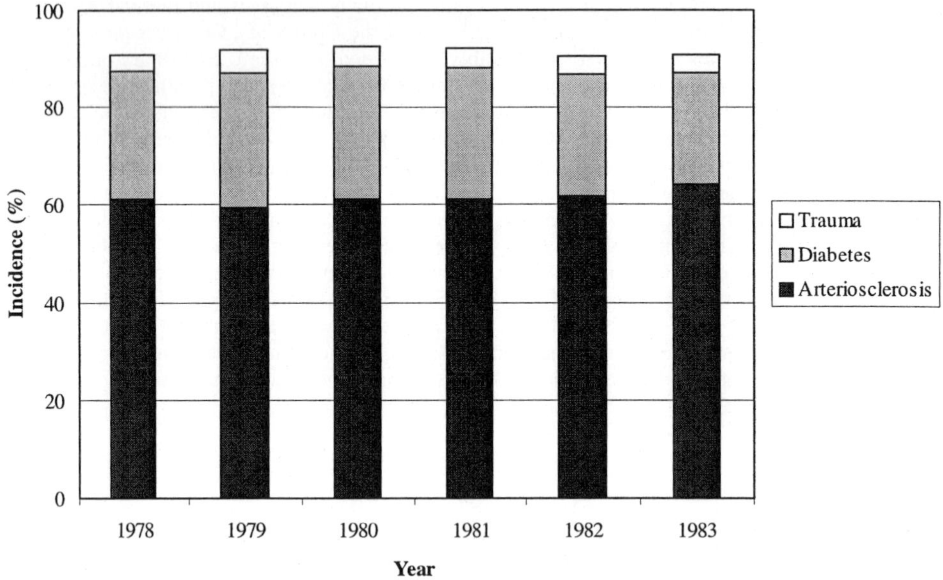

FIGURE 21.3 Trends in lower extremity amputation. These data are from Denmark, but comparable trends are expected in other developed countries. (*Adapted from Ref. 16, Table 1.1 and Figs. 1.3* and *1.4.*)

the diagnostic utility of these techniques and measures.) Amputation levels of lower extremity (Fig. 21.4) include

- Partial foot: transmetatarsal, metatarsal disarticulation (Lisfranc), disarticulation between the talus and the rest of the foot (Chopart), and transcalcaneal amputations (Pirogoff, Boyd)
- Ankle disarticulation or Syme's amputation

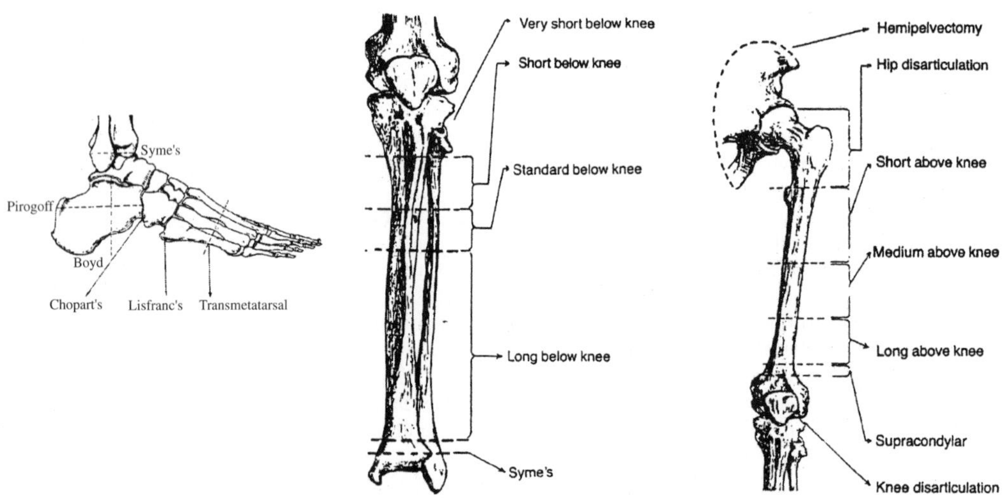

FIGURE 21.4 Lower extremity amputation levels of the foot (*left*), leg (*center*), and pelvis and femur (*right*). (*Adapted from Ref. 12.*)

- Transtibial or below-knee amputation
- Knee disarticulation
- Transfemoral or above-knee amputation
- Hip disarticulation
- Hemipelvectomy

The two primary goals of amputation surgery are the ablation of the diseased or traumatized tissues and reconstruction of the remnant or residual limb.[7] Generally, surgeons want to save as much length as possible while providing a residual limb that can tolerate stresses induced by the prosthesis and ambulation. To minimize the incidence of large, painful neuromas, the major nerves are pulled firmly distally, resected sharply, and allowed to retract into the soft tissue. Amputation is typically a closed technique in which skin flaps are used for primary closure. In cases of infection or when all devitalized tissue has not been removed by debridement, open amputation may be performed. Skin traction is then used to pull the skin and muscle distally over the end of the bone until the wound heals.

When a muscle is severed, it loses its distal attachment. Without attachment at both ends, a muscle is unable to function. If left loose, the muscle will retract, atrophy, and scar against adjacent structures. To improve future muscle function, surgeons have investigated both myodesis and myoplasty to secure the distal muscle. Myodesis involves attaching the distal muscle to the bone. While myodesis attempts to prevent excessive muscle shortening and resulting muscle weakness, it is not commonly practiced because it may "tether" the stump and contribute to bone spur formation. Instead, myoplasty is often performed. The muscles are regrouped about the bone to create distal padding. This procedure secures the distal muscle and improves future muscle function. It also serves to counter the tendency for development of joint contractures.

In addition to the loss of motor function of the amputated joints, the amputee is also deprived of sensory information present in the intact limb. This lack of sensory information is important in the lower extremity but is likely more important in the upper extremity, where lack of sensation is a major factor limiting the effective use of artificial hands and hooks.[3]

Because the artificial limb is attached to the residual limb by a prosthetic socket that encompasses the remnant limb tissues, there is a false joint between the skeletal system and the prosthesis. This insecure attachment often results in perceived instability and uncertainty in control of the prosthesis. The unstable attachment to the skeletal system contributes to the perception that the artificial limb is heavier than the intact limb, even though it may, in fact, be considerably lighter.[3]

The prosthetic socket is fitted over tissues that do not normally bear weight. As such, secondary problems are often observed, including edema from a socket that is too tight proximally, osteoporosis due to reduced skeletal weight bearing, allergic reactions to the socket (or socks, inserts), reduced blood flow, and development of bone spurs, cysts, and/or infections. In addition, many amputees experience phantom sensation (awareness of missing limb, often described as tingling, pressure sensation, or numbness) and/or phantom pain (cramping or squeezing sensation, shooting or burning pain in the missing extremity). Phantom sensation is frequently experienced, whereas phantom pain is reported less commonly.[8,9]

21.4 PROSTHETIC CLINIC TEAM

Following amputation surgery, the patient is often referred to physical therapy for education regarding proper limb positioning and residual limb care and to a prosthetic/amputee clinic. The clinic team typically includes a physician, a physical therapist, and a prosthetist. It may also include a social worker and/or vocational counselor. These multidisciplinary teams were first established after World War II to provide evaluation, prescription, delivery, and follow-up prosthetic services.[10]

21.4.1 Rehabilitation

The earlier the onset of rehabilitation, the greater is the potential for prosthetic success. The longer the delay, the more likely is the development of complications such as joint contractures, general debilitation, and depressed psychological state.[5] The postoperative rehabilitation program includes preprosthetic and prosthetic phases. The preprosthetic or early postoperative residual limb management includes the time between surgery and fitting with a prosthesis. As such, it involves minimizing edema, enhanced healing of the residual limb, prevention of joint contractures and other secondary complications, maintaining or regaining strength in the affected lower extremity, initiating adjustment to the loss of a body part, regaining independence in mobility and self-care, and learning proper care of the intact extremity. The prosthetic phase begins with prosthetic prescription, proper prosthetic fitting, and training and follow-up in a prosthetic or amputee clinic.

Preprosthetic Treatment. A postoperative dressing is often used to protect the incision and residual limb and control edema. It may involve an immediate postoperative fitting, a rigid or semirigid dressing, a controlled environment, or a soft dressing. The use of an immediate postoperative dressing greatly limits postoperative edema, thereby reducing postoperative pain and enhancing wound healing. It allows early bipedal ambulation with the attachment of a pylon and foot and allows early fitting of a definitive prosthesis by reducing the length of time to shrink the limb. However, it requires careful application and close supervision during early healing and does not allow daily wound inspection and dressing changes.[5] Soft dressings such as an elastic wrap and/or an elastic shrinker (a socklike garment of knitted rubber-reinforced cotton) are relatively inexpensive, readily available, and washable. Elastic wraps require frequent rewrapping. Shrinkers may be used after the sutures have been removed and drainage has stopped. Semirigid dressings provide better control of edema than the elastic wrap and shrinker but may loosen with time.

The dimensions of the residual limb vary with time (Fig. 21.5). The decrease in stump size results from the reduction of edema, wasting of soft tissues from prosthetic stresses, disuse atrophy of the residual limb musculature, and decrease in fatty tissue with overall weight loss. Initial prosthetic fitting often begins 1 to 2 weeks after surgery, following early compression wrapping. The time

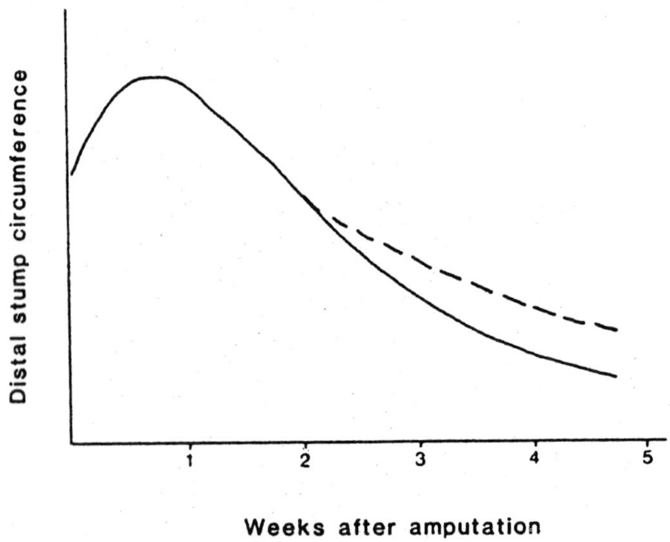

FIGURE 21.5 Residual limb circumference as a function of time. (*Adapted from Ref. 16, Fig. 9.1.*)

between amputation and definitive prosthetic fitting is at least 6 weeks because definitive fitting requires an approximately stable limb volume for 2 to 3 weeks.[5]

Prosthetic Prescription. The director of the prosthetic clinic (e.g., orthopedist or physiatrist) typically writes the prosthetic prescription, with input from the physical therapist and prosthetist team members. *Prosthetic prescription* refers to specification of the prosthetic socket design, commercial componentry (foot, knee units), suspension, and interface materials (insert, stump socks). Prosthetic selection is influenced by the age and general condition of the patient, his or her skin and vascular status, the presence or absence of disease, and any limitations imposed by such disease.

There are two primary types of prostheses: preparatory and definitive prostheses. The purpose of a *preparatory prosthesis* (Fig. 21.6) is to allow early ambulation at an efficient and safe level and yet allow for rapid changes in limb volume that often occur in the days and weeks postoperatively. Preparatory prostheses may also include temporary prostheses or permanent prostheses that lack the cosmetic cover. Preparatory prostheses are typically endoskeletal, facilitating the interchange of components as may be necessary before finalizing the limb design.

Permanent prostheses may be either endoskeletal or exoskeletal (external support, often used synonymously with crustacean or an outer-shell design). Most permanent endoskeletal prostheses are covered by a soft cosmetic outer covering. Exoskeletal prostheses are less versatile in terms of interchangeability of components and alignment variations but may be indicated for clients with a large build or excessive loading, prior experience with such designs, or use in environments in which the cosmetic cover (foam and stocking) of an endoskeletal prosthesis would be torn or stained.

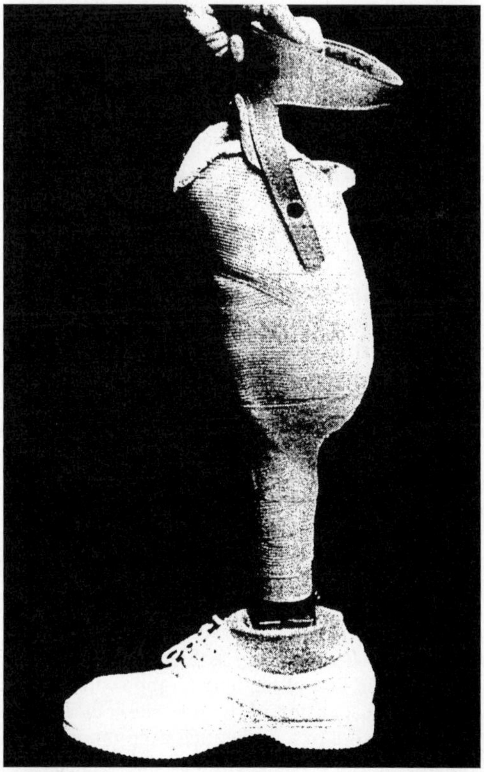

FIGURE 21.6 Preparatory transtibial prosthesis. (*Adapted from Ref. 49, Fig. 3.4.*)

Due to the limited success of direct skeletal attachment, prosthetic sockets form the interface between the residual limb and prosthesis. The socket fits over and encloses the residual limb tissues. The more intimate the fit, the less need there is for supplemental suspension, and the more control the amputee has over the prosthesis. However, a tightly fitting socket often makes greater demands on the skin, which must be tough enough to tolerate pressure and some slippage and healthy enough to withstand the confining environment. The intimately fitting socket does not merely mirror the residual limb. Rather, its contours are designed so as to provide a comfortable and functional connection between the residual limb and the prosthesis under dynamic loading.

21.5 PROSTHESIS DESIGN

Prosthetic design involves making a replacement of a missing body part of the appropriate shape and size. The prosthesis must be comfortable, functional, and cosmetic (appearance of the prosthetic device, including visual appearance, smell, sound). The prosthesis should take into account the client's general health, weight, activity level, and motivation so as to set realistic goals. The patient's residual limb length, shape, skin condition, circulation, range of motion, and maturation should also be taken into account. Since prostheses are expensive and many insurance companies provide limited reimbursement or a single artificial limb, cost may also be a factor.

The principal function of the residual limb is to serve as the lever to power and control the prosthesis. The prosthetic socket must support the patient's body weight and hold the residual limb firmly and comfortably during all activities. As such, the prosthetic socket should be designed to support the residual limb tissues, facilitate control of the prosthesis during stance and swing, provide suspension during swing, and facilitate alignment of the artificial limb. Near-total contact between the distal limb and socket is required to aid proprioceptive feedback and prevent edema and skin problems.

Since the design of the prosthesis varies with amputation level, prosthetic design will be reviewed for the aforementioned lower extremity amputation levels. Since the primary levels of lower extremity amputation are transtibial (54 percent[11]) and transfemoral (33 percent[11]), the prostheses for these amputation levels will be presented in greater detail.

Partial Foot Amputation Prostheses. The significance of partial foot amputation includes (1) the loss of the anterior lever arm of the foot, thereby affecting the base of support and stability, (2) the functional loss of ankle dorsiflexion, (3) the tendency for the ankle to be fixed in equinus or plantarflexed, (4) a bony anterior residual limb that has poor skin coverage and is therefore difficult to fit and prone to tissue breakdown, and (5) potentially poor cosmetic replacement for prostheses that extend above the shoe. For the more distal levels of partial foot amputations (e.g., transmetatarsal, Lisfranc), prosthetic replacement is minimal, involving the use of a toe filler and arch support. The toe/shoe fillers prevent anterior migration of the foot, provide resistance to creasing of the shoe vamp, and provide shoe-size symmetry. These fillers are typically fabricated from wool, cotton, Silastic foam, synthetic rubber, Plastazote, or Kemblo. More proximal partial foot amputations may have prosthetic replacements that include a slipper or boot, extending to an ankle-foot orthosis (AFO) for Chopart, Boyd, and Pirogoff amputations[12] (Fig. 21.7).

Syme's Amputation Prostheses. A Syme's prosthesis must compensate for the loss of foot and ankle motion and the loss of leg length (approximately 2 in), as well as provide adequate support during stance and suspension of the prosthesis during swing. The primary difficulty with Syme's prostheses is the design of a socket that accommodates the relatively bulbous distal residual limb and yet remains durable and facilitates donning. Syme's prostheses include the leather-socket Symes, the posterior-opening Symes, the medial-opening Symes, and the hidden-panel Symes (Fig. 21.8).

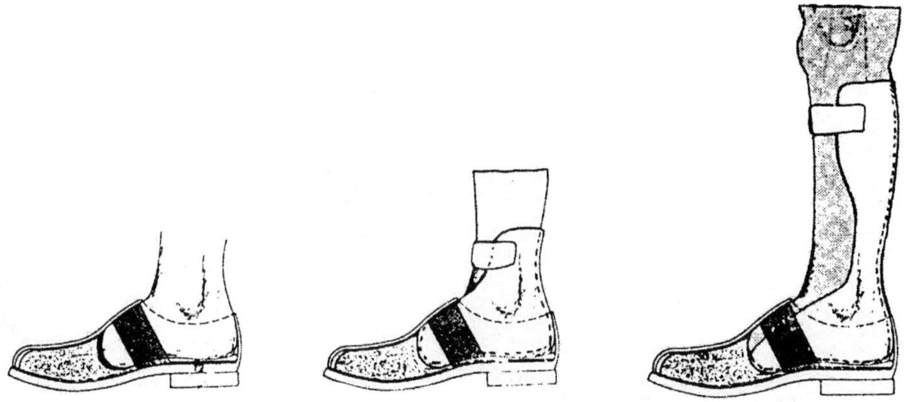

FIGURE 21.7 Prostheses for partial foot amputation: transmetatarsal amputation or amputations resulting in an intact functional ankle (*left*), Lisfranc or amputations resulting in an ankle requiring some support (*center*), and Chopart amputation or amputations resulting in an unstable ankle (*right*). (*Adapted from Ref. 4, Fig. 4.3.*)

Transtibial (Below-Knee) Amputation Prostheses. By definition, the residual limb of a functional transtibial amputee includes the tibial tubercle into which the quadriceps tendon inserts so as to retain knee extension capability. The prosthesis for a transtibial amputee, in general, consists of a socket with an optional insert, adapter hardware to attach the socket to the shank, and an artificial foot. In addition, the prosthesis often includes some means of auxiliary suspension.

There are two primary transtibial prosthetic designs: the historic design (dating back to 1696), which incorporates a thigh corset, side joints, and an open-ended wood socket, and the patellar-tendon-bearing (PTB) design (Fig. 21.9). In the historic design, the thigh corset takes load off the residual limb, the side joints prevent knee hyperextension and provide medial-lateral stability, and

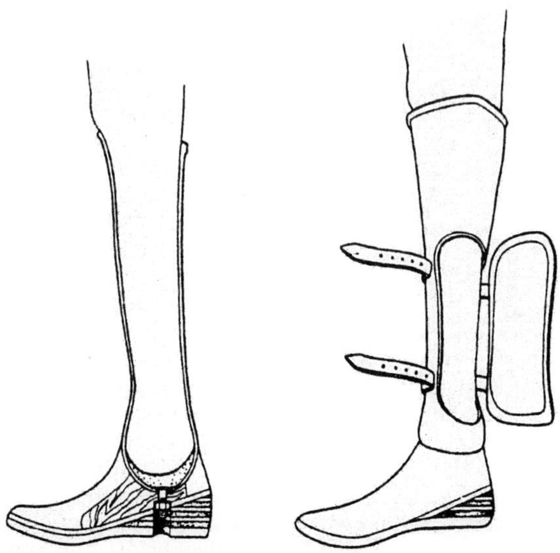

FIGURE 21.8 Hidden-panel (*left*) and medial-opening (*right*) Syme's prostheses. (*Adapted from Ref. 3, Fig. 4.3.*)

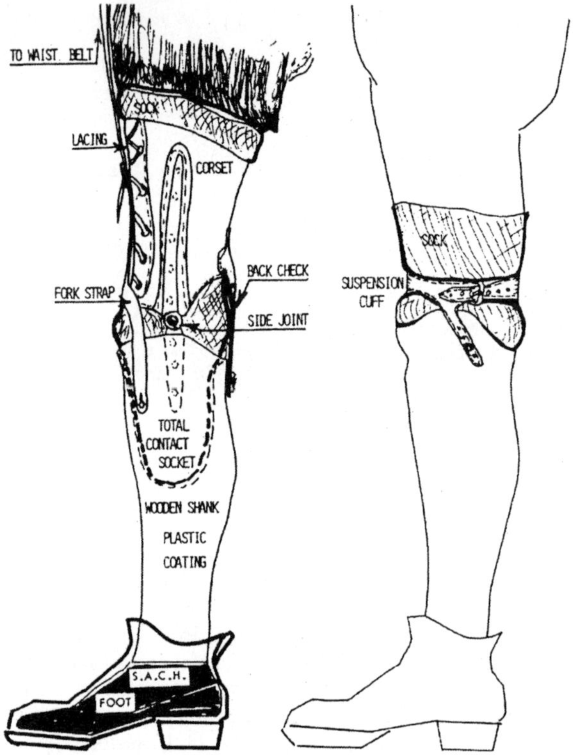

FIGURE 21.9 Transtibial prostheses: historic design (left) and patellar tendon bearing (right). (*Adapted from Ref. 10, Fig. 4.4.*)

the open-ended socket may provide a cooler environment for the residual limb. However, this historic prosthetic design is bulky, heavy, and noncosmetic and may cause distal edema due to the lack of total contact. In addition, this design contributes to thigh atrophy and may result in limb pistoning within the socket. In contrast, the PTB design is nearly total contact. As such, the PTB design may increase proprioception and decrease edema.

The soft tissues of the lower extremity residual limb are not well suited for load bearing. The load-bearing potentials of the residual limb soft tissues are not uniform and vary between individuals. Some tissues, such as the patellar tendon that is relatively avascular, can accept higher loads for a longer period of time without tissue degradation. As such, the patellar tendon is well suited to handling compressive load. The tissues over both the medial and lateral flares of the tibial condyles and shaft are also well suited for load bearing. However, the tissues covering the anterior crest of the tibia cannot assume load without tissue breakdown. Similarly, the tissues over the distal ends of the tibia and fibula cannot tolerate compressive stresses. Finally, due to the presence of the peroneal nerve below the head of the fibula, very low stresses are tolerated in this region.

The PTB socket design, initially developed at the University of California at Berkeley in the late 1950s, accommodates the nonuniform load-bearing tolerances of the residual limb. The basic concept of the PTB socket is to distribute the load over areas of the residual limb in proportion to their ability to tolerate load. Therefore, the majority of the load is to be borne on the patellar tendon (hence the name), medial and lateral flares of the tibia, and the popliteal area. The PTB socket precompresses the residual limb tissues in these load areas so that forces are transmitted comfortably and movement of the socket relative to the skeleton is minimized.[13,14] The socket is thus a replica of the residual limb, with appropriate shape modifications or rectifications such that the pressure-tolerant areas bear the majority of the load and the pressure-sensitive areas are largely relieved of load.

While the PTB socket design remains the default socket design today, several variants exist that enhance medial-lateral stability and/or socket suspension. The nominal suspension for a PTB prosthesis is the supracondylar cuff. (This design can be augmented by a waist belt and modified fork strap for improved suspension.) The PTB prosthesis is therefore indicated for individuals with good ligamentous structure or medial-lateral stability of the knee. Alternative PTB designs include suspension sleeves, the PTB-supracondylar (PTB-SC) socket, the PTB-suprapatellar (PTB/SP) socket, and the PTB-supracondylar-suprapatellar (PTB-SC/SP) socket (Fig. 21.10).

The suspension sleeve may be silicone, latex, neoprene, or elastic. Since this sleeve does not provide medial-lateral stability, it requires inherent knee stability. The sleeve provides excellent suspension and helps mask the prosthetic socket trimlines. However, the sleeve is warm and may induce excessive perspiration and contribute to dermatological problems. As such, suspension sleeves may not be indicated for vascular patients.

The medial and lateral walls of the PTB-SC design are extended proximally so as to enhance medial-lateral stability and provide suspension. This design in indicated for individuals with transtibial amputation who require increased medial-lateral stability and indicate dissatisfaction with the supracondylar strap. Since the anterior socket brimline is lowered, this socket does not provide a

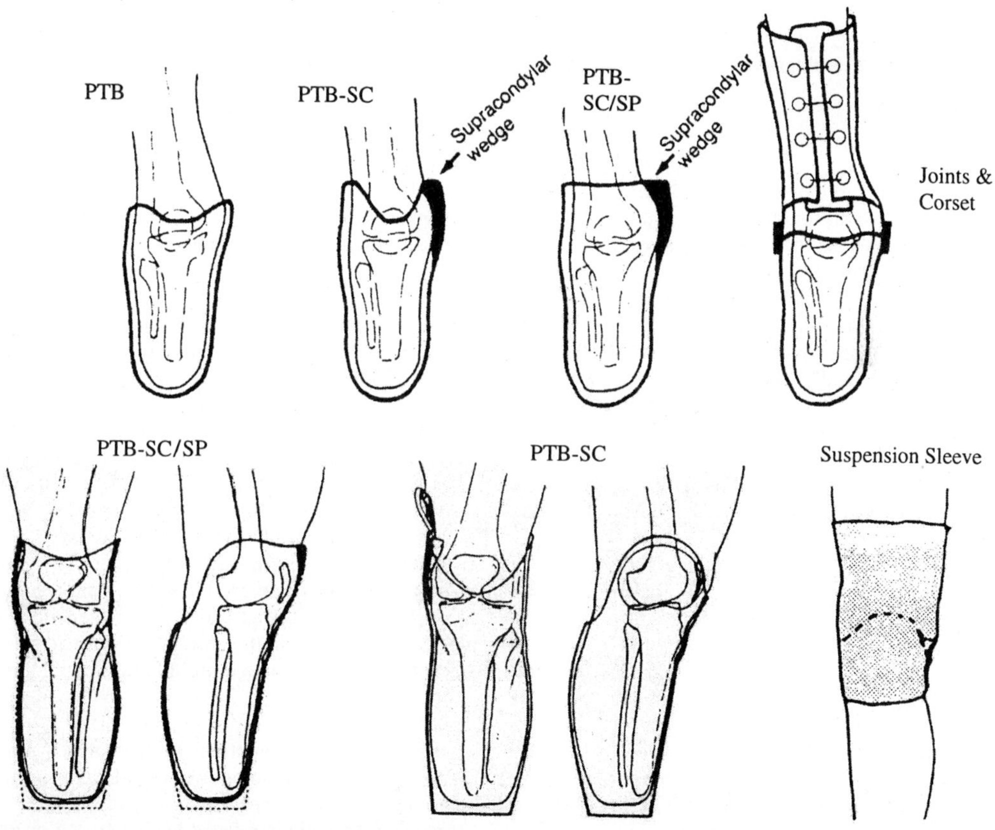

FIGURE 21.10 Alternative means of suspending transtibial prostheses: PTB, PTB-SC, PTB-SC/SP, joints and corset, PTB-SP, removable medial wedge, and suspension sleeve. (*Adapted from Ref. 49, Fig. 5.11, and Ref. 4, Fig. 4.11.*)

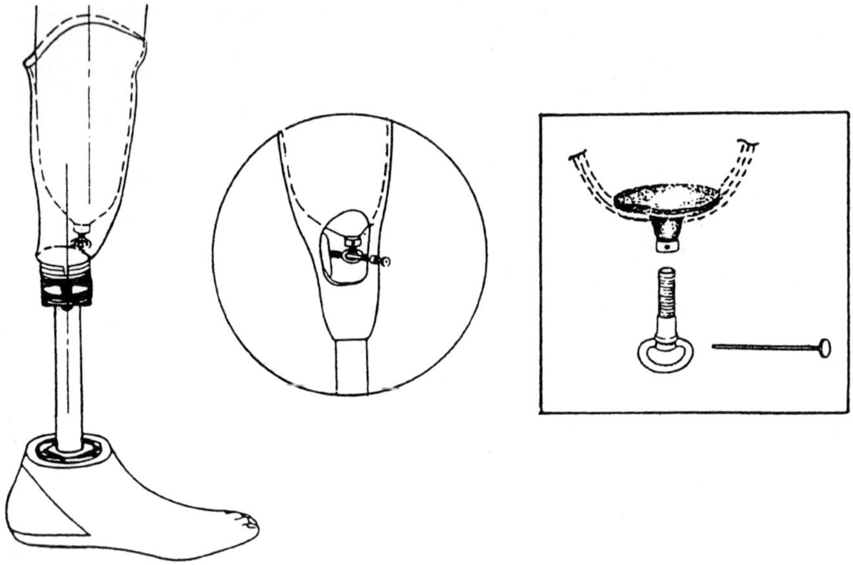

FIGURE 21.11 Suction socket for transtibial amputees. The flexible inner liner is held in place by the outer socket through the use of a locking pin. (*Adapted from Ref. 4, Fig. 4.12.*)

rigid hyperextension stop. A variation of the PTB-SC design incorporates a medial supracondylar wedge or detachable medial brim. These variations facilitate donning and suspension for individuals whose femoral dimensions do not otherwise permit donning and suspension via the supracondylar brim.

The PTB socket may also be modified to extend the anterior brimline so as to enclose the patella. This PTB-SP design does not provide inherent medial-lateral stability but provides a hyperextension stop. Finally, the PTB-SC/SP design extends the proximal socket brimlines anteriorly and medial-laterally, providing the hyperextension stop as for the PTB-SP design and the medial-lateral stability offered by the PTB-SC design.

An alternative means of suspension that has become increasingly common for transtibial amputees is suction. Suction has been used routinely for individuals with transfemoral amputation for some time. Its use in transtibial prostheses has increased through the use of a shuttle locking pin, such as incorporated in the Silcone Suction Socket (3S, Durr-Fillauer, Chattanooga, Tenn.) (Fig. 21.11).

While transtibial prostheses may be worn without an insert, such practice is less common. Silicone or foam (e.g., Pelite, Spenco, Plastazote) inserts are often used to cushion the residual limb and potentially absorb and redistribute some of the compressive and shear forces generated during ambulation. In addition, the transtibial amputee typically wears cotton, wool, or synthetic socks, 1 to 15 ply, to absorb or wick perspiration and accommodate residual limb volume fluctuations often observed throughout the day.

Knee Disarticulation Prostheses. The knee disarticulation amputation, while relatively rare in the United States (more common in Europe), is generally fitted as a long transfemoral amputation. Since this long residual limb has a bulbous end due to the retention of the femoral condyles, the socket is similar to that for a Symes amputee. The prosthesis may include a laced leather socket or anterior-opening socket with side joints and a posterior check strap.

Transfemoral Amputation Prostheses. The femur of functional transfemoral amputees must extend distal to the ischial public ramus, providing some lever arm for hip extension and flexion. The prosthesis for a transfemoral amputee includes a prosthetic foot, a shank that may be endo- or exoskeletal in design, a knee unit, a socket, and a means of suspension (Fig. 21.12).

General concepts of transfemoral socket design include (1) proper contouring to facilitate remnant muscle function, (2) stabilized force application so as to apply load to the skeletal structures as much as possible, (3) stretching the hip muscles for improved functionality (i.e., length-tension relationship for muscle[15]), (4) maximized contact area so as to minimize soft tissue pressures, and (5) adequate contact between the distal limb and socket walls so as to prevent edema.

There are three common types of sockets for transfemoral amputees. Plug fit (wood) is the more historic design in which the conical socket interior mirrors that of the residual limb. This design was replaced by the quadrilateral socket,[1] designed by Radcliffe and Foort at University of California at Berkeley in the early 1960s (Fig. 21.13). This socket design provides total contact but not end bearing. This socket design reportedly allows better muscle control and limb comfort by contouring the socket walls and adducting and flexing the femur within the socket. The adducted lateral wall provides support for the femoral shaft and allows the hip abductors to contract effectively during gait. The anterior wall pushes the residual limb onto the posterior ischial seat, whereas the posterior wall provides a major area for weight bearing on the ischial tuberosity and gluteus maximus. The socket also serves to support the femoral shaft so that the hip extensors can contract effectively. The quadrilateral socket design has since evolved to the ischial-containment socket design.

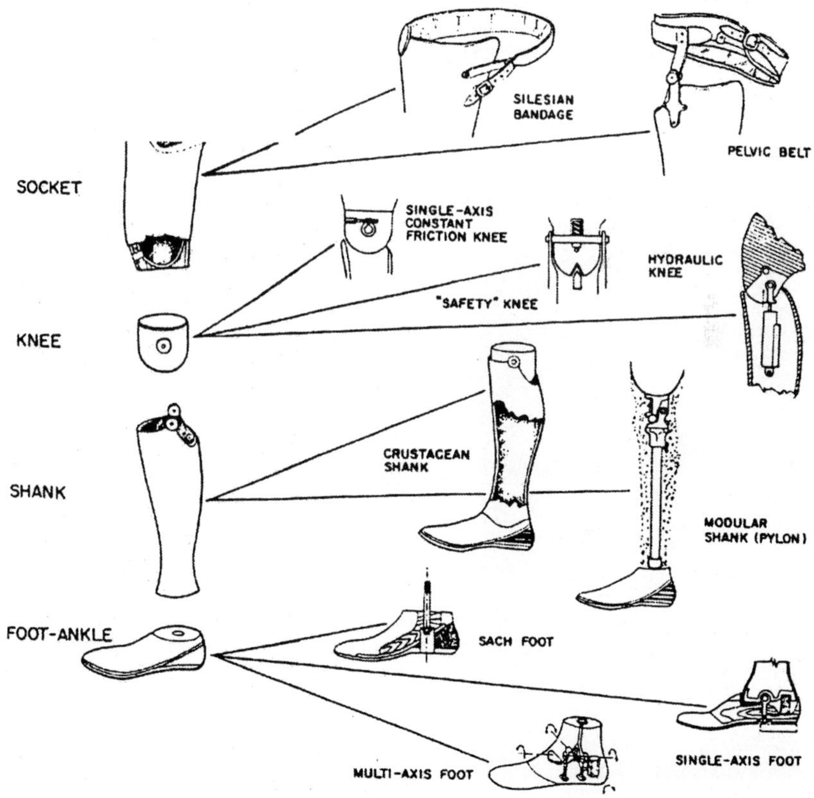

FIGURE 21.12 Prosthetic prescription options for individuals with transfemoral amputation. (*Adapted from Ref. 4, Fig. 4.14.*)

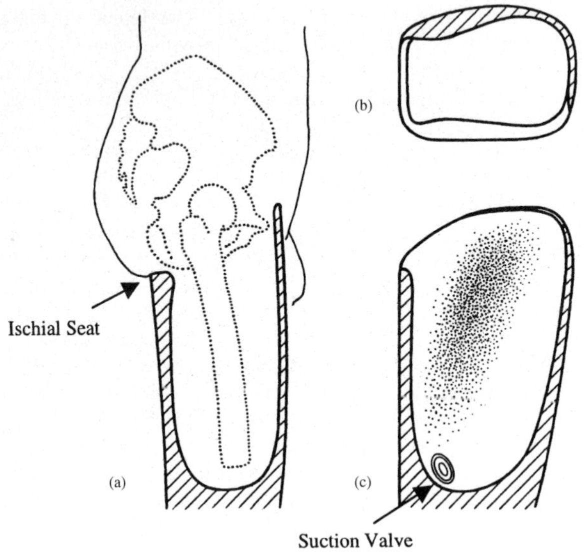

FIGURE 21.13 Quadrilateral ischial seat transfemoral suction socket with total contact: lateral view (*a*), cross section (*b*), and suction valve on medial aspect (*c*). (*Adapted from Ref. 50, Fig. 43.*)

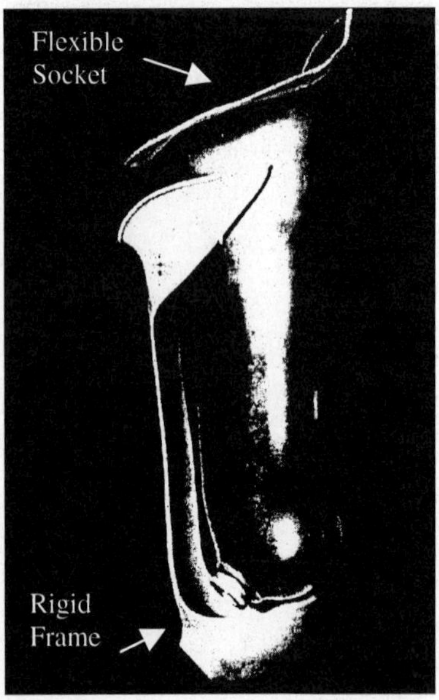

FIGURE 21.14 Flexible socket and rigid frame for transfemoral amputees. (*Adapted from Ref. 16, Fig. 18.1.*)

The ischial-containment socket [e.g., normal shape, normal alignment (NSNA), contoured adducted trochanter controlled-alignment method (CAT-CAM), skeletal CAT-CAM (SCAT-CAM)] contains the ischium within the socket and attempts to provide a bony lock to maintain femoral geometry within the socket. This socket design reportedly provides better mechanical support of the pelvis by restoring the normal pelvic/femoral angle. The ischial lock acts to prevent pelvic shift. In contrast to the quadrilateral socket, the ischial-containment socket is narrower in the medial-lateral dimension, wider in the anterior-posterior dimension, and of course, contains the ischium within the socket. However, this socket design has increased cost, and the fitting and fabrication procedures are not as well documented.

Transfemoral sockets are typically rigid. Flexible sockets fabricated using a malleable thermoplastic [low-density polyethylene and Surlyn (Thermovac)] have recently been incorporated within a rigid or semirigid frame[16] (Fig. 21.14). The potential advantages of these flexible sockets include increased perceived comfort due to the flexible walls, improved proprioception, accommodation of minor volume changes, and enhanced suction suspension.

Suspension of the transfemoral socket and prosthesis is typically achieved through suction (expulsion valve or roll-on gel liner with shuttle lock), a total elastic suspension (TES) belt, a Silesian belt, or a hip joint/pelvic band/waist belt. In rare instances, suspenders may also be used. Suction is believed to reduce pistoning

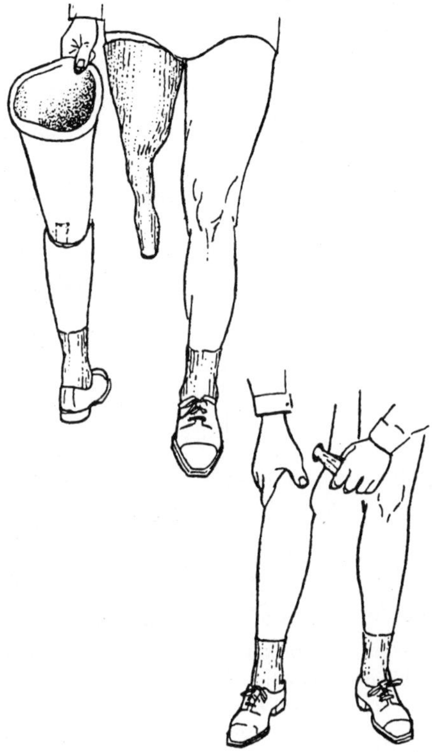

FIGURE 21.15 Common donning procedure for a transfemoral prosthesis incorporating a suction (expulsion valve) socket. (*Adapted from Ref. 4, Fig. 6.1.*)

of the residual limb within the socket, improve proprioception, provide total contact fit, and result in a lighter prosthesis. However, suction requires that the residual limb maintain constant limb volume and shape. Suction sockets are also hot and, for expulsion systems, may be difficult to don. (As seen in Fig. 21.15, socket donning for an expulsion-valve system requires that a stockinet or nylon stocking be pulled over the residual limb. The residual limb is inserted into the socket. The soft tissues are drawn into the socket by pulling the stockinet out through the valve opening before closing the valve. No sock is worn between the skin and the socket.) The TES belt is a wide neoprene band lined with nylon tricot that can be used with suction or as a primary suspension mechanism. The Silesian belt is typically an auxiliary means of suspension, often augmenting suction. The Silesian belt provides rotational stability but no medial-lateral stability. In contrast, the hip joint/pelvic band/waist belt provides medial-lateral stability and is easy to don, although it is quite cumbersome.

Hip Disarticulation Amputation Prostheses. The Canadian hip disarticulation prosthesis, introduced in the United States in 1954, is still used almost universally today. It consists of a foot, a shank, a prosthetic knee, a "thigh," a hip joint/bumper/control strap, and a socket (Fig. 21.16). The hip disarticulation socket is essentially a bucket, providing a seat for the ischial tuberosity, medial-lateral stability, suspension, and support for weight bearing.

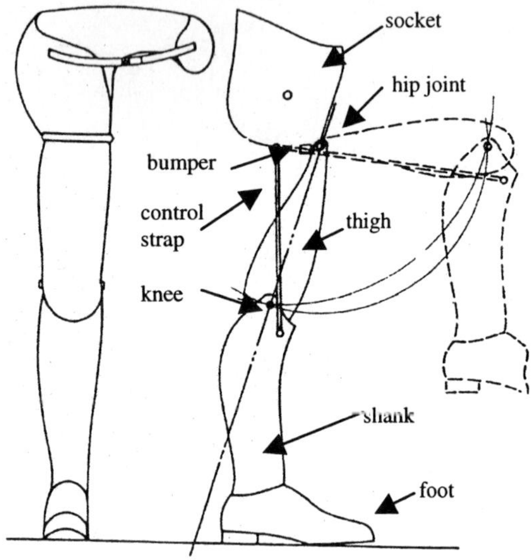

FIGURE 21.16 Alignment principle of the hip disarticulation prosthesis. (*Adapted from Ref. 12.*)

Hemipelvectomy Prostheses. The prosthesis for an individual with a hemipelvectomy is similar to that of the hip disarticulation prosthesis. However, the residuum of an individual with a hemipelvectomy no longer contains the ischial tuberosity. The socket must therefore provide distal support solely through the soft tissues. To minimize soft tissue pressures, the socket may extend more proximally using the iliac crest, distal ribs, and gluteal muscles for support. Suspension may be augmented by shoulder straps. This prosthesis is typically endoskeletal so as to minimize the weight of the prosthesis.

Although the modified Canadian-type hip disarticulation prosthesis can be successfully fitted, many hemipelvectomy amputees prefer crutches for speed and agility in ambulation and use the prosthesis for cosmetic purposes on special occasions.[1]

21.5.1 Prosthetic Socket Fabrication

Lower extremity prostheses are custom devices. While the connective componentry, joints (knees, feet/ankles), and suspension are commercially available, the socket that encases the residual limb is custom-designed. The socket design may or may not involve a computer, as in CAD-CAM.

Many prosthetic facilities now use central fabrication to allow use of complex and expensive CAD-CAM technology without the need for each facility to purchase and maintain such equipment. With central fabrication, patient evaluation, casting, fitting, and delivery continue to be conducted in the prosthetist's office. The fabrication of the socket itself is done off-site and minimizes noise, dust, odors, and potential zoning law difficulties. As such, there is less need to hire technicians and theoretically more efficient use of the practitioner's time. Disadvantages of central fabrication include potential communication problems between the prosthetic and central fabrication facilities, shipping delays, and quality control.[3,7]

PTB Socket for Transtibial Amputees. Prosthetic socket fabrication for transtibial amputees includes some means of residual limb shape sensing (casting or digitizing), socket design (plaster positive or digital representation), and manufacture (vacuum forming or lamination). Specific methodologies for both hand-rectification and CAD-CAM techniques are detailed below.

Sockets for transtibial amputees were originally carved from wooden blocks.[17] However, very few prosthetists use this medium today, and exceedingly few amputees request wooden sockets. Most transtibial sockets are fabricated using thermoplastics (e.g., polypropylene, copolymer) or laminated resins (e.g., acrylic, epoxy, polyester).

Hand-rectified PTB sockets for transtibial amputees involve donning a stockinet over the residual limb, identifying anatomic landmarks (patellar ligament, tibial flares, fibular head) with an ink pen, and casting the residual limb with plaster bandages. This cast is then removed and filled with plaster to create a positive model of the residual limb. The inked bony landmarks are thus transferred to this plaster model. The plaster model is then modified or rectified such that plaster is built up over areas of intended socket relief. A rasp is used to remove plaster over regions of preferential loading. The socket is then vacuum-formed or laminated over this modified plaster positive.

The plaster casting and rectification procedures in current prosthetic practice require skill and experience, as well as considerable time. In an attempt to eliminate factors relating to manual dexterity both in the casting and rectification processes, Murdoch[18,19] developed the Dundee socket in which hydrostatic pressure is used during casting. Unlike the PTB socket design, the entire surface of the residual limb theoretically bears the same load with this design. A similar procedure was recently documented by Lee et al.[20] for use in developing countries.

Successful hand-rectified socket designs cannot be easily duplicated. In addition, such designs do not facilitate documentation of residual limb shape over time. The introduction of CAD-CAM into prosthetics was motivated by the desire to improve the accuracy and quality of socket design, as well as reduce the amount of time for socket manufacture.

CAD-CAM for transtibial prosthetic sockets generally emulates the procedures used in conventional hand-rectified PTB socket fabrication. Starting with a replica of the residual limb, changes are made such that the majority of weight bearing will be borne on the pressure-tolerant areas of the residual limb. As such, the first step of CAD involves obtaining a digital representation of the residual limb, a process known as *shape sensing*. Computer software is then used to modify the digital socket, generally mimicking the rectification procedure of the plaster positive. The final stage, CAM, involves transfer of the proposed socket design to a computerized milling machine so that either a positive mold suitable for vacuum forming is produced or a socket is directly fabricated.

Both contact and noncontact methods of shape sensing of the residual limb have been developed. In general, contact methods are susceptible to errors due to soft tissue deformation. Current commercial shape-sensing technologies include contact techniques such as casting with subsequent cast digitization [Provel d1L ShapeMaker, Seattle Limb Systems (Model + Instrument Development Corporation), Poulsbo, Wash.; CMM and Compression Probe, Active Life Sciences, Troy, Mich.; CANFIT-PLUS, Vorum Research Corporation, Vancouver, British Columbia, Canada], and direct limb shape sensing (TracerCAD, Tracer Corporation, Miami, Fla.; Virtual Casting, BioSculptor Corporation, Coral Gables, Fla.). Noncontact methods typically involve optical or laser scanning techniques [ShapeMaker 3000, Seattle Limb Systems (Model + Instrument Development Corporation), Poulsbo, Wash.; Delta Systems II, Clynch Technologies, Inc., Calgary, Alberta, Canada; CAPOD Systems, CAPOD Systems, South Lyon, Mich.].

The design of the socket is implemented using CAD. In CAD, the sculpting tools of conventional socket rectification are replaced by a computer, graphics terminal, mouse, and on-screen cursor. Modifications typically include scaling, addition or removal of ply, patching or local rectification, and smoothing. Quantification of the rectifications allows direct comparison between various socket designs. In addition, the permanent record of the residual limb geometry provides the capability of monitoring residual limb shape over time (local atrophy or edema, volume changes), as well as the capability of producing duplicate sockets.

As stated previously, CAM of transtibial sockets typically involves use of a computer numerically controlled (CNC) milling machine to carve the equivalent of the positive plaster socket mold. Fabrication of the socket is again performed by vacuum forming or laminating the socket over this mold. A recent development in CAM of prosthetic sockets that obviates the plaster positive is direct fabrication of the prosthetic socket using rapid prototyping techniques (e.g., SQUIRT Shape, Northwestern University Prosthetics Research Laboratory and Rehabilitation Engineering Research

Program).[21] Such methods have resulted in successful fitting but are limited to some extent by the materials available for deposition and stereolithography.

Regardless of the rectification and fabrication technique, the prosthetic socket is then trimmed proximally by hand to either allow complete or limited motion of the knee.

Socket Fabrication for Transfemoral Amputees. Fabrication of the transfemoral socket is similar to that for a transtibial socket. Information regarding the residual limb shape is obtained using casts. A Berkeley or Hosmer brim frame is used to shape the proximal socket and provide the ischial seat for quadrilateral sockets. If the patient is unable to stand during casting, CAD-CAM techniques may be used. For transfemoral amputee sockets, CAD involves residual limb shape sensing based on discrete measures (e.g., limb length, limb circumference at specific levels, select anterior-posterior and medial-lateral dimensions). The socket design is then based on scaling of an appropriate socket template. As before, the final socket is vacuum formed or laminated over a plaster positive.

21.5.2 Prosthetic Componentry

The transtibial prosthesis incorporates one of the aforementioned prosthetic socket designs and suspension methods, a spacer (shank), and an artificial foot. The transfemoral prosthesis is similar, with the inclusion of a prosthetic knee unit and an additional spacer for the thigh. The spacer is usually made of wood, plastic, or metal, depending on whether the design is exo- or endoskeletal.

Prosthetic Feet. With the exception of partial foot amputees, the prostheses for all lower extremity amputees require a prosthetic foot. The prescription criteria for these feet take into consideration the amputation level, residual limb length, subject activity level, cosmetic needs, and the weight of the individual. Prosthetic feet range from the SACH (solid ankle cushioned heel) foot, which is relatively simple and inexpensive, to dynamic-response or energy-storing feet that are more complicated and considerably more costly. Note that prosthetic feet are often foot and ankle complexes. As such, prosthetic feet may replace plantarflexion/dorsiflexion, pronation/supination, and inversion/eversion. Prosthetic feet are typically categorized in terms of the function(s) they provide or replace and whether or not they are articulated.

Nonarticulated feet are typically the simplest and least expensive. The foot and ankle are combined in a single component, and shock absorption and ankle motion are provided by the materials and structure of the foot. Since these feet are nonarticulated, they are quiet and typically require little maintenance. These feet are also cosmetic, lightweight, and provide good shock absorption and limited inversion/eversion on uneven terrain. Disadvantages of nonarticulated feet are the limited range of plantarflexion/dorsiflexion, difficulty with inclines due to heel compression, lack of adjustability for different heel heights, and little torque-absorption capability.

The SACH foot is the most common nonarticulating foot. As the name implies, this foot contains a rigid wooden keel with a compliant or flexible heel and forefoot (Fig. 21.17). The heel wedge of the SACH foot compresses to emulate plantarflexion; the forefoot flexes to emulate dorsiflexion. This foot is contraindicated for active amputees and amputees who require torque-absorption and/or inversion/eversion capabilities.

Single-axis feet/ankles are articulated to allow plantarflexion and dorsiflexion (see Fig. 21.17). The range of motion is maintained by bumpers or stops and typically ranges from 15 degrees of plantarflexion to 6 degrees of dorsiflexion. The amount of plantarflexion and dorsiflexion can be adjusted by changing the durometer of the bumpers. These feet do not permit inversion/eversion or transverse rotation. As such, ambulation on uneven terrain with these feet results in transmission of torques and shears to the residual limb. This type of articulated foot is typically heavier and less cosmetic than the SACH foot, and the moving parts may become noisy with use and may necessitate bumper replacement.

Multiaxis feet incorporate a "fully" functional ankle (e.g., Greissinger, Otto Bock, Minneapolis, Minn.; College Park, College Park Industries, Inc., Fraser, Mich.; Genesis II, MICA Corp., Kelso,

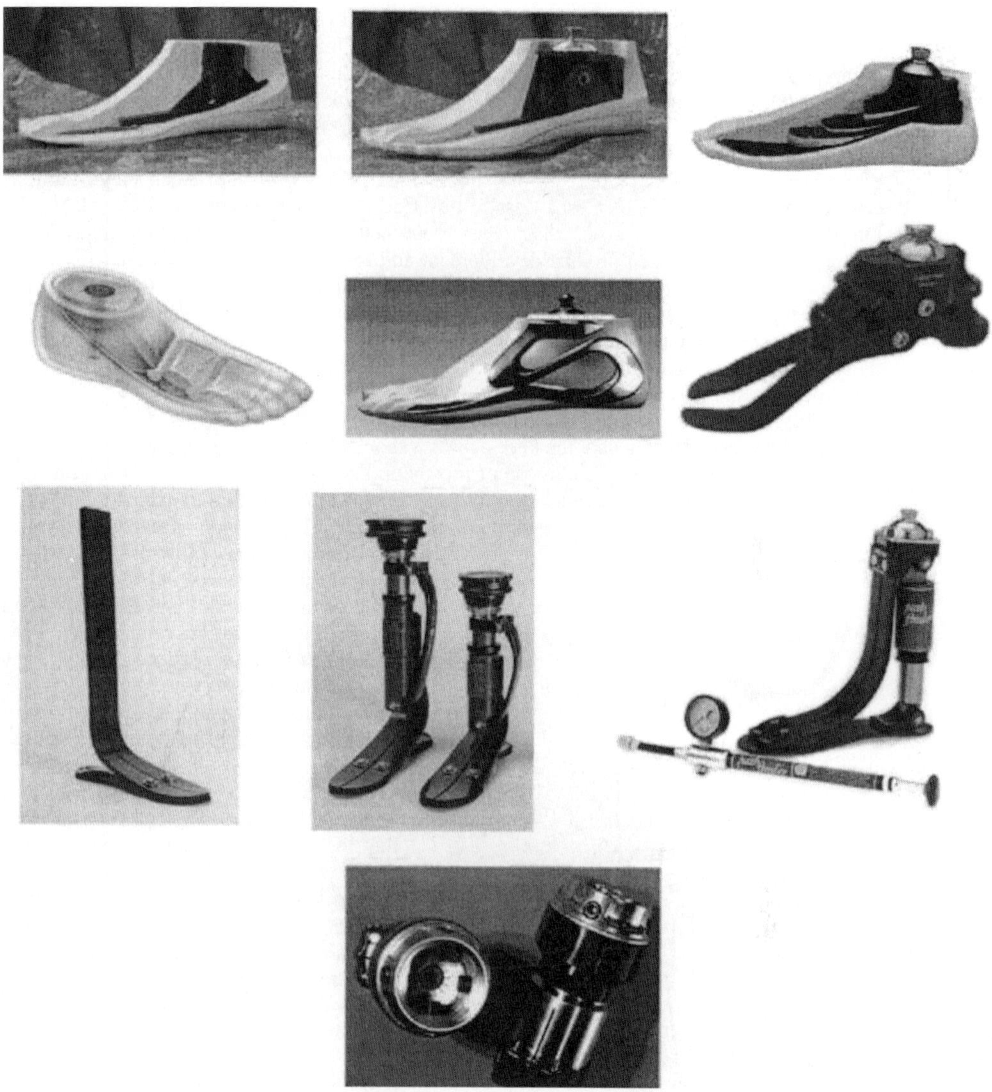

FIGURE 21.17 Prosthetic feet and ankle units: SACH, single-axis, Carbon Copy HP, STEN flexible keel foot, 1D25 dynamic plus foot, TruStep, Modular III, Re-Flex VSP, and Pathfinder. Also shown is a torsion adapter.

Wash.). Degrees of freedom include plantarflexion/dorsiflexion, inversion/eversion, and transverse rotation and may be invoked with mechanical joints and/or composite structures (see Fig. 21.17). While such feet may be bulky, heavy, noisy, and expensive and may require frequent repair, they accommodate uneven terrain and therefore reduce shear and torsional forces that might otherwise be transferred to the residual limb.

While rotators are not explicitly a foot or an ankle, they act to reduce the torque/shear forces on the residual limb due to ambulation over uneven terrain by allowing the socket to rotate independent of foot position. This component may be positioned anywhere in the prosthesis, not just at the ankle, where inertial effects may be problematic (see Fig. 21.17). Since this component adds mass and complexity to the prosthesis, its inclusion may necessitate improved or auxiliary suspension. Another component that is again not a foot or an ankle is shock absorbers. As for the rotators, shock absorbers, which decrease the effective length of the shank during loading, are typically positioned in the shank.

One of the most common areas of prosthetic development is recent years involves dynamic-response or energy-storing feet (e.g., Flex Foot, OSSUR/Flex Foot, Inc., Aliso Viejo, Calif.; STEN, Kingsley Manufacturing Co., Costa Mesa, Calif.; Carbon Copy II, Ohio Willow Wood, Mt. Sterling, Ohio) (see Fig. 21.17). This research and the exceptional performance of disabled athletes using such technology have motivated product development and research assessing the utility (energy-storing capabilities, optimality of energy release) of such technology.[22–36] These feet store energy via heel/forefoot compression during stance, with partial energy release during heel-off and/or toe-off. Some of these feet are multiaxial, accommodating inversion/eversion and rotation. The advantage of these feet include potentially reduced energy expenditure and decreased mass. However, such feet are expensive and may not accommodate children and large adults.

Prosthetic Knees. During gait, the knee acts as a shock absorber and a support structure and shortens the limb during swing. The purpose of prosthetic knee units is to restore normal function (i.e., quadriceps and hamstring function[37]) and the appearance of gait with minimal energy expenditure. Factors influencing prosthetic prescription include the client's ability to voluntarily control the knee during stance based on their hip musculature and residual limb length and the inherent stability of the knee unit itself. Prosthetic knee units may be classified in terms of their control, such as no mechanical knee control (locked knee), stance phase control only, swing phase control only, and swing and stance phase control.

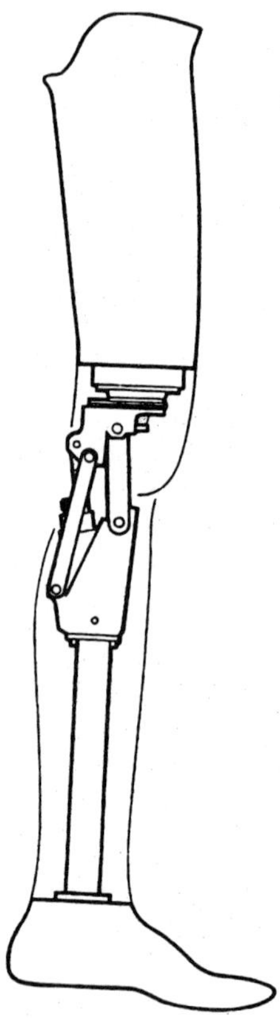

FIGURE 21.18 Four-bar polycentric knee in a transfemoral prosthesis. (*Adapted from Ref. 50, Fig. 36.*)

Stance-phase-control knees include (1) manual locking knees that prevent knee motion until the locking mechanism is manually disengaged, (2) knee units that are alignment controlled such that knee axis is positioned posterior to the weight line from heel strike to midstance such that an inherently stable knee extension moment is provided, (3) friction brakes that "lock" the knee on weight bearing, (4) polycentric linkages, and (5) fluid-resistive devices. A knee unit that is inherently stable requires little voluntary control of the hip musculature for function. Manual-locking knees provide the most inherent stability, followed by many polycentric knees (e.g., Stability Knee, DAW Industries, San Diego, Calif.), weight-activated friction knees, constant-friction knees, and lastly, outside hinges. The manual-locking knee, which can be unlocked for sitting, provides maximum stability during stance but results in an unnatural gait. Polycentric knees (typically four-bar linkages; Fig. 21.18), by definition, have a moving center of rotation that may result in an extremely stable knee. This design is relatively compact, thereby minimizing leg-length discrepancies for knee disarticulation and long transfemoral amputees. Weight-activated stance-control knees (e.g., Stabilized Knee, Ohio Willow Wood, Mt. Sterling, Ohio) function as a single-axis knee during swing and a braked knee during stance. Most weight-activated knees lock as axial load is applied following foot contact and remain locked until the weight has shifted to the sound limb after heel-off, just prior to toe-off. Such knees can lock at 20 to 30 degrees of flexion and may be used in conjunction with a knee-extension assist to initiate swing. Problems such as increased noise, frequent maintenance, and difficulty in jackknifing on stairs have been noted with these knee units. Conventional constant-friction knees are durable, easy to maintain and repair, and relatively inexpensive, but they provide little inherent knee stability. Thus these knees require good voluntary control of the hip musculature. Outside hinges may be used for individuals with knee disarticulation amputation because they do not add length to the femoral section of the prosthesis. They provide little inherent knee stability (but the very long residual limb of a knee disarticulation amputee typically has good hip musculature), with any stability provided via alignment.

Swing-phase-control knees may have constant resistance, variable resistance, or cadence-responsive resistance during swing.[7] The resistance of a constant-resistance swing-phase-control knee, as the name implies, does not vary during swing, regardless of knee angle or cadence. The amount of resistance can be preset by the prosthetist. The resistance of variable-resistance swing-phase-control knees varies as a function of knee flexion angle. In contrast, the resistance of cadence-responsive resistance swing-phase-control knees varies (multiple preset options) as a function of knee angular velocity.

Knee-resistance mechanisms include sliding mechanical friction and fluid mechanisms. The sliding mechanical friction is contact friction, usually applied by a clamp around a knee bolt. It is relatively simple and inexpensive, but since the friction does not vary with cadence, an amputee wearing a prosthesis incorporating this type of knee unit is able to walk at only one cadence with optimal security and ease. The fluid mechanisms consist of a fluid-filled cylinder joined to the knee bolt by a piston, typically located in the posterior aspect of the shank. The resistance to knee flexion during swing is produced as the piston in the cylinder pushes against air or oil. The resistance to swing triggers a knee extension bias that then assists the prosthetic knee into extension. All stance phase control is achieved by alignment and muscle contraction of the hip extensors during stance.

The fluid in these cadence-responsive knee units may be oil (hydraulic) or air (pneumatic). For hydraulic knees, the fluid is incompressible. The resistance to piston motion results from fluid flow through one or more orifices. As such, the resistance is dependent on the fluid viscosity and density, the size and smoothness of the channel, and the speed of movement. In contrast, for pneumatic knees, the fluid is compressible. The resistance is again due to fluid flow through the orifice(s) but is also influenced by fluid compression. Since air is a gas, potential leaks in pneumatic knee units will not result in soiled clothing, unlike what may occur with hydraulic knees. In addition, since air is less dense than oil, pneumatic units tend to be lighter than hydraulic units. However, since air is less dense and less viscous than oil, pneumatic units provide less cadence control than hydraulic units. Note that since viscosity is influenced by temperature, hydraulic (and pneumatic) knee units may perform differently inside and outside in cold weather climates. An example of a hydraulic cadence-responsive knee unit is the Black Max (USMC, Pasadena, Calif.). Additional examples include the Spectrum Ex (pneumatic, Hosmer, Campbell, Calif.), Pendulum (pneumatic, Ohio Willow Wood, Mt. Sterling, Ohio), and Total Knee (hydraulic, Model 2000, Century XXII Innovations, Jackson, Mich.), which combine a cadence-responsive resistance swing-phase-control knee with a four-bar polycentric stance control knee.

21.5.3 Prosthetic Fit

The prosthetist also evaluates prosthetic fit, or the comfort (pressure distribution), stability, suspension, alignment, and function of the prosthesis. The fitting of a prosthesis is an empirical process. The prosthetist has no quantitative information regarding the load distribution of the soft tissues and must rely on experience, feedback from the amputee, and indirect indications of tissue loading to assess socket/prosthesis fit. To assist this process, the prosthetist often fits a test or check socket. This test socket is transparent and is typically fabricated by vacuum forming a polycarbonate sheet over the plaster positive model. After the amputee dons the test socket, the prosthetist provides distal resistance, or the amputee stands in an alignment rig. Skin blanching during loading and subsequent redness (reactive hyperemia) on removal of the prosthesis are used to identify areas of excessive pressure. If a prosthetic sock is worn, areas of excessive pressure are indicated by the compression of the prosthetic sock or sock weave impressions on the residual limb. Other means of estimating tissue loading include the use of chalk, talcum powder, clay, or lipstick to assess distal end bearing and the presence of calluses on the residual limb. These methods provide some basis on which to qualitatively assess comfort and the weight-bearing pressure distribution.

Fitting also includes assessment of prosthetic suspension, the adequacy of the proximal trim lines in terms of comfort and the associated mobility of the proximal joint, and the alignment of the prosthesis itself (see Sec. 21.5.4).

As alluded to earlier, knowledge of the interface stress distribution between the residual limb and the prosthetic socket enables objective evaluation of prosthetic fit. It is this desire for quantitative description of the prosthetic interface stress distribution that has motivated many experimental and numerical investigations of prosthetic interface stress.

Several groups have investigated the stress distribution between the residual limb and prosthetic socket for both transtibial and transfemoral amputees in laboratory and clinical settings. Investigation of the effects of prosthetic alignment, relative weightbearing, muscle contraction, socket liners, and suspension mechanisms on the interface pressure distribution have been conducted (for review, see Ref. 38). These experimental stress measures have been limited to specific sites on the limb, since measurements can only be obtained at transducer locations. Comparison of the results of these investigations is difficult because the interface pressure measures are highly dependent on both the means of measurement (transducer type) and the transducer calibration method employed. Ferguson-Pell[39,40] has reviewed several key factors in transducer use and selection relevant to stress measures between human soft tissues and a support structure.

Many of the interface pressure-measurement techniques involve research applications and methodologies that are not appropriate for clinical use. However, the relatively recent development of commercial systems using force-sensitive resistors and capacitive sensors to measure interface loading for seating systems and prosthetic sockets provides a diagnostic tool that can be incorporated into prosthetic fitting. These systems have clinical potential and may facilitate creation of prosthetic databases such that interface pressures, whether measured in research settings or clinical settings or estimated with computer models, may be properly interpreted.

Polliack et al.[41] recently compared the accuracy, hysteresis, drift, and effect of curvature on sensor performance for these commercial prosthetic systems (force sensitive resistors: F-Socket Measurement System, Tekscan, Inc., Boston, Mass.; and Socket Fitting System, Rincoe, Golden, Colo; prototype capacitive sensor, Novel Electronic, Minneapolis, Minn.). These authors concluded that the current systems were more appropriate for static use because the hysteresis, drift, and large standard deviations become more problematic during dynamic and long-term loading.

In contrast to the experimental techniques, computer models of the residual limb and prosthetic socket have the potential to estimate interface pressures for the entire residuum and indeed are not limited to the interface but can also provide information regarding the subcutaneous tissue stresses. Nola and Vistnes[42] and Daniel et al.[43] have found that initial pathological changes in pressure sore formation occur in the muscle directly overlying the bone and then spread outward toward the skin. Therefore, the subcutaneous stresses may be important when evaluating long-term prosthetic success. These subcutaneous stresses are particularly difficult to measure in vivo.

Several groups have used computer models of the residual limb to investigate the residual limb–prosthetic socket interface.[44,45] Many investigators have also used finite-element modeling of the residual limb and the prosthetic socket of lower extremity amputees to investigate residual limb–prosthetic socket biomechanics and to estimate the interface stress distribution (for review, see Refs. 38, 46, and 47).

Two primary limitations of these modeling efforts involve the representation of tissue properties across the entire limb and the interface condition between the residual limb and prosthesis. The ability of current finite-element models to estimate prosthetic interface stresses, while performing reasonably well in some cases, has not been highly accurate. Nevertheless, the methodology has potential. Advances in finite-element software enabling nonlinear elastomeric formulations of bulk soft tissue, contact analysis, and dynamic analysis may help address some of the current model limitations. Corresponding advances in pressure-transducer technology will help validate the computer models and facilitate interpretation of the analyses.

Finally, finite-element models have potential applicability in CAD of prosthetic sockets. Current prosthetic CAD systems emulate the hand-rectification process, whereby the socket geometry is manipulated to control the force distribution on the residual limb. Incorporation of the finite-element technique into future CAD would enable prescription of the desired interface stress distribution (i.e., based on tissue tolerance). The CAD would then compute the shape of the new socket that would theoretically yield this optimal load distribution. In this manner, prosthetic design would be directly based on the residual limb–prosthetic socket interface stresses.

21.5.4 Prosthetic Alignment

Prosthetic alignment refers to the orientation of the various components of a lower extremity prosthesis such that the user has optimal physical security, the best possible gait, minimum energy expenditure during walking, and a generally comfortable leg, resulting in good posture without injury to the residual limb even when used for comparatively long periods of time. Good alignment begins with proper fit of the residual limb in the socket (see Sec. 21.5.3). The adapter hardware used to connect the socket to the endoskeletal components, and to the foot and knee, facilitates alignment changes.

Alignment of the prosthesis consists of static and dynamic stages. For transtibial amputees, static alignment places the knee in approximately 5 degrees of flexion to prevent hyperextension and increase pressures on the anterior surface of the limb.[13] The pylon is vertical, and alignment in the sagittal plane is such that a plumb line at the center of the greater trochanter intersects the medial-lateral axis of the knee and aligns with the anterior surface of the pylon so that there is no tendency for the knee to buckle during stance. Additional modifications may be invoked during dynamic alignment based on observation of amputee gait in the frontal and sagittal planes. (Sanders,[1] Chap. 20, reviews static and dynamic alignment of the transtibial prosthesis and identifies malalignment symptoms.)

Zahedi and Spence[52] found that a transtibial amputee can adapt to several alignments, ranging from as much as 148-mm shifts and 17-degree tilts. This tolerance of alignment variability was attributed to the degree of control that an amputee has over the prosthesis. For a transtibial amputee, for example, the retention of the knee joint allows the body to compensate more readily to malalignments. In addition, Zahedi and Spence[52] hypothesized that the nonuniform distribution of alignment data about the mean was indicative of an optimum alignment configuration not readily achieved by current alignment procedures.

For transfemoral amputees, the socket is mounted on an alignment rig. The desired height of the prosthesis is determined, as is the relative position of the knee and foot with respect to the socket/limb. This bench alignment is such that the center of the heel falls just under the ischial seat, with the trochanter-knee-ankle (TKA) line passing through the knee and ankle axes of rotation. As for alignment of transtibial prostheses, this bench alignment is modified based on static and dynamic observations of amputee gait in the frontal and sagittal planes.

In general, prosthetic socket fit and alignment are dependent. Prosthetic alignment depends on the length of the residual limb (lever arm), strength of the remnant musculature, and the amputee's balance and control. For the hip disarticulation prosthesis, alignment *defines* prosthetic stability because there are no knee extensors to prevent the knee from buckling during stance. For stability, the weight line during stance must go through the base of support, be posterior to the hip so as to provide an inherently stable hip extension moment, and be anterior to the knee so as to provide a knee extension moment. As such, the prosthetic hip joint is located distal and anterior to the axis of the anatomic hip (see Fig. 21.16). (The position of the hip joint also determines the length of the thigh when sitting.) The posterior bumper, which controls the amount of hip extension, is mounted well forward of the weight line so as to produce a hip extension moment during stance. The stride-length control strap is positioned posterior to the hip and anterior to the knee. This strap is a critical feature of the hip disarticulation prosthesis, acting as the quadriceps muscle—preventing excess hip extension and excess knee flexion while assisting in knee extension.

21.6 AMPUTEE GAIT

Since one of the goals of lower extremity prosthetics is to replace function, much attention is given to the restoration of gait or ambulation. While some argue that optimal gait for a lower extremity amputee need not be symmetric, symmetry in ambulation is cosmetic. As such, the prosthetist and physical therapists attempt to restore normal, symmetric gait—given constraints such as joint contractures, weak hip/knee musculature, poor balance, and the potential need for an assistive device.

Another primary factor that influences ambulation and prosthetic use is tissue pain. The residual limb soft tissues are routinely loaded during ambulation. As such, these tissues are stressed, unlike prior to amputation. These stresses are the direct result of load transfer from the prosthetic foot through the residual limb soft tissues and subsequently through the skeleton. Thus, while symmetric gait may be desired, tissue sensitivity and pain due to the presence of neuromas and local stress concentrations may mandate altered gait.

The residual limb–prosthetic socket stresses are influenced by the fit of the socket and the alignment of the prosthesis. For transtibial amputees, medial-lateral stability is influenced by foot placement. Foot inset (or outset) may result in varus (or valgus) moments applied to the limb. Similarly, anterior-posterior stability is influenced by the fore-aft position (extension-flexion moment) of the foot, foot plantarflexion/dorsiflexion (extension-flexion moment), and heel durometer (soft heel increases foot plantarflexion). For transtibial amputees with normal knee extensors, knee flexion moments on heel strike are desired, as for individuals without amputation.

Since most prosthetists do not have motion-analysis systems, they cannot quantitatively evaluate lower limb kinematics nor measure lower extremity kinetics. Therefore, prosthetists rely on visual assessment of limb kinematics and indirect measures of tissue loading and joint moments. Joint moments are inferred from the relative position of a weight line with respect to the ankle, knee, and hip axes of rotation. Muscle activity that may be required to oppose such joint moments for stability is similarly inferred. While such moment estimation ignores inertial factors, it provides a visual estimate for evaluation of prosthetic fit and alignment. These visual estimates are only be applied during stance, since stance phase dictates stability and tissue loading. Analysis of swing is restricted to kinematic analysis in the frontal and sagittal planes.

For transfemoral and knee disarticulation amputees, the remnant hip musculature is vital to normal gait and prosthetic stability. As noted previously in the discussion of transfemoral socket design, the thigh is adducted in the socket so as to position the hip abductors at an appropriate functional length. The hip abductors play an important role in stabilizing the pelvis in the frontal plane during single-limb support. Since individuals with a short transfemoral residual limb may have weak hip abductors, their pelvis may dip excessively to the swing side during single-limb support. The hip adductors are important during weight transfer. The hamstrings (hip extensors) act to decelerate the limb during swing in anticipation of heel strike. If the hip extensors are weak, lumbar lordosis may be observed as a common compensatory mechanism. To maximize the efficiency of the hip extensors, the residual femur is routinely flexed within the socket. The amount of hip flexion is dictated by the length of the residual limb, the lever arm for hip extension.

Note that many individuals with transfemoral amputation choose not to wear a prosthesis and walk with crutches. The use of these assistive devices may facilitate faster and more efficient (per distance traveled) ambulation.

Gait analysis of the hip disarticulation amputee will not be discussed due to the relative rarity of this level of amputation and the fact that the excessive cost of ambulation often dictates that such amputees do not routinely use a prosthesis for ambulation. Many individuals with hip disarticulation prefer to use forearm crutches for ambulation and don their prosthesis for cosmetic purposes only. However, as discussed previously in the design of the prosthesis for individuals with this level of amputation, the stride-length control strap and hip bumper are critical to prosthetic limb stability and function during ambulation.

As alluded to earlier, energy consumption during ambulation is higher for amputees than for nonamputees.[7] While energy cost (energy consumption per distance traveled) is comparable for unilateral traumatic transtibial amputees and normal individuals, energy cost increases substantially as the level of amputation becomes more proximal (Fig. 21.19). These energy costs tend to be higher for vascular amputees than for individuals who have lost their limbs due to trauma. As one might expect, the energy cost of ambulation for individuals with bilateral lower extremity amputation is higher than for unilateral amputees. Finally, the natural velocity of individuals with amputation is typically less than for normal individuals, with the velocity decreasing for the more proximal levels of amputation (see Fig. 21.19). Assessment of amputee performance is further confounded by age, since the majority of lower extremity amputations are due to vascular complications, prevalent in older individuals.

21.7 RECENT DEVELOPMENTS

As indicated throughout this chapter, many advances in lower extremity prosthetics are due to technological advances in materials. This has facilitated fabrication of markedly lighter prostheses, stronger prosthetics sockets, and composite feet with energy-storing capabilities. Prosthetic liners for transtibial amputees have also benefited from such technology. The OrthoGel liners (Otto Bock, Minneapolis, Minn.) incorporate polyurethane gel and provide enhanced comfort for individuals whose residual limb tissues are very sensitive and/or prone to breakdown.

In terms of recent innovations, it is worth acknowledging advances in lower extremity prosthetics with respect to suspension. Historic suspension mechanisms such as hip and waist belts and fork straps and supracondylar cuffs for transfemoral and transtibial amputees, respectively, have been largely replaced by suction. Suction has been induced using neoprene suspension sleeves, TES belts, and shuttle-locking mechanisms.

Sabolich Research and Development (Oklahoma City, Okla.) recently has developed commercial systems for the upper and lower extremities that attempt to supplement sensation lost by amputation. Their Sense of Feel leg provides sensory feedback to the residual limb. Output from force transducers in the sole of the foot is transmitted to the residual limb via electrodes in the prosthetic socket. The amplitude of the "tingling" sensation is proportional to the force measured at the foot, thereby providing direct feedback to the amputee regarding the relative loading of the forefoot versus the heel. Such information is hypothesized to improve lower extremity balance. Clinical trials are currently underway.

Another new commercial product is the 3C100 C-Leg (Otto Bock, Minneapolis, Minn.) (Fig. 21.20). This transfemoral leg incorporates a microprocessor-controlled hydraulic knee with swing and stance phase control. The controls are adjusted for the individual subject. The knee angles and moments are measured at 50 Hz, and the prosthesis facilitates ambulation at various speeds on inclines, declines, stairs (step over step), and uneven terrain. The rechargeable lithium-ion battery provides sufficient power for a full day (25 to 30 h). Similar microprocessor-controlled pneumatic knees are also available from Endolite (Intelligent Prosthesis Plus, Centerville, Ohio) and Seattle Limb Systems (Power Knee, Poulsbo, Wash.)

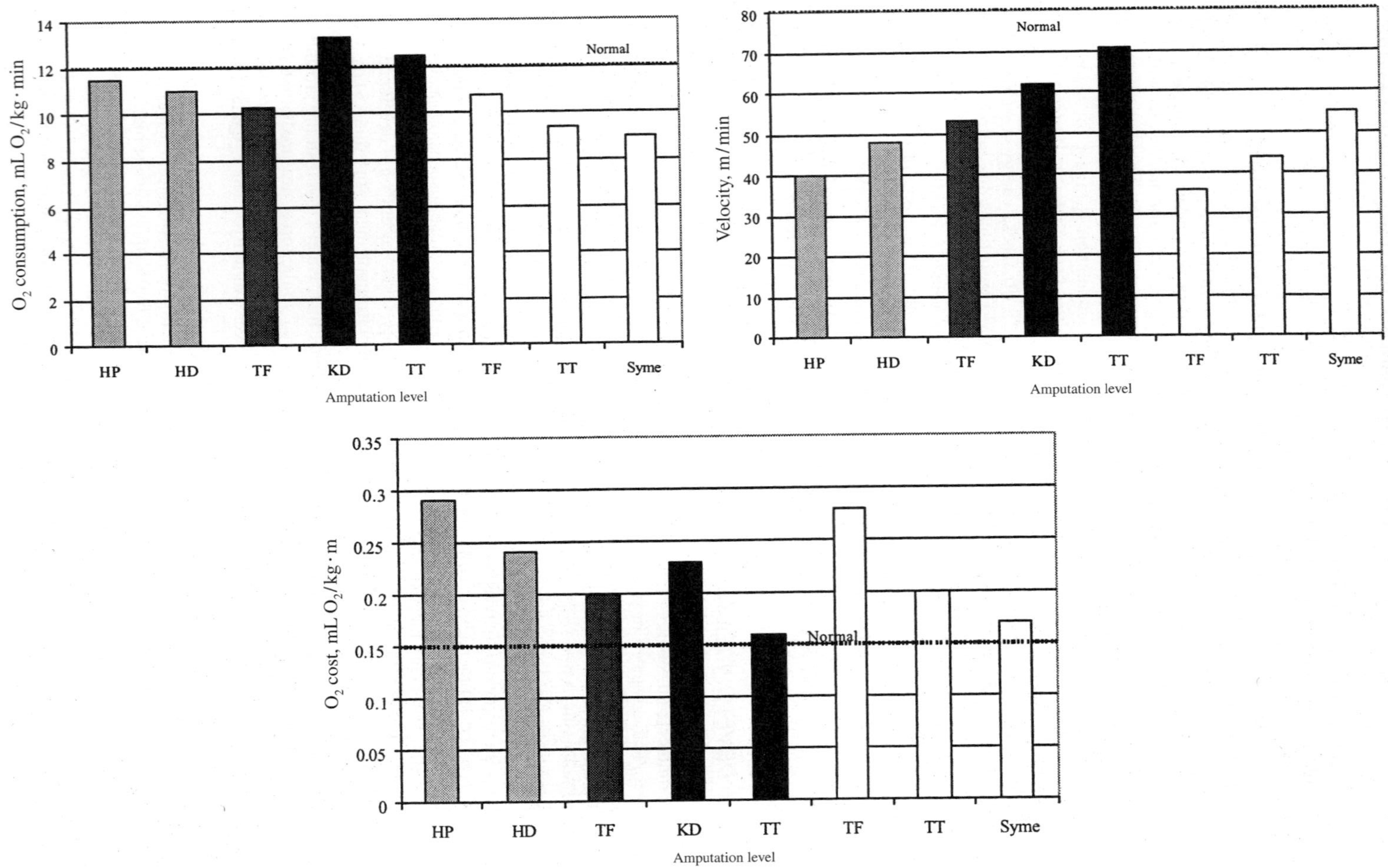

FIGURE 21.19 Rate of oxygen consumption and walking speed for surgical (gray), traumatic (black), and vascular (white) amputees for various levels of amputation (HP = hemipelvectomy, HD = hip disarticulation; TF = transfemoral; KD = knee disarticulation; TT = transtibial). (*From Ref. 6.*)

One final noteworthy lower extremity development in that of shock-absorbing pylons and shock-absorbing feet (Re-Flex VSP, OSSUR/Flex-Foot, Inc., Aliso Viejo, Calif.) (see Fig. 21.17). These pylons and feet alter the effective length of the shank during loading and introduce new fitting issues and potential problems. The shock absorption or vertical compliance serves to spare the residual limb tissues during high-impact activities.

Some of the latest technology with respect to artificial limbs was recently highlighted in a medical device journal.[48] Many of these developments involve the use of robotics and/or smart materials in lower (and upper) extremity prostheses. A transfemoral prosthesis is under development at Biedermann Motech (Schwennigen, Germany) that incorporates sensors in the prosthetic knee to measure the force and moment exerted on the prosthesis, as well as the angular orientation of the knee. The knee of this prosthesis incorporates a magnetorheological fluid in its damper that reportedly results in improved response times over conventional hydraulic knee units. The BioRobotics Laboratory at the University of Washington in Seattle is investigating use of the McKibben artificial muscle (pneumatically operated actuators) to power a lower extremity prosthesis. After development of the functional prototype of the powered prosthesis, these researchers will compare their active design with conventional limbs in terms of function (gait) and energy expenditure.

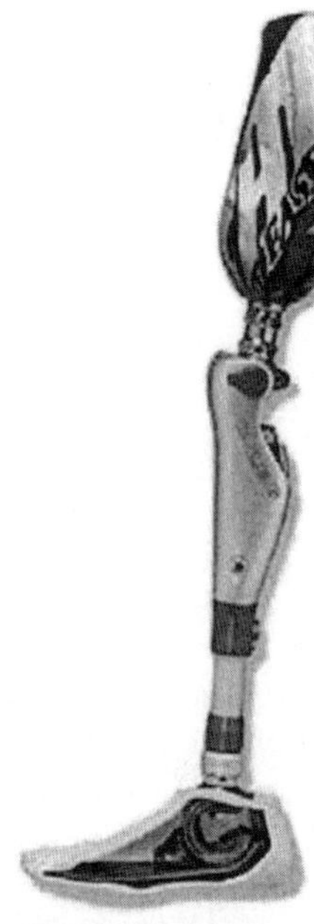

FIGURE 21.20 C-leg system with microprocessor-controlled hydraulic knee with stance and swing phase control.

Prosthetics research is also being conducted in a collaborative effort by researchers at Sandia National Laboratories (Albuquerque, N.M.), the Seattle Orthopedic Group (Poulsbo, Wash.) and the Russian nuclear weapons laboratory at Chelyabinsk-70. A recent project involves the design of a lower extremity prosthetic limb that can adjust to an amputee's gait/environment (incline, decline, and irregular terrain) and compensate for changes in residual limb shape. The first initiative involves the use of microprocessor controls for the hydraulic joints and piezoelectric motors governing the ankle and knee mechanisms. The latter initiative is based on sensors in the socket that monitor the diameter of the residual limb over the course of the day. Difficulties reportedly involve the development of a robust, lightweight power source for the entire system.

As prostheses improve, amputee function improves. Such improved function is often accompanied by increased desire to participate in additional activities and/or further improvements in performance, especially with respect to athletics and recreation. As such, there have been continued developments regarding task-specific prostheses and adaptive equipment. Amputee athletes' prowess with respect to running has received considerable press. These amputees post amazing times, supported by energy-storage prosthetic feet—with dorsiflexed alignment specific for running. Many lower extremity amputees also ski. Individuals with transfemoral amputations often ski without a prosthesis and may use outriggers (adapted ski poles that are a cross between a crutch and a miniski). Transtibial amputees, on the other hand, typically ski with a prosthesis that has been modified (e.g., alignment that accommodates skiing; step-in, rear-entry boots). Individuals with lower extremity amputations may also swim and again may opt to use or not use a prosthesis. Modifications for swimming include a prosthetic socket with a distal fin, peg legs for the beach, and/or a swim leg that does not float but provides some functionality. As for snow skiing, individuals with lower extremity amputation may also waterski, typically using a single ski; they may or may not use a prosthesis. Finally, amputee golfing has gained in popularity. For transfemoral amputees, shear on the residual limb is minimized by the inclusion of a rotator.

Finally, future developments in CAD of prosthetic sockets are also likely to be influenced by alternative shape-sensing methodology and finite-element model development that will enable timely evaluation of residual limb geometry and/or material properties.

REFERENCES

1. G. T. Sanders, B. J. May, R. Hurd, and J. Milani (1986), *Lower Limb Amputations: A Guide to Rehabilitation,* F. A. Davis, Philadelphia, Pa.
2. C. L. Thomas (ed.) (1993), *Taber's Cyclopedic Medical Dictionary,* 17th ed, F. A. Davis, Philadelphia, Pa.
3. D. G. Shurr and T. M. Cook (1990), *Prosthetics and Orthotics,* Appleton & Lange, East Norwalk, Conn.
4. A. B. Wilson (1989), *Limb Prosthetics,* 6th ed., Demos Publications, New York, N.Y.
5. B. J. May (1996), *Amputations and Prosthetics: A Case Study Approach,* F. A. Davis, Philadelphia, Pa.
6. W. S. Moore and J. M. Malone (1989), *Lower Extremity Amputation,* Saunders, Philadelphia, Pa.
7. J. H. Bowker and J. W. Michael (eds.) (1992), *Atlas of Limb Prosthetics: Surgical, Prosthetic, and Rehabilitation Principles,* Mosby–Year Book, St Louis, Mo.
8. S. W. Levy, M. F. Allende, and G. H. Barnes, Skin problems of the leg amputee, *Arch. Dermatol.* **85**:65–81.
9. R. A. Sherman (1996), *Phantom Pain,* Plenum Press, New York, N.Y.
10. S. Banerjee (ed.) (1982), *Rehabilitation Management of Amputees,* Williams & Wilkins, Baltimore, Md.
11. H. W. Kay and J. D. Newman (1975), Relative incidences of new amputations: Statistical comparisons of 6000 new amputees, *Orthot. Prosthet.* **29**(2):3–16.
12. *Lower- and Upper-Limb Prosthetics and Orthotics,* 1992, Northwestern University Medical School, Prosthetic & Orthotic Center, Chicago, Ill.
13. W. Barclay (1970), Below-knee amputation: Prosthetics, *Prosthetic and Orthotic Practice* 70–78.
14. J. Hughes (1970), Below-knee amputation: Biomechanics, *Prosthetic and Orthotic Practice* 61–68.
15. T. A. McMahon (1984), *Muscle, Reflexes, and Locomotion,* Princeton University Press, Princeton, N.J.
16. G. Murdoch and R. G. Donovan (eds.) (1988), *Amputation Surgery and Lower Limb Prosthetics,* Blackwell Scientific, Boston, Mass.
17. P. E. Klopsteg and P. D. Wilson (1986), *Human Limbs and Their Substitutes,* Hafner Publishing, New York, N.Y.
18. G. Murdoch (1964), The "Dundee" socket: A total contact socket for the below-knee amputation, *Health Bull.* **22**(4):70–71.
19. G. Murdoch (1968), The "Dundee" socket for below-knee amputation, *Prosthet. Int.* **3**(4–5):15–21.
20. J. G. P. Lee and S. Cheung (2000), Biomechanical evaluation of the pressure cast (PCAST) prosthetic socket for trans-tibial amputee, in *World Congress on Medical Physics and Biomedical Engineering,* Chicago, Ill.
21. J. S. Rolock (1998), *Capabilities,* Northwestern University Prosthetics Research Laboratory & Rehabilitation Engineering Research Program, Chicago, Ill. **7**(1):1–2, 8–9.
22. D. H. Nielsen, D. G. Shurr, J. C. Golden, and K. Meier (1989), Comparison of energy cost and gait efficiency during ambulation in below-knee amputees using different prosthetic feet–a preliminary report. *J. Prosthet. Orthot.* **1**(1):24–31.
23. A. P. Arya, A. Lees, H. C. Nirula, and L. Klenerman (1995), A biomechanical comparison of the SACH Seattle and Jalpur feet using ground reaction forces, *Prosthet. Orthot. Int.* **19**:37–45.
24. D. G. Barth, L. Schumacher, and S. S. Thomas Gait analysis and energy cost of below-knee amputees wearing six different prosthetic feet, *J. Prosthet. Orthot.* **4**(2):63–75.
25. A. M. Boonstra, V. Fidler, G. M. A. Spits, P. Tuil, and A. L. Hof (1993), Comparison of gait using a Multiflex foot versus a Quantum foot in knee disarticulation amputees, *Prosthet. Orthot. Int.* **17**:90–94.
26. J. M. Casillas, V. Dulieu, M. Cohen, I. Marcer, and J. P. Didier (1995), Bioenergetic comparison of a new energy-storing foot and SACH foot in traumatic below-knee vascular amputations, *Arch. Phys. Med. Rehabil.* **76**:39–44.
27. E. G. Culham, M. Peat, and E. Newell (1986), Below-knee amputation: A comparison of the effect of the SACH foot and single axis foot on electromyographic patterns during locomotion, *Prosthet. Orthot. Int.* **10**:15–22.

28. N. E. Doane and L. E. Holt (1983), A comparison of the SACH and single axis foot in the gait of unilateral below-knee amputees, *Prosthet, Orthot. Int.* **7**:33–36.

29. Y. Ehara, M. Beppu, S. Nomura, Y. Kunimi, S. Takahashi (1993), Energy storing property of so-called energy-storing prosthetic feet, *Arch. Phys. Med. Rehabil.* **74**:68–72.

30. J. C. H. Goh, S. E. Solomonidis, W. D. Spence, J. P. Paul (1984), Biomechanical evaluation of SACH and uniaxial feet, *Prosthet. Orthot. Int.* **8**:147–154.

31. J. F. Lehmann, R. Price, A. Boswell-Bessette Dralle, and K. Questad (1993), Comprehensive analysis of elastic response feet: Seattle ankle/Lite foot versus SACH foot, *Arch. Phys. Med. Rehabil.* **74**:853–861.

32. J. F. Lehmann, R. Price, A. Boswell-Bessette Dralle, K. Questad, and B. J. deLateur (1993), Comprehensive analysis of energy storing prosthestic feet. Flex foot and Seattle foot versus standard SACH foot, *Arch. Phys. Med. Rehabil.* **74**:1225–1231.

33. M. R. Menard, M. E. McBride, D. J. Sanderson, and D. D. Murray (1992), Comparative biomechanical analysis of energy-storing prosthetic feet, *Arch. Phys. Med. Rehabil.* **73**:451–458.

34. R. D. Snyder, C. M. Powers, and Perry J. Fontaine (1996) The effect of five prosthetic feet on the gait and loading of the sound limb in dysvascular below-knee amputees, *J. Rehabil. Res. Dev.* **32**(4):309–315.

35. L. Torburn, J. Perry, E. Ayyappa, and S. L. Shanfield (1990), Below-knee amputee gait with dynamic elastic response prosthetic feet: A pilot study, *J. Rehabil. Res. Dev.* **27**(4):369–384.

36. J. L. Van Leeuwen, L. A. W. Speth, H. A. Daanen (1990), Shock absorption of below-knee prostheses: A comparison between the SACH and Multiflex foot, *J. Biomechanics* **23**(5):441–446.

37. V. T. Inman, H. J. Ralston, and F. Todd (1981), *Human Walking,* Williams & Wilkins, Baltimore, Md., 129–148.

38. M. B. Silver-Thorn, J. W. Steege, and D. S. Childress (1996), A review of prosthetic interface stress investigations, *J. Rehabil. Res. Dev.* **33**(3):253–266.

39. M. W. Ferguson-Pell, F. Bell, and J. H. Evans (1976), Interface pressure sensors: existing devices, their suitability and limitations, (1976), R. M. Kennedy and J. H. Cowden (eds.), *Bedsore Biomechanics,* University Park Press, Baltimore, Md., 189–197.

40. M. W. Ferguson-Pell (1980), Design criteria for the measurement of pressure at body/support interface, *Eng. Med.* **9**(4):209–214.

41. A. Polliack, S. Landsberger, D. McNeal, R. Sieh, D. Craig, and E. Ayyappa (1999), Socket measurement systems perform under pressure, *Biomechanics* 71–80.

42. G. T. Nola and L. M. Vistnes (1980), Differential response of skin and muscle in the experimental production of pressure sores, *Plast. Reconstr. Surg.* **66**(5):728–733.

43. R. K. Daniel, D. L. Priest, and D. C. Wheatley (1981), Etiological factors in pressure sores, *Arch. Phys. Med. Rehabil.* **62**:492–498.

44. M. Nissan (1977), A simplified model for the short-below-knee stump, *J. Biomechanics* **10**:651–658.

45. D. J. Winarski and J. R. Pearson (1990), First-order model for the analysis of stump stresses for below-knee amputees, *J. Biomech. Eng.* **112**:475–478.

46. S. G. Zachariah and J. E. Sanders (1996), Interface mechanics in lower-limb external prosthetics: A review of finite element methods, *IEEE Trans. Rehabil. Eng.* **4**(4):288–302.

47. M. Zhang, A. F. T. Mak, and V. C. Roberts (1998), Finite element modelling of a residual lower-limb in a prosthetic socket: A survey of development in the first decade, *Med. Eng. Phys.* **20**:360–373.

48. W. Loob (2001), Robotics and electronics research aid building "smart" prostheses, *in Medical Device and Diagnostic Industry,* Jan., 64.

49. L. A. Karacoloff (1986), *Lower Extremity Amputation,* Aspen Systems Corporation, Rockville, Md.

50. S. W. Levy and H. Warren (1983), *Skin Problems of the Amputee,* Green, Inc., St. Louis, Mo.

51. American Academy of Orthopedic Surgeons, (1981), *Atlas of Limb Prosthetics: Surgical and Prosthetic Principles,* Mosby, St Louis, Mo.

52. M. S. Zahedi and W. D. Spence (1986), Alignment of lower-limb prostheses, *J. Rehabil. Res. Dev.* **23**(2):2–19.

CHAPTER 22
WEAR OF TOTAL HIP AND KNEE JOINT REPLACEMENTS

Mohsen Mosleh
Howard University, Washington, DC

Jorge F. Arinez
General Motors, Research and Development Center, Warren, Michigan

22.1 INTRODUCTION

The *wear phenomenon* is a normal consequence of systems with components in relative motion. That component surfaces must be in contact and thus experience wear is an unavoidable reality of being able to provide motion and carry load. While wear is something that engineers strive to reduce in all systems, for artificial joints that function in a biological system, the negative effects of wear are especially harmful since they directly impact the patient's health. In particular, wear in artificial joints causes implant failure for two reasons. First, because a large number of small wear particles are produced both from the articulating and nonarticulating surfaces, an adverse biological response is triggered. Secondly, wear causes changes in nominal dimensions leading to degradation in joint function and performance, resulting in the failure of the artificial joint. The biological response to foreign body wear particles involves a cascading series of events leading to osteolysis and periprosthetic bone resorption, resulting in aseptic loosening of the implant. Currently, the average life span of a total hip replacement in patients over the age of 60 is approximately 15 years, with only 10 percent of implants requiring revision after 10 years. Such an average life span presents serious concerns in implant longevity for hip replacement patients younger than 60 years old with high level of physical activities. Due to the increasing number of overall candidates receiving total joint replacements in the near future, much research has been conducted to better understand wear phenomena, namely, the factors that contribute to wear, and their undesirable consequences. This chapter seeks to review our current understanding of wear in total joint replacements. Although there are various types of joint prostheses including elbow, ankle, wrist, and shoulder joints, our focus is on total hip and knee joint replacements because of the large numbers of people receiving such implants. Also, the failure of total joint replacements due to nonwear-related factors such as implant fracture, infection, or implant loosening due to pure mechanical effects is not discussed.

22.2 HISTORICAL PERSPECTIVE

The earliest recorded attempt for hip replacement dates back to 1881 when T. Gluck developed an ivory ball and socket joint that was fixed to bone with nickel-plated screws.[1] The use of mixtures of plaster and pumice with a resin for fixation was also considered. For the next several decades, new implant materials, designs, and surgical procedures were tried by numerous surgeons and researchers whose clinical results were highly variable and largely unsatisfactory.[2] In 1950s, the development rate and success of total joint replacement was accelerated by incorporating such design features as flared collar stems by F.R. Thompson, textured surfaces on implants for bone ingrowths by A. Moore, press fit stainless steel components by P. Wiles, and metal-on-metal articulating components by K. McKee and P. Ring, some of which produced good clinical results after long periods of follow up.[1,3,4] The knowledge base and clinical results generated in preceding decades set the stage for the arrival of the modern age of successful total joint replacements ushered in by Sir John Charnley in the mid 1960s.[5] Charnley utilized fundamental tribological principles and testing methodologies along with medical skills to introduce cemented metal ball-on-polyethylene cup hip replacements that also motivated the development of other joint replacements. Today, total joint replacement (TJR) is considered to be one of the most successful types of orthopedic surgeries.

22.3 INTERFACES AND WEAR MECHANISMS

Modern total hip and knee implants consist of several components shown in Fig. 22.1. Each implant may be thought of as a system consisting of a number of interfaces, one of which is the designed articulating interface where the majority of wear occurs. Specifically, the articulating surface pairs in the hip and knee prostheses are the ball/cup and femoral implant/insert interfaces, respectively. The minimum number of interfaces for such geometrical configurations that could be imagined for each of these joints is three. However, because increased modularity provides more intraoperative flexibility in surgery, modern hip and knee joint replacements consist of at least five and four interfaces, respectively.

The nonarticulating interfaces in total joint replacements are either fixed to the surrounding bones, such as the stem/femur and tray/tibia interfaces, or mated to other components, such as the cup/shell or the tray/insert interfaces. In each case, these interfaces are subjected to cyclical loading and unloading. Because of the incompatibility in material properties, minute relative moments between the contacting components at these interfaces occur. The amplitude of the movements can be as small as a few micrometers and as big as few hundred micrometers. The relative motion even at these small amplitudes can generate wear and cause failure of the implant. The mechanisms by which wear at the articulating and nonarticulating interfaces occurs are described here.

22.3.1 Wear of Articulating Interfaces

The underlying cause for wear is either chemical or mechanical in nature. The former involves chemical interactions of surfaces or the surrounding environment with the surfaces, resulting in separation of minute matter as surfaces slide past one another. Two of the most well-known chemical mechanisms for wear are corrosion and adhesion. Since materials used for total joint replacements are corrosion resistant, the dominant wear mechanism chemical in nature is adhesion. Wear due to purely mechanical effects is either cycle-dependent, known specifically as *fatigue and delamination wear*, or is noncycle-dependent, in which case it is called *abrasion*. Abrasion wear also includes wear by impact known as *erosion* and is not applicable to wear in total joint replacements. The major wear mechanisms pertaining to total joint replacements are abrasion, adhesion, and fatigue and delamination.[6,7]

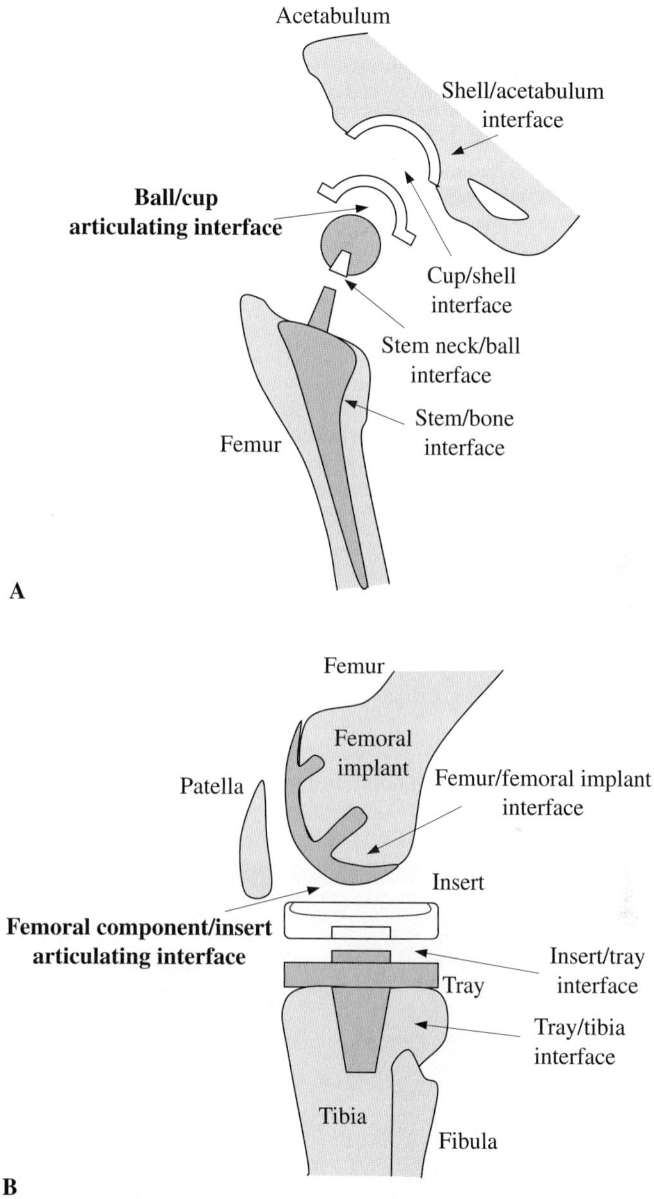

FIGURE 22.1 Components of modern (*a*) total hip replacements and (*b*) total knee replacements showing both articulating and nonarticulating interfaces.

Abrasion. In this wear mechanism, the softer articulating joint surface is plowed by either the asperities of the harder surface or by the particles/wear particles that migrate into the interface. The particles from the surrounding environment can include cement particles, fractured bone particles, and wear debris. The abrasion caused by the asperities of the harder surface is known as *two-body abrasion* and that caused by particles/wear particles is called *three-body abrasion*. The use of smooth, hard counterfaces in total joint replacements significantly reduces two-body wear. Also, three-body wear is minimized when particles are prevented from entering the sliding interface or eliminated from the sliding interface if generated there.[8,9] Terms such as gouging,[10,11] scratching,[7] embedded third bodies,[12,13] and indentation[7,11] frequently mentioned in the literature concern the end result of this type of wear in TJR.[14]

Adhesion. The junctions formed between the asperities of sliding surfaces are continuously broken due to the shear forces of articulation. When fragments of the softer material are pulled off one surface while adhered to the other surface, adhesive wear occurs. Fragments may either come off the surface on which they are adhered to form loose particles at the interface or be transferred to the original surface.[15,16] Terms such as burnishing,[17,18] smears and pulls,[17,19] and polishing[11] in the artificial joint refer to the effects caused by adhesive wear.[14]

Fatigue and Delamination. This form of wear is related to the fatigue of materials under cyclic loading and includes two mechanisms, namely surface fatigue and delamination wear. The former occurs mostly in rolling applications where surface cracks develop under repetitive stress cycles and results in spalling of particles from the surface and its subsequent deterioration.[20] However, in delamination wear[21] repeat loading and unloading by the hard asperities causes plastic deformation of the subsurface. This cyclic stress experienced by the subsurface consequently results in the nucleation of cracks and their propagation beneath the surface. When these cracks join and shear to the surface, thin, large sheet-like wear particles are formed. The articulating motion found both in hip and knee joint replacements consists of sliding and rolling, and therefore, both of these mechanisms cause wear. Terms such as cracks,[22] pitting,[23,24] flaking,[19] and delamination[25,26] in the TJR literature refer to the effects of this type of wear.[14]

One or a combination of several wear mechanisms can cause severe wear in the softer articulating surface, resulting in wear through the entire thickness. The polyethylene acetabular cup in Fig. 22.2 shows the effects of severe three-body wear from cement particles entrapped at the articulating interface. Also, the polyethylene knee insert in Fig. 22.3 has experienced severe fatigue and delamination wear.

Complete or significant wear of one of the articulating surfaces necessitates surgical revisions. However, the cause of majority of TJR revisions is not the complete wear of one of the articulating surfaces. Instead, the majority of revisions can be attributed to the adverse biological response to wear particles.

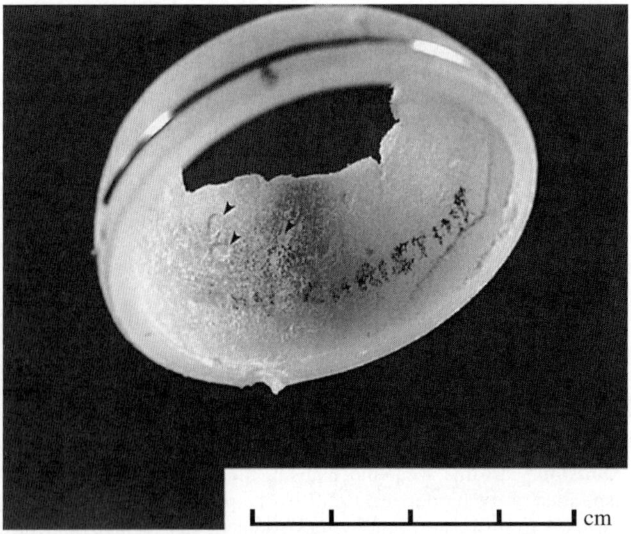

FIGURE 22.2 A cemented acetabular implant revised for aseptic loosening. Severe wear is associated with three-body abrasion caused by cement particles found at the articulating interface. (*Printed with permission from Ref. 27.*)

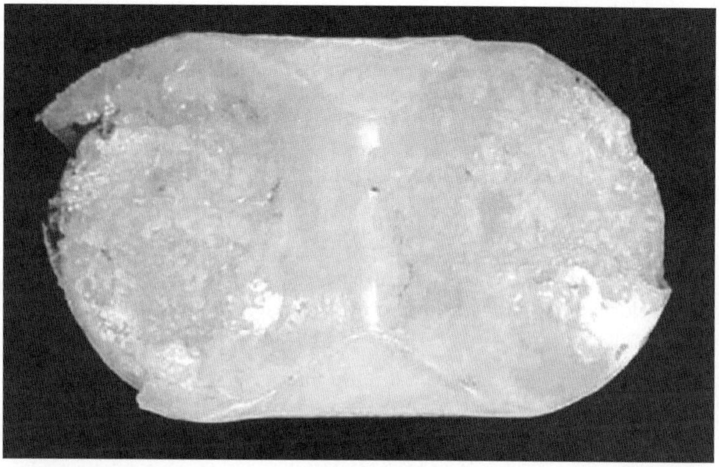

FIGURE 22.3 Severe wear of a total knee insert.[28]

22.3.2 Wear of Nonarticulating Interfaces

The nonarticulating interfaces of artificial joints are not designed to experience wear. However, some retrieved total joint replacements have shown considerable wear in interfaces such as stem neck/ball (Fig. 22.4), tray/insert in knee prostheses and cup/shell in hip replacements.[29,30] The type of wear associated with these interfaces is specifically known as *fretting wear*.

Fretting. This form of wear is not a distinct mechanism of wear. Instead, fretting wear is the application of other mechanisms of wear to sliding conditions with small-amplitude oscillations. The magnitude of these oscillations is very small, with a typical maximum range of a few hundred micrometers.[31] With fretting, if the formed asperity junctions move elastically, there will be no wear and no energy dissipation and is referred to as a *closed cycle*. If one surface slips and the other sticks, crack initiation and propagation at the surface dominates and is referred to as an *elliptical cycle*. Finally, when the entire surface slips, abrasive wear dominates and is described as a *parallelogram cycle*.[32]

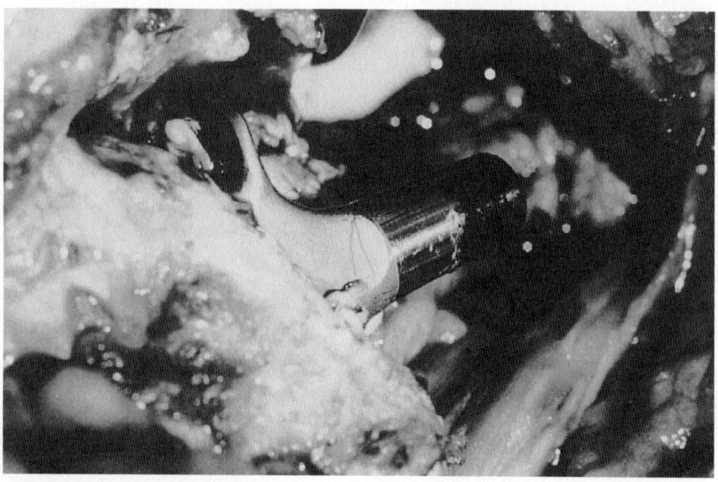

FIGURE 22.4 Fretting corrosion of the titanium Morse taper of a femoral component at revision surgery showing extensive wear.[29]

Fretting wear can be combined with corrosion in oxygen-rich biological environments and cause fretting corrosion.[33] The fretting wear in total joint replacements can occur at the implant/bone interface as in cementless fixations, implant/cement interface as in cemented fixation, and implant/implant interface as between tray and insert in knee and stem neck and ball in hip replacements.

Fretting and/or fretting oxidation leads to the production of bone particles, metallic particles, bone cement particles, and polyethylene wear particles. When harder metallic and cement particles migrate to the articulating interface, they can cause severe three-body wear and accelerate the wear rate in polymer-on-metal total joint replacements. The severely worn polyethylene cup shown in Fig. 22.2 is an example of three-body wear caused by cement particles. Softer polyethylene wear particles produced by fretting action at the cup/shell interface of hip implants and insert/tray interface of knee implants add both to the volume and quantity of wear particles produced at the articulating interfaces and contribute to the biological response. This type of wear is referred to as *backside wear* in the literature[24,34–37] and raises questions about the benefits of modular metal-backed implants, especially in total knee replacements.

22.4 CONSEQUENCE OF WEAR

Wear of the articulating surfaces of total joint replacements results in a decrease in the nominal dimensions of the softer surface. If the dimensional reduction is excessive, as shown in Fig. 22.2, revision surgery is needed to replace the worn component. The percentage of this type of artificial joint failure (totally worn polyethylene component), compared to the number of total joint failures from other causes, is small. The UHMWPE (ultrahigh molecular weight polyethylene) component of a polymer-on-metal total hip replacement historically wears at a rate of approximately 0.1 mm per year. Therefore, it would normally take several decades to wear through UHMWPE components having thicknesses ranging from 5 to 10 mm.

A more critical consequence of wear in total joint replacements is the production of a very large amount of wear particles. The wear particles generated in UHMWPE-on-metal joints have been found to range in size from tens of nanometers to a few millimeters. Specifically, particles having a size in the range of 0.1 to 1 μm have been found to be clinically important as a wealth of evidence suggests that such particles activate macrophages.[38–40] Activated macrophages in the periprosthetic tissue produce different cytokines and other mediators of inflammation that eventually lead to osteolysis and bone resorption. Bone resorption undermines the prosthetic bed and results in aseptic loosening and eventually failure of the total joint replacement. Figure 22.5 shows severe osteolysis in the pelvis, tibia, and femur of a patient with a total joint replacement. Such patients often undergo revision surgery to repair the loose implant and reduce pain.[41,42]

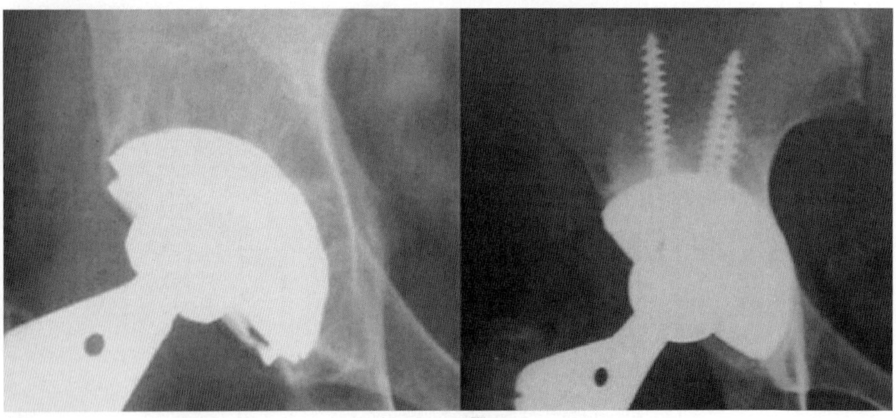

A B

FIGURE 22.5 A radiograph of a hip that shows pelvic severe osteolysis (*a*) and the following revision surgery using cementless acetabular cup and screws (*b*). (*Printed with permission from Ref. 41.*)

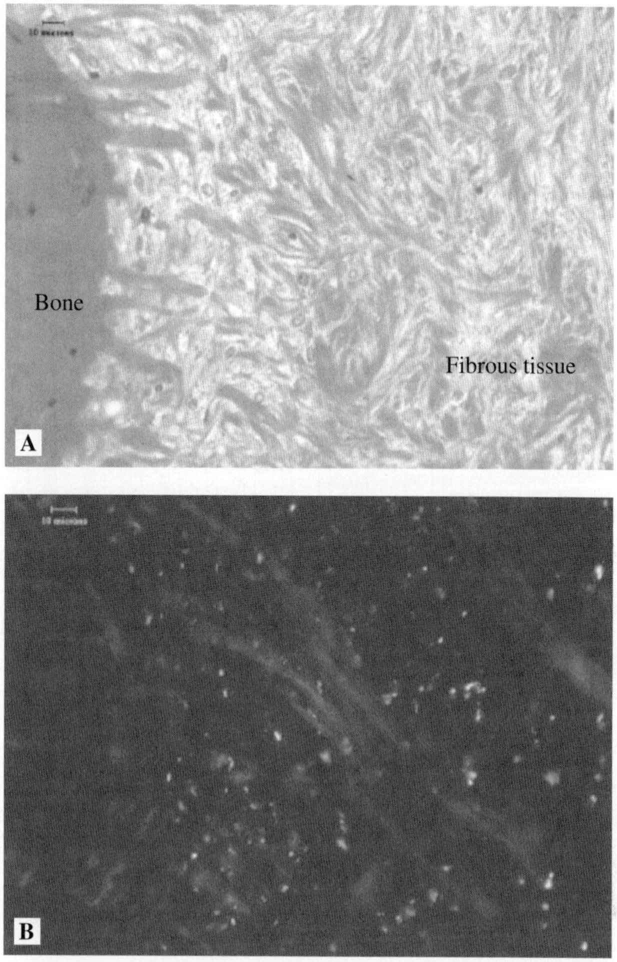

FIGURE 22.6 Fibrous tissue adjacent to the rim of a loose acetabular component (*a*) and birefringent polyethylene particles (white particles) within tissue adjacent to the implant under polarized light (*b*). The magnification was 20×. (*Printed with permission from Ref. 43.*)

Furthermore, the surrounding tissues of total joint replacements also have been widely examined in the literature. The existence of wear particle of UHMWPE in the periprosthetic tissue and the elicitation of biological response is well established.[44,45] Figure 22.6 shows polyethylene wear particles within tissue adjacent to implants under polarized light. Two characteristics of wear particles are known to affect the biological responses. These two characteristics are particles size distribution and particle concentration in the surrounding tissue.

22.4.1 Wear Particle Size Distribution

The retrieval and subsequent analysis of UHMWPE wear debris from the surrounding tissue in vivo and from the lubricant of the in vitro wear tests is a challenging task. Also, the examination of wear debris with only polarized light microscopy[41,45] is difficult due to its limited resolution, and therefore submicron wear particles may be overlooked. When atomic force microscopy

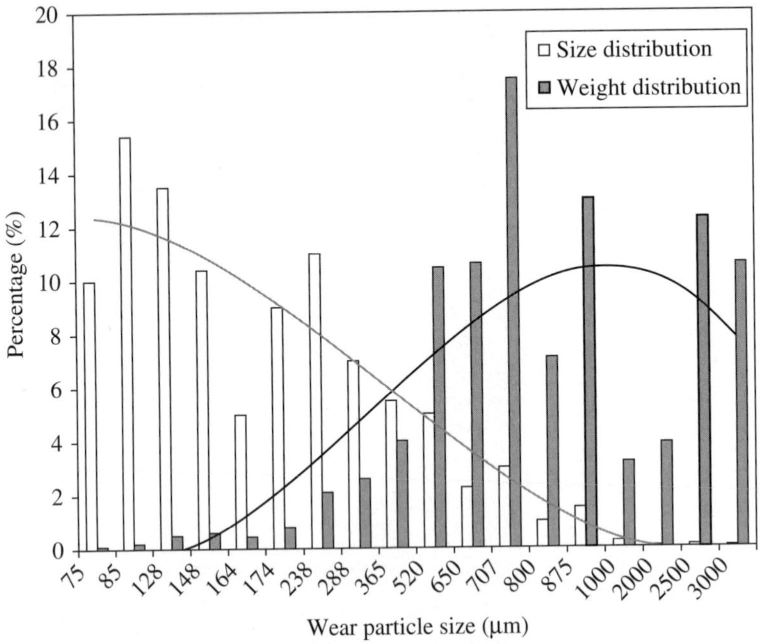

FIGURE 22.7 Size and wear distribution of UHMWPE wear particles in laboratory testing.[47]

was utilized to study wear particle distribution generated in vitro,[46,47] it was found that the majority of UHMWPE particles have an average size of 240 nm or less as shown in Fig. 22.7. In particular, wear debris with sizes of 85 to 128 nm accounted for 29 percent of the total number of UHMWPE wear debris. Yet, the total weight of these submicron particles was negligible compared with the weight of larger particles because the weight is proportional to the cubic power of the radius. Similar findings with respect to the size of UHMWPE wear particles were obtained using a hip simulator.[48]

The isolation of wear debris from periprosthetic in vivo tissue is normally done through hydrolysis of tissues with acid,[49] alkali,[50] and by the use of enzymes.[51] Using scanning electron microscopy, UHMWPE debris from low-contact-stress knees has yielded two-peaked size distributions[52] as illustrated in Fig. 22.8. The first peak occurs at 200 nm and the second peak at 5 μm. Other characterization tools such as modified infrared spectroscopy method have revealed the existence of UHMWPE wear particles with sizes of 0.1 to 10 μm in the periprosthetic tissues around the total joint replacements.[53]

22.4.2 Wear Particle Concentration

It has been clinically shown that total joint replacement cases with a high volumetric wear rate also experience a higher incidence rate of osteolysis, implant migration, and revision.[54] In contrast, THR patients with minimal formation of wear particles, such as patients having a lesser degree of activity or those with ceramic-on-ceramic implants, had shown little or no bone loss during long-term follow-ups.[55,56] A recent survey of several reports in the literature has found follow-up periods of 1 to 15 years, indicating that in wear rate groups of 80, 80 to 140, and >140 mm^3/year, osteolysis was rare, 6 to 32 percent, and 21 to 100 percent, respectively.[57] In other in vitro studies, it was found that as the ratio of particle concentration/macrophage cell number is increased, so to does the number of proinflammatory mediators (such as IL-1β and TNF-α) that are suspected to activate osteoclasts that lead to bone resorption.[58]

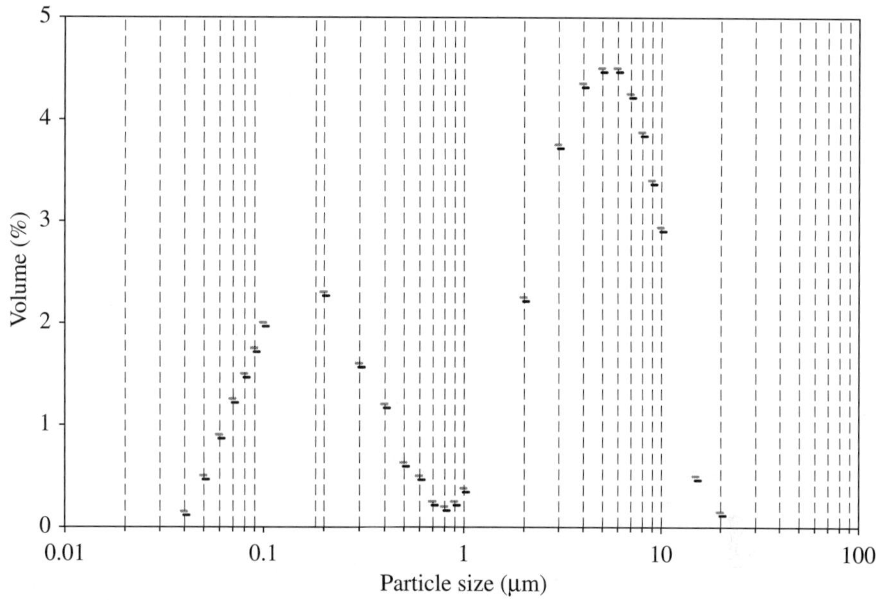

FIGURE 22.8 The particle size distribution of UHMWPE in low-contact-stress knees. (*Plotted from data obtained from Ref. 52 with permission.*)

Other wear debris characteristics such as shape, aspect ratio, surface characteristics have been studied in the literature. However, there is no significant clinical evidence regarding the effect of these characteristics on osteolysis and bone resorption.

22.5 FACTORS AFFECTING WEAR IN TOTAL JOINT REPLACEMENTS

Metals, polymers, ceramics, and composites have been used for various components of total joint replacements. The properties of some of these materials are shown in Table 22.1.

The most dominant material pair for the articulating components has been the polymer/metal system used during the past four decades. The choice of materials is one of the most important factors that affect the wear rate of articulating and nonarticulating interfaces. In addition, important factors such as the topographical design of surfaces, the geometry of implants, the fixation method and surgical procedure, and the operating conditions of the implants all are known to affect the wear rate. These factors are discussed in this chapter.

22.5.1 Materials

Polymer-Metal and Polymer-Ceramic Systems. Ultrahigh molecular weight polyethylene (UHMWPE) is widely used as the acetabular cup and as the insert in hip and knee joints during the last four decades, respectively. The articulating counterface, that is, the hip ball and the femoral component in the knee, is a metallic component that has been made of stainless steel, titanium, or cobalt-chromium alloys. However, Co-Cr alloys are the dominant choice of counterface materials. UHMWPE possesses extremely long molecular chains that exhibit high wear resistance compared to that of other polymers.

TABLE 22.1 Mechanical Properties of Biomaterials Used in Total Joint Replacements

Material	Density (kg/m^3)	Yield strength (MPa)	Ultimate tensile strength (MPa)	Modulus (GPa)	Component (Fig. 22.1)
Co-Cr-Mo (austenite)	8280	848	600–1795	200–230	Ball, femoral implant, stem, cup
Ti-6Al-4V (α'/β)	4430	1100	960–970	110	Stem, shell, tray
SS-316-L (austenite)	8030	621	465–950	200	Ball, stem
UHMWPE (GUR 1120)	932	22	43.1	0.689–0.720	Cup, insert
UHMWPE (GUR 4150)	934	23.3	33.8	1.39	Cup, insert
PMMA	1190	65.5	21	4.5	Stem to bone Shell to bone
Alumina	3790	292	300	380	Ball, cup
Zirconia	5740	430–725	820	220	Ball, cup

Source: Refs. 60–63.

TABLE 22.2 Wear Rate of Acetabular UHMWPE Cup Against a Variety of Femoral Ball Material

Femoral ball	Diameter (mm)	UHMWPE wear rate (mm/year)	Reference(s)
Co-Cr	32	0.04–0.1	65, 66
	28	0.08–0.14	65, 67
Stainless steel	28	0.08	65
	22	0.13–0.14	65, 67
Alumina	32	0.03	68
	28	0.03–0.08	66, 67

The processing, manufacture, sterilization, and crosslinking of UHMWPE for total joint replacements affect its mechanical and wear properties and are extensively addressed in the literature.[62] The in vivo wear rate of UHMWPE against several counterfaces is shown in Table 22.2.[64]

Polyethylene components of total joint replacements need to be sterilized for bacterial eradication. The sterilization techniques employed also affect the wear rate of UHMWPE and is described in the following along with the role of crosslinking caused by high doses of gamma irradiation.

Sterilization. In recent years, sterilization of UHMWPE with a gamma irradiation dosage of 2.5 to 4 Mrad in air has been utilized successfully to annihilate bacteria, which may cause infection and premature revision. When UHMWPE is exposed to gamma irradiation, several phenomena occur in varying amounts, including formation of free radicals, chain scission, oxidation, and crosslinking.[69,70] There is mounting evidence that suggests irradiation in the presence of oxygen (in air) promotes chain scission over crosslinking. Chain scission leads to a decrease in molecular weight and lower wear resistance and mechanical properties.[71,72] Also, irradiation sterilization in air-permeable packaging of UHMWPE components of TJR leads to the oxidative degradation during shelf-storage prior to implantation and during in vivo use.[73,74] The maximum extent of oxidation is approximately 1 to 2 mm below the surface, which is where the severe contact stresses that can cause delamination wear, especially in knee inserts, are experienced.[75] Therefore, the new sterilization method that has been adopted is the irradiation in a reduced oxygen environment, such as in a nitrogen environment and in vacuum or sterilization with nonionizing radiation techniques using ethylene oxide (EtO) or gas plasma. The long-term clinical data on the effects of these improved sterilization methods on the wear of UHMWPE is beginning to emerge. Based on limited retrieval studies, UHMWPE components (acetabular and tibial) that were sterilized using EtO showed significantly less surface damage and delamination than those sterilized by gamma irradiation in air.[76,77]

Crosslinking. The nonair irradiation and nonionizing techniques both improve wear of UHMWPE in TJR. However, the former can also increase UHMWPE crosslinking, which is shown in some studies to improve abrasion and adhesive wear mechanisms. For instance, in simulated hip wear tests, it has been shown that as the irradiation dosage increases from 2.5 to 10 Mrad, the wear rate of UHMWPE decreased by approximately 85 percent. In a knee simulator, the decrease in the wear rate was approximately 44 percent.[78] The three-body abrasion resistance of 9.5 Mrad gamma-irradiated UHMWPE is also shown in laboratory simulated-wear testing to increase significantly.[79] Overall, in vitro studies point to the fact that high levels of crosslinking (up to 100 Mrad) lead to a decrease in the UHMWPE wear rate, while it also causes a noticeable drop in tensile strength and tensile elongation at fracture.[80] On the other hand, the in vivo wear data on highly crosslinked UHMWPE is rather limited and inconsistent. For instance, the mean steady wear rate of 100-Mrad gamma-irradiated UHMWPE cups against alumina heads was 0.098 mm/year which is not significantly higher than that of noncrosslinked UHMWPE cup reported as 0.072 mm/year.[81] On the other hand, crosslinking yielded an 80 percent lower wear rate when Co-Cr balls were used.[82]

Owing to the much higher hardness of the metal part, only UHMWPE-articulating components experienced noticeable wear in total joint replacements. However, the counterface material may also experience three-body wear. The ability of several counterface materials to resist scratching by the bone or cement particles is shown in Table 22.3 indicated by the change in arithmetic roughness (R_a) after prolonged in vivo operations.[18–20] The Co-Cr counterface shows the highest scratch resistance.

The highest wear resistance to three-body wear by Co-Cr alloys was also reflected in the least amount of ion release compared with that of other metallic counterfaces in simulated laboratory tests used to determine the material consistency of particulates produced from several counterfaces.[21]

Metal-on-Metal (MOM) Systems. The first series of MOM total hip replacements were performed in the 1960s.[83] However, due to the high occurrence of impingement and clinical observation of high wear volumes and inferior fixation, their use was abandoned in favor of Charnley's polyethylene-metal bearings by the 1970s.[84,85] However, in recent years, MOM total hip arthroplasty and MOM resurfacing ideas are remerging because of significantly improved mechanical and wear properties of metallic alloys that introduced new candidates for MOM-articulating surfaces.

Although the use of MOM TJR significantly reduces the volume of wear particles compared with UHMWPE-metal joints, there is a concern that these bearings may release a high concentration of metal ions and particulates that may cause cellular toxicity, hypersensitivity, and carcinogenicity. Some clinical studies indicate that patients with MOM prostheses had significant elevations in serum chromium and serum cobalt levels compared with control patients.[86,87] Other clinical studies do not show such a significant difference in serum chromium concentration between metal-on-metal bearings and polyethylene-on-metal bearings in midterm studies.[88]

One tribological concern on long-term wear of MOM joints is that when the initial highly polished articulating surfaces are damaged by three-body abrasion, the wear rate on both surfaces can accelerate

TABLE 22.3 Increase in Roughness of Metallic Counterfaces as a Result of In Vivo Articulation

Material	Hardness (DHP)	Wear depth (μm)	Increase in R_a (μm)	Number of cycles
316L SS	230	48	0.74	0^6
Ti-6Al-4V	330	28	4.09	10^6
Ti-6Al-4V (nitrogen ion implanted)	700	31	3.25	10^6
Co-Cr-Mo (nitrogen ion implanted)	400	1	0.1	10^6

Source: Ref. 18.

significantly. Since, the relative hardness of MOM articulating surfaces cannot be very high, as in the case of UHMWPE/Co-Cr bearings, the possibility of both the harder and softer surface being severely abraded by three-body abrasion is high.

Ceramic-on-Ceramic Systems. Ceramic-on-ceramic articulating surfaces have been tried in total joint arthroplasty since 1970s. Due to the high hardness, extremely smooth surfaces, and improved wettability, a new generation of all-ceramic joint prostheses made of alumina have exhibited good short-term clinical results.[89,90] The major advantages of all-ceramic bearing systems are that they produce the lowest wear volume compared with other prostheses material combinations, and in addition, ceramic wear debris is bio-inert. As a result, decreased levels of osteolysis are observed with these prostheses.[91]

A key concern with ceramic-on-ceramic prostheses is that of fracture due to the low ductility of ceramics under tensile or impact stresses.[92–94] Also squeaking has been reported in 1.4 percent of patients with this type of prostheses.[95]

The same tribological concern surrounding long-term wear MOM prostheses, that is, small hardness ratio between articulating surfaces, also exists in all-ceramic bearings. The low relative hardness makes such bearings vulnerable to severe three-body abrasion once hard particulates are trapped in between their articulating interfaces.

22.5.2 Design

All design parameters, including geometry, dimensions, and topography, of total joint replacement components affect the long-term performance and survival of these joints. Some of the design factors that directly affect wear are addressed here.

Surface Topography. The roughness characteristics of articulating surfaces affect friction and wear rate in all circumstances, especially at the onset of sliding where abrasion is dominant. When one of the surfaces is significantly harder that the other, as is the case in UHMWPE/Co-Cr bearings, it is highly desired to achieve the lowest possible roughness on the harder surface to obtain the lowest wear rate. In vitro simulated wear testing of UHMWPE against Co-Cr balls has shown that the wear factor is proportional to the mean arithmetic roughness of the Co-Cr counterface to the power of 0.41.[96] Similar correlations between wear rate and counterface roughness have been reported in clinical studies of the wear of UHMWPE against Co-Cr balls in TJR with a power exponent of 0.54.[97]

Ceramic materials offer the possibility of achieving lower surface roughness than metals and therefore may reduce wear of the softer counterpart as was shown in Table 22.2. Cost considerations and technological limitations are the barriers that dictate the lower limit of counterface roughness.

Ball Radius. As the radius of the hip ball increases two parameters simultaneously change. The siding distance increases because it is proportional to the radius and the contact stress decreases because the load bearing area has increased. The increase in the sliding distance results in higher wear. Some clinical wear results indicate that as the diameter of the ball increased from 22 mm to 32 mm, the UHMWPE volumetric wear rate increased between 70 to 200 percent.[98,99] On the other hand, if the ratio of volumetric wear rate to the ball diameter is calculated in these studies, one can be found in a narrow range of 2.3 to 3.0. Therefore, the linear penetration depth of the UHMWPE remains relatively unchanged as the ball diameter varies.

The increased ball diameter adds to joint stability, which is highly desirable for the patient. However, the higher volumetric wear rate increases the concentration of wear particles, which adversely affect the biological response.

Clearance. The clearance of ball-in-socket hip bearings affects their lubrication and the uniformity of joint rotation. It has been found that a small radial clearance results in lower coefficients of friction under various loading, and therefore less wear.[100] A clearance of 20 μm for 28-mm balls has been shown to retain a fluid film with a thickness of 0.02 μm that is able to provide elastohydrodynamic lubrication in ceramic bearings. When the radial thickness is increased above 30 mm, the lubrication film is squeezed out.[101] Increasing radial clearance is also shown to increase the contact stresses for the cup inclination in a range of 35 to 60°, which corresponds to physiological implantations.[102]

Locking Mechanisms in Modular Systems. The increased modularity of total joint replacement designs introduces additional nonarticulating interfaces. These additional interfaces introduce surfaces that can experience wear and generate wear particles that contribute to the failure of TJR. Therefore, the mechanism designs that lock nonarticulating surfaces together should maximize the hold of one component on the other to minimize fretting. Also, tight tolerances created by precision machining should eliminate gaps and pockets that potentially allow plastic deformation and stress concentration to occur and also provide a seal that prevents particles from entering the interface.[103,104]

22.5.3 Fixation and Placement

Total hip and knee replacement components experience significant cyclic loads of tension, compression, bending, and shearing generated during normal daily activities and other physically demanding exercises. These loads tend to shear the implant/bone interfaces, cause fretting wear, produce wear debris, and ultimately cause implant loosening. Adding to this complexity is the critical role played by placement of components, surgical techniques and tools, and finally the skill and experience of the surgeon.

For fixation of total joint replacement components to the bone, two methods of cemented and cementless fixations have been employed. Both methods have yielded highly durable fixation for long-term follow-ups. Each of these methods is described along with their advantages and disadvantages.

Cemented Fixation. Even though use of cement for improved fixation of implants dates back to the nineteenth century, the use of polymethyl methacrylate (PMMA) bone cement for fixation of total hip prostheses was introduced and popularized by Charnley.[105] The chemical composition of bone cement has remained basically the same since its introduction. However, there has been much improvement in the cementation techniques to provide better long-term fixation. Because the bone cement is a grout with little adhesion, fixation is obtained by mechanical interlocking of the implant in the bone bed. New improved cementation methods include cleaning of the endosteal surfaces for better cement intrusion into bone,[106] pressurization of cement for enhanced penetration into the bone interstices and adequate and complete cement mantle,[107] and sustaining pressure for improved interlock at the asperity level of interfaces. These methods have been shown to improve the tensile and shear strengths at the bone/cement/implant interfaces. The geometry of implants (stem or acetabular cup) also plays a significant role in the performance of cemented fixation. The surface of these implants is typically smooth and their shape is optimized for load distribution on the surrounding bone. Survival rates of 100 percent have been reported for some cemented stems at 10-year follow-ups with aseptic loosening at the end point.[108]

One of the main shortcomings limiting the long-term performance of PMMA cement for fixation is the formation of cement particles by fragmentation through fatigue fracture and fretting. Both in vivo and in vitro studies have shown that these particles can elicit biological response, leading to osteolysis and bone resorption with little evidence of polyethylene wear.[109–113] This problem is referred to as *cement disease* in the literature.[114]

Cementless Fixation. This type of fixation relies solely on a biological substrate's ingrowth into the implant surface. The ability to remodel actively and to repair over time are characteristics sought to obtain the benefits of this type of fixation.[115] Poor survival results with cemented acetabular fixation have prompted surgeons to consider biologic fixation. The cementless orthopedic porous coatings, roughened surfaces, or beaded textures are areas potentially receptive to bone tissue ingrowth at the implant surface. The biological stabilization in the bone can take several months.[105] The long-term survival for uncemented acetabular cups is inferior to the cemented ones. However, the data for uncemented stems is good.[116]

The major wear-related advantage of uncemented fixation is the lack of particle problems associated with the PMMA cement, as described in the previous section. However, the frequency of pain experienced by the recipient of a cementless femoral implant has been high.[117]

Placement. Inaccurate positioning and placement of total joint replacement components can also result in increased wear, instability, and an enhanced possibility of dislocation.[118–120] The positioning of the implant can also adversely alter the loads on the articulating and nonarticulating interfaces. Studies have revealed that if the safe range of acetabular inclination and radiographic anteversion angles are exceeded, the risk of dislocation is significantly increased.[121] Because of the human factors involved in preparation for surgery, surgical procedure, and alignments, the possibility of improper cup alignment remains. Computational navigation methods and computer-assisted surgical tools have been examined to help surgeon in accurate three-dimensional positioning of implants and improved results have been reported.[117,122,123] These tools offer reproducible, more accurate results compared with freehand techniques.

22.5.4 Operating Conditions

The operating conditions of total joint replacements affect the load and sliding distance at the articulating and nonarticulating surfaces, and therefore directly affect their wear performance. These patient-dependent operating conditions include gender, age, physical attributes such as height and weight, and activity level. Therefore, such factors are impossible to be controlled by designers and researchers of total joint replacement. Survival data from the Swedish National Hip Arthroplasty Register suggest that age is the most important factor that determines the operating conditions on recipients of TJR as it is a good indication of activity level, and therefore the intensity of loading and use of joints (Fig. 22.9).[124]

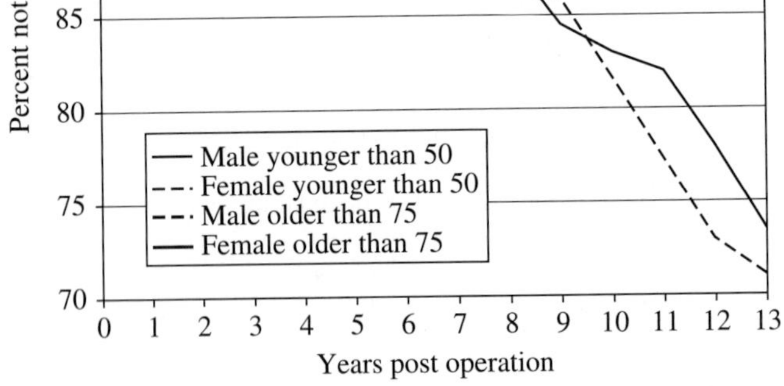

FIGURE 22.9 All hip arthroplasty revisions in patients younger than 50 and older than 75 years. (*Plotted from data obtained from Ref. 124 with permission.*)

22.6 CONCLUSION

The first three major factors (materials, design, fixation, and placement) affecting wear in total joint replacements can be controlled by materials scientists, tribologists, biomedical engineers, and surgeons to produce TJRs that last beyond what Sir John Charnley thought possible, that is beyond 30 years. In moving toward that goal, ongoing research to introduce new material combinations with lowest possible wear, bulk and debris biocompatibility, and other desired mechanical properties is the most critical task at hand. However, design factors are also extremely important. One major development will be the consideration of custom-designed implants technologies. In today's engineering and manufacturing era where a tooth crown is custom fitted, so can be the design process of a total joint replacement whose cost is an order of magnitude higher. Finally, the significance of surgical alignment in wear of total joint replacements should prompt the development of computer-assisted TJR surgical technologies to enhance the consistency of implant alignment.

REFERENCES

1. Rang, M., *Anthology of Orthopaedic,* Edinburgh, London, New York: Churchill Livingstone, (1966).
2. Gomez, P.F. and Morcuende, J.A., "Early attempts at hip arthroplasty," *Iowa Orthop J,* **25**:25–29, (2005).
3. McKee, G.K. and Watson-Farrar, J., "Replacement of arthritic hips by the McKee-Farrar prosthesis," *J Bone Joint Surg* (*Br*), **48**(2):245–259, (1966).
4. Ring, P.A., "Replacement of the hip joint," *Ann R Coll Surg Engl,* **48**(6):344–355, (1971).
5. Charnley, J. and Cupric Z., "The nine and ten year results of the low-friction arthroplasty of the hip," *Clin Orthop,* **95**:9–25, (1973).
6. Brown, K.J., Atkinson, J.R., et al., "The wear of ultra-high molecular weight polyethylene with reference to its use in prostheses," *Plast Med and Surg*, London: Plastics and Rubber Institute, pp. 2.1–2.5, (1975).
7. Trent, P.S., Walker P.S., "Wear and conformity in total knee replacement," *Wear*, **36**:175–187, (1976).
8. Burwell, J.T., "Survey of possible wear mechanisms," *Wear*, **1**:119–141, (1957).
9. Sin, H.C., Saka, N., and Suh, N.P., "Abrasive wear mechanisms and the grit size effect," *Wear*, **55**:163–190, (1979).
10. Weightman, B.O., Paul, I.L., Rose, R.M., Simon, S.R., and Radin, E.L., "A comparative study of total hip replacement prostheses," *J Biomech*, **6**(3):299–311, (1973).
11. Rostoker W., Chao, E.Y.S., and Galante, J.O., "The appearances of wear on polyethylene—a comparison of in vivo and in vitro wear surfaces," *J Biomed Mat Res*, **12**(3):317–335, (1978).
12. Bradford, L., Baker, D.A., Graham, J., Chawan, A., Ries, M.D., and Pruitt, L.A., "Wear and surface cracking in early retrieved highly cross-linked polyethylene acetabular liners," *J Bone Joint Surg (Am)*, **86-A(6)**: 1271–1282, (2004).
13. Kurtz, S., van Ooij, A., Ross, R., de Waal Malefijt, J., Peloza, J., Ciccarelli, L., and Villarraga, M., "Polyethylene wear and rim fracture in total disc arthroplasty," *Spine J*, **7**(1):12–21, (2007).
14. McKellop, H.A., "The lexicon of polyethylene wear in artificial joints," *Biomaterials*, **28**:5049–5057, (2007).
15. Bowden, F.P., and Tabor, D., *The Friction and Lubrication of Solids*, Pt. I, Clarendon Press, Oxford, (1954).
16. Archard, J.F., "Contact and rubbing of flat surfaces," *J Appl Phys*, **24**:981–988, (1953).
17. Landy, M.M., and Walker, P.S., "Wear of ultra-high-molecular-weight polyethylene components of 90 retrieved knee prostheses," *J Arthroplasty*, Suppl (**3**):S73–S85, (1988).
18. Puloski, S.K.T., McCalden, R.W., MacDonald, S.J., Rorabeck, C.H., and Bourne, R.B., "Tibial post wear in posterior stabilized total knee arthroplasty. An unrecognized source of polyethylene debris," *J Bone Joint Surg (Am)*, **83-A(3)**:390–397, (2001).
19. Dowling, J.M., Atkinson, J.R., Dowson, D., and Charnley, J., "The characteristics of acetabular cups worn in the human body," *J Bone Joint Surg*, **60B**:375–382, (1978).
20. Rabinowicz, E., *Friction and Wear of Materials*, John Wiley & Sons, Inc., (1965).

21. Suh, N.P., "The delamination theory of wear," *Wear*, **25**:111–124, (1973).
22. Williams, I.R., Mayor M.B., and Collier, J.P., "The impact of sterilization method on wear in knee arthroplasty," *Clin Orthop Relat Res*, **356**:170–180, (1998).
23. Bradford, L., Baker, D.A., Graham, J., Chawan, A., Ries, M.D., and Pruitt, L.A., "Wear and surface cracking in early retrieved highly cross-linked polyethylene acetabular liners," *J Bone Joint Surg (Am)*, **86-A(6)**: 1271–1282, (2004).
24. Conditt, M.A., Stein J.A., and Noble, P.C., "Factors affecting the severity of backside wear of modular tibial inserts," *J Bone Joint Surg (Am)*, **86-A(2)**:305–311, (2004).
25. Berzins, A., Jacobs, J.J., Berger, R., Ed, C., Natarajan, R., Andriacchi, T., and Galante, J.O., "Surface damage in machined ram extruded and net-shape molded retrieved polyethylene tibial inserts of total knee replacements," *J Bone Joint Surg (Am)*, **84-A(9)**:1534–1540, (2002).
26. Surace, M.F., Berzins, A., Urban, R.M., Jacobs, J.J., Berger, R.A., Natarajan, R.N., Andriacchi, T.P., and Galante, J.O., "Coventry award paper. Backsurface wear and deformation in polyethylene tibial inserts retrieved postmortem," *Clin Orthop Relat Res*, **404**:14–23, (2002).
27. McGee, M.A., Howie, D.W., Costi, K., Haynes, D.R., Wildenauer, C.I., Pearcy, M.J., and McLean, J.D., "Implant retrieval studies of the wear and loosening of prosthetic joints: a review," *Wear*, **241**(2):158–165, (2000).
28. Huang, C.H., Liau, J.J., and Cheng, C.K., "Fixed or mobile-bearing total knee arthroplasty," *J Orthop Surg Res*, **2**:1, (2007).
29. Learmonth, I.D., and Cunningham, J.L., Factors Contributing to the Wear of Polyethylene in Clinical Practice," *Proceedings of the Institution of Mechanical Engineers*, p. 211, Part H, (1997).
30. Crowninshield, R.D., Wimmer, M.A., Jacobs, J.J., and Rosenberg, A.G., "Clinical performance of contemporary tibial polyethylene components," *J Arthroplasty*, **21**(5):754–761, (2006).
31. Blau, P.J., Fretting-Wear, ASM Handbook No. 1, *Friction, Lubrication and Wear Technology*, ASM Int. Edit. pp. 242–256, (1992).
32. Geringer, J., Forest. B., and Combrade, P., "Fretting-corrosion of materials used as orthopaedic implants," *Wear*, **259**:943–951, (2005).
33. Tritschler, B., Forest, B., and Rieu, J., "Fretting corrosion of materials for orthopaedic implants: a study of a metal/polymer contact in an artificial physiological medium," *Tribol Int*, **32**:587–596, (1999).
34. Collier, J.P., Mayor, M.B., Jensen, R.E., Surprenant, V.A., Surprenant, H.P., McNamar, J.L., and Belec, L., "Mechanisms of failure of modular prostheses," *Clin Orthop*, **285**:129–139, (1992).
35. Furman, B.D., Schmieg, J.J., Bhattacharyya, S., and Li, S., "Assessment of backside polyethylene wear in three different metal backed total knee designs," *Trans Orthop Res Soc*, **24**:149, (1999).
36. Wasielewski, R.C., Parks, N., Williams, I., Surprenant, H., Collier, J.P., and Engh, G., "Tibial insert undersurface as a contributing source of polyethylene wear debris," *Clin Orthop*, **345**:53–59, (1997).
37. Huk, O.L., Bansal, M., Betts, F., Rimnac, C.M., Lieberman, J.R., Huo, M.H., and Salvati, E.A., "Polyethylene and metal debris generated by non-articulating surfaces of modular acetabular components," *J Bone Jt Surg (Br)*, **76**:568–574, (1994).
38. Howling, G.I., Barnett, P.I., Tipper, J.L., Stone, M.H., Fisher J, and Ingham, E., "Quantitative characterization of polyethylene debris isolated from periprosthetic tissue in early failure knee implants and early and late failure Charnley hip implants," *Biomed Mater Res*, **58**:415–420, (2001).
39. Ingham, E., and Fisher, J., "Review: The role of macrophages in osteolysis of total joint replacement," *Biomaterials*, **26**:1271–1286, (2005).
40. Neale, S.D., and Athanasou, N.A., "Cytokine receptor profile of arthroplasty macrophages foreign body giant cells and mature osteoclasts," *Acta Orthop Scand*, **70**:452–458, (1999).
41. Chang, J.D., Yoo, J.H., Hur, M., Lee, S.S., Chung, Y.K., and Lee, C.J., "Revision total hip arthroplasty for pelvic osteolysis with well-fixed cementless cup," *J Arthroplasty*, **22**(7):987–992, (2007).
42. Berquist, T.H., "Imaging of joint replacement procedures," *Radiol Clin N Am*, **44**:419–437, (2006).
43. Coathup, M.J., Blackburn, J., Goodship, A.E., Cunningham, J.L., Smith, T., and Blunn, G.W., "Role of hydroxyapatite coating in resisting wear particle migration and osteolysis around acetabular components," *Biomaterials*, **26**(19):4161–4169, (2005).
44. Al-Saffar, N., Ma, J.T.L., Kadoya, Y., and Revell, P.A., "Neovascularisation and the induction of cell adhesion molecules in response to degradation products from orthopaedic implants," *Ann Rheum Dis*, **54**:201–208, (1995).

45. Goodman, S., "Wear particulate and osteolysis," *Orthop Clin N Am*, **36**:41–48, (2005).

46. Mosleh, M., Arinez, J., and Suh, N.P., "Nanometer particles produced by the wear of polyethylene: atomic force microscopy in the Tapping mode," *Proceedings of the 41st Annual Meeting*, Orthopedic Research Society, Orlando, Fa., (1995).

47. Mosleh, M., and Suh, N.P. "Wear particles of polyethylene in biological systems", *Tribol Trans*, **39**:843–848, (1996).

48. Tipper, J.L., Firkins, P.J., Besong, A.A., Barbour, P.S.M., Nevelos, J., Stone, M.H., Ingham, E., and Fisher, J., "Characterisation of wear debris from UHMWPE on zirconia ceramic metal-on-metal and alumina ceramic-on-ceramic hip prostheses generated in a physiological anatomical hip joint simulator," *Wear*, **250**:120–128, (2001).

49. Scott, M., Widding, K., and Jani, S., "Do current wear particle isolation procedures underestimate the number of particles generated by prosthetic bearing components?" *Wear*, **251**:1213–1217, (2001).

50. Shanbhag, A.S., Jacobs, J.J., Glant, T.T., Gilbert, J.L., Black, J., and Galante, J.O., "Composition and morphology of wear debris in failed uncemented total hip replacement," *J Bone Joint Surg*, **76-B**:60–67, (1994).

51. Maloney, W.J., Smith, R.L., Schmalzried, T.P., Chiba, J., Huene, D., and Rubash, H., "Isolation and characterization of wear particles generated in patients who have had failure of a hip arthroplasty without cement," *J Bone Joint Surg*, **77-A**:1301–1310, (1995).

52. Huang, C.H., Ho, F.Y., Ma, H.M., Yang, C.T., Liau, J.J., Kao, H.C., Young, T.H., and Cheng, C.K., "Particle size and morphology of UHMWPE wear debris in failed total knee arthroplasties—a comparison between mobile bearing and fixed bearing knees," *J Orthop Res*, **20**:1038–1041, (2002).

53. Slouf, M., Pokorny, D., Entlicher, G., Dybal, J., Synkova, H., Lapcikova, M., Zlata, F., Marcela, S., Vesely, F., and Sosna, A., "Quantification of UHMWPE wear in periprosthetic tissues of hip arthroplasty: description of a new method based on IR and comparison with radiographic appearance," *Wear*, In Press.

54. Sochart D.H., "Relationship of acetabular wear to osteolysis and loosening in total hip arthroplasty," *Clin Orthop*, **363**:135–150, (1999).

55. Griffith, M.J., Seidenstein, M.K., Williams, D., and Charnley, J., "Socket wear in Charnley low friction arthroplasty of the hip," *Clin Orthop*, **137**:37–47, (1978).

56. Yoon, T.R., Rowe, S.M., Jung, S.T., Seon K.J., and Maloney, W.J., "Osteolysis in association with a total hip arthroplasty with ceramic bearing surfaces," *J Bone Joint Surg (Am)*, **80**(10):1459–1468, (1998).

57. Oparaugo, P.C., Clarke, I.C., Malchau, H., and Herberts, P., "Correlation of wear debris-induced osteolysis and revision with volumetric wear-rates of polyethylene—a survey of 8 reports in the literature," *Acta Orthop Scand,* **72**(1):22–28, (2001).

58. Green, T.R., Fisher, J., Stone, M., Wroblewski, B.M., and Ingham, E., "Polyethylene particles of a 'critical size' are necessary for the induction of cytokines by macrophages in vitro," *Biomaterials*, **19**:2297–2302, (1998).

59. Catelas, I., Huk, O.L., Petit, A., Zukor, D.J., Marchand, R., and Yahia, L., "Flow cytometric analysis of macrophage response to ceramic and polyethylene particles: effects of size, concentration, and composition," *J Biomed Mater Res*, **41**:600–607, (1998).

60. Katti, K.S., "Biomaterials in total joint replacement," *Colloids Surf B Biointerfaces*, **39**:133–142, (2004).

61. Barbour, P.S.M., Stone, M.H., and Fisher, J., "A study of the wear resistance of three types of clinically applied UHMWPE for total replacement hip prostheses," *Biomaterials*, **20**:2101–2106, (1999).

62. Kurtz, S.M., *The UHMWPE Handbook: Ultra-High Molecular Weight Polyethylene in Total Joint Replacement*, Elsevier Inc., (2004).

63. Material Property Data, http://www.matweb.com.

64. Buford, A., and Goswami, T., "Review of wear mechanisms in hip implants: Paper I–General," *Mater Des*, **25**:385–393, (2004).

65. Livermore, J., Listrup, D., and Morrey, B., "Effect of femoral head sizes on wear of the polyethylene acetabular component," *J Bone Joint Surg (Am)*, **72**(5):518–528, (1990).

66. Ohashi, T., and Kajikawa, K., The Clinical Wear Rate of Acetabular Component Accompanied with Aluminum Ceramic Head," In: Oonishi H., Aoli H., and Sawai K., eds. *Bioceramics*. St. Louis: Ishiyaku EuroAmerica, p. 278, (1989).

67. Okumura, H., Yamamuro, T., and Kurmar, T., "Socket Wear in Total Hip Prosthesis with Alumina Ceramic Head, In: Oonishi H., Aoli H., and Sawai K., eds. *Biomedics: Proceedings of the First International Symposium on Bioceramics*. St. Louis: Ishiyaku Euro-America, p. 284, (1989).

68. Schuller, H.M., and Marti, R.K., "Ten year socket wear in 66 hip arthroplasties. Ceramic versus metal heads," *Acta Orthop Scand*, **61**:240–243, (1990).

69. Kurtz, S.M., Muratoglu, O.K., Evans, M., and Edidin, A.A., "Advances in the processing, sterilization, and crosslinking of ultra-high molecular weight polyethylene for total joint arthroplasty," *Biomaterials*, **20**:1659–1688, (1999).

70. Rimnac, C.M., and Kurtz, S.M., "Ionizing radiation and orthopaedic prostheses," *Nucl Instrum Methods Phys Res B*, **236**:30–37, (2005).

71. Edidin, A.A., Jewett, C.W., Kwarteng, K., Kalinowski, A., and Kurtz, S.M., "Degradation of mechanical behavior in UHMWPE after natural and accelerated aging", *Biomaterials*, **21**:1451, (2000).

72. Edidin, A.A., and Kurtz, S.M., "Influence of mechanical behavior on the wear of 4 clinically relevant polymeric biomaterials in a hip simulator," *J Arthroplasty*, **15**(3):321–331, (2000).

73. Rimnac, C.M., Klein, R.W., Betts, F., and Wright, T.M., "Post-irradiation aging of ultra-high molecular weight polyethylene," *J Bone Joint Surg*, **76A**:1052, (1994).

74. Streicher, R.M., "Ionizing irradiation for sterilization and modification of high molecular weight polyethylenes," *Plast Rubber Proc Appl*, **10**:221, (1988).

75. Currier, B.H., Currier, J.H., Collier, J.P., Mayor, M.B., and Scott, R.D., "Shelf life and in vivo duration: Impacts on performance of tibial bearings", *Clin Orthop Relat Res,* **342**:111, (1997).

76. Sutula, L.C., et al., "Impact of gamma sterilization on clinical performance of polyethylene in the hip," *Clin Orthop*, **319**:28–40, (1995).

77. White, S.E., Paxson, R.D., Tanner, M.G., and Whiteside, L.A., "Effects of sterilization on wear in total knee arthroplasty," *Clin Orthop*, no. 331, 164–171, (1996).

78. Wang, A., Essner, A., Polineni, V.K., Stark, C., and Dumbleton, J.H., "Lubrication and wear of ultrahigh molecular weight polyethylene in total joint replacements," *Tribol Int*, **31**:no. 1–3, 17–33, (1998).

79. Bragdon, C.R., Jasty, M., Muratoglu, O.K., O'Connor, D.O., and Harris, W.H., "Third-body wear of highly cross-linked polyethylene in a hip simulator," *J Arthroplasty*, **18**:5, (2003).

80. Lewis, G., "Properties of crosslinked ultra-high-molecular-weight polyethylene," *Biomaterials*, **22**:371–401, (2001).

81. Wroblewski, B.M., Siney, P.D., Dowson, D., and Collins, S.N., "Prospective clinical and joint simulator studies of a new total hip arthroplasty using alumina ceramic heads and cross-linked polyethylene cups," *J Bone Joint Surg*, **78-B**:280–285, (1996).

82. Oonishi, H., Saito, M., and Kadoya, Y., "Wear of high-dose gamma irradiated polyethylene in total joint replacement-long term radiologic evaluation," In *Transactions of the 44th Annual Meeting of the Orthopaedic Research Society*, New Orleans, LA., pp. 97–117, (1998).

83. McKee, G.K., and Watson-Farrar, J., "Replacement of arthritic hips by the McKee-Farrar prosthesis," *J Bone Joint Surg (Br)*, **48**:245, (1966).

84. Clarke, I.C., Donaldson, T., Bowsher, J.G., Nasser, S., and Takahashi, T., "Current concepts of metal-on-metal hip resurfacing," *Orthop Clin N Am*, **36**:143–162, (2005).

85. Gispert, M.P., Serro, A.P., Colaco, R., Pires, E., and Saramago, B., "Wear of ceramic coated metal-on-metal bearings used for hip replacement," *Wear*, **263**:1060–1065, (2007).

86. Jacobs, J.J., Skipor, A.K., Doorn, P.F., Campbell, P., Schmalzried, T.P., Black, J., and Amstutz, H.C., "Cobalt and chromium concentrations in patients with metal on metal total hip replacements," *Clin Orthop Relat Res*, **329S**:256, (1996).

87. Brodner, W., Bitzan, P., Meisinger, V., Kaider, A., Gottsauner-Wolf, F., and Kotz, R., "Elevated serum cobalt with metal-on-metal articulating surfaces," *J Bone Joint Surg (Br)*, **79**:316, (1997).

88. Saito, S., Ryu, J., Watanabe, M., Ishii, T., and Saigo, K., "Midterm results of metasul metal-on-metal total hip arthroplasty," *J Arthroplasty*, vol. 21, no. 8, (2006).

89. Hamadouche, M., Boutin, P., Daussange, J., Bolander, M.E., and Sedel, L., "Alumina-on-alumina total hip arthroplasty: a minimum 18.5-year follow-up study," *J Bone Joint Surg (Am)*, **84-A**:69, (2002).

90. Bierbaum, B.E., Nairus, J., Kuesis, D., Morrison, J.C., and Ward, D., "Ceramic-on-ceramic bearings in total hip arthroplasty," *Clin Orthop Relat Res*, 158, (2002).

91. D'Antonio, J., Capello, W., Manley, M., and Bierbaum, B., "New experience with alumina-on-alumina ceramic bearings for total hip arthroplasty," *J Arthroplasty*, **17**(4):390–397, (2002).

92. Barrack, R.L., Burak, C., and Skinner, H.B., "Concerns about ceramics in THA," *Clin Orthop Relat Res*, no. 429:73–79, (2004).

93. Rosneck, J., Klika, A., and Barsoum, W., "A rare complication of ceramic-on-ceramic bearings in total hip arthroplasty," *J Arthroplasty*, **23**(2), (2008).

94. Stewart, T.D., Tipper, J.L., Insley, G., Streicher, R.M., Ingham, E., and Fisher, J., "Severe wear and fracture of zirconia heads against alumina inserts in hip simulator studies with microseparation," *J Arthroplasty*, **18**(6):726–734, (2003).

95. Murphy, S.B., Ecker, T.M., and Tannast, M., "Incidence of squeaking after alumina ceramic-ceramic total hip arthroplasty," *J Arthroplasty*, **23**(2):327–327, (2008).

96. Wang, A., Essner, A., Polineni, V.K., Stark, C., and Dumbleton, J.H., "Lubrication and wear of ultrahigh molecular weight polyethylene in total joint replacements," *Tribol Int,* **31**(1–3):17–33, (1998).

97. Hall, R.M., Unsworth, A., Siney, P., and Wroblewski, B.M., "Wear in retrieved Charnley acetabular sockets," *Proc Inst Mech Engrs, Part H: J Eng Med*, **210**:197–207, (1996).

98. Kabo, J.M., Gebhard, J.S., Loren, G., and Amstutz, H.C., "In vivo wear of polyethylene acetabular components," *J Bone Joint Surg (Br)*, **75B**:254–258, (1993).

99. Hall, R.M., Siney, P., Unsworth, A., and Wroblewski, B.M., "The association between rates of wear in retrieved acetabular components and the radius of the femoral head," *Proc Instn Mech Engrs*, **212**:Part H, (1998).

100. Wang, A., Essner, A., and Klein, R., "Effects of contact stress on friction and wear of ultra high molecular weight polyethylene in total hip replacement," *J Engl Med*, **215**(2):133–139, (2001).

101. Mabuchi, K., Sakai, R., Ota, M., and Ujihira, M., "Appropriate radial clearance of ceramic-on-ceramic total hip prostheses to realize squeeze-film lubrication," *Clin Biomech*, **19**:362–369, (2004).

102. Rixratha, E., Wendling-Mansuya, S., Flecherb, X., Chabranda, P., and Argenson, J.N., "Design parameters dependences on contact stress distribution in gait and jogging phases after total hip arthroplasty," *J Biomech*, **41**:1137–1142, (2008).

103. Kurtz, S.M., Ochoa, J.A., White, C.V., Srivastav, S., and Cournoyer, J., "Backside nonconformity and locking restraints affect liner/shell load transfer mechanisms and relative motion in modular acetabular components for total hip replacement," *J Biomech*, **31**:431–437, (1998).

104. Williams, V.G.N., Whiteside, L.A., White, S.E., and McCarthy, D.S., "Fixation of ultrahigh-molecular-weight polyethylene liners to metal-backed acetabular cups," *J Arthroplasty*, **12**:25–31, (1997).

105. Learmonth, I.D., Young, C., and Rorabeck C., "The operation of the century: total hip replacement," *Lancet*, **370**:1508–1519, (2007).

106. Majkowski, R.S., Miles, A.W., Bannister, G.C., Perkins, J., and Taylor, G.J., "Bone surface preparation in cemented joint replacement," *J Bone Joint Surg (Br)*, **75**:459–463, (1993).

107. Krause, W.R., Krug, W., and Miller, J., "Strength of the cement-bone interface," *Clin Orthop Relat Res,* **163**:290–299, (1982).

108. Williams, H.D., Browne, G., Gie, G.A., Ling, R.S., Timperley, A.J., and Wendover, N.A., "The Exeter universal cemented femoral component at 8 to 12 years: a study of the first 325 hips," *J Bone Joint Surg (Br),* **84**:324–334, (2002).

109. Goodman, S., "Wear particulate and osteolysis," *Orthop Clin N Am*, **36**:41–48, (2005).

110. Horowitz, S.M., Frondoza, C.G., and Lennox, D.W., "Effects of polymethylmethacrylate exposure upon macrophages," *J Orthop Res*, **6**:827–832, (1988).

111. Herman J.E., Sowder, W.G., Anderson, D., Appel, A.M., and Hopson, C.N., "Polymethyl-methacrylate-induced release of bone-resorbing factors," *J Bone Joint Surg*, **71**:1530–1541, (1989).

112. Gonzales, O., Smith, R.L., and Goodman, S.B., "Effect of size, concentration, surface area, and volume of polymethylmethacrylate particles on human macrophages in vitro," *J Biomed Mat Res*, **30**:463–473, (1996).

113. Maloney, W.J., Jasty, M.J., Rosenberg, A., and Harris, W.H., "Bone lysis in well-fixed, cemented femoral components," *J Bone Joint Surg*, **72B**:966–970, (1990).

114. Jones, L.C., and Hungerford, D.S., "Cement disease," *Clin Orthop Relat Res*, **225**:192–206, (1987).

115. Sporer, S.M., and Paprosky, W.G., "Biologic fixation and bone ingrowth," *Orthop Clin N Am*, **36**:105–111, (2005).

116. Kearns, S.R., Jamal, B., Rorabeck, C.H., and Bourne, R.B., "Factors affecting survival of uncemented total hip arthroplasty in patients 50 years or younger," *Clin Orthop Relat Res,* **453**:103–109, (2006).

117. Bourne, R.B., Rorabeck, C.H., Ghazal, M.E., and Lee, M.H., "Pain in the thigh following total hip replacement with a porous-coated anatomic prosthesis for osteoarthrosis: a five-year follow-up study," *J Bone Joint Surg (Am),* **76**:1464–1470, (1994).

118. Haaker, R., Tiedjen, K. , Ottersbach, A. ,Rubenthaler, F., Stockheim, M., and Stiehl, J., "Comparison of conventional versus computer-navigated acetabular component insertion," *J Arthroplasty*, **22**(2), (2007).

119. Giurea, A., Zehetgruber, H., Funovics, P., Grampp, S., Karamat, L., and Gottsauner-Wolf, F., "Risk factors for dislocation in cementless hip arthroplasty—a statistical analysis," *Z Orthop*, **139**:194, (2001).

120. Kennedy, J.G., Rogers, W.B., Soffe, K.E., Sullivan R.J., Griffen, D.G., and Sheehan, L.J., "Effect of acetabular component orientation on recurrent dislocation, pelvic osteolysis, polyethylene wear and component migration," *J Arthroplasty*, **13**:530, (1998).

121. Lewinnek, G.E., Lewis, J.L., Tarr, R., Compere, C.L., and Zimmerman, J.R., "Dislocations after total hip replacement arthroplasties," *J Bone Joint Surg (Am)*, **60**:217, (1978).

122. Zheng, G., Marx, A., Langlotz, U., Widmer, K.H., Buttaro, M., and Nolte, L.P., "A hybrid CT-free navigation system for total hip arthroplasty," *Comput Aided Surg*, **7**:129–145, (2002).

123. Digioia, A.M., Jaramaz, B., Nikou, C., Labarca, R.S., Moody, J.E., and Colgan, B.D., "Surgical navigation for total hip replacement with the use of HipNav," *Oper Tech Orthop*, **10**:1, 3–8, (2000).

124. Herberts, P., Kärrholm, J., and Garellick, G., *The Swedish National Hip Arthroplasty Register: Annual Report 2004*. Sahlgrenska: Sahlgrenska University Hospital, Available at: http://www.jru.orthop.gu.se/documents. htm, (2005).

P · A · R · T · 5

CLINICAL ENGINEERING

CHAPTER 23
CLINICAL ENGINEERING OVERVIEW

Alfred Dolan
University of Toronto, Toronto, Canada

23.1 BIOMEDICAL ENGINEERING

23.1.1 Historical Background

No discussion of what is now referred to as *clinical engineering* can begin without considering first the development of biomedical engineering, and, in turn, engineering.

In the past, *engineering* was defined as "the facility to direct the sources of power in nature for man's use and convenience."[1] Today, modern engineering involves the application of scientific techniques, theories, and technology for the solution of societal needs. That definition has implications which all engineers, and clinical engineers in particular, must address.

As professionals, who wish to consider society's problems, engineers must first address three issues. It is essential that engineers must possess skills that are appropriate to the problem being addressed or else exempt themselves from that work. Second, engineers must ensure that the solutions they propose do not impose new and more serious problems for society. Third, engineers must meet the real needs of society and must be instrumental in defining those needs. These issues are of particular relevance for biomedical engineers and clinical engineers, as we shall see.

Biomedical engineering, rather than limiting the range of engineering brought to bear on a societal problem, limits the range of problems addressed to those in the medical and biological area. Indeed, we increasingly recognize the field more as the integration of engineering with medicine and biology for better understanding and solutions of societal needs.

Although we may feel that this recognition may seem progressive, history shows that the established boundaries of the various professional and scientific fields, and the medical and engineering sciences in particular, are of modern origin. Indications are that the giants of scientific engineering investigation throughout history were either ignored or insensitive to these boundaries. More likely, they recognized that the same scientific and engineering laws applied to all of natural phenomena, whether in the physical or biological world.

The origin of biomedical engineering, while obscure, can be traced to ancient times. We know that Alcmaeon, a student of Pythagoras, in the period around 500 B.C., became interested in applying mathematics to the study of physiology. That propensity for crossing boundaries and recognizing common scientific principles persisted throughout most of recorded history. Both Plato (427 to 347 B.C.) and Aristotle (384 to 322 B.C.) investigated, observed, and systematized the world they studied around them. Their study of the human body included detailed explanation of the pumping action of the heart and function of other organs. Galen, who was the son of an architect and mathematician in Roman times, developed theories on hemodynamics, which persisted to the time of the great physician Maimonides 1200 years later. Certainly, this integration of sciences and mathematics is consistent with modern biomedical engineering.

Leonardo da Vinci, one of the greatest engineers in history, also applied physical principles and experimental analysis to the study of physiology and medicine. Santorio invented an instrument to count the pulse—the *pulsilogium*, which was almost certainly the first recorded medical instrument. In addition, for his study of metabolic physiology, he built a metabolic balance chair to monitor body weight over long periods. Robert Hooke, who was a student of Boyle, studied respiratory phenomena as he investigated the relationship between pressures and volumes. Was this work biomedical engineering?

Stephen Hales, an English clergyman and physicist, carried out a classic experiment in 1732 to determine blood pressure. He connected a "U" tube to the carotid artery of a mare and observed the height that blood rose in the tube. Then, using fluid dynamic principles he calculated the velocity of blood in the aorta, force of contraction, and stroke volume.[2] This work has been the foundation of modern hemodynamics and was used by Bernoulli in his quite accurate calculation of cardiac output in 1737.

Lavoiser (1747 to 1794), during his studies of oxygen, extended that work to respiration. Galvani, recognized as a pioneer in electrical engineering, observed in 1780 the contraction of a frog's leg muscle when stimulated electrically. Alessandro Volta, also a physical scientist, worked extensively with the "animal electricity" that Galvani had observed. Was this work biomedical engineering?

In the mid-nineteenth century, several fields of science saw explosive activity. Men like Orstead, Gauss, Weber, Laplace, Lagrange, Carnot, Faraday, Maxwell, and Helmholtz were contemporaries in physics and chemistry. Divergence and segregation of the fields gradually occurred at this time, but some such as Helmholtz crossed these boundaries.

Helmholtz, with his early interests in physics and mathematics, undertook a career in medicine in 1838. He applied his knowledge of thermodynamics to the study of conservation of energy and metabolic physiology in 1847. He estimated the velocity of nerve transmission, invented the ophthalmoscope, and investigated the physiology and psychology of hearing, a topic of investigation to this day. Surely, Helmholtz was a biomedical engineer.

In 1837, Samuel Haughton quite clearly applied mechanical engineering principles and contemporary engineering technology to acquire new knowledge about biomechanics and cardiovascular physiology.[3] In his preface, he referred to ". . . the mutual advantages obtainable by Anatomists and Geometers from a combination of the Sciences they cultivate." Using tools, which we would consider hopelessly inadequate, he quite accurately deduced the velocity of blood in an artery, capillary resistance, blood pressure, cardiac work, and the time required for the circulation of the blood.

These investigators, scientists, and engineers like Helmholtz and Haughton recognized that the same laws apply to studies of physics, engineering, or biology—the unity of the sciences. That understanding represents the greatest challenge and potential both on the research and development side and on the applied side of the field of biomedical engineering today. That fact makes clear why developments in fields such as DNA sequencing and communications theory, which we think of as separate fields, can be successfully melded to yield outstanding gains in our understanding and treatment of disease. It also should make clear to us that techniques and technology, and not just instrumentation, which may derive from traditional engineering applications, are equally applicable in health care. This application side defines that portion of biomedical engineering which has come to be called *clinical engineering*, where all aspects of engineering and technology come to play directly in provision of patient care in the healthcare field.

23.2 CLINICAL ENGINEERING

23.2.1 Development

Clinical engineering developed in healthcare facilities around the world over the last four decades of the twentieth century. There was widespread recognition in professional and government circles of the technological explosion, which had affected society in general, and health care in particular.[4] A series of workshops held in 1972 provided a forum for the discussion of the need for an engineering approach to effect some control on this technology.[5,6] Let us consider four of the factors, which can be cited as having had a great influence on the way in which clinical engineering has developed in the hospital:

1. The rapid influx of technology and its resultant instrumentation into the hospital primarily in the 1960s and 1970s.
2. The recognition of an electrical safety issue associated with the increase in clinical instrumentation coming in contact with the patient.
3. The move to develop a certification process for engineers in hospital clinical settings.
4. The rapid influx of information technology into the healthcare technology environment.

The first three factors served to encourage the development of the field, while at the same time served to define the field itself. The field is now further redefining itself as the integration of information technology and networks, with medical devices has become ubiquitous.[7–9]

The increased prevalence of technology and medical instrumentation in hospitals meant that hospital organizations had to develop ways to take care of those devices. With that rapid proliferation of what were primarily electrical devices in the vicinity of the patient, some assurance of the electrical safety of the patient needed to be provided. Now that same assurance needs to be provided for information technology networks. At an early stage, the skills, training, and education of engineers and technologists who were to become involved in those activities needed to be vetted. Finally, the revolution in the capabilities of computer and communications technology has resulted in medical devices universally being dependent on that technology for acquisition and utilization of physiological data and patient information.

Perhaps the start of the new field, which was to become clinical engineering, can be attributed to the establishment, in January 1942, of the U.S. Army Medical Equipment Maintenance Course.[10] This developed into the Army Medical Equipment School in Denver, Colorado, and the Air Force Training Wing at Sheppard Air Force Base in Texas. Thus, maintenance of medical equipment became the first of the defined functions of what was to become the clinical engineering field.

Others recognized other problems in health care, that were associated with this rapid influx of technology and that could be amenable to an engineering approach. Robert Rushmer[11] understood the need for engineering involvement, not just in maintenance, but in all parts of health care. He emphasized the need for optimization and improvement of the effectiveness, safety, and benefit of existing technologies as a means for their more efficient and appropriate use by healthcare professionals and the resultant improved patient care. He further recognized the need for medical engineers to help to define the technological applications beyond the critical care applications of the day. He understood the need for the engineering approach and involvement in all parts of health care from hospitals to home care.

T. D. Kinney[12] in 1974 broadened the role of biomedical engineering in the hospital as he anticipated the potential for savings in chemistry laboratories through the work of biomedical engineering. He estimated that 90 percent of advanced laboratories were automated in some way at that time.

Raymon D. Garret specifically addressed the computing needs of the hospital.[13] While the solutions available in 1973 clearly were inadequate, the analysis of the hospital as a system remains valid today and serves as an excellent description of an opportunity for clinical engineering involvement today.

This brief survey illustrates that there was recognition of the problems, which existed in health care in that time period, and that there was recognition of the potential for biomedical engineering to effect solutions for those problems. It is interesting to note that the initial understanding of the role engineering could play in health care did not come necessarily or solely from engineers. Rather that broader understanding came from visionaries such as Robert Rushmer, a cardiovascular research scientist, and Cesar Caceres, a clinical cardiologist, whose recognition of what the range of engineering involvement in health care could be defines, in essence, the role of clinical engineering.

Cesar Caceres offered perhaps the most insightful description of clinical engineering:

> ". . . An engineer who is trained for and works in a health service facility where he or she is responsible for the direct and immediate application of engineering expertise to health and medical care."[14]

Except for the constraint this definition places on the practice of clinical engineering to that being within the precincts of the hospital, this definition accurately outlines the role of clinical engineering. It is important to notice that this definition assumes both appropriate engineering expertise, and direct benefit to patient care or health care, which are two of the important issues previously cited that engineers must address.

The next step in the beginning of what has been called clinical engineering can be traced back to the late 1950s and a convergence of the first two factors. Concern arose over electrical safety for patients in hospitals, resulting from the proliferation of electronic equipment in the vicinity of the patient devices.[15,16] The results of a number of reports and analyses[17,18] were that the need for biomedical engineering expertise in the hospitals centred for many years on the electrical safety aspect.[19] S. Powers and D. G. Gisser, in discussing the issues related to monitoring of trauma patients in 1974, again brought forward the electrical safety issues.[12] Indeed some clinical engineering departments were built on the electrical safety testing. Even today, the concern for safety sometimes masks other arguably more important clinical engineering functions in some hospitals. The recognition that such things as, for example, usability of medical devices profoundly affects the effectiveness of medical devices is being more widely recognized.[20]

The other great influence on the development of the field of clinical engineering was provided by the efforts to establish a peer recognition of this new group of engineers who practised in the healthcare institution. In the early 1970s, Cesar Caceres and Tom Hargest coined the name *clinical engineering* to describe the new field of engineering practice, which had gradually been developing in hospitals over the previous decade. Since it was directed toward the improvement of patient care in the clinical environment, the somewhat curious name clinical engineering stuck. They also can be considered as pioneers in developing a certification program for vetting the competence of engineers wishing to practice this new field. Modeled after other speciality fellowship training and certification programs in other medical fields such as cardiovascular surgery, a certification commission was set up in 1974 with the Association for the Advancement of Medical Instrumentation agreeing to serve as secretariat.

Initially two boards of examiners were established, which reported to a certification commission. Subsequently other boards of examiners were established starting in Canada in 1979. The bylaws and terms of reference of each board, such as the U.S. Board of Examiners for Clinical Engineering and the U.S. Board of Examiners for Biomedical Technicians, were subject to review and approval by the certification commission. The boards, in turn, had the responsibility of establishing the examination process, setting appropriate examinations, and conducting the examinations for clinical engineering and biomedical technician applicants. Following the completion of that process, the boards of examiners made recommendations to the certification commission and certification was approved or not approved by the commission.

In parallel, the American Board of Examiners for Clinical Engineering set up a similar, albeit much smaller, certification program. The two programs were merged in July 1983 to form the International Certification Commission.

Certification influenced development of clinical engineering in three ways. First, it established and crystallized the name of the field as clinical engineering. Second, it provided some assurance of the competency of clinical engineering practitioners to the healthcare facilities where they practised. Third, however, it tended to result in clinical engineers defining themselves in terms of the certification process. The examination process, in particular, which in the U.S. Boards of Examiners was heavily oriented toward electronics, had an effect on both the type of engineering people who went in to the field as well as the educational programs, which provided the training. The wide range of management and broad healthcare issues identified by people like Rushmer and Caceres tended not to have as heavy an emphasis.

Over the past two decades, the integration and merging of information technology departments in hospitals and clinical engineering has changed the face of the field yet again. Modern healthcare diagnostic instrumentation consists largely of signal and data processing systems coupled with input devices that perform physiological transduction. Processors are further linked through small or large networks as required for diagnosis or therapy.

This background provides a basis for the understanding of the role clinical engineering occupies in health care today. Clinical engineering developed with an early large emphasis on the maintenance, electrical safety, and electronics aspects of medical equipment. Some people such as Scott[15] and Rushmer[11] encouraged the consideration of broader safety aspects in health care. Gordon repeatedly emphasized that the assessment, evaluation, and management of healthcare technology rather than of medical equipment was key.[10] Caceres consistently outlined the broadest possible role for clinical engineering in health care to include all aspects of management of technology and the impact on patient care throughout the spectrum of healthcare delivery.[21] Let us then consider that role.

23.3 ROLE OF CLINICAL ENGINEERING

The application of engineering techniques, technology, and theory to the solution of healthcare problems and a management of technology in health care is, by definition, clinical engineering. The American College of Clinical Engineering emphasizes both patient care and management by defining a clinical engineer as "a professional who supports and advances patient care by applying engineering and management skills to health care technology."[22] More than three decades ago, Scott and Caceres separately identified a number of clinical engineering responsibilities, which remain valid today.[23,24] Their combined list of clinical engineering responsibilities includes development and management of medical systems, education, maintenance, safety, clinical research and development, and analysis and development for the more effective patient care systems. Betts, in considering the changing role of clinical engineering in the 1980s, emphasized the need for management skills in addition to the requisite technical knowledge.[25] More recently, Bronzino identified technology management, risk management, technology assessment, facilities design and project management, and training as the key functions for a clinical engineering department.[16] The clinical engineer must be directly involved with solutions in any of these problem areas at the delivery level, if available solutions are to be effected.

He/she must provide education for nursing, medical, and paramedical staff to facilitate their understanding of present technology and future trends. In consultation with medical and administrative staff, he/she must ensure that equipment purchases and hospital designs and systems are optimal, and technology acquisitions are appropriate. He/she must engage in applied research and development at all levels to improve patient care and make provisions for the safe and effective utilization of technology. Accordingly, the following functions can be taken as descriptive of the role of clinical engineering.

23.3.1 Education

- Prime responsibility for making provisions for training and education associated with technology and instrumentation used in the hospital
- Education of clinical engineering staff
- Education of healthcare facility staff

The objective is to provide to all medical equipment users the understanding and knowledge necessary for the proper use of all patient care equipment, calibration, routines, instrument errors, safety procedures, and possible hazards.

23.3.2 Clinical Research/Development

- Design of new equipment, patient aids, and techniques for the provision of effective patient care
- Assistive devices

While the old adage "don't build if you can buy" certainly should apply in all clinical engineering departments, it is clear that in most hospitals there is a continuing need for what we could call customized devices. A clinical engineering department in a rehabilitation healthcare facility might be heavily involved in the design or modification of assistive technologies. Other examples arise from the particular type of patient care or particular procedures encountered in a specific hospital. These may be as simple as the need to provide electrical isolation for an amalgam of devices, which would require an understanding of medical electrical system standards. More commonly, it would involve providing assistance to other departments in clinical research projects and the development of solutions to current clinical problems unique to the facility. Whatever the application, it is important that clinical engineering have the facility or be able to serve as an interface, so that specialized devices, techniques, or accessories can be made available for more effective patient care.

23.3.3 Information Technology Applications

- Development and management of hospital and patient information and physiological data acquisition systems
- Development and responsibility for patient care networks
- Integration of medical devices with IT networks

Certainly, the ubiquitous presence of computing and data processing in all functions of the hospital is well recognized. Those range from what we recognize as mainframe computers and servers to word processors or personal computers and handheld devices, and finally to processors incorporated within diagnostic and therapeutic devices. It is incumbent on the hospital, therefore, that some management of computing in the hospital is established. Traditionally, that constituted establishment of a department with that function starting with large-scale accounting computing. Increasingly, it is understood that the overlap of other computing needs such as patient records, patient information systems, medical device data and storage systems, or diagnostic and direct patient care computing require a much broader approach. Such an approach is consistent with the role of clinical engineering. Furthermore, medical devices almost universally incorporate computing or processing functions which generate or utilize data for the provision of patient care. It is imperative that the integration of multiple medical devices as part of IT networks be carefully planned and maintained. There is currently a major international standards development project set up within the International Electrotechnical Commission aimed at addressing the risks associated with the incorporation of IT networks within medical devices.[26] The planning that must take place for the effective implementation and operation of these networks will be discussed in a later chapter of this book.

23.3.4 Facility Planning

- Advising and consulting with administrative and healthcare staff on matters related to the impact of technological developments in healthcare facility planning
- Standards and regulations

Botz has emphasized that the application and proper use of technology entails the appropriate management of all resources, including equipment, manpower, supplies, and space.[27] It is obviously important then that the requirements placed on a healthcare facility by a particular technology become part of the considerations for the technology and related equipment. However, it must also be reflected at a very early stage in the planning process in the planning and design of the facility itself. This may be as simple as the planning for an appropriate electrical power supply or adequate heating and ventilation for the installation of a device. Ensuring that relevant standards are met is assumed. It may be the much more intensive planning required to ensure the proper integration of the technology and all associated equipment in the architectural design.

23.3.5 Systems Management

- Systems analysis
- Design and evaluation of healthcare systems
- Quality management
- Risk management

System analysis and synthesis has long been a well-established engineering approach that has been used in many different branches of engineering. This formal way of examining the inputs, outputs, and the transfer functions applied to a healthcare system or portion thereof has provided some important insights and identified opportunities for improvement.[28] In a similar way, the relatively recent recognition of the applicability of quality management approaches long used in engineering offers the same potential.[29] Formal risk management procedures and analytical methods, while providing a focus on criticality (severity) and probability of occurrence, are assuming more prominent roles as engineering methodologies for adding value. The ISO 14971-2007 standard on risk management for medical devices shows how manufacturers must use risk management principles for the provision of safe and effective medical devices for hospitals.[30] That standard can also serve as a model for clinical engineering departments in hospitals. Clinical engineering departments are uniquely positioned for involvement in these activities.

23.3.6 Equipment Management

- Consultation with other healthcare staff in the planning and purchase of equipment
- Prime responsibility for maintenance and modification of equipment

The large number of individual devices in modern hospitals present a unique set of problems in management and represent a major role for clinical engineering. That set can broadly be segregated into:

- Planning—Functional program review
  - Technology planning
  - New equipment planning
  - Renewal equipment planning
- Acquisition—Definition of clinical requirements
  - Survey of available equipment
  - Specification writing
  - Equipment evaluation
  - Generation of purchase documents
  - Vendor selection
  - Acceptance testing
- Control—Inventory management
  - Maintenance
  - Repair
  - Test and calibration procedures
  - Scheduled inspection
  - Safety program

The technology planning function is one of the most cost-effective roles for clinical engineering.[31] Equipment planning, which includes planning for new and renewal of equipment, is an important subset of that technology planning process. It begins at the functional programming stage of planning. It involves continuing participation in the organizational-wide strategic planning process so that equipment-related issues can be appropriately identified. Those issues include life cycle, new technology, obsolescence, capital costs, personnel and training requirements, maintenance requirements, operating costs, and facility design considerations. The hospital needs to have all the information to make a decision on the economic and technical viability of either new or existing equipment.

The acquisition of equipment is the next major part of effective equipment management. It follows and is indeed part of the equipment-planning phase. Flowing from definition of requirements, specifications are developed. Based on those specifications, a subset of possible equipment is evaluated for conformance to those specifications or standards, and purchase of the most appropriate equipment is initiated. When the equipment arrives at the hospital, the acceptance or incoming inspection of the equipment is a very common function which clinical engineering fulfils. Clinical engineering acts as a technical conduit between the hospital and the vendor(s).

For all those devices deemed necessary by the hospital to be utilized effectively, an inventory of those devices needs to be in place. Such a system, therefore, however it is maintained, must be able to provide for the hospital the type of device, the capability of each device, the location, status and some way to ensure its availability at the point of care. To meet these requirements in turn, the devices must be adequately maintained and calibrated. All these functions are routine clinical engineering functions. To ensure that takes place, some sort of inventory, tracking, maintenance and repair log, and calibration activity has to be provided. Typically, safety testing is part of that process.

23.3.7 Patient Safety/Risk Management

- Prime responsibility for safety of medical equipment and systems in-patient care areas
- Prime responsibility for risk management of systems, networks, and devices

The management of the safety risk associated with the use of medical devices is an important function for clinical engineering. While in some facilities this may be incorrectly confined to incident investigation, the broader understanding of the function includes identification of hazards, establishing realistic estimates of the risks associated with those hazards, and instituting suitable control measures to minimize those risks. While the concepts of risk management are more than 400 years old, Leeming was the first to specifically apply the concepts to the clinical engineering field.[32] His work in the electrical safety field allowed realistic estimates of the risk associated with the use of multiple electrical devices in the patient care vicinity and provided a basis for a rational deployment of resources and choice of risk control measures. Much more recently, there is an increasing recognition of the risk management approach in clinical engineering for in technology management as well as in safety applications.[33]

Risk management is a widely deployed term that has different meanings to different departments and functional areas. Clinical engineers must be able to operate within the context of the risk management activities of the various functional areas. Often, this means discriminating between enterprise risk management and risk management associated with patient/operator health and safety.

Enterprise risk management typically defines risk as the uncertainty in meeting the objectives of the organization. This definition drives a managerial approach to risk management and ensures that the enterprise considers factors such as financial, inventories, policies, procedures, strategies, values, asset management, and any other element of the organization. Typically, there are many different tools utilized to control risk within the context of enterprise risk management (ERM).

Risk management associated with patient/operator health and safety has been the focus of many consensus standards (such as ISO 14971 for medical devices), regulatory agencies such as the Joint Commission, and various improvement initiatives within the hospital. *Risk* here is defined as the combination of probability of occurrence of harm and the severity of the harm. The objective is to manage risk using appropriate risk assessment and mitigation methods. Tools typically used for assessment include FMEAs and FMECAs, fault trees, probabilistic risk assessment, and other formal methodologies. The two key functions of risk management, risk assessment and risk mitigation, include, respectively, risk estimation and risk evaluation against set acceptability criteria, and risk control to bring the risk down to meet that set acceptability criteria.

FMEAs and FMECAs are failure mode and effects analysis and failure mode and effects criticality analysis, respectively. These are typically considered as bottom-up methodologies in that the components and subsystems are individually evaluated for the impact of failures on the whole system. Often the distinction between the two is academic and the terms are used interchangeably.

Fault tree and event tree methods relate to focusing on the relationships between elements, components, and processes of a system. By focusing on the relationships, Boolean algebra may be applied through the use of operations such as "and," "or," and "not." By plotting and analyzing the system, significant insights are often made which augment decision making. Fault trees often focus on undesirable system performance, while event trees are more generalized in nature.

Probabilistic risk assessments seek to determine an actual value for probability of occurrence of faults, hazards, and ultimately harm. Through research, testing, and experimentation, values are established and confidence intervals defined. These values can be evaluated against separate risk acceptability criteria established by the organization and decisions made regarding the risk.

There are many other formal methodologies to evaluate risk. Most tools available to statisticians are also appropriate for risk management. Tools such as hypothesis testing, Monte Carlo analysis, and acceptance sampling OC curves are useful. Explanations for tools such as HACCP and HAZOP are beyond the scope of this chapter, but can be applied to risk management activities in the context of the hospital environment with significant utility.

23.3.8 Regulatory Activities

- Codes
- National and international standards
- Regulations and accreditations

Health care in all countries operates subject to a broad variety of standards and regulations. In many cases, these are technological in nature and should come under the purview of clinical engineering. Feinberg emphasized the importance of this point in hospitals in the United States in listing some of the codes and standards pertaining to the clinical engineer.[34] In all jurisdictions, regulations such as municipal, provincial, or national building codes have an impact on health facility design, for example. Furthermore, technical standards affect every device in the hospital. These standards are increasingly international standards but may also be developed by a national or local standards body. Finally, in most countries such as in the United States of America, extensive federal regulations govern virtually all aspects of medical devices design, distribution, and application. Clinical engineering, the department responsible for those devices must be conversant with the appropriate standards and regulations.

Educational programs for clinical engineers and biomedical engineering technicians and technologists reflect the need for training specific to the perceived role of clinical engineering. Figure 23.1 illustrates a set of guidelines and matrix of duties for graduate students during internship periods in one such program. It is provided as an example only.

With this background, of the current role of clinical engineering in health care, we can consider the future role for the field and the way it will address the three issues cited earlier:

- Defining and meeting societal needs
- Ensuring that technological solutions are responsible solutions
- Continuing development of required professional skills

Clinical engineering role	Internship activities
Equipment design	Circuit design, fabrication Circuit modification Mechanical design, modification Pneumatic/hydraulic design, modification Computer hardware, software
Facility planning	Assessment of applicable standards Assessment of facility plans
Information systems	System design Programming Network integration Integration with medical devices
Professional affairs	Associations/societies Government
Education	Education CE staff Education healthcare facility staff
Equipment planning	Functional program strategic planning Capital planning Renewal
Equipment acquisition	Definition of clinical requirements Assessment available equipment Specification writing Equipment evaluation Vendor selection Acceptance testing
Equipment control	Inventory control Test and calibration procedures Scheduled inspection Repair
Safety program	Hazard report management Risk evaluation Incident investigation
System analysis	
Regulatory affairs	Codes Standards Regulations

FIGURE 23.1 Example of experience matrix guidelines for clinical engineering students in one clinical engineering master's training program. (*University of Toronto, Institute of Biomaterials and Biomedical Engineering, Internship Guidelines, 2007.*)

Clinical engineering role	Internship activities
Research	Literature review Experimentation Clinical trials
Continuing education	Courses, conferences, site visits Literature, journals Practice and lab
Departmental management	Policy and services Supervision personnel Healthcare facility meetings Coordination activities Budgeting
Documentation	Reporting
Technology planning	Strategic Short term Personnel planning
Technology assessment	Components Materials Methodology Systems

FIGURE 23.1 (*Continued*)

23.4 FUTURE DEVELOPMENT OF CLINICAL ENGINEERING

In keeping with our definition of clinical engineering as supporting and advancing patient care through application of engineering management and technology, it is important to recognize that the field of clinical engineering will need to continue to develop as health care develops. This will include developments both in sophistication, such as physiological functional imaging or highly integrated information systems, and in scope, such as in wellness care or in distributed clinical care. Moreover, it will be important that every clinical engineering program or department obeys the laws of entropy. Those laws describe the natural tendency for systems to run "down hill" rather than evolve to something bigger and better. Very active development by individual departments and by the field will be required for the field to keep abreast of changes and issues in health care. Let us first consider some of those changing healthcare issues and how they might influence the role of clinical engineering in the future.

In a later chapter of this book, J. Currie carefully discusses the impact that technology and other factors have on healthcare facility design. Figure 23.2 lists some of those factors. Advances in science and technology will lead to continuing developments in diagnosis and therapy. The ubiquitous and expanding presence of information technology applications in health care is widely accepted. New modalities for treatment stemming from current research in areas such as tissue engineering and biomaterials will come to fruition. The incursion of new or newly important disease entities coupled with shifts in population composition will present challenges to healthcare systems everywhere. Finally, the economic impact of all these factors on healthcare systems needs to be taken into account.

Context for the hospital of the future
- Advancing science and technology
- Diagnosis and therapy developments
- Information technology
- New modalities of treatment
- Closer role for research
- External healthcare challenges
- Epidemiological shifts
- Changing economics
- Electronic records
- IT networking of equipment
- Risk management
- Quality assurance/quality improvement

FIGURE 23.2 Issues affecting design for hospitals in the future. (*Adapted from The Hospital of the Future, J. Currie, Smith Group, 2001.*)

Nearly two decades ago, Robert Rushmer described some of these same health technology issues for the twenty-first century.[35] In reviewing research and development at the Imaging Research Centre at the University of Washington, he provided a summary of sophisticated new imaging techniques ranging from three-dimensional confocal microscopy for displaying cellular structure to the more common Doppler imaging of flow (Fig. 23.3). These examples in just this one area of technology serve to illustrate three important related healthcare issues, which were also brought out in Currie's work, mentioned earlier. Those key issues are the rapid development of new technology, ubiquitous incorporation of computing technology, and the communication and information technology imperative.

Imaging technique
Scanning, tunneling microscopy
Biosensors
X-ray microanalysis
High-resolution optical/electron microscopy
3D confocal microscopy
CT, MRI, PET, SPECT
Metabolic and flow imaging
Burn depth imaging
Ultrasound monitoring trauma
Monolayer analysis
Microtonometry
Cancer karyotyping
Quantitative cytometry
Doppler flow
3D cardiac reconstruction
Ultrasound endoscopy
Impedance imaging

FIGURE 23.3 Applications of imaging analysis. [*Adapted from Rushmer (IEEE Engineering in Medicine and Biology, 1990.)*]

First, each of these new imaging techniques is based on either new or newly applied scientific principles in health care. Information on the structure, chemical composition, physiological function, and metabolic function of organs or cells can be generated. Imaging of the current density distribution in living muscle or neurological tissue provides a representation of the electrophysiologic function of tissues.[36] Healthcare practitioners at all levels, including clinical engineering practitioners, will need to become conversant with these underlying scientific principles if the new technique is to be introduced and utilized effectively. Current examples can be drawn from the differences in three of the commonly available scanning techniques, magnetic resonance imaging (MRI), positron emission tomography (PET), and single positron emission computed tomography (SPECT). Since each is based on the recording of different emissions from tissues generated in different ways, each, therefore, has different clinical capabilities. This requires an ongoing educational and training effort by healthcare facilities as well as consistent assessment of the suitability of the new technology in each particular healthcare environment.

Second, the previously cited examples of MRI, PET, or SPECT imaging are obvious examples of technologies, which require extensive computing power for transduction, manipulation, and display of information. Less obvious is the ubiquitous presence of digital processors in virtually all medical devices which may be serving as either input or output stages, or be running algorithms to generate diagnostic data. The signal from a finger or ear transducer requires the application of an algorithm to convert it to a representation of oxygen saturation. An appreciation by clinical engineering of the computational requirements for any of these devices is essential.

Finally, the data and information generated in all the imaging examples used as examples must be converted to usable information and communicated effectively to care providers around the healthcare facility if patient care is to be affected positively.[28] Information must be accurate, timely, and appropriate to the user. This demands not only that the technological infrastructure be provided for moving and storing information but that new, innovative user-friendly ways of presenting information must be available. Computer systems must be appropriately designed, developed, installed, and operated to meet the needs of the functional departments of the hospital.

The integration of multiple computer systems in the hospital environment has yielded new solutions and better customer service while significantly increasing the complexity of the systems architecture and expanding the opportunity for critical systems failure. To meet the needs of customers and competitive performance pressures, novel solutions and aggressive teamwork has been required. IEC document 80001 is under development to address these issues and to provide solutions for IT networking of medical devices, ISO 80001.[26] Equipment manufacturers, the hospital, system integrators, and IT staff personnel all must work jointly to ensure success for the creation and maintenance of these complex systems.

Mack, in discussing the development of minimally invasive and robotic surgery, brought out similar issues.[37] The development of high-resolution CCD chips, together with high-intensity lighting and high-precision miniaturized handheld surgical instruments, has allowed the application of minimally invasive techniques for a wider variety of procedures. The further development into robotic and computer-assisted surgery will place a great reliance on communications and telemetry in particular. Griffith and Grodzinsky also recognized engineering advances in these same areas of microinstrumentation and virtual surgery techniques.[38] New challenges will be presented for clinical engineering not only in keeping abreast of these new surgical technologies but also in integrating the related communications and computer technology into the hospital environment.

While these changes in health care are occurring, there are other external factors which will also affect the clinical engineering field.

Internationalization of Science and Technology. The science and technology used in health care is universal. Coupled with global manufacturing and international companies, it is clear that science and technology is worldwide in application.

Integration of Technology. In the examples provided by some of the previous authors, it is evident that healthcare technology is sophisticated and cross disciplinary. The application of communications theory for improving the accuracy and speed of DNA sequencing is such an example.[39] In addition, devices are increasingly interdependent and intercommunicate freely as they are combined into systems.

Communications Technology. Information is the new currency of modern healthcare delivery. The data generated at the instrument site must be transformed into information usable for diagnosis and therapy. The healthcare facility or system must have the ability to move that information to the patient care site. Considerations of information storage, transfer, and the protocols for making that transfer are all now part of healthcare technology management decisions.

Regulation of Healthcare Technology. The healthcare medical device field is heavily regulated in all countries in the world. The impact this has on the application of technology at an individual or hospitals level varies with the sophistication of the hospital(s). However, three examples of international standards, which influence the safety and effectiveness of every medical device in the hospital, illustrate the pervasive nature of these standards and regulations. These three standards are the ISO risk management standard, ISO 14971; the medical electrical standard, IEC 60601; and the ISO quality management standard, ISO 13485. Clinical engineering needs to be fully informed about each of these standards and the impact they have on their hospital.[30,40,41]

With the changing healthcare environment both within and without the hospital, what can we say about the future role that clinical engineering should play? Enderle et al. have offered some helpful insight into the possible future role for clinical engineering, including computer support, telecommunications, facilities operation, and strategic planning.[42] It is perhaps most appropriate, however, first to return to the definition of clinical engineering as being the application of engineering techniques, technology, and theory to the solution of healthcare problems and management of technology in health care. While the environment is changing, this definition is not. We understand there is a moving technological horizon in clinical engineering. In the 1960s, the concern was electrical patient safety; in the 1970s and 1980s, it was equipment acquisition; in the 1990s, planning came more to the fore. Moving into the twenty-first century, risk management and quality assurance initiatives are increasingly common. Success is measured in terms of improving patient outcomes through teamwork and the application of the scientific method, meeting the needs of the organization, and eliminating activities that are not essential. Gordon has consistently strongly emphasized that clinical engineering must concentrate on management.[10] Botz voiced a similar theme stating that management of technological resources necessitated the management of equipment, manpower, supplies, and space.[27] Technology management then must be the overriding theme for clinical engineering departments in the future, whatever the technology that evolves. Within that broad theme, we can identify four key roles that clinical engineering must play, which are consistent with those of Enderle et al. and which will ensure that the field deals effectively with the factors that have been previously cited in the changing healthcare field.

Strategic Planning. As new scientific advances are considered for implementation, a clear understanding of the resource, economic, and technical implications must be developed by the hospital planning team. Clinical engineering needs to be involved in all those aspects of planning for the hospital system from the generation of the functional program to the final implementation of the technology within the hospital. Some firms are utilizing formal risk management tools to augment strategic planning activities. For example, corporate leadership may utilize a polling approach starting at the department level and working through division and corporate functions to compile risks (both positive and negative) to the organization. Enterprise risk management considers risk to be both positive and negative as opposed to the approach typically utilized by safety and health risk management, which considers risk related to hazards and harms. For enterprise risk management, negative risk would be any issue that could have an adverse impact on meeting the objectives of the organization. Positive risk would be those opportunities that are available to the organization for the enhancement of meeting objectives. Taken together, the management of positive and negative risk can be a beneficial tool in providing focus and direction in the development of strategic plans.

Technology Management. Once a technology is in place in a healthcare system, it must be managed in the best interests of the patient, the users, and the hospital. This management function includes all the traditional maintenance and safety considerations, but will increasingly include more advanced management functions such as benefit analysis, reliability, risk management techniques, and sustainability. Industrial programs such as Six Sigma and lean manufacturing are migrating into the hospital sector and will play a more significant role in the future. Six Sigma activities were initially considered to be related to industrial processes, but have expanded to include service activities and are well positioned to provide significant operational improvements for hospitals in the twenty-first century.

Information Technology. The overwhelming presence of information and communications technology in health care will only increase. Incorporated in this broad role is computing support, network support, integration of systems, data transmission and storage considerations, and telemedicine. It is imperative that clinical engineering play a part in this key aspect of modern health care. Clinical engineering has a significant role in the implementation of new technologies associated with the automation of patient records. Most importantly, it takes a lead role in ensuring that patient data are correctly transferred around the hospital and correctly used and interpreted to ensure better patient care.

Standards and Regulatory Activity. Health will continue to operate in a highly regulated environment. Standards and the regulations and accreditations, which implement those standards, affect the hospital explicitly or implicitly. Quality management and risk management are important aspects of technology management, which are now very well defined in national and international standards as well as in many accreditation processes. Technical standards now cover virtually every device used in the hospital. Effective utilization of these standards and regulations as part of the hospital management will be essential. The reuse of medical devices has become a significant regulatory issue in the hospital environment. Clinical engineering has a significant role in providing technical support and guidance to various departments to ensure medical devices that are reused are safe, meet regulatory requirements, and meet manufacturer's requirements.

Health care and the technology supporting health care will continue to develop. This accelerating trend in scientific developments in health care will, in turn, drive the development in clinical engineering. Active development in clinical engineering will be required if the field is to continue to thrive.

REFERENCES

1. Dolan, A. M., Wolf, H. K., and Rautaharju, P. M., Medical; Engineering—Past Accomplishments and Future Challenges, *Journal APENS*, 1973.
2. Hales, S., *Statistical Essays Containing Haemostatics*, Inn and Manley Publishers, 1733.
3. Haughton, S., *Principles of Animal Mechanics*, Longmans, Green and Company, London, 1873.
4. *Biomedical Engineering and Biophysics*, Report of the Ontario Council of Health, 1974.
5. Hopps, J. A., (Ed.), First International Biomedical Engineering Workshop Series, *I: Biomedical Equipment Maintenance Service Programs,* The American Institute of Biological Sciences, Bio Instrumentation Advisory Council, April 1972.
6. Craig, J. L., (Ed.), First International Biomedical Engineering Workshop Series, *I: Biomedical Equipment Maintenance Service Programs,* The American Institute of Biological Sciences, Bio Instrumentation Advisory Council, April 1972.
7. Hu, F., et al., Privacy–Preserving Telecardiology Sensor Networks: Toward a Low-Cost Wireless Hardware/Software Co-Design, *IEEE Transactions Information Technology in Biomedicine*, Volume **11**(6):619–27, 2007.
8. Moran, E. B., et al., Mobility in Hospital Work: Towards a Pervasive Computing Hospital Environment, *International Journal Electronic Healthcare*, Volume **3**(1):72–89, 2007.
9. Schrenker, R. A., Software Engineering for Future Healthcare and Clinical Systems, *IEEE Computer*, Volume **39**(4):26–32, 2006.
10. Gordon, G. F., Hospital Technology Management: The Tao of Clinical Engineering, *Journal of Clinical Engineering*, Volume **15**:111, 1990.
11. Rushmer, R. F., *Medical Engineering, Projections for Health Care Delivery*, Academic Press, 1972.
12. Brown, J.H.U., and Dickson, J. F., III, (Eds.), *Advances in Biomedical Engineering*, Volume **4**, 1974.
13. Garret, R. D., *Hospitals—A System Approach*, Auerbach Publishers Inc., 1973.

14. Caceres, C. A., (Ed.), *Management and Clinical Engineering*, Artech House Books, 1980.
15. Scott, R. N., and Paasche, P. E., Safety Considerations in Clinical Engineering, *CRC Reviews in Biomedical Engineering*, Volume **13**(3):201–26, 1986.
16. Bronzino, J. D., (Ed.), *The Biomedical Engineering Handbook*, CRC Press, 1995.
17. Dalziel, C. F., Effects of Electric Shock on Man, *IEEE Professional Group on Medical Electronics 5, Transactions*, July 1956.
18. Weinberg, D. I., Artley, J. L., Whalen, R. I., and McIntosh, H. D., Electric Shock Hazards in Cardiac Catheterization, *Circulation Research*, **11**:1004, 1962.
19. Todd, J. S., (Guest Ed.), *Symposium on Intensive Care Units,* The Medical Clinics of North America, Volume **55**(5), September 1971.
20. IEC 62366:2007, *Medical Devices—Application of Usability Engineering to Medical Devices.*
21. Caceres, C. A., (Ed.), *The Management of Technology in Health and Medical Care*, Artech House Inc., 1980.
22. *Enhancing Patient Safety: The Role of Clinical Engineering,* American College of Clinical Engineering, White Paper, 2001.
23. Scott, R. N., Portrait of Clinical Engineering—the Report of a Study of the Role of the Professional Engineer in Health Care, CMBES Monograph 1976-1, vi+85, Ed. A. M. Dolan; CMBES, Ottawa, Canada, 1976.
24. Caceres, C. A., *Clinical Engineering: A Model Development in Medical Personnel Utilization*, Medical Instrumentation, Volume **15**(1):8, 1981.
25. Betts, W., The Changing Role of the Clinical Engineer: The Need to Develop Management Skills, *AAMI 18th Annual Meeting*, Dallas, Tex., May, 1983.
26. IEC Project No. 80001 Ed. 1.0: Application of Risk Management to Information Technology (IT) Networks Incorporating Medical Devices.
27. Botz, C. K., Technology Resource Management in Hospitals, a New Opportunity, *AAMI 18th Annual Meeting*, Dallas, Tex., May, 1983.
28. Gordon, D. B., *A Strategic Information System for Hospital Management,* PhD. Thesis, University of Toronto, 1998.
29. White Paper. International Workshop Agreement (IWA 1)—Quality Management Systems—Guidelines for Process Improvements in Health Service Organizations, Based on ISO 9004:2000, 2d ed., 2000-12–15, reference number IWA 1:2001(E).
30. ISO 14971:2007, *Medical Devices—Application of Risk Management to Medical Devices* (reference number ISO 14971:2007 (E)).
31. Bauer, S., Dolan, A. M., and Ramirez, M. R., Technology Planning Programs for Clinical Engineering Departments, *18th CMBEC Conference*, Toronto, 1992.
32. Leeming, M. N., A Probabilistic Approach to Safety Design: The Two Element Environment, *Medical Instrumentation,* Volume **10**(1):2, 1976.
33. Brewin, D., *Design of an Optimization System for a Medical Engineering Device Maintenance Program,* MHSc. Thesis, University of Toronto, November 2001.
34. Feinberg, B. N., *Applied Clinical Engineering*, Prentice Hall Inc., 1986.
35. Rushmer, R. E., Technologies and Health in the 21st Century, *IEEE Engineering in Medicine and Biology*, Volume **9**(2):50, June 1990.
36. Joy, M. L. G., Lebedev, V. P., and Gati, J. S., Imaging of Current Density and Current Pathways in Rabbit Brain During Transcranial Electrostimulation, *IEEE Transactions on Biomedical Engineering*, Volume **46**(9):1139, 1999.
37. Mack, J. M., Minimally Invasive and Robotic Surgery, *JAMA*, Volume **285**(5):568, 2001.
38. Griffith, L. G., and Grodzinsky, A. J., Advances in Biomedical Engineering, *JAMA*, Volume **285**(5), 2001.
39. Davies, S., Davies, W., Eizenman, M., and Pasupathy, S., Optimal structure for automatic processing of DNA sequences, *IEEE Transactions on Biomedical Engineering*, Volume **46**(9):1044–56, Sept. 1999.
40. ISO 13485:2003, *Medical Devices—Quality Management Systems—Requirements for Regulatory Purposes* (reference number ISO 13485:2003 (E)).
41. IEC 60601-1:2005, *Medical Electrical Equipment—Part 1: General Requirements for Basic Safety and Essential Performance.*
42. Enderle, J. D., Blanchard, S. M., and Bronzino, J. D., *Introduction to Biomedical Engineering*, Academic Press, 1999.

CHAPTER 24
RISK MANAGEMENT IN CLINICAL ENGINEERING

Alfred Dolan
University of Toronto, Toronto, Canada and Center for Applied Health Science, Virginia Tech, Blacksburg, Virginia

Stan Mastrangelo
Center for Applied Health Science, Virginia Tech, Blacksburg, Virginia

24.1 INTRODUCTION

The word *risk* has become one of the most ubiquitous terms in use in the twenty-first century. Managing risk has become synonymous with making decisions and achieving objectives.

Risk is a romance language term that was popularized in the Renaissance era and derived from early Italian word, *risicare*, meaning to dare.[1] The evolution of the understanding of risk paralleled the development of modern scientific thought, and the evolution is continuing today. The field of risk management continues to develop and evolve today.

In the past, it was often said that certain leaders were lucky, insightful, or had good decision-making instincts. While these dependencies may have been adequate explanations for making decisions in the past, the public currently expects decisions to be made via the application of appropriate scientific methods, using objective evidence, and with communication to the appropriate stakeholders. The field of risk management provides the processes, tools, and techniques to meet these needs.

Risk management has become a very broad field and, as a result, the word risk has taken on a wide spectrum of meanings. For example, *risk* has been variously defined as "possibility of loss or injury,"[2] "the chance of something happening that will have an impact on objectives,"[3] and "a combination of the probability of occurrence of harm and severity of that harm."[4] While these may appear to be quite different to the casual reader, all of the definitions are facets of the same fundamental concept of an unknown future condition. The differences in the definitions are actually related to the subject under study and the method of study, not actual differences in the fundamental concept.

As a result, there may be multiple departments or organizational elements that bear the term risk or risk management and yet are doing significantly different activities. For example, a risk manager may work in the nursing department, the legal department, the accounting department, or the board of directors. All of these personnel would be doing very different things, for example, improving patient outcomes, containing costs due to litigation, complying with Sarbanes-Oxley regulations, or establishing an organization's strategic direction, respectively. Yet, the concepts, tools, and techniques in managing risk are quite portable and universal between the various disciplines. The main difference between these apparently disparate roles is actually the goal or objective under study, not the processes used. These processes, tools, and techniques, once learned, may be applied to a wide variety of activities and issues.

In order to understand the appropriate application of risk management in healthcare settings, it is important to understand the basic principles underlying risk management science. These basic principles will be explored in this chapter through a description of a risk management life cycle model, with the understanding that these basic principles are applicable to risk management in a broad spectrum of organizations and industry sectors.

This chapter explores the application of risk management primarily in the context of clinical settings. There will be several approaches taken to perform this exploration:

- Modeling the risk management process
- Reviewing tools and techniques
- Improving patient outcomes
- Managing the organization

Biomedical engineering has a significant role in managing risks associated with patient outcomes. Patient outcomes are the *raison d'être* for hospitals and other clinical settings. Engineers of all disciplines utilize risk management methods to solve problems, make decisions, and control risks. Biomedical engineers, through a combination of education, training, and experience, are well poised to be significant leaders of risk management activities in the clinical setting.

Throughout this chapter, the term *hospitals* will be used to describe all manner of clinical settings. Medical devices are key to the appropriate delivery of many forms of health care in the modern hospital. Related to medical devices, hospitals have multifaceted roles, including, but not limited to, developing, manufacturing (or remanufacturing), installing, calibrating, and maintaining these systems. Additionally, hospitals have networked medical devices into various systems. These networks may collect data from devices, control device operations, or a combination of these.

The third approach for this exploration of risk management is the body of knowledge related to enterprise risk management (ERM). ERM is a function of organizational leadership and is likely to impact biomedical engineering when these activities are rolled out at the hospital site. This chapter explores the current state of the art for ERM, methods for ERM, and how to appropriately integrate ERM with other risk management approaches.

This chapter also discusses various methods, tools, and techniques in the toolbox of the risk management practitioner. This chapter does not serve as a primer in the detailed implementation of the tools. Technical literature is replete with instructions and examples on these various tools, and the references used in this chapter contain additional information regarding the tools and techniques. Good risk management practice entails an understanding of what tools are generally available, and using the correct tool for the right job. Various considerations for these concepts have also been included in this chapter.

To conclude this brief introduction, risk management is an important field of study. A basic understanding of risk management will be beneficial for biomedical engineers in the hospital of the future. As a part of a multifunctional team in the hospital setting, biomedical engineers are key team members for achieving organization objectives and ensuring the safety and health of patients.

24.2 MODEL FOR THE RISK MANAGEMENT PROCESS—MEDICAL DEVICES

In order to understand the appropriate application of risk management in healthcare settings, it is important to understand the basic principles underlying risk management science. These principles are applied throughout a broad spectrum of industrial sectors from the space industry to the financial industry to the foods industry. Each of these sectors favour the use of certain tools for identifying hazards and analyzing risks. Common to all these sectors is the need for a thorough understanding of what we mean by hazard and risk and what systems must absolutely be in place if risks are to be effectively managed. First let us consider the development of risk management science.

The development of the risk management concepts and science we understand today has had a long history of at least 400 years. During the seventeenth and early eighteenth centuries, numerous renowned scientists including Galileo, Pascal, and Bernoulli were instrumental in developing these concepts, which, at the time, were revolutionary.

The following individuals were noteworthy in that time period:

- Galileo—probability theory
- Blaise Pascal—probability theory and risk acceptability
- Pierre de Fermat—probability theory
- John Graunt—mortality statistics
- Edmund Halley—mortality tables
- Edward Lloyd—shipping information
- Daniel Bernoulli—acceptability

The concept of chance and the mathematical description of the most likely outcome of an event was the subject of some of Galileo's research, work that was further extended by Pascal. Graunt studied the mortality tables of the city of London and interpreted those tables and related mortality to age. Halley, apparently building on this work, applied the results to the issuing of annuities based on an applicant's age. Lloyd provided the very important service of providing weather and storm data to shipping captains from his seaside coffee house. Pascal and Bernoulli introduced the signally important concept of risk acceptability and how it depended on the individual or organization accepting that risk. Bernoulli and Pascal discussed the relationship between the actual risk and a subject's willingness to accept that risk.

Modern risk management science has evolved as a result of the work of these early scientists and mathematicians. Risk management is now recognized to be, first and foremost, a management activity.

The medical device industry is unique as an industrial sector due to the fact that there is one international standard (IS) for the management of risks related to device safety and health that has been recognized around the world. This standard is ISO/IEC 14971, *Medical Devices—Application of Risk Management to Medical Devices*.[5] The final vote for this international standard was unanimous by all participating countries around the world, including the United States, Canada, Europe, China, and Japan. The IS has been used to fulfill a wide range of regulatory (US FDA recognized standard) and legal (national law in Japan) needs throughout the world. The standard has also been referenced by other industrial sectors such as the pharmaceutical industry, as noted in the International Conference for Harmonization Standard Q9, *Quality Risk Management*.[6] ISO/IEC 14971 was first published in 2000 and is a life-cycle standard that describes a holistic approach to managing related safety and health risks in the organization.

The concept of hazard is the starting point for any understanding of risk. In the world standard for medical devices, ISO/IEC 14971,[7] a *hazard* is defined as a "potential source of harm." *Harm* is defined in turn as "physical injury or damage to the health of people, or damage to property or the environment." Since this standard is a medical safety standard, those definitions are taken in the narrow context of safety and health, especially the definition for harm. However, we can extrapolate those definitions to encompass harm beyond safety considerations such as failure to achieve expected outcome or loss of something of value. Later in the chapter, we will explore the use of enterprise risk management (ERM) in the healthcare industry.

It is important to emphasize that a hazard simply exists as a condition, which could produce harm under certain circumstances. How likely are those circumstances to exist and how serious might the resultant harm be? That brings up the concept of risk as the next fundamental concept that must be clear. Once again, according to ISO/IEC 14971, *risk* is defined as a "combination of the probability of occurrence of harm and the severity of that harm."[8] It is imperative that these concepts be clearly separated since it is risk that we seek to manage so that a hazard which is identified does not lead to a harm that cannot be tolerated. Note that there is no detection term in the definition of risk; *detection* is a function of the probability of occurrence of harm. *Detection* is the difference between the inherent failure probability of a component, accessory, therapy, or medical device and the probability of harm being inflicted. *Severity* is the extent of the harm anticipated and may range, for example, from minor to moderate to catastrophic.

The IS is a good example of the key elements of a successful risk management process. As biomedical engineers work closely with medical device suppliers in the normal course of their duties, a good understanding of medical device risk management theory will be of practicable utility.

Management responsibility is identified as the initial—and the key—requirement for successful management of risks. The senior management of any organization or project must

- Establish a risk management process, which includes defined elements
- Establish a policy that identifies acceptable risk levels
- Provide adequate resources for the risk management team
- Provide appropriate personnel to carry out the process
- Review the process on a regular basis

Establishing the policy by which risk acceptability will be set is a key responsibility of top management. Managing risks simply cannot occur if the policy for setting the criteria for accepting risk within the organization is not established and well understood throughout the organization. As Bernoulli correctly observed, the level of risk that an individual is prepared to accept varies from person to person. So too that level of risk acceptance varies from project to project and from organization to organization. This is key because it is the basis for determining which risks are acceptable and which are not, and, therefore, which will need to be addressed and which need not be addressed.

The IS describes four principle activities in conducting the risk management process:

1. Risk analysis
2. Risk evaluation
3. Risk control
4. Production and postproduction information

Risk analysis is often used to mean risk management, but the two terms are not interchangeable. *Risk analysis* is usually limited to identification and characterization of risks while *risk management* is considered to be the whole life-cycle endeavour, including management involvement, defining risk acceptability, and closing the loop. Thus, risk analysis is only one element, albeit a significant element, in the comprehensive process of managing risks.

The risk management process that must be defined has to include the following elements:

- Risk analysis, which involves gathering information about the types of hazards that exist, the likelihood that those hazards will result in harm, and the severity of that harm to make an estimate of the risk to the project, organization, or clinical setting.
- Risk evaluation, which involves comparing that risk to a predetermined level of acceptability for that organization or project or clinical setting.
- Risk control, which involves mitigation of those risks which are deemed to be not acceptable based on the predetermined acceptability criteria.
- Ongoing monitoring of the effectiveness and continuing suitability of the risk management process.

Step 4 above refers to production and postproduction information. This step ensures that the life-cycle concept is executed in the risk management process in a manufacturing environment. Information is gathered during the manufacturing phase and subsequent phases and is fed back into the risk management process to close the loop. Information may be in many forms, for example, new failure modes, product complaints, reliability data, and service data. This information may be compared to the predicted information during product design and fed back into the risk assessment process to determine if the risk continues to be considered acceptable or additional risk control measures are necessary. In the clinical environment, while there is no production phase, the concept of life cycle is similarly appropriate. After the RM team has made and implemented the clinical risk controls, the RM team, with management oversight, then monitors the effectivity of the risk controls. This information is fed back into the risk management process as appropriate, thereby closing the life-cycle loop.

The need for top management to provide adequate resources includes both financial and human resources. Ensuring that the knowledge and experience of personnel involved in risk management are appropriate is a critical success factor.

Finally, it is imperative that top management consistently reviews the results and the effectiveness of the risk management system. Are the resources available adequate? Has the risk acceptability policy been properly applied throughout the organization? Has the risk management process been properly implemented? Have all steps of the process been carried out? Does there need to be changes in the risk management process? These are the types of questions that need to be addressed in reviewing the implementation of a full risk management system. It is that overview of the risk management system by top management that ensures effective management of the risks in a healthcare organization.

The medical device ISO standard for risk management was used as a model for risk management activities in the clinical environment.[9] It is a good model for demonstrating the core concepts of risk management theory from an industrial sector closely related to biomedical engineering.

24.3 TOOLS AND TECHNIQUES

There are many tools and techniques that are utilized to perform formal risk management activities. These formal risk management methods are universal in application and may be adapted to a wide variety of risk management problems. The following is a nonexhaustive overview of methods used in the field:

- FMEA—Failure mode and effects analysis is the most common method used, but is actually a spectrum of methods, as there are so many variations in the literature. FMEA is often referred to as a *bottom-up* methodology as the approach is to analyze the elements of a process individually to determine the local effects for a given failure mode. Then the individual effects, or local effects, are considered for impact on the overall process (system effects). A single failure mode becomes a line item of the FMEA. The FMEA is compiled and often becomes a multipage detailed analysis of the system.
- FMECA—Failure mode and effects criticality analysis is an explicit descriptive term where the criticality of the failure mode is determined. Criticality is usually determined by analyzing severity and/or probability of occurrence. The two terms of FMEA and FMECA are often used by practitioners interchangeably.
- Event tree analysis (ETA)—Another spectrum of methods, the ETA typically starts with an initiating event and then describes the consequences or the subsequent steps. Branches on the tree demonstrate alternatives. Event trees are typically displayed graphically and range from simplistic to quite complex. Event trees are of utility in risk communication and are a good method to demonstrate various options in decision-making. The risk management practitioner may use this method to communicate to management, patients, and other staff members of the organization.
- FTA—Fault tree analysis can be viewed as a specialized type of event tree where faults or failures are the focus of the analysis. Fault trees are often termed as *top-down* analyses because the team often starts with the end result or the outcome and then documents various alternatives to achieve (or avoid in the case of a safety issue) the end result. If probabilities are known, mathematical projections may be made to obtain rigorous probabilities of the system faults.

- HACCP—Hazard analysis and critical control points is a method that has been embraced by various regulatory agencies (e.g., Center for Food Sanitation, U.S. FDA). In HACCP, a hazard analysis is performed and significant risks are determined. Critical control points are applied to the process to ensure that the significant risks are adequately controlled.
- HAZOP—Hazard and operability studies is a technique used in the chemical and nuclear industry. Deviations from the intended process are systematically determined, hazards are identified, and controls are established. The controls are reduced to procedures, and the procedures are readily accessible to operators. When the operators are confronted with a deviation, the operator refers to the procedure and follows the appropriate instructions to return the process to a state of control.
- Analysis of safety functions—There are many methods and techniques available to the practitioner to describe, analyze, and control the safety characteristics of a system. Typically, the team starts with comprehensively documenting the existing safety functions of the system. Depending on the type of system and the focus of the team, various specific methods are available to assess the adequacy of the system versus the team objectives. For example, a general strategy would be to perform a safety function survey to assess the overall safety of the system as a team exercise. Such a survey may be as simple as a listing of the safety functions and a brainstorming session to consider additional safety functions. As a result of the survey, a safety barrier analysis may be performed to understand the adequacy of the safety barriers. The safety barrier analysis may lead the team to perform an energy analysis, which may be used to trace the electrical energy applied to and used by a system.
- Human factors analyses—Human factors analyses, in recent years, has been the subject of significant scientific inquiry in the field of medical risk management. The study of human factors is a multidisciplinary field of science with a rapidly expanding body of literature. Analyzing the tasks that personnel perform in operating equipment is one of many techniques used by human factors professionals.

This brief overview should provide the biomedical engineer with an appreciation for the diverse and powerful tools and techniques available to the risk management team. Many of the tools do not require specialized knowledge to derive benefit. While one tool may be emphasized at a site over the others, no single tool should be used to the exclusion of others. Indeed, proper use of multiple tools is likely to lead to better risk management results over time. Experienced risk management practitioners will be familiar with the multiple tools. The practitioner should support the team with recommendations for specific tools and techniques to solve problems and meet team objectives.

24.4 RISK MANAGEMENT FOR IMPROVING PATIENT OUTCOMES

Risk management for safety and health is a powerful tool in the process of improving patient outcomes in the clinical environment. A multifunctional representative team utilizing formal analytical methods within a life-cycle risk management framework is a powerful tool for a hospital department to identify, control, and monitor risks associated with health and safety.

Various organizations have embraced the concept of clinical risk management. The Joint Commission requires hospitals to manage risks such as risks of infection, reduce the risk of harm from patient falls, identify patients at risk for suicide, and identify safety risks to the patient population.[10] For some hospitals, Joint Commission requirements precipitated the initial experiences with performing formal risk assessments. Another example of an organization embracing risk management is the Center for Patient Safety of the Veterans Administration. This group has developed the Healthcare FMEA™.[11]

For risk management of safety and health, *risk* may be defined as the combination of severity and frequency. *Safety* may be defined as the freedom from harm. Hazards are sources of harm.

There are several key elements necessary to ensure the effectiveness of a clinical risk management process: management support, clear objectives, appropriate technical representation, an effective risk management process, appropriate use of risk management analytical tools, monitoring for effectiveness, and life-cycle approach.

Effective clinical risk management for health and safety should be predicated on the use of good scientific methods. Objectivity in evaluating the issues is essential. Even though the application of good scientific methodologies is often considered simplistic compared to more advanced methods of risk management, it is extremely important to utilize good science. The risk management team should utilize the following techniques as appropriate: hypothesis testing, calibration, quantitative data (where available), positive and negative controls, validation of results, duplication of results, and use of statistics, including hypothesis testing, ANOVA (analysis of variance), DOEs (design of experiments), and SPC (statistical process control).

There are many risk management tools available to the biomedical engineer today. Some of the more common tools include: hazard analysis, FTA (fault tree analysis), HAZOP (hazard and operability studies), HACCP (hazard analysis and critical control points), RCA (root cause analysis), and FMEA (failure modes and effects analysis). FMEAs are ubiquitous today and are considered to be a fundamental analytical tool for various disciplines.

Due to the plethora of FMEA models in the public domain, there are many variations on the basic theme of FMEA. For example, FMECA is failure modes and effects criticality analysis. Most FMEAs look at failures as the combination of a severity measure, a frequency measure, and a detection measure. By estimating each measure, failures (risks) may be ranked and evaluated against defined acceptability criteria. Risks that require mitigation are controlled and reranked after controls to determine if the improvement in risk is appropriate.

It is beyond the intent of this chapter to delve into the subtle nuances of FMEAs in the clinical environment. There is extensive literature on this in the public domain (much of it readily available with simple searches on the Internet). The casual searching reader is often struck by the fact that there are many different FMEA methodologies in use. FMEAs are a spectrum of techniques, not a single method.

The following are practical considerations related to FMEAs and similar analyses:

- Pick the right tool for the job. For example, don't use a complex procedure for a simple analysis.
- Consider the scales that will be used for severity, frequency, and detection before starting the analysis. For example, a 10 × 10 × 10 scale needs a lot of data to support the difference between values (such as between 5 and 6, for example). Whereas a 5 × 5 × 5 or a 3 × 3 × 3 needs much less data to discriminate between the levels.
- Establish the weighting of the scales chosen. Does severity have more weight than probability or does it depend on the hazard under consideration?
- Understand the criteria for when failure modes will be controlled. This is commonly referred to as the *risk acceptance criteria*. Understand how differences in severity, frequency, or detection may affect, whether a failure is controlled or not. Review the risk acceptance criteria with the team, review boundary conditions and various permutations, and ensure that there is a good consensus that the criteria are adequate and defendable. Be careful about copying another organization's risk acceptance criteria. Is the rationale for that risk acceptance criteria available and is it appropriate?
- Detection may be considered to be a modifier of frequency. If this is acceptable to the team, then failure modes may be assessed as a combination of severity and frequency only. This makes the process even simpler for the team and makes the risk acceptance criteria more transparent for all.
- Software may be managed with only one scale—severity. This is because frequency goes to 100 percent whenever the conditions are recreated, so the only decision to make is how severe is the failure mode. In safety and health risk management, the single most important component of risk is the severity of the failure. Severity should be the focus on much activity of the team.
- FMEAs are good tools for iteration. Only those issues that have changed need to be managed in the subsequent iteration (unless risk acceptance has been redefined).
- Use caution addressing financial considerations or availability of treatment in safety and health risk management activities. It is especially sensitive not to use cost as a determinant to whether patients receive care or the type of care that they receive at the clinical level. Analyses of cost versus patient care are typically the domain of healthcare policy institutions such as governmental

agencies (e.g., Centers for Medicare and Medicaid) and academia. Failure mode controls should be practical and reasonable. Science can predict how decisions will affect the future, but science cannot make the policy decision, only people can. This is why it is vitally important to have all stakeholders represented on the team; the voice of the customer should be strong for risk management to be effective.

- Annotate decisions such that they can be justified at a future date if necessary.
- Where data are used to make estimates, annotate the source of the data and the values considered.
- Develop a process for handling differences of opinion.
- Accumulate data. The power of a risk management process lies in its iterative nature. Make sure the process captures subsequent data.

Many of these considerations are valid for other risk management analytical tools such as fault trees. If the use of a tool or process does not lead the user to a better understanding of risk management clinical issues, then the tool is of minimal utility. Tools should be adapted to meet the needs of the organization and should be well understood by the assessment team members and the management team of the organization.

While effective risk management is often conducted with simple tools, there is a place for sophisticated analyses such as computer simulations and modeling. However, the sophistication should be in the simulation, not in the evaluation of the acceptability of risk. People make risk acceptance determinations. The tolerance for accepting a particular risk may be modified by the risk culture of the organization, the experience of the department and the individuals performing the assessment, state of the science, alternative therapies, and the incremental benefit of the studied therapy versus no therapy.

A chapter on risk management would not be complete without discussing potential problems that may be encountered in implementing and executing an effective clinical risk management process. Potential problems include, but are not limited to, the following: failure to involve representatives from all stakeholders, failure to use the appropriate analytical tool, lack of focus, inadequate information, inadequate documentation, incorrect risk acceptance criteria, failure to monitor risk control measures, and failure to use a life-cycle approach. It is the responsibility of top management to ensure that these issues are addressed.

After risk controls have been implemented, and the residual risks are deemed to be acceptable, risk communication should be considered. Are there stakeholders who should receive the results of the risk mitigation? Affected stakeholders may include top management, patients, relatives, the legal department, employees, vendors, practitioners, and regulators. The results of the risk management should be communicated in a manner that facilitates clear communication with each group of stakeholders.

The diagram shown in Fig. 24.1 is similar to the risk management process for medical device manufacturers.[7] Note that there are two additional boxes in the diagram labeled "evaluation of overall residual risk acceptability" and "risk management report." These two boxes are reminders for medical device manufacturers that it is necessary to consider the totality of accumulated residual risks before the device is ready to move to production and that a report is necessary to ensure that the risk management activities have been appropriately documented. Another key element of the diagram is that the whole process is a loop and not a single pass.

The iterative nature of risk management has been discussed throughout this chapter. The life-cycle concept is a key element in successful risk management. There are several reasons for this. Information improves over time, and an ongoing evaluation of the information is necessary to determine if further risk control may be necessary. Once a device is on the market, risk control activities may include field repairs, additional risk communications to users or patients, software upgrades, field corrections, or recalls. In clinical risk management, as procedures are implemented, risks will be modified and the risk profile will change (including the possibility that new risks may be introduced).

When a new device is developed or an existing line of devices is extended, the manufacturer will typically review the risk management file on the predicate devices and consider the risk management history of similar devices. Much information related to product safety is available through public

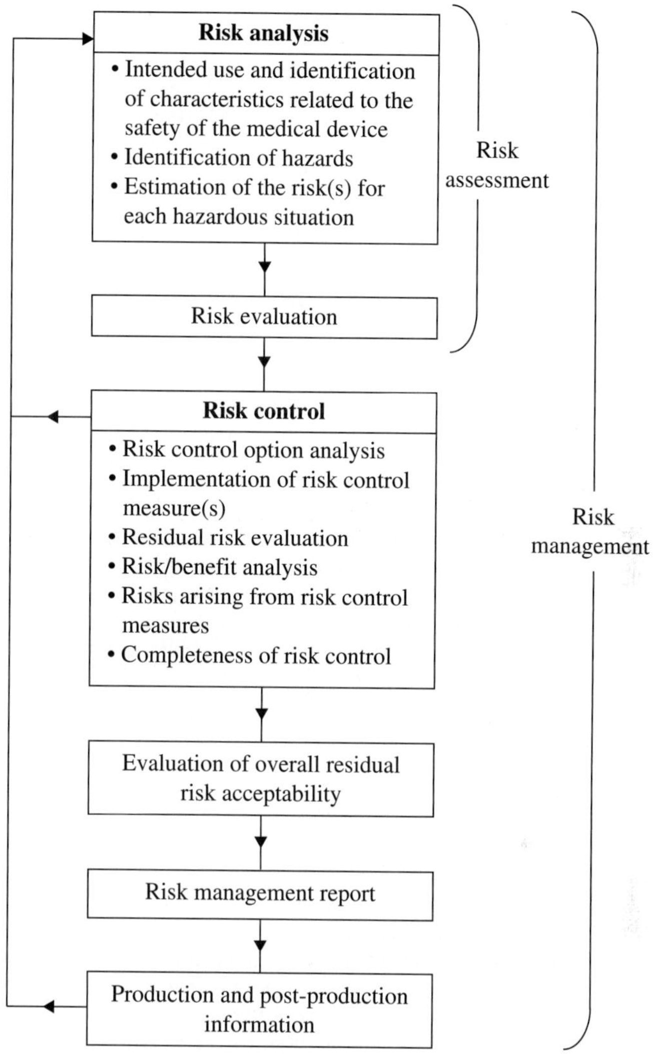

FIGURE 24.1 A schematic representation of the risk management process.

sources, especially the Internet. Literature searches can illuminate device development and provide significant insights to the medical device manufacturer about competitive devices. Similarly, in clinical risk management, consider the impact of risk controls under consideration based on previous experiences of your organization, and other organizations based on literature reviews.

It is important that risk management becomes a part of the routine activity of personnel. Risk management should be part of the organizational culture. Gateways to the risk management process should exist in routine documentation of the department so that risk considerations are made when other departmental decisions are made. For example, the change control form for departmental procedures may have questions pertaining to whether the change in consideration has patient (or user) safety and health considerations. If so, then attach the risk assessment to the change form for management review.

Another example would be a risk assessment of new technology that is implemented in the clinical setting. Does the new technology improve patient safety? Are there key safety features in the technology being replaced that are under revision in the new technology and requiring special training of user personnel to make the transition? Is the acclimation process and transition time for the new technology appropriate to the significance (to safety and health) of the change? Are adequate support services in place to make a smooth transition to the new technology? Is calibration equipment available for the new technology?

Technology transition is not a new topic to biomedical engineering per se. The point is that individual risk management activities should be comprehensive, iterative, and integrated processes that are tuned to the day-to-day operations of the department.

A new area of regulatory interest is evolving related to computer networking of medical devices. The FDA has issued draft regulations related to computer networking of medical devices in the clinical setting.[12] These networks will likely be considered as medical devices and the developers of these networks will be considered medical device manufacturers. While the definitions and specifics may vary from country to country, a common set of processes will likely develop related to the integration of medical devices into networks. New standards are in development to define the integration process in the clinical setting; these standards will be the IEC 80000 series. In the interim, investigations may be conducted by the FDA in the event there is a perceived risk to public health caused by these systems.

One of the new concepts under discussion by the Joint Working Group 7 working on the IEC 80000 series is the creation of an IT network risk manager role.[13] This risk manager role would be responsible for the overall risk to safety and health of the computer network. This role is not necessarily the responsibility of a single individual, but may be a committee composed of various personnel from associated functional areas. The risk manager role would include responsibility for change control management of an existing system as well as approval of a new computer system. Another role under consideration is the systems integrator who is functionally the project manager for a specific implementation. This role may be internal or external to the clinical organization.

24.5 RISK MANAGEMENT FOR MANAGING THE ENTERPRISE

In many institutions, the risk management department is an extension of the legal department. Typically, these departments are tasked with limiting liability. These departments may or may not utilize formal risk management analytical methods. When risk management methods are utilized to meet the needs of the organization, these are considered to be enterprise risk management (ERM). Enterprise risk management considers risk as the probability of meeting objectives.[14] Obviously, these are the objectives of the enterprise.

Enterprise is a neutral term that describes a complete range of human endeavours. An enterprise may be anything from a single individual or two people to a large multinational corporation. ERM provides tools and methods useful for making both tactical and strategic decisions. ERM may be employed at all levels of the organization: department, group, division, and corporate. ERM may be used to control a single issue, to address a spectrum of risks, or to provide the foundation for a comprehensive management process such as for a board of directors of a large organization.

As opposed to risk management for safety and health, *risk* may be defined in the ERM arena as the probability of meeting objectives. Risk may be positive or negative. Positive risk may be thought of as an opportunity. For ERM, risk management may be considered to be the pursuit of positive risk and the avoidance of negative risk. Both types of risks may be used to develop tactical and strategic plans for the enterprise.

Normal considerations for ERM include costs, availability of goods and services, crisis management and avoidance, external and internal threats, risk appetite, financial controls, and public stewardship. Even though ERM appears on the surface to be different from risk management of medical products or clinical outcomes, the processes and tools are identical.

Key risk management concepts are just as appropriate here as in the safety and health arena: risk communication, risk acceptability criteria, multidisciplinary team, involvement of top management, appropriate use of tools, objective assessment of data, scientific approach, good documentation, and iterative process. Tools such as FMEAs, statistical analyses, and FTAs, are easily and appropriately utilized in the ERM environment.

In clinical settings, biomedical engineers are well positioned to assist the organization in the performance of ERM assessments. ERM assessments can be conducted as separate and discrete projects or as an ongoing, evolving, and overarching set of management procedures and processes. Biomedical engineers often act as the interface between administration and clinical employees, so they are well suited to facilitate risk management and maintain these same communication pathways.

It should be stressed that ERM goals may be very different from clinical outcome goals and that it is very difficult to perform both of these analyses concurrently without some loss of focus on the particular objectives of each of the activities. It is best to treat these as separate ventures with different goals and objectives. The risk controls arising from clinical risk management may be considered as input into the ERM process. Thus, if a safety risk control entails the purchase of a piece of equipment costing $100,000 (for example); the clinical risk control recommendation may enter into the ERM process and be subsequently addressed. Note that the ERM process input takes the output from the safety and health process (the risk control recommendation).

As stated earlier, it is not good risk management practice to mix the enterprise risk considerations into the safety and health risk management decision-making at the team level and to try to accomplish all decisions in a single step. Risk management activities should utilize the appropriate personnel, including considerations such as the role in the organization and the technical specialties needed to make the decision. Where capital costs may be significant and exceed defined thresholds (e.g., exceed department approval levels), it is appropriate to take the safety and health risk control recommendations to a divisional or corporate team utilizing an ERM approach to the issue. The ERM team considering a safety-related capital request will often use the organization's vision, values, mission, objectives, key goals, and strategic plan to facilitate decision-making related to the capital request. It is clear that the ERM team is likely to be a different group of specialists within most organizations and with different roles than the safety team (although some individuals may likely serve on both teams and act as liaisons).

One key consideration of the management team is how to document ERM decisions. Legal department members in the team will likely weigh in on how to document these issues, including the level of detail to support the team and the enterprise. Well-documented, good decisions, with good rationales protect the enterprise and provide a platform for good future decisions and good tactical and strategic planning. Mistakes also provide a basis for good future decision-making. Inadequate documentation does not support planning, decision-making, or organizational management of knowledge. *Organizational memory*[16] (OM) is the concept that there is a body of knowledge which is utilized by members of the organization to meet its objectives. This memory is both organic (and subject to rapid change during employee turnover or retirements) and inorganic (such as policies and procedures). Often the OM is a small subset of the total body of knowledge available. OM includes the concepts of formal and informal processes and considers the roles of technical process owners, where key information is stored, and who makes what decisions at different levels of the organization. After surveying the OM, revision or addition of management controls may occur to convert organic and inorganic OM and to institutionalize good, yet informal, practices.

There is an ISO standard under development in 2008 that establishes an ERM process for use by all organizations, that is, ISO 31000.[17] The current committee draft of this standard provides significant insight for individuals with an interest in ERM.

24.6 CONCLUSION

Risk management has been regarded as one of the defining elements of modern society.[17] The box of tools available to personnel performing risk assessments is growing as new techniques are developed. Tools are multifunctional and general in nature, and the user(s) is left with the responsibility to ensure the tools used are appropriate to the application.

Risk management is not a fully mature applied science. There remains considerable *art* in the science as the body of knowledge continues to mature and expand. As such, there are many experts advertizing risk management services.

Risk management principles have universal application. Tools are readily portable and adaptable. There are more experienced practitioners available now than ever, but may be parochial with respect to tools, techniques, and subject matter applications.

Good risk management personnel have special skills: can communicate with top management as well as personnel at all levels of the organization, have a wide range of risk management experience, utilize a scientific approach, and have a panoramic view of the risk management field. As stated above, biomedical engineering specialists have the unique combination of education, skills, and experience to fulfill these roles in the modern clinical organization. These uniquely qualified individuals will move our institutions successfully into the twenty-first century.

REFERENCES

1. Peter Bernstein, *Against the Gods: The Remarkable Story of Risk*, John Wiley & Sons, 1996.
2. Risk, In *Merriam-Webster Online Dictionary*. Retrieved June 12, 2008, from http://www.merriam-webster.com/dictionary/risk.
3. AU/NZS 4360:1999, *Australian Standard on Risk Management*, Standards Australia, 1999.
4. ISO/IEC Guide 51:1999, *Safety Aspects—Guideline for the Inclusion in Standards*, 1999.
5. ISO 14971:2007, *Medical Devices—Application of Risk Management to Medical Devices* [reference number ISO 14971:2007 (E)].
6. ICH Q9 *Quality Risk Management*, International Conference for Harmonization, 2005. Retrieved on June 12, 2008 from http://www.ich.org/cache/compo/276-254-1.html.
7. ISO 14971:2007, *Medical Devices—Application of Risk Management to Medical Devices* [reference number ISO 14971:2007 (E)].
8. *Ibid.*
9. *Ibid.*
10. *2008 National Patient Safety Goals, Hospital Program*. Retrieved June 12, 2008, from http://www.jointcommission.org/PatientSafety/NationalPatientSafetyGoals/08_hap_npsgs.htm.
11. *Basics for Healthcare Failure Mode and Effects Analysis*, VA National Center for Patient Safety. Retrieved June 12, 2008, from http://www.va.gov/ncps/SafetyTopics/HFMEA/HFMEAIntro.doc.
12. FR Doc E8-2325, Federal Register, February 28, 2008, *Devices: General Hospital and Personal Use Devices; Reclassification of Medical Device Data System, Proposed Rule.*
13. IEC 80001 Committee Draft, *Application of Risk Management for IT-Networks Incorporating Medical Devices*, International Electrotechnical Commission, 2007.
14. AU/NZS 4360:1999, *Australian Standard on Risk Management*, Standards Australia, 1999.
15. Stan Mastrangelo, *Proceedings from Congress on Global Approaches to Risk Management, Current and Future Developments*, Enterprise Risk Management for Healthcare Industries—A Panoramic View, Virginia Tech, 2006.
16. ISO 31000 Committee Draft, *Risk Management—Guidelines on Principles and Implementation of Risk Management,* International Standards Organization, 2007.
17. Stan Mastrangelo, *Proceedings of Second Congress on Global Approaches to Risk Management,* Through Product Life Cycles, Challenges of Integrating Risk Management into the Pharmaceutical Industry, Virginia Tech, 2007.

CHAPTER 25
TECHNOLOGY PLANNING FOR HEALTH-CARE INSTITUTIONS

John M. Smith
Consultant, Gormley, Canada

Daniela Crivianu-Gaita
The Hospital for Sick Children, Toronto, Canada

25.1 PRELUDE

While the basic principles and processes of technology planning remain intact, during the past 5 years advances in technology, as defined in the context of this chapter, have made it necessary to reexamine how those processes can continue to be effectively applied. During this time, technology has changed both in the enhanced capabilities, broader application of existing technologies and the introduction of new technologies. This comes together with the increasing costs of delivering health care that in turn places a greater emphasis on the need for the critical analysis, assessment, and evaluation of technologies in a framework that ultimately must focus on efficacy and cost effectiveness for improving patient outcomes and quality of life.

As decisions among health technologies become more difficult, there is an increasing reliance on health technology assessments to inform these decisions. Such assessments typically examine the efficacy of technologies and their contribution to improved clinical decision making and patient outcomes. Because of the effort involved, such assessments are usually conducted by national or provincial jurisdictions in support of associated health policy. They also provide an important input to the technology-planning process. Of particular importance is the assessment of technologies applied to population screening, where inappropriate application can significantly increase costs.

Of particular note is the tighter relationship and the expansion of common ground between the domains of medical devices and information technology. Both domains have traditionally had distinct custodians, introducing territorial prerogatives that distract attention from the bigger picture. From a technology planning perspective, it is appropriate to address the technology continuum, bringing together rational expertise from both domains into a coherent planning framework. This means breaking down barriers and reaching beyond traditional boundaries. For example, basic devices and systems such as patient monitors and infusion pumps have now become part of the information technology infrastructure, and planning for such systems can no longer take place in isolation.

Integrated planning must be supported by the interoperability of devices and systems from different manufacturers. Thus, the development and compliance with interoperability standards is becoming an essential tool upon which planning assumptions are based. Further, this must be balanced with the availability of integrated applications from a single vendor, where proprietary internal standards will usually apply.

Technology planning is a process that cannot be encapsulated in a set of deterministic rules and procedures; rather, it is a process that involves the intelligent and informed application of information from many sources adapted to a particular environment. This chapter attempts to provide stimulation and guidance for clinical engineers who decide to embark on this journey.

25.2 INTRODUCTION

In health care, in common with many industries, the application of technology to advance business objectives is essential in order to remain competitive. It is clear that technology can enable, and even facilitate, the creation of business objectives; however, unless the business objectives are themselves sound, successful outcomes cannot be guaranteed. Thus, the concept that technology alone is sufficient to sustain a business model has serious flaws. This serves to emphasize the importance of technology planning as an integrated component of developing and implementing business strategies.[1]

The same principles apply to health care, which, by its nature, is very much a social industry catering to the needs of people in times of ill health and the stresses this condition brings. Health care has many facets, many of which deal with the need for emotional support, allaying the fears and anxieties that are associated with modern treatments and therapies. Technology often exacerbates these fears, presenting a harsh and unfriendly environment, while at the same time providing diagnostic information or enabling the administration of therapies that can dramatically change the course of disease processes. The affordability of technology is a significant factor in its application, and this will vary from country to country[2] and even among jurisdictions within countries. In fact, technology drivers may themselves cause dramatic changes in the way health-care facilities are structured and organized.[3]

Health-care technology in its broadest sense includes drugs, therapies, surgical procedures, interventions, as well as devices and systems. As such, health-care technology is the domain of a large number of practitioners, including physicians, surgeons, radiologists, pharmacists, laboratory scientists, nurses, and therapists. Clinical engineers have primary expertise in the subset of technology that centers on instrumentation, devices, and systems, and in this context, they are usually separated from the patient by an intervening practitioner or caregiver who uses the applicable technology to deliver a treatment or to perform a diagnosis. It is with this model in mind that the concepts and ideas in this chapter have been developed.

Successful technology planning in health care on the part of clinical engineers requires definition of the technology domain, a clear understanding of health-care processes and technology stakeholders, and how such technologies can enable and enhance these processes and the activities of stakeholders. It also requires establishing working relationships with key technology stakeholders such as those with specific expertise and training in technology management, medical physics, information technology, and technology utilization. It is facility with the processes associated with technology planning that is equally, if not more, important than knowledge and expertise relating to the inner workings of technology. The position that clinical engineers are able to take will determine whether they are drivers of the planning process, or participants along with the many other stakeholders.

25.3 STRATEGIC PLANNING

In recent times, the proliferation of medical technology and its associated costs has placed health-care institutions in a position where choices are necessary. This is in contrast to earlier times when the availability of technology was such that choices were limited to essential technologies, and decisions were much easier to make. Today, it is necessary to have a framework in which technology decisions can be made, and this framework is most commonly found as a strategic plan. This is developed in a wider organizational context, defining the broad directions of the organization, the communities that will be served, the type of diseases that will be treated, therapies that will be administered, areas for research focus, and the interactions with external organizations and funding agencies, be they governments, insurance providers, or benevolent organizations. Once these fundamental strategies have been defined, it becomes a lot easier to determine the human resources that will be necessary, the facilities that will be required, the nature of the specific clinical programs, and the technology that will be necessary to support the strategic goals.

Technology planning cannot be performed in isolation, and a logical first step is to study, understand, and participate in the development and maintenance of the strategic plan for the organization. If such a plan exists, actively determine the technology needs that arise from it, and integrate these into a technology plan. If no such plan exists, facilitate the development of such a plan by identifying key technologies and challenge the organization to define how they can facilitate the achievement of its goals.

Examples of strategic plan components which drive technology are many. For instance, a strategic initiative to be a regional cardiac center[4] has immediate technology implications. It defines a basic need for a cardiac catheterization facility, recognizing the contemporary shift from diagnostic to interventional procedures. For adults, this means at least single plane angiography, cardiac echo ultrasound, and an ECG and stress system. In a broader context, it might imply the implementation of emerging cardiac modalities such as cardiac MRI, the implementation of information and image archives, communication with related organizations using communication technologies for the real-time transmission of cardiac angiography and ultrasound, and the sharing of common patient records across referring institutions.

As a basic principle, strategy drives technology; however, at the same time it must be recognized that technology can enable strategy. It is therefore essential that technology planning is an integral part of strategic planning. A careful balance can avoid the trap of technology push, wherein technologies are implemented simply because they exist, primarily driven by market forces.

To be successful, clinical engineers must take time to understand the strategic planning processes of the organization, and bring to bear technology planning skills which enhance this process.

25.4 TECHNOLOGY PLANNING PRINCIPLES

Technology planning is a process, of which the assessments of the particular attributes of a technology are only a part. It is clearly distinguishable from technology management, which relates to the acquisition, application, utilization, education, distribution, safety, maintenance, and repair of technologies once they are in place. Technology management is, in fact, a consequence of the technology planning process. An analogy can be found in the facilities planning area, where planners develop master program plans, and the functional plans arising from them. Architects and consulting engineers take these inputs and realize them in the form of physical buildings and infrastructure.

The outputs of the technology management domain serve as valuable feedback into the technology planning process, as they represent the experience associated with the implementation of previous technology plans. Important feedback paths apply to the replacement and sustainability of existing technologies, a clearer understanding of risks, and influences relating to the effectiveness of managing the technologies, which result from the implementation of technology plans. As technology managers, it can be argued that clinical engineers are one of the key stakeholders, as well as key participants, in the technology planning process.[5] The relationship between technology planning and technology management is illustrated in Fig. 25.1.

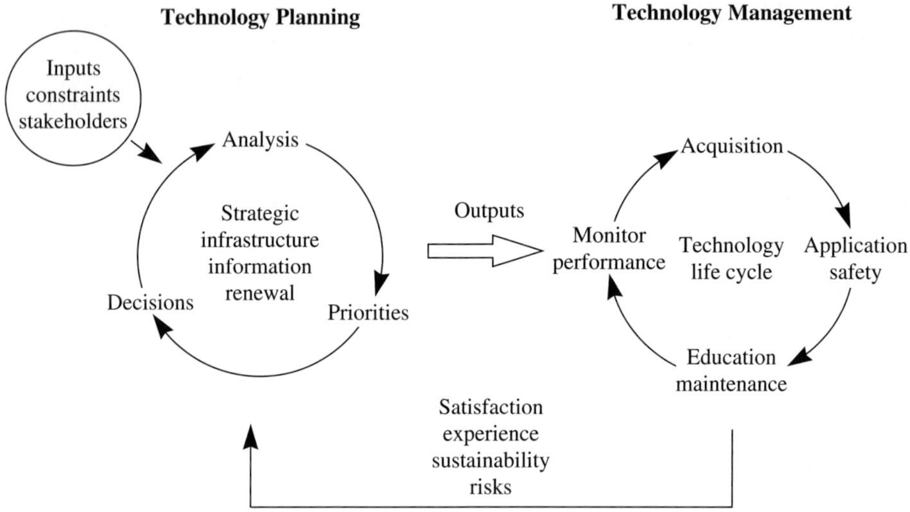

FIGURE 25.1 A schematic representation of the technology planning process and its relationship to technology management.

Acceptance of technology planning as a process allows identification of process components. As with any process, these include inputs, outputs, constraints, stakeholders, and transformation components that are internal to the process, which essentially modify inputs to create outputs. Table 25.1 lists the key components of the technology planning process.

The key outputs of the process are specific requirements for each of four technology categories, strategic technologies, information technologies, technology infrastructure, and renewal of existing technologies, together with priorities and implementation plans that typically involve a project management component. Further details are provided in the following sections.

TABLE 25.1 Key Components of the Technology Planning Process

Inputs	Constraints	Stakeholders	Internal process	Outputs
• Strategic plan • Experience: internal and external • Available technologies • Health technology assessments • Priority assessments[46] • Maturity of technologies • Corporate stability • Standards: internal and external	• Government regulation[47] • Privacy legislation • Financial • Return on investment efficacy • Technology risks • Sustainability of current technologies • Facilities	• Corporate • Providers • Physicians • Nurses • Clinical Engineering • Allied health professionals • Support services	• Analysis • Impact • Setting priorities • Phasing • Assessment of benefits and risks • Satisfaction of input criteria • Satisfaction of stakeholders • Impact on workflow	• Technology plan priorities • Strategic technologies • Information technologies • Technology Infrastructure • Renewal of existing technologies • Implementation • Project management

Strategic technologies are those arising from the initiatives described in the strategic plan. They typically characterize the need for an organization to be leading edge in particular clinical disciplines, thus providing state-of-the-art care. They typically represent a large financial commitment, may involve the renovation or development of facilities, and may address either new opportunities or the renewal, in the context of contemporary technology, of existing strategic equipment and facilities.

Information technologies support strategy, and are essential for the operation of any contemporary organization. Health care is no exception. In fact, the particular complexities of health-care systems, even though they differ from country to country, incorporate a blend of specialized professionals, corporate administration, security and privacy, and funding agencies or insurance providers, each of which present particular challenges for effective information systems.

Technology infrastructure is a term which applies to those technologies which provide a foundation for other technologies, or which are technologies fundamental to contemporary organizations. As technologies move from stand-alone devices to devices which are integrated into systems, the need for infrastructure becomes more important. In the digital world, networked and interoperable systems are no longer luxuries, and at a basic level, a good sustainable network infrastructure is essential. At a higher level, information and communication infrastructures, wherein data can be exchanged among systems are becoming more and more important. As many institutions strategically strive toward an electronic patient record, the ability to receive and present information from disparate sources in a common context is essential. Further, communication systems such as e-mail, voice mail, and voice communications using VoIP (voice over Internet protocol) are components of infrastructure.

Maintenance of existing technologies is often placed at a priority lower than newer technologies until such time as an emergency arises, in which case the problem will be dealt with in the absence of any coordinated planning. Existing technologies typically include devices on which the daily operations of the organization depend, for example, typically include basic surgical tools, patient-monitoring devices, life-support systems, and laboratory instrumentation through to personal computers which are found on every desktop.

According to this model, the deliverable from the technology planning process is a plan that can be executed in the technology management domain. It is here that the details associated with acquisition, installation, acceptance, and ownership responsibilities relating to maintenance, education, safety, and utilization can be appropriately managed. The strategies and processes associated with these activities are beyond the scope of technology planning, and are well known to clinical engineers.

The important message is that technology planning and technology management cannot exist in isolation. There are critical feed forward and feedback links which must be exercised for assurance of success.

Successful execution of the technology planning process requires active executive sponsorship. Typically, this should exist at the vice presidential level in an organization, for example, the chief technology officer (CTO), common in many organizations. The CTO should be the champion for all technologies, including both medical devices and information technologies. Separation of these two components in contemporary environments will lead to inappropriate emphasis upon one or the other. Notwithstanding the above, executive sponsorship must be an intelligent interface between technology push and the true strategic needs of the organization. Failure of this interface can result in significant failures, and examples of significance are documented in the literature.[8]

In the technology planning context, it is clear that the environment will not adapt to clinical engineers; therefore, clinical engineers must adapt to the environment, an adaptation that is a matter of challenge and choice.

25.5 THE FOUR CATEGORIES OF TECHNOLOGY PLANNING

As described earlier, technology requirements can be subdivided into four primary categories. Each of these will be dealt with in turn. The extent to which these apply will vary according to the environment. For example, the strategic requirements of a large academic organization will be quite different from those of a community-based health-care organization.

A key planning concept is to balance strategic needs, information systems requirements, infrastructure needs, and technology renewal needs, within a sustainable funding framework. Consideration should be given to the allocation of separate funding categories for each of the components. For example, individual budget line items for each of strategic projects, information technologie's, technology infrastructure, and maintenance of existing technologies will avoid the common problem of higher-cost technologies financially overwhelming the maintenance of existing technologies to the extent that the latter are deferred or indefinitely postponed. Where overlap occurs, decisions regarding particular budget allocations will be required, which is an example for the need of a single executive champion.

25.5.1 Strategic Technologies

Strategic technologies in the domain of devices and systems typically have the following characteristics:

- A consequence of the organization strategic plan
- Necessary to achieve the strategic goals of the organization
- Frequently in the early stage of maturity and dissemination
- Require a significant investment in either facilities, equipment, or both
- Require long-term planning cycles
- Subject to some risk

Examples of strategic technologies are provided in Table 25.2. Rather than representing the interests of particular constituencies, they should represent the strategies of the organization.

It is important to note that each of these areas has its own set of stakeholders and specialists whose domain of expertise can individually address each in significant detail. It is unreasonable to expect clinical engineers to have both a broad and in-depth knowledge with respect to all strategic initiatives, and to many, this may at first glance appear to be a significant weakness. However, the strength that clinical engineers can bring to the planning process is that they can operate at a level above the domain experts, bring together the relative strengths and weaknesses of each domain into a broader planning framework, look for common elements, and provide assessments based on the outcomes that particular technologies promise. The role is one of facilitation, and requires a special blend of technical and administrative skills. If domain experts are not available within a particular

TABLE 25.2 Examples of Contemporary Strategic Technologies

Imaging	Surgery	Clinical laboratories	Monitoring and diagnosis
• Positron-emission tomography (PET) • Magneto-encephalography • Integrated image archiving systems • Cardiac applications of CT • Interventional radiology • Functional MRI and spectroscopy • Interventional MRI[6,7] • Cardiac MRI • Radiation oncology	• Endoscopy • Laparoscopy • Minimally invasive surgery and surgical robotics • Image-guided surgery • Tissue engineering[8] • OR of the future[9] • Virtual endoscopy[10] • Virtual reality[11] • Catheter guidance systems	• Molecular diagnostic systems • Automated laboratory systems • Electron microscopy • Mass spectrometry • Therapeutic drug monitoring	• Epilepsy-monitoring systems • Signal processing applied to monitoring • Cardiac-mapping systems • Tele-medicine[12] • "Smart" infusion systems

institution, the clinical engineer may be called upon to fill this gap to the extent possible, or to facilitate the provision of external consulting expertise. In an alternate model, the clinical engineer may fulfill a role as an external consultant, where particular expertise exists.[16]

The planning cycle for strategic technologies incorporates the following components:

- Identification and assessment[17–19] of the applicability of the technology, its efficacy, maturity, reliability, and impact on patient outcomes[20–21] based on, where possible, clinical evidence.
- Development of a functional plan incorporating the use of the technology. Such a plan includes the patient population that will be served, personnel resources required, impact on workflow,[22] impact on other services, definition of resources that will be displaced, facility requirements, and generic technology requirements. This plan will also incorporate preliminary budget estimates. At this time, it is appropriate to perform a life-cycle cost-analysis so that impacts on operating budgets are clearly understood.
- Development of detailed capital requirements, including equipment specifications, specification of special-purpose facilities, and specification of the costs of implementation.
- Development of a business case, which details net cash flows over the life of the equipment, based on capital and operating costs and addresses less financially tangible criteria such as patient outcomes and quality of life.
- Incorporation of the above information into a detailed proposal suitable for presentation to key decision makers at the executive level; solicitation of support for the proposal among key stakeholders and decision makers.
- Presentation and justification of the proposal at the appropriate executive level, seeking approval for moving forward with the project. The likelihood of success will, to a large extent, depend on the strategic importance, the strength of the proposal, and the relevance of the arguments that are presented.

Health Technology Assessment. A useful primer on the first point, health technology assessment, is available from the National Information Center on Health Services Research and Health Care Technology (NICHSR).[23] With reference to diagnostic imaging, Fryback and Thornbury[24] described a six-level hierarchical model for the assessment of medical imaging technology, which can also be applied to other medical technologies. Level 1 concerns technical quality of the images; level 2 addresses diagnostic accuracy, sensitivity, and specificity associated with interpretation of the images. Next, level 3 focuses on whether the information produces change in the referring physician's diagnostic thinking. Such a change is a logical prerequisite for level 4, which concerns the effect on the patient-management plan. Level 5, efficacy studies measure or compute the effect of the information on patient outcomes. Finally, level 6, analysis examines societal costs and benefits of a diagnostic imaging technology. In this model, the satisfaction of lower levels is a prerequisite for entry to the higher levels. Typical health technology assessments focus on levels 3 through 6, and in many cases, are retrospective studies based on available published information.

Assessments can focus on technologies requiring devices for their implementation, for example, negative pressure wound therapy,[25] or on the application of a technology for a particular purpose, for example, the use of computed tomography for (a) screening for coronary artery disease[26,27] and (b) evaluating coronary artery disease in symptomatic patients.[28,29] The assessments in the referenced cases generally were not favorable. It is noted that the assessments were based upon 64-slice CT technology, which has recently been superseded by 320-slice technology,[30] thus providing a salient example of the moving target problem.[23] Application of this finding would not preclude the acquisition of a multislice CT, but may prompt deferral of the acquisition of a cardiac option until such time as the newer CT technologies have been appropriately assessed. A further example is the use of CT colonography for the detection of colorectal cancer both as a population screening tool for at risk asymptomatic patients and diagnostic testing of symptomatic patients.[31] Use of a technology for asymptomatic screening for a particular condition requires demonstration of high sensitivity and specificity in order to reduce false positive and false negatives to an acceptable level with respect to the occurrence of the condition in the screened population.[32]

Applicable health technology assessments provide a valuable input to the technology planning process and need to be intelligently interpreted for the context in which the technology will be applied. For a routine application, a negative assessment should preclude the acquisition of the technology or its use for a specific diagnostic test. Often retrospective health technology assessment studies rely on data of varying quality, with the result that the reports do not satisfy the criteria established by the International Network of Agencies for Health Technology Assessment (INAHTA),[33] and this does not allow a definitive conclusion to be reached. This has been identified as a problem,[34–36] and in these cases, some health technology assessment bodies are facilitating funding for more appropriate studies, particularly if they have authority for withholding approval for dissemination.[37]

Assessments may also include the evaluation of technologies to achieve a clinical objective. An example is catheter steering technology that finds application in cardiac catheterization facilities. Alternatives available include magnetic steering[38] involving substantial infrastructure in the form of magnets, magnetic shielding and control systems, and automated mechanical steering systems that do not require any infrastructure.[39] In this case, the assessment of catheter steering is influenced by approaches to its realization.

A Strategic Technology Example: Interventional Radiology or Image-Guided Therapy. Interventional radiology or image-guided therapy embraces the use of imaging modalities such as x-ray angiography, ultrasound, computed tomography, endoscopy, laparoscopy, and magnetic resonance imaging. In an appropriate setting, and with the appropriate clinical skills, these technologies can be used for a variety of procedures, where using conventional surgical techniques are either difficult or impossible. These include line and shunt placements, biopsies, lineograms, venograms, cecostomies, abscess drainage, tumor removal, correction of vascular malformations, and image-assisted minimally invasive surgery.

The obvious benefits of performing procedures using image-guided techniques include improved patient outcomes; reduced patient trauma, when compared to open procedures; reduction in operating room hours, allowing reallocation to other procedures; reduction in patient stay; improved administration of intravenous therapies; and a potential reduction in delivery costs. In its broadest sense, it impacts the way in which surgical services are delivered, and requires a new relationship between interventional radiologists and surgeons.

The technology that is required is significant, and it is probable that existing facilities may require significant renovation in order to meet the requirements for the integration of imaging modalities and patient support, especially where sedation, general anesthesia, and recovery is required. This translates into a significant financial commitment.

From a planning perspective, a proposal for the implementation of this technology must include a master and functional plan which addresses technology, facilities, staffing, patient benefits, patient flow, displacement of existing procedures, and quantitative financial projections, all of which must be combined into a coherent and plausible framework for presentation and approval. It is only upon approval that detailed technology planning can take place, resulting in a detailed set of requirements for the imaging modalities that can be passed on to the acquisition process.

25.5.2 Information Technologies

Information technologies are an accepted part of contemporary health-care enterprises. A recent survey[40] gives an impression of the diffusion and use of information technology in hospitals, and an assessment of benefits in the context of return on investment is explored in a detailed report.[41]

They are characterized by their diversity as many vendors provide niche products directed to meeting the needs of individual professions, while others provide comprehensive systems geared to meeting the needs of complete organizations.[42] Quite often, the niche products conflict with corporate needs, whereas the comprehensive systems fail to adequately meet niche requirements. Thus, a sound management strategy is required. For operational systems, in-house software development is not a viable option, which leaves basically two approaches: one vendor fits all, or best of breed in conjunction with integration and interoperability. Interestingly, this is a moving target, as vendors, through acquisitions, assemble what they consider to be best of breed and present them to the marketplace as a one-vendor solution. This simply shifts the task of integration from the health-care organization to the vendor community, and at the same time requires adaptive strategies from a planning perspective.

Information technology serves to automate existing processes, and to add value to existing processes by providing data input to quality improvement and management processes, data and facilitation for decision support at the point of physician orders, and data for research and analysis. The diversity of needs, the available systems on the market represented as meeting those needs, and the varying status of legacy systems makes it virtually impossible to specify one universal solution. However, planning strategies can be generalized, and these will be summarized in the remainder of this section.

Information technologies are themselves sufficiently complex and diverse that is wise to develop a specific strategic plan for information technologies which best serve the needs of the organization. Derived from and consistent with the strategic plan of the organization, such a plan should address the strategic information technology needs of particular organizational units, including both administrative and clinical, and the data links and relationships that exist between them.

On the clinical side, the plan should specify key organizational units that through information technology can contribute to the strategic goals of the organization. Typically these will include laboratories, radiology, cardiology, pharmacy, critical care units, operating rooms, surgery, anesthesia, health records, emergency departments, professional service departments such as physiotherapy, and outpatient or ambulatory departments. Within organizational units, key considerations relate to key stakeholder needs, transactional and analytical requirements, workflow, and desirable data sets. Across organizational units, key considerations are data integration and interoperability, workflow integration, coordinated scheduling, and consistent data access and presentation. The desirability and scope of an electronic patient record,[43,44] and the manner and timeframe in which this can be realized should be analyzed, and the results of the analysis incorporated into the plan.

It is not unusual that within organizational units, there will be pressure to acquire systems that are geared to particular needs, and that these be implemented before a master plan can be realized. If this can be justified, it is important to include such systems in an integration strategy, which allows connection of best-of-breed systems. The most appropriate method for dealing with this problem is to implement an integration engine which can translate and map data elements, within a non–plug-and-play standards environment, such as HL-7, thus ensuring compatibility between applications from different vendors. Over time, the availability of IHE profiles with specifically defined interfaces will assume the function of the integration engine.

From the time a patient is admitted to the health-care organization until the time the patient is discharged, there are many transactions that take place. These may include assessments, medications, laboratory tests, and diagnostic and therapeutic procedures. Each transaction generates a result, which may be in the form of numbers, images, reports, or the administration of a therapy. Transactions may be interdependent in that subsequent transactions are based on the results of previous transactions. Such processes generate a longitudinal record which profiles the activities and results associated with a particular patient. In a paper world, this is the patient chart, which, if implemented in an electronic context, becomes the electronic patient record.

Transactions arise from an order from qualified practitioners, and each transaction triggers a series of support activities. An order for a medication results in a request to the pharmacy, where it may be screened for correctness, formulated and delivered to the patient caregiver for administration. An order for an image results in a request to radiology for scheduling the patient to an imaging modality, wherein a series of images is generated, forwarded to a radiologist for reporting, and the resulting report directed back to the responsible physician for assimilation with data from other sources. In these examples, the management of activities within the pharmacy and radiology departments can be met by information systems which address the specific needs of each specialty. In the latter case, this typically comprises a radiology information system (RIS) and a picture archiving and communication system (PACS).[45] In each case, there is a requirement for the bidirectional communication of information between involved systems, and an important part of the planning process is to determine what will be communicated and the means by which it will be communicated.

Systems integration at the point of care is an essential goal, especially where best-of-breed system with integration is the chosen strategy. The concept of a universal clinical workstation, where orders can be placed, results reviewed, images and reports viewed, all accessed in the same patient context is the answer to the problem of requiring many workstations running different applications. The evolution of web technology is perhaps the most significant advance which makes this objective achievable. The planning, specification, and acquisition of any contemporary system should include this functionality.

Transactional systems serve to automate the many transactions that are part of health-care delivery. These alone are not sufficient to realize the full potential of information technology, and any comprehensive plan should include an analytical system, which allows detailed analysis and queries across patient longitudinal records for the purposes of quality improvement, evaluation of patient outcomes, and other research. Such systems are usually classified as data warehouses and are founded on architectures which facilitate analysis and activities such as data mining in response to ad hoc queries.

Decision support systems,[46] wherein transactions are screened according to a set of rules, add an additional layer of value to transactional systems. To be effective, such systems require that rules be invoked in real time and draw upon data relevant to the transaction. For example, drug order may be contraindicated based on allergies, or a laboratory order may be contraindicated by the results of previous tests, or applicability in the context of the patient's condition as recorded in the electronic chart. The implementation of decision support technology requires significant effort in the development of acceptable rules, and the processing power to process them in real time.

Typically, information technologies in health-care systems are either underfunded, or place an unreasonable emphasis upon administrative systems. An allocation in the range of 6 to 8 percent of the annual operating budget for information systems is not unrealistic and is consistent with information-intensive industries in other sectors.

A summary of contemporary information systems is included in Table 25.3.

Many contemporary medical device systems now have a significant information technology component. For example, networked patient-monitoring systems communicate with hospital information systems such as laboratory information systems and electronic health records. Smart infusion pump systems require access to pharmacy formularies, and surgical navigation systems need to communicate with enterprise PACS systems. In fact, many contemporary medical devices are essentially computers with signal processing front-ends where analog signals are digitized as soon as possible. Data are generated and passed to other systems or stored for later analysis or review. From an external point of view, the device is really a manifestation of information technology, and as such many of the information technology paradigms apply—implementation processes, server management, upgrade procedures, security and privacy issues, storage management, and disaster recovery.

In the past, such devices could be plugged in and become immediately operable but they now have to be integrated into the information technology fabric. Although the situation is gradually improving, many device vendors are accustomed to selling hardware, and are having difficulty adapting to the

TABLE 25.3 Examples of Contemporary Health-Care Information Systems Required for Clinical and Administrative Purposes

Clinical systems		Administrative systems	Infrastructure systems
• Image archiving systems[14] • Radiology information systems • Cardiology information systems • Neurology information systems • Laboratory systems electronic patient record	• Electronic patient chart • Computer provider order entry • Decision support systems • Patient-monitoring networks • Charting systems • Pharmacy systems • Telehealth • Data warehouse	• Financial systems • E-mail • Communications systems • Voice mail • Human resources and payroll • Inventory systems • Scheduling systems • Hospital information system • Logistics systems	• Wired network • Wireless network • Nurse call systems • Alarm paging systems • Voice over IP • Enterprise storage • Central server facility • Applications servers • Integration engines • Desktop computers

information technology environment. When planning the acquisition and implementation of these hybrid systems, it is useful to have an understanding of the information technology relationships. It is in situations such as these that the technology must be treated as a continuum notwithstanding process or organizational barriers. A recent article[47] proposes that interoperability standards will reduce information technology to a utility. While there may be some truth in this for infrastructure, the proposition reinforces the barriers that need to be removed.

The increasing complexity of information systems and the associated accumulation of data that is an essential asset of any organization, together with the strengthening relationship with medical devices, require particular attention during the planning stages. In this context, there are a number of important factors to consider: compliance with standards, interoperability both intra- and inter-enterprise, sustainability, workflow and ergonomics, software licensing, maintainability, disaster recovery, backup and restore, security and privacy, implementation processes, and compatibility with enterprise infrastructure such as networks and storage.

Standards and Interoperability Within the Enterprise. An integral part of technology planning is the incorporation and recognition of standards. Standards-based systems improve the probability of compatibility for upgrades, additions, and replacements independent of vendor. Standards for medical devices, such as those relating to safety and performance, are relatively well known in the clinical engineering community; however, information systems standards tend to be better known in the information technology community. Two important standards in this arena at the applications level are HL-7 and DICOM 3.0, the former applying to the communication of patient information, and the latter applying to images generated from diagnostic imaging modalities. Neither standard is plug-and-play in the sense that a direct seamless connection can be made, and interoperability immediately achieved; however, they do define a framework in which prescribed data elements can be exchanged between devices from different manufacturers. In each standard, it is necessary to know message content, as opposed to format, before a reliable interface can be achieved. Once content can be rationalized between two systems, communication can take place. The task of rationalizing content can usually be efficiently achieved through an integration engine connecting the two systems. In the case of DICOM 3.0, the task of establishing connectivity involves the matching of DICOM 3.0 conformance statements, statements wherein each device discloses the content of the messages available for communication. Conformance is categorized by class, with separate classes being established for query/retrieve, store, and print, for example.

Despite the evolution of health-care information technology, issues associated with integration and interoperability continue to remain. A recent report[48] indicates that complete enterprise integration still requires a lot of effort. However, initiatives such as integrating the health-care enterprise (IHE) framework,[49] now 10 years old, are building upon existing HL7 and DICOM 3.0 standards to define specific workflow-related messaging between applications from different vendors; thus in theory, decoupling decisions relating to interoperability from those relating to vendor selection. Initially driven from a medical imaging perspective, the number of IHE domains has been gradually expanding as has the number of integration profiles attached to each domain. An important component is the IT Infrastructure domain that addresses application infrastructure issues such as consistent time, single sign on, patient identification, patient context, and various levels of document exchange. A recent addition includes a domain for patient-care devices (PCD)[50] and the development of an integration profile that defines messaging between a PCD and an electronic health record via a configurable filter that can define the subset of available data, if necessary, to be communicated. Some standards development organizations have stepped beyond IHE by defining specific messaging for domains not currently addressed, for example, drug prescription.[51]

The IHE framework is designed for communication between actors from different vendors, but does not require these to be applied between actors that are defined within a particular vendor's system. For institutions that had already developed interfaces using HL7 messaging through interface engines and have established DICOM 3.0 compatibility between vendors, prior to IHE, IHE will not offer any immediate benefit, but as systems get replaced, migration to the IHE framework should be considered. To facilitate the use of IHE, the organization publishes user handbooks which document the application of IHE profiles in a clinical environment.[52]

While IHE is not perfect, and is subject to continuing development, the IHE framework is an important consideration in technology planning processes as it makes it easier to move data between disparate applications where the communication of such data can have a positive impact on patient outcomes. Thus, it allows the choice of different vendors for systems that must share data. The framework does define workflow, so it is important that these definitions be understood in the context of assumptions concerning connectivity. Normally, this should not be a problem as the integration profiles are the subject of significant expert peer review prior to the release of the final document. In any event, any specification documents relating to the acquisition of systems where connectivity is required should include conformity with the applicable published integration profile, even if they may not be immediately implemented. In order to take advantage of the IHE framework in a planning context, the following steps should be considered:

- Assess the enterprise needs for systems and data integration. Base this assessment on realistic outcomes criteria such as quality improvement, productivity, error reduction, stakeholder satisfaction, and cost reduction.
- Develop a plan for the integration of enterprise systems and data.
- Understand the currently available IHE profiles and consider how they meet the established enterprise requirements; reassess needs in this context.
- Determine the availability of systems and devices that have implemented the required profiles.
- Evaluate the functionality of these systems and devices to determine how well they meet the enterprise requirements.
- Incorporate findings into a technology plan.

IHE provides user guidance with respect to the application of the framework in an enterprise. One example is the *IHE Radiology User's Handbook*.[52] The use of the IHE framework, where available and applicable, will avoid the need for the development of custom interfaces, thus avoiding both development and maintenance costs. Further, establishment of an IHE framework will make future acquisitions easier to plan and to allow for the incorporation of profiles that become available in the future.

Where legacy systems use custom-developed interfaces, there is no need to consider phasing them out until the systems they support become obsolete, or unless there is a business case supporting their replacement. Where IHE profiles do not exist for required interoperability, there are two options, wait for their development or implement custom interfaces as per past practice.

The interoperability offered by IHE and its applicability to integration in a particular enterprise should be well understood by institutional stakeholders, and become part of the information technology strategic planning framework. The availability of interoperability standards such as IHE does not excuse the need for critical due diligence when planning and acquiring or upgrading enterprise systems. There is no substitute for rigorous interoperability testing as part of acceptance. There are many reports in the popular technical press regarding successful implementation of IHE frameworks in particular situations; however, it is probably premature for critical evidence-based reviews. Caveat emptor always applies.

Standards and Interoperability Beyond the Enterprise. For the purposes of this discussion, an *enterprise* is defined as an entity with the one governance, and as such could include a single institution or a group of institutions under the same governance. Interoperability across governance boundaries is becoming more important as the electronic health record for mobile individuals is seen to be a significant benefit in reducing duplication and costs and improving access and quality of care. In this context, it is useful to consider planning approaches from within a governance unit that will address interoperability beyond the governance unit.

Since a governance unit is responsible for delivering health-care services within its jurisdiction, a more pragmatic approach is to permit each governance unit to define their own needs in a framework of predetermined cross-enterprise data and information requirements. Cross-enterprise connectivity should specify interoperability requirements that can be addressed in the context of available interoperability standards, such as IHE. If these are not available, data required for cross-enterprise purposes can be provided by custom interfaces based on HL7 messaging to an external database representing cross-enterprise interests. Using this approach, data can be normalized, security and privacy requirements can be implemented, and there is no interference with the source systems. A system based on this approach links 151 hospitals, pediatric treatment centers and community-care organizations, and 600 physician offices in Ontario.[53] In all, there are 5000 registered clinical users. Using this approach, enterprise systems can be planned and implemented according to enterprise needs, without compromising the cross-enterprise interoperability and functionality that may be required. It does need appropriate accountability mechanisms and quality skills and commitment within the enterprise in order to be successful.

An alternative approach is to use web portal technology to provide access to patient information maintained in enterprise systems for authorized stakeholders, including physicians, clinical personnel, and patients. The portals typically provide a view data available attached to sign on privileges, and may include functionality for secure e-mail to care providers and appointment scheduling, for example. Portals do not provide access to the underlying functionality of applications, but do play a useful role in extracting and making data available through a web browser from any location. Portals rely on the extraction of data by query from a variety of sources, which have to be polled to determine the availability of that data. Many transactional systems are not optimized for ad hoc queries of this nature with the result that portal queries can impact the performance and reliability of the source systems. Further, data from sources with different standards with respect to nomenclature and data interpretation, such as measurement units or methodology, need to be normalized before presentation. Finally, privacy legislation may require restrictive access based on data subsets as defined by the patient. Currently portals have a role to play within a homogeneous environment, for example, a single enterprise; however, portals that require information across enterprise boundaries have many issues that need to be resolved before they are a viable alternative to systems such as that described in the previous paragraph. It is noted that portals are only as good as the underlying enterprise systems, and are therefore not a substitute for them.

The alternative cross-enterprise approach of one system for all is typically sponsored by large government or jurisdictional agencies,[54] and there are few, if any, examples of successful implementations. The approach lacks the robustness of diversity and hybrid vigor, and is usually encumbered by large consultant and project management overheads that overpromise and underdeliver. Further it works against stakeholder buy-in at the enterprise level, failing to recognize that most IT systems have a significant organizational cultural component.

The primary benefits of interoperability, as specified by the IHE framework, will be flexibility in the choice of vendors for different information technology applications within an enterprise, without having to purchase or develop and maintain custom HL7 interfaces. Even though the offerings of a particular vendor are becoming more diverse, through additional development or acquisitions, there will always be decisions as to where to draw the line between vendors. Vendors tend to optimize their offering, which means that there will always be overlapping functionality. For example, modality vendors tend to migrate their available products upward into the traditional domain of enterprise information technology vendors. Likewise, enterprise information technology vendors tend to migrate downward into the tradition domain of modality vendors. For example, it is possible to purchase a RIS/PACS system from an enterprise vendor, and it is possible to purchase an electronic health record system from a modality vendor. The flexibility of choice requires criteria on which to base a decision, and this is best supported by intelligent planning.

Sustainability. Sustainability implies the expectation of a reasonable technological lifetime from any set of applications. In the past, there have been many examples of new versions of applications being incompatible with older versions, even though they come from the same vendor. In these situations, upgrading can involve extensive data migration efforts which, upon completion, add no intrinsic value. While architectures and database technologies do evolve, providing improved performance, prudent planning should minimize the impact and cost by proactively addressing these issues with prospective vendors. Further, it is not uncommon for modules of the same system to be operating on different database platforms with back-end interfaces linking them together. While this can be a short-term solution, one should expect a seamless transition to a common database at some time in the future.

In addition to the capital costs, the cost of ownership for any IT system includes the cost of resources required to maintain the system, together with the cost of downtime associated with maintenance activities. Maintenance costs usually exceed capital cost over time.[41] Proactive consideration of these requirements can help to minimize these costs. Where system uptime is important, server architectures that provide redundancy require consideration. Where there are many workstations connected to these servers, thin clients are typically easier to maintain, and a means of distributing upgrades to each workstation from a central location is essential. Responsibility for the installation of security patches and service packs required for server and workstation operating systems is often contentious, in particular where such updates may impact the performance of the application. Ensure prospectively that the vendor takes responsibility for the security of their systems.

Key operational components of an information technology plan include provision for the costs associated with the maintenance of current systems: software maintenance costs that can typically range from 18 to 22 percent of software list prices, and the costs associated with qualified human resources necessary to support installed systems.

Workflow and Ergonomics. Workflow describes the processes necessary to complete a prescribed task. Since many of these processes are incorporated into and constrained by information systems, it is useful to examine the relationship. Contemporary approaches include the development and implementation of use case scenarios,[55] which identify and implement workflow for particular applications, and an evolution of Six Sigma,[56] known as lean manufacturing.[57,58] The latter technique is based on the removal of waste from the process stream by first identifying the value to the user, followed by identification of the value stream; that is, the activities that contribute to that value. The next step is to improve flow by removing steps that do not contribute to value, and finally to work toward perfection by reiteration through the above processes. The end result is an optimized workflow. From a planning perspective, identification of the optimized workflow, to the extent possible, is a key consideration in adopting a particular technology or a particular instance of a technology.

Examples where workflow is important are specimen processing in a clinical laboratory, where lean is finding application[59] and the processes associated with the acquisition and processing of images from an imaging modality such as computed tomography. Prospective analysis of workflow during the planning phase may influence the choice of particular technologies and devices.

The majority of significant medical devices use software or firmware to control functions and, in this context, can be considered as a subset of the workflow issue. Perhaps more familiar as a component of ergonomics, it involves navigation through menus, the probability of user errors and inefficiencies, such as the number of actions that are required to execute a given task.

Software Licensing. Approaches to software application licensing have important implications, both with respect to cost and availability to appropriate users. Unfortunately, licensing approaches used by vendors are often constrained by the licensing management tools built into the software applications. Fixed seat licensing means that the license is attached to a particular workstation, which means that the number of workstations cannot exceed the number of licenses. This can be restrictive where users are mobile and need access to applications from different locations. A preferable approach is to use a concurrent license model wherein the use of a license defines a number of users, and is independent of the number of workstations or access points to the application. This has the advantage that it is based on the statistical use patterns of the application, and the number of licenses can be determined accordingly. In turn, it requires the use software to monitor usage which is not necessarily supported by all vendors. Software application providers, in contrast to modality vendors, are more likely to provide this option.

Disaster Recovery. While the occurrence of a disaster that significantly affects operations dependent on information technology is a low-probability event, it will have a high impact, and therefore requires consideration during planning processes. Disasters could include partial or catastrophic loss of servers or storage associated with critical systems through electrical power or hardware failure or loss due to fire or flood or other natural disaster.[60] Two criteria, business continuity and no permanent loss of data, are important. In the first case, an acceptable downtime should be established and backup systems planned accordingly. At the very least, this would require an uninterruptible power system (UPS) and hardware replication providing redundancy, automatic failover, and fault notification for critical server and storage systems. Consolidation of assets in a well-designed data center is appropriate, as it facilitates the implementation of risk mitigation strategies such as fire and flood protection; however, the loss or partial loss of such a center would require the existence of second data center adequately replicating critical systems with both servers and accessible data storage in order to reasonably maintain business continuity. Backup storage, for example, does not require the same performance as the primary storage as long as it is adequate to meet the business continuity criteria. In the case of the loss of data storage systems, recovery from a remotely located tape archive, for example, would typically not meet reasonable business continuity requirements because of the volume of data that may be involved, even though it would satisfy the requirement for no loss of data. Irrespective of whether the planning and management of data center services are maintained in house, or outsourced to a third party, careful consideration should be given to the allocation of resources or the exercise of appropriate due diligence in order to reduce risks to an acceptable level. Such strategies are not without cost, so the engagement of a qualified consultant may be appropriate as these issues are addressed. Any disaster recovery process is only as good as the data backup systems and the procedures in place to restore this data to an operational environment. Typically, disaster recovery procedures will not be invoked very often, so it is important that they are thoroughly tested upon implementation and periodically reviewed and evaluated so that they will be available when needed.

Security and Privacy. Security of data from unauthorized access is of particular concern for personal health data where privacy is a key consideration.[61] Many jurisdictions have enacted privacy legislation[62,63] that mandates requirements that impose security constraints on information systems. Any applications that gather and distribute patient data must meet the legal requirements for the jurisdiction in which they are used, and as such become part of the system specification. Such privacy legislation may prevent the storage of patient data outside national boundaries, which becomes an important consideration when services are outsourced to providers in a different country. Should any services, ranging from simple remote access to outsourcing the storage of data, be performed from outside the health-care organization, it is important that there are adequate clauses in the contract to ensure compliance with the applicable privacy legislation.

In Canada PHIPA, for example, identifies the patient or the patient's legal representative as the owner of the information, and the person who can assign rights of access. Access restrictions can apply to selected subsets of the data or all the data. There is a "break the glass" provision whereby restricted information can be accessed if it is essential for the care of the patient. It also has provision for access to images or other data by practitioners who will generate a report on the images or data. Once the report is signed, it, together with the source data, is protected according to the legislation. Unfortunately, many information systems do not intrinsically meet the current requirements of the legislation, and in the absence of suitable alternatives, it will be necessary to perform a gap analysis and consideration of other means to address these gaps.

Privacy legislation will generally require the adoption of specific policies and procedures that, together with the technical framework, provide a secure environment, to the extent possible, in compliance with the legislation. Security requirements need to be recognized at all stages of the planning process, including sustainability after implementation.

Implementation Processes. Virtually all information systems, or devices with an information technology component, require implementation prior to being placed into production. Tasks involved include server configurations, integration with enterprise infrastructure, security, privacy, incorporation of geographical and personnel data, data normalization and the configuration of specific workflows. A detailed implementation plan is essential, and the stage at which such a plan is developed is critical to avoid cost overruns and scope creep.

Ideally, a detailed implementation plan should be developed and included as part of the contract at a negotiated price. Incremental changes can then be handled by a predetermined change management process where costs can be controlled. Open-ended implementation plans introduce exposure to billable hours, which represents a conflict of interest between increasing revenues and completing the job. It is difficult to control the productivity and efficiency with which tasks are performed and the quality of skills that are assigned to the job. Beware also of costs associated with extensive consultant-based reengineering of processes promoted as being necessary to obtain value from the application, as these primarily represent the self-interest of vendors.

Every implementation plan will include a requirement for testing. This process should be well documented, and test every operational mode of the system in a test environment. Consideration should also be given to the loads that the system will experience in operational use, and where possible, these should be simulated in the test environment. Once the system has been turned over to production (go-live), performance under load should be assessed prior to final acceptance of the system. In short, take ownership, define what is needed, stay with the plan, define change management, and negotiate firmly but fairly with vendors to contractually define scope and cost.

A Planning Example: Reduction of Medication Errors. Application of planning principles is demonstrated by the following example relating to the technology for the reduction of medication errors, where a patient fails to receive the correct drug or the correct dose and adverse drug events, where an injury occurs related to the use of a drug, associated with intravenous administration. This example illustrates that technology should be considered as a continuum that includes devices, technology infrastructure, and information technologies.

Analysis of the problem reveals that there are several points in the drug administration process where technology can be implemented: at the point of provider order, at the point of dispensing, at the point of delivery to the patient and at the point of administration. Contributions to a medication error from each of these stages appear to vary according to the experience of different authors.[64,65] This most probably has its origins in behavior rather than technology. Each of the above steps has a technology solution: computerized provider order entry (CPOE), robotic dispensing systems, bar coding, and smart infusion pumps. The first steps in the planning process are therefore to characterize the drug administration process and evaluate the technologies that can be applied to each stage of the process. A Pareto chart[66] developed using process improvement techniques will serve as an aid to determine which technologies, in conjunction with behavior modification, can have the greatest impact in addressing the root causes.

Assume that one of the outcomes of this process is a decision to implement smart infusion pump technology. This is another example of a medical device technology that has a significant information technology component. Recent evaluations of this technology[67,68] provide information on appropriate functionality, and there are reports showing that it does reduce medication error. However, it is important to remember that this technology is part of a larger process, and therefore should be interoperable with other components of this process. Current systems keep the pump updated with drug information from the pump system server; however, from a systems point of view, it would be better if the pump was updated with information from the same database on which the orders are based, resident in the CPOE system. This interoperability is no different to that being provided in the IHE framework in other domains, and if it was available it would avoid errors arising from the two sources of data becoming asynchronous. It would also avoid the cost associated in maintaining the pump database. Further, extensions of the smart pump technology in the future should involve automatic (bar code) identification of the patient and the medication with the pump and loop closure back to the order, keeping in mind that the pump should be able to safely operate autonomously in case of network or server failure. Finally, behavioral factors[69] must be addressed if the pumps are to achieve their potential. Planning in the broader context identifies gaps in the interoperability of the technology, and facilitates assessment of the impact on the problem at hand.

Since this technology is typically server based, it can use a wireless network infrastructure to keep pumps up to date. As it is required on a 24/7 basis, it should be fault tolerant, and be located in the institutions data centre. In addition, if the server uses a commercial operating system, there will need to be a process for managing security and security patch and service pack updates, which should be consistent with the information technology policies of the organization. There will also be a requirement for software upgrades to the server and the clients (pumps), which require consideration of downtime, testing, and go-live procedures. Such procedures are well established in the information technology environment and do not need to be reinvented.

The consideration of smart pump technology in the broader context does not preclude the requirement for conducting due diligence on the performance and safety of the pumps themselves. These evaluation processes are well documented[70] and familiar to clinical engineers.

Several key points related to device technologies can be drawn from this example:

- Technology typically addresses processes; keep the immediate and related processes in mind during the assessment phase.
- Integration into an existing environment is an essential consideration.
- Technology is a continuum; devices can no longer be considered in isolation.
- In order to achieve the desired outcomes, positive user acceptance and potential behavior modification is required.
- Cooperative involvement of information technology skills and resources are mandatory to ensure success and sustainability.
- Medical device planning and acquisition decisions are now broader in scope, and require very different approaches.

25.5.3 Technology Infrastructure

Assuming that information technology resources are maintained in house, integration into an existing environment may be required at a number of levels, typically involving hardware, data communications, network utilization, and storage. Responsible application suppliers should be vendor agnostic with respect to choice of hardware, allowing clients the benefits of standardization of hardware within their facility. This flexibility assumes increasing importance with the introduction of blade server and virtual server architectures that are becoming part of contemporary data center design.[71] This technology has significant promise; however, there are issues relating to single points of failure affecting multiple applications, the intensity of use by a particular application, and the functionality of server alerts that require critical assessment. At the application level, there will typically be a requirement to exchange data with existing legacy systems. Traditionally, this has been achieved through HL7 or DICOM interfaces, which require development and adaptation as they are not plug-and-play. The introduction of the IHE framework, discussed earlier, facilitates this integration, assuming that the integration profiles are compatible with data exchange and workflow requirements. In any event, some workflow adaptation will inevitably be necessary and this will require negotiation with stakeholders.

Technology infrastructure warrants independent planning cycles. It refers to infrastructure that is designed to support the introduction of new technologies in the present and the future. Infrastructure includes data networks, data centers and enterprise storage, and the hardware and software that are necessary to support these functions. Examples of technology infrastructure are listed in Table 25.3.

Data Network Infrastructure. All server-based applications will require access to a network for connectivity with clients, and it is now commonly accepted that such applications should run on a well-designed and stable enterprise network with a minimum of Cat 5, 5e, or 6 (100 Mbit/s to 1 Gbit/s) terminal connections, a gigabit backbone incorporating logical segmentation, redundant data pathways, quality of service support, and 24/7 reliability. Application suppliers will argue that performance specifications such as response times will be compromised by the performance of client networks, and while this is not generally true, a high-performance, well-managed network is the best defense. This includes the provision for the protection against intrusions that can generate malicious traffic and severely degrade network performance. Every monitored bedside, operating room, clinic location, physician's office, laboratory workstation, and general office should have network connectivity, even if there is not an immediate need. In fact, a strategy of two or more network connections for each location is not excessive.

For example, at a critical care bedside, network connections may be required on a permanent basis for patient-monitoring network and a clinical information system, and on a temporary basis for connection of an ultrasound machine or other networked diagnostic device. In an operating room, at each anesthesia location, similar connections would be needed. Unless integrated with the bedside systems, additional network connections will be utilized for connection to institution-wide systems such as hospital information systems and PACS. With an appropriate network infrastructure in place, it becomes much easier to introduce networked systems into the environment, and avoids the addition of significant cabling costs for each application. Note that in some cases, it may be desirable to provide logical separation, for example, in the case of clinical systems and facilities maintenance systems.

In addition to a wired network infrastructure, it is becoming essential to implement a wireless network infrastructure, providing the advantage of device and personnel mobility. Applications include wireless patient networks, voice over IP for mobile communications, and communication with handheld information terminals carried by caregivers. Emerging technologies extend to nurse call systems and alarm paging systems under the umbrella term "unified communications." A wireless infrastructure requires careful planning with attention being paid to access points, data rates, and electromagnetic compatibility with medical devices. Factors favoring wireless networks are increased data rates with the introduction of 802.11n and improvements in security management with the centralization of wireless access point servers. Integrated wired/wireless networks are becoming available, and these architectures should be seriously considered. The mobility enabled through use of wireless devices enhances communication as long as due consideration is given to potential interference with clinical telemetry systems that may operate in the same region of the frequency spectrum.

Data Centers. The development of a central computer facility is an important part of an infrastructure plan. An adequately sized room with appropriate environmental controls, UPS protection against power failure, fire protection and security, combined with 24-h, 7-day-a-week operations support, should be considered a minimum requirement. With an appropriate network infrastructure in place, this facility can house enterprise storage and all servers, including those for all clinical, administrative, communication, and networking applications. This strategy facilitates data backup and data security.

Data center design is usually based on the ability of cooling systems to manage the heat load generated by the installed hardware. With more efficient cooling systems,[71] higher power densities can be achieved. This is particularly important with the adoption of blade servers, where the heat load per rack can reach 18 kW. Further, virtualization wherein more than one application runs on a physical server can impact the number of servers required, and therefore the overall power consumption. High-density rack systems with built-in cooling and UPS support are worthy of consideration when conventional data center space is at a premium. Assuming that data center operations are maintained in house, when planning the introduction of new systems, it is important to plan for adequate data center capacity with a lead time that allows for remedial action.

Enterprise Storage. All information technology applications and many clinical applications require data storage. Traditionally, storage solutions will be provided by the application vendor, which does not make good sense because storage is not their core business. The evolution of storage technology makes enterprise storage an essential consideration. This involves the centralization of storage for all major information technology applications in an enterprise, including data-intensive clinical applications such as digital EEG and epilepsy monitoring. Enterprise storage is supported by major storage system manufacturers. In particular, virtualization of storage, which provides logical abstractions of physical storage systems, permits transparent management of storage, and matching of performance requirements and cost of storage hardware with that required by the applications using the storage. It also simplifies backup, redundancy, and disaster management strategies. While unit storage costs are decreasing this is offset by the demand for greater storage capacity that increases the cost of storage infrastructure overheads, such as redundancy, disaster recovery, and those associated with virtualization. However, if enterprise storage is not already in place, it should be an essential component of any technology plan.

25.5.4 Renewal of Existing Technologies: Capital Equipment

In any organization, technology planning must include the appropriate maintenance of existing technologies. This activity ranges from direct replacement to upgrading the technologies associated with continuing functional requirements. This category may also include the introduction of new technologies, which contribute to operational requirements, but do not qualify as strategic initiatives.

It is a fundamental axiom that if stakeholders are polled with respect to their technology needs, the value of requests will exceed any reasonable budget allocations. This is more evident if planning is performed on a renewable annual basis as stakeholders see each year as a new competition.

While funding formulas differ across jurisdictions, two key planning principles can avoid a lot of problems. First, develop a rolling plan that extends over a period between 3 and 5 years, and second, secure a fixed annual budget allocation for maintenance of existing technologies based upon the multiyear plan. Once these have been implemented, rational planning that meets both stakeholder expectations and financial constraints becomes possible.

Dependent on the type of care provided by the organization, there will always be a need for fundamental technologies. These include patient monitoring, patient thermal support, anesthesia technologies, ventilatory support, infusion therapy, laboratory instrumentation, surgical tools, and diagnostic imaging tools such as ultrasound. Typically, these technologies will already exist in the organization, and will be at some stage in their life cycle. An analysis of this situation will allow the development of a replacement plan, extending over the selected timeframe. The key driver for replacement is obsolescence, which can either be based on the technology or serviceability, both of which can be addressed in the planning and acquisition process. An important resource for the development of replacement strategies is an inventory of existing equipment, coupled with knowledge of the performance expected from the equipment, the risks associated with continuing use, and the status of current technologies providing similar functions. Each of these falls within the knowledge and resource domain of clinical engineering.

Typically, organizations will structure the equivalent of an enterprise capital equipment committee to oversee the equitable distribution of funds for the maintenance of existing technologies, with the exclusion of information technologies. Membership of such a committee will comprise key equipment stakeholders, such as physicians from clinical and surgical services, clinical laboratories, and diagnostic imaging. In addition, there will usually be representatives from the administration, financial, and purchasing constituencies. The mandate of such a committee can range from the simple allocation of available annual funds allocated for renewal of technologies based on submitted equipment requests to the management of a technology maintenance plan. The latter is obviously more effective, and should be an explicit mandate of the group. Clinical engineers can play a variety of roles, from that of a technology consultant to that of a technology planner. They are uniquely qualified to bring a balanced impartial viewpoint, and can take a leadership role in facilitating the development of the plan through the committee. Planning decisions, particularly those related to the introduction of new technologies, can be difficult, and should be supported by inputs, where available, from health technology assessments. While this function can be integrated into the committee structure, devices and systems are typically a small subset of health technology assessment domain.

Key inputs to the planning process are

- A current inventory of equipment in categories that will be included in the plan.
- An assessment of risks associated with the continuing use of current equipment. Risks include those associated with safe operation, precision, and efficacy, when compared with contemporary technologies.
- An assessment of the current point in the life cycle (e.g., technological and serviceability). This will be a function of the particular technology and the particular product.
- An assessment of technologies, falling within the context of the plan that can enhance operations. New technologies may impact productivity, or allow new tests, that directly impact patient care, to be performed.

Key processes in the development of a plan are

- Categorization of key stakeholder groups. It is important that stakeholder groups, usually best defined along organizational lines, have some ownership in the specification and prioritization of their respective internal requirements.

- Development of equipment and systems groups which can be handled collectively. For example, an organization-wide patient-monitor plan is more effective than addressing individual requirements and partial replacement strategies.
- Balancing the plan across multiyear timeframe. Several iterations of the plan may be necessary to provide a balanced annual cash flow within the set budget allowance.
- Establishment of an acceptable annual budget allocation to sustain operations. The plan, once established and balanced and determined as meeting organizational needs, can be used to determine a proposal for an annual budget.
- Establishment of a fund for small-cost items and assignment of management to stakeholders. Responsibility for minor items, below some predetermined cost threshold, can be delegated to organizational units, together with an annual budget allowance. This relieves the committee of the task of prioritizing and approving such items.
- Establishment of a contingency allowance. A contingency allowance provides for unexpected needs. However, consideration can be given to inserting contingency items into plan priorities, in which case such items would displace planned items.
- Establishment of a fund for new and innovative technologies. An allowance for technologies which are innovative and subject to some risk may be included in the plan. Typically, this allowance would be subject to rules of competition.

A key output of the planning process is a plan that

- Provides flexibility across multiple years. A multiyear view minimizes the possibility of current year funding cuts, as the impact in future years is readily visible.
- Allows ready consolidation of a plan for the current planning year and coordination with annual operating plans. Typically operating plans should be supported by technology, and presenting both the operating plan and the capital plan in the same context reinforces this position.
- Facilitates discussion and approval at the committee and executive level.
- Can be effectively managed during its implementation. Execution of the plan involves specification, tender, selection, delivery, acceptance, and payment.
- Allows metering of cash flow in a particular implementation year. Cash flow at the time of payment represents the end point of implementation, and the timing of acquisitions can be driven by an annual cash-flow plan.
- Is fair and acceptable to stakeholders. Stakeholder requirements are often independent; therefore equity across stakeholders is a desirable outcome.

The multiyear planning process for the maintenance of existing technologies is a framework that has been found to be effective in practice. It avoids traditional problems associated with single year planning cycles, and allows the capital equipment committee to operate at appropriate executive level, avoiding the need to deal with item-by-item detail. The process is defined independently of particular professional expertise; however, it is apparent that expertise and experience of clinical engineers are well suited to playing a leadership role. Assertion of this role in a manner consistent with the goals of the process remains a situational challenge in each environment.

It is wise for a planning process such as this to establish an evaluation component, so that experience gained during implementation can be fed back into the process in order to introduce improvements. For example, once equipment has been purchased, installed and used for a period of time, a discussion with users to determine whether the original goals have been achieved can provide valuable information.

Capital Equipment Example: Patient Monitors. Patient monitors are a technology staple for critical care units. More recently, there has been emphasis on subacute monitoring, which is used for surveillance of patients being cared for outside of critical care units.

Typically, supply of monitors to these areas has been ad hoc, with no coherent strategy. The introduction of planning principles for these technologies facilitates the identification of the rationale for monitoring, the selection of the most appropriate parameters for monitoring, the protocols to be used for these parameters, and the education necessary to ensure that maximum benefits are achieved.

For example, if the primary reason for monitoring patients is to determine changes in physiological condition due to cardiac or respiratory difficulties, oxygen saturation monitoring alone is probably appropriate. This parameter, by its nature, is subject to artifact due to movement and low perfusion states, which can be the cause of excessive false-positive alarms. An assessment of the current state of oxygen saturation monitoring reveals that current generation algorithms, which take advantage of advanced signal processing techniques, can reduce false-positive alarm rates, making them suitable for single parameter monitoring of subacute patients. A decision to use saturation monitoring alone for this purpose precludes the need for ECG monitoring and the application of electrodes, even though this parameter may be available in the device.

A subacute patient-monitoring plan should start with requirements based on patient needs, and choosing an appropriate technology offering, which meets these needs.

A particular point arising from this example is alarm management. The problems with false alarms are well documented[72] and have been well known for many years. Despite this the problem persists, but can be minimized through proper planning. The analysis of false alarms for pulse oximetry using sensitivity and specificity determinations presented as a receiver operating characteristic (ROC) has promoted the development of pulse oximetry technologies where false-alarm rates are significantly reduced.[73]

False-alarm rates can be increased by monitoring unnecessary parameters. Further, false-alarm rates propagate through the system by creating false alarms at central stations or through alarm paging systems, creating adverse behavioral responses that can result in missing a critical event. Further, high false-alarm rates promote a sense of complacency that results in real alarms being ignored.

In this instance, appropriate planning resulting in the identification of appropriate technologies, can significantly impact the mitigation of a clinical problem.

25.6 TECHNOLOGY AND EQUIPMENT PLANNING FOR NEW FACILITIES

The requirement to equip a new facility with medical devices and systems provides an opportunity to begin with a new technology plan rather than sustain and adapt an existing plan. Despite this, the principles already discussed still apply. It is quite likely that the new facility will be occupied by an existing organization with existing strategic plans, or with a restructured organization arising from amalgamation for example, in which case one would expect strategies underlying the new structure to already be in place. Thus from a planning perspective, the primary difference is the fact that the plan is zero based.

Equipment planners, who may not necessarily be clinical engineers, provide planning services, which typically include pro forma databases which list typical equipment requirements by category for particular functions. For example, a critical care unit will require life-support equipment, thermal support systems, patient monitors and monitor networks, infusion therapy devices, patient beds and stretchers, sterilizers, laboratory instruments down to commodity items such as IV poles, suction systems, flowmeters, and resuscitation equipment. Such databases are a key asset of equipment planners, and are a key starting point of any new facility planning process. Technology planning is a precursor to equipment planning as it provides the framework on which equipment lists are based.

A typical strategy is through an appropriately structured equipment committee to solicit input from stakeholders in the new facility and to modify and update the database, resulting in equipment lists which represent the detailed requirements. At this time, a budget allowance for each line item is also developed. The list is then refined on the basis of available funding and priorities.

As with any technology planning initiative, success depends on the participation of a team of professionals with particular areas of expertise. An effective core committee for new facility equipment planning should include a materials management professional, a clinical engineer, an equipment planner, and an architectural planner. Each plays a role as follows:

Materials Management. Familiar with all aspects of procurement, including suppliers, pricing, lead times, and logistics.

Clinical Engineer. Familiar with performance requirements, detailed specifications, safety, efficacy, and aspects of systems integration.

Equipment Planner. Familiar with generic specialty requirements, equipment databases, and list management.

Architectural Planner. Familiar with the interface between equipment and facilities. They may draw upon more detailed information from electrical and mechanical consultants.

Each profession brings a particular expertise and working together as a team can produce a more effective result.

25.7 PROJECT MANAGEMENT

The complexity of many technology projects is such that an implementation process is required. Elements are the relationship with facilities, system configuration, integration with existing systems, commissioning, and acceptance procedures. Most vendors will assign a project manager and a project team to coordinate processes from the vendor side, and to protect the vendor's interest in the context of the contract. Most responsible vendors expect a similar structure to exist on the customer side, and the establishment of a project team, including a project manager is essential. Such a team provides a liaison with the stakeholders in the organization, and protects the organization's interest in the context of the governing contract. Project management is a specific skill,[74,75] and if such duties are assumed by a clinical engineer, it is appropriate that the individual has formal project management training or prior relevant experience.

There are many examples of systems, particularly information systems, that either do not meet expectations or are outright failures. Many of these outcomes can be attributed to inadequate project and expectation management that is people issues, rather than the inadequacies of the underlying technical attributes of the system. Failures are rarely documented in detail for obvious reasons; however, there are isolated examples where this issue is critically examined.[8] Examination of the root causes of failures and assimilation of the lessons presented is a major step toward ensuring future success.

25.8 FACILITY COMPONENTS

Many technology-based systems will have a facility component. This can range from the supply of special-purpose power and network connections to the renovation of a space for a particular need, requiring new electrical and mechanical infrastructures. It is important that the facilities component be incorporated into any technology plan.

Facilities can be designed for general or particular use. For example, operating rooms or critical care units have generic requirements, which are usually defined by standards and codes relating to facilities systems. These include electrical and mechanical systems such as normal and emergency power systems, medical gas systems, air-handling systems, and fire protection systems. This is in contrast to special procedure rooms which are generally designed to accommodate special-purpose systems such as x-ray and other imaging systems, display systems, and surgical microscopes.

The implementation of a facilities plan requires the establishment of an internal project team coordinated by a project manager representing the interests of the organization. The project manager can either be an employee of the organization, or acquired through an outsourcing contract. The project manager engages a health facilities architect who acts as a coordinator for other design consultants who will become involved in the development of detailed plans.

The project manager assumes responsibility for coordinating and facilitating discussions between the internal stakeholders and the design consultants in order to ensure that needs are translated into specific requirements that can be incorporated into a preliminary design. Typically, this will be at the architectural level, defining structural constraints, clearances, room layouts, the physical location of key functional elements, traffic flows, and points of access. Completion of the architectural design may take several iterations, and once complete leads to stakeholder sign off. The project manager keeps detailed minutes of all discussions in case of later disputes.

Once the architectural plans are finalized, the architectural consultants coordinate the detailed design in conjunction with the electrical and mechanical consultants who have been retained for the project. In the case of a renovated facility, this will involve the integration and connection with existing building systems. The end point of this process is a detailed set of design drawings, which are suitable for submission to a tender process. Where special-purpose equipment is required, the specification of the equipment requirements that impact on the facility, and that are not intended to be part of the contract need to be available for incorporation into design drawings and documents. Equipment, which is part of the construction contract, is supplied by the contractor and is included in the response to the tender call.

Interested contractors respond to the request for tenders, and from these submissions a successful general contractor is chosen. A contract is developed between the bidder and the organization. Typically, this will be done using contract documents which are standardized within the industry.

Once construction starts, the appointed project manager assumes responsibility for the project on behalf of the organization, and through the general contractor utilizes the architects and the electrical and mechanical consultants as appropriate for the duration of the project.

Upon completion, a commissioning phase is entered, wherein the installed systems are checked and calibrated according to the design specifications, at which point, subject to minor deficiencies, the facility can be turned over to the owner.

Installation of special-purpose systems can then take place, which, when completed, is handed over to the owner for acceptance testing prior to being placed into clinical use. In practice, some of the above processes may be run in parallel, subject to cooperation among the parties involved. Such coordination is the responsibility of the project manager.

It is important for clinical engineers to understand the construction processes, and their relationship to the final performance of the installed equipment. There is ample opportunity for involvement during each stage of the project, particularly in the initial planning stages, and in the final commissioning stages, and full advantage should be taken of these opportunities to add value to the process. clinical engineers, with special expertise relating to equipment and systems, are in a unique position to ensure that the interface with the facility is functional, safe, and effective. The key liaison is with the project manager representing the organization.

25.9 BUSINESS CASES

Assuming that a given project fits with the strategic plan, before approval, the development of a business case[41,76,77] is an important planning tool which provides a measure of affordability. The validity and structure of business cases will vary from jurisdiction to jurisdiction and the financial basis on which the health-care organization is structured. Business cases in systems where revenue is available on a case-by-case basis from insurance providers will differ from those where health-care systems are globally funded.

In general, business cases provide an analysis of positive and negative cash flows, which can be expected during the lifetime of the technology. This lifetime will depend on the technology under consideration, and in today's environment is closely related to the expected lifetime of the platform on which the technology is based. During the product lifetime, there will be negative cash flows associated with its use, and positive cash flows arising from revenue generated, or more tenuously, from costs avoided. One approach to quantify a business case is to calculate a net present value based on the net cash flows over the life of the technology, discounted to the present time at an interest rate typical for a secure investment, and to compare this value with what the technology is worth in the context of the patients served by the organization. This approach also allows comparisons between technologies where choices must be made. In a strict business environment, the net present value should be positive to represent a financial reward for effort expended. In a globally funded environment, the magnitude of the contributions required from the global budget required to balance the plan becomes an important consideration. Excellent cost of ownership information for clinical laboratory analyzers, for example, is provided by ECRI.[70]

Typical negative cash flows are

- The capital cost, usually occurring in year one, or in the case of a lease payments over the lease period
- Maintenance costs, on a quarterly, semiannual, or annual basis
- Cost of technology upgrades as these become available
- Salary costs for operating personnel
- Cost of supplies required to operate the equipment

Typical positive cash flows are

- Revenues earned through use of the technology
- Cost avoidance for personnel and supplies that can be realized through use of the technology
- Cost avoidance relating to reduction in patient stay, for example
- Disposal value of equipment, which the technology replaces

Net cash flows are the difference between positive and negative cash flows and can be calculated using a spreadsheet format and the net present value function available in most spreadsheet applications. This approach is useful to compare different technologies where return on financial investment is a key decision criterion.

While business cases have some value, there will always be technology where the business model does not apply. Typically, these are infrastructure technologies such as networks, computer communications (e-mail, voice mail, VoIP), and in these cases, investment decisions must be made on the basis of broader organizational criteria.

Business cases are built on assumptions, and one is not complete without an assessment of the risks associated with each assumption. Typically where risks are significant, mitigating strategies need to be included. Finally, it is difficult for business cases to incorporate the less quantifiable issues such as the impact of a technology on quality of life, family life, and other social factors. Those that are applicable should be explicitly articulated and qualitatively factored into the business plan.

25.10 PRIORITIES AND FUNDING

Technology costs money, and it is clear that among the available technologies choices will have to be made. Technologies represent an investment, and the criteria that will determine whether such investments should be made and their associated priorities will depend on the type of health-care system in which the organization operates. In a for profit system, decisions are more likely to be influenced by financial business plans driven by return on investment. In a social system, priorities may be set according to community or regional needs or in some cases by a central authority. Whatever the system, the ultimate goal is the delivery of quality patient care, and it is certain that technology will play a role in achieving this goal. Organizations that do not take a proactive approach to technology investment may have an uncertain future.[3]

At the very least, allocating funding for the replacement of the current technology infrastructure is essential. An annual allowance consistent with industry benchmarks for investment in information technology is also a basic necessity. This, at least, maintains the status quo. For organizations keen to develop new strategic initiatives, funding on a project-by-project basis is necessary.

Allocation of appropriate funding for technology plans will almost always require a technology advocate at the executive level, as it is there that the allocation of resources and the setting of priorities is usually decided. To play a meaningful role in technology planning, the clinical engineer needs to have a direct line of communication to the decision makers, and if this does not exist, it should be actively cultivated.

25.11 OUTSOURCING

The complexity of systems, particularly those involving software requiring integration with other systems, places specialized demands on the skills of the individuals charged with the responsibility of managing these systems. Developing an in-house resource requires a critical mass that may only be cost-effective within larger institutions. Under these conditions, outsourcing to a vendor or a third-party supplier is an option. This may be extended to include technology planning and technology management functions, and may even involve off-site transaction management and data storage. The advent of service-oriented architectures potentially facilitates the opportunity for outsourcing at the application level, but should be approached with caution.

Some advantages of outsourcing are

- Qualified personnel with appropriate skills should be available
- Backup resources are available as required
- Day-to-day management of resources becomes the responsibility of the provider
- Costs of services are capped for appropriately structured contracts

Some disadvantages of outsourcing are

- Possible loss of control of internal assets, such as data and information.
- Critical systems are dependent on a third party. Their failure is the organization's failure.
- Completion for provider resources may result in the assignment of inexperienced personnel.
- Lack of ownership for problems that may arise.
- It requires a major effort to revert if outsourcing does not perform.
- Costs can escalate because of dependencies.

A study[78] has shown that outsourcing of information services can improve the revenue of health-care organizations, but this must be considered in the context of the size of the organization and the quality of people in the organization on which the comparison is based.

Once the risks are understood, problems with provider screening and selection can be minimized, and performance expectations can be contractually developed. Good legal advice, preferably grounded in the practical aspects of technology rather than nonexistent risks, in developing a contract is essential. Once a relationship is established, success will depend on the quality of the contract management, and the assignment of a qualified contract manager is highly recommended. Here again, the clinical engineer may have or acquire the skills necessary for this function.

25.12 CORPORATE RELATIONSHIPS

Technologies will generally be acquired from the industrial sector. While make-or-buy decisions may have been appropriate in the past, in contemporary times with the availability of a broad range of technology from industry, these are no longer particularly relevant, except in the case of special-purpose research applications. For example, an organization that undertakes the development of complex software-based systems assumes the risks associated with continuing support, dependence on particular individuals, adaptation to changing technologies, organizational dependence on the system, and sustainability. Also assumed are the responsibilities in dealing with the regulatory environment.

The contemporary medical industry is currently characterized by consolidation of diverse technologies under a small number of corporate umbrellas. It is now possible to acquire from one vendor, technologies ranging from diagnostic imaging systems, monitoring systems, cardiovascular systems, and information systems. Similar consolidation is taking place in technologies such as intravenous therapy systems.

From a technology planning perspective, this environment can provide opportunities in the context of developing strategic corporate partnerships to meet needs across a variety of technology sectors. Such relationships must, however, be approached with appropriate caution. From the point of view of the health-care organization, the advantages include definition of a consistent set of generic contractual relationships and performance expectations across products. Within this framework, specific equipment or device specifications and requirements can be developed.

Contractual agreements defining relationships can range from those which require preferential purchasing of specific technologies during the term of the agreement, subject to those technologies meeting clinical requirements, to supply agreements which define the supply of specific goods from a particular vendor over a specified period of time. The degree in which an organization is bound to a particular vendor will define the benefits that accrue. The most frequent examples are favorable pricing structures, access to new and developing technologies, support for research, favorable delivery terms, and favorable access to service options and spare parts. Intangible benefits include the opportunity to standardize on technologies from one vendor, consolidated service agreements, and a consistent performance level based on the extent of the relationship.

Criteria on which such agreements should be evaluated include the match between the vendor's offerings and organization requirements, trends for future developments, flexibility with respect to alternative choices, cultural synergies between the organizations, and the extent of favorable contractual conditions. Once established, such agreements require sustained commitment on the part of both parties to make them work. Such agreements should anticipate that issues of disagreement will arise, and to the extent possible contain language that addresses these possibilities. In the event of disagreement and dispute, the ability to work these out will be defined by the strength of the agreement and the depth of the respective commitments.

While corporate agreements do have advantages, situations do arise where the technology of a corporate partner is adequate, but alternatives better suited to the needs of the organization exist elsewhere. While this situation can be dealt with contractually, it will generally trigger conditions that dilute the strength of the agreement. As with any agreement of this nature, the risks and benefits that will accrue over the life of the agreement deserve careful precontractual consideration.

Qualified technology-based legal advice in developing the original contract is strongly recommended. Time and effort invested in the development of such agreements prior to signing offsets risks, and will yield dividends when difficulties arise.

Such corporate agreements should be driven and executed at the executive level, and the solicited participation of internal stakeholders will depend on management styles that exist at that level. The probability of success is enhanced when internal stakeholders are part of the process. Despite this obvious observation, it will be necessary for clinical engineers to assert their presence in the context of the value that they can contribute to the process along with other stakeholders. Certainly, they will be affected by the outcome, and as such should be in a position to influence contributing factors.

25.12.1 Forms of Corporate Agreement

Corporate agreements, should they be appropriate, can take a number of forms. One model, which has been found to be effective, includes two separate agreements, the first specifying the relationship between parties, such as purchase obligations, and benefits that accrue from the discharge of these obligations.

A second agreement, in the form of a master purchase agreement, defines conditions of purchase, including obligations of the vendor with respect to supply, and obligations of the purchaser with respect to acceptance and payment. Conditions and remedies for nonperformance are also included in this agreement.

For each individual purchase, a schedule to the master purchase agreement is generated. This schedule details specifications and requirements for the individual item or system, and provides the opportunity to override or extend the conditions contained in the master agreement.

If necessary and desirable, a third agreement, relating to service of items purchased on individual schedules can be negotiated. Such an agreement contains conditions that would normally be found in any service contract.

25.13 SUMMARY

Technology planning in health care is a process which provides a framework for the identification of technology needs for health-care organizations. There are many stakeholders and professionals involved in this process, one of which is clinical engineering. The role that clinical engineers play will be situational, and can vary from one of leadership in the process, that is, as a process facilitator, to one of active participation, ensuring that the technology is appropriate, efficacious, and optimized with respect to its environment.

Technology has been subdivided into four distinct categories: strategic technologies, information technologies, technology infrastructure, and renewal of existing technologies. The rationale for each and a discussion of approaches are provided. It is proposed that each be allocated a separate technology budget to avoid the particular problems of large-cost items financially overwhelming lower-cost items. The total technology budget will be a measure of the extent to which an organization is prepared to invest in technology in order to achieve its strategic objectives.

The gap between significant medical devices and information systems is gradually closing, and will continue to do so, to the point where it is now appropriate to consider the technology continuum. Information technology being the integrating technology will tend to dominate. An emphasis has been placed on the relationship between clinical engineering and information technology with the message that organizational interests are best served through a cooperative approach.

Even though the technology plan is driven by the strategic plan, it is subject to the same scrutiny and challenge as any other plans requiring allocation of resources. It therefore requires careful preparation and advocacy throughout the review process. Technology requires scrutiny in the context of the key end-point parameters, of which the most important is the extent to which it improves patient outcomes. Measurement of patient outcomes is a developing science, which in itself requires information technology to provide the necessary data.

A clear distinction is drawn between technology planning and technology management. The domains are interdependent with clearly defined links between them. The more familiar domain for clinical engineers is that of technology management, and a transition to technology planning requires the adoption of new skills or cooperation with other professionals where these skills are already available.

Finally, the success of any technology-based endeavor is significantly dependent on the skills of people who will be involved in the strategy, planning, implementation, and use of the technologies. The need for quality people cannot be overemphasized, for without such people the probability of success is significantly diminished.

In times of fiscal restraint, the first casualty is often technology-based capital spending. A well-structured technology plan clearly defines the consequences of such actions, and permits rational choices to be made.

REFERENCES

1. Mathews P, "Leveraging technology for success," *J Health Care Manag*, 2000 Summer;**14**(2): 5–12.

2. Weil TP, "Comparisons of medical technology in Canadian, German and U.S. hospitals," *Hosp Health Serv Adm*, 1995 Winter;**40**(4):524–33.

3. Prince TR, Sullivan JA, "Financial viability, medical technology, and hospital closures." *J Health Care Finance,* 2000 Summer;**26**(4):1–18.

4. Sheldon WC, "Trends in cardiac catheterization laboratories in the United States," *Catheter Cardiovasc Interv,* 2001 May;**53**(1):40–5.
5. Patail BM, Arahana AN, "Role of the biomedical engineering department in William Beaumont Hospital's technology assessment process," *J Clin Eng*, 1995 July-August;**20**(4):290–6.
6. Singer PA, Martin DK, Giacomini M, Purdy L, "Priority setting for new technologies in medicine: qualitative case study," *BMJ,* 2000 Nov. 25;**321**:1316–1318.
7. Perleth M, Busse R, Schwartz FW, "Regulation of health related technologies in Germany," *Health Policy*, 1999 January;**46**(2):105–26.
8. Handbook: *Case Studies—How Boards and Senior Management Have Governed ICT Projects to Succeed (or Fail)*, Standards Australia HB 280-2006; ISBN 0733777082.
9. Manninen PH, Kucharczyk W, "A new frontier: magnetic resonance imaging-operating room," *J Neurosurg Anesthesiol*, 2000 April;**12**(2):141–8.
10. Jolez FA, Nabavi A, Kikinis R, "Integration of interventional MRI with computer assisted surgery," *J Magn Reson Imaging*, 2001 January;**13**(1):69–77.
11. Nerem RM, "Tissue engineering: confronting the transplantation crisis," *Proc Inst Mech Eng [H]*, 2000;**214**(1):95–9.
12. Broeders IA, Niessen W, van der Werken C, van Vroonhoven TJ, "[The operating room of the future]," *Ned Tijdschr Geneeskd,* 2000, Apr. 15;**144**(16):773–4. [Article in Dutch].
13. Allan JD, Tolley DA, "Virtual endoscopy in urology," *Curr Opin Urol,* 2001 March;**11**(2):189–92.
14. Tronnier VM, Staubert A, Bonsanto MM, Wirtz CR, Kunze S, "[Virtual reality in neurosurgery]," *Radiologe,* 2000 March;**40**(3):211–17. [Article in German].
15. Tanriverdi H, Iacono CS, "Diffusion of telemedicine: a knowledge barrier perspective," *Telemed J*, 1999 Fall;**5**(3):223–44.
16. Rogers TL, "Hospital–based technology assessment," *J Clin Eng*, 2002 Fall;276–9.
17. Valk PE, "Clinical trial of cost effectiveness in technology evaluation," *Q J Nucl Med,* 2000 June;**44**(2):197–203.
18. Papatheofanis FJ, "Health technology assessment," *Q J Nucl Med,* 2000 June;**44**(2):105–11.
19. Crepea AT, "A systems engineering approach to technology assessment," *J Clin Eng,* 1995 July-August;**20**(4):297–303.
20. Roberts, G, "Supporting children with serious health care needs. Analyzing the costs and benefits," *Eval Health Prof*, 2001 March;**24**(1):72–83.
21. Thompson DI, Sirio C, Holt P, "The strategic use of outcome information," *Jt Comm J Qual Improv*, 2000 October;**26**(10):576–86.
22. Mira A, Lehmann C, "Pre-analytical workflow analysis reveals simple changes and can result in improved hospital efficiency," *Clin Leadersh Manag Rev,* 2001 January-February;**15**(1):23–9.
23. "HTA 101: II. Fundamental concepts," National Information Center on Health Services Research and Healthcare Technology (NICHSR). Available at http://www.nlm.nih.gov/nichsr/hta101/ ta10104.html; accessed, 2008 Mar. 3.
24. Fryback DG, Thornbury JR, "The efficacy of diagnostic imaging," *Med Dec Making,* 1991; **11**(2):88–94.
25. Gregor S, Maegele M, Sauerland S, Krahn JF, Peinemann F, Lange S, "Negative pressure wound therapy a vacuum of evidence," *Arch Surg*, 2008 February;**143**(2):189–196.
26. Waugh N, Black C, Walker S, McIntyre L, Cummins E, Hills G, "The effectiveness and cost-effectiveness of computed tomography screening for coronary artery disease: systematic review," *Health Technol Assess*, 2006;**10**(39).
27. "Multidetector computed tomography for coronary artery disease screening in asymptomatic populations," The Medical Advisory Secretariat Ministry of Health and Long Term Care, Ontario, Canada, 2007 May, ISBN 9781424952632.
28. "Contrast-enhanced cardiac computed tomographic angiography for coronary artery evaluation," Blue Cross and Blue Shield Association Assessment Program, 2006 May, **20**(4).
29. Matchar DB, Mark DB, Patel MR, Hurwitz LM, Orlando LA, McCrory DC, Sanders GD, "Non-invasive imaging for coronary artery disease duke evidence-based practice center," Agency for Healthcare Research and Quality, 2006 Oct. 3.

30. *Dynamic Volume CT*, Toshiba, Tokyo, Japan, 105–8001.
31. Broadstock M, "Computed tomographic (CT) colonography for the detection of colorectal cancer–a technical brief," *N Z Health Technol Assess*, 2007 June, **6**(6).
32. Loong TW, "Understanding sensitivity and specificity with the right side of the brain," *BMJ*, 2003;**327:**716–719.
33. INHTA Secretariat, Stockholm, Sweden, "A checklist for health technology assessment reports," 2001, July 1–9.
34. Stevens AJ, Raftery J, Roderick P, "Can health technologies be assessed using routine data?" *Int J Technol Assess Health Care*, 2005;**21**(1):96–103.
35. Parzsolt F, Kajnar H, Awa A, Fassler M, Herzberger B, "Validity of original studies in health technology assessment reports: significance of standardized assessment and reporting," *Int J Technol Assess Health Care,* 2006;**21**(3):410–3.
36. Kamerow D, "Paying for promising but unproven technologies," *BMJ*, 2007;**335:**965.
37. Levin L, Goeree R, Sikich N, Jorgensen B, Brouwers MC, Easty T, Zhan C, "Establishing a comprehensive continuum from an evidentiary base to policy development for health technologies: the Ontario experience," *Int J Technol Assess Health Care*, 2007;**23**(3):299–309.
38. James CH, CHU WCH, Hubbard L, Yankee Z, Bernard D, Reeder P, Lopes D, "Performance of magnetic field-guided navigation system for interventional neurosurgical and cardiac procedures," *J App Clint Med Phys*, 2005;**6**(3):143–9.
39. Technology and Trends, "Robotic Platform for Catheter Mapping Improves Access to Areas of the Heart," *J Clin Eng,* 2007 July/September, 94.
40. American Hospital Association, *Continued Progress Hospital Use of Information Technology,* 2007:1–20.
41. Menachemi N, Brooks RG, "Exploring the return on investment associated with health information technologies," College of Medicine, Center on Patient Safety, Florida State University, 2007 February.
42. Austin CJ, Hornberger KD, Shmerling JE, "Managing information resources: a study of ten healthcare organizations," *J Health Care Manag*, 2000 July-August;**45**(4):229–38.
43. Souther E, "Implementation of the electronic medical record: the team approach," *Comput Nurs*, 2001 March-April;**19**(2):47–55.
44. Dansky KH, Gamm LD, Vasey JJ, Barsukiewicz CK, "Electronic medical record: are physicians ready?" *J Health Care Manag*, 1999 November-December;**44**(6):440–54.
45. Unkel PJ, Shelton PD, Inamdar R, "Picture archiving and communications system planning: a methodology," *J Digit Imaging,* 1999 August;**12**(3):144–9.
46. Rivers JA, Rivers PA, "The ABCs for deciding on a decision support system in the health care industry," *J Health Hum Serv Adm,* 2000 Winter;**22**(3):346–53.
47. Hyman WA, "Is the 800-lb information technology gorilla a permanent resident, or is it just visiting?" *J Clin Eng,* 2008 January/March;43–45.
48. Healthcare Information and Management Systems Society, *Enterprise Integration: Defining the Landscape*, 2007.
49. www.ihe.org. Accessed, 2008 Mar. 3.
50. IHE Patient Care Device Technical Framework, Year 1: 2006-2007: Volume 1 Integration Profiles, 2006;**08**:15.
51. "Implementation of health level 7 (HL7) version 2.4, part 3 electronic messages for exchange of information on drug prescription," Standards Australia, AS 4700.3-2005.
52. "Integrating the Healthcare Enterprise," *IHE Radiology User's Handbook*, 2005 June 20.
53. Electronic Child Health Network (eCHN), Toronto, Ontario, Canada, www.echn.ca, accessed, 2008 Mar. 3.
54. "The national programme for IT in the NHS," National Audit Office UK, 2006 June 15. Available at http://www.nao.org.uk/publications/0506/department_of_health_the_nati.aspx. Accessed, 2008 Mar. 3.
55. Gregoriades A, Sutcliffe A, "Workload prediction for improved design and reliability of complex systems," *Reliability Engineering and System Safety*, 2008;**93**(4):530–549.
56. Blaha J, White M, "Power of Lean in the Laboratory: A Clinical Application," 2005, Available at www.healthcare.isixsigma.com/library/content/c051207a.asp. Accessed, 2008 Mar. 3.

57. Herasuta M, "A 'lean' laboratory," *Labmedicine*, 2007 March;**38**(3):143–4.

58. Hurley B, Taylor T, Levett J, Huber C, Hahn E, "Implementation of six sigma and lean methodology into the anticoagulation management process," *J Thromb Thrombolysis,* 2008;**25**(1):106.

59. Greig HE, "Using LEAN thinking in staffing a new clinical laboratory," Presentation B-94, *XIX International Congress of Clinical Chemistry/2005 AACC Annual Meeting*.

60. Khorasani R, "Business continuity and disaster recovery: PACS as a case example," 2008 February; **5**(2):144–5.

61. McClanahan K, "Balancing good intentions: protecting the privacy of electronic health information," *Bull Sci Technol Soc*, 2008;**28**(1):69–79.

62. "Health Insurance Portability and Accountability Act of 1996," Public Law 104-191, 104th U.S. Congress.

63. "Personal Health Information Protection Act, 2004," Government of Ontario, Canada, 2004.

64. Manno MS, "Preventing adverse drug events," *Nursing,* 2006;**36**(3):56–61.

65. Fields M, "Intravenous medication safety system avers high-risk medication errors and provides actionable data," *Nurs Admin Q*, 2005;**29**(1):78–87.

66. Simon K, "Pareto Chart," Available at http://healthcare.isixsigma.com/library/content/ c010527a.asp, Accessed, 2008 Mar. 3.

67. ECRI Institute, "Evaluation general purpose infusion pumps," *Health Devices,* 2007 October; **36**(10):307–29.

68. ECRI Institute, "Evaluation syringe infusion pumps with dose error reduction systems," *Health Devices*, 2008 February;**37**(2):31–56.

69. Booth ME, Philip G, "Information systems management: role of planning, alignment and leadership," *Behav Inf Technol*, 2005;**24**(5):391–404.

70. ECRI Institute, 5200 Butler Pike, Plymouth Meeting, PA, 19462-1298, U.S.A.

71. Rasmussen N, "Guidelines for specification of data center power density," White Paper No. 120, 2005, American Power Conversion.

72. ACCE Healthcare Technology Foundation, "Impact of clinical alarms on patient safety," *J Clin Eng,* 2007 January/March:22–33.

73. Barker SJ, "'Motion-resistant' pulse oximetry: a comparison of new and old models," *Anesth Analg*, 2002;**95:**967–72.

74. Carr JJ, "Requirements management: keeping your technology acquisition project under control," *J Nurs Admin*, 2000 March;**30**(3):133–9.

75. Zimmer BT, "Project management: a methodology for success," *Hosp Mater Manage Q,* 1999 November;**21**(2):83–9.

76. Abendshien J, "Managing the future," *Health Forum J,* 2001 January-February;**44**(1):26–8, 46.

77. Neumann CL, Blouin AS, Byrne EM, "Achieving success: assessing the role of and building a business case for technology in healthcare," *Front Health Serv Manage,* 1999 Spring; **15**(3):3–28.

78. Thoiin MF, Hoffman JJ, Ford EW, "The effect of information technology investment on firm-level performance in the health care industry," *Health Care Manag Rev*, 2008;**3391**:60–8.

CHAPTER 26
AN OVERVIEW OF HEALTH CARE FACILITIES PLANNING

John Michael Currie
EwingCole, Washington, DC

26.1 INTRODUCTION

26.1.1 Health Care Facilities Planning

The business of health care facility design is all about the future. We cannot plan well simply to correct today's facility shortcomings. In dealing with the future of health care, the future of technology is critical.

The process of planning and design is made up of several sequential steps. Each step builds on the information created and the decisions made in the preceding one. The process is often not linear. Alternative ideas are tested and the results combined. This chapter concentrates on the work leading up to commencement of the construction activity on site. This chapter also assumes that the process of planning for and including medical technology and equipment is an intrinsic part of designing a health facility in a responsible manner. Separate consultants can help in this process, provided they are brought into the project from the beginning. As the work progresses, the opportunity to positively influence its direction with valuable input on medical technology consideration diminishes. Hospital technology specialists need to take a place at the table at the beginning of the process and must monitor the design for compliance with the technology plans of the institution.

26.1.2 Historical Overview

> "The building or buildings should be simple in style and designed to make a pleasing impression upon the patients . . . Hospital planning demands the same careful thought that is the foundation of any modern successful business enterprise. . . . The hospital planner must seek to eliminate here all lost motion or unnecessary work."
>
> EDWARD F. STEVENS, *The American Hospital of the Twentieth Century*

In these few simple statements, made in 1918, architect Edward F. Stevens has captured ideas that are still central today in hospital planning. While Stevens could not anticipate the enormous growth in medical knowledge, technique, and technology that would come to bear in the fullness of the twentieth century, his works have covered four important goals of hospital facility planning today:

1. Simplicity of design
2. Focus on the patient
3. Understanding of function
4. Design to support medical activities

Early hospital architectural designs, the Greek Asklepieion and the Roman Valetudinarium, were forms adapted from buildings already in use. The Asklepieion (Fig. 26.1) was simply a stoa or public business arcade put to medical use. The Valetudinarium (Fig. 26.2) was a military barracks building modified for the sick. These plans are derived from other uses, and the planner had few opportunities to introduce design for the specific needs of the medical staff.

Early Christian monasticism and the constant flow of travelers and pilgrims brought the first hospices into being. The hospice of Turmanin (475 AD) in Syria received all travelers, sick or well, in the convent building, with nursing care provided for those in need. This building contains an early example of the open ward with deep porticos on all four sides.

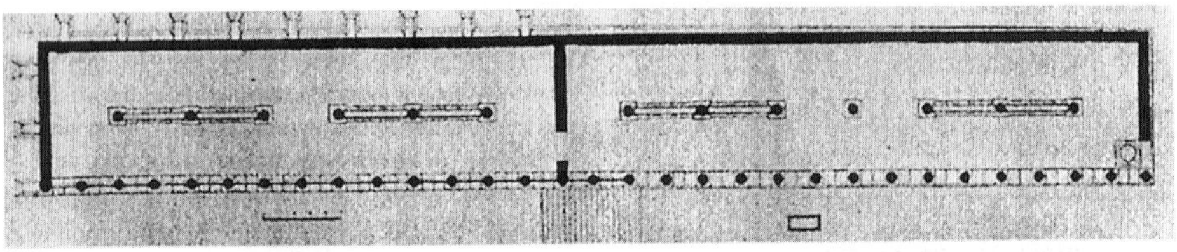

FIGURE 26.1 Stoa plan (Greek Asklepieion).

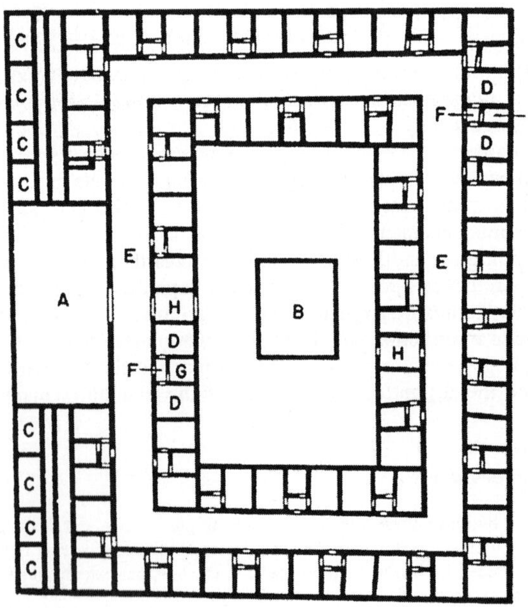

FIGURE 26.2 Valetudinarium plan (Roman).

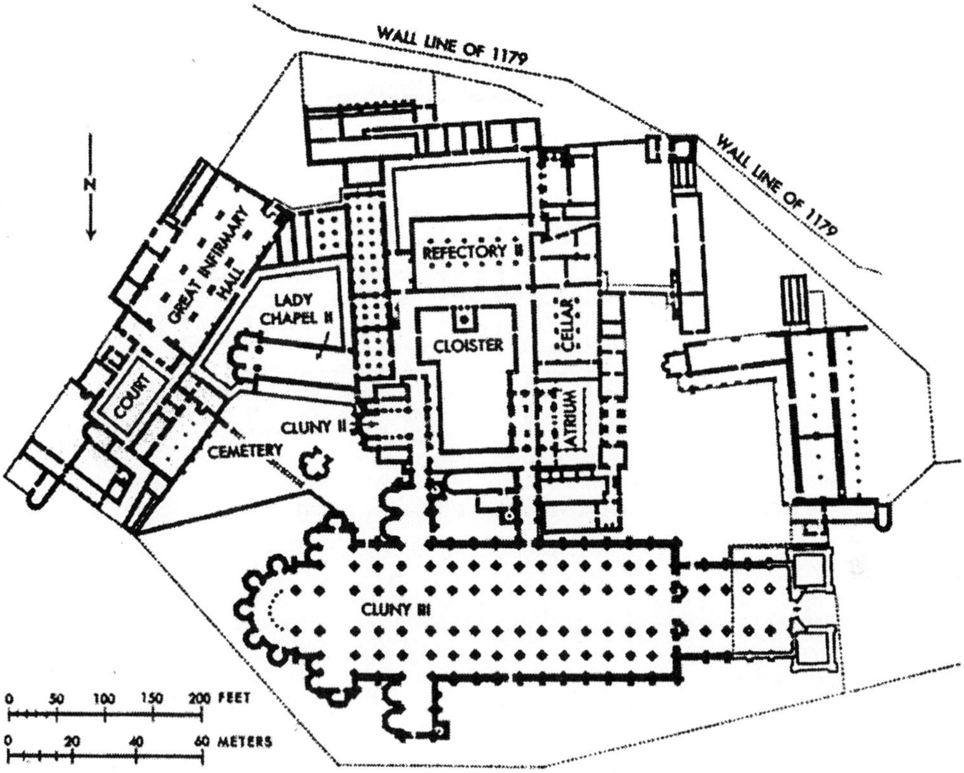

FIGURE 26.3 Cluny Monastery plan.

The famous monastery of St. Gall in Switzerland (820 AD) had more specific portions of the overall plan devoted to medical care and medical staff. Its plan clearly shows separate facilities for bloodletting, physician housing, infirmary, kitchens, bathing facilities for the sick, and medicinal herb garden.

Many other important European monastic centers cared for patients throughout the Middle Ages. Notable among these are the Great St. Bernard Hospital (960 AD) in Switzerland and Cluny (1050 AD) in France (Fig. 26.3).

The era of the hospital began in the twelfth century when the sick were to be housed in separate buildings designed for medical care. Examples include St. Bartholomew's Hospital (London, 1123 AD) and St. Thomas' Hospital (London, 1200 AD). Both hospitals are in service today, having been founded again in the mid-1500s due to the dissolution of the monasteries in England in 1536 AD.

Early general hospitals were established throughout Europe during the sixteenth and seventeenth centuries. The pavilion plan was developed in the mid-nineteenth century. This concept was supported by the writings of Florence Nightingale (*Notes on Hospitals,* 1859). These hospitals, arranged into an interconnected series of small patient care buildings, were designed to help control infection, provide separation of various types of patients, and promote natural light and ventilation.

Three main causes influenced the development of specialist hospitals:

1. A growing patient population excluded from general hospitals, such as pregnant women, children, people suffering from contagious disease, and patients requiring a long length of stay
2. Emerging medical and nursing specialties
3. Individual entrepreneurs founding their own hospitals and clinics to promote their private practices

Key
1 Ward
2 Nurse's room
3 Mess room
4 Matron's sitting-room
5 Scullery
6 Board room
7 Bedroom
8 Waiting-room for midwives
9 Pantry

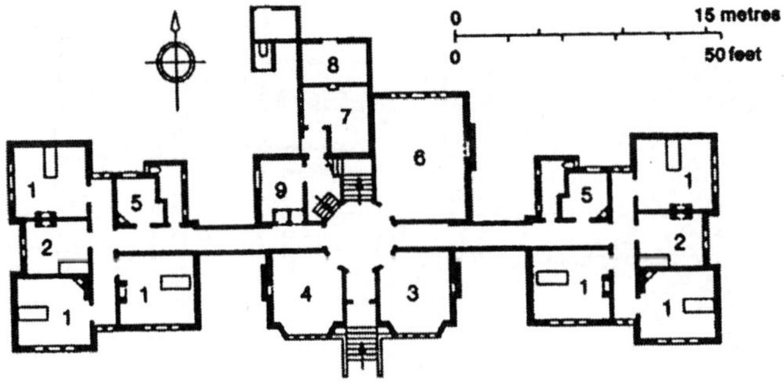

FIGURE 26.4 Plan of Liverpool Lying-In Hospital (1880s).

Key
1 Ward
2 Duty-room
3 Operating room
4 Stove
5 Examination room
6 Consulting-room
7 Dressing-room
8 Dispensary
9 Matron's sitting-room
10 Board room
11 Secretary's room
12 Bedroom
13 Waiting-room
14 Entrance hall
15 Medical Institute

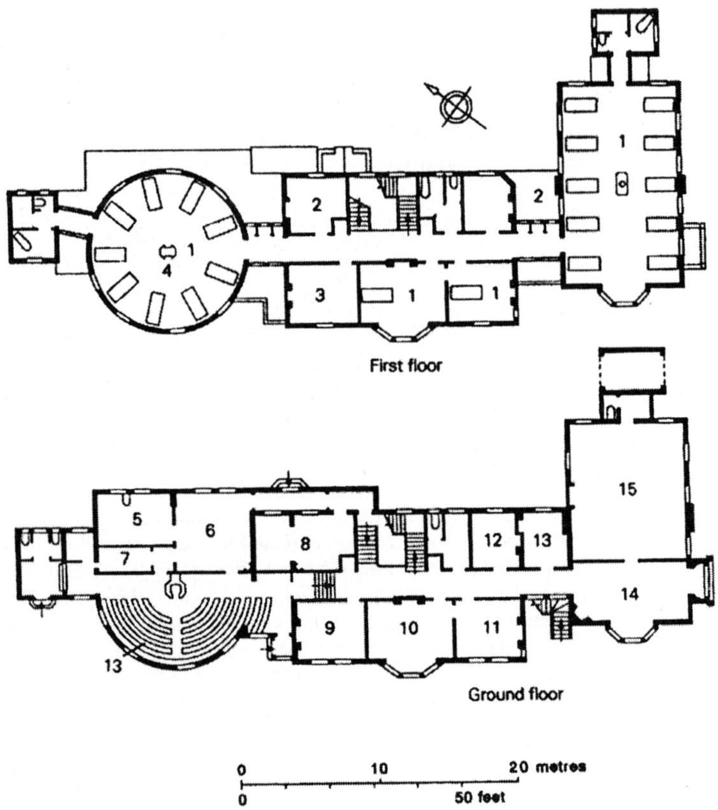

FIGURE 26.5 Plan of Anderson Hospital (London, 1889).

Maternity or lying-in hospitals were among the earliest of specialty hospitals. The Liverpool Lying-In Hospital (Fig. 26.4) was separated from the Hospital for Women to help control infection, again supported by Nightingale's recommendations. One can see from the plan of this building that the architect has created separation between nursing and support functions.

Looking at the plan of the Anderson Hospital in London (1889) (Fig. 26.5), the ward area is seen as a circular room supporting ease of nursing and good visualization of patients but not much privacy for those in bed.

The work of John Shaw Billings, MD, at Johns Hopkins Hospital in the late 1870s and 1880s is shown in Fig. 26.6. Collaborating with the architect, Billings proposed plans that took into account the control of infection, growth and flexibility, separation, natural light, and ventilation. Billings clearly saw that whatever design was built, continuing scientific advantages would necessitate change:

> . . . no matter what plan is adopted . . . it will appear that it can be improved and a certain amount of funds should be reserved for that purpose. The general principles which I have tried to state . . . are in accordance with the present condition of our knowledge of the subject, but that knowledge is imperfect, and too much of the teaching of books on the subject of hospital construction is theoretical only (J. S. Billings, MD, 1875).

Dr. Billings was right, and today we continue to follow his advice when developing facility plans for health care facilities.

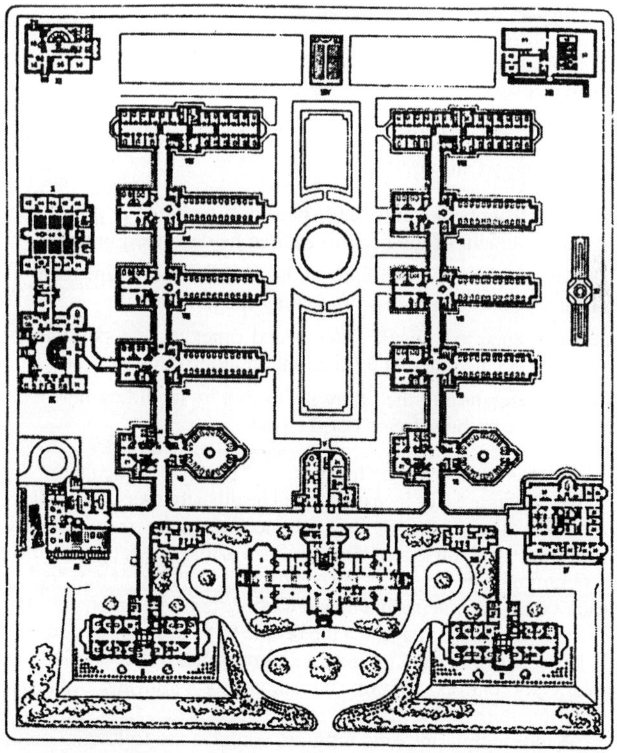

FIGURE 26.6 John Shaw Billings plan for Johns Hopkins Hospital (Baltimore, 1870s) (modified by Architect John Niernsee for the Johns Hopkins trustees).

26.2 HEALTH CARE FACILITIES PLANNING AND DESIGN

The planning of health care facilities is a unique area of endeavor. The unique character of this work comes from the fact that the patient and family are silent users of the space represented by all the members of the planning and design team. This responsibility to uphold the future well-being of these patients gives the process an added dimension.

It is useful to discuss this process by describing it in phases. These phases or steps are given different names by various groups, but the activities are common to all projects. The American Institute of Architects, as an industry standard, is the source for terms describing the various phases of planning and design through construction and occupancy. In this chapter, I will confine my discussion to the work leading up to construction activities.

The health facility planning and design phases are

- Programming
- Schematic design
- Design development
- Construction documents

Each succeeding phase builds on the preceding one as decisions are made and the design solution is refined. In order for this process to produce good results, all participants should be completely clear in their understanding of the decisions to be made. This is a process of interaction and challenge. All ideas to improve the design solution and all relevant facts must be openly and honestly sought out, discussed, and evaluated.

26.2.1 Programming

Programming is the first major phase of work that the project team undertakes. Programming has several important purposes:

1. Input from health care facility users is gathered in this phase. By preparing a thorough program, each element of the department can be described in detail.
2. Communication with and guidance from the entire team are recorded to be used and refined throughout the process of creating the new facility.
3. Adherence to budget, criteria, and other project parameters can be checked and controlled as space is calculated and functional relationships recorded.
4. An orientation to the future is ensured by including new technology considerations and avoiding reliance of the solutions of the past.

Programs are prepared for the use of the team by health facility architects, by consultants who specialize in this area, or by experienced health care users. Regardless of the authorship source, it is imperative that the programmer be a full member of the planning team who stays with the work of creating the project. The program will be refined as the project goes forward, and continuity is important when programming decisions are reconsidered in the light of developing design solutions. Programs consider each space, each department, and each system to be included. Programs describe (1) the activity to be carried out in each space, (2) the people to be accommodated, (3) the technical and support equipment to be included, (4) the furniture and furnishings to be supplied, (5) the physical environment (and environmental controls), (6) critical relationships within and among spaces, (7) the size and makeup of each department, (8) relationships among departments, and (9) the size and makeup of the entire project.

A thoroughly prepared program contains the following components:

- Space listings and area tabulations
- Diagrams

SPACE PROGRAM DRAFT

Room #	Room name	Number of spaces	Net area each space	Total net area	Remarks
	CHEMOTHERAPY				
	Patient/Family Waiting	1	300	300	
	Reception	1	120	120	
	Toilets	2	60	120	
	Patient Treatment - Private	8	100	800	with toilet
	Patient Treatment - 4 Patient	4	280	1120	with toilet
	Patient Treatment - 8 Patient	2	480	960	with toilet
	Nurse Work Area	1	200	200	
	MD Work Area	1	200	200	
	Admin Office	1	120	120	
	Clean Utility	1	100	100	
	Soiled Utility	1	100	100	
	Housekeeping Closet	1	50	50	
	Pharmacy	1	500	500	
	Research Pharmacy	1	500	500	
	Research Office	1	100	100	
	Research Nurse/QA	1	100	100	
	Interview/consult Room	1	100	100	
	subtotal				5490
	Pheresis Unit	1	2000	2000	program to be determined
	subtotal				2000

FIGURE 26.7 Sample space listing.

- Room data sheets
- Equipment and furniture
- Technical data sheets on critical equipment systems
- Written functional statements

Space listings and area tabulations are the heart of the program. A number of forms are possible. Commonly, these listings are organized into functional groupings, and then quantities are added. These space listings (Fig. 26.7) must be established using some mutually agreed on forecast of future workload. This can take the form of procedures, visits, or operating room minutes. It is essential that the need for space be directly linked to and driven by a disciplined forecast of future activity.

The areas shown are net, that is, exclusive of walls, doors, structure, and sometimes cabinetry. The areas need to be based on serious discussions among the users plus attention paid to codes and standards that apply to the project. The areas shown need to include full consideration to equipment and other technology that will operate within these rooms. Allowances for departmental gross area must be included to provide appropriate circulation, walls, doors, cabinetry, mechanical and electrical systems, and other items. The remarks column within the space listing spreadsheet can contain cues for designers and planners to read further or to refer to functional diagrams included in other sections of the program document.

The inclusion of room and department diagrams increases the usefulness of the program document. The facility planning and design process is highly dependent on graphics, drawings, and other visual items and is conducted largely by professionals who use graphics to record and communicate ideas. Not every space is so demanding that a diagram such as that in Fig. 26.8 is required, but it is clear that words and numbers alone would not completely explain the complexities of the operating room.

Department organization and critical relationships between spaces can be illustrated simply by an adjacency matrix diagram, as shown in Fig. 26.9. This information provides critical guidance for the design team.

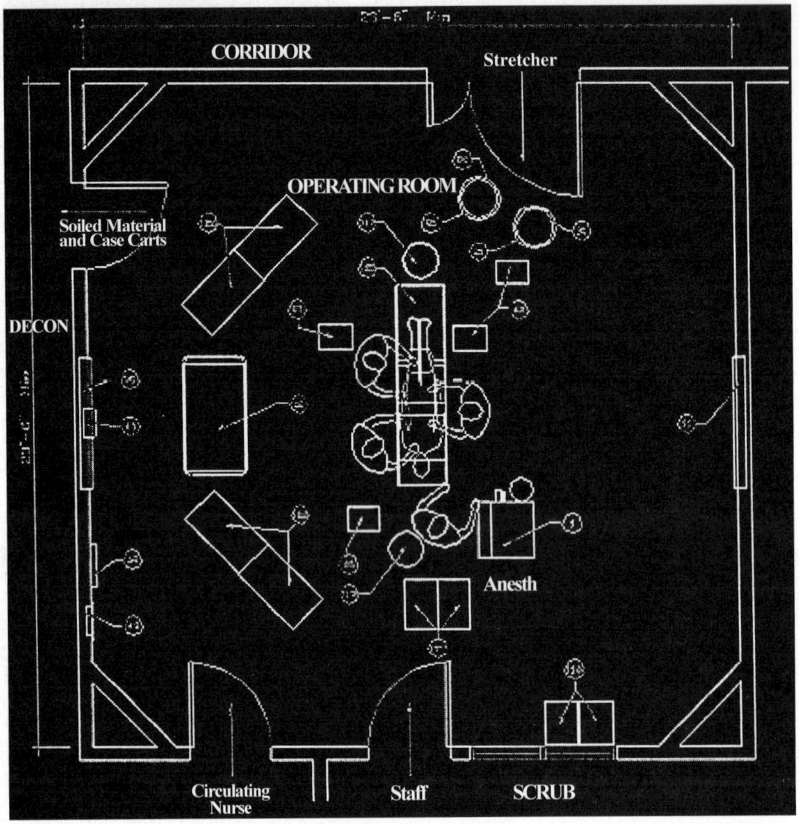

FIGURE 26.8 Sample operating room diagram.

Room data sheets are extremely valuable vehicles for carefully recording information about each space. An example, shown in Fig. 26.10, demonstrates the range of facility information that can be shown for the designers and engineers working on the project.

Space programs are concerned with describing rooms/spaces that contain technical equipment. Equipment and furniture lists are important to guide designers and to create a complete picture of the project budget. A preliminary list, such as shown in Fig. 26.11, can be modified as design and knowledge progress on the project. Including this type of information is an important notice to designers that equipment/systems must not be added in later (or forgotten entirely).

If understanding a particular equipment item is critical to the successful layout of the room or must be considered in developing engineering systems, then a technical data sheet can be added to this part of the program document. It is unlikely that a specific choice of equipment will be made in final form at the programming stage of a project, but including the technical data sheet as an example will ensure that appropriate space, floor loading, HVAC, and other provisions are made. Manufacturer-supplied material can be used and marked as "Preliminary—subject to change."

Each programmed department should be described in writing by including a written functional statement. Department health care staff members are well equipped to supply this information, which should include

- An overall summary of the department
- Staffing and hours of operation
- Workload history and forecasts

	RECEIVING	BULK STORES	PROCESSED STORES	DECONTAM	LINEN	PACK AND STERILIZATION	PHARMACY
RECEIVING		1	2	3	1	3	1
BULK STORES			1	2	2	1	1
PROCESSED STORES				1	1	1	2
DECONTAM					1	2	2
LINEN						1	3
PACK AND STERILIZATION							3
PHARMACY							

LEGEND	
Directly Adjacent	1
Corridor Connection	2
Indirect	3

FIGURE 26.9 Sample adjacency matrix.

- Descriptions of activities, procedures, and processes
- Any unique planning considerations, including technology issues

26.2.2 Design Phases

Schematic Design Phase. The American Institute of Architects' *Handbook of Professional Practice* describes the schematic design phase of a project as having the following purpose:

> Schematic Design establishes the general scope, conceptual design, scale, and relationships among the components of the project. The primary objective is to arrive at a clearly defined, feasible concept and to present it in a form that achieves understanding and acceptance. The secondary objectives are to clarify the project program, explore the most promising alternative design solutions, and provide a reasonable basis for analyzing the cost of the project.

Schematic design often begins with the creation of block diagrams that address the overall relationships between and among the various departments of the project. Block diagrams (Fig. 26.12) are established for each type of traffic. Circulation routes are studied on each floor to carefully separate traffic. Vertical circulation (stairs, elevations, service lifts, etc.) is planned.

At this very early stage of design, provisions for the communications and data technology must be considered and included within the block diagrams. Allowances for information technology (IT) equipment and cabling pathways within the building must be shown with sufficient accuracy that technology professionals can judge their adequacy. This is not a planning element that can be added in at a later stage of design.

Block diagrams should be drawn using a planning grid that will reflect a structural grid system. This will facilitate planning in later stages and avoid conflicts between desired floor plan arrangements and the structural system.

HEALTH CARE FACILITY ROOM DATA SHEET

PROJECT NAME

Project Number

Date | Prepared By

DEPARTMENT

ROOM NAME

ROOM NUMBER

GENERAL

Net Area | Occupant Count

Ceiling Height | Door Size and Type

Room Function

ROOM FINISHES

Floor | Walls

Base | Ceiling

Finish Notes

ROOM ACOUSTICS

Level of Speech Privacy | Absorption

Wall/Ceiling Performance | Other

Acoustics Notes

MECHANICAL REQUIREMENTS

Air Changes/Hour | Pressure Relationships | Filtration | Humidity

O/A Required | Exhaust Requirements | Temperature Control | Other

Equipment Connections

Mechanical Notes

ELECTRICAL and TELECOMMUNICATIONS REQUIREMENTS

Duplex Outlets | Special Outlets | Special Cabling

Room Illumination | Special Lighting | Telecom and Data Outlets

Equipment Connections | Other

Electrical Notes

PLUMBING AND PIPED SYSTEMS

HW | CW | Direct Drain | Special Waste

Floor Drain

Gas Outlets

Equipment Connections

Plumbing and Piped Systems Notes

EQUIPMENT NOTES

FIGURE 26.10 Sample room data sheet.

SPACE: 24.2004000 INFANT RESUSCITATION QTY. OF SPACES: 2

CAT.NUMBER	ITEM NAME	UNIT COST	QTY	EXT.COST	GRP	CAT	INST.COST
MAS CLK0500	CLOCK ELAPSED TIME	$ 0	1	$ 0	1	E	$ 0
MAS HDW0900	HEADWALL UNIT INTENSIVE	$ 0	1	$ 0	1	B	$ 0
MAS ICC0000	INFANT CARE CENTER	$ 0	1	$ 0	2	B	$ 0
MAS ILL0200	ILLUMINATOR, X-RAY FILM 2 PANEL	$ 0	1	$ 0	2	B	$ 0
MAS LTS0500	LIGHT EXAMINATION	$ 0	1	$ 0	2	B	$ 0
MAS OTS0000	OTOSCOPE/OPHTHALMOSCOPE SET	$ 0	1	$ 0	2	B	$ 0
MAS RSS1600	RESUSCITATOR PEDIATRIC	$ 0	1	$ 0	2	E	$ 0
MAS SCL0900	SCALE INFANT	$ 0	1	$ 0	3	B	$ 0
MAS SNK1900	SINK SCRUB	$ 0	1	$ 0	1	A	$ 0
MAS STD1300	STAND MAYO	$ 0	1	$ 0	3	B	$ 0
MAS STL0100	STOOL ANESTHETIST'S	$ 0	1	$ 0	3	B	$ 0
MAS TBL0900	TABLE INSTRUMENT	$ 0	1	$ 0	3	B	$ 0

FIGURE 26.11 Sample equipment list.

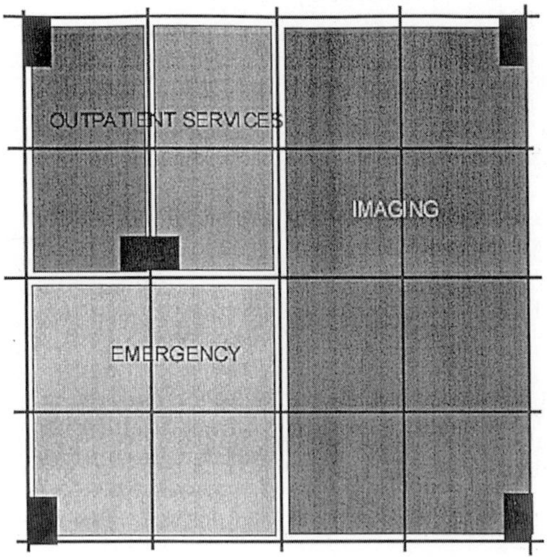

FIGURE 26.12 Sample block plan.

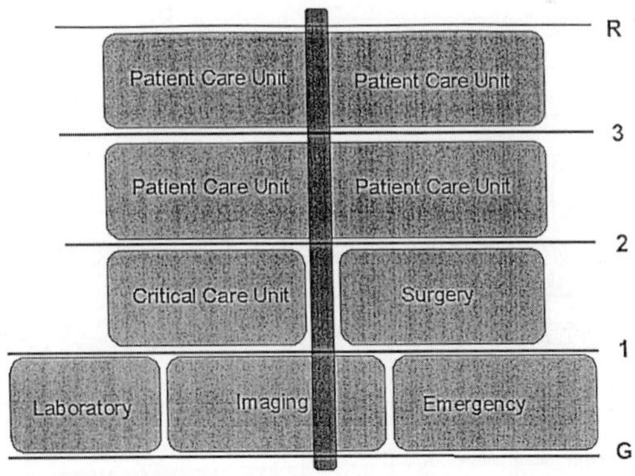

FIGURE 26.13 Sample blocking and stacking plan.

Block diagrams will also be considered in section showing vertical relationships (Fig. 26.13) from one floor to the next. The building height will be defined in this phase, and issues of floor-to-floor height can be decided. Departments that have high levels of engineered systems can be located so as to allow maximum space overhead, which will allow easy routing of ducted and piped systems without conflict.

Once all alternative block diagrams have been thoroughly considered and reviewed with hospital personnel, a single direction can be established for more detailed schematic design. Alternative

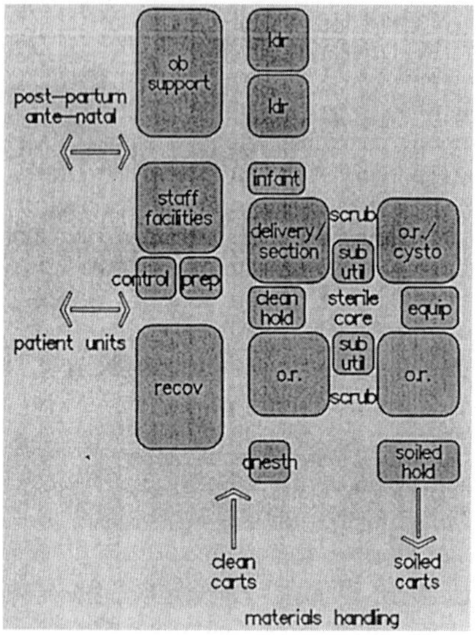

FIGURE 26.14 Sample department bubble diagram.

layouts for each department are studied using drawings called *bubble diagrams*.

Figure 26.14 shows a typical bubble diagram. Normally, several alternative arrangements are studied using diagrams such as these. Bubble diagrams can help the team study by showing

- Room-to-room relationships
- Circulation of staff and patients
- The basic size and shape of key spaces
- Provisions for critical support spaces
- Engineering and technology requirements

The success of the planning at this level depends in part on the completeness of the program documents prepared in the programming phase. Program material will guide the team as it studies and evaluates alternative layouts. Bubble diagrams are drawn to scale and also follow the planning grid. The selected diagram layout will be developed in more detail as single-line schematic drawings.

Figure 26.15 shows a typical single-line plan. Note that many details are left out, such as door swings and furniture and equipment placement. These important considerations will be relatively easy to add as plans are refined if they have been well described in the program and if those program data are kept in mind as the plan work progresses.

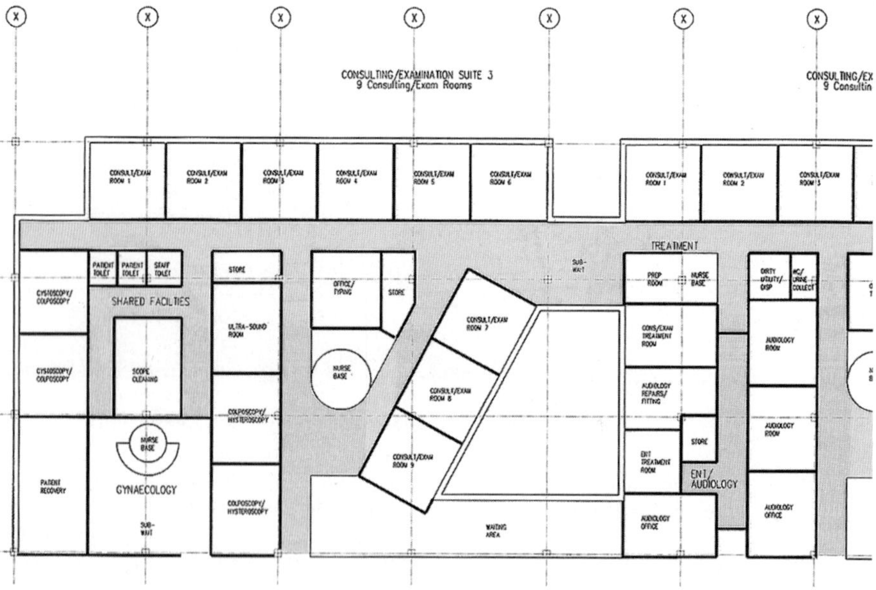

FIGURE 26.15 Sample single-line plan.

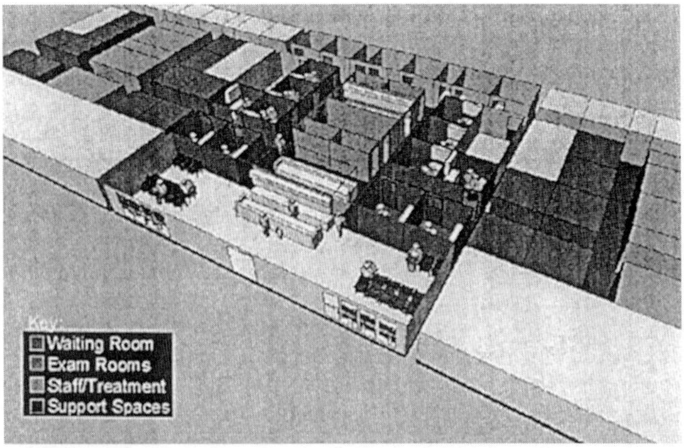

FIGURE 26.16 Sample 3D sketch.

Schematic plans are often difficult to fully interpret, and so three-dimensional (3D) sketches are quite useful in judging the success of the plan in meeting the objectives set out in the program. Figure 26.16 shows a 3D sketch drawn with a computer graphics program that very clearly demonstrates the various elements of the plan. Physical models also can be employed to illustrate elements of the schematic plan, but their usefulness is somewhat limited by the comparative lack of detail available.

During schematic design, it is also useful to prepare documents called outline specifications. *Outline specifications* describe the various construction contract elements in words citing industry standards, methods, and levels of quality. These documents provide an opportunity to clearly spell out each part of the construction, and they form an important part of the basis for estimating the cost of the project. The program-based equipment listings can be carried forward to be included within the outline specifications so that adequate consideration of the cost of equipment is made a part of the job. Further, these specifications should include clear technical provisions for

- Special piping systems
- Special wiring/cabling systems
- Information technology support
- Communications systems
- Critical environmental controls
- Other fixed items such as casework

Schematic design documents must be submitted together for a formal approval by all the user groups and to be accepted as the basis for moving ahead into the next phase of design.

Design Development Phase. *Design development* is the project phase in which the design is refined and coordinated among all the disciplines involved on the team. The schematic design work carried out in the preceding phase is brought forward, and detailed information is added. Each element of the project is worked out at a larger scale, and changes are incorporated as the team members see more detail and can arrive at additional decisions.

Design development begins with plans and sections drawn at increased scale so that users can see the functional and technical details of each space. As information is added, each room in the project should be assigned a unique identification number. This allows the team to track the refinement of the design of each room. Room data sheets prepared during programming can now be brought forward and keyed to these unique numbers. Similarly, equipment lists and technical data sheets are also keyed to the room numbering system. Each room or space will then have a data

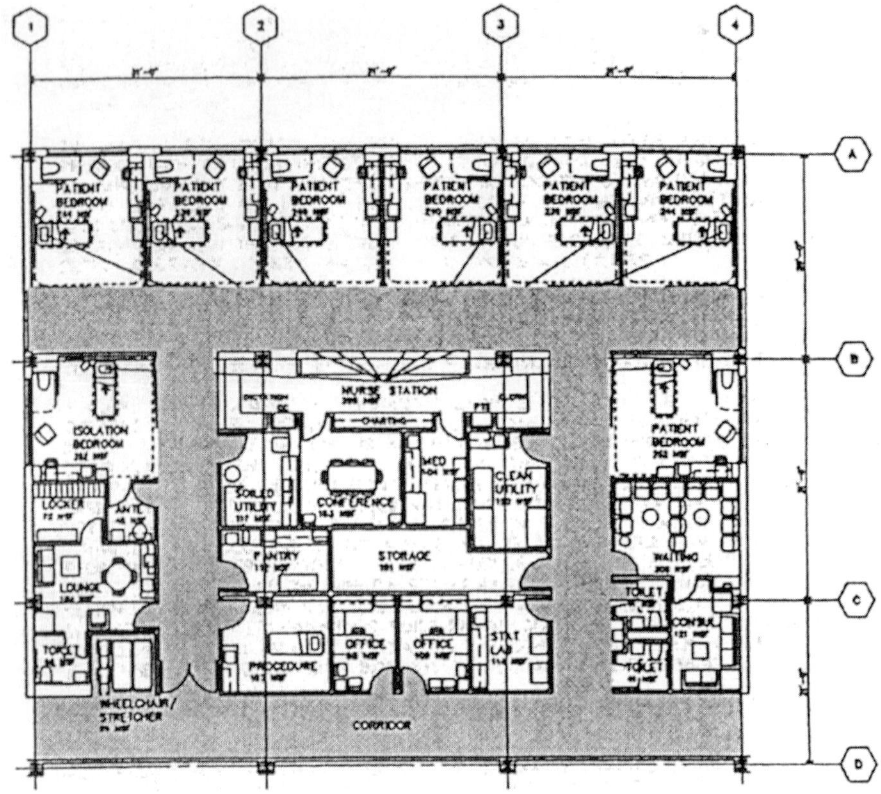

FIGURE 26.17 Sample design development drawing.

file that architects and engineers can use for design. Users will use the data file for monitoring the progress of the design and measuring the success of the design of each space in meeting functional and technical needs.

Design development floor plans, such as that shown in Fig. 26.17, contain the details that were not shown in schematic design. These include

- Wall thickness and special wall construction, including shielding or structural support
- Code-required construction for control of smoke spread, fire stopping, etc.
- Doors
- Fixed elements such as plumbing fixtures, cabinetry, etc.
- Equipment placement
- Furniture placement
- Building structure and engineering spaces

Design development also should include drawings that illustrate all wall and ceiling surfaces. Elevation drawings of wall surfaces, such as shown in Fig. 26.18, will illustrate the placement of electrical, piping, communication, and data outlets to scale, giving mounting heights above the floor and clearances for convenient use by hospital staff. These elevation drawings also show equipment (fixed and movable) to be attached or connected to ensure that the equipment will function and that adequate clearance is provided for service access.

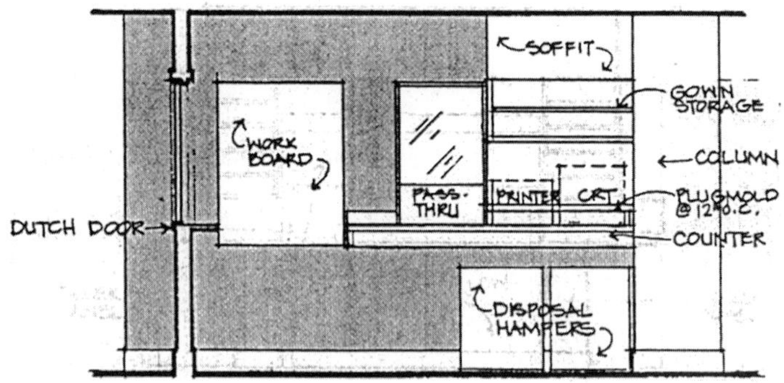

FIGURE 26.18 Sample interior elevation.

Reflected ceiling plans are useful in controlling the design of the ceiling plane. Figure 26.19 shows that each element (lighting, HVAC, fire-protection sprinkler heads, special systems, and ceiling-mounted equipment) can be installed and can operate properly.

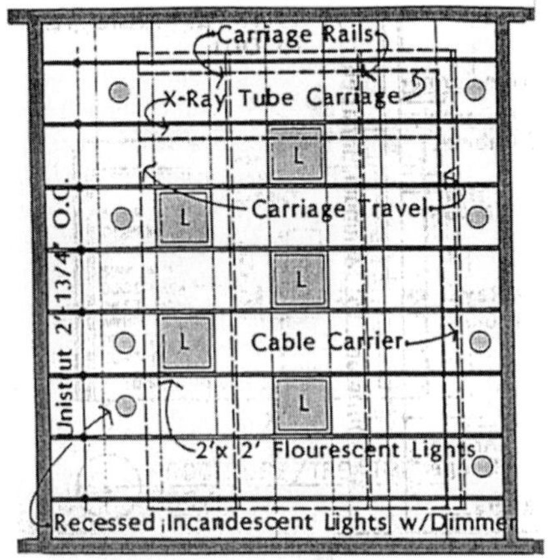

FIGURE 26.19 Sample ceiling plan.

During design development, additional information and detail are created. These are interior finish materials selection and casework and workstation design.

Each space or room will have materials assigned by the design team to be reviewed by users. One method of managing this new information is with a finish schedule. Much of these data can come directly from the room data sheets created during programming. This information will now need to be updated and refined. The finish schedule will eventually become an important component of the construction process. The design and placement of casework, workstations, shelving, and other cabinetry are an important part of design development. Each user must be satisfied that the patient care and other work processes to be supported by these items are thoroughly understood by the designers. Each element must be carefully considered. Computers, displays, benchtop equipment, and other critical elements must be drawn to scale and included in the design. It is quite common to build full-sized mockups or models of these workstations so that users can try out the new design before it is built. Workstations should be tested for user comfort, success in accommodating equipment, visual access to patients, and more.

There is no satisfactory substitute for a full-size mockup in discovering and correcting flaws in the design. The same can be said for critical full-room mockups as well. These have been used to produce excellent results in developing designs of rooms that contain critical new technology features.

Design development also addresses the full coordination of all the design disciplines involved in producing a complete architectural and engineering design for the project. Each department, each space, and all physical elements of the project are brought up to a similar level of design refinement. All systems (HVAC, structural, site/civil) and all specialty areas must be carefully designed and coordinated to avoid conflict. Design development leans heavily on the work done during programming and schematic design.

Design development documents must be published for user and hospital approval. Prior to this approval being obtained as notice to proceed into final working drawings, a cost estimate based on the design development package must be prepared. This is a critical juncture of the project effort, and the completeness of the work done to this point will help to avoid serious problems later in the project.

26.2.3 Construction Documents Phase (Working Drawings)

Most design issues will have been answered during the preceding phases of work. The construction documents phase is principally concerned with the creation of drawings and written instructions to be used by the various building trades in constructing the project. These documents become part of the contract between the owner and the builder. They have important legal consequences. They must be clear, accurate, and free from ambiguity.

The construction documents consist of three basic elements:

1. Specifications (discussed in earlier sections)
2. Drawings
3. Written contract provisions

Each element makes reference to the other and must be consistent, using similar language to mean the same in each instance. Each element is briefly discussed here.

Specifications generally fall into two categories. Descriptive specifications use words and make reference to industry standards to describe a method of construction or to describe a building product/material. Performance specifications use words and make reference to industry standards to make clear how a part of the construction is to perform. Both types are used successfully in health care facility construction. The project's final specifications are developed from the earlier outline specifications prepared during schematic design and design development. Specification writing is a highly specialized endeavor that is the responsibility of the design team and typically is carried out by a design professional with special qualifications in this area.

In medical facility construction, it is very common to have unresolved issues even this late in the design. An example of this is the procurement of certain types of equipment such as medical imaging systems that will be attached to the building but will be supplied by a third-party vendor. Such issues will need to be dealt with in the specifications so that the builder is fully aware that these late decisions will be coming and that funds must be included to accommodate the work to be done.

Certain items to be specified may be covered by proprietary specifications. These are items where no competitive alternative exists, and the owner is willing to state an exact make, model, or product name to be used exclusively.

Drawings will be prepared during this phase that will become a legal part of the contract for construction. These drawings are based on the work of earlier phases. The intended audience is the builder and individual trade workers, so the drawings focus on providing the data needed to successfully construct the building. Each element to be constructed is drawn in detail, with all dimensions and explanatory notes shown. In the case cited earlier of a delayed decision regarding equipment (say, for imaging), the drawings must show how the work is to be undertaken to allow for a later decision.

Written documents called General Conditions, Special Conditions, and Supplemental Conditions are included as important parts of the contract. These set down the various procedures to be followed by the contract parties in constructing the project. The American Institute of Architects publishes a model of these documents (AIA document A201) that is the standard of the construction industry.

26.2.4 Codes, Standards, and Industry Data

There are literally thousands of documents published by more thousands of authorities that provide information, best practices, professional criteria, and otherwise control every part of a project from inception to completion. We will deal here in outline form with those that influence the medical or technical aspects of planning the project.

Building codes that have been adopted by a government body have the force of law over the project. The team must comply with the provisions of the building code applied by the authority having jurisdiction over the project. This is usually a building department at the municipal or state level. Building codes often include sections of or references to other documents, most notably the Life Safety Code published by the National Fire Protection Association. Three code-making bodies publish codes in the United States, and several significant U.S. cities publish unique code for their municipalities.

- Building Officials and Code Administrators International (BOCA), publishers of the BOCA National Building Code
- International Conference of Building Officials (ICBO), publishers of the Uniform Building Code
- Southern Building Code Congress International (SBCCI), publishers of the Standard Building Code

These model codes, together with additional expert work of technical committees, have formed the basis for the building codes in force around the United States and have all been subsumed by the International Code Council (ICC). The ICC was established in 1994 as a nonprofit organization and is dedicated to developing and perfecting a single set of comprehensive and coordinated national model construction codes. There are advantages in combining the efforts of the existing code organizations to produce a single set of codes. Code enforcement officials, architects, engineers, designers, and contractors have access to consistent requirements throughout the United States.

In additional to the state-controlled building codes, a number of other important codes having legal standing are in force. These cover areas of architectural and engineering practice, such as

- Mechanical systems
- Plumbing and piped systems
- Fire protection and life safety
- Energy conservation
- Electrical systems
- Signage

Most code documents refer to a large body of construction industry standards. The American National Standards Institute and the American Society for Testing and Materials publish enormous volumes of important standards to be followed in designing a building, specifying products, and carrying out construction activities.

The National Fire Protection Association (NFPA), headquartered in Quincy, Massachusetts, is an international nonprofit (tax-exempt) membership organization founded in 1896. The mission of NFPA is to reduce the worldwide burden of fire and other hazards on the quality of life by developing and advocating scientifically based consensus codes and standards, research, training, and education. NFPA activities generally fall into two broad, interrelated areas: technical and educational. NFPA's technical activity involves development, publication, and dissemination of more than 300 codes and standards. NFPA codes and standards are developed by nearly 250 technical committees. The Health Care Section of NFPA comprises individuals with a focus on the protection of patients, visitors, staff, property, and the environment from fire, disaster, and related safety issues.

Other regulations influence facility design as well. In health care, the requirements for licensure by the states invoke an additional body of criteria to be followed plus other standards by reference. The Joint Commission on Accreditation of Healthcare Organizations conducts surveys of hospitals using criteria that refer to the American Institute of Architects' Guidelines for Design and Construction of Hospital and Health Care Facilities. These guidelines, in turn, refer to other sources that govern planning and design. The 2006 edition of the guidelines covers most health care departments and functions and contains a brief chapter on medical equipment.

Federal regulations strongly influence the design of buildings. The provisions of the Occupational Safety and Health Act (OSHA) of 1970 control many of the conditions found on construction sites. Failure to comply with OSHA can involve stiff penalties. In 1990, the Americans with Disabilities

Act (ADA) was passed, governing the provision of reasonable access to people with disabilities. This act covers all buildings, both existing and new construction. The Department of Justice (DOJ) administers this act. DOJ has developed accessibility guidelines for use by design professionals. Further, the federal government, in regulating the design of its own health facilities, has developed full collection of codes, regulations, and other criteria to follow.

Important standards are published in addition to all the preceding by the following organizations that directly or indirectly influence the design of health care facilities:

- Association for the Advancement of Medical Instrumentation (AAMI)
- American Society of Heating, Refrigerating, and Air Conditioning Engineers (ASHRAE)
- Centers for Disease Control and Prevention (CDC)
- College of American Pathologists (CAP)
- Compressed Gas Association (CGA)
- General Services Administration (GSA)
- Illuminating Engineering Society of North America
- National Association of Plumbing, Heating, and Cooling Contractors
- National Bureau of Standards (NBS)
- National Council on Radiation Protection (NCRP)
- National Fire Protection Association (NFPA)
- Underwriters Laboratories, Inc. (UL)

Health care industry data are an important part of this library of criteria that influence design. Each manufacturer or supplier is a useful (and usually willing) source of up-to-date information on products or systems to be included in the project. Some of these have profound effects on the design of spaces and on building systems. During the life of a project, this material must be updated and verified as new items are introduced or as variations are made by the manufacturer.

26.2.5 The Importance of Project Management

The key to successfully mobilizing a health facility planning effort lies in the strength of the work of a team of professionals. Designing a health care facility is a complex task. The team needed to carry out this task is large and multidisciplinary.

Project management has emerged as an important area of special experience and training within the architectural profession. Project managers not only pull together the efforts of the architectural and engineering staff but also must coordinate the efforts of the hospital staff and ensure that all the various points of view are included in the effort.

> "The Joint Commission [on Accreditation of Healthcare Organizations] expects . . . a collaborative design process. This process should team department direction, medical staff, and individuals having special knowledge. . ."

The project manager needs information in a timely manner and will come to rely on the hospital's technology managers to provide it. No other group is more completely aware of the hospital's capital equipment program. No other group is more completely engaged with the medical equipment industry. This unique knowledge, properly applied, as suggested here, will help ensure a successful, responsive, and flexible design result.

26.2.6 The Value of Evidence-Based Design (EBD)

Testing clinical interventions for efficacy has been practiced since the time of Avicenna's The Canon of Medicine in the eleventh century, but it was only in the twentieth century did this effort come to involve almost all fields of health care. The term "evidence based" was first used in 1990 by Dr. David Eddy and the term "evidence-based medicine" first appeared in the medical literature in 1992.

Evidence-based medicine (EBM) is the conscientious, explicit, and judicious use of current best evidence in making decisions about the care of the individual patient and the integration of clinical expertise, patient values, and the best evidence into the decision-making process for patient care. Evidence-based medicine requires new skills of the clinician, including efficient literature-searching, and the application of formal rules of evidence in evaluating the clinical literature.

Evidence-based design is not the natural analog of evidence-based medicine or evidence-based nursing but the principles of EBD can transform the ordinary health care environment and help improve treatment outcomes. Using these principles can

- Enhance patient safety
- Reduce stress for patients, families, and staff
- Promote healing
- Take the form of practical, affordable design practices

Design for Privacy the recent AIA guidelines on single patient rooms help with this. Speech privacy and family privacy must be provided to make privacy possible and comforting. Designers need to note that a sense of isolation is not the same as a sense of privacy.

Help staff avoid errors and accidents through logical, standardized organization for the health care workplace by putting instruments and supplies in expected locations relative to patients in the care setting.

Design to eliminate environmental sources of infection and accident, including improved indoor air quality, practical choices for environmental surfaces and details, elimination of cross trafficking, and thoughtful placement of support and ambulation devices for recovering patients.

Design for access to the outside world by enhancing the use of day lighting and creating views of well-designed outdoor spaces. Study accessible physical outdoor spaces for patient and family use and bring appropriate plant materials, water features, and other landscaping devices into the building.

Design for comfort and clarity using best practices in planning and interior design for patients, families, and staff spaces.

Design around a clear, precise understanding of all processes of direct and indirect patient care and support activities.

Two overall beliefs are central to successfully employing these design practices.

1. Designers must bring knowledge to the design effort. Designers should use what they have observed working well in real patient care environments, not just what they have read about.
2. Owners and users must view the building for health care as assets in the care process and understand their critical contribution to solid design decision making.

26.3 KEY POINTS OF INFLUENCE—CHECKLIST FOR MEDICAL TECHNOLOGY INPUT INTO THE HEALTH CARE FACILITIES PLANNING PROCESS

26.3.1 During Project Inception

Prior to beginning any formal work, review and evaluate capital purchasing plans for 3 to 5 years into the future to check for possible deferrals. Evaluate leases and maintenance contracts. Evaluate technology staff. Survey technology-intensive departments for upcoming changes or anticipated new technology. Coordinate with information technology (IT) group.

It would be useful if a technology master plan were in place.

Prepare (or gather together) all existing medical equipment listings, showing details useful for programming and later planning. Identify key individuals to serve on programming and design user groups to represent medical technology management.

Organize materials by department or cost center or other hospital organizational entity for ease of use by planners.

26.3.2 During Programming

Direct participation in or authorship of

- Key room sizing and diagramming
- Room data sheets
- Equipment listing
- Manufacturer technical data sheets

Representation on user groups

Review, comment on, or refine programming documents

26.3.3 During Schematic Design Development

Continued representation on user groups and continued responsibility for review and input to design products

Liaison with manufacturers and clinical staff for equipment and systems decision-making

Testing critical room layouts with real templates for equipment (plans, elevations, ceiling plans)

Mockup room design and evaluation

26.3.4 During Construction Document Preparation

Continued liaison for design team and clinical staff regarding equipment and systems questions

Liaison with manufacturers for updated accurate installation template and diagrams

Prepare a logistics work plan for specification, procurement, receipt, storage, and placement of equipment to be purchased outside of construction contract

Provide coordination for vendor workforces if access to construction site is necessary for rough-in or for equipment placement

REFERENCES

Allison, David J. (ed.) (1997), *Planning, Designing, and Construction of Health Care Environments*, Joint Commission on Accreditation of Healthcare Organizations, Oakbrook, Ill.

Bronzino, Joseph D. (ed.) (1992), *Management of Medical Technology: A Primer for Clinical Engineers*, Butterworth-Heinemann, Boston, Mass.

Facilities Guidelines Institute (2006), *Guidelines for Design and Construction of Hospital and Health Care Facilities*, The American Institute of Architects, Washington, D.C.

Galison, Peter, and Thompson, Emily (eds.) (1999), *The Architecture of Science*, MIT Press, Cambridge, Mass.

Haviland, David (ed.) (1994), *The Architect's Handbook of Professional Practice*, Vol. 2, American Institute of Architects Press, Washington, D.C.

Haynes, Marion E. (1996), *Project Management from Idea to Implementation*, Crisp Publications, Menlo Park, Calif.

Howell, Joel D. (1995), *Technology in the Hospital: Transforming Patient Care in the Early Twentieth Century*, Johns Hopkins University Press, Baltimore, Md.

Kostof, Spiro (1985), *History of Architecture: Settings and Rituals*, Oxford University Press, New York, N. Y.

Lewis, James P. (1997), *Fundamentals of Project Management*, AMACOM, New York, N. Y.

Marberry, Sara O. (ed.) (1997), *Healthcare Design*, Wiley, New York, N. Y.

Masson, Madeleine (1985), *A Pictorial History of Nursing*, Hamlyn Publishing, London, England.

Reiser, Stanley Joel (1978), *Medicine and the Reign of Technology*, Cambridge University Press, Cambridge, England.

Risse, Guenter B. (1999), *Mending Bodies, Saving Souls: A History of Hospitals*, Oxford University Press, New York, N. Y.

Russell, Louise B. (1979), *Technology in Hospitals: Medical Advances and Their Diffusion*, The Brookings Institution, Washington, D.C.

Stevens, Edward F. (1918), *The American Hospital of the Twentieth Century*, Architectural Record Publishing Company, New York, N. Y.

Tomasik, Kristine M. (ed.) (1993), *Plant Technology and Safety Management Handbook: Designing the Environment of Care*, Joint Commission on Accreditation of Healthcare Organizations, Oakbrook, Ill.

CHAPTER 27
HEALTHCARE SYSTEMS ENGINEERING*

Sandra K. Garrett
Clemson University, Clemson, South Carolina

Barrett S. Caldwell
Purdue University, West Lafayette, Indiana

27.1 INTRODUCTION

The relationship between healthcare delivery and the technologies developed by engineers is pervasive in modern society. However, in much the same way that there are different general practice and specialty areas of healthcare, there are multiple disciplines of engineering that can be applied to healthcare systems engineering. As described in other chapters of this book, including the focus on clinical engineering, there are numerous practical applications of engineering and technology development in the practice of healthcare. There is a difference, however, between the engineering tools and methods used in improving a diagnostic or clinical procedure, and those tools used to improve the system performance of flows of care that may include combinations of diagnostic or clinical procedures.

The term *healthcare systems engineering* is used to encompass a broad field with a variety of facets. For the purposes of this chapter, the term has been used in the sense of systems engineering applied to healthcare delivery. Thus, this chapter provides an overview of the general and unique issues of systems engineering in the healthcare context, followed by a systems approach to describing the communication and coordination processes between teams of healthcare providers. That description also addresses how the communication strategies of healthcare providers can influence the efficiency and effectiveness of patient care. The focus of this chapter is distinctly different from a focus on diagnostics or other engineering approaches to improve the capabilities of implementing

**Portions of this chapter were included in the primary author's dissertation in a prepublication format.*

outcomes of biomedical science research. Instead, the emphasis here is on the coordination and collaboration of human activities that enable diagnostics or clinical procedures to be integrated in a more timely, cost-effective, and appropriate manner.

27.2 SYSTEMS ENGINEERING

Healthcare systems engineering can be described as the application of systems engineering principles and techniques to the healthcare industry. As such, the healthcare industry is viewed as a complex system, made up of interrelated parts which create a larger entity, or unified whole, with properties not evident from the study of the individual components, and which produce results not obtainable by the elements alone (INCOSE, 2006). Systems engineering is both a holistic perspective and an interdisciplinary approach utilized throughout the entire development process, integrating all disciplines to enable the realization of successful systems (INCOSE, 2006). One of the primary objectives of the systems engineer is to define and characterize the relevant systems and subsystems, including the interactions among them, which is intrinsically complicated because the behavior and interactions of the system components are often inadequately defined or misunderstood (Systems Engineering, 2006).

The systems engineering process is composed of seven fundamental tasks, which "are preformed in a parallel and iterative manner" (INCOSE, 2006). Several variations of these task descriptions exist; however, the general purpose and concepts remain the same throughout each version. These seven tasks, as described by the International Council on Systems Engineering (INCOSE), include

1. Define the system objectives (user's needs)
2. Establish the functionality (functional analysis)
3. Establish performance requirements (requirements analysis)
4. Evolve design and operations concepts (architecture synthesis)
5. Select a baseline (through cost/benefit trades)
6. Verify the baseline meets requirements (user's needs)
7. Iterate the process through lower-level trades (decomposition) (INCOSE, 2003)

As previously stated, these steps are not implemented in a strict linear, sequential method, but rather iteratively, with the outcome of any particular step having the ability to feedback to a previous step. Since the types of systems that are investigated and produced through systems engineering are highly diverse, no one formula or set of steps will fit all processes. Thus, the systems engineer must tailor the process to the problem at hand.

27.2.1 System-of-Systems

Systems engineering has proven itself to be an effective method for studying complex problems. However, because of the increasing complexity of today's systems, many of which can be thought of as the integration of independent smaller systems, engineers are now faced with the difficulty of designing effective interfaces between systems to create complex metasystems. The concept of *system-of-systems engineering* (SoSE) is emerging as an attempt to address integrating complex metasystems (Keating et al., 2003, p. 36). While still in the early stages of development, SoSE is beginning to progress into a more mature discipline that is capable of addressing problems that are moving beyond the capabilities of traditional systems engineering. Keating et al. (2003) specifically addresses three such areas where SoSE is demonstrating the potential to manage areas beyond the effective bounds of systems engineering: complex systems problems of high ambiguity and uncertainty; situations where context dominates the success of a particular solution; and the need to deploy partial or incomplete system solutions (p. 38). Section 27.3 demonstrates the complexity of the healthcare-delivery environment, which suggests that a SoSE approach may be appropriate for further investigation.

Boustany (2007) defines healthcare facilities in the SoSE context, with a specific focus on classifying relationships between layers of healthcare facility interactions, as well as different policy, economic, and bureaucratic functional roles of the facility that affect the implementation of flows of care. This definition emphasized interrelationships of healthcare coordination of information, physical objects, and knowledge between providers, providers and technology systems, and purely among technology systems. Through this approach, Boustany suggests the ability to more effectively study communication and coordination links between healthcare providers, as well as characteristic processes of information and resource flow in healthcare facilities at multiple levels of analysis.

27.2.2 Systems Engineering: Tools and Techniques

Significant progress has been found in both manufacturing and service industries when systems engineering tools have been applied. In these sectors, improvements have been made in the quality, efficiency, safety, and customer-centeredness through the use of systems engineering. The National Academy of Engineering (NAE) and the Institute of Medicine (IOM) call for the use and application of systems engineering to healthcare delivery, supporting the collaboration between engineers and healthcare providers in order to "transform the U.S. health care sector from an underperforming conglomerate of independent entities . . . into a high-performance 'system' in which every participating unit recognized its dependence and influence on every other unit" (National Academy of Engineering and Institute of Medicine, 2005, p. 2). And yet, even though case studies have shown that these same systems-engineering tools which have proven to be beneficial in other industries can produce substantial enhancements in healthcare organizations, they have not been widely applied throughout the healthcare sector (National Academy of Engineering and Institute of Medicine, 2005).

Many of the tools and techniques used in systems engineering overlap with those found in industrial engineering. In fact, many academic programs, such as those at the University of Arizona, University of Florida, North Carolina State University, and Virginia Polytechnic Institute and State University, combine the fields into an "industrial and systems engineering program." (See http://www.sie.arizona.edu/, http://www.ise.ufl.edu/, http://www.ise.ncsu.edu/, and http://www.ise.vt.edu/main/index.php, e.g., academic programs.) Other names associated with engineering professionals, often with an industrial engineering background, working in healthcare include: quality improvement engineer, continuous improvement engineer, process engineer, and management engineer.

The NAE/IOM report, *Building a Better Delivery System: A New Engineering/Health Care Partnership*, was written to create a framework and plan for how to establish a systems approach to healthcare delivery, with the foundations built on a partnership between engineers and healthcare professionals (2005). This report identified a number of systems engineering tools that they believed would contribute the highest gain in healthcare delivery. Of these tools, almost all of them are taught in traditional industrial engineering settings, which gives rise to the apparent overlap in the two fields. High-level examples of systems engineering tools that have either been applied in a healthcare context, or have been suggested as being applicable for use in such an area include

- *Concurrent engineering* is the process of doing cross-functional design-engineering tasks in parallel in order to address all aspects of the product's development process at an early stage, rather than using the traditional, sequential, and department-specific approach. Concurrent engineering is used to "overcome silos of function and responsibility" by creating a team of specialists from all relevant areas in an organization to design a product or process from beginning to end (National Academy of Engineering and Institute of Medicine, 2005, p. 28).

- *Quality functional deployment* (QFD) is a concept and a methodology that focuses on the needs of the customer throughout the design process and "relates the factors for design, including the customer requirements, to the quality characteristics" in order to ensure that the desired performance is achieved (Moen et al., 1991, p. 296). The House of Quality is a pictorial method, which is one part of QFD, for illustrating the relationship between the customer's requirements and the design capabilities. "Customer satisfaction is the primary goal in QFD," and while the House of Quality is often used to determine which product characteristics to emphasize, "other tools such as matrices, tables and tree diagrams are also utilized" (Tague, 2005, p. 17).
- *Human factors engineering* describes the discipline and method of applying the knowledge of human limitations and capabilities to the design of tasks, products, and systems. One way to think about this approach is that it strives to optimize the relationship between the technology and the human. Human factors focuses on integrating the human element in design and analysis to increase the effectiveness and efficiency of work processes, while improving safety and satisfaction, and reducing fatigue, error, and stress. Human factors engineering provides methods for human and system performance assessment, knowledge elicitation, rapid prototyping, and usability evaluation (FAA Human Factors Workbench). Human error analysis, human reliability, and risk assessment are also key techniques utilized by human factors engineers. Some of the specific tools and techniques used in human factors engineering include: cognitive task analysis, decision action diagrams, subjective workload assessment technique, and social network analysis (Stanton, et al., 2005).
- *Tools for failure analysis,* such as failure modes and effects analysis (FMEA), are used to determine how a product or procedure can fail or deviate from a desired level of performance in a variety of scenarios. The failures identified through FMEA are prioritized based on frequency and consequence seriousness in order to determine which actions to reduce failures should be taken first (Tague, 2005). The cognitive reliability and error analysis method (CREAM) has been developed as a method of identifying human error, to both predict and retrospectively analyze error (Hollnagel, 1998 as cited in Stanton et al., 2005). CREAM specifically focuses on how tasks depend on the reliability of human cognition, the conditions under which that reliability may be reduced, and identifies ways to reduce the associated risk. The human factors analysis and classification system (HFACS) is a theoretically based tool for investigating and analyzing human error associated with accidents and incidents (Wiegmann and Shappell, 2003). Drawing upon Reason's (1990) concept of latent and active failures, HFACS describes human error at each of four levels: (1) organizational influences, (2) unsafe supervision (i.e., middle-management), (3) preconditions for unsafe acts, and (4) the unsafe acts of operators (e.g., aircrew, maintainers, air traffic controllers). These three methods are just a brief glimpse of the quantity of tools available for failure analysis, and yet they also begin to demonstrate the wide range of techniques that are available in this area.
- *Simulation,* specifically computer simulation, is the technique used in designing a model of an actual or theoretical physical system in order to scientifically study the system behavior through experimentation. Discrete-event simulation is often used to evaluate different alternatives by modeling a system as it evolves over time, through a representation of how the variables of interest (state variables) "change instantaneously at separate points in time," during an event (Law and Kelton, 2000, p. 6). "Simulation is the process of designing a model of a real or imagined system and conducting experiments with that model" (Smith, 1998); and thus simulation is specifically useful as a way of comparing possible results from different strategies or choices, and for studying the relationships and interactions within complex systems.
- *Data mining* (also known as *knowledge discovery in databases*) is the process of sorting through large amounts of data to select and retrieve relevant information. Data mining allows individuals to analyze large databases from various points of view to find correlations, patterns, or predictive trends within the data sets. Data mining has been utilized for customer relationship management, market research, security screening, and medical diagnostics. (For healthcare related examples of data mining applications, see Breault et al., 2002; Brossette et al., 1998; Delen et al., 2005).
- *Statistical process control* (SPC) utilizes statistical techniques to monitor a process by measuring and analyzing the process variation, and thus helps determine the consistency of the process. Control charts are typically used to monitor a specific process attribute, such as quality or number

of events (defects), to maintain a predetermined level or target goal. Control charts also have the ability to help detect whether variation is due to a common cause, "causes that are inherent in the process over time, and thus affect all outcomes," or a special cause, "variation that arises because of a specific circumstance that is not part of the process all the time" (Moen et al., 1991, p. 25). SPC has the ability to enable early detection and prevention of problems before a process deviates too much from nominal. (See Benneyan, 1998a; 1998b, for a more detailed discussion of applying SPC methods to infection control and hospital epidemiology.)

- Lean/Six Sigma are actually two distinct business improvement methodologies, but they tend to be described and utilized together. Although they both originated in statistical analysis, they are now considered broader techniques used for the management of systems and organizational culture change. The concept of lean originates in manufacturing with its basic philosophy of eliminating waste (nonvalue-adding activities) and enhancing process flow being derived from the Toyota Production System. Just-in-time processes and short cycle times create lean organizations which are "efficient, flexible, and highly responsive to customer needs" (Tague, 2005, p. 30). Six Sigma, on the other hand, is product centered and focuses on the elimination of defects. "It is best focused on reducing variation in any major process from the production floor to headquarters offices" (Tague, 2005, p. 27). The improvement process utilized in Six Sigma has five general steps: define, measure, analyze, improve, and control. The success of both lean and Six Sigma is attracting the attention of CEOs in a wide range of industries, who are now grabbing on to these concepts as management philosophies.

27.2.3 Successful Systems Engineering Tool Implementation Examples

As just discussed, systems engineering tools have been used extensively in both manufacturing and service industries, demonstrating gains in both productivity and efficiency. The healthcare industry is becoming aware that it needs to catch up to these other industries, and thus some of the more innovative facilities have taken the lead in implementing systems engineering techniques. While only sparse pockets of the healthcare industry have taken this forward-thinking approach, there are enough examples that only a few will be illustrated here.

Ventilator-associated pneumonia (VAP) is a very common infection acquired by patients in hospitals, causing these patients to have up to a sevenfold increase in the number of days spent on mechanical ventilation (Schleder et al., 2002). Similarly, methicillin-resistant *Staphylococcus aureus* (MRSA) is another very serious hospital-associated infection as it is resistant to most commonly used antibiotics. Statistical process control (SPC) methods have been used to track and thus reduce the quantity of VAP and MRSA cases in a number of hospitals (see Curran et al., 2002; Schleder et al., 2002). Specifically, Curran et al.'s (2002) work found that utilizing annotated control charts to track MRSA cases in a hospital ward, and regularly providing that feedback to medical staff, led to almost a 50 percent reduction in MRSA cases when compared to before the program started. Even more remarkably, those results have been sustained through continued surveillance and process feedback.

Lean has not only been used in manufacturing, but has also proven successful in the service sector. In just the past few years, lean principles have been shown to have similar successes in healthcare environments, from large urban hospitals (Gabow et al., 2008) and smaller rural hospitals (Cross, 2008) to outpatient clinics (Endsely et al., 2006) and radiology departments (Workman-Germann and Hagg, 2006). The key lean tools and techniques that have been applied in many of these settings include value stream mapping, 5S, and visual controls. Example productivity improvements from applying lean methodologies in healthcare include: a significant reduction in the time taken to locate respiratory therapy equipment, reclaiming 6 percent of a laboratory's space for value-added processes, reducing overall inventory, and decreasing laboratory procedure turnaround time by over 11 percent (Gabow et al., 2008).

A third systems engineering tool that has been used for a wide array of purposes in healthcare is simulation. Two of the common ways simulation has been used include modeling process flow or throughput in a hospital or clinic, and to study the effect of various scheduling and staffing strategies (Guo et al., 2004; Lowery and Davis, 1999; Rossetti et al., 1999). Simulation can be helpful when determining whether proposed changes, such as remolding a facility, are feasible and an improvement over the current system. For example, Lowery and Davis (1999) used discrete event simulation to examine the impact of remodeling a hospital's surgical suite to have two fewer rooms than were currently available. Even with a number of simplifying assumptions, the simulation model was able to predict that the new operating suite would be feasible when combined with modifications to the block scheduling. Similarly, Guo et al. (2004) used a simulation approach to optimize the scheduling strategies in an outpatient clinic, improve efficiency of patient flow, and serve as a decision-support system to assist management's decision in hiring and making operational changes.

And finally, data mining techniques allow researchers to examine immense quantities of data to detect patterns and predictive relationships. Data mining has been used to address a range of issues in healthcare, from infection control surveillance (Brossette et al., 1998) and the genomic discovery of genes associated with Alzheimer's disease (Walker et al., 2004) to predicting breast cancer survivability (Delen et al., 2005) and diabetic care and comorbidity factors (Breault et al., 2002). A unifying theme in each of these application areas is that the amount of data available for investigation is too large to be probed manually. In this way, computers with faster processing power and new information technology are enabling medical researchers to investigate areas not even imaginable in the past.

27.3 THE HEALTHCARE DELIVERY ENVIRONMENT

Healthcare delivery has become the focus of much societal and professional scrutiny in recent years. As highlighted in multiple sources, the processes of healthcare delivery are highly complex, convoluted, and riddled with inefficiencies and errors that increase costs unnecessarily. These increased costs include "money wasted on overuse, underuse, misuse, duplication, system failures, unnecessary repetition, poor communication and inefficiency" (Lawrence, 2005, p. 99). Since these problems have been raised and elaborated elsewhere [Bogner, 1994; Institute of Medicine (U.S.) Committee on Quality of Health Care in America, 2000; Leape, 1994], they will not be covered in detail here. Nonetheless, there is little debate that these issues are critical priorities to be addressed. One feature of healthcare delivery that is often cited as a vital element of effective care is that of successful communication and coordination, which in turn impacts the efficiency of care delivery. Consequently, the communication and coordination strategies of healthcare providers will specifically be dealt with in more detail later in this chapter.

27.3.1 Complexity of the Healthcare System

Healthcare delivery encompasses a wide range of resources such as providers, facilities, and agencies. The complexity in healthcare delivery is in large part due to the "different kinds of personnel working in a variety of settings using many resources and generating and using multiple flows of information" (Robert Wood Johnson Foundation, 2005, A.2). The types of healthcare providers range from nurses and medical assistants to physicians, surgeons, and specialists. Other staff directly involved in the care-delivery process include: translators, pharmacists, laboratory technicians, registration personnel, and medical billing clerks. Healthcare facilities include outpatient or ambulatory clinics, hospitals, emergency care facilities, long-term care facilities, hospice care sites, and public health departments. The range of healthcare agencies include hospital systems, insurance agencies, and state and federal agencies such as the South Carolina Department of Health and Environmental Control (DHEC), the Department of Health and Human Services (DHHS), the Centers for Disease Control and Prevention (CDC), the National Institute of Health (NIH), and the Centers for Medicare and Medicaid Services (CMS). In addition, there are numerous healthcare technology and medical equipment vendors who impact the care provided in various facilities. To further complicate matters, these vendors do not work together to create compatible products, thus creating an unnecessary level of complexity that could be avoided.

To emphasize the complexity and diversity found within the healthcare-delivery environment, a brief comparison of healthcare facilities provides an important educational example. The range of healthcare-delivery facilities and locations has similar superficial goals to improve the health and well-being of patients. These facilities can, however, vary substantially on a variety of factors such as number of expected appointments per day, stability and predictability of appointment numbers, expected waiting times, and time patients spend with providers. Facilities also differ greatly in the health status risk and urgency of the patient when the visit takes place. For example, a general outpatient clinic can be considered a less time-constrained or risky setting than an emergency department. The time scales associated with particular healthcare environments depend on both the types of healthcare events that are processed at the facility and the providers who deliver care in that environment.

As a complex, dynamic system, healthcare delivery can begin looking toward the systems engineering strategies and technologies that have revolutionized other industries to initiate improvement throughout the entire system. "A major reason for some of these [system] shortfalls is the lack of involvement from the systems engineers and researchers who have done so much to improve the effectiveness of global manufacturing and distribution operations" (Sick System, 2006, p. 12). However, as most healthcare practitioners and administrators are not trained to systematically study healthcare delivery as a system, nor are they prepared to work with engineers to utilize systems-engineering tools, a consorted effort will be required in order to effectively merge the disciplines (National Academy of Engineering and Institute of Medicine, 2005).

27.3.2 Characteristics of Healthcare Environments

The application of systems engineering to healthcare is affected by a number of conditions unique to the healthcare environment. Although there has been much discussion of the application of production systems and lean manufacturing tools to healthcare, there are several critical caveats. One of the most obvious is that, in many healthcare settings, the workers (physicians and nurses) have a great deal more autonomy and power over the scheduling and organization of work; thus labor shortages and increased competition for improved working conditions are a growing concern among these classes of "skilled labor." Hospital administration has less cultural control over physician tasks and work design, and individual surgeons can create and maintain their own schedules.

In most healthcare settings, the mission of profit is less clear-cut than in traditional production settings. The hospital priorities of saving lives are very inelastic to changes in demand or marginal profitability—our society is intolerant of patient deaths due to economic evaluations of the relative cost of treatment compared to the benefit of patient recovery. Furthermore, hospital "losses" (in terms of adverse events leading to patient deaths or other catastrophic healthcare outcomes) in one economic quarter cannot be recovered or balanced by additional profits in a future quarter. Even the concept of foregoing unprofitable activities can be challenged in the healthcare environment. While there have been reports of a disproportionate fraction of healthcare costs expended in the final days of a patient's life (U.S. Congress. Office of Technology Assessment, 1987), society as a whole is not willing to consider reducing overall healthcare expenditures by denying such care. As a result, many economic valuation calculations that are commonplace in production systems environments and other branches of industrial engineering and operations research cannot be translated effectively into the healthcare environment.

Attempts to model healthcare provider activities as production systems flows can also fail because of a fundamental modeling error: healthcare providers do not provide sequential care to only one patient at a time until that patient's care is finished. Providers may be forced to handle simultaneous case loads with multiple patients, whose care experiences or visits are dynamic based on historical (patient presentation), logistical (availability of requested lab results), or case load (patients arriving early or late, or unexpectedly canceling appointments) factors. In some cases, tolerance for patient waiting becomes extremely limited (such as emergency arrivals or sudden patient "coding"), requiring rapid and multifaceted reprioritizing and rescheduling that can be beyond the capability of long-term scheduling software systems.

Of course, the components that are the production outputs of a manufacturing system—"widgets"—rarely care how they are treated or change their behavior in unexpected ways that change their interactions with the factory. The issue of patient compliance is a sometimes euphemistic reference to the challenge that patients won't always do what is best for them, but will still desire good outcomes. Compliance cannot be forced on patients for ethical reasons, and some patients will intentionally engage in behaviors other than what their physicians or nurses request as a proactive effort to improve their own care beyond that which is prescribed.

Fundamentally, the outputs of hospitals (or other healthcare-delivery environments) as production systems are humans whom we expect to be better, not damaged, by the production system. In summary, the healthcare environment is subject to many challenges and unique characteristics that affect the application of systems engineering tools, including the following:

- Healthcare providers are not always tolerant or responsive to work design or organizational changes imposed by "management" and are uniquely able to resist such changes.
- Healthcare settings are subject to nonrational, and sometimes irrational, cost and benefit evaluations.
- Production losses (adverse events leading to patient deaths or catastrophes) in one time period cannot be balanced by profits or successes in later time periods.
- Healthcare providers conduct dynamic, multitasking performance efforts with frequent needs for reprioritization and retasking based on conditions not always known in advance.
- Patients will significantly affect their own care and their interactions with providers, either in effective (proactive patients who develop advanced learning skills and technical expertise relevant to their condition) or ineffective (failed patient compliance, self-destructive health habits) ways that affect paths of patient care.
- Healthcare provider activities operate over multiple overlapping time scales, with distinct operational sequence cycles and system behaviors that occur differently at each time scale.

This last issue, changing time scales and sequence cycles, lies at the heart of a discussion of healthcare event rates and response capabilities. Some operations research approaches to systems engineering may examine performance over the time scale of weeks, with the unit of analysis as the facility as a whole. However, an awareness of event rates at different time scales helps enable and support a system-of-systems engineering examination of healthcare environments. Production planning and scheduling tools, for example, may ensure that a hospital as a whole does not run low on latex gloves or tongue depressors due to weekly order management. However, these levels of analysis are insufficient to examine and improve the performance of individual physicians and nurses on the time scales of minutes as they move between patient treatment rooms.

These smaller-scale logistics and resource coordination processes are described as "foraging" in the healthcare environment (Caldwell and Garrett, 2006; Garrett, 2008). Foraging at this level of analysis is making sure that individual physicians, nurses, or other healthcare professionals have the specific information and resources that they need at particular points of patient care. In this context, then, healthcare resource foraging can be seen as a type of lean process management, minimizing waste and time loss associated with not having what a provider needs at the time of patient care delivery. Provider capabilities for resource foraging are also dependent on time scales of events: resources that can be gathered when there is an hour of time available may well be effectively "out of range" for events that only have 5 to 10 min separating life and death.

At the level of team communication and integration, resource foraging may be a form of task and team coordination that includes active and passive interactions between providers. Depending on task loads, time available, or relative expertise, it may be more efficient for one provider to wait for a colleague to provide information and expertise, or even delegate another individual to procure resources that might be needed. Some of these team coordination issues will be addressed in the following section.

27.4 COMMUNICATION AND COORDINATION ISSUES

The complexity of healthcare delivery in today's society necessitates a team of healthcare providers working together to perform basic care-delivery tasks. Thus, a systems engineering approach must consider the healthcare-delivery team as one level in the system that should be studied to determine interactions with other parts of the system. These interactions should be considered when changes to staffing ratios, task/job allocation, or training occur, as they will all have an effect on the effectiveness and efficiency of the healthcare provider team.

As a first step, creating a common language to describe healthcare objects, outcomes, and best practices, will go a long way toward facilitating communication and collaboration between disciplines. In addition to a common language, sharing more information and training about what tools and techniques are available through a systems engineering approach will build a greater understanding and appreciation for how healthcare and engineering disciplines can work together. New educational programs are starting to focus on healthcare systems engineering and may help bridge the gap in each of these disciplines. The Regenstrief Center for Healthcare Engineering at Purdue University, the partnership between the University of Wisconsin, Madison, and several hospitals, and Clemson University's engagement with the Medical University of South Carolina (MUSC) through the Bio-Engineering Alliance are examples of these new classes of programs.

27.4.1 Team Coordination Level Focus

In the United States, the common perception of how to improve the effectiveness of patient care has historically been to study the individual providing that care, and to optimize his or her interactions with the patient. Often this viewpoint has lead to studies which focus on a single healthcare provider, such as the physician, rather than the team of providers, which actually works together to care for the patient. This single provider perspective has been illustrated in papers focusing on the complexity of nurse work (Ebright et al., 2003; Potter et al., 2005), ambulatory clinic physicians (Overhage et al., 2001), emergency department physicians (Friedman et al., 2005), and anesthetists (McDonald and Dzwonczyk, 1988; McDonald et al., 1983). Even in a study designed to explore the communication patterns in an emergency department, the "nurse in charge" was the primary focus of the study, and thus interactions with other providers were recorded solely in relation to that nurse (Woloshynowych et al., 2007).

A significantly different approach has been published in the *Scandinavian Journal of Information Systems,* which described research conducted in radiology departments in three European countries (Lundberg and Tellioglu, 1999). The focus of this research was very much centered on the coordination processes and the interdependencies of work activities performed by radiological teams. In the course of focusing on complex coordination processes, this study also considered relevant work context issues so that future technologies implemented to improve coordination would also fit the needs of the user in various situations. In a similar manner, more recent work has studied the healthcare-delivery team as the primary unit of focus in studying healthcare providers' resource foraging strategies (Garrett, 2008; Garrett and Caldwell, 2006a), or managed to inadvertently study the entire team of providers through a study of communication facilitated by visual artifacts such as white boards in a trauma center operating suite (Xiao et al., 2007).

The NAE/IOM report on *Building a Better Delivery System* (2005) presents an adapted model to show the structure and dynamics of the healthcare-delivery environment. This model illustrates the healthcare-delivery environment as a four-level system, nested within each other like the layers of an onion, which includes (starting from the center): the patient, the care provider team, the organization, and the environment. Much current research has been focused on the individual patient level, or even an individual provider, as was described earlier. A substantial amount of research has also been directed at the organizational, or infrastructure, level. Currently there is significantly less research that concentrates on the role and coordination issues of the healthcare provider teams (Realff, 2005). The care team level is essential, not only because it connects the two more heavily researched levels, but also because it is the direct link between the healthcare-delivery system and the patient. Since team coordination processes are so complex, it is also an area where there is a high chance for system breakdown, which can lead to either a near-miss or an adverse event. Therefore, finding ways to improve the information and task synchronization within a healthcare-delivery team may result in the discovery of "low-hanging fruit" which may substantially improve overall patient care.

Patient safety is directly affected by the effectiveness of team coordination and effective resource foraging. Emergency facilities and critical care units are well-stocked and well-labeled precisely because delays or confusion in resource access can prove fatal to the patient. Even in less consequence-laden situations, the ability to sustain high-quality information flow and resource coordination in healthcare-delivery reduces opportunities for adverse events and increases the probability for recovery from those events.

As previously stated, teams of healthcare providers must work together to deliver effective patient care. Given the number of individuals involved in this care delivery, issues related to communication and distributed coordination must be highlighted.

27.4.2 Team Communication

It is well recognized that communication is essential for effective, efficient, and safe healthcare delivery (e.g., see Woloshynowych et al., 2007; Xiao et al., 2007). Effective communication is important "for several reasons: it sets the pace for a quick resolution; it makes better control of information possible; it earns public trust; keeps the flow of information consistent and accurate; and may even avert a crisis elsewhere" (Strohl Systems, 2007). In contrast, poor communication is both a waste of time (Gosbee, 1998), and can lead to errors or adverse events, including "higher mortality rates, longer lengths of stay and higher nurse turnover in intensive care units, and greater postoperative pain" (Mills et al., 2008). And yet, even knowing the criticality of effective communication, communication in healthcare is challenged by interruptions, background noise (Xiao et al., 2007), misalignment of situational awareness, concurrent task work, and steep role hierarchies between staff.

In a systematic review of work involving the study of the physician–nurse relationship and roles in providing care, Fagin (1992) describes provider collaborative models as more patient-centered since they promote autonomy, establishing complementary roles for both physicians and nurses rather than a hierarchical relationship structure. Within this review, Fagin highlights hospitals that had a "high degree of coordinated care between physicians and nurses, and the most comprehensive nursing education support system . . ." also experienced lower than predicted death rates for patients with AIDS (p. 297). Studies on care for the elderly which have looked at using a team approach to outpatient geriatric care over that of a general internist found that the group approach reduced the length of hospital stays, as well as creating a net reduction in costs. In spending a shift shadowing a nurse, an associate chief medical officer became more acutely aware of the value of collaborative communication between physicians and nurses. He noted that "when physicians and nurses worked together on a plan, physicians benefited from the nurse's assessment and received more complete information about the patient's daily activities, responses to medications, and home and family situations" (Goldszer, 2004, p. 166). Nurses also received more complete information from this interaction, enabling them to better communicate care plans to the patients and their family members. All in all, the connection between nurse–physician collaboration and the effect on patient outcomes is becoming widely accepted (Jones, 1994); thus, it is important to examine how various strategies, tools, and information technologies can be used to improve communication and collaboration between healthcare providers.

Team Communication Support Tools. The first communication tool examined here is one that is often overlooked when studying communication patterns in healthcare delivery, the patient chart. The patient chart, while seemingly a very basic part of healthcare delivery, serves a very important set of information storage and team communication functions. Healthcare team members consider the patient chart an indispensable tool for locating the information required to do their work. Consequently, a significant problem arises when team members are not able to consistently access the chart, or are forced to go "chart hunting" in order to locate it (Lingard et al., 2007, p. 661). The process of chart hunting, or "foraging for this information resource" (Garrett and Caldwell, 2006b), is time consuming and serves to destabilize one very important communication aspect in collaborative care (Lingard et al., 2007). Oral communication produces a positive system redundancy, that is, when used to supplement and not replace formal charting. Thus, while the patient chart is a crucial element in care-delivery coordination, additional methods can be used to enhance teamwork such as electronic records that can be accessed by multiple individuals simultaneously and are not limited by physical location/unpredictable availability (Bernstein et al., 2005).

A second common tool is that of a "whiteboard," which serves as a visual display within a department to increase group situational awareness (Wears et al., 2007). Whiteboards have been used as a "lean healthcare" tool to increase status visibility for issues such as bed allocation and patient discharge status. Whiteboards have also been studied to determine how these information-rich artifacts impact communication and workflow in trauma operating suites (Xiao et al., 2007), urban emergency departments, and a general pediatric ward (Wears et al., 2007). Xiao et al. identified eight ways that whiteboards facilitated collaborative work among healthcare providers: "task management, team attention management, task status tracking, task articulation, resource planning and tracking, synchronous and asynchronous communication, multidisciplinary problem solving and negotiation, and socialization and team building" (2007, p. 387).

A final example of how information technology has been implemented to improve the communication and collaboration between healthcare providers is that of the electronic medical record. Electronic medical records (EMRs) have the capability of dramatically altering the way in which healthcare providers record, retrieve, organize, and manage medical information, and provide a means for improved care by augmenting the clinician's expertise with a database of best practice examples to compare with any given case. EMRs have been shown to improve the quality of patient care and safety when utilized appropriately. For example, the implementation of electronic medical records was shown to improve the communication in an inner-city women's (prenatal) clinic, between the outpatient office, the ultrasonography unit, and the labor floor (Bernstein et al., 2005, p. 607). More specifically, the availability of prenatal charts during hospital admission for delivery was significantly increased (from 84 to 98 percent) and the median length of time between the last documented prenatal visit and delivery was reduced after EMR implementation (Bernstein et al., 2005, p. 609).

However, even with the enhanced abilities to manage medical information, EMRs have not always created better, more efficient care delivery, since many clinicians are not using them to their full capabilities or are duplicating efforts by maintaining a hard copy record which is later transcribed into the computer records (Garrett, 2008). EMR implementation is hindered when it is put into practice without understanding how the new technology will impact organizational culture and how to adapt previous practice techniques to fit the new technology (Crosson et al., 2005). Relatively few primary care practices (in comparison to hospital systems) have currently adopted the use of electronic medical records, yet that number is growing. While much can still be done to augment the capabilities of the EMR, such as integrating it with clinical decision support systems (Sim et al., 2001) and workflow management techniques (Schadow et al., 2001), they are still valuable in their current state when employed properly. As more work is done to understand the impact of using EMRs on healthcare delivery and how they can be implemented smoothly to enhance current processes, it is expected that electronic medical records will become an integral part of clinical practices and as such will serve to coordinate information between providers, improving medical communication and provider collaboration.

27.4.3 Group Coordination

Indexical Coordination. One aspect of efficient coordination among team members is the ability to apparently anticipate or otherwise respond to information or task coordination needs without being explicitly asked to do so. This type of coordination can be described as *indexical* coordination, a form of implicit coordination where one actor derives meaning from another actor's activity based on understanding of the work context and intended goals (Stahl, 2006). Thus, as members of a work team become more familiar with each other's work patterns and roles, they can observe and recognize intentions and the initiations of relevant actions. Indexical coordination is most often provided through direct (unmediated) observation, because the richness of contextual data is restricted by information technology. However, just the use of specific information technologies, or "listening in" on communications not directly addressed to an actor, can be seen as a source of indexical coordination. For instance, NASA flight controllers will all listen in on general "party line" voice communications so that, if a problem related to their area of specialty arises, they are able to recognize their need for action and begin to respond before anyone directly instructs them to do so (Caldwell, 2006).

In all cases, though, indexical coordination helps us to do more with less: you understand and respond to what I'm doing from having a contextual and experiential understanding of the task, and from observing me work, rather than explicit requests for coordination.

Communication Configurations. The variety of disciplines addressing interpersonal communications helps to explain the complex, and sometimes confusing, terminology and analysis of team-level communications. Thus, we must be able to recognize and distinguish three aspects of communication configurations that affect healthcare team coordination: *structure*, *process*, and *technology constraints*.

Structure. At the most basic level, patterns of communication within teams may be seen as distinguishing one-to-one, one-to-many, and many-to-many communication pathways. This distinction is most frequently used in discussions of computer-supported collaboration, because it helps to distinguish different types of information technology systems (Borghoff and Schlichter, 2000). This description of communication configuration helps to define individual-based, one-to-one coordination paths (one doctor coordinates patient treatment options with the attending nurse) based on face-to-face or telephone conversations; broadcast-based, one-to-many instructions or commands (a public address "code" announcement or grand rounds lecture); or group discussion-based, many-to-many coordination (such as a physician specialist discussion board or staff meeting). A need for well-defined and structured coordination becomes imperative in both geographically distributed teams and teams composed of members with heterogeneous subject matter expertise, in order for them to achieve optimal functionality (Garrett et al., 2009).

A more complex view of the structure of communication is that of the communication net (McGrath, 1984; Shaw, 1981), which describes the communication paths that are available among members of a team or group. The communication net can be affected by the number of connection paths to other team members that a team member may have, or the number of "hops" it may take for a communication to get from one person to another. There can be concern that excessively centralized or *saturated* communications nets (ones where the total communications task load through a specific person overloads their ability to complete all communications or their own individual tasks) are subject to single points of breakdown. However, completely independent paths in a sparsely connected network can be seen to lose efficiency due to the additional time required, and lack of context sharing or knowledge coordination, for each communication hop. A multiphysician hospital ward may find it difficult to have a single coordinating receptionist or duty nurse attempting to manage a period of high workload and needs for coordination. However, the advantages of such coordination become evident when a single person can be the effective communicator to multiple physicians with a minimum of confusion about the right person to contact, or provide additional indexical coordination by understanding and responding to coordination needs between physicians without being explicitly requested to do so.

Process. A frequent issue in studies of group and team dynamics is that not all groups are created for the same purpose, or to do the same sorts of tasks. While much of the group dynamics literature is focused on the processes of group decision making, healthcare provider teams have a number of other different requirements. Sundstrom and colleagues highlight surgical teams as a prototypical example of "action/negotiation" teams, where the team goal is to complete a goal-oriented performance in a dynamic and complex task setting (Sundstrom et al., 1990). In addition, such teams have high levels of role differentiation and integration, allowing different team members with distinct areas of expertise to effectively share information and resources to achieve team-level goals. As a result, it is goal-directed performance outcomes, and not simply achieving a "winning" position in a debate or decision choice, that marks execution tasks such as those conducted by healthcare teams (McGrath, 1984).

Another set of considerations raised by both McGrath and Sundstrom is that teams in such complex environments rarely have a single, purely sequential set of tasks to complete in order to achieve overall task goals. "Heal the patient" is not simply a linear sequence of events, and also importantly, most healthcare providers do not focus their attention solely on one patient. Thus, there are critical issues involved in management and shifting among multiple tasks, and how communications and actions are developed in order to support complex and dynamic task loads. Here, indexical coordination also becomes important, as the number of possible references for any given act increases, and further resolution of context is required to recognize for whom or what a particular activity was intended. Some authors specifically distinguish "taskwork" and "teamwork" or other terms that emphasize the relative focus on task completion compared to team coordination process efforts (Caldwell, 2005, 2006; Cooke et al., 2001a, 2001b; Garrett and Caldwell, 2002; Helmreich and Merritt, 1998; Helmreich et al., 1980; Spence, 1985). The long-term application of crew resource management (CRM) techniques, originally developed in aviation, to healthcare provider teams is also a recognition of the critical role of effective coordination process in performing important dynamic tasks in the healthcare environment (Helmreich and Merritt, 1998).

Technology Constraints. In the 1980s and 1990s, some researchers developed models of media richness to discuss the relative capabilities and constraints of emerging electronic information and communication technologies (ICTs) (Rice, 1992; Rice and Shook, 1990). However, it cannot be assumed that unmediated, face-to-face communication is always the best form of interaction, especially in high workload, physically distributed settings such as healthcare. Instead, a more proper focus is on the relative advantages of specific ICT options, and the situational conditions under which an ICT is effective (Caldwell and Paradkar, 1995). Here, the issues of both coordination structure and coordination process can be paramount in determining which technologies can be effectively integrated in a healthcare setting, and how technological constraints or limitations can affect the strength of provider coordination. Some constraints may be as straightforward as sensory persistence and availability in a complex environment—persistent communications (such as history functions on chat or e-mails that are not deleted) can provide support for healthcare personnel who need to refer back to previous actions or decisions when reliance on memory is not sufficient. However, persistence can also provide reference context, or the ability to reconstruct the conditions and interactions that contributed to past activity regarding a patient or healthcare resource.

Again, the importance of indexical coordination becomes clear when discussing ICT implementations that support effective healthcare task performance. As described above, indexical coordination is coordination and information sharing that comes from one provider being aware of the context, actions, and information available to the other provider. It is not impossible for modern ICTs to provide shared awareness and indexical coordination—the design of NASA mission control centers can be seen as specifically intended to support such visual as well as auditory coordination (Caldwell, 2005). To the extent that ICT systems are implemented to promote one-to-one instead of many-to-many communication paths, these shared and synchronized contexts can be lost. Some examples exist of new technologies introduced into emergency room settings that did not provide sufficient shared display awareness, and led to breakdowns in local as well as hospital-level coordination (Wears et al., 2007).

27.5 CONCLUSION

As engineering capabilities evolve in the healthcare setting, the probability grows that different functional groups or units in a large facility will be using incompatible or misaligned technologies. For instance, different groups in a hospital may all have patient scheduling software systems or electronic patient records, but those technologies may not easily or reliably pass required data between them. In addition, organizational processes and policies do not evolve nearly as quickly as the state of the art in a new diagnostic tool capability or clinical equipment design. As a result, healthcare delivery facilities can be especially vulnerable to information misalignment between organizational processes, information systems, and critical outputs (healthy patients).

The system-of-systems Engineering (SoSE) approach is one potentially promising method to reduce these problems of misalignment and instability. A core feature of SoSE is its ability to analyze flows of information and resources simultaneously within and across multiple layers of the healthcare facility, ranging from the individual treatment area to the multibuilding integrated healthcare campus with ancillary radiology, pharmacy, and laboratory professionals providing inpatient as well as outpatient services. The SoSE approach can help avoid breakdowns of integration of healthcare delivery flows of care that may be missed when focusing on and trying to separately optimize the tasks and processes of individual providers. It is suggested that this SoSE framework, combined with an appropriate multilevel analysis of healthcare events and time scales, can help identify systems engineering opportunities for improving efficiency and reducing waste in coordinated, distributed healthcare settings.

REFERENCES

Benneyan, J. C. (1998a). Statistical quality control methods in infection control and hospital epidemiology, part 1: introduction and basic theory. *Infection Control and Hospital Epidemiology,* **19**(3), 194–214.

Benneyan, J. C. (1998b). Statistical quality control methods in infection control and hospital epidemiology, part 2: chart use, statistical properties, and research issues. *Infection Control and Hospital Epidemiology,* **19**(4), 265–283.

Bernstein, P. S., Farinelli, C., and Merkatz, I. R. (2005). Using an electronic medical record to improve communication within a prenatal care network. *Obstetrics & Gynecology,* **105**(3), 607–612.

Bogner, M. S. (1994). Human Error in Medicine: A Frontier for Change. In M. S. Bogner (ed.), *Human Error in Medicine* (pp. 373–383). Hillsdale, NJ: Lawrence Erlbaum Associates.

Borghoff, U. M., and Schlichter, J. H. (2000). *Computer-Supported Cooperative Work: Introduction to Distributed Applications.* Berlin: Springer.

Boustany, K. C. (2007). *A System-of-Systems Examination of Humans in Multi-Site Healthcare Coordination Under Nominal and Degraded Conditions.* Unpublished Thesis, Purdue University, West Lafayette, IN.

Breault, J. L., Goodall, C. R., and Fos, P. J. (2002). Data mining a diabetic data warehouse. *Artificial Intelligence in Medicine,* **26**(1–2), 37–54.

Brossette, S. E., Sprague, A. P., Hardin, J. M., Waites, K. B., Jones, W. T., and Moser, S. A. (1998). Data mining in hospital infection control and public health surveillance. *Journal of the American Medical Informatics Association,* **5**(4), 373–381.

Caldwell, B. S. (2005). Multi-team dynamics and distributed expertise in mission operations. *Aviation, Space, and Environmental Medicine,* **76**(6), B145–B153.

Caldwell, B. S. (2006). Group Performance and Space Flight Teams. In C. A. Bowers, E. Salas, and F. G. Jentsch (eds.), *Creating High-Tech Teams: Practical Guidance on Work Performance and Technology* (pp. 161–182). Washington, D.C.: American Psychological Association.

Caldwell, B. S., and Garrett, S. K. (2006). Coordination of Healthcare Expertise and Information Flow in Provider Teams. In R. N. Pikaar, E. A. P. Koningsveld, and P. J. M. Settels (eds.), *Proceedings of the 16th World Congress of the International Ergonomics Association* (pp. 3565–3570). Maastricht, Netherlands, July 10–14.

Caldwell, B. S., and Paradkar, P. V. (1995). Factors affecting user tolerance for voice mail message transmission delays. *International Journal of Human-Computer Interaction,* **7**(3), 235–248.

Cooke, N. J., Kiekel, P. A., and Helm, E. E. (2001a). Comparing and Validating Measures of Team Knowledge, Paper presented at the *Proceedings of the Human Factors and Ergonomics Society 45th Annual Meeting.* Minneapolis, MN.

Cooke, N. J., Kiekel, P. A., and Helm, E. E. (2001b). Measuring team knowledge during skill acquisition of a complex task. *International Journal of Cognitive Ergonomics,* **5**(3), 297–315.

Cross, C. S. (2008). *Lean reaches rural hospital.* Institute of Industrial Engineers. Retrieved March 20, 2008, from the World Wide Web: http://www.iienet2.org/Details.aspx?id=10808.

Crosson, J. C., Stroebel, C., Scott, J. G., Stello, B., and Crabtree, B. F. (2005). Implementing an electronic medical record in a family medicine practice: communication, decision making, and conflict. *Annals of Family Medicine,* **3**(4), 307–311.

Curran, E. T., Benneyan, J. C., and Hood, J. (2002). Controling methicillin-resistant *Staphylococcus aureus*: a feedback approach using annotated statistical process control charts. *Infection Control and Hospital Epidemiology,* **23**(1), 13–18.

Delen, D., Walker, G., and Kadam, A. (2005). Predicting breast cancer survivability: a comparison of three data mining methods. *Artificial Intelligence in Medicine,* **34**(2), 113–127.

Ebright, P. R., Patterson, E. S., Chalko, B. A., and Render, M. L. (2003). Understanding the complexity of registered nurse work in acute care settings. *Journal of Nursing Administration,* **33**(12), 630–638.

Endsely, S., Magill, M. K., and Godfrey, M. M. (2006). Creating a lean practice. *Family Practice Management*, pp. 34–38.

FAA Human Factors Workbench (n.d.). The Federal Aviation Administration. Retrieved April 26, 2008, from the World Wide Web: http://www2.hf.faa.gov/workbenchtools/.

Fagin, C. M. (1992). Collaboration between nurses and physicians: no longer a choice. *Academic Medicine,* **67**(5), 295–303.

Friedman, S. M., Elinson, R., and Arenovich, T. (2005). A study of emergency physician work and communication: a human factors approach. *Israeli Journal of Emergency Medicine,* **5**(3), 35–42.

Gabow, P. A., Albert, R., Kaufman, L., Wilson, M., and Eisert, S. (2008, February). Picture of health: Denver Health uses 5S to deliver quality, safety, efficiency. *Industrial Engineer,* **40**, 44–48.

Garrett, S. K. (2008). *Provider Centered Coordination, Resource Foraging, and Event Management in Healthcare Tasks.* Dissertation Abstracts International, **68**(10), 177B. (UMI No. 3287211)

Garrett, S. K., and Caldwell, B. S. (2002). Describing functional requirements for knowledge sharing communities. *Behaviour & Information Technology,* **21**(5), 359–364.

Garrett, S. K., and Caldwell, B. S. (2006a). Task Coordination and Group Foraging in Healthcare Delivery Teams, *Proceedings of the Human Factors and Ergonomics Society 50th Annual Meeting* (pp. 1059–1063). San Francisco, CA.

Garrett, S. K., and Caldwell, B. S. (2006b). Team Resource Foraging in Event-Driven Task Environments, *Proceedings of the Human Factors and Ergonomics Society 50th Annual Meeting* (pp. 1514–1518). San Francisco, CA.

Garrett, S. K., Caldwell, B. S., Harris, E. C., and Gonzalez, M. C. (2009). Six dimensions of expertise: a more comprehensive definition of cognitive expertise for team coordination. *Theoretical Issues in Ergonomics Science*. **10**(2), 93–105.

Goldszer, R. C. (2004). My day shadowing a nurse: learning about teamwork in health care. *Journal of Clinical Outcomes Management,* **11**(3), 165–166.

Gosbee, J. (1998). Communication among health professionals: human factors engineering can help make sense of the chaos. *British Medical Journal,* **316**, 642.

Guo, M., Wagner, M., and West, C. (2004). Outpatient Clinic Scheduling—A Simulation Approach. *Proceedings of the 2004 Winter Simulation Conference,* 1981–1987.

Helmreich, R. L., and Merritt, A. C. (1998). *Culture at Work in Aviation and Medicine: National, Organizational and Professional Influences*. Hampshire, UK: Ashgate Publishing Ltd.

Helmreich, R. L., Wilhelm, J. A., and Runge, T. E. (1980). Psychological Considerations in Future Space Missions. In T. S. Cheston and D. L. Winter (eds.), *Human Factors of Outer Space Production.* Boulder, CO: Westview Press.

INCOSE. (2003, September 1). *INCOSE Handbook SE Process Model.* Retrieved April 5, 2008, from the World Wide Web: http://g2sebok.incose.org/app/mss/asset.cfm?ID=INCOSE%20G2SEBOK%203.60&ST=F.

INCOSE. (2006, October 2). *A Consensus of the INCOSE Fellows*. Retrieved April 5, 2008, from the World Wide Web: http://www.incose.org/practice/fellowsconsensus.aspx.

Institute of Medicine (U.S.). Committee on Quality of Health Care in America. (2000). *To Err Is Human: Building a Safer Health System*. Washington, D.C.: National Academy Press.

Jones, R. A. P. (1994). Nurse-physician collaboration: a descriptive study. *Holistic Nurse Practitioner,* **8**(3), 38–53.

Keating, C., Rogers, R., Unal, R., Dryer, D., Sousa-Poza, A., Safford, R., Peterson, W., and Rabadi, G. (2003). Systems of systems engineering. *Engineering Management Journal,* **15**(3), 36-45.

Law, A. M., and Kelton, W. D. (2000). *Simulation Modeling and Analysis*. Boston, MA: McGraw-Hill.

Lawrence, D. (2005). Bridging the Quality Chasm. In P. P. Reid, W. D. Compton, J. H. Grossman, and G. Fanjiang (eds.), *Building a Better Delivery System: A New Engineering/Health Care Partnership* (pp. 99–101). Washington, D.C.: The National Academies Press.

Leape, L. L. (1994). Error in medicine. *Journal of the American Medical Association,* **272**(23), 1851–1857.

Lingard, L., Conn, L. G., Russell, A., Reeves, S., Miller, K.-L., Kenaszchuk, C., and Zwarenstein, M. (2007). Interprofessional information work: innovations in the use of the chart on internal medicine teams. *Journal of Interprofessional Care,* **21**(6), 657–667.

Lowery, J. C., and Davis, J. A. (1999). Determination of Operating Room Requirements Using Simulation. *Proceedings of the 1999 Winter Simulation Conference*, 1568–1572.

Lundberg, N., and Tellioglu, H. (1999). Understanding complex coordination processes in health care. *Scandinavian Journal of Information Systems,* **11**, 157–182.

McDonald, J. S., and Dzwonczyk, R. R. (1988). A time and motion study of the anaesthetist's intraoperative time. *British Journal of Anaesthesia,* **61**(6), 738–742.

McDonald, J. S., Peterson, S. F., and Hansell, J. (1983). Operating room event analysis. *Medical Instrumentation,* **17**(2), 107–108.

McGrath, J. E. (1984). *Groups: Interaction and Performance*. Englewood Cliffs, NJ: Prentice-Hall.

Mills, P., Neily, J., and Dunn, E. (2008). Teamwork and communication in surgical teams: implications for patient safety. *Journal of the American College of Surgeons,* **206**, 107–112.

Moen, R. D., Nolan, T. W., and Provost, L. P. (1991). *Improving Quality Through Planned Experimentation*. Boston, MA: McGraw-Hill.

National Academy of Engineering, and Institute of Medicine. (2005). *Building a Better Delivery System: A New Engineering/Health Care Partnership*. Washington, D.C.: The National Academies Press.

Overhage, J. M., Perkins, S., Tierney, W. M., and McDonald, C. J. (2001). Controlled trial of direct physician order entry: effects on physicians' time utilization in ambulatory primary care internal medicine practices. *Journal of the American Medical Informatics Association,* **8**(4), 361–371.

Potter, P., Wolf, L., Boxerman, S., Grayson, D., Sledge, J., Dunagan, C., and Evanoff, B. (2005). Understanding the cognitive work of nursing in the acute care environment. *Journal of Nursing Administration,* **35**(7/8), 327–335.

Realff, M. J. (2005, November 21). *NSF and Service Enterprise Engineering: An Overview.* Paper presented at the Purdue University Regenstrief Center for Healthcare Engineering Presentation Series, West Lafayette, IN.

Reason, J. (1990). *Human Error*. Cambridge, UK: Cambridge University Press.

Rice, R. E. (1992). Task analyzability, use of new media, and effectiveness: a multi-site exploration of media richness. *Organization Science,* **3**(4), 475–500.

Rice, R. E., and Shook, D. E. (1990). Voice Messaging, Coordination, and Communication. In J. Galegher, R. E. Kraut, and C. Egido (eds.), *Intellectual Teamwork: Social and Technological Foundations of Cooperative Work* (pp. 327–350). Hillsdale, NJ: Lawrence Erlbaum Associates.

Robert Wood Johnson Foundation. (2005, December 13). *Using Systems Engineering to Improve the Health Care Delivery System*. Retrieved March 23, 2008, from the World Wide Web: http://www.rwjf.org/programareas/resources/product.jsp?id=20980&pid=1142&gsa=1.

Rossetti, M. D., Trzcinski, G. F., and Syverud, S. A. (1999). Emergency Department Simulation and Determination of Optimal Attending Physician Staffing Schedules. *Proceedings of the 1999 Winter Simulation Conference*, 1532–1540.

Schadow, G., Russler, D. C., and McDonald, C. J. (2001). Conceptual Alignment of Electronic Health Record Data with Guideline and Workflow Knowledge. *International Journal of Medical Informatics,* **64**, 259–274.

Schleder, B., Stott, K., and Lloyd, R. C. (2002). The effect of a comprehensive oral care protocol on patients at risk for ventilator-associated pneumonia. *Journal of Advocate Health Care,* **4**(1), 27–30.

Shaw, M. E. (1981). *Group Dynamics: The Psychology of Small Group Behavior* (3d ed.). New York, NY: McGraw Hill Book Company.

Sick System. (2006, August). *Industrial Engineer,* **38**, 12.

Sim, I., Gorman, P., Greenes, R. A., Haynes, R. B., Kaplan, B., Lehmann, H., and Tang, P. C. (2001). Clinical decision support systems for the practice of evidence-based medicine. *Journal of the American Medical Informatics Association,* **8**(6), 527–534.

Smith, R. D. (1998). *Simulation Article*. Model Benders, LCC: Encyclopedia of Computer Science. Retrieved April 12, 2008, from the World Wide Web: http://www.modelbenders.com/encyclopedia/encyclopedia.html.

Spence, J. T. (1985). Achievement and achievement motivation: a cultural perspective. In J. T. Spence and C. E. Izard (eds.), *Motivation, Emotion, and Personality* (pp. 65–75). New York, NY: Elsevier Science Publishers.

Stahl, G. (2006). *Group Cognition: Computer Support for Building Collaborative Knowledge*. Cambridge, MA: MIT Press.

Stanton, N. A., Salmon, P. M., Walker, G. H., Baber, C., and Jenkins, D. P. (2005). *Human Factors Methods: A Practical Guide for Engineering and Design.* Aldershot, Hampshire, England: Ashgate.

Strohl Systems. (2007). *The Need for Efficient Communications in Healthcare.* Retrieved April 14, 2008, from the World Wide Web: http://www.strohlsystems.com/Software/_files/NotiFind/NotiFind_Healthcare.pdf.

Sundstrom, E., DeMeuse, K. P., and Futrell, D. (1990). Work teams: applications and effectiveness. *American Psychologist,* **45**(2), 120–133.

Systems Engineering. (2006). [Web site]. Wikipedia. Retrieved October 27, 2006, from the World Wide Web: http://en.wikipedia.org/wiki/Systems_engineering.

Tague, N. R. (2005). *The Quality Toolbox* (2d ed.). Milwaukee, WI: ASQ Quality Press.

U.S. Congress. Office of Technology Assessment. (1987). *Life-Sustaining Technologies and the Elderly.* Washington, D.C.: U.S. Government Printing Office.

Walker, P. R., Smith, B., Liu, Q. Y., Famili, A. F., Valdés, J. J., Liu, Z., and Lach, B. (2004). Data mining of gene expression changes in Alzheimber brain. *Artificial Intelligence in Medicine,* **31**, 137–154.

Wears, R. L., Perry, S. J., Wilson, S., Galliers, J., and Fone, J. (2007). Emergency department status boards: user-evolved artefacts for inter- and intra-group coordination. *Cognition, Technology & Work,* **9**(3), 163–170.

Wiegmann, D. A., and Shappell, S. A. (2003). *A Human Error Approach to Aviation Accident Analysis: The Human Factors Analysis and Classification System.* Aldershot, Hants, England: Ashgate.

Woloshynowych, M., Davis, R., Brown, R., and Vincent, C. (2007). Communication patterns in a UK emergency department. *Annals of Emergency Medicine,* **50**(4), 407–413.

Workman-Germann, J., and Hagg, H. W. (2006). Implementing Lean/Six Sigma methodologies in the radiology department of a hospital healthcare system. Paper presented at the *American Society for Engineering Education Annual Conference.*

Xiao, Y., Schenkel, S., Faraj, S., Mackenzie, C. F., and Moss, J. (2007). What whiteboards in a trauma center operating suite can teach us about emergency department communication. *Annals of Emergency Medicine,* **50**(4), 387–395.

CHAPTER 28
ENCLOSED HABITAT LIFE SUPPORT

Tom Filburn
University of Hartford, West Hartford, Connecticut

Joe Genovese
Hamilton Sundstrand (retired), Windsor Locks, Connecticut

John Graf
NASA Johnson Space Center, Houston, Texas

28.1 INTRODUCTION

Space exploration has pushed the frontiers of human knowledge for our planet, our moon, and beyond. This exploration initiative has expanded our understanding by providing new information obtained from both robotic and human-occupied missions. Both types of missions have their own requirements and constraints; however, this chapter focuses on those requirements necessary to keep humans alive inside enclosed habitats such as in human-supported space missions. The systems included in this chapter are capable of operating in a gravity or microgravity environment.

The foundations of life-support systems requirements were established by naval submersible operations. This broad database was then used to extend man's presence into space. The United States Navy along with those of the United Kingdom, France, and Russia operate nuclear-powered submarines. These vessels contain crews of ~100 individuals with mission durations lasting months. These warfare platforms are designed to keep their crew isolated from our atmosphere for periods up to the entire mission length.

The space programs of the United States and Russia have launched astronauts into near-earth orbit and to our moon. These missions also require their crews to be isolated from our sustaining atmosphere for periods of 8 h (space suit) to 6 months (visit to the International Space Station).

When maintaining human life safe inside of enclosed spaces, three major parameters are typically the first to be considered. The number one parameter is air quality. Humans have a small tolerance band for certain contaminants and we need oxygen in sufficient quantity to support our metabolic functions. The second parameter considered is thermal. Again, humans have a small tolerance for their ambient temperature. This thermal tolerance is narrow with a definite minimum and maximum. Along with an ambient temperature limit, both humans and equipments require a limit to water vapor in the air stream. The final parameter is liquid water, and the ability to recycle it. Short missions can simply supply clean fresh water, longer mission durations can frequently reduce the overall mission supply weight by incorporating systems to recycle the water. Therefore, this chapter deals with systems to achieve human comfort inside enclosed habitats via

1. Removing gaseous contaminants and providing a life-sustaining oxygen partial pressure
2. Maintaining a comfortable thermal environment with a reasonable water vapor content
3. Providing methods to recover safe drinking water from metabolically produced water (sweat, urine) for longer duration missions

As we have already discussed, we will focus on three types of systems, providing safe breathable atmosphere, keeping within appropriate thermal and humidity limits, and recycling water for long-duration missions. We will need to understand the specific limits for each of these parameters in order to design appropriate systems for use in maintaining an enclosed habitat.

28.2 HUMAN COMFORT

Comfort is important in enclosed habitats for a variety of reasons, including crew productivity, health, and under extreme circumstances, it may be a life-threatening issue. Unfortunately not one single index can be used to provide a measure of comfort. Dry bulb temperature, relative humidity, clothing, crew activity, and the external environment can all factor into the determination of comfort.

Different researchers have attempted to provide a single index for environmental comfort. One indicator is the mean radiant temperature, which relies on global temperature (a function of convective and radiant inputs), ambient air temperature, air velocity, and a constant in the following equation:[1]

$$T_{\mathrm{mrt}}^4 = T_{\mathrm{g}}^4 CV^{1/2}(T_{\mathrm{g}} - T_{\mathrm{a}})$$

where T_{mrt} = mean radiant temperature, R or K
T_{g} = global temperature, R or K
T_{a} = ambient temperature, R or K
$C = 0.103 \times 10^9$ (R), 0.247×10^9 (K)
V = air velocity, ft/min or m/s

While the mean radiant temperature is one attempt to provide a single indicator of thermal comfort, other factors will still influence an individual's perception. Figure 28.1 shows the comfort box proposed by NASA for crew members on the ISS. The box is bounded by the 25 percent and 70 percent relative humidity lines.

28.2.1 Enclosed Habitat Air Quality

Many HVAC handbooks provide a wealth of information regarding indoor air quality and potential contaminants. Most of these treatises assume the air is at 1 atm. For most terrestrial applications this is correct; however, for NASA and many aerospace installations this is not accurate. The operating pressure for most commercial airliners is in the range of 10.9 to 11.8 psia. NASA's Apollo capsule operated at 3.7 psia, while today's Extravehicular Mobility Unit (EMU) uses an atmosphere at 4.3 psia; both these NASA applications specify a pure oxygen atmosphere.

These various (typically subatmospheric) pressures from aerospace-enclosed habitats increase the difficulty of maintaining acceptable indoor air quality. The lower pressure decreases the mass flow rate through air-handling equipment (fans, reactors, etc.). In addition, the specialty gas mixture of the space suit (pure oxygen) creates added constraints for hypoxia and hyperoxia as well as raising material concerns about ignition.

Assuming that a pressure boundary is available to maintain a habitable atmosphere with sufficient oxygen content and pressure, the next item of concern with indoor air are contaminants. Carbon dioxide

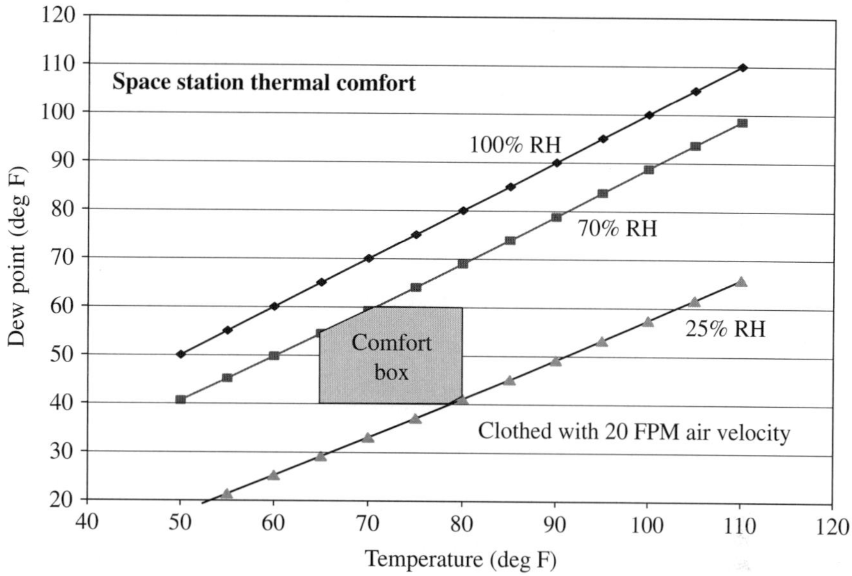

FIGURE 28.1 Space station thermal comfort (dry bulb vs. wet bulb temperatures).[2]

becomes the first contaminant of concern for enclosed habitats when human metabolism is the predominant mechanism for producing contaminants. This is due to our low tolerance for CO_2 and our relatively high metabolic production rate of this gas. Other gaseous contaminants in the atmosphere need to be controlled along with carbon dioxide. The much lower production rate of these other species makes our capture system for these trace contaminants less urgent (lower capture quantity) compared to CO_2.

28.2.2 Oxygen Sources

In an enclosed habitat, the oxygen consumed by metabolic processes must be replaced to maintain a viable atmosphere. The options for storing the replacement oxygen vary from storage via compressed gas or cryogenic liquid to solid and liquid chemical reactors. The choice of the storage method depends on usage factors and habitat characteristics, such as the duration of the storage period, the quantity of stored oxygen required, and the desired ratio of oxygen mass to total storage mass.

Using typical lightweight tank and system mass values from the literature, a comparison can be made between storage methods for increasing closed habitat operation. The value of the calculated ratio of the required mass of oxygen to the mass of the storage system is given in Table 28.1. The table shows that for short operational periods, the solid storage or compressed gas storage options provide the best ratio of stored oxygen. When larger quantities of oxygen are needed, cryogenic storage provides high mass ratios. The water electrolysis system requires a substantial fixed system mass, and therefore only becomes a viable option for very long-term applications.

TABLE 28.1 Oxygen Mass Divided by System Mass for Various O_2 Delivery Methods

Mission days	O_2 need lb	Chlorate candles	Compressed gas	Cryogen	Water electrolysis
0.5	3.8	0.33	0.25	0.19	
7	53.2	0.33	0.63	0.61	0.06
30	228	0.33	0.69	0.70	0.19
90	684	0.33	0.71	0.72	0.39
180	1368	0.33	0.71	0.73	0.53

Chemical Storage. Chemical oxygen generators are found most suitable for applications with long dormancy and short operating periods. This is the technology that is used for passenger emergency oxygen onboard commercial airliners. The most common formulation generates oxygen using a mix of sodium chlorate and iron powder. When ignited, the mixture smolders at about 600°C. The heat released by the oxidation of iron powder [Eq. (28.1)] supports the decomposition reaction of sodium chlorate [Eq. (28.2)]:

$$NaClO_3 + Fe \rightarrow FeO + NaCl + O_2\ (600°C) \tag{28.1}$$

$$2NaClO_3 + Heat \rightarrow 2NaCl + 3O_2 \tag{28.2}$$

The candles have an indefinite shelf-life, if stored properly, and have a good safety record when operated correctly. They are used in submarines, planes, and spacecraft. However, the candles have been involved in three high-profile incidents in the past 20 years:

1. On May 11, 1996, a U.S. airliner en route from Miami to Atlanta exploded when a case of the candles accidentally ignited. The oxygen released by the candles led to a fire in the aircraft's hold, killing all 110 passengers on board.
2. On February 23, 1997, during the exchange of an air filter on the MIR space station, a chlorate candle malfunctioned and spewed molten metal and sparks across one of the space station modules. It burned for 14 minutes blocking the escape route to one of the Soyuz spacecraft. There were no injuries.
3. On March 21, 2007, a chlorate candle, used to produce oxygen on board a nuclear submarine, exploded during a training exercise. Two British sailors were killed and another injured in the resulting explosion.

Compressed Gas. The most common form of gas storage for both commercial and military applications is in the form of a compressed gas. The storage tanks may be all metal or be a composite of a thin metal bladder with carbon or glass fiber over-wrap. Typical storage pressures vary from 2500 to 6000 psi. The compressed gas systems consist of the high pressure tank, shut-off and relief valves, and a gas pressure regulation method, as shown in Fig. 28.2.

When compressed oxygen is used, great attention to materials of construction and scrupulous system cleanliness must be maintained to avoid compression ignition within the system.

Cryogenic Storage of Liquid Oxygen. When large quantities of oxygen are required, cryogenic storage becomes an attractive option. Oxygen is stored in a supercritical condition in thermally insulated double-walled vacuum annulus tanks. The storage temperature of –176°C requires highly efficient insulation to limit the boil-off of oxygen. The NASA Space Shuttle presently uses a cryogenic oxygen storage system. It contains 320 L of oxygen in lightweight tanks with Inconel 718 inner shell and aluminum 2219 outer-shell construction. The lightweight construction permits the storage of 4 kg of oxygen per kg of tank. These cryogenic tanks were added during a redesign effort in the 1990s, which provided an extension to the duration of on-orbit stay time. The original orbiters relied on pressurized oxygen to replenish that lost through leakage and consumed metabolically.

Water Electrolysis Oxygen Generators. When sufficient quantities of water and electrical energy are available oxygen, can be generated on a demand basis using water electrolysis cells. This approach avoids the need for storage of large quantities of compressed or liquid cryogenic oxygen. The U.S. Navy pioneered the use of this technology for use aboard nuclear submarines. Early Navy electrolysis systems used a potassium hydroxide electrolyte retained within a porous asbestos matrix. This electrolyte was also used for the Elektron oxygen generator on the Russian MIR space station. Current technology replaces this electrolyte system with a very stable perfluorosulfonic acid membrane that resists oxidative degradation and is capable of sustaining differential pressures across the membrane wall. The basic electrolysis cell is presented in Fig. 28.3.

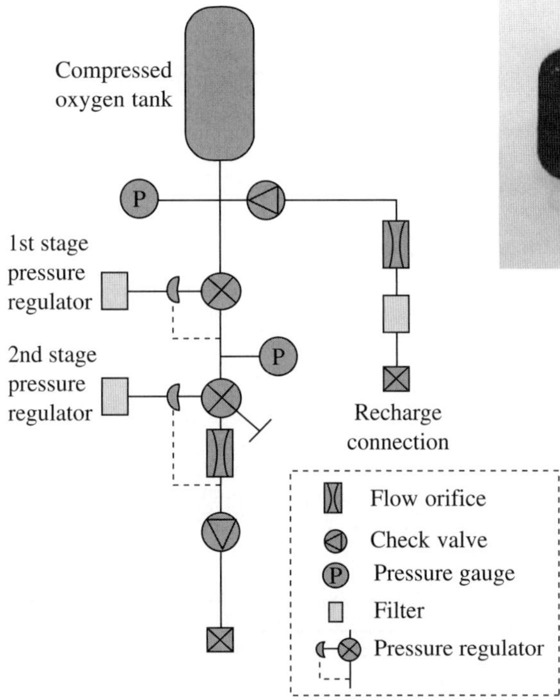

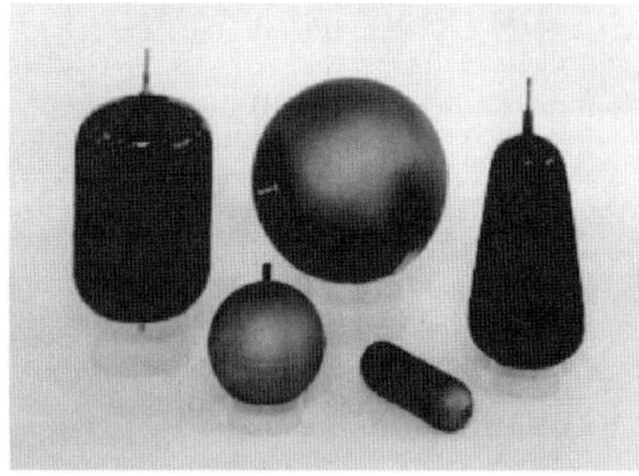

FIGURE 28.2 Typical compressed oxygen system schematic.

The current necessary to pass the ions through a solution is governed by Faraday's second law. The current (I) equals the Faraday constant multiplied by the mass flow of ions and the number of electrons per ion and divided by the molecular weight of the ion.

A polymer electrolysis membrane (PEM)-based oxygen generator has been installed in the International Space Station and has begun operation. It is capable of generating 2.3 to 9.1 kg of oxygen per day and consumes 300 to 3300 W.

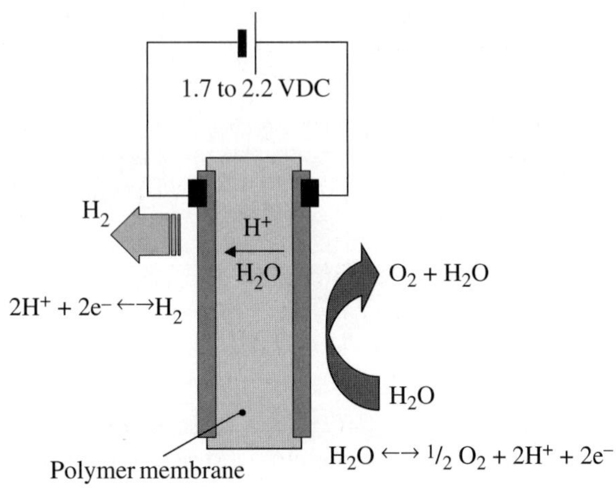

FIGURE 28.3 Basic water electrolysis cell.

28.3 AIR CONTAMINANTS

In any habitat, as air exchange and air leakage is reduced in an effort to reduce energy consumption, contaminant levels can build to unhealthy or unsafe levels. The term *sick building syndrome* is applied to these problem habitats where the amount of clean fresh air being introduced is unable to counter the materials of construction and/or environmental factors favorable to mold growth that have led to unhealthy contaminant levels in the living space. The presence of humans and large amounts of electronic support equipment add to the contaminant levels found in a habitat. A closed habitat exacerbates all of these issues and requires specific contaminant removal or destruction approaches.

To design a system that maintains a safe breathable atmosphere for humans, contaminant standards need to be set. The National Research Council, together with NASA, has developed a set of standards called *spacecraft maximum allowable concentrations* (SMACs). The SMAC is the maximum concentration that will not cause adverse health effects, significant discomfort, or degradation of crew performance for continuous exposures of 7 to 180 days. Detailed information on the toxicological basis for the SMAC levels can be found in Refs. 3 through 5, and a complete listing of the NASA standards is presented in Ref. 6. Table 28.2 presents the SMAC values for four important trace contaminants. The four representative contaminants in this table were selected based on their level of impact to human health and their average generation rate.

To maintain human life and support basic human metabolic processes, Fig. 28.4 shows the material balances, which need to be maintained, and which will vary with the activity level (metabolic rate) of the inhabitants.

TABLE 28.2 Spacecraft Maximum Allowable Concentrations for Some Typical Compounds

	Spacecraft maximum allowable concentration (mg/m^3) exposure time				
Compound	1 h	24 h	7 days	30 days	180 days
Ammonia	20	14	7	7	7
Carbon monoxide	63	23	11	11	11
Formaldehyde	0.5	0.12	0.05	0.05	0.05
Methanol	40	13	9	9	9

Source: Reference 3.

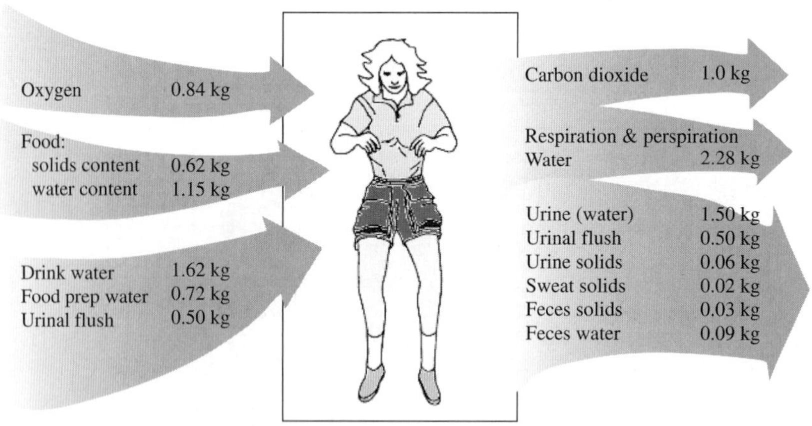

Metabolic Rate = 2,677 kcal/person/day

Respiratory quotient (RQ) = 0.87 (molar ratio of CO_2 production to O_2 consumption)

FIGURE 28.4 The human life-support material balance.

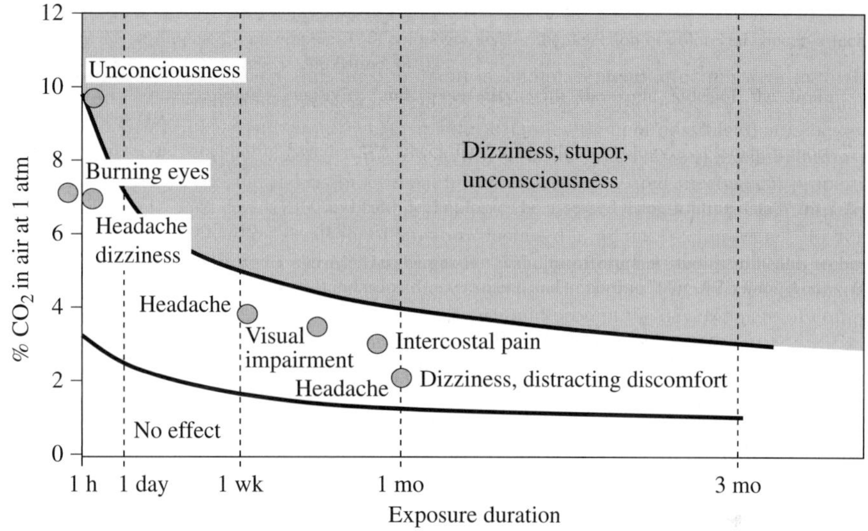

FIGURE 28.5 Effects of carbon dioxide exposure on humans.

The most significant output components are seen to be carbon dioxide and water vapor. Allowable levels of carbon dioxide have been established based on physiological testing and U.S. Navy submarine experience. Figure 28.5 presents data on carbon dioxide concentration in air and physiological effects experienced for increasing exposure time. The data are taken from Ref. 7 and is in good agreement with the long-term exposure guidelines calling for control between 0.5 percent and 1.0 percent CO_2 in air. Carbon dioxide is generated at a significant rate and is not treated as a trace contaminant but rather as a dedicated removal system, as described in Sec. 28.4.

28.3.1 Trace Contaminant Sources

Trace gases are evolved at low rates from many sources within the habitat. Humans are responsible for the bulk of the production for a significant number of the trace gases of concern. Trace gaseous and vaporous contaminants generated by occupants include a range of organic compounds such as acetone, butyric acid, acetic acid, methyl alcohol, and ethyl alcohol, as well as ammonia, methane, and hydrogen sulfide. The total generation rate of these compounds can exceed several hundred milligrams per day per person. In addition to the metabolic processes, activities related to food preparation, hygiene, and sanitary practices introduce other contaminants. The habitat itself often contributes to the problem. Plastics and other polymers, used in furnishings, off-gas processing solvents or degradation products over time. The thermal and acoustic insulation used within the habitat can have a profound effect on trace contaminant levels. Foam materials can evolve low levels of formaldehyde and foaming or blowing agents like pentane. An emergency event, such as a fire, will obviously trigger the release of significant levels of contaminants from nonmetallic materials, but thermal excursions are also possible in proximity to electrical components and can result in release of low levels of ammonia, carbon monoxide, and even hydrogen cyanide. The habitat may also house experiments that may vent or be subject to accidental release of contaminating gases. The inclusion of electronic controllers, computers, and electromechanical actuators leads to out-gassing of carbon monoxide and low-molecular-weight solvents. Thermal gradients through the wall insulation and humidity levels in the living space may form a favorable environment for microbial growth. Microbial metabolism and spores can then add to the gaseous and particulate contamination levels.

TABLE 28.3 Contaminant Generation Rates for Some Typical Compounds

Compound	30-day SMAC (mg/m^3)	Molecular weight (gm/mol)	Contaminant generation rate: Equipment (mg/kg/day)	Contaminant generation rate: Metabolic (mg/person/day)
Ammonia	7	17.00	8.46×10^{-5}	321
Carbon monoxide	11	28.01	2.03×10^{-3}	23
Formaldehyde	0.05	30.03	4.4×10^{-8}	0
Methanol	9	32.04	1.27×10^{-3}	1.5

There are also factors that attenuate the buildup of contaminant levels. Cabin leakage, however small, can serve to control a great many of the low-generation-rate contaminants. The humidity control system may include a condensing heat exchanger that absorbs water-soluble contaminants like ammonia, while the carbon dioxide system may include an absorbent that also removes low levels of contaminants. A sample of the equipment out-gassing and metabolic contaminant generation rates found in Ref. 8 is shown in Table 28.3.

28.3.2 Trace Contaminant Control Methods

The literature referenced for SMAC levels contains a great many compounds found at very low trace levels and with low generation rates. For short, closed-operation durations, those contaminants often do not build up to levels close to the SMAC limits, especially if a small level of habitat leakage exists. The "time-to-SMAC" value should be evaluated to reduce the list to compounds of concern. An example of that calculation is presented here for carbon monoxide: Assuming a habitat volume of 12 m^3, housing 4 persons and containing 1000 kg of electronic equipment, the SMAC level for 30-day exposure (from Table 28.2) is 11 mg/m^3 and the equipment generation rate is 2.03×10^{-3} mg/kg/day while the metabolic rate is 11 mg/person/day. For this problem, the total generation rate is then 2.03×10^{-3} (1000 kg) + 11 (4 persons). So, total generation rate = 46 mg/day. The SMAC level for this particular volume is 11 mg/m^3 (12 m^3) = 132 mg.

Therefore, assuming zero leakage, it takes 2.9 days to reach the SMAC level. This indicates that it would only be safe for four people to occupy the habitat for less than 68 h without a trace contaminant control system for carbon monoxide. Each contaminant must be checked to find the limiting constituent. If the desired occupation time exceeds the shortest time to reach SMAC, a control method must be considered.

When implementing an active contaminant removal system, the airflow rate must be adequate to deliver the trace contaminants to the removal bed for adsorption or destruction. The method of calculation for required flow rate is described in Fig. 28.6.

Several options exist for the removal of trace contaminants from an air stream.

Activated Charcoal. One of the most commonly used approaches for trace contaminant control, activated charcoal provides a high surface area and a varied pore size for adsorption of contaminants. It is most effective for medium- to high-molecular-weight compounds and provides very low capacity for volatile organic compounds. The granular material is typically packed in a cylinder with retaining screens and filters on the inlet and outlet. It is considered an expendable absorbent material and is replaced prior to the calculated bed breakthrough time for the contaminants. Charcoal beds must be protected from significant humidity excursions, as the charcoal will desorb the contaminants back into the air stream in order to preferentially adsorb water. The steady-state humidity level will also affect the charcoal's total capacity for adsorbing contaminants.

Treated Charcoal. Activated charcoal is also available treated with an acid (typically phosphoric acid). The charcoal acts as a carrier for the acid as well, retaining some of its adsorption capacity.

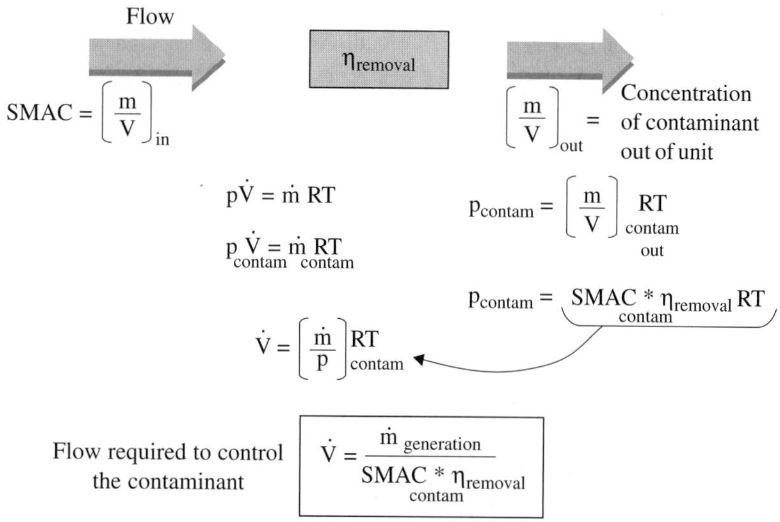

FIGURE 28.6 Calculation of airflow for a contaminant-removal system.

The presence of the acid makes the material effective against high pH gases such as ammonia. It is also an expendable material that is sensitive to humidity.

Granular Alkaline Adsorbent. When acid gases are present (especially downstream of an oxidation reactor), a high pH adsorbent material is required. Granular lithium hydroxide is the material of choice for this application. The material is also contained in a packed bed and will remove sulfur dioxide and oxides of nitrogen.

Catalytic Reactors. The removal of some combustible gases and hydrocarbon gases from the air stream is best accomplished by a catalytic bed. A substrate of activated charcoal is impregnated with a noble metal to catalyze the reaction with the oxygen in the air stream. High-activity catalysts permit hydrogen and carbon monoxide oxidation to water vapor and carbon dioxide at ambient temperature.

The destruction of methane requires a high-temperature catalyst bed. Typical systems use a Hopcalite base metal catalyst operating at 600°F. Because methane is one of the most refractive gases, this system provides protection against a wide range of contaminants. A high-temperature bed requires pretreatment of the air stream to remove ammonia (to prevent conversion to NO_x) and post-treatment with an alkali bed to remove acid gases that are products of combustion. When using a high-temperature catalyst bed, steps must be taken to prevent the flow of air until the bed is at full operating temperature. Reduced temperature operation can create harmful or toxic by-products.

A new technology for air purification is the application of ultraviolet light catalyzed with titania. These systems operate at ambient temperature and have been demonstrated to be effective against carbon monoxide, hydrogen, ethanol, and benzene.

28.4 CO_2 CONTROL SCHEMES

Research completed by NASA[9] and the U.S. Navy[7] have indicated that CO_2 levels should be maintained at or below 3.8 mmHg partial pressure for typical missions, and excursions to 1 percent are tolerable for shorter periods (e.g., 8-h EVA). Over a 24-h day, the average human produces about 1 kg of CO_2. CO_2 production may vary by a 5:1 ratio between maximum of rigorous exercise and the minimum production rate of sleep. Habitats with little free volume (e.g., the EMU) need CO_2 capture systems that can handle the maximum CO_2 production rate. More traditional habitats can size their CO_2 control system for the average rate, relying on the greater free volume to limit CO_2 concentrations.

Research has been ongoing for over 50 years to remove CO_2 from a gas stream. The bulk of this work has been investigating methods to "sweeten" natural gas. Natural gas typically contains large quantities of CO_2 and other acid gases; these contaminants must be removed to produce the commercial gas supplied via pipelines.

Methods to remove CO_2 from gas streams can be either a physical or chemical sorbent. Chemical absorbents rely on the acid nature of CO_2, reacting it with a base chemical to remove it from the gas stream. Reversing the acid-gas base reaction can be accomplished by increasing the temperature of the mix (temperature swing absorption, TSA) or reducing the CO_2 partial pressure (pressure swing absorption, PSA).

A variety of physical sorbents have been used to remove CO_2 from gas streams. Some of these physical sorbents (Selexol) simply use changes in CO_2 solubility to remove the gas at a low temperature and release it at a higher temperature. Other physical sorbents rely on cage-like openings to selectively capture the CO_2 molecule (e.g., molecular sieves). The majority of these sorbents rely on either temperature or partial pressure changes to capture CO_2 and release it into a different space. These methods (temperature swing absorption, TSA, or pressure swing absorption, PSA) are popular for the regenerable nature of the sorbent. Natural gas sweetening as well as CO_2 capture from submarine atmospheres has been accomplished by pumped aqueous amine solutions like that shown in Fig. 28.7. These systems use a large contacting tower to expose the CO_2-laden gas to the amine sorbent. A second tower is then used to heat the CO_2-rich mixture and regenerate the amine solution.

In addition to the regenerable sorbents and their systems, other single use sorbents are also available such as potassium, sodium, or lithium hydroxide.

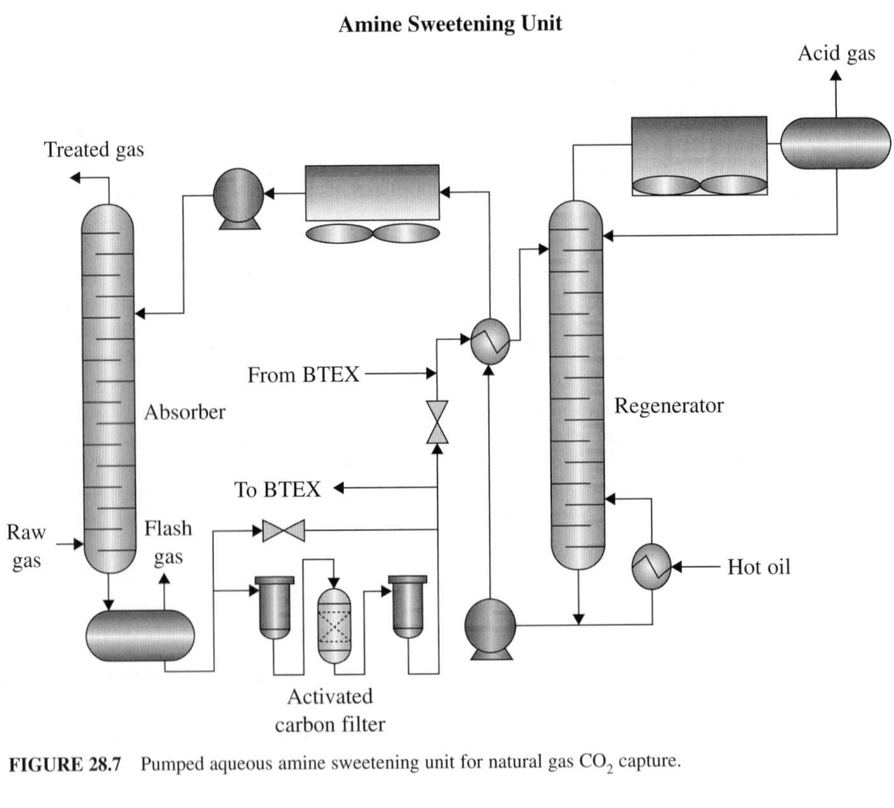

FIGURE 28.7 Pumped aqueous amine sweetening unit for natural gas CO_2 capture.

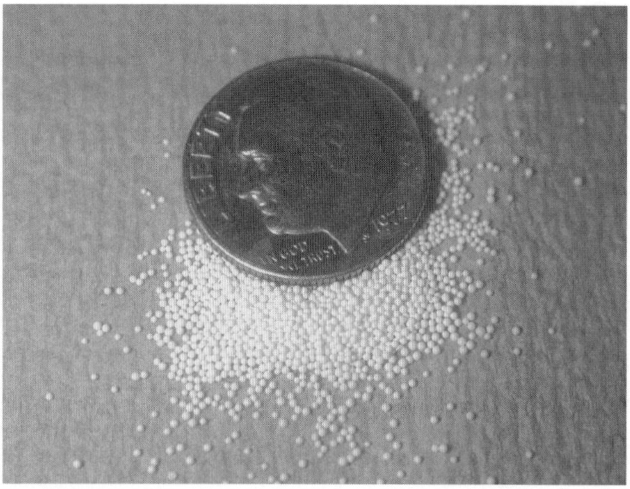

FIGURE 28.8 Solid amine beads spread across flat surface.

28.4.1 Solid Amines

NASA has relied on a novel material that combines the high pH of liquid amines (basicity) with a porous commercial support bead. The liquid amine is impregnated into the pores of the support creating a *solid* amine. The liquid amine is held within the pores of the support by surface tension forces. The final product behaves as a solid CO_2 absorbent. This solid amine system removes the shortcoming of operating liquid amines in microgravity environments. Terrestrial liquid amine CO_2 capture systems use gravity to separate the liquid absorbent from the gas phase. However, the microgravity environment of many NASA missions makes this liquid/gas separation step difficult. Instead the gas phase is passed through the bed of solid particles, relying on a simple screen to perform the bead (solid)/gas separation. Figure 28.8 shows these solid amine beads loosely arrayed on a flat surface. Actual applications will use the beads in a packed bed with fine mesh screen retaining the beads within the bed.

In addition to their utility for NASA, the solid amine sorbents may offer other advantages over conventional aqueous amine systems. The porosity of the support allows for high amine loadings, which is limited in aqueous systems due to the corrosive nature of the amine. Other additives (e.g., antifoaming) are not required for these solid amine systems as well.

The solid amines operated by NASA are used in a two-bed semicontinuous fashion with one bed online absorbing CO_2 from the gas stream while the second bed is off-line regenerating by exposure to space vacuum. This PSA system makes use of the very low CO_2 partial pressure available in space to reject the carbon dioxide. Figure 28.9 is a simplified schematic of this system proposed for the new crew exploration vehicle (CEV). The solid amines also offer some utility in controlling the relative humidity of an enclosed habitat. The amines and their support are hygroscopic, thereby reducing the moisture in the gas stream.

28.4.2 Molecular Sieves

Zeolites, more commonly referred to as molecular sieves, are crystalline materials that can be synthetic or naturally occurring. These materials have a microporous cage-like structure that allows for the segregation (sieving) of different liquid- or gas-phase species. These materials have been found and manufactured with a variety of pore openings, thus permitting the capture of specific molecules based on their

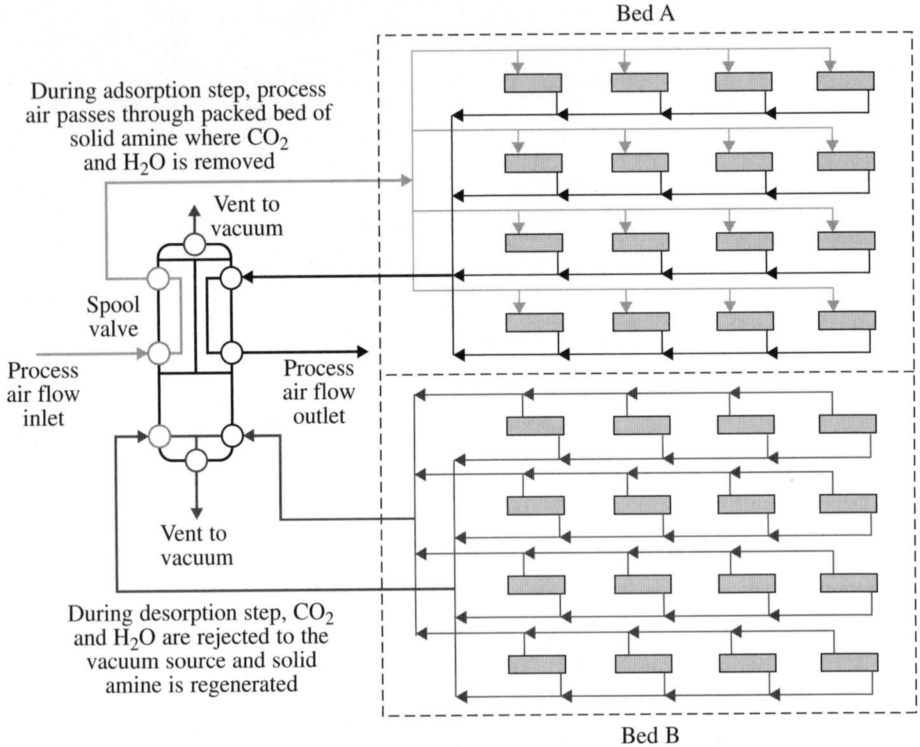

FIGURE 28.9 Two-bed solid amine operation proposed for crew exploration vehicle.

size. One feature that all of the zeolites share is a large affinity for water vapor. Therefore, any system incorporating a zeolite absorbent needs to provide a mechanism for dehydrating the gas stream prior to entering the CO_2 capture bed. The United States' first space station (Skylab) and the International Space Station rely on two zeolite beds to continuously remove CO_2 from the cabin atmosphere.

Figure 28.10 shows a schematic of the four-bed mole sieve system used on board the ISS. This system uses four beds which combine two beds of desiccants with two beds of molecular-sieve material (sized to capture CO_2, generally 5 Å). These four beds are arranged so that one desiccant bed is on-line removing moisture, while the second is regenerating and sending moisture back into the cabin. The two zeolite beds are operated in a similar fashion, one bed is off-line regenerating (either sending CO_2 overboard or to a CO_2 reduction system), while the second bed is online removing CO_2 from the cabin atmosphere (via delegated airflow through both the desiccant and CO_2 capture beds).

28.4.3 Nonregenerable Absorbents

A wide variety of solid absorbents are commercially available for removing carbon dioxide from a gas stream. The majority of these materials are not practically regenerable; therefore they must be replaced after reaching their removal limit. These materials include hydroxides of several metals, including LiOH, NaOH, KOH, and $Ca(OH)_2$. The granular form of these materials are typically used in commercial applications relying on the high pH of the material to capture the acid gas CO_2. The individual granules are sieved to between 4 and 12 mesh (US) to limit the pressure drop when loaded into a packed bed. Due to the caustic nature of the granules dusting can be a concern, so efforts are needed to retain the granules within the bed. Loading and operating with these materials should also be done to minimize the creation of dust.

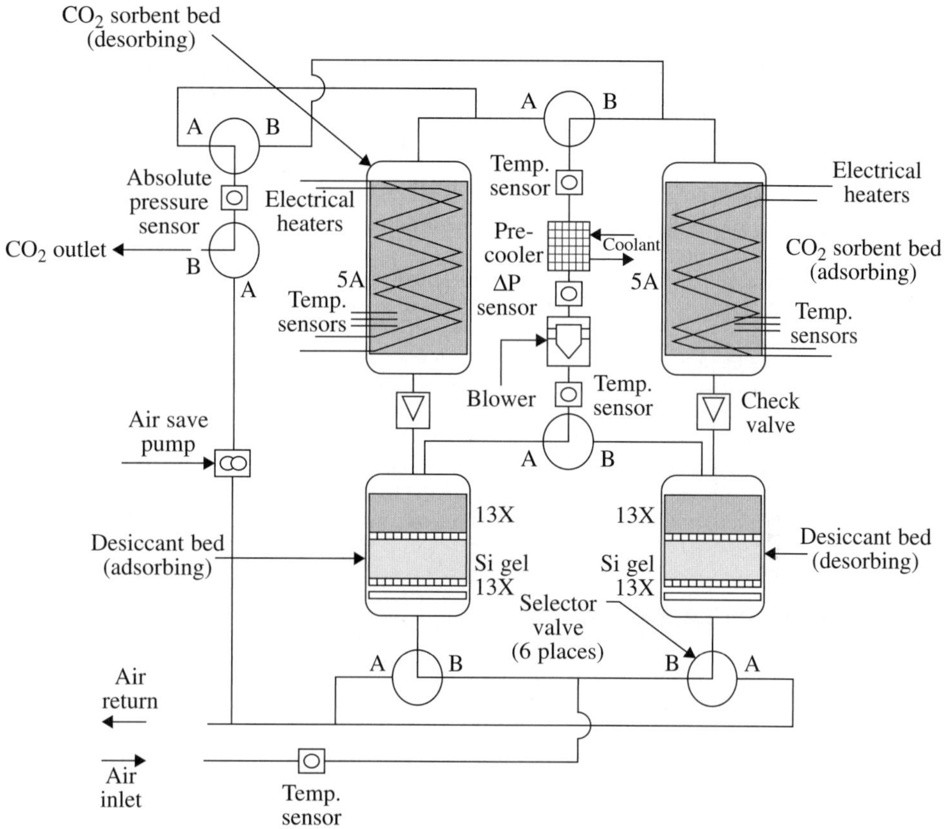

FIGURE 28.10 Four-bed MS system for CO_2 capture on the International Space Station.

28.4.4 Membranes and Electrochemical Methods

While not commercially available, membranes and electrochemical systems are being investigated for the removal of CO_2 from gas streams. Membrane systems still must rely on a partial pressure gradient across the membrane wall to achieve CO_2 removal from a gas stream. These membranes may offer lower pressure drop and smaller systems in the future when research has produced the combination of selectivity and CO_2 permeability. *Selectivity* refers to the membrane wall's ability to limit the transmission of other gaseous species. For instance, a low total pressure providing the driving force for the permeation of carbon dioxide through the membrane wall will also generate a potential for other gaseous species. The ability of the membrane to limit the transmission of these other molecules is a measure of its selectivity. The permeability is simply a measure of the ease of passage for CO_2.

28.4.5 Electrochemical Methods

Electrochemical cells have been investigated for removing CO_2 from gas streams. These cells, like the electrochemical depolarized CO_2 concentrator (EDC) cell, offer some advantages over traditional towers or packed-bed absorbents. The EDC operates by passing the gas stream over the cathode of an electrochemical cell with an aqueous electrolyte. The CO_2 diffuses into the electrolyte due to the availability of free hydroxyl ions (OH^-). These ions react with the CO_2 to form carbonate or bicarbonate ions. The CO_2 is released from the carbonate or bicarbonate at the anode.

Electrochemical cells can achieve lower pressure drop with their hardware due to the open nature of the cell assembly. The cathode can be a broad flat surface so that high volumetric flow rates can be reached with very low pressure drops. This open architecture and low ΔP mean that low ambient CO_2 concentrations can be reached directly from the high air throughput rate.

There are several disadvantages to these electrochemical systems, including difficulty in maintaining the electrolyte concentration, dryout, and retention of the electrolyte between the cathode and anode.

28.4.6 Regeneration Methods

Several methods are available to regenerate the CO_2 sorbents listed in the aforementioned sections. Temperature swing absorption (TSA) is a very popular method frequently used in natural gas sweetening. In the pumped aqueous systems used in natural gas sweetening, a large tower is used to contact the aqueous amine solution with the natural gas containing CO_2 at ambient temperatures. The caustic amine solution removes CO_2 from the gas stream due to the acidic nature of carbon dioxide. This same amine solution is then warmed (typically through regenerative heat exchanger) to an elevated temperature (~250°F, depending on amine, loading, etc.). This high-temperature liquid passes through a second contactor column which can use steam to further increase the temperature of the CO_2-rich liquid. The CO_2 capacity of the liquid is greatly reduced due to these elevated temperatures, thereby driving the equilibrium reaction toward releasing CO_2 from the amine.

28.5 WATER RECLAMATION

Water constitutes the greatest expendable mass for life support in a closed habitat. As shown in Fig. 28.4, the basic water needs for keeping a person hydrated, including thermoregulation and waste flushing, as well as food preparation, amount to 2.84 kg/person/day. The life-support system must therefore be capable of storing and delivering usable water. If one adds hygiene and wash water for showers, dishwasher, and clothes washer, the total water need increases to over 18 kg/person/day. Based on this large mass, water is therefore the first expendable resource to be reclaimed, even for moderate durations of closed habitat operation. In addition to collecting and storing the wastewater, the processor must then purify and return a potable water stream.

28.5.1 Wastewater Characteristics

The various wastewater streams that must be processed each have different contaminant characteristics. Table 28.4 presents the contaminant concentration and daily generation rate for the common wastewater streams. The urine waste is a smaller volume and contains contaminants at a much higher concentration than the other waste streams. This supports the typical strategy of using a separate and specific treatment system for the urine waste while mixing the waste from the other sources.

The composition of urine is complex with many trace compounds that vary with diet and fluid intake. The major substances are presented in Table 28.5. Urine contains a large concentration of urea as well as a high level of inorganic salts. A complete list of constituents can be found in Ref. 10.

TABLE 28.4 Wastewater Sources and Characteristics

Source	Concentration (mg/L)	Rate (kg/person/day)
Urine (treated and untreated)	37,057	1.5
Hand and oral wash	1,018	4.44
Crew shower	945	2.72
Humidity condensate	248	1.83

TABLE 28.5 Major Constituents of Human Urine

Item	Formula	Min%	Max%
Urea	$(NH_2)_2CO$	0.9	2.3
Chloride	Cl^-	0.2	0.8
Sodium	Na+	0.1	0.4
Potassium	K+	0.08	0.3
Creatinine	$C_4H_7N_3O$	0.07	0.2
Sulfur	S	0.02	0.18
Hippuric acid	$C_6H_6CO \cdot NHC_2O \cdot CO_2H$	0.005	0.17
Phosphorus	P	0.05	0.1

The urea readily decomposes to form ammonia which contaminants water vapor. The salts tend to precipitate and form calcifications and carbonates, jamming pumps, and valves. A high acid capacity with a pH of approximately 4 is required to prevent precipitates and scale from forming in the system. If flushing alone is used, flush volume should provide for clearing the urine transfer tube as a minimum. The urine waste also posseses the greatest psychological barrier to reuse and so requires the most aggressive treatment technology, usually a distillation-based approach. The collected condensate is then added to the other wastewater streams for further processing or may be used for oxygen generation in an electrolysis unit (as was done on the Russian MIR space station).

28.5.2 Processor Options

Distillation. The power demand of simple ambient pressure distillation usually rules out this approach. The typical urine reclamation system uses vapor compression distillation (VCD) instead. This technology uses subatmospheric boiling inside a rotating drum. Vapor is boosted in pressure and condensed on outside of the drum to recover energy. The VCD technology, like simple distillation, is effective in separating the inorganic and low vapor pressure contaminants from the condensate, but permits the carryover of volatile contaminants and gaseous decomposition products into the product water. The vapor phase catalytic ammonia removal (VPCAR) system operates in the same basic manner as the VCD technology, but includes a catalytic reactor operating on the generated water vapor in order to destroy the ammonia and volatile organic compounds that are carried over with the vapor.

In summary, distillation processes

- Offer a high degree of water recovery
- Are energy intensive due to the phase changes
- Incorporate regenerative techniques to try and minimize energy requirements
- Do not remove volatile organic (e.g., ethanol and acetone) and inorganic (e.g., ammonia) species

Membrane Separation (Filtration). Membrane separation avoids the high-energy input required for distillation systems but results in less of a separation between the waste stream (retentate) and the product water (permeate). As membrane processes rely on molecular weight (molecule size) separation, volatile organic compounds tend to permeate along with the product water. Because both the contaminated water and product water are in contact with a porous membrane, there exists a danger of bacterial "grow-through" into the product water. Postprocessing such as aqueous phase catalytic oxidation is required to produce potable water with a total organic content (TOC) reading below 2 mg/L. The membrane separation processes include: forward osmosis (FO), reverse osmosis (RO), micro/ultrafiltration, and electrodialysis.

Reverse Osmosis (RO). The waste stream represents a concentrated solution, and the natural osmotic gradient is for pure water to permeate through the membrane to dilute the solution. By application of a pressure force that overcomes the natural osmotic pressure, water can be made to reverse its flow and permeate into the product water stream. The extraction of water from the waste stream increases its concentration and decreases the applied pressure gradient. The process is halted at this point and the concentrated brine stream is purged from the membrane by a fresh batch of wastewater. The requirement for high pressure (hence high power) and the wide range of contaminants in the waste stream result in membrane-fouling issues for this approach.

Forward Osmosis (FO). In a forward osmosis system, the waste stream is retained by an osmosis membrane and exposed to a highly concentrated working solution. The concentration gradient will then pull water through the membrane and into the working solution. The working solution is concentrated using reverse osmosis, and the permeate from that step is the product water. Because the FO process operates at ambient conditions without a large pressure gradient, there is less of a tendency for contaminant molecules to be driven into the pores of the membrane, fouling the system. The use of a known concentrated working solution minimizes the risk of fouling and blockage in the RO stage of the process.

Micro/Ultrafiltration. Membranes are selected on the basis of pore size to provide a molecular cut-off on size. The wastewater is pressurized to force the solution through the filtration membrane. Like RO, this process is subject to fouling as the rejected contaminants accumulate on the retentate side of the membrane.

Electrodialysis. Wastewaters containing ionic species can be processed using electrodialysis. In this process, the solution is placed in a chamber bounded by two semipermeable membranes. An electrical potential between two electrodes causes electric current to pass through the solution and create a migration of cations toward the negative electrode and a migration of anions to the positive electrode. The ions then pass through the cation- and anion-permeable membranes, causing formation of concentrated and dilute salt solutions. Wastewater is pumped through membranes that are separated by spacers and assembled into stacks.

In summary, membrane processes

- Provide lower energy requirements than distillation process.
- Produce concentrated brine that must be either treated using an additional process or disposed of as a waste.
- Exhibit a process efficiency that decreases as brine concentration increases.
- Have a separation efficiency that depends on the membrane selected. RO membranes are more selective than microfiltration membranes, but still allow small molecules and ionic solutes to pass through with permeate water.
- Are consumables because they eventually foul and must be replaced.

Adsorption. Adsorption is a process of accumulating substances that are in solution on a suitable interface.

Activated Carbon. Activated carbon is prepared by making a char from organic materials (almond, coconut, coal) by heating material at less than 700°C in an oxygen-deficient environment (i.e., pyrolysis process).

Activated carbon effectively removes organic species from water that have a higher affinity for carbon surface than water, but has a finite amount of adsorption capacity. Carbon is an expendable item because it needs to be replaced once it reaches its usable capacity.

Ion Exchange. This is a unit process in which ions of a given species are displaced from an insoluble exchange material by ions of a different species in solution. This process is most commonly used for domestic water softening where sodium ions from a cationic exchange resin replace calcium and magnesium ions in the water, thus reducing the hardness. Naturally occurring ion-exchange materials (zeolites) are used for water softening and ammonium ion removal. There is a large selection of synthetic resins available for water purification. They are classified as: strong-acid cation, weak-acid cation, strong-base anion, and weak-base anion resins, as well as heavy-metal selective chelating resins. An ion exchange resin effectively removes the targeted ions from solution; however, the resin bed has a finite capacity and either needs to be replaced or regenerated. Regeneration results in a concentrated brine solution that needs to be reprocessed. Because ion exchange is an "exchange" process, the resin needs to be selected so that the exchanged ion does not adversely affect the quality of the water.

Aqueous Phase Catalytic Oxidation. Catalytic oxidation processes can be used to oxidize low-molecular-weight volatile organic species that are not removed by distillation or carbon adsorption. Highly effective catalysts have been developed to effectively oxidize volatile organic species completely to carbon dioxide and water at a temperature of 120 to 135°C and provide up to a 6 log reduction in bacterial colony-forming units. The oxidation of greater than 10 ppm TOC requires the addition of oxygen to the input water. The resulting two-phase solution must be passed through the packed bed of catalyst. A gas/liquid separator is required downstream of the catalytic reactor to remove excess gaseous oxygen and carbon dioxide from the product stream. The use of a regenerative heat exchanger increases the energy efficiency of process.

ISS Water Processor. Input waste stream is a mixture of humidity condensate, hygiene wastewater, and recovered distillate from the ISS urine processor.

Space Station water processor uses a combination of filtration, adsorption, ion exchange, and catalytic oxidation to produce water to the NASA potable standard. Main challenges facing the processor is the hygiene soap which can agglomerate and clog filters.

Microbial Control. Microbial control is a critical element of all potable water systems. It is necessary in order to maintain the water in a condition that is safe for consumption. There are several options for microbial control and they need to be rated based on four main factors:

1. Effectiveness
2. Stability (shelf-life of potable water)
3. Safe for crew to consume
4. Must be compatible with all materials

Chlorine. Many municipal water systems use chlorination to maintain the safety of the water. When dealing with closed habitats, chlorine poses a corrosion danger as both a concentrated additive and in the diluted water supply. It also tends to interact with bladder materials in positive expulsion tanks. It does persist in the stored water and has only a mild effect on the taste of the water.

Iodine. This is not in general use for municipal water systems. Its action is similar, but not as drastic as chlorine; however, iodine needs to be removed prior to consumption. NASA has developed a convenient resin cartridge system that provides the needed iodine dose on input and can remove the iodine prior to use.

Silver. Silver is an active microbial agent that does not need to be removed prior to consumption. Silver does tend to react with metals in the system and loose effectiveness over time. NASA is performing analysis and testing to confirm its effectiveness as a biocide and to determine the materials compatibility for its use in water systems.

28.6 NASA SPACE FLIGHT EXPERIENCES

28.6.1 CO_2 Capture

As previously described, the high generation rate and low tolerance for carbon dioxide make this contaminant removal a top priority, typically relying on a dedicated system simply for CO_2

capture. The early space flight experience of NASA started with U.S. Navy experiences for identifying potential capture agents. The low-molecular-weight of lithium made lithium hydroxide (LiOH) ideal for CO_2 capture in these Mercury/Gemini and Apollo missions. Canisters filled with granular LiOH were used throughout these missions for both cabin CO_2 control and capture within the space suit while performing extravehicular activity (EVA). While two LiOH molecules are required to capture one CO_2 molecule, no material has been proven to be more effective in CO_2 capture on a mass basis. The equation below shows this process and the equimolar generation of water from the CO_2 capture:

$$2LiOH + CO_2 \rightarrow Li_2CO_3 + H_2O$$

While LiOH has been routinely used for the CO_2-capture mission in these previously identified missions, it cannot be practically regenerated within the constraints of a space mission. Therefore, each used cartridge must be replaced on a regular basis with new, fresh sorbent.

After, using LiOH for all human-occupied space missions throughout the 1960s, NASA began the design, construction, and operation of the Skylab orbiting space station. This mission would place a three-person crew into Low Earth Orbit, for lengthy stay times, approaching 90 days (the third and final Skylab crew stayed on-board for 84 days). The combination of crew size and mission length, provided for an opportunity to save overall system weight by incorporating a regenerable CO_2 capture system versus the single-use LiOH used up until that point. Skylab used a two-bed zeolite absorbent for both water vapor removal and CO_2 control. The predrier section (Zeolite 13X) is required to remove moisture from the gas stream prior to entering the CO_2 absorbing section due to the very affinity for water vapor from the CO_2 capture material (Zeolite 5A). The two-bed system placed one bed online with cabin air circulating through the predrier and CO_2 capture section. The second bed relied on valves to isolate it from cabin air, but was instead exposed to space vacuum where the captured species (predominantly water vapor and carbon dioxide, but also some trace contaminants) were vented overboard. Figure 28.11 is a schematic of this two-bed system that operated successfully for three complete missions and over 170 mission days while on-orbit.

The Space Shuttle Orbiter began its operation with granular LiOH as its sole CO_2 capture sorbent. The short mission length meant that system weights would be minimized by relying once again on this single-use sorbent. During the 1990s when NASA introduced the Extended Duration Orbiter (EDO), a regenerable two-bed solid amine system provided the primary CO_2-capture agent during the Low Earth Orbit missions. This two-bed solid amine system provided humidity control as well as CO_2 capture for these missions. Figure 28.12 shows a simplified schematic of this system, which used an ullage save compressor, to limit the gas lost overboard when the bed functions (online absorbing CO_2, off-line vacuum regeneration) switched.

28.6.2 O_2 Generation/Storage

As previously described generically, the oxygen supply for enclosed habitats will usually be stored in high-pressure tanks (along with separate nitrogen tanks if a mixed gas system is being used) for short-duration missions. Longer missions and larger crew sizes may reduce overall system weight and volume by generating oxygen as required by chemical candles or the electrolysis of water.

The oxygen supply for the Mercury capsule was provided by two 1.8-kg capacity tanks pressurized with pure oxygen to 7500 psi with regulators to maintain the capsule pressure at a nominal 5-psi O_2 pressure. The tanks were constructed of AISI 4340 carbon steel with electroless nickel plating. One tank was the primary supply while the second tank served as a backup.

The Gemini capsule and crew used oxygen that was stored as a supercritical cryogen in tanks at 850 psi. These tanks supplied the metabolic oxygen load and were used to generate electricity in the on-board fuel cell. The capsule was maintained at 5 psi in a pure oxygen state.

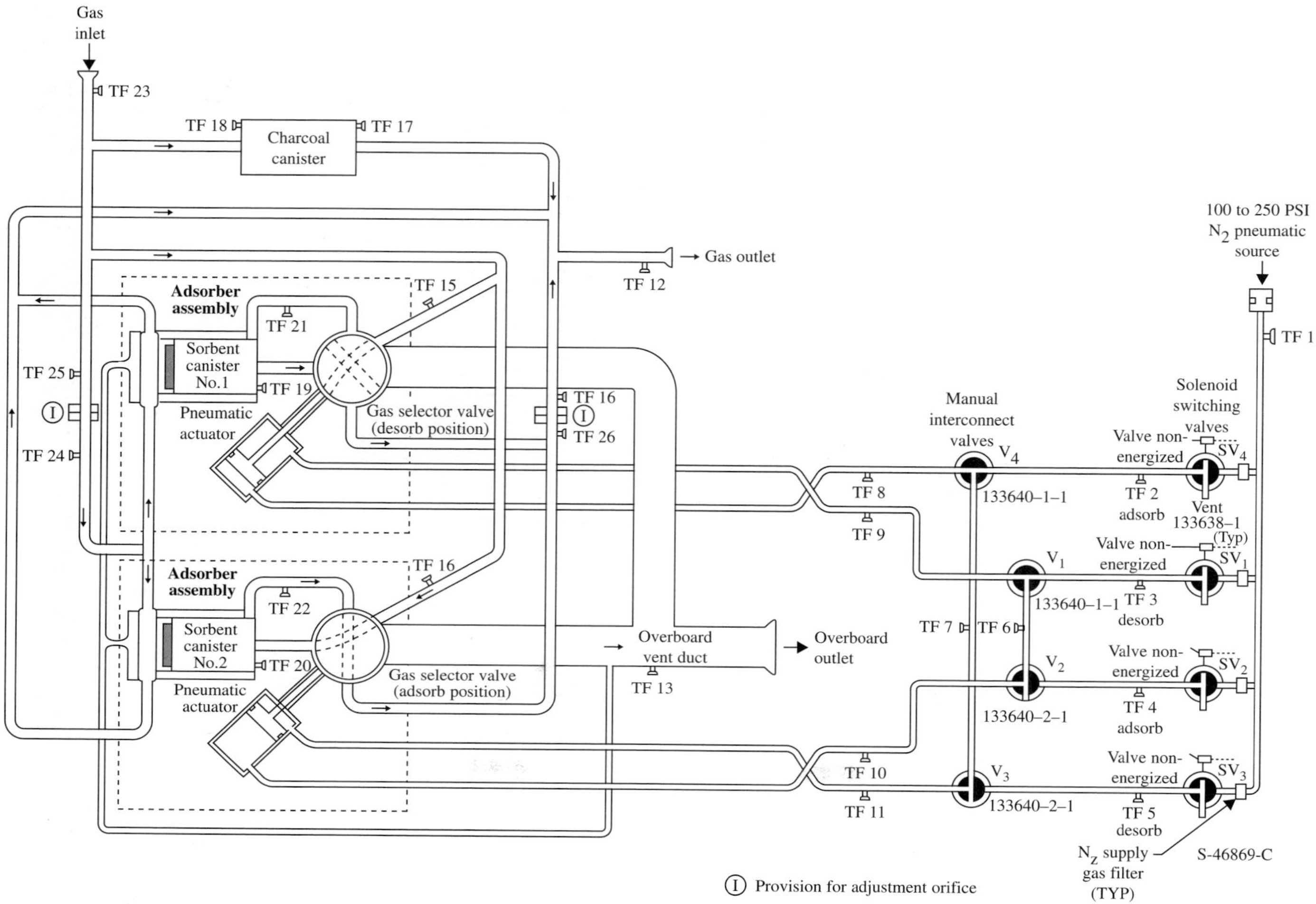

FIGURE 28.11 Skylab two-bed zeolite CO_2 capture system.

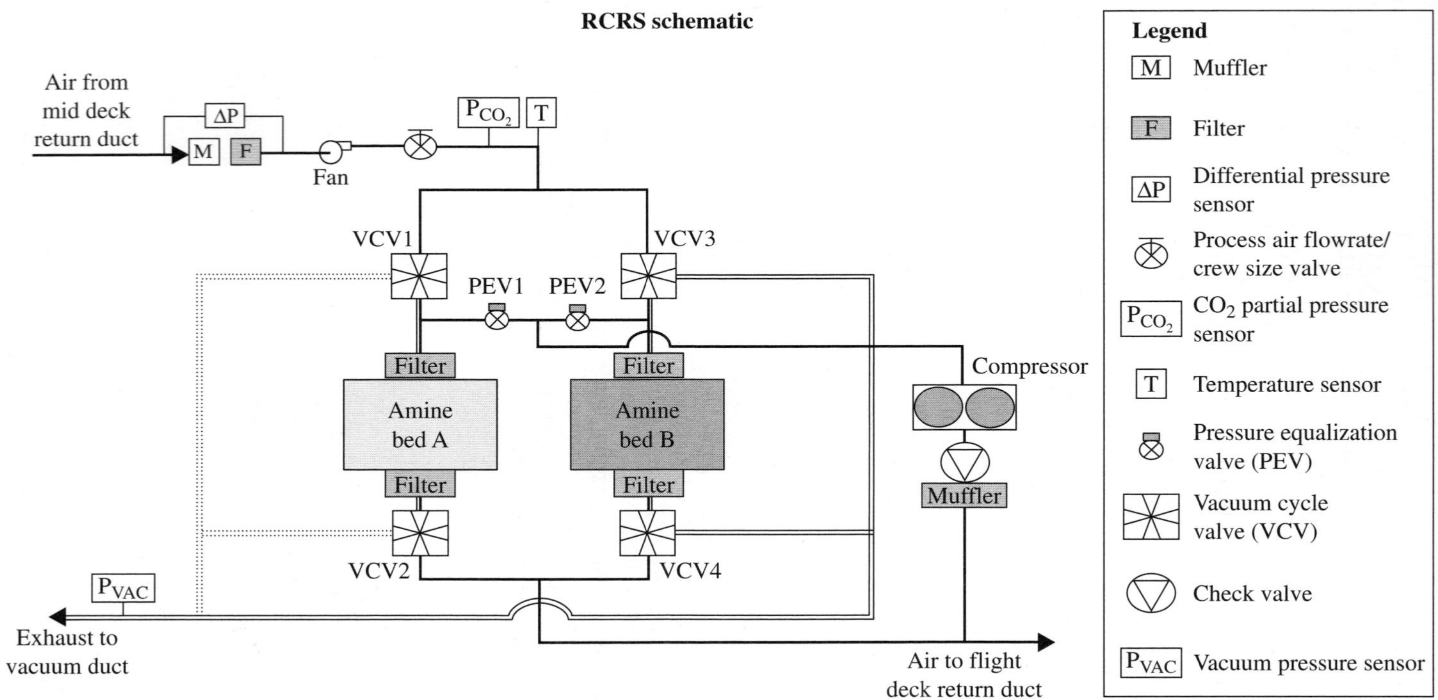

FIGURE 28.12 Two-bed solid amine system used on the EDO shuttle orbiter.

The Apollo mission used a cryogenic oxygen tank to supply gaseous oxygen to maintain a pure oxygen environment within the Crew Module. These same cryogenic tanks were used to supply gaseous oxygen to the fuel cell which supplied electricity for all of the systems on-board the vehicle. Storing oxygen as a cryogen allowed for reducing the mass and volume of the storage system for the expected 1 to 2 week duration of the Apollo missions.

Skylab used a N_2/O_2 gas mixture that was set to 26 percent N_2 and 74 percent O_2 and maintained at a total pressure of 5 psia. The lower than atmospheric pressure (~1/3 atm) provided for reduced overboard leakage. The nitrogen gas was a diluent to reduce flammability dangers. Both the nitrogen and oxygen were supplied from tanks filled during the initial vehicle launch.

The Space Shuttle Orbiter uses cryogenic oxygen and gaseous oxygen to maintain its cabin pressure. This vehicle typically maintains an earthlike atmosphere of 14.7 psia with a nominal composition of 21.7 percent oxygen and 78.3 percent nitrogen. A high-pressure spherical tank holds nitrogen at 3300 psi while the metabolically required oxygen is supplied from a cryogenic tank. Similarly, the International Space Station uses stored supplies of oxygen and nitrogen to maintain the atmosphere at 14.7 psia (21.5 percent O_2, 78.5 percent N_2). Future resupply missions will rely on the electrolysis of water to generate the oxygen lost through metabolic processes and leakage.

28.6.3 Trace Contaminant Control

Activated charcoal has been a mainstay of trace contaminant control (TCC) systems for most of NASA's human-occupied missions. This high surface area, granular material has been used in the Mercury, Gemini, Apollo, and Skylab missions to control odors and remove low concentrations of gaseous contaminants. The space shuttle also employs activated charcoal to remove trace contaminants. It is located downstream of the LiOH beds and is combined with an ambient temperature catalyst to convert CO to CO_2. For the International Space Station, a combination of activated charcoal, treated charcoal, and a high-temperature catalyst is used to control trace contaminants.

Most of the NASA vehicles operating prior to the launch of the International Space Station (ISS) had mission profiles that allowed the use of a nonregenerable sorbent for the capture of trace contaminants from the habitable atmosphere. However, the ISS has had a crew on-board since 2000 with continued operation expected for many more years. This long-duration mission has been able to reduce the mass and volume of resupply by incorporating a catalytic oxidation system as part of the trace contaminant control system. Figure 28.13 is a simplified schematic of this system that combines an activated charcoal bed with a catalytic oxidizer.

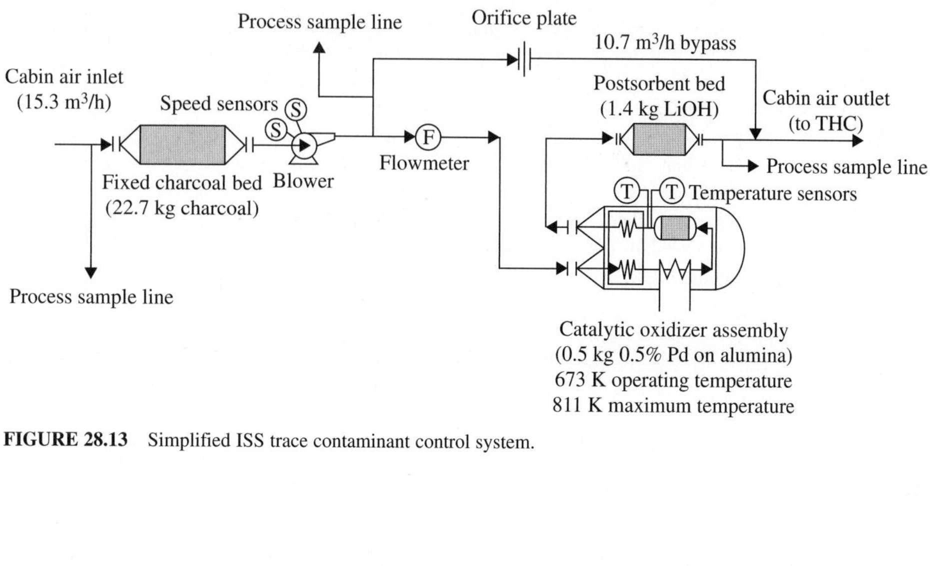

FIGURE 28.13 Simplified ISS trace contaminant control system.

28.7 SUMMARY

This chapter has provided a variety of technologies that are presently available to maintain a habitable atmosphere for an enclosed habitat. These techniques include methods to control temperature and moisture and keep gaseous contaminants at levels below those deemed safe for long-term human exposure.

Thermal control is important (i.e., dry bulb temperature), but radiation heat transfer as well as water vapor level (i.e., wet bulb temperature) also provide input into overall human comfort. Other factors can influence the ultimate crew comfort measure, including, air velocity, habitat pressure, and the clothing worn by the crew.

To maintain a habitable atmosphere within a sealed enclave, several systems are available. Generally, the first system is centered on O_2 control, maintaining the concentration above hypoxic and below hyperoxic limits. The second system found in enclosed cabin life-support systems (ECLSS) is a method to remove CO_2 from the atmosphere. Several chemical-based systems are available which generally rely on caustic chemicals to react with the acid gas CO_2. These systems can be single-use materials or regenerable via pressure change or temperature swing methods. While CO_2 is usually the contaminant with the highest generation rate, due to metabolic processes, other gaseous contaminants can impact the health of a cabin atmosphere. Therefore, a trace contaminant control system (TCCS) is usually required to hold these contaminants below there maximum allowable concentration.

Longer-mission scenarios may actually benefit from systems that reclaim water. Therefore, systems have been implemented that recover water from humidity and urine, process this water, and return it to potable standards.

REFERENCES

1. McQuiston, Parker, and Spitler: *Heating, Ventilating and Air Conditioning Analysis and Design*, 6th Edition, John Wiley & Sons, 2005.
2. Wieland, P.: *Designing for Human Presence in Space: An Introduction to Environmental Control and Life Support Systems*, NASA Reference Publication 1324, 1994.
3. *Spacecraft Maximum Allowable Concentrations for Selected Airborne Contaminants*, Volume 1. National Academy Press: Washington D.C.; 1994.
4. *Spacecraft Maximum Allowable Concentrations for Selected Airborne Contaminants*, Volume 2. National Academy Press: Washington D.C.; 1996.
5. *Spacecraft Maximum Allowable Concentrations for Selected Airborne Contaminants*, Volume 3. National Academy Press: Washington D.C.; 1996.
6. James, J.T.: Spacecraft Maximum Allowable Concentrations for Airborne Contaminants. JSC 20584. Lyndon B. Johnson Space Center: Houston, TX; February 1995.
7. *The Toxic Effects of Chronic Exposure to Low Levels of Carbon Dioxide*, Naval Submarine Medical Research Laboratory, Report Number 973, January 1982.
8. *Advanced Life Support Program, Requirements Definition and Design Considerations*. CTSD-ADV-245. Crew and Thermal Systems Division. December 1996. NASA Lyndon B. Johnson Space Center, Houston, Texas.
9. Seter, A.: *Allowable Exposure Limits for Carbon Dioxide During Extravehicular Activity*, NASA Technical Memorandum 103832, April 1993.
10. Schmidt, J.M., Alleman, J.E.: Urine Processing for Water Recovery via Freeze Concentration, *International Conference on Environmental Systems*, SAE 2005-010-3032, July 2005, Rome, Italy.

INDEX